As a part of Mosby's continuing effort to provide you with the most current information possible, here is the most recent regimen for prophylactic use of antibiotics for dental procedures. This information was released by the American Heart Association in December 1984. It replaces Table 36-7 on p. 536.

Dosage regimens for prophylactic use of antibiotics for dental procedures

Regimen	Adults	Children*
Use of penicillin acceptable		
Standard		
Oral	Penicillin V 2 gm 1 hour before procedure	Penicillin V 1 gm 1 hour before procedure†
	FOLLOWED BY	FOLLOWED BY
	Penicillin V 1 gm 6 hours later	Penicillin V 500 mg 6 hours later
Parenteral	Aqueous crystalline penicillin G 2 million units IV or IM 30 to 60 minutes before procedure	Aqueous crystalline penicillin G 50,000 units/kg IV or IM 30 to 60 minutes before procedure
	FOLLOWED BY	FOLLOWED BY
	Aqueous crystalline penicillin G 1 million units IV or IM 6 hours later	Aqueous crystalline penicillin G 25,000 units/kg IV or IM 6 hours later
Highest risk of endocarditis‡		
	Ampicillin 1 to 2 gm plus gentamicin 1.5 mg/kg both IM or IV ½ hour before procedure	Ampicillin 50 mg/kg plus gentamicin 2 mg/kg both IM or IV ½ hour before procedure
	FOLLOWED BY	FOLLOWED BY
	Penicillin V 1 gm orally 6 hours later	Penicillin V 1 gm orally 6 hours later
	OR	OR
	Above parenteral regime repeated 8 hours later	Above parenteral regime repeated 8 hours later
Use of penicillin not acceptable because of patient allergy		
Standard		
Oral	Erythromycin 1 gm 1 hour before procedure	Erythromycin 20 mg/kg 1 hour before procedure
	FOLLOWED BY	FOLLOWED BY
	Erythromycin 500 mg 6 hours later§	Erythromycin 10 mg/kg 6 hours later
Highest risk of endocarditis‡		
	Vancomycin 1 gm IV *slowly* over 1 hour starting 1 hour before procedure‖	Vancomycin 20 mg/kg IV *slowly* over 1 hour starting 1 hour before procedure

This information is taken from a statement prepared by the Committee on Rheumatic Fever and Bacterial Endocarditis of the Council on Cardiovascular Diseases in the Young of the American Heart Association, released in December 1984.

*Doses for children should not exceed the maximum adult doses.

†Children weighing more than 60 lb (27 kg) should be given the adult regimen.

‡This category includes most patients with prosthetic heart valves and patients who require extensive dental procedures (e.g., exodontia or other surgical procedures).

§Patients unable to tolerate oral erythromycin may be helped by changing to a different erythromycin preparation. If the patient cannot tolerate either penicillin or erythromycin, cephalosporin 1 gm 1 hour before the procedure followed by cephalosporin 500 mg 6 hours later may be substituted, but the available data do not allow specific recommendation of this regimen. Tetracyclines are *not* recommended for this purpose.

‖A repeat dose of vancomycin is not necessary because of the drug's long plasma half-life.

Pharmacology and therapeutics
for dentistry

Pharmacology and therapeutics
for dentistry

SECOND EDITION

Enid A. Neidle, Ph.D.

Professor and Chairman, Department of Pharmacology, Director of Research,
New York University College of Dentistry, New York, New York

Donald C. Kroeger, M.S., Ph.D.

Professor and Chairman, Department of Pharmacology,
University of Texas Health Science Center at Houston,
Dental Branch, Houston, Texas

John A. Yagiela, D.D.S., Ph.D.

Professor, Section of Oral Biology, School of Dentistry,
Department of Anesthesiology, School of Medicine, University of
California at Los Angeles, Center for the Health Sciences,
Los Angeles, California

with 183 illustrations

The C. V. Mosby Company

ST. LOUIS • TORONTO • PRINCETON   1985

MOSBY

A TRADITION OF PUBLISHING EXCELLENCE

Editors: Samuel E. Harshberger and Darlene Warfel
Editing supervisor: Lin Dempsey
Manuscript editor: Sheila Walker
Book design: Jeanne Bush
Cover design: Kathleen A. Johnson
Production: Jeanne A. Gulledge

SECOND EDITION

The C.V. Mosby Company
11830 Westline Industrial Drive, St. Louis, Missouri 63146

Library of Congress Cataloging in Publication Data

Neidle, Enid Anne.
    Pharmacology and therapeutics for dentistry.

    Bibliography: p.
    Includes index.
    1. Dental pharmacology. I. Kroeger, Donald C.
II. Yagiela, John A. III. Title. [DNLM: 1. Dentistry.
2. Pharmacology. QV 50 N397p]
RK701.N44 1984   617.6′061   84-6782
ISBN 0-8016-3743-0

GW/MV/MV 9 8 7 6 5 4 3 2 1   02/A/248

CONTRIBUTORS

Roy Aston, Ph.D.
Professor of Physiology and Pharmacology,
University of Detroit School of Dentistry;
Adjunct Associate Professor of Anesthesiology,
Wayne State University School of Medicine,
Detroit, Michigan

Stephen A. Cooper, D.M.D., Ph.D.
Associate Dean for Research and Post Graduate
Studies, Professor of Biodental Sciences and Oral
Surgery, University of Medicine and Dentistry,
New Jersey Dental School,
Newark, New Jersey

Paul J. Desjardins, D.M.D., Ph.D.
Assistant Professor,
Department of Biodental Sciences,
Oral and Maxillofacial Surgery,
University of Medicine and Dentistry,
New Jersey Dental School,
Newark, New Jersey

Roger R. Deuben, M.S., Ph.D.
Associate Professor and Chairman,
Department of Physiology and Pharmacology,
University of Detroit School of Dentistry,
Detroit, Michigan

Frank Dowd, D.D.S., Ph.D.
Associate Professor and Chairman,
Department of Pharmacology,
Creighton University School of Medicine,
Omaha, Nebraska

Samuel Dreizen, D.D.S., M.D.
Professor and Chairman, Department of Oral
Oncology; Professor, Department of Pathology,
University of Texas Health Science Center at Houston,
Dental Branch; Professor, University of Texas Dental
Science Institute; Consultant, University of Texas
M.D. Anderson Hospital and Tumor Institute,
Houston, Texas

Harold R. Englander, D.D.S., M.P.H.
Formerly Chief of Clinical Trials,
National Institute of Dental Research,
National Institutes of Health,
Bethesda, Maryland

Leslie P. Felpel, Ph.D.
Associate Professor, Department of Pharmacology,
University of Texas Health Science Center at
San Antonio, San Antonio, Texas

Gerald F. Gebhart, Ph.D.
Professor, Department of Pharmacology,
University of Iowa College of Medicine,
Iowa City, Iowa

Glenn T. Housholder, Ph.D.
Professor, Department of Pharmacology,
University of Texas Health Science Center
at Houston, Dental Branch, Houston, Texas

Wyatt R. Hume, B.D.S., Ph.D.
Associate Professor,
Department of Restorative Dentistry,
University of Adelaide,
Adelaide, Australia

Donald C. Kroeger, M.S., Ph.D.
Professor and Chairman, Department of
Pharmacology, University of Texas Health
Science Center at Houston,
Dental Branch, Houston, Texas

Vahn A. Lewis, Ph.D.
Associate Professor, Department of Pharmacology,
University of Texas Health Science Center at
Houston, Dental Branch, Houston, Texas

Stanley F. Malamed, D.D.S.
Associate Professor of Anesthesia and Medicine,
Division of Surgical Sciences,
Section of Anesthesia and Medicine,
University of Southern California
School of Dentistry,
Los Angeles, California

James L. Matheny, Ph.D.
Professor, Department of Oral Biology,
University of Kentucky, Albert B. Chandler
Medical Center, College of Dentistry,
Lexington, Kentucky

Edward H. Montgomery, M.S., Ph.D.
Associate Professor, Department of Pharmacology,
University of Texas Health Science Center at
Houston, Dental Branch, Houston, Texas

Enid A. Neidle, Ph.D.
Professor and Chairman, Department
of Pharmacology, Director of Research,
New York University College of Dentistry,
New York, New York

Thomas E. Nelson, Jr., M.S., Ph.D.
Professor of Pharmacology and Chairman of
Biomedical Sciences, Southern Illinois University at
Edwardsville School of Dental Medicine,
Edwardsville, Illinois

Anthony Picozzi, B.S. (Pharm.), D.D.S.
Professor, Department of Pharmacology,
Director, Oral Health Research Center,
Fairleigh Dickinson University School of Dentistry,
Hackensack, New Jersey

Norton M. Ross, D.D.S., M.A.
Director, Department of Dental/Oral Clinical
Research, Warner-Lambert Company,
Morris Plains, New Jersey; Clinical Professor,
Department of Pharmacology,
Fairleigh Dickinson University School of Dentistry,
Hackensack, New Jersey

Joel D. Schiff, Ph.D.
Associate Professor, Department of Physiology,
New York University College of Dentistry,
New York, New York

Clarence L. Trummel, D.D.S., Ph.D.
Professor, Department of Periodontology,
University of Connecticut, School of Dental
Medicine, Farmington, Connecticut

William Warner, Ph.D.
Associate Professor, Department of Pharmacology,
New York University College of Dentistry,
New York, New York

Robert R. White, Ph.D.
Professor, Department of Microbiology,
University of Texas Health Science Center at
Houston, Dental Branch, Houston, Texas

John A. Yagiela, D.D.S., Ph.D.
Professor, Section of Oral Biology, School of
Dentistry, Department of Anesthesiology, School of
Medicine, University of California at Los Angeles,
Center for the Health Sciences, Los Angeles,
California

PREFACE

Although revised to include all the important drug developments that have occurred since the first edition went to press, the second edition of *Pharmacology and Therapeutics for Dentistry* remains essentially unchanged in its philosophy and goals. We set out in the first edition to write a thorough and professional textbook of pharmacology that would be especially responsive to the needs of the dental student, resident, and practitioner. Judging from the positive acceptance of the first edition, we believe that we succeeded in meeting that challenge.

By using the book in courses on pharmacology, therapeutics, and pain and anxiety control, and with the aid of helpful comments from colleagues, the editors and contributors have all gained insights into what changes would make the book even better for teaching purposes. Thus, there is now a separate chapter on diuretics, reorganized chapters on antimicrobial agents and on psychoactive drugs, and completely new chapters on geriatric pharmacology and toxicology. A glossary of abbreviations used in the book (and in the scientific world as well) has also been added.

Some of the most significant changes are in the end-of-chapter drug lists, which serve collectively as a fairly complete catalog of drugs available in the United States at the time of publication, and in the index, which lists all drugs mentioned in the text or in the drug lists by proprietary and nonproprietary names. All pathologic conditions referred to in the book are also carried in the index. These enrichments should bring us closer to our goal of providing a freestanding textbook, one that is not only comprehensive in its coverage of pharmacology but also complete as a therapeutic guide to the dental applications, implications, and uses of drugs.

A number of individuals deserve our gratitude. First and foremost, we thank our contributors, without whose efforts this book would never have been written. We are also indebted to our colleagues who contributed unofficially by offering constructive criticisms, answering questions of fact and style, and providing other forms of support. Ms. Irene Petravicius deserves our thanks for preparing the new illustrations for this edition. Finally, we are indebted to our families for their patience and understanding.

Enid A. Neidle
Donald C. Kroeger
John A. Yagiela

CONTENTS

ix

Pharmacology and therapeutics
for dentistry

Introduction

Pharmacology may be defined as the science of drugs, their preparation, uses, and effects. The term derives from *pharmakon*, the Greek word for drug or medicine, and *logia,* the Latin suffix traditionally used to designate a body of knowledge and its study. As an organized discipline, pharmacology is of recent origin, but the study of medicinal substances is as old as civilization itself.

HISTORY

Sir William Osler once said, ''The desire to take medicine is perhaps the greatest feature which distinguishes man from animals.'' Although this argument has been vitiated by experiments involving self-medication in rats and other laboratory species, it nevertheless serves to illustrate the historic relationship between drugs and humankind. The use of natural products to cure disease and alter mentation dates back to the dawn of recorded time. By the writing of the Ebers papyrus (ca. 1550 B.C.), more than 700 prescriptions for various ailments were known. Many of the ingredients incorporated in these preparations—lizard's blood, virgin's hair, fly excreta—are humorous by modern standards, but also included were many compounds recognized today as pharmacologically active. A summary of folk remedies and other medicinals that have withstood scientific scrutiny would list such substances as opium (morphine), belladonna (atropine), squill and foxglove (digitalis), cinchona bark (quinine and quinidine), coca leaves (cocaine), and ma huang (ephedrine). The empirical study of plant derivatives and animal products must have been quite extensive to have been so fruitful.

A major hindrance to the effective use of these drugs, however, was the large number of materials usually present in apothecary formulations. For example, the most popular drug of the fifteenth century, triaca, contained over 100 separate components. Aureolus Paracelsus (1493-1541) was the first to recognize that the indiscriminate mixing of numerous substances did little but dilute whatever effective compounds may have been present initially. The focus of Paracelsus on single agents was refined by Felice Fontana (1720-1805), who deduced from his own experiments that each crude drug contains an ''active principle'' that, when administered, yields a characteristic effect on the body. One of the greatest scientific achievements of the nineteenth century was the isolation and objective evaluation of such active principles.

In 1803, a young German pharmacist, Frederick Sertürner (1780-1841), extracted the alkaloid morphine from opium. This singular achievement not only marked the beginning of pharmaceutical chemistry; it also led to a revolution in experimental biology. The availability of newly purified drugs and the standardization of existing biologic preparations encouraged pioneers like François Magendie (1783-1855) and Claude Bernard (1813-1878) to employ pharmacologic agents as probes in the study of physiologic processes. The use of curare by Bernard for the elucidation of the neuromuscular junction is but one example of the successes obtained with this approach. Perhaps because drugs became associated with several biologic sciences and were of course considered under the domain of the various medical specialties, the development of pharmacology as a separate discipline was delayed.

Rudolf Buchheim (1820-1879) and Oswald Schmiedeberg (1838-1921) were the two individuals most responsible for establishing pharmacology as a science in its own right. Buchheim organized the first laboratory exclusively devoted to pharmacology and became the first professor of his discipline. A student of Buchheim's, Schmiedeberg founded the first scientific journal of pharmacology. More importantly, through his tutelage Schmiedeberg helped spread acceptance of pharmacology throughout the world. One protégé of Schmiedeberg was John Abel (1857-1938), generally regarded as the father of American pharmacology.

Once an obscure experimental science, the purview of pharmacology has expanded to such an extent that the subject has become an important area of study for all health professionals and holds certain interests for the lay public as well. In dentistry, the impact of pharmacology was formally recognized by the American Dental Association in 1934 with publication of the first edition of *Accepted Dental Remedies.*

SCOPE OF PHARMACOLOGY

Pharmacology is one of the few medical sciences that straddles the division between the basic and the clinical. The scope of pharmacology is so extensive that several subdivisions have come to be recognized. *Pharmacodynamics* is the study of the biologic activity that a drug has on a living system. It includes a study of the mechanisms of action of the drug and the exact processes that are affected by it. The influence of chemical structure on drug action (the structure-activity relationship) is also a concern of this branch of pharmacology. *Pharmacokinetics* deals with the magnitude and time course of drug effect, and it attempts to explain these aspects of drug action through a consideration of dosage and the absorption, distribution, and fate of chemicals in living systems. *Pharmacotherapeutics* is the proper selection of an agent whose biologic effect on a living organism is most appropriate to treat a particular disease state. It requires a consideration of, among many other things, dose, duration of therapy, and side effects of drug treat-

ment. The practice of *pharmacy* involves the preparation and dispensing of medicines. Although pharmacists today are rarely called on to actually prepare drug products, they can serve as a useful source of drug information for both the clinician and the patient. *Toxicology* is that aspect of pharmacology dealing with poisons, their actions, their detection, and the treatment of conditions produced by them. The importance of toxicology to modern life is continually underscored by new discoveries of chemical hazards in the environment. A final subdivision, *pharmacognosy,* is now a somewhat vestigial science. Essential at a time when most drugs were derived from plants, it literally means "drug recognition" and deals with the characteristics of plants and how to identify those with pharmacologic activity. Most drugs today are synthesized chemically, but phytochemistry, especially the synthesis of complex chemical structures by plants, remains of interest.

After a description of how the study of drugs is classified, it is appropriate to discuss what is meant by the word *drug*. To the pharmacologist, a drug is any chemical agent that has an effect on the processes associated with life. This definition is obviously quite broad and ill-suited for many parties who define the term more restrictively to better serve their particular needs. The therapist, for example, considers as drugs those chemicals that are effective in treating disease states. To the lay public, drugs generally connote those substances that cause mental and psychologic alterations. Finally, governmental agencies are concerned with the revenue derived from the taxes levied against the sale of certain substances or with public health problems associated with their use. Some of these agents, such as tobacco and alcohol, are legally sequestered; that is, by law they are considered "nondrugs." While pharmacologists have long recognized these agents as potent drugs, they are exempted from the usual governmental restraints and are not subject to normal scrutiny by the Food and Drug Administration. There are other substances that have gained such special status not by historical accident as did the above but by considerations of public health. Examples of these include chlorine and fluoride added to community water supplies and iodides mixed in with table salt. Lawsuits over the question of whether these public health measures constitute an illegal form of "mass medication" have been resolved by the courts, at least in part, through the categorization of these chemicals as legal nondrugs when they are employed in a specified manner for the public good.

Drugs to be covered in this text will include almost exclusively only those substances with a known therapeutic application. Even so, the potential number of agents for consideration is large—several thousand drugs marketed in a multiplicity of dosage forms and, in some instances, in a bewildering variety of combinations. To limit confusion, emphasis will be placed on single, prototypical agents that are representative of their respective drug classes. By this approach, an understanding of the properties of related agents can be more readily achieved; at the same time, differences that may exist between them can be highlighted. Finally, it is important to recognize that there are certain generalizations which apply to all drugs. These principles of drug action are the subject of the first four chapters of this text. A mastery of the concepts presented in these chapters is necessary for a thorough understanding of pharmacology, for the rational use of therapeutic agents, and for the objective evaluation of new drugs.

PRINCIPLES OF PHARMACOLOGY

1 Pharmacodynamics: mechanisms of drug action

John A. Yagiela

DRUG-RECEPTOR INTERACTIONS

The actions of most therapeutic agents are imbued with a certain degree of specificity. In conventional doses, for example, drugs are generally selective in action; that is, they influence a narrow spectrum of biologic events. The pharmacologic profile of such agents is, in addition, often markedly dependent on chemical structure; thus, simple molecular modifications may drastically alter drug activity. These attributes of drug action suggest that the tissue components with which drugs interact to cause observable effects are uniquely individualized. Such tissue elements must have highly ordered physicochemical properties to permit particular compounds to combine with them while prohibiting all others from doing so. Furthermore, they must be intimately involved with discrete processes of life in order for drug interactions to exert specific physiologic influences. These "biologic partners" of drug action are given the term *receptors*.

Receptor characterization

For many years after their postulation around the turn of this century,[6,10] receptors remained an enigma to pharmacologists. Little was known about them other than the probability that they were complex macromolecules. With development of biochemical methods for the isolation, solubilization, and characterization of proteins, however, enzymes became available as model systems for the study of drug-receptor interactions. Enzymes exhibit many of the properties that are ascribed to receptors. They are, for example, macromolecules having measurable biologic functions and possessing specific reactive sites for selected substrates. The close association between enzymes and receptors

was underscored in the early 1940s when it became apparent that some enzymes are, in fact, drug receptors.[1] The list of drugs that alter known enzymatic activities is fairly extensive and includes the sulfonamides, anticholinesterases, carbonic anhydrase inhibitors, monoamine oxidase inhibitors, trimethoprim, disulfiram, and various antimetabolites used in cancer chemotherapy.

Besides enzymes (including coenzymes) and certain other easily solubilized proteins, there are at least two additional classes of receptors that have been identified and are of clinical significance: nucleic acids and membrane constituents. Nucleic acids serve as receptors for a limited number of agents. Certain antibiotics and antineoplastic compounds interfere with replication, transcription, or translation by binding, sometimes irreversibly, to the nucleic acids involved. Other drugs, such as phenobarbital and some steroids, may induce protein synthesis, but it appears that the affected DNA acts as part of a receptor complex or becomes derepressed as a consequence of drug interaction with a structurally separate receptor inside the cell.

By far the most common receptors of drugs are those located on or within the various membranes of the cell. These receptors unfortunately have resisted characterization. A brief description of some of the difficulties involved in their isolation and study should help to explain why tissue-bound receptors are still largely enigmatic. Even when prevalent, membrane receptors are sparsely distributed. It is estimated, for example, that each intestinal smooth muscle cell contains about 16,000 receptors for acetylcholine (ACh), the major transmitter of the peripheral nervous system.[16] Assuming that these receptors are scattered over a smooth plasma

Table 1-1. Selected drug-receptor interactions

Drug	Receptor (type)	Mechanism of action	Therapeutic effect
Trimethoprim	Dihydrofolate reductase (enzyme)	Inhibition of tetrahydrofolate synthesis	Cure of infection
Pargyline	Monoamine oxidase (enzyme)	Inhibition of catecholamine metabolism	Mood elevation
Dactinomycin	DNA (nucleic acid)	Transcription blockade	Tumor regression
Bleomycin	DNA (nucleic acid)	DNA fragmentation	Tumor regression
Epinephrine	Adrenergic receptor (membrane-bound)	Alteration of membrane permeability	Vasoconstriction
Atropine	Cholinergic receptor (membrane-bound)	Receptor blockade	Xerostomia

membrane, only 0.002% of the available surface area is involved with the binding of ACh. Calculations with other drugs, such as histamine, epinephrine, ouabain, and atropine, also show them to occupy an equally small fraction of the cell surface when present at effective concentrations.[13] Although a considerable number of enzymes have been solubilized and consequently made accessible for further study, few tissue-bound receptors have. Attempts to remove the receptor macromolecule from its natural setting may inactivate it. Even if inactivation does not occur, a problem is always posed by isolation of the receptor per se, since in the isolated state the usual method of measuring its response (muscle contraction, etc.) is no longer possible. Finally, although receptors bind drugs selectively, drugs often adhere to other tissue constituents rather indiscriminately. Plasma proteins, especially albumin, represent a common binding site for pharmacologically active molecules. In high concentrations, drugs can also be taken up nonselectively by a wide range of tissues. Since binding of this type is not saturable, the total amount of drug sequestered can be large. Fortunately, this nonspecific uptake can be differentiated from specific (e.g., receptor) binding because the latter is capacity-limited and operates at low drug concentrations.

In spite of these impediments, it has become possible to study membrane receptors directly through the isolation and purification of macromolecules that have many, if not all, of the properties of specific drug receptors. Because these receptors are tightly bound to tissues, it is first necessary to disrupt the cellular elements.[9] The chemical dissection of membranes and the release of receptor moieties is accomplished through the use of chelating agents, salts, phospholipases, and detergents. The mixture of macromolecules so derived must then be purified. An important technique for this process is affinity chromatography, in which a ligand (a compound that is complementary to the receptor and binds to it) is attached covalently to an insoluble polysaccharide matrix. Ligands that have proved useful in this regard include specific and potent drugs, snake toxins, and monoclonal antibodies.[9,19] When passed through a column of this matrix, the receptors become bound to their ligands. After several washings to remove contaminants, the receptors are eluted by one of several methods, including the addition of free ligand. The recovered receptors can then be studied in vitro, but special methods are needed because they are no longer in their native environment.

The characterization of drug receptors, though difficult, holds great promise for pharmacology. For the scientist, the examination of receptors and their distribution can, for instance, provide insight into the existence of previously unidentified neurotransmitters. For the clinician, receptor investigations can lead to a deeper understanding of disease states and to new methods of drug treatment. The isolation of opioid receptors in the central nervous system and the subsequent discovery of endogenous morphine-like compounds is but one example of how the study of receptors can yield basic scientific information while concurrently opening new avenues for drug therapy.[7]

Table 1-1 lists representatives for each of the three categories of receptors described above. Drugs that act on the receptors listed are included along with their mechanisms of action and resultant therapeutic effects.

Drug-binding forces

Implicit in the interaction of a drug with its receptor is the chemical binding of that drug to one or more specific sites on the receptor molecule. There are four basic types of bonding that may be involved (Figure 1-1).

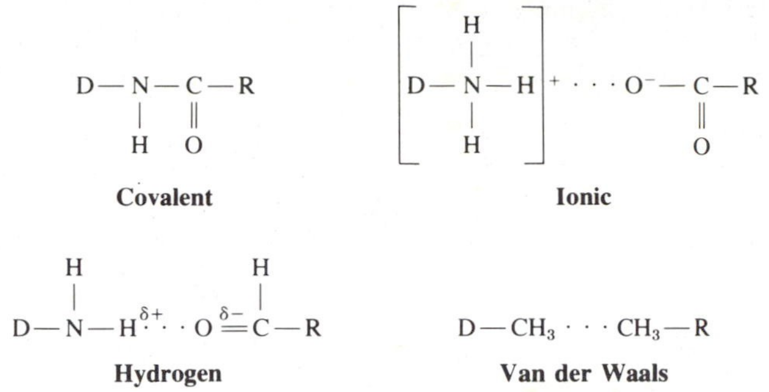

```
        H                               H
        |                               |
D — N — C — R              [ D — N — H ]+ · · · O⁻ — C — R
    |   ||                      |                    ||
    H   O                       H                    O
      Covalent                          Ionic


    H           H
    |           |
D — N — H δ+· · ·O δ— C — R            D — CH₃ · · · CH₃ — R
   Hydrogen                              Van der Waals
```

Figure 1-1. Major chemical bonds associated with drug-receptor interactions, where D = drug and R = receptor.

Covalent bonds. Covalent bonds arise from the sharing of electrons by a pair of atoms. Although covalent bonds are required for the structural integrity of molecules, they are generally not involved in drug-receptor interactions. Most drugs reversibly associate with their receptors. As described in Chapter 2, the duration of action of these agents is related to how long an effective drug concentration remains in the vicinity of the drug receptors. This time may vary from minutes to days but usually is on the order of several hours. With bond energies of 50 to 100 kcal/mole, the stability of covalent linkages is so great that, once formed, drug-receptor complexes are often irreversible. In these instances, the duration of action is not influenced by the concentration of unbound drug vicinal to the receptors. Instead, it may depend on the synthesis of new receptors or on the turnover of the affected cells, processes that often take days to weeks. When the receptors happen to compose the genetic material of a cell, drug effects may be permanent.

Ionic bonds. Ionic bonds result from the electrostatic attraction between ions of opposite charge. Such associations are relatively weak, having bond energies of approximately 5 kcal/mole. Nevertheless, many drugs have a formal charge at physiologic pH, and it is likely that ionic bonds are commonly made with ionized groups located at receptor sites. Because the attraction between ions is inversely proportional to the square of the distance separating them, ionic influences operate over much greater distances than do other interatomic forces. It is reasonable to assume, therefore, that ionic bonds initiate many drug-receptor combinations.

Hydrogen bonds. The hydrogen bond represents a special type of interaction between polar molecules. When a hydrogen atom is covalently attached to a strongly electronegative atom such as oxygen or nitrogen, it becomes partially stripped of its electron and takes on some of the characteristics of a bare proton. Strongly electropositive and with an exceedingly small atomic radius, the hydrogen nucleus is able to associate closely with a second electronegative atom. Hydrogen linkages are slightly weaker than ionic bonds and are more sensitive to interatomic separation. However, functional groups capable of forming hydrogen bonds are common to both drugs and receptor sites, and should multiple unions occur, the resultant stabilizing force would far outweigh that of a single ionic bond.

Van der Waals forces. Van der Waals forces collectively describe the weak interactions that develop when two atoms are placed into close proximity. The electrostatic attractions that compose these forces result from reciprocal perturbations in the electron clouds of the atoms involved. These ''bonds'' are the weakest of the four types described; in addition, they decrease in strength according to the seventh power of the interatomic distance. Paradoxical as it may seem, van der Waals forces are of primary importance in conferring specificity to drug-receptor interactions. Since even electroneutral carbon atoms can participate in such associations, the number of these bonds that connect a drug to its receptor may be large and the total binding force considerable. When minor steric influences prevent an exact fit between a drug and its receptor, the sensitivity of van der Waals forces to interatomic separation forestalls their development, and drug-receptor stability markedly suffers.

Cooperation of binding forces. The binding of a drug to its receptor is generally not related to a particular attractive force but results from the conjoint action of ionic, hydrogen, van der Waals, and (rarely) covalent linkages. Each type of association contributes differently to the drug-receptor complex. When random movement causes a drug molecule to approach or collide with the receptor surface, ionic attractions are the first to develop. Unable to convey specificity or stability to a drug-receptor union by themselves, ionic forces nevertheless serve to draw in and partially orient the drug to its receptor. As the intermolecular separation diminishes, hydrogen bonding and subsequently van der Waals forces become prominent. In concert, these bonds provide for the specificity of drug action; without an exact fit, binding is impaired, and the drug cannot adhere long enough to influence receptor function. Covalent linkage confers a high degree of permanency to the drug-receptor complex. It is fortunate, however, that irreversible binding is uncommon in therapeutics. Many agents are employed to produce a single, temporary effect; covalent attachment would preclude such use. Furthermore, covalent bonding would, in many instances, make drug regimens more difficult to administer and adverse reactions more troublesome to treat.

Structure-activity relationships

Examination of structure-activity relationships (SAR) is a time-honored method of studying drug-receptor interactions. In SAR investigations, specific features of the structure of a drug molecule are identified and then altered systematically to determine their influence on pharmacologic activity. The chemical features that are most often involved in these considerations are the presence and type of ionic charge, the effect of neighboring groups on the degree of ionization, hydrogen bonding capability, and steric factors such as the size of alkyl side chains, the distance between reactive groups, and the three-dimensional configuration of such groups. SAR studies of closely related agents (congeners) not only have led to an understanding of the chemical prerequisites for pharmacologic activity but have, on a very practical level, made possible the molecular modification of drugs to provide enhanced or even novel therapeutic effects while reducing the incidence and severity of toxic reactions. In addition, they serve to illustrate how

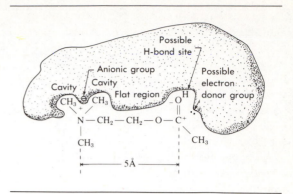

Figure. 1-2. Postulated interaction of acetylcholine (ACh) with its receptor (dotted area). The partial ionic character of the carbonyl group is shown by the symbols for positive and negative charges. (From Goldstein, A., Aronow, L., and Kalman, S.M. Principles of Drug Action: The Basis of Pharmacology, ed. 2. New York, John Wiley & Sons, Inc., 1974.)

the combined action of the various bonding forces described above are necessary for maximal drug activity and yield certain clues concerning the physicochemical properties of the receptor sites involved.

A typical example of SAR is provided by the study of ACh.[8] The ACh molecule is composed of an acetyl residue connected by a two-carbon intermediate chain to a trimethylated quaternary nitrogen terminus. Figure 1-2 summarizes the various features involved in the attachment of ACh to its receptor. The presence of a positively charged ionic group at the nitrogen locus is essential for full activity; loss of the positive charge by replacing the quaternary amino group with an uncharged but similarly shaped isobutyl structure virtually eliminates drug action. By inference, the receptor for ACh must have a negatively charged site that accepts the cationic group. The nitrogen-bound methyl groups are also involved in binding, but the tetrahedral configuration of the quaternary amino structure suggests that all three methyls cannot be accommodated at the same time. In fact, only two of the three methyl groups need to be present in order to obtain near maximal activity. With only one methyl group, even though the cationic nature of the nitrogen is maintained, activity is greatly diminished. Since alkyl moieties do not form hydrogen or ionic bonds, this finding implies that van der Waals forces contribute significantly to ACh binding. As with a single hydrogen substitution, replacement of one methyl group by an ethyl side chain has essentially no effect on activity, presumably because free rotation of the cationic terminus allows the two remaining methyls to fit into the receptor site. Considerations analogous to these indicate that ACh action also depends on the presence of an ester capable of participating in a hydrogen bond. The distance separating the esteratic and cationic positions of the molecule is likewise critical for full activity.

An important source of support for the concept of specificity in drug-receptor interactions comes from the differences so often observed in the activity of optical isomers, such as *d*- and *l*-epinephrine. It is common for virtually all the activity in a racemic mixture to reside in one of the two stereoisomers. In the case of epinephrine, the levorotatory isomer is highly active while the other member of the pair is almost devoid of activity. The presence of only a single atom with an opposite configuration is apparently sufficient to bring about dramatic differences in binding efficiency. Such critical sensitivity can occur only if the drug and receptor fit together with some degree of precision. The optical isomers quinine and quinidine are of interest because both are used therapeutically but for different purposes.[3] Quinidine (dextro) and quinine (levo) differ from each other only in the configuration of a single secondary alcohol group that serves as the connector of the two halves of the molecule. Both isomers are approximately equal in antimalarial activity, a property that depends on the drug reacting with the DNA of the plasmodial parasites responsible for the disease. The antiarrhythmic action on cardiac muscle, however, is greater for quinidine than for quinine. The enantiomers of D-mannose are another example of two molecules that differ only in the spatial arrangement of a single hydroxyl group and yet vary in their biologic activity. α-D-Mannose is sweet when applied to chemoreceptors of the tongue whereas β-D-mannose is bitter.[18]

Consequences of drug binding

The combination of a drug with its receptor represents the incipient event in a series of reactions that culminate in a pharmacologic effect. Of prime importance is the second step in this chain—the receptor response to drug binding. Drugs generally are not highly reactive compounds in the chemical sense; they exert their influences indirectly by altering (through receptor attachment) the activity of an important regulator of a biologic process. The mechanism of action of a drug refers to this initial perturbation of normal function.

Of the various receptor-based mechanisms of drug action, perhaps the most readily observed are those involving enzymes. Certain drugs are analogues of natural enzyme substrates. These antimetabolites compete with the substrate for the same catalytic site on the enzyme molecule, the result of this competition being a decrease in the rate of product formation. As a general rule, however, such inhibitions are likely to be of little biologic consequence unless the magnitude of inhibition approaches 50%. This phenomenon appears to be explained best by the concept that the number of enzyme molecules present usually exceeds that which is necessary for adequate catalysis. A 20% inhibition, therefore, might produce no observable response because the remaining fraction of uninhibited enzyme is still capable of providing enough product. The enzyme carbonic anhydrase represents an extreme example of this situation. To reduce by half the enzymatic hydration of carbon dioxide, 99.7% of the carbonic anhydrase activity must be abolished.[12] Another consideration related to antimetabolites is the oftentimes greater affinity of the reactive site for the natural substrate. This difference may be as much as thousandfold and has some significance for pharmacology. If the substrate to be interfered with is abundant, like glucose, the dose of inhibitor needed to obtain a body fluid concentration a thousand times that of the metabolite would be formidable indeed. Substrates that are in more limited supply, such as vitamin derivatives or chemical mediators, are more reasonable targets for therapy based on this form of inhibition.

Many drugs that influence enzyme activity are not structurally related to native substrates. These drugs affect catalysis by serving as allosteric regulators; that is, by binding elsewhere on the enzyme surface they induce conformational changes at the active center. These disturbances may lead to an increased affinity for the substrate, but it is more likely for the effect to be one of inhibition. Although the basis of drug-induced allosteric changes in enzymes is poorly understood, the surrounding hydration layer appears to be involved. As with other macromolecules, enzymes are covered by a surface film of water. When a drug is bound to its receptor, it upsets the microenvironment around the binding site. Alkyl groups common to many drugs are especially proficient at disturbing the hydration layer; as a result, they promote conformational changes in the drug-receptor complex so as to minimize their impact. It should be noted that the quaternary structure of proteins is greatly influenced by the state of the surrounding water molecules and that enzymes subject to allosteric regulation have quaternary structures of exceptional conformational sensitivity. The requirement described above that a certain percentage of enzyme be affected before an observable effect is achieved also holds for allosteric regulation, but the need for the drug concentration to be in excess of the substrate does not, because the two compounds are not in direct competition for binding.

The concept of allostericism may be of particular relevance to membrane-bound receptors. This class of receptors normally translates the binding of endogenous chemical messengers (hormones or neurotransmitters) into cellular responses. The action of many drugs is dependent on the mimicry of chemical messengers involved in cellular communication. The allosteric concept suggests that a receptor, whether stimulated by its natural effector or by a drug substitute, becomes distorted morphologically. This disturbance then causes a change in a particular enzyme activity or transport mechanism or an alteration of membrane permeability. An illustration of the consequences of drug binding is provided by epinephrine. Incorporated into local anesthetic solutions to prolong the duration of anesthesia, epinephrine mimics the action of the neurotransmitter norepinephrine. As a result of epinephrine attachment to the adrenergic receptor of vascular smooth muscle cells, the ionic permeability of the plasma membrane is altered, free calcium ions accumulate within the cytoplasm, muscle contraction becomes activated, and vasoconstriction ensues. The binding of epinephrine can also affect enzyme activities. In the heart, for example, receptors for norepinephrine are associated functionally with adenylate cyclase, the enzyme responsible for the conversion of adenosine triphosphate into the intracellular mediator 3'-5'-adenosine monophosphate (cAMP). Epinephrine, by inducing a conformational change in the receptor, indirectly activates adenylate cyclase to produce large quantities of cAMP. In turn, the cyclic nucleotide influences, through allosteric mechanisms of its own, a number of metabolic events inside the cell.

Drugs can directly alter processes controlled by membrane-bound receptors without resorting to mimicry of natural messengers. As is the case with enzymes, drugs can act either by physically interfering with messenger binding or by adjusting receptor affinity for the messenger through an allosteric mechanism.

DOSE-RESPONSE RELATIONSHIPS

One of the most fundamental aspects of drug action is the relationship between the dose administered and the effect obtained. Common experience dictates that the magnitude of a chemical's effect on a system is positively correlated with the quantity or concentration of that chemical present. To increase the saltiness of a food, for example, more salt must be added. Within certain limits, the addition of salt yields a graded response, but very small increments have no effect on taste, and if the food is quite salty to begin with, further additions, no matter how great, will have no effect either. There is reason to expect, therefore, that the dose-effect relationship of a drug is not a linear function throughout the entire dose range. Below a minimum threshold there can be no incremental effect from a dose, since there is no observable effect to begin with. Above a certain ceiling, even a large dose will exert no demonstrable influence because the maximal effect has already been reached.

Occupation theory

Recognizing the close correspondence between dose-response relationships and enzyme kinetics, A. J. Clark attempted in the 1920s to quantitate drug effects through application of the law of mass action.[5] Out of his efforts and the contributions of others emerged the occupation theory of drug action.[11] The occupation theory holds that the magnitude of a pharmacologic response elicited by a drug that reversibly combines with its receptor is directly proportional to the number (or fraction) of receptors occupied by the drug. The relationship can be written as:

$$D + R \underset{k_2}{\overset{k_1}{\rightleftharpoons}} DR \overset{k_3}{\rightarrow} \text{Effect}$$

where D is the drug and R the receptor. This reaction is analogous to the interaction of an enzyme with a single substrate yielding a single product. Hence, a derivative of the Michaelis-Menton equation can be used to quantify drug effects:

$$\text{Effect} = \frac{\text{Maximal effect} \times [D]}{K_D + [D]}$$

where $K_D = k_2/k_1$.

This mathematical relationship between the dose (or concentration) of a drug and its response may be demonstrated graphically by an experiment in which an isolated muscle is exposed to increasing concentrations of a drug while the force of contraction is measured (Figure 1-3). When a drug is introduced into a tissue, it binds to its receptor in accordance with the dissociation constant (K_D). For various reasons, very small quantities will not elicit a measurable response: each muscle cell may require a minimal number of receptors to be occupied before it contracts; technical difficulties in detecting small contractions may make such determina-tions inaccurate or impossible to obtain. The lowest dose to elicit a measurable response is termed the *threshold dose*. As higher doses are administered, the number of receptors occupied rises, as does the intensity of response. An increase in the fraction of receptors occupied necessarily reduces the number available for subsequent binding, so that at high doses each increment produces progressively smaller additions to the magnitude of contraction. At very high concentrations, the receptor population becomes saturated, and further drug admin-istration will no longer influence contraction.

The most useful dose range for a drug is that which falls between the threshold and the ceiling. By expressing data as the logarithm of the dose versus the degree of response, this important, nor-mally hyperbolic segment of the dose-effect rela-tionship becomes a sigmoid curve with a linear central portion extending over a tenfold concentra-tion range. The advantage of plotting with the log dose instead of the arithmetic dose is that it greatly simplifies drug study. For example, the ED_{50} of a drug (the dose that produces a half-maximal re-sponse) is often used in comparisons with like agents. When data from several experiments are expressed on a single graph using the log dose, this value can be accurately determined for each drug from the linear portion of the respective curve. If the dosage data were not logarithmically trans-formed, statistical analysis would become more complex and less reliable. Figure 1-4 illustrates the difficulties encountered if two drugs differing only in receptor affinity are examined on an arithmetic dose scale. The curve for drug A is so compressed that the ED_{50} cannot be accurately ascertained, yet

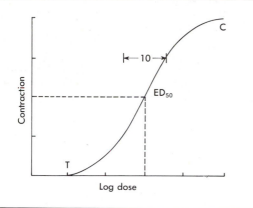

Figure 1-3. Theoretical log dose-response curve for a smooth muscle stimulant. The threshold and ceiling effects are repre-sented by T and C, respectively. As shown, the linear portion of the sigmoid curve, extending from 25% to 75% of the max-imal effect, is encompassed by a tenfold dose range. A range of 10,000 times is required, however, to depict the curve in its entirety (from 1% to 99% of the maximum effect).

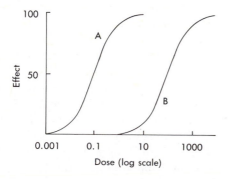 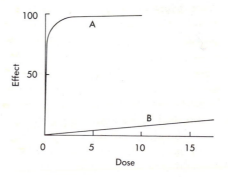

Figure 1-4. Dose-effect curves for two drugs differing in receptor affinity by a factor of 1000. At left, a log dose scale, note the identical shapes of the two dose-effect relationships. At right, an arithmetic dose scale, the lack of correspondence between the two curves hinders drug comparison.

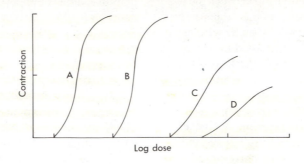

Figure 1-5. Effects of four catecholamines on muscle contraction in the vas deferens of the rat. Drugs A and B differ in affinity but not in intrinsic activity. Drugs C and D differ from each other and from A and B in both affinity and intrinsic activity. (Adapted from Ariëns, E.J., Simonis, A.M., and van Rossum, J.M. Drug-receptor interactions: interaction of one or more drugs with one receptor system. In Ariëns, E.J., ed. Molecular Pharmacology: The Mode of Action of Biologically Active Compounds. New York, Academic Press, Inc., 1964.)

the ED_{50} for drug B cannot even be represented on the same page. Indeed, to portray the dose-response relationship of drug B in its entirety, as are the other curves (to within 99% of the maximal effect), the graph would need to extend some 83 feet.

Agonists

Drugs that elicit a response from a tissue are known as agonists. Agonists that produce ceiling effects, effects that are not exceeded by other drugs, are called *full agonists*, and drugs whose maximal effects are less than those of full agonists are referred to as *partial agonists*. It should be stressed that the distinction between full and partial agonists does not merely reflect variances in receptor affinity; the relatively low ceiling effect of a partial agonist cannot be raised by increasing its dose. The difference between these two classes of agonists lies in their unequal intrinsic activities. *Intrinsic activity* (or efficacy) is an empirical term introduced as a modification of occupation theory to describe the ability of a drug to activate a receptor once the drug-receptor complex has formed. Drugs with a low intrinsic activity (a small k_3) not only have relatively low ceiling effects, but each fraction of receptors occupied elicits a response that is smaller than that produced by a similar degree of receptor binding by a full agonist. In other words, the log dose-response curve of a partial agonist has a lower maximum and a smaller slope than does that of a full agonist.

These principles are demonstrated in Figure 1-

5, which presents data from a study of four agonists of muscle contraction.[2] The muscle to be investigated was removed from an animal, placed in a bath containing an oxygenated physiologic salt solution, and attached to a strain gauge to measure isometric contractions. In such experiments, conditions can be manipulated to ensure that each drug tested has equal access to the receptor. (This condition, which greatly simplifies the interpretation of experimental results, cannot be duplicated in whole-animal investigations.) The most potent drug shown is A, with drugs B, C, and D exhibiting progressively decreasing potencies. The potency of a drug is the dose required to elicit an arbitrarily determined level of response. Potency is usually a matter of little importance, since a drug that is very potent with respect to its desirable effects is often equally potent with respect to those that are undesirable. In the intact animal (or patient), potency is influenced not only by the affinity of a drug for its receptor and by its intrinsic activity but also by its ability to reach the receptor (determined by the rate of absorption and the patterns of distribution and elimination). A very active drug will appear to have low potency if it is not well absorbed, becomes bound to nonspecific sites, or cannot reach the target organ.

Drugs A and B are full agonists (assuming no other drug with an affinity for this particular receptor can produce a greater ceiling effect), and drugs C and D are partial agonists. Drug D has the smallest intrinsic activity. Note that the consequences of the low potency of drug B can be com-

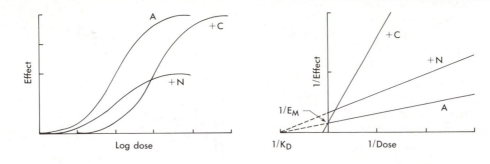

Figure 1-6. Modification of a pharmacologic effect by drug antagonism. At left, a log dose-response graph: curve A depicts the dose-effect relationship of a full agonist; curves C and N represent, respectively, the influences of a competitive and a noncompetitive antagonist. Note the shift to the right of the agonist log dose-response curve by the competitive inhibitor and its downward displacement by the noncompetitive variety. At right, a double-reciprocal plot of the same curves, the competitive antagonist increases the dissociation constant (K_D) without influencing the maximum effect obtainable by the agonist (E_M). The reverse is true for the purely noncompetitive inhibitor.

pletely overcome by increasing its dose. This characteristic suggests that drug B exhibits a lower potency than drug A solely because it has a weaker affinity for its receptor. Drugs C and D represent a more complex problem. Obviously, these agents are less potent than A and B, which suggests that they possess lesser affinities. Part of their reduced potency, however, is a consequence of their lower intrinsic activities.

Antagonists

Drugs that bind to a receptor but have an intrinsic activity of zero (no receptor activation; $k_3 = 0$) are competitive antagonists. By making receptors less available for agonist binding, a competitive antagonist will depress the response to a given dose of agonist. The result is a parallel shift to the right of the agonist dose-response curve. The most important aspect of this type of inhibition is that it is completely surmountable by a high enough dose of agonist. As in enzymology, the presence of a competitive antagonist produces an apparent reduction in the affinity of a drug for its receptor. Such a reduction can occur, though, not only through competition by the antagonist for the receptor site itself but also via allosteric distortion of the site so as to reduce binding efficiency for the agonist. Competitive antagonisms are very common in pharmacology, and numerous examples will be cited in succeeding chapters: histamine versus antihistamines, morphine versus naloxone, acetylcholine versus atropine, epinephrine versus propranolol. By virtue of their small intrinsic activi-

ties, partial agonists can also serve as competitive antagonists of fully active drugs.

Another type of antagonism that is commmonly encountered is the noncompetitive variety. The noncompetitive blockade is insurmountable in that the ceiling effect of an agonist can never be reattained, regardless of the dose administered. A noncompetitive antagonist decreases the effective number of receptors, either by irreversibly binding to the receptor site or by binding elsewhere and eliminating receptor sites through allosteric influences. In neither case can the agonist successfully "compete" against the block, and the result is a downward displacement of the agonist log dose-response curve. For drugs that display aspects of both competitive and noncompetitive antagonisms, the dose-response curve is shifted to the right and depressed. Figure 1-6 reviews the dissimilarities between the two major types of drug blockade.

Limitations of occupation theory

Basic to the foregoing discussion are several assumptions about the interactions between a drug and its receptor:

1. One drug molecule reversibly combines with a single receptor.
2. All receptors are identical and equally accessible to the drug.
3. Only a small portion of the total drug is involved in forming complexes with the receptor.
4. The biologic response is proportional to the degree of receptor occupancy.

Although these assumptions are often valid, there are situations where they do not apply and where the dose-response curves vary from the expected. One such case involves the inhibition of ACh by atropine. Atropine is classified as a competitive antagonist of ACh. It binds to the ACh receptor and causes an inhibition that can be surmounted by increasing the concentration of agonist present. Surprisingly, the association of atropine with the receptor site is practically irreversible; neither ACh nor extensive washing will remove the drug once it is bound. To explain the paradox presented by atropine, pharmacologists have borrowed from the phenomenon of enzyme excess to postulate the existence of spare receptors.[17] This amendment to the occupation theory states that, for some drugs at least, there are more receptors available than are required to yield a maximal response. Although atropine completely blocks a number of receptors from binding ACh, a sufficient quantity remains to produce a ceiling effect, albeit at a higher agonist concentration. As one might predict, the competitive inhibition obtained with a conventional dose of an antagonist like atropine gradually takes on the characteristics of a mixed competitive-noncompetitive blockade as larger doses of the antagonist deplete the spare receptor pool.[14]

In addition to the fact that pharmacologic responses are not always proportional to receptor occupancy, it is likely that situations exist in which the receptors to a drug are not identical to one another. As is true with ion channels, receptors may exist in at least two configurations: active and inactive. According to the "allosteric model" of drug action these forms of the receptor are in equilibrium, and drugs act by altering their relative distributions.[11] Figure 1-7 illustrates a simple, two-state version in which the equilibrium greatly favors the inactive state. In this model, full agonists combine only with active receptors. Partial agonists combine with both forms of the receptor but have greater affinity for the active species. Competitive antagonists bind to the inactive receptor at least as well as they do to the active form. The major attractions of the allosteric model are that it provides a physical explanation for differences in intrinsic activity between congeners and that it affords a simple mechanism for the pharmacologic response elicited by drug binding. On the other hand, it is by no means certain that drug receptors generally exist in more than one conformational state.

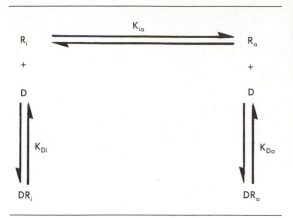

Figure 1-7. Allosteric two-state model of drug-receptor interaction. The receptor can exist in an active (R_a) or inactive (R_i) state, as governed by the equilibrium constant K_{ia}. Unless the receptor mediates a tonically active process, K_{ia} greatly favors the inactive form. Drugs (D) may bind to R_a, R_i, or both. Drug binding does not directly affect receptor function; instead, it may alter, through mass action, the proportion of active ($R_a + DR_a$) to inactive ($R_i + DR_i$) receptors.

Another example of the limitations of the classical occupation theory is provided by nicotine. This natural alkaloid exhibits a complex pharmacologic activity. Initially, nicotine acts like an agonist: it stimulates ACh receptors at autonomic ganglia and in skeletal muscle. The stimulation is temporary, however, and in a matter of minutes the action of nicotine transforms from that of excitation to one of antagonism. This metamorphosis cannot be adequately explained by occupation theory. To account for such anomalies a rate theory of drug action has been proposed.[15] The rate theory is based on the premise that drug effects arise not from the occupation of receptors but from the process of occupation. Each time a drug interacts with a receptor, a "quantum" of excitation is produced. According to this view, drugs that are agonists have high rates of both association (k_1) and dissociation (k_2), features that permit the generation of many quanta per unit time. Antagonists, on the other hand, have very low rates of dissociation, and their occupancy of the receptor prevents the agonist from acting at that site with a high rate of association. Finally, a drug like nicotine is accounted for by having a large k_1, permitting an initial stimulation, and a small k_2, prohibiting further instances of new binding. Although the rate theory provides a neat solution for certain properties of partial agonists and antagonists, it cannot explain the common observation that congeneric drugs often yield the same maximal response, even in the face of substantially divergent potencies. The theory also cannot apply to enzyme receptors, which are known to be influenced by the occupancy of a drug and not by the process of association. When these caveats are considered, it becomes difficult to accept the rate theory as a general description of drug action.[8]

Probably the most significant limitation of occupation theory arises from the gulf that can separate the binding of a drug by its receptor and the resultant development of a biologic effect. Even if the assumptions basic to occupation theory hold for the initial action of a drug, they often do not apply to an observed effect that is removed from the incipient response by several intermediate events. The spare receptor concept described above represents one case in which a rate-limiting intermediate step in the drug action/pharmacologic effect sequence invalidates the assumption that the magnitude of drug effect is uniformly proportional to the degree of receptor occupancy. There are many other mechanisms that can also modify the dose-response relationship. As illustration of this point, consider a drug that increases blood pressure by causing vasoconstriction in selected vascular beds. As increasing doses of the drug are administered, various cardiovascular reflexes will be evoked that will tend to reverse the drug effect. The build-up of lactate and other metabolites in the affected tissues will also limit vasoconstriction. Should the drug have multiple actions, for example, on the heart or on the vasomotor centers of the central nervous system, additional drug influences will be superimposed on the vasoconstriction-induced hypertension as well. Obviously, the blood pressure increases obtained with various doses of the drug will most likely not be determined by a simple occupancy relation that ignores all of these other factors.

The occupation theory, then, offers for many drugs and receptors a quantitative description of the dose-response relationship, provided that the effect measured closely follows the initial consequence of drug binding. However, assumptions basic to the occupancy theory do not always hold, and other models of drug action may at times be more appropriate.[11] Finally, the occupation theory cannot account for drugs whose actions are temporally dependent; these agents are described better by a function dependent on the kinetics of drug binding and not by the association itself.

RECEPTOR-INDEPENDENT DRUG ACTIONS

No description of drug action would be complete without a consideration of those agents that exert pharmacologic effects through receptor-independent mechanisms. Aside from the fact that these drugs act without the benefit of receptor intermediaries, there are no common traits serving to link this diverse array of compounds. For the sake of discussion, therefore, these drugs will be grouped arbitrarily into three categories: (1) chemically reactive agents, (2) physically active agents, and (3) counterfeit biochemical constituents.

Chemically reactive agents

Chemically reactive drugs include a wide variety of compounds, some of which interact with small molecules or ions, others that attack proteins and other macromolecules. Gastric antacids and metallic ion chelators are two kinds of drugs that combine with inorganic substances within the body. Of particular importance to dentistry is dimercaprol, a chelating agent capable of forming coordination complexes with mercury and other heavy metals. Drugs affecting macromolecules include most germicides and the antineoplastic alkylating agents. Sodium hypochlorite solutions provide antisepsis and facilitate canal debridement during endodontic therapy because they release hypochlorous acid, a potent chemical disruptor of biologic matter. In general, these compounds can be readily distinguished from drugs that are receptor mediated. With the exception of certain chelating agents, they lack specificity and may individually react with a variety of substances, organic or otherwise. Minor structural modifications also do not usually influence drug activity. Finally, the reactions of these drugs rely heavily on covalent bonding or on strong ionic attachments; they are not usually dependent on hydrogen bonding and van der Waals forces.

Physically active agents

Physically active agents, in contrast, are often useful therapeutically because they are chemically inert. Thus, magnesium sulfate is an effective cathartic because it is not absorbed from the gastrointestinal tract. The salt exerts an osmotic effect, retaining large amounts of water within the intestinal lumen. The colon becomes distended and is stimulated to undergo expulsive contraction. Through a similar osmotic mechanism, mannitol promotes diuresis and serves to prevent kidney damage during episodes of acute renal failure. A totally unrelated physical mechanism is evoked by hydrogen peroxide. Although highly reactive, hydrogen peroxide finds use in periodontics because of its effervescent action. The release of gas bubbles promotes the physical removal of debris from periodontal tissues. Perhaps the most important drugs of this category, however, are the volatile general anesthetics. Through physicochemical influences on plasma membranes, brain neurons become reversibly depressed, and sensations are blocked. The inhalation anesthetics, in particular, and the physically active agents, in general, exhibit a surprising lack of structural specificity. The major requirements for activity appear to consist of a certain pharmacologic inertness coupled with the ability to be administered in high concentrations (compared with most other drugs) without causing undue toxicity.

Counterfeit biochemical constituents

The counterfeit biochemical constituents resemble antimetabolite drugs inasmuch as they are artificial analogues of natural substrates. Hence, they have to meet the same rigid structural requirements as do their receptor-based counterparts. Counterfeit agents, however, do not affect enzymes; they are instead incorporated into specific macromolecules by the cell. The resulting drug effects arise from an altered biologic activity of the affected macromolecules or from their increased susceptibility to destruction. The thymine analogue 5-bromouracil is representative of this group.[4] The effect of 5-bromouracil incorporation into the genetic material of a cell is an elevation in the mutation rate and an increased frequency of chromosomal disturbances. Agents of this type are used therapeutically in the treatment of several neoplasias and microbial infections.

It should now be clear that it is impossible to derive a quantitative description of responses to receptor-independent drugs akin to that presented for receptor-based agents. As a group, the very diversity of these drugs precludes any unifying relationship between dose and effect. Nevertheless, log dose-response curves similar to those previously discussed are often obtained with these drugs, and the general concepts of potency and efficacy still apply.

CITED REFERENCES

1. Albert, A. Relations between molecular structure and biological activity: stages in the evolution of current concepts. Annual Review of Pharmacology and Toxicology **11**:13-36, 1971.
2. Ariëns, E.J., Simonis, A.M., and van Rossum, J.M. Drug-receptor interactions: interaction of one or more drugs with one receptor system. In Ariëns, E.J., ed. Molecular Pharmacology: The Mode of Action of Biologically Active Compounds. New York, Academic Press, Inc., 1964.
3. Bigger, J.T., Jr., and Hoffman, B.F. Antiarrhythmic drugs. In Gilman, A.G., Goodman, L.S., and Gilman, A., eds. Goodman and Gilman's The Pharmacological Basis of Therapeutics, ed. 6. New York, Macmillan, Inc., 1980.
4. Brockman, R.W., and Anderson, E.P. Pyrimidine analogues. In Hochster, R.M., and Quastel, J.H., eds. Metabolic Inhibitors, vol. 1. New York, Academic Press, Inc., 1963.
5. Clark, A.J. The Mode of Action of Drugs on Cells. London, Edward Arnold & Co., 1933.
6. Erlich, P. Chemotherapeutics: scientific principles, methods, and results. Lancet **2**:445-451, 1913.
7. Goldstein, A. Opioid peptides (endorphins) in pituitary and brain. Science **193**:1081-1086, 1976.
8. Goldstein, A., Aronow, L., and Kalman, S.M. Principles of Drug Action: The Basis of Pharmacology, ed. 2. New York, John Wiley & Sons, Inc., 1974.
9. Laduron, P.M., and Ilien, B. Solubilization of brain muscarinic, dopaminergic and serotonergic receptors: a critical analysis. Biochemical Pharmacology **31**:2145-2151, 1982.
10. Langley, J.N. On the contraction of muscle, chiefly in relation to the presence of ''receptive'' substances. Part IV. The effect of curari and of some other substances on the nicotine response of the sartorius and gastrocnemius muscles of the frog. Journal of Physiology (London) **39**:235-295, 1909.
11. Mackay, D. A critical survey of receptor theories of drug action. In van Rossum, J.M., ed. Kinetics of Drug Action. Handbook of Experimental Pharmacology, vol. 47. Berlin, Springer-Verlag, 1977.
12. Maren, T.H. The relation between enzyme inhibition and physiological response in the carbonic anhydrase system. Journal of Pharmacology and Experimental Therapeutics **139**:140-153, 1963.
13. Miller, J.W., and Lewis, J.E. Drugs affecting smooth muscle. Annual Review of Pharmacology and Toxicology **9**:147-171, 1969.
14. Nickerson, M. Receptor occupancy and tissue response. Nature **178**:697-698, 1956.
15. Paton, W.D.M. A theory of drug action based on the rate of drug-receptor combination. Proceedings of the Royal Society of London; B: Biological Sciences **154**:21-69, 1961.
16. Paton, W.D.M., and Rang, H.P. The uptake of atropine and related drugs by intestinal smooth muscle of the guinea pig in relation to acetylcholine receptors. Proceedings of the Royal Society of London; B: Biological Sciences **163**:1-44, 1965.
17. Stephenson, R.P. A modification of receptor theory. British Journal of Pharmacology **11**:379-393, 1956.
18. Stewart, R.A., Carrico, C.K., Webster, R.L., and Steinhardt, R.G., Jr. Physicochemical stereospecificity in taste perception of α-D-mannose and β-D-mannose. Nature **234**:220, 1971.

19. Venter, J.C., Fraser, C.M., Soiefer, A.I., Jeffrey, D.R., Strauss, W.L., Charlton, R.R., and Greguski, R. Auto-antibodies and monoclonal antibodies to β-adrenergic receptors: their use in receptor purification and characterization. Advances in Cyclic Nucleotide Research **14:**135-143, 1981.

GENERAL REFERENCES

Gilman, A.G., Mayer, S.E., and Melmon, K.L. Pharmacodynamics: mechanisms of drug action and the relationship between drug concentration and effect. In Gilman, A.G., Goodman, L.S., and Gilman, A., eds. Goodman and Gilman's The Pharmacological Basis of Therapeutics, ed. 6. New York, Macmillan, Inc., 1980.

Goldstein, A., Aronow, L., and Kalman, S.M. Principles of Drug Action: The Basis of Pharmacology, ed. 2. New York, John Wiley & Sons, Inc., 1974.

Hair, M., ed. The Chemistry of Biosurfaces, vol. 1. New York, Marcel Dekker, Inc., 1971.

Levine, R.R. Pharmacology: Drug Actions and Reactions, ed. 2. Boston, Little, Brown & Co., 1978.

Von Rossum, J.M., ed. Kinetics of Drug Action. Handbook of Experimental Pharmacology, vol. 47. Berlin, Springer-Verlag, 1977.

2 Pharmacokinetics: the absorption, distribution, and fate of drugs

John A. Yagiela

When the magnitude of a drug's pharmacologic effect is quantified as a function of dose, it is tacitly assumed that the drug concentration vicinal to the site of action is linearly related to the amount administered. While this assumption may strictly apply to an in vitro test, it ignores the temporal factors that modify drug effects in vivo. Drug concentrations are rarely static; they rise and fall as dictated by the processes of absorption, distribution, metabolism, and excretion. The following discussion will examine these processes (Figure 2-1) and how they influence the sojourn of drugs in the body.

PASSAGE OF DRUGS ACROSS MEMBRANES

In order for a drug to be absorbed, reach its site of action, and eventually be eliminated, it must cross one or more biologic membrane barriers. These may consist of a single plasma membrane or comprise a layer of closely packed cells. Since such barriers to drugs behave similarly, the cell membrane can serve as a prototype for all. The plasma membrane is about 100 Å thick. It is composed of a bimolecular sheet of lipids (primarily cholesterol and phospholipids) and a variety of proteins. Although early models depicted the protein as covering essentially the entire membrane surface,[10] subsequent observations suggest a more fluid model with globular proteins interspersed throughout and extending beyond the lipid phase of the membrane (Figure 2-2).[32] The presence of protein molecules spanning the entire thickness of the membrane provides a necessary link between the extracellular environment and the cell interior,

which is consistent with the concept that drug activation of a membrane-bound receptor on the external surface of a cell can be directly translated into an intracellular response.

Passive diffusion

The passage of drugs across membranes can involve several different mechanisms. Of these, passive diffusion is the most commonly encountered. Studies by Overton and Meyer at the turn of this century demonstrated that the cell membrane acts for the most part as a lipoid barrier. As shown by Collander and Bärlund (Figure 2-3),[7] the rate of transfer of nonelectrolytes across a membrane is directly proportional to the lipid/water partition coefficient. (The partition coefficient is a measure of the relative solubility of an agent in a fat solvent versus its solubility in water.) A drug with a high partition coefficient will readily enter the lipid phase of the membrane and pass down its concentration gradient to the aqueous phase on the other side. More molecules are then free to enter the membrane and continue the transfer process. With poorly lipid-soluble compounds, however, few molecules enter the membrane per unit time, and the rate of passage is depressed.

The absence of an ionic charge is one major factor favoring lipid solubility. Drugs with a fixed charge, such as those containing a quaternary nitrogen atom, permeate membranes slowly, if at all. The reason for the relative solubility of nonionized molecules in lipids relates to their exclusion from polar media. Simple ions and charged molecules are stabilized in water by the hydration shells that

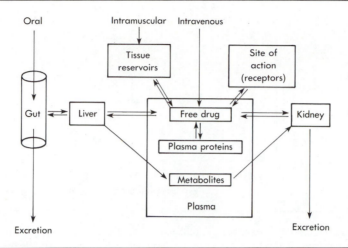

Figure 2-1. Outline of the major pathways of absorption, distribution, metabolism, and excretion of drugs. Compounds taken orally must pass through the liver before reaching the systemic circulation. Once in the bloodstream, agents are distributed throughout the body and come in contact with their respective sites of action. Drugs are filtered by the kidney, only to be reabsorbed if lipid soluble. Metabolism of many drugs occurs primarily in the liver, after which the metabolites are excreted via the bile or urine. Some agents eliminated in the bile are subject to reabsorption and may participate in an enterohepatic cycle.

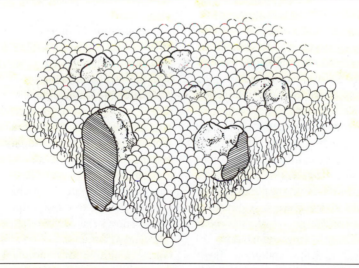

Figure 2-2. Schematic drawing of a section of cell membrane depicting the phospholipid bilayer, with the hydrophilic heads as circles and the fatty acid chains as wavy lines. Globular proteins dispersed throughout the membrane penetrate the lipid phase, providing channels of communication between the external environment and the cell interior. (From Singer, S.J., and Nicolson, G.L. The fluid mosaic model of the structure of cell membranes. Science **175:**720-731, Feb. 18. 1972. Copyright 1972 by the American Association for the Advancement of Science.)

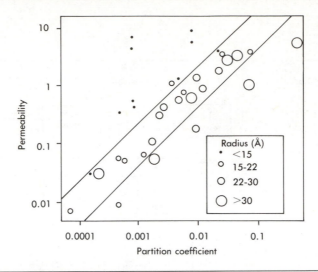

Figure 2-3. Relationship between membrane permeability and lipid (olive oil)/water partition coefficient in *Chara certatophylla*. Each circle represents a single nonelectrolyte with a molecular radius as indicated in the key. Small compounds permeate more readily than their partition coefficient would indicate; the reverse is true for large molecules. (Adapted from Collander, R. Physiologia Plantarum **2:**300-311, 1949.)

surround them, a consequence of the tendency of charged species to orient polar molecules. This process excludes nonpolar substances, and the resulting segregation causes them to coalesce in a manner analogous to the formation of oil droplets at the surface of water. The term *hydrophobic bonding* refers to the tendency for water-insoluble molecules to be drawn together, and it is this behavior that is responsible for the preferential tendency of lipid-soluble drugs to penetrate cell membranes via the lipid components. Ionized compounds, on the other hand, are so stabilized by their interaction with water that movement into a lipid phase is markedly restricted. Many therapeutic agents are weak electrolytes; depending on the pH of their aqueous environment, they can exist in both ionized and neutral forms. Since charged molecules penetrate membranes with considerable difficulty, the rate of movement of these drugs is governed not only by the partition coefficient of the neutral species but also by the degree of ionization. As illustrated in Figure 2-4, acidic conditions favor the transport of weak acids, and the opposite holds true for basic compounds.

The same concept of water interaction used to explain the aqueous solubility of ions also applies to many nonionic molecules. Although unsubstituted aliphatic and aromatic hydrocarbons have no tendency to react with water, affinity for water molecules is not restricted to structures with a formal charge. Organic residues possessing electronegative atoms such as oxygen, nitrogen, and sulfer can interact with water through the formation of hydrogen bonds to provide some degree of aqueous solubility.

Examination of Figure 2-3 reveals that lipid solubility is not the only factor influencing the passive diffusion of drugs across cell membranes; molecular size is also important. Many small molecules permeate much more readily than would be predicted from their partition coefficients. This finding, plus the rapid penetration of water and small ions, has led to the postulation of channels extending through the plasma membrane. These pores are about 4 Å in diameter; compounds small enough to penetrate these channels can enter cells without having to cross a lipoid barrier. Figure 2-3 also shows that large organic molecules diffuse more slowly than expected. Nonelectrolytes containing a number of hydrophobic groups are often so insoluble in water that their transit across the lipid/water interface may be retarded despite a favorable partition coefficient.[21]

The foregoing discussion of large nonelectrolytes should indicate that some degree of water solubility is necessary for the passive diffusion of

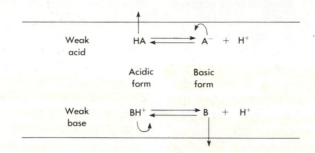

Figure 2-4. Membrane penetration by weak electrolytes. The nonionic species of drugs (HA, B) permeate membranes much more efficiently than do the charged forms (A⁻, BH⁺). Acidic conditions shift the dissociation curves to the left, favoring the diffusion of weak acids. An increase in pH favors the loss of hydrogen (H⁺) and the diffusion of weak bases.

drugs across membranes. No matter how lipid-soluble an agent is, it will never cross a membrane if it cannot first dissolve in the extracellular fluid and be carried to the structure. Thus, benzocaine, an active local anesthetic when applied directly to nerves, is ineffective after injection because its water insolubility precludes significant diffusion away from the administration site and toward its locus of action within the neuronal membrane. Once inside the membrane lipids, a drug with an extremely high partition coefficient may be so soluble that it has little tendency to diffuse outward down its concentration gradient.[30]

In summary, the passive diffusion of drugs across lipoid barriers is largely a function of their lipid/water partition coefficients. A modicum of water solubility is required, though, for drugs to reach and to cross membranes in concentrations sufficient to permit a reasonable rate of diffusion. Because ions do not generally penetrate membranes well, except those small enough to traverse membrane pores, the passage of weak electrolytes is further governed by their degree of ionization.

Specialized transport processes

Several mechanisms besides passive diffusion are responsible for the movement of drugs across membranes. Many hydrophilic compounds too large for 4 Å diameter channels nevertheless migrate through membranes without difficulty. These anomalies are especially prevalent in tissues specialized for the transport of chemicals and fluids (e.g., intestinal mucosa, capillary endothelium, choroid plexus, renal tubule). Drugs resembling important endogenous compounds (metabolites,

neurotransmitters, etc.) are the most likely to receive special handling.

Carrier-mediated transport. A number of lipid-insoluble substances are shuttled across plasma membranes by forming complexes with specific membrane constituents called carriers. Carriers are like receptors in many ways: they are proteins, quite selective in the agents they combine with, and subject to competitive inhibition. Since the number of carriers is finite, carrier-mediated transport can be saturated at high drug concentrations. *Facilitated diffusion* is the term given to carrier-based transfer when the driving force is simply the concentration difference of the drug across the membrane. Frequently, however, carriers move substances against their electrochemical gradients. This *active transport*, in addition to exhibiting selectivity and saturability, requires the expenditure of energy and may be blocked by inhibitors of cellular metabolism. Active transport permits the efficient absorption of materials vital for cellular function and the selective elimination of waste products. The sodium pump, by maintaining a large sodium gradient across the membrane, indirectly serves as the energy source for the active transport of many drugs.

Filtration. The endothelial lining of most capillaries behaves as if it were fenestrated by holes up to 80 Å in diameter. Fluids move through these holes by bulk flow according to the pressure differential across the membrane. Since materials are excluded from passage only on the basis of size, this type of drug transfer is, in fact, a form of filtration. Filtration is involved in the distribution and elimination of virtually all drugs and is often the only mechanism of membrane penetration available to large, lipid-insoluble compounds.

Pinocytosis. Probably the least important but most complex method of drug transport is pinocytosis. Certain cells have the capacity to absorb soluble substances by vesiculation. The process begins when the substance to be transported stimulates the membrane to form a depression around the solute. The invagination deepens with time and is sealed over as the membrane fuses. The newly formed vesicle is then pinched off and free to migrate into the cell interior. Eventually, the membrane surrounding the engulfed material is dissolved, and the contents are released into the cytoplasm. Pinocytosis is probably responsible for the absorption of antigenic proteins and certain toxins from the small intestine, but it currently plays a very minor role in the transport of drugs.

ABSORPTION

Absorption refers to the transfer of a drug from its site of administration into the bloodstream. Obviously, the particular route of administration selected will greatly influence the rate and perhaps even the extent of drug absorption.

Oral ingestion

Oral ingestion was the first and is still the most commonly used method for the administration of therapeutic agents. The major advantages of the oral route lie in three areas: convenience, economics, and safety. Patient acceptance of oral medication is good, since the technique itself is painless, and trained personnel are not required for its accomplishment. The convenience and low cost with respect to other modes of therapy are especially prominent for drugs that must be given several times daily on a long-term basis. The oral route is relatively safe because drug absorption is comparatively slow. Sudden high blood concentrations are not nearly as likely to be achieved by the ingestion of drugs as they are by parenteral injection. Allergic reactions are also less likely to occur, especially those of a serious nature. The oral route, however, does have some drawbacks. Because self-administration is the rule, patient cooperation, or compliance, is required for optimal therapy. Drug absorption is likely to be delayed (on a clinical average of 30 to 60 minutes) and may be incomplete. Metabolic inactivation or complex formation may also occur before the drug has a chance to reach the systemic circulation. These limitations to the oral route translate into an increased variability in patient response. Finally, the spectrum of adverse reactions caused by oral medication can extend from one end of the gastrointestinal tract to the other.

Drugs taken orally may be absorbed along the entire alimentary canal, but the relative degree of contact with the mucosa will determine the amount of uptake in each segment. Variables affecting absorption include the duration of exposure, the concentration of the drug, and the surface area available for absorption. Under normal circumstances, the oral and esophageal mucosae are exposed too briefly to a drug during the process of swallowing for any absorption to take place. The colon normally plays no role in the absorption of orally administered compounds because little nonabsorbed drug usually reaches it. By exclusion, the bulk of drug absorption must take place in the stomach and small intestine.

Influence of pH. As previously discussed, absorption is favored when the drug ingested is lipid soluble. For weak electrolytes, the pH of the surrounding medium will affect the degree of ionization and, therefore, drug absorption. Because the hydrogen ion concentrations of the stomach and small intestine diverge widely, the two structures appear to be qualitatively dissimilar in their respective patterns of drug absorption. Figure 2-5 illustrates this difference and its effect on the commonly used analgesic combination of aspirin plus codeine. Aspirin is an organic acid, with a pK_a of 3.49. In gastric juice (pH 1 to 3), aspirin will remain nonionized, and its passage across the stomach mucosa and into the bloodstream will be favored. The plasma, however, has a pH of 7.4. On entering this environment, the acid will become ionized to such an extent that return of the drug to the gastrointestinal tract will be prevented by the low lipid solubility of the anionic species. When equilibrium is established, the concentration of nonionized aspirin molecules on both sides of the membrane will be the same, but the total amount of drug (ionized plus neutral forms) will be much greater on the plasma side. This unequal distribution of drug molecules based on the pH gradient across the gastric membrane is an example of ion trapping. The biologic process that sustains this partitioning is the energy-consuming secretion of hydrogen ions by the gastric chief cells. Since there are few organic acids with a pK_a low enough to permit significant ionization at stomach pH, almost

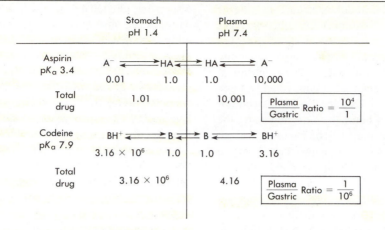

Figure 2-5. Gastric absorption of aspirin, a weak acid, and codeine, a weak base. The absorption of aspirin is promoted by ion trapping within the plasma; the low pH of stomach fluid favors gastric retention of codeine. (The 3.49 pK_a of aspirin was truncated to 3.4 for purposes of illustration.)

all acidic drugs will be effectively absorbed by the gastric mucosa.

For bases like codeine (pK_a 7.9) the opposite applies. Codeine is almost completely ionized in the acidic environment of the stomach; hence, absorption will be negligible. At equilibrium virtually all of the drug would remain within the stomach. Only very weak bases will be nonionized at gastric pH and available for absorption. The ion trapping of basic compounds within the gastric lumen is sometimes useful in forensic medicine. Many drugs subject to abuse are organic bases (e.g., morphine, cocaine, and amphetamine). Even when injected intravenously, they will tend to accumulate in the stomach by crossing the gastric mucosa in the reverse direction. Questions of intravenous overdosage can often be answered from the analysis of stomach contents.

When the gastric fluid passes into the small intestine, it is quickly neutralized by pancreatic, biliary, and intestinal secretions. The pH of the proximal one fourth of the intestine varies from 4.0 to 6.0, but it reaches neutrality in more distal segments. Under these more alkaline conditions, aspirin converts to the anionic form, while a significant fraction of the codeine molecules give up their positive charge. Although basic drugs will be favored for absorption over acids in the small intestine, ion trapping is not extensive because the pH differential across the intestinal mucosa is small. Therefore, differences in intestinal absorption based on pH are more concerned with the rate of

uptake than with the extent. As one might expect, neutralization of gastric contents by the administration of antacids removes the qualitative disparity in electrolyte absorption normally observed between the stomach and the small intestine.

Mucosal surface area. A second major difference between absorption in the stomach and the small intestine relates to the intralumenal surface areas involved in drug uptake. Aside from certain mucosal irregularities (rugae) the stomach lining approximates that of a smooth pouch. The mucosa of the small intestine, however, is uniquely adapted for absorption. Contributions by the folds of Kerckring, villi, and microvilli combine to increase the effective surface area 600-fold.[37] Assuming a small intestine 280 cm in length and 4 cm in diameter, about 200 m^2 is available for drug absorption. The surface/volume ratio in the small intestine is so great that drugs ionized even to the extent of 99% may still be effectively absorbed. Many studies have shown, in fact, that acidic drugs with pK_as greater than 3.0 and basic compounds with pK_as less than 8.0 readily pass from the intestinal fluid into the plasma.[18] Although pH considerations favor the gastric absorption of aspirin, as much as 90% of the drug when given in tablet form is actually absorbed from the small intestine in vivo.[8] Experimentally, nonelectrolytes like ethanol are also absorbed from the intestine many times faster than from the stomach.[24]

Gastric emptying. Since virtually any substance that can penetrate the gastrointestinal epithelium is best absorbed in the small intestine, the rate of gastric emptying can significantly affect drug absorption, particularly for organic bases that are not absorbed at all from the stomach. Gastric emptying is accomplished by contraction of the antrum of the stomach, an event that occurs roughly three times per minute. A mixed meal of solids and liquids requires about 4 hours to completely leave the stomach, but liquids alone will be removed in about 1½ hours. As a general rule, approximately 10 ml of liquid will be passed into the duodenum per minute.

A major variable in delaying gastric emptying is the presence of fat. Unless there is a need to avoid drug-induced irritation of the gastric mucosa, it is often best to take oral medications in the absence of food but with a full glass of water. This procedure will speed drug entry into the small intestine and provide maximum access to the gastrointestinal mucosa. Occasionally, the presence of a fatty meal will promote the absorption of a drug that has a high lipid but low water solubility. The antibiotic griseofulvin and the fat-soluble vitamins are examples of substances that are better absorbed in the presence of lipids. In these instances, the delay in gastric emptying produced by the high fat content of the chyme is compensated for by a more complete absorption.[34]

Additional situations in which food enhances drug uptake have been reviewed by Melander.[27] Nevertheless, because gastric emptying is often a limiting factor in the rate of drug absorption, it is not surprising that many unrelated drugs exhibit latency periods (the lag phase between oral ingestion and onset of drug effect) of a similar magnitude.

Influence of dosage form. While the times required for gastric emptying and for diffusion across the mucosal barrier undoubtedly contribute to the delayed onset of action of drugs taken orally, situations exist in which these events are not rate-limiting. Most drugs intended for oral use are marketed in the form of capsules or solid tablets. Unlike solutions, these preparations must first dissolve in the gastrointestinal fluid before absorption can occur. If dissolution is very slow, it can become the controlling factor in drug absorption.

The first step in the dissolution process is the disintegration of the tablet (or the capsule and its granules) to yield the primary drug particles. Various excipients are usually included in solid drug preparations to promote disintegration and particle dispersion. Obviously, should disintegration be impaired, drug absorption will be depressed accordingly. The dissolution of drug particles occur by a diffusion-limited mechanism. The diffusion layer of solvent surrounding each particle becomes saturated very quickly with drug molecules escaping from the solid. Since saturation of the diffusion layer occurs far more rapidly than does diffusion from it into the bulk solution, the entire process proceeds no faster than the rate of drug diffusion. Several methods can be employed, however, to accelerate the dissolution rate. Because the total surface area of the particles determines the area available for diffusion, reducing the mean particle size through the process of micronization will promote solubilization. A decrease in particle size of 85% with a compensating increase in particle number will, for example, double the rate of dissolution.[22] Another useful approach is to manufacture drugs in the form of water-soluble salts. The concentration of drug in the dissolution layer will be enhanced (often many-fold) and the rate of diffusion increased.

The dissolution process may be considered rate-limiting whenever a drug solution produces a systemic effect faster than does a solid formulation of the same agent. Sometimes, discrepancies in absorption between dosage forms are of such magnitude that clinical differences are noted. With aspirin, the concentration of drug in the plasma 30 minutes after administration can be twice as high for a solution as for a solid tablet.[22] Although it is not clear whether this difference is due solely to drug dissolution or to other factors as well, such as the more rapid gastric emptying typical of liquids, it is probable that dissolution is at least partially responsible.

The influence of dosage form on drug absorption is quite often taken advantage of by drug manufacturers. For instance, some drugs (e.g., erythromycin) are unstable at low pH and others (e.g., ammonium chloride) are irritating to the gastric mucosa. To avoid release of these drugs within the stomach, they are often prepared in the form of enteric-coated tablets. An enteric coat consists of a film of shellac or some polymeric substitute. The covering is insoluble under acidic conditions but does break down to permit tablet disintegration in the more alkaline environment of the small intestine. Although these preparations are often beneficial, their usefulness nevertheless suffers from an increased variability in patient response. Since drug absorption cannot begin until the tablet passes into the duodenum, the time required for gastric transit becomes an important variable. The passage of a single insoluble tablet from the stomach into the intestine is a random event that can take anywhere from several minutes to over 6 hours.[14]

Sustained-release preparations represent another method of capitalizing on the influence of formulation on drug absorption. These products are designed to release a steady amount of drug within the gastrointestinal tract for a period of 12 to 24 hours. In addition, some preparations also provide an initial loading dose that is readily available for absorption. Sustained release may be accomplished by using a porous matrix, with the drug located in the interior spaces as well as on the external surface. An alternative is to make spheres of drug which will dissolve at different rates because of various coatings. Advantages claimed for these drug products include greater patient compliance and smaller fluctuations in blood concentration between dosages. Studies with some preparations, however, have documented a greater variability in performance than is normally encountered with conventional dosage forms. Because sustained-release products contain several conventional doses of medication, a danger exists that a too rapid release of drug from these preparations might cause unexpected toxic concentrations. Conversely, inordinately slow or incomplete release could lead to inadequate drug therapy. Uncertainty over the effects of these formulations is recognized by the Food and Drug Administration which regards them as new drugs and requires that both efficacy and safety be demonstrated before they can be marketed. In general, orally administered agents are taken three or four times each day, rarely a hardship for most patients. The additional cost of sustained-release preparations may also influence decisions about their use in place of more conventional forms.

The sensitivity of gastrointestinal absorption to variations in drug formulation is best exemplified by the concern over bioavailability. In a number of instances, chemically identical drugs have proved to be biologically inequivalent. In one study of tetracycline hydrochloride, for example, nine preparations of different manufacture were compared with an aqueous solution of the same drug.[23] Although seven brands produced blood concentrations ranging from 70% to 100% of the reference solution, two products exhibited relative bioavail-

abilities of only 20% to 30%. Differences in bioavailability are most likely to be clinically important with drugs that are poorly absorbed, have low margins of safety, and are inactivated by capacity-limited processes. Bioavailability considerations related to drug selection are considered further in Chapter 49.

Drug inactivation. One of the shortcomings of oral ingestion is the inactivation of drugs before they reach the systemic circulation. The destruction of some agents (e.g., epinephrine and insulin) is sufficiently great to preclude their administration by this route. With other drugs (e.g., penicillin G), losses may be smaller but still large enough to make oral administration inefficient. Gastric acid is undoubtedly one of the principal causes of drug breakdown within the gastrointestinal tract, but degradation is also due to enzymatic activity. Isoproterenol, for instance, is metabolized by conjugation with sulfate under the catalytic control of mucosal enzymes. Likewise, vasopressin, insulin, calcitonin, and other polypeptides are subject to hydrolysis by pancreatic and intestinal peptidases. Enteric bacterial enzymes may also destroy certain ingested agents, such as chlorpromazine. Finally, intestinal contents can alter the effectiveness of many orally administered drugs. Binding to constituents of chyme, chelation with divalent cations, or formation of insoluble salts may decrease the amount of drug available for absorption.

Aside from intralumenal inactivation, a special fate exists for substances absorbed from the gastrointestinal tract. The venous drainage of the stomach, small intestine, and colon is routed by the hepatic portal system to the liver. A first pass of high drug concentration through this enzyme-laden organ can significantly reduce the quantity of agent reaching the systemic circulation. Lidocaine, in fact, is metabolized so rapidly in the liver that virtually all of an oral dose is destroyed during its first pass. Although less pronounced, disparities in opioid analgesic and antibiotic efficacies observed between the oral route and other modes of administration are of clinical importance to the practice of dentistry.

Other enteral routes. The oral and rectal mucosae are occasionally used as the site of drug absorption. Sublingual administration, in which a tablet or troche is allowed to dissolve completely in the oral cavity, takes advantage of the permeability of the oral epithelium and is the preferred route for a few drugs, such as nitroglycerin, oxytocin, and testosterone. The oral and intestinal mucosal layers do not differ qualitatively as absorbing surfaces, and comparable absorption has been shown for many agents.[5] One reason for selecting the sublingual route is to avoid drug destruction. Since gastric acid as well as intestinal and hepatic enzymes are bypassed, sublingual absorption can be more efficient overall for certain drugs than is intestinal uptake. Rectal administration may be employed when other enteral routes are precluded, as in the unconscious or nauseated patient. Although a significant fraction of absorbed drug enters the circulation without having to pass through the liver, uptake is often unpredictable. Several drugs irritating to the gastric mucosa (e.g., xanthines) may be given rectally; for some others, rectal sensitivity prohibits administration by this route.

Inhalation

The alveolar membrane is an important route of entry for some drugs and many noxious substances. Although the alveolar lining is highly permeable, it is accessible only to those agents that are in a gaseous state or are sufficiently divided to reach the deepest endings of the respiratory tree. Included in the first category are the therapeutic gases, carbon monoxide, the inhalation anesthetics, and a number of volatile organic solvents. These compounds gain entry into the bloodstream by virtue of their high lipid/water partition coefficients and small molecular size. The second category of alveolar membrane penetrants are collectively described as aerosols. This term refers to liquid or solid particles small enough (usually 10 μm or less in diameter) to remain suspended in air for prolonged periods of time. Particles of this sort include bacteria, viruses, smoke, pollens, sprays, and dusts. Any such finely divided material, when inhaled, will reach some portion of the respiratory tree and become impacted by the processes of sedimentation and inertial precipitation. Most aerosols contain a mixture of particle sizes. Relatively large particles (greater than 4 μm) impact on the terminal bronchioles and larger branches of the respiratory tree and are removed from the lungs by a cilia-driven blanket of mucus flowing continuously toward the pharynx. Smaller particles, which do reach the alveolar sacs, can be absorbed through the lining cells into the bloodstream, taken up by the process of phagocytosis, or carried by an aqueous film covering the alveolar cells to the terminal bronchioles where they join the mucous blan-

ket. Although two of these three possible fates involve particle uptake, the mechanism for removing solids is remarkably efficient. Only a minute portion of the inhaled dusts of a lifetime fails to be removed by ciliary transport.

Therapeutic use of aerosols is not widespread, but some emergency medications are prepared in this form. Since the onset of effect is extremely rapid following inhalation of an aerosol drug, this route can provide a means of quick self-medication for individuals in danger of acute allergic reactions to venoms or drugs. Epinephrine is one such emergency agent that is marketed as an aerosol. Many respiratory drugs are also prepared in aerosol form, but the rapidity and efficiency of alveolar membrane absorption can, on occasion, pose problems for therapy. The use of pressurized aerosols containing isoproterenol is illustrative. Although up to 97% of an isoproterenol spray is swallowed under normal conditions and inactivated by hepatic enzymes, overmedication can produce toxic effects. Data gathered over a 7-year period in the United Kingdom suggested that the undisciplined use of these preparations produced an increased death rate in asthmatic patients. Restriction of over-the-counter sales and warnings to physicians were accompanied by a fall in mortality.[19] Findings like these not only reflect the hazards of aerosols when abused but also provide a caveat for uncontrolled self-medication with any potentially dangerous drug. Concern over aerosols is also related to questions of toxicology, the absorption of lead from gasoline exhaust being one example.

Parenteral injection

Drugs are frequently given by parenteral injection when oral ingestion is precluded by the patient's condition, when a rapid onset of effect is necessary, or when blood concentrations in excess of those obtainable with the enteral route are required. The method of injection selected will vary with the particular drug and therapeutic need of the patient.

Intravenous route. The administration of drugs by infusion or injection directly into the bloodstream is particularly useful when immediate effects or exact blood concentrations are desired. Because absorption is bypassed, intravenous injection circumvents the delays and variations in drug response characteristically associated with other modes of administration. Rapid dilution in the bloodstream and the relative insensitivity of vascular walls to drugs often permit the successful administration of compounds or solutions too irritating for other routes (e.g., nitrogen mustards and hypertonic fluids). Also, through the technique of titration, the intravenous route provides an avenue for the controlled administration of drugs that have a very narrow margin of safety between therapeutic and toxic concentrations. The infusion of lidocaine to prevent ventricular arrhythmias and the incremental injection of antianxiety drugs during intravenous sedation are two examples in which titration is used to achieve a desired effect while avoiding adverse reactions. Although many intravenous agents do not require titration and may be given in standardized doses, it is still necessary that they be injected slowly. If administered too quickly, a dose may move initially through the heart, lungs, and major arteries as a bolus of high drug concentration. Nonspecific but potentially disastrous cardiopulmonary side effects may result, even from the rapid injection of simple salt solutions. For most drugs, it is best to administer them over a period of 1 minute, which approximates the circulation time of blood through the body. This procedure will avoid high, transient concentrations and permit discontinuance should any untoward effect be observed during the course of injection.

A major disadvantage of the intravenous route is that once the drug is injected, very little can be done to remove it from the bloodstream. When an adverse response is noted with another route, further absorption can usually be delayed or perhaps even prevented. Toxic reactions to drugs given intravenously are often instantaneous and severe. Life-threatening anaphylactic events are also more likely because of the possibility of a massive antigen-antibody reaction occurring. Other complications of intravenous injection include vasculitis and embolism (either from drug irritation, particulate matter in the injected solution, or needle trauma), fever (from injection of pyrogens such as bacterial lipopolysaccharides), infection, and hematoma formation.

Intramuscular route. The intramuscular route is often selected for drugs that cannot be given orally because of slow or erratic absorption, high percentage of drug inactivation, or lack of patient cooperation. The rate of absorption from an intramuscular site is governed by the same factors influencing gastrointestinal uptake: lipid/water partition coefficient, degree of ionization, molecular size, and so on. Many drugs, however, are absorbed at about the same rate, regardless of these factors. The only barrier separating a drug deposited intramuscularly from the bloodstream is the capillary endothelium, a multicellular membrane with large intercellular pores. Many lipid-insoluble substances can enter the vascular compartment through these pores, and even proteins are capable of being absorbed. In these circumstances, it is not surprising that blood flow through the tissue is often the primary determinant of the rate of drug absorption. Thus, muscles with high blood flows (e.g., deltoid) provide faster absorption rates than do muscles with lesser flows (e.g., gluteus maximus). In general, 10 to 30 minutes is required for the onset of drug effect, but this latency period can be controlled to some extent. Exercise will markedly speed absorption by stimulating local circulation. Conversely, uptake may be minimized by the application of ice packs or (in an emergency) tourniquets.

With the exception of a few drugs that are relatively insoluble at tissue pH (diazepam, phenytoin, etc.), absorption from an intramuscular injection is usually rapid and complete. Formulations have been developed, therefore, to provide for prolonged and steady drug release. These depot preparations consist of drugs manufactured as insoluble salts or dispensed in oil vehicles, or both, such as procaine penicillin suspended in peanut oil. Relatively large volumes of solution may be given by this route, but soreness at the injection site is frequent, and some drugs (e.g., tetracyclines) are too irritating to be administered in this manner.

Subcutaneous route. Injection of drugs into the subcutaneous connective tissue is a widely used method of administration for agents that can be given in small volumes (2 ml or less) and are not locally damaging. Subcutaneous absorption is similar to that of resting muscle, and onset times are often comparable. As with the intramuscular route, absorption can be delayed by diminishing blood flow, either through the application of pressure or by surface cooling. Pharmacologic interruption of circulation with vasoconstrictors is also a common strategy, especially in local anesthesia. Because of the ease of subcutaneous implantation, compressed pellets of drugs, sometimes mixed with insoluble matrix material, can be inserted to provide nearly constant drug release for weeks or months. Testosterone and several progestational contraceptive agents have been successfully administered by this approach. Slow absorption can be achieved, too, through the use of depot forms as described for intramuscular injections.

When subcutaneous administration is chosen for a systemic effect, it is sometimes advantageous to hasten drug absorption. Toward this end, warming the tissue will promote drug uptake by improving local circulation. Massage of the injection site, in addition to stimulating blood flow, will help spread the drug and provide an increased surface area for absorption. This latter effect can also be accomplished through the coadministration of hyaluronidase, an enzyme that breaks down the mucopolysaccharide matrix of connective tissue. The lateral spread of aqueous solutions is so enhanced, in fact, that hyaluronidase is sometimes employed to permit the injection of large fluid volumes in situations in which continuous intravenous infusion is difficult or impossible.

Other parenteral injection routes. Intraarterial injections are occasionally performed when a localized effect on a particular organ or area of the body is desired. Injections of radiopaque dyes for diagnostic purposes and antineoplastic agents for the control of localized tumors are the most commonly encountered examples. Intrathecal administration is used when the direct access of drug to the central nervous system is necessary. Indications for injection into the subarachnoid space include the production of spinal anesthesia with local anesthetics and the resolution of acute central nervous system (CNS) infections with antibiotics. The intraperitoneal infusion of fluids is a useful substitute for hemodialysis in the treatment of drug poisoning. Although the intraperitoneal injection is commonly employed in animal experimentation, the risk of infection usually precludes such use in humans.

All of these specialized injection techniques are potentially dangerous to the patient. They should be performed only when expressly indicated and then only by qualified personnel.

Topical application

Drugs are often applied to epithelial surfaces for local effects and less frequently for systemic absorption. Penetration of drugs across the epithelium is strongly influenced by the degree of keratinization.

Skin. The epidermis is a highly modified tissue serving to isolate the body from the external environment. The outer layer of skin (stratum corneum) is densely packed with the protein keratin.

Not only is this layer impervious to water and therefore water-soluble drugs, its relative thickness and paucity of lipids in contrast to other biologic membranes retards even the diffusion of strongly lipophilic agents. The impermeable nature of skin to water-soluble drugs often requires that agents (antibiotics, fungicides, etc.) intended for dermatologic conditions be administered by a systemic route, in spite of the obvious accessibility of the skin. For lipid-soluble drugs, however, the percutaneous route is often successful for local problems. Moreover, when the keratinized layer is disrupted, drug absorption, especially of hydrophilic compounds, is markedly enhanced. The underlying connective tissue (dermis) is as permeable as are mucosal surfaces, although it differs in having an abundant supply of arteriovenous shunts, which may cause absorption to be particularly sensitive to changes in temperature.

The general resistance of the intact skin to drugs does not invalidate the need for caution when dealing with potentially toxic chemicals. Sufficient documentation of epidermal absorption of foreign substances has established that certain compounds may readily penetrate the skin to cause systemic effects. These drugs include organic solvents, organophosphate and nicotine-based insecticides, and some nerve gases. Severe poisoning has also resulted from the excessive application of sunburn creams containing local anesthetics. Even lipid-insoluble substances such as inorganic mercury can diffuse across skin if exposure is prolonged.

The obvious benefits of improving and sufficiently controlling percutaneous absorption to make it a reliable route of drug administration have prompted several strategies. For example, a "transdermal therapeutic system" has been developed to provide continuous systemic uptake of nitroglycerin and scopolamine for the respective prophylaxis of angina pectoris and motion sickness. The system is a complex patch that consists of an outer impermeable backing, a reservoir containing the drug in a suspended form, a semipermeable membrane, and an inner adhesive seal. In the early 1960s, it was discovered that the industrial solvent dimethyl sulfoxide (DMSO) promotes the percutaneous absorption of water-soluble drugs. The potential that this drug carrier offered of simplified therapy for arthritic and other patients generated much enthusiasm. Subsequent reports of adverse reactions in animals caused interest to wane, however, until the late 1970s when DMSO was repopularized as an effective agent for the symptomatic relief of a wide variety of musculoskeletal and collagen disorders. Currently, DMSO is restricted by the FDA to the treatment of interstitial cystitis. Another approach to improving drug penetration through the epidermis is the use of occlusive dressings. These dressings retain moisture and break down the horny layer through the process of maceration. A final technique, iontophoresis, is covered below.

Mucous membranes. The topical application of drugs to mucous membranes offers several potential advantages for local therapy. The tissues can often be visualized by the clinician, permitting accurate drug placement. The use of this route generally minimizes systemic effects while providing an optimal concentration of drug in the area being treated. Unlike the case with skin, drugs have little trouble permeating mucous membranes to affect localized conditions. Indeed, as previously discussed in connection with sublingual administration, absorption of drugs across mucous membranes occurs readily. Before this fact was widely appreciated, the topical application of tetracaine to the pharyngeal and tracheal mucosae was a leading cause of local anesthetic overdose.[1] In dentistry, the use of corticosteroids to ameliorate inflammatory conditions has also given rise to systemic responses, such as the suppression of adrenocortical function by triamcinolone.[20] Although these effects are generally mild and transient, they could create problems for patients with hypertension, diabetes mellitus, or peptic ulcer. Local therapy can also affect systemic health by serving as antigenic stimulants and, in the case of antibiotics, by disturbing the normal microbial ecology and promoting the emergence of resistant microorganisms.

Iontophoresis. Iontophoresis is the electrical transport of positively or negatively charged drugs across surface tissues. The technique involves passing a direct electrical current of appropriate polarity through the drug solution and patient. Permeation of mucous membranes and even skin and hard tissues is possible with this approach, yet the total dose delivered is small and systemic toxicity unlikely. In dental therapeutics, iontophoretic application of drugs has been used in several situations. Loose deciduous teeth have been extracted successfully following the iontophoretic administration of lidocaine with epinephrine for soft tissue anesthesia.[12] For the treatment of herpes orolabialis, galvanic current increases the tissue concentration of idoxuridine up to three times that ob-

tainable with topical application alone.[13] Probably the most common use of iontophoresis in dentistry, however, is the promotion of fluoride uptake into exposed ''hypersensitive'' dentin. A 1% solution of sodium fluoride administered in this manner produced better results than did a 33% paste.[28] Further employment of this technique in dental practice can be expected in view of the frequent necessity for topical and local treatment. However, the prolonged treatment period sometimes required may limit patient acceptance.

DISTRIBUTION

Distribution refers to the movement of drugs throughout the body. The rate, sequence, and extent of distribution depends on many factors: the physicochemical properties of the drug, cardiac output and regional blood flows, anatomic characteristics of membranes, transmembrane electrical and pH gradients, binding to plasma proteins and tissue reservoirs, and sometimes active transport or facilitated diffusion. For all but the very few drugs that act intravascularly, the capillary membrane constitutes the first tissue barrier to be crossed in the journey of a drug from the bloodstream to its site of action.

Capillary penetration

Once a drug gains access to the systemic circulation, it becomes diluted by the plasma volume of the entire vascular compartment. For a compound administered intravenously, this process requires only several minutes for completion; for drugs given by other routes, intravascular distribution takes place concurrently with absorption. The transfer of drugs out of the bloodstream is governed by the same factors that control its entrance. Lipophilic drugs, for example, diffuse across the capillary membrane extremely rapidly. The transfer is so expeditious, in fact, that equilibrium with interstitial fluid is practically instantaneous. Under these conditions, the rate of drug uptake is determined by the blood flow through the tissue under consideration. Thus, well-perfused organs are saturated with drug long before many other tissues have had a chance to reach even a fraction of the equilibrium concentration. Water-soluble drugs diffuse through pores located within or between adjacent endothelial cells. With these agents, transcapillary movement is slower than for drugs that enjoy high lipid/water partition coefficients and is inversely proportional to molecular weight.

As drug size increases, aqueous diffusion becomes less important, and filtration takes over as the primary motive force behind drug transport. Substances with molecular weights greater than 60,000 pass across capillary membranes very slowly. Electron microscopic evidence suggests that pinocytosis is involved in their translocation.[15]

Entry of drugs into cells

As previously discussed, the cell membrane acts as a semipermeable barrier, admitting some drugs into the cell while excluding others. Nonpolar, lipid-soluble compounds distribute evenly across plasma membranes, but distribution of weak electrolytes at equilibrium is somewhat more complex. The intracellular pH is approximately 7.0, differing slightly from the pH 7.4 of extracellular fluid. Acids with pK_as less than 8.0 will tend to remain outside the cell while basic drugs with pK_as greater than 6.0 will tend to accumulate within. Because the concentration differential across the cell membrane based on a pH gradient of 0.4 can equal 2.5/1, the acid-base status of a patient can significantly affect the dose response of weak electrolytes acting intracellularly. (The influence of pH on the distribution of local anesthetics across nerve membranes is described in Chapter 17). Ions, unless very small in size (molecular weights of 60 or less) or transported by membrane-bound carriers, penetrate cell membranes with difficulty or not at all. Charged drugs that do gain access to the cell by passive diffusion are distributed at equilibrium according to the electrical gradient across the membrane.

Distribution into special fluid compartments

In some tissues or organs, anatomical components permit the sequestration of interstitial or transcellular fluids from the general extracellular space. The most important examples for therapeutics involve the central nervous system, the fetal circulation, and, insofar as dentistry is concerned, saliva.

Central nervous system. Entry of drugs into the central nervous system is unusually dependent on lipid solubility. Drugs with high lipid/water partition coefficients are taken up very fast, as exemplified by the immediate onset of general anesthesia following the intravenous injection of thiopental. The rapid distribution of lipophilic drugs into the brain and spinal cord arises from the fact that the central nervous system receives about 15%

of the cardiac output yet composes only 2% of the body weight. Despite this favorable blood supply, drugs sparingly lipid soluble are largely excluded from the extracellular space of the brain. In contrast to capillaries elsewhere, the endothelial cells of the central nervous system are nonfenestrated, are joined together by tight junctions, and limit the entry of water-soluble drugs to those with an effective molecular radius of 8 Å or less. Thus, relatively large molecules (e.g., inulin, with a molecular weight of 5000) that normally pass without difficulty into the interstitial space are completely barred, and most other drugs dependent on aqueous channels for penetration are slowed considerably. A second impediment to the transfer of ions and other water-soluble substances is the cellular sheath that surrounds the capillaries of the brain. This investing layer is composed of processes extending from connective tissue astrocytes. Although the area of capillary surface coverage is not complete, it nevertheless is sufficient to retard the diffusion of all but highly lipid-soluble compounds. Together, the modified capillary endothelium and the astrocytic sheath constitute the blood-brain barrier.

Drugs may also gain access to the central nervous system by way of the choroid plexuses. Each choroid plexus is composed of a network of small blood vessels and capillaries projecting into a ventricular space and covered by a layer of epithelial cells specifically adapted for the secretion of cerebrospinal fluid. Diffusion of drugs across the choroid plexus and into the cerebrospinal fluid is largely restricted to highly lipid-soluble drugs. The close correspondence in drug transfer with other brain capillaries indicates the analogous existence of a barrier between blood and cerebrospinal fluid. The choroid plexus and cerebrospinal fluid are actually more closely involved with the removal of drugs from the central nervous system than with their entry. Secreted into the third, fourth, and lateral ventricles, the cerebrospinal fluid moves by bulk flow through the ventriculocisternal system to bathe the surfaces of the brain and spinal cord before exiting by way of the arachnoid villi. Drugs present in the extracellular fluid of the central nervous system are free to diffuse into the cerebrospinal fluid. Because the total quantity of cerebrospinal fluid (150 ml) approximates the volume of the interstitial space and because it has a moderately fast turnover rate (10% per hour), the removal of drugs by bulk flow through the arachnoid villi can prevent an agent in the brain from ever reaching equilibrium with the blood. The active transport of organic ions from the cerebrospinal fluid back into the systemic circulation by the lining cells of the choroid plexus also promotes the removal of many drugs from the brain.

The selective distribution of compounds into the central nervous system has several important therapeutic ramifications. Alkaloids intended for peripheral nervous system effects, for example, can cause CNS disturbances on entry into the brain. Conversion of such drugs (e.g., scopolamine) to positively charged quaternary ammonium derivatives (e.g., methscopolamine) will prevent central influences yet allow essential peripheral activity. Conversely, drugs used for their central effects may benefit by molecular modifications that enhance their entry into the brain. Lower total doses can then be given and peripheral effects minimized. Sometimes the blood-brain barrier is a hindrance to therapy. Penicillin G, a water-soluble organic acid with a pK_a of 2.6, diffuses slowly into the central nervous system and is subject to active removal by the choroid plexus. For individuals suffering from bacterial encephalitis, this lack of drug penetration can complicate treatment. (It is fortunate that capillary permeability in the brain often increases during meningeal inflammation.) A clever approach to circumventing the blood-brain barrier is embodied in the treatment of parkinsonism. This disease is associated with a deficiency of dopamine within selected portions of the brain. Replacement therapy with dopamine is ineffective, however, because the drug is excluded by the blood-brain barrier. To avoid this problem, levodopa, the amino acid precursor of dopamine, is used instead. Levodopa readily enters the brain, where it is subsequently decarboxylated to the active drug.

Placental transfer. Obstetrical delivery of conscious infants from anesthetized mothers was once misconstrued as evidence for a unique placental barrier excluding even lipid-soluble drugs from the fetus. It is now understood that such observations result merely from the finite rate of drug transfer from the maternal circulation to fetal tissues. Fetal blood vessels projecting into sinuses filled with maternal blood are covered by a single layer of cells called trophoblasts. The movement of drugs across the placenta is limited by the trophoblastic membrane, which is qualitatively no different from plasma membranes elsewhere. Although trophoblasts are known to actively secrete amino acids and other nutrients into the fetal circulation, the entry of most drugs depends on passive diffusion across the lipoid barrier. For highly lipophilic drugs like thiopental, distribution is retarded only by the rate of maternal blood flow through the placenta and by peculiarities in the fetal circulation that limit tissue perfusion. It has been calculated that at least 40 minutes is required for fetal tissues to attain 90% of equilibrium (thus explaining the misinterpreted observations made during childbirth).[15] Limited by a sluggish transmembrane diffusion, the transfer of water-soluble compounds is so inefficient that virtually no drug from a single administration may gain access to the fetus. Nevertheless, even sparingly lipid-soluble agents will eventually accumulate in the fetus if administered to the mother in multiple doses.

Concern over the placental transfer of drugs arises from the possibility of inducing toxic manifestations in the newborn and developmental defects in the embryo and fetus. These topics are considered further in Chapter 3.

Salivary secretion. The distribution of drugs into saliva is of pharmacologic interest in two respects. First, drugs gaining access to the oral environment from the systemic circulation can affect microorganisms or tissue surfaces within the mouth. Although these influences are usually undesirable, it is conceivable that a drug developed for a local effect, like caries prevention, could be administered systemically to achieve a sustained therapeutic concentration in the saliva while obviating the necessity for repeated mouth rinsings. The second pharmacologic interest in saliva stems from the fact that salivary drug determinations can provide a noninvasive measure of the free plasma concentration of drugs. Since the free drug concentration in plasma is normally the primary determinant of patient response, the benefit of salivary drug quantitation to therapeutics is potentially great. However, clinical studies have documented a complex relationship between plasma and salivary drug titers, one that must be fully understood before salivary monitoring can be successfully used.[4,31]

Drugs may enter the oral fluids from several sources: (1) passive diffusion across the alveolar and ductal cells of salivary glands, (2) passive diffusion across the oral epithelium, and (3) bulk flow of fluid from the gingival crevice. Of these avenues, the first is the most important and the third is the least (except for drugs that cannot gain entry

Table 2-1. Distribution of drugs into saliva

Drug	L*	Protein binding (%)	pK_a	Saliva/plasma ratio[†] Resting	Saliva/plasma ratio[†] Stimulation
Quinidine	3000	89	8.8b‡	3.1	1.3
Sulfamerazine	0.4	88	7.1a	0.69	0.55
Acetaminophen	1.8	0	10.1a	1.0	0.66
Diazepam	820	96	3.3b	1.0	1.0
Ethanol	0.5	0	—	1.0	1.0

Adapted from Feller, K., and le Petit, G. On the distribution of drugs in saliva and blood plasma. International Journal of Clinical Pharmacology and Biopharmacy **15:**468-469, 1977.

*L = lipid/water partition coefficient (*n*-octanol as the lipid).
†Refers to the unbound drug.
‡a = acid; b = base.

by either of the other two routes). As exemplified in Table 2-1, the salivary concentration of a drug is influenced by many factors.[11] Agents that are relatively lipid soluble (diazepam) or very small in size (ethanol) encounter little difficulty in equilibrating with saliva. Since only the unbound portion of a drug is involved in distribution across membranes and the salivary compartment is quite small with respect to the total intravascular space, protein binding does not affect the saliva/plasma ratio of the free drug (diazepam and acetaminophen). Regarding weak electrolytes, the disparity in pH between the plasma and the more acidic saliva results in the concentration of bases with pK_as greater than 5.5 in saliva (quinidine) and an opposite effect on acids with pK_as less than 8.5 (sulfamerazine). Finally, the rate of salivary flow can alter intraoral concentrations in at least two ways. Increased salivary production may outpace the diffusion rate of drugs with moderate to low lipid solubility (acetaminophen), thus lowering the saliva/plasma ratio. Additionally, the pH of stimulated saliva tends to approach 7.4, thus eliminating the unequal distribution of drugs based on pH (quinidine). With some weak acids, these two influences on drug concentration may tend to cancel each other out (sulfamerazine).

Volume of distribution

It should be obvious from the foregoing discussion that drugs are not distributed equally throughout the body. Although lipophilic substances tend to penetrate all tissue compartments (provided they have a modicum of water solubility), hydrophilic compounds are often disseminated more restrictively. The volume of distribution is a useful indicator of how drugs are dispersed among the various body fluids. In its simplest form, the volume of distribution (V_d) is calculated from the equation $V_d = Q/C$, where Q is the quantity of drug administered and C is the plasma concentration of drug at equilibrium. The volume of distribution, then, is the amount of water by which a particular dose would have to be diluted in order to produce a given plasma concentration, assuming that no drug has been lost through incomplete absorption or by metabolism or excretion.

The dye Evans blue is typical of the very few drugs that are distributed only within the vascular space. Several minutes after an intravenous injection, Evans blue becomes thoroughly mixed within the blood, and a V_d of 3 L is obtained. This value represents the total plasma volume of a 70 kg man of average build. Most compounds, however, pass readily from the vascular tree into the interstitial compartment. At equilibrium, these drugs will be distributed in an extracellular volume of 12 L, which includes the vascular and interstitial fluids. Ionic drugs (e.g., decamethonium) are generally contained in this volume of distribution. Molecules that can freely penetrate all membranes will be diluted by the water of the entire body, approximately 41 L. Figure 2-6 depicts the major body fluid volumes, and Table 2-2 provides a list of agents with representative V_d values.

It is apparent from the bottom half of Table 2-2 that the V_d of many compounds does not correspond to any definable anatomic fluid compartment. Accepting that the measurements were made correctly and that problems in drug absorption and elimination were successfully avoided, there remain several explanations for these results. The V_d equation actually provides only an apparent distribution, partly because it assumes that drugs are

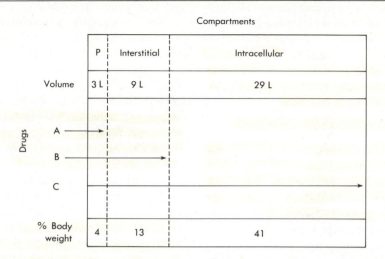

Figure 2-6. Diagram of body water compartments. The membrane barriers that separate plasma from interstitial fluid and interstitial fluid from intracellular water are indicated by dashed lines. The upper set of figures are the respective volumes for a 70 kg man; the lower set are percentages of total body weight. Of the drugs shown, A is restricted to the plasma, B is distributed within the extracellular compartment (plasma + interstitial fluid), and C is disseminated throughout the total body water.

Table 2-2. Volumes of distribution of various agents

Agent	V_d	Corresponding fluid compartment
Evans blue	3	Plasma water
[131]I-albumin	3	
Mannitol	12	Extracellular water
Inulin	11	
Urea	41	Total body water
Barbital	40	
Sodium ion	18	
Tetracycline	90	
Meperidine	300	
Chlorpromazine	1500	

ent in fluids of different pH, or drugs are actively transported into or out of a water space.

The enormous volumes of distribution recorded for drugs like meperidine and chlorpromazine generally result from tissue binding. The sequestration of compounds within cells or certain tissues necessarily reduces the concentration of drug in the plasma, leading to an abnormally high calculation of V_d. (Obviously, no drug can have a true volume of distribution greater than about 41 L.) Plasma protein binding can also affect V_d determinations. Since the total drug in plasma is usually measured, binding will artificially inflate the drug concentration and depress V_d. If free drug is measured, significant binding by plasma proteins will have the same effect as binding at extravascular sites.

Drug binding and storage

The sojourn of drugs in the body is considerably influenced by binding to proteins and other tissue components. Reduction in the concentration of free solute causes a decrease in the rate of passage across membrane barriers and may, as reflected in V_d determinations, alter drug distribution at equilibrium as well. Drug sequestration can also affect the processes of absorption and elimination.

Plasma protein binding. Many drugs become associated with plasma proteins, especially albu-

evenly dispersed. To illustrate this point, sodium ions are present in all body fluids (with an actual V_d of 41 L), but the apparent (calculated) V_d for sodium is only 18 L. This discrepancy arises because sodium is actively but incompletely extruded from intracellular water. Dissimilarities between true and calculated volumes of distribution based on unequal compartment concentrations arise whenever ions are distributed across electrically polarized membranes, weak electrolytes are pres-

min. The predominant protein in plasma, albumin contains roughly 200 ionized functional groups per molecule and has the capacity to bind a number of different substances concurrently. The reversible attachment of drugs to plasma proteins is reminiscent of drug-receptor combinations in that the reaction obeys the law of mass action:

Drug + Protein ⇌ Drug-protein complex

Since the number of binding sites is finite, the fraction of drug bound varies inversely with the concentration of drug in the plasma. The percentage of bound drug usually does not change over the dosage ranges employed clinically, however, and it is permissible to assign to most drugs a fixed value (e.g., 96% for diazepam; Table 2-1). The percentage of drug bound can range from zero to 100%.

The binding of agents within the vascular compartment reduces the concentration gradient of free drug across the capillary membrane and slows egress from the plasma into the extravascular space. As free molecules leave the circulation, a portion of the bound drug dissociates according to the law of mass action and becomes available for further transport. Hence, the rate but not the extent of distribution is generally altered by plasma protein binding. There are, of course, exceptions. The attachment of Evans blue is so tight, for example, that the compound is retained virtually in toto within the bloodstream. For a drug that is 95% bound in plasma, a little over half of the total dose will remain intravascular, assuming that the agent is not sequestered elsewhere.

The reversibility of binding causes the plasma proteins to act as a kind of drug reservoir. Agents must occasionally be administered in large loading doses to saturate binding sites as a prelude to achieving therapeutic concentrations at the site of action. Once accommodated, though, reservoirs of bound drug can provide certain benefits. For instance, fluctuations in drug concentration resulting from intermittent dosage schedules are kept to a minimum. As the dose is absorbed, a portion becomes bound, only to be released later as metabolism and excretion lower free drug titers. Drug binding additionally often prolongs the duration of action, which may permit administrations to be spaced more conveniently than would otherwise be possible. Both hepatic uptake and glomerular filtration are ineffective against the bound fraction; significant binding, therefore, may depress the me-

tabolism and excretion of drugs. When compounds are actively taken up by these organs, however, the instantaneous reversibility of binding can lead to a faster than normal elimination rate. Penicillin G, for example, is secreted into the urine so efficiently that blood flowing through the kidney is almost completely cleared of the antibiotic in a single pass. Because albumin binding presents the kidney with more total drug per unit time, secretion is quicker than would be the case if the drug were more evenly distributed throughout the body.

Two primary clinical concerns related to plasma protein binding involve patient variability in binding efficacy and the possibility for drug interaction. Differences in drug binding will affect the concentration of free drug within the bloodstream and may lead to insufficient therapy on the one hand and overdosage on the other. The unusual susceptibility to diazepam exhibited by patients with hypoalbuminemia should be considered when that drug is used for conscious sedation in dental practice.[16] Inasmuch as the attachment of drugs to albumin is generally less selective than are drug-receptor associations, competition between drugs for binding sites is relatively common. Such interactions take on clinical significance, though, only when the drugs are highly bound, administered in large doses, and have narrow margins of safety or small volumes of distribution.

Tissue binding. Drugs capable of associating with plasma proteins are also likely to bind to tissue elements. Such binding does not impede the movement of drugs out of the bloodstream, but it does slow the rate of elimination. By virtue of its aggregate size, muscle tissue is a significant reservoir for many drugs. Fat is also quantitatively important, especially for highly lipid-soluble compounds. Although uptake into fat is limited by a parsimonious blood supply, adipose tissue constitutes from 10% to over 50% of the total body weight, and most of an administered dose of a lipophilic drug may accumulate in fat over the course of several hours. Certain tissues display unusual affinities for particular drugs. The antimalarial agents chloroquine and quinacrine are heavily concentrated in the liver. Guanethidine and other quaternary ammonium compounds adhere to negatively charged residues in mucous secretions of the gastrointestinal tract.

The attachment of drugs to drug receptors deserves special comment. Obviously important in the pharmacologic sense, the contribution of drug-receptor interactions to the total amount of binding is usually quite small. When distribution throughout the body and the various types of sequestration are considered, it becomes clear that the percentage of drug administered that actually reaches its receptor to evoke a response is quantitatively negligible.

Storage. The association between drugs and tissue elements is sometimes so stable that it becomes appropriate to discuss such binding in terms of storage. When drugs are stored, they are not readily available for release and thus do not effectively prolong the duration of action. Some of the most common examples of storage involve mineralized tissues and fat. Bone-seeking elements such as fluoride and lead, and calcium chelators like the tetracyclines, may be deposited with bone salts during mineralization or become associated with existing hydroxyapatite crystals. Essentially in an insoluble state, these substances are difficult or impossible to remove completely. Bone and tooth mineralization may benefit from appropriate concentrations of fluoride, but most drug-induced alterations are detrimental. In the case of radioactive metals (e.g., strontium-90 and radium), storage in bone can lead to the development of leukemia, osteogenic sarcoma, and other neoplasias. Several general anesthetics (e.g., halothane) and some lipophilic insecticides (e.g., DDT) are commonly sequestered in fat. Although not usually dangerous when stored, the slow release of these substances has been linked to a variety of health problems, including carcinogenesis.[15,25] Plasma proteins are generally not associated with drug storage, yet the now obsolete radiocontrast medium 3-hydroxy-2,4,6-triiodo-α-ethylhydrocinnamic acid exhibited a binding half-life to albumin of about 2.5 years.[3]

Redistribution

Strongly lipophilic drugs administered intravenously in bolus form characteristically go through two phases of distribution: an initial transfer into vessel-rich organs (brain, heart, kidney, liver, and lungs) followed by redistribution to less highly vascularized tissues (muscle, skin, and eventually fat). When the target organ of a drug happens to enjoy a high blood flow per unit mass, redistribution can result in the abrupt termination of drug effect. Thiopental has been extensively studied in this regard.[26] The onset of anesthesia with thiopental is almost instantaneous; however, consciousness is lost only temporarily, and the patient normally awakens in about 15 minutes. The quick onset and brief duration of thiopental reflect the rapidity by which the agent equilibrates between the blood and the central nervous system. Soon after a peak brain titer is reached (in 30 to 90 seconds), the concentration begins to fall as thiopental continues to be absorbed by the relatively large mass of muscle. Consciousness returns at about the same time muscle reaches equilibrium with the blood. Thereafter, both the brain and muscle concentrations parallel the plasma decay curve as the drug slowly passes into adipose tissue. With a metabolic half-life of 3 to 8 hours, thiopental would be a relatively long-acting drug were it not for redistribution. Indeed, when repetitive injections saturate the fat reservoir, thiopental assumes the characteristics of a long-duration anesthetic.

METABOLISM

Metabolism is a major pathway for the termination of pharmacologic effects of drugs and is often a prerequisite for the excretion of lipid-soluble chemicals. From an evolutionary standpoint, mechanisms for the biotransformation of lipophilic substances to compounds with reduced lipid/water partition coefficients appear necessary for terrestrial vertebrate life. The constraint imposed on land animals to eliminate waste products in limited volumes of water precludes the excretion of drugs with high lipid solubility. In humans, the kidney represents the major pathway for drug excretion. All drugs that exist free in the plasma are present in the glomerular filtrate. But, whereas polar compounds tend to remain within the renal tubule during the resorptive phase of urine formation, lipophilic chemicals diffuse back into the systemic circulation. Since the urinary concentration of a lipid-soluble nonelectrolyte should theoretically equal the free plasma titer, the rate of renal excretion (given a normal urinary output of 1000 to 1500 ml/day) would be very small for a drug having a reasonably large volume of distribution. Creatures in an aquatic habitat, however, experience little difficulty in eliminating lipophilic chemicals. Substances with a high lipid/water partition coefficient will readily diffuse across the gill membrane and be lost to the surrounding water. It is not surprising, therefore, that highly developed enzyme systems for metabolizing drugs in terrestrial species are often absent in marine and fresh-water organisms.

Historically, the term *detoxification* was used in reference to drug metabolism. Although it is true that many compounds are rendered pharmacologically inert by metabolic attack, this is not always the case. Numerous drugs yield metabolites with full or partial activity, and some provide derivatives with novel or highly toxic drug effects. A few agents even require chemical activation in order to be of therapeutic benefit (e.g., cyclophosphamide, mercaptopurine, mephobarbital, and sulindac). The best generalization that can be drawn concerning drug metabolism is that agents are eventually converted to polar, relatively lipid-insoluble compounds that are susceptible to renal or biliary excretion, or both.

Drug metabolism can be categorized according to the types of reactions involved and where they take place. *Nonsynthetic reactions* include the various transformations of molecular structure: oxidation, reduction, and hydrolysis. These events are also called *phase I reactions* because they often represent the initial stage of biotransformation. *Synthetic*, or *phase II*, *reactions* consist of the conjugation of drugs or their metabolites with functional groups provided by endogenous cofactors. Drugs may be metabolized by virtually any tissue of the body, but quantitatively the most important enzyme systems for the biotransformation of exogenous substances are located in the liver.

Hepatic microsomal metabolism

Each hepatocyte contains an extensive network of smooth endoplasmic reticulum which catalyzes the metabolism of a variety of endogenous chemicals (e.g., bilirubin, thyroxine, and steroids). Studies of fragmented reticular elements isolated along with other membrane structures in the form of microsomes have demonstrated that numerous drugs are also chemically altered by enzymes located within this subcellular organelle. The greatest number of reactions involve oxidation; however, reduction, hydrolysis, and conjugation with glucuronic acid also occur.

Oxidation. The oxidation of drugs results in compounds that are more polar, relatively more hydrophilic, and less likely to penetrate cells and bind to tissue elements. Microsomal oxidations are catalyzed by a set of mixed-function oxidases, so named because one atom of an oxygen dimer is incorporated into the drug while the other is converted to water through the addition of two hydrogen atoms. Of particular significance to microsomal oxidation is the component that actually binds the drug during metabolism, cytochrome P-450. This hemoprotein (or group of closely related he-

moproteins), designated P-450 because of its absorption peak at 450 nm when combined in the reduced state with carbon monoxide, constitutes in its various forms up to 20% of the total protein content of liver microsomes. It acts as the terminal acceptor of electrons in a transport chain that also includes the reduced coenzyme nicotinamide adenine dinucleotide phosphate (NADPH) and the flavoprotein NADPH-cytochrome P-450 reductase. A unique ability of cytochrome P-450 is its capacity to react with a diverse array of chemicals. In fact, the only identified requirement for microsomal oxidation is that the drug have sufficient lipid solubility to penetrate the cell membranes and reach the hemoprotein.

The general pathway for oxidation of drugs by the hepatic microsomal enzyme system is depicted in Figure 2-7. (Similar mechanisms exist in other organs, such as the kidney and the adrenal gland, but they are quantitatively much less important than those of the liver.) The drug initially attaches to an oxidized (Fe^{+++}) cytochrome P-450 unit. This complex then accepts an electron from the flavoprotein-catalyzed oxidation of NADPH. A ternary structure is produced next by the inclusion of molecular oxygen, and finally the addition of a second electron and two protons causes the complex to break down, yielding cytochrome P-450, a water molecule, and the oxidized drug.

The oxidation of an agent may lead to several different derivatives. Oxygen may be incorporated in the form of an alcohol, aldehyde, epoxide, ketone, or carboxylic acid in such structures as aliphatic residues, aromatic rings, amino groups, and sulfur moieties. Oxygen may also replace a sulfur atom (desulfuration) or an amino group (deamination), or it may not appear in the metabolite at all but become attached to a hydrocarbon unit released during the dealkylation of nitrogen, oxygen, or sulfur. How a single enzymatic pathway can generate such a diversity of compounds is best explained by the postulate that oxidations dependent on cytochrome P-450 create hydroxylated intermediates that are converted, either spontaneously or by enzyme catalysis, to the final products.[15] To illustrate, Figure 2-8 shows how the O-demethylation of codeine to morphine is thought to occur. The various types of microsomal oxidations are reviewed along with other phase I reactions in Table 2-3.

Reduction. The microsomal reduction of drugs is limited to molecules with nitro groups or azo

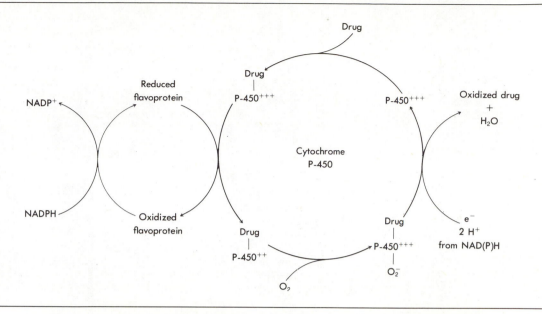

Figure 2-7. Microsomal enzyme oxidation system. In the electron transport chain, the initial electron is passed from nicotinamide adenine dinucleotide phosphate (NADPH) by the flavoprotein NADPH-cytochrome P-450 reductase to the complex of drug and cytochrome P-450. The second electron and two hydrogens may also come from NADPH or from nicotinamide adenine dinucleotide (NADH) via the cytochrome b_5 pathway.

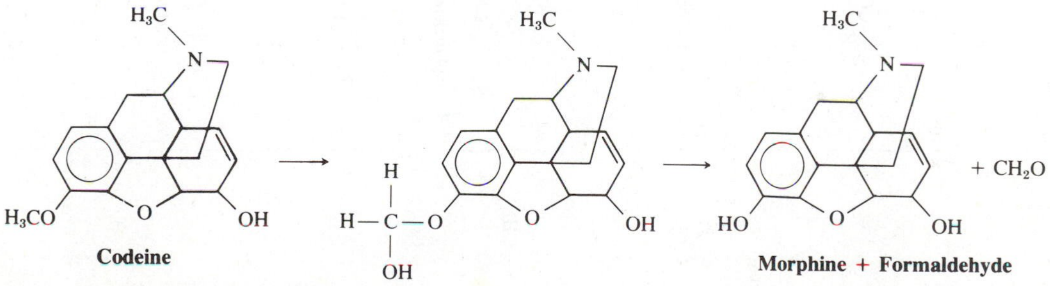

Figure 2-8. Microsomal oxidation of codeine. The O-methyl group is initially hydroxylated and then is cleaved off the molecule in the form of formaldehyde.

linkages. Similar reactions may also be mediated by nonmicrosomal enzymes of the body, but most reductions of this variety appear to result primarily from the action of enteric bacteria. In cases in which reduction occurs at one site in a molecule, oxidation usually takes place elsewhere, and the final product is more polar in spite of the initial addition of hydrogen atoms.

Hydrolysis. The hydrolysis of ester or amide compounds resulting in the production of two smaller entities, each with a polar end, is occasionally dependent on microsomal enzymes. The hydrolysis of the ester meperidine and the cleavage of amide local anesthetics and their oxidized metabolites are two important examples of microsomal hydrolysis.

Dehalogenation. Various compounds, such as the insecticide chlorphenothane (DDT) and some volatile general anesthetics (e.g., halothane and methoxyflurane), are dehalogenated by microsomal enzymes. The reactions are complex, may involve oxidative as well as reductive steps, and may result in the information of potentially toxic metabolites.[25]

Table 2-3. Phase I reactions—metabolic transformations

Reaction	Example
Microsomal enzyme system *Oxidation*	
$RCH_2R' \rightarrow RCHR'$ (OH) **Aliphatic hydroxylation**	Acetanilid $\xrightarrow{[O]}$ Acetaminophen
$R\text{-}C_6H_4 \rightarrow R\text{-}C_6H_4\text{-}OH$ **Aromatic hydroxylation**	
$RNHR' \rightarrow RNR'$ (OH) **N-hydroxylation**	
$RCH{=}CHR' \rightarrow RCH\overset{O}{-}CHR'$ **Epoxidation**	Naphthalene $\xrightarrow{[O]}$
$RNHR' \rightarrow RNH_2 + R'{=}O$ **N-dealkylation**	
$ROR' \rightarrow ROH + R'{=}O$ **O-dealkylation**	Phenacetin $\xrightarrow{[O]}$ Acetaminophen $+ CH_3CHO$
$RSCH_3 \rightarrow RSH + CH_2O$ **S-dealkylation**	
$(R)_3N \rightarrow (R)_3N{=}O$ **N-oxidation**	
$RSR' \rightarrow RSR'$ ($=O$) **Sulfoxidation**	$\xrightarrow{[O]}$

Deamination

$$C_6H_5-CH_2CHNH_2-CH_3 \xrightarrow{[O]} C_6H_5-CH_2C=O-CH_3 + NH_3$$
(with side CH_3 group)

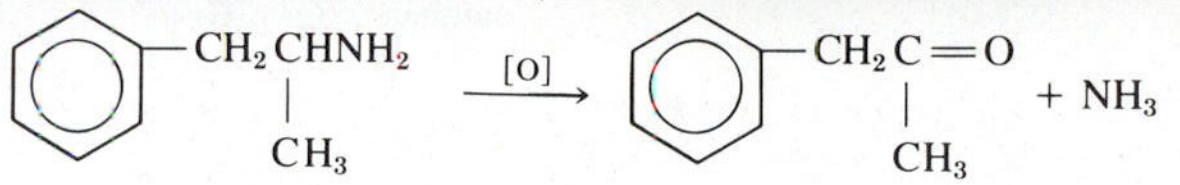

Amphetamine

$RSH \rightarrow ROH$
Desulfuration

Reduction

$RNO_2 \rightarrow RNH_2$
Nitro reduction

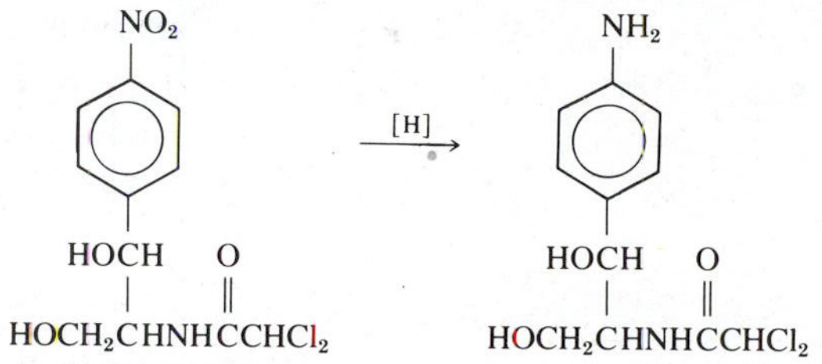

$RN=NR' \rightarrow RNH_2 + R'NH_2$
Azo reduction

Chloramphenicol: $O_2N-C_6H_4-HOCH-CHNHCCHCl_2(O)-HOCH_2 \xrightarrow{[H]} H_2N-C_6H_4-HOCH-CHNHCCHCl_2(O)-HOCH_2$

Chloramphenicol

Hydrolysis

$RCOOR' \rightarrow RCOOH + R'OH$
Ester hydrolysis

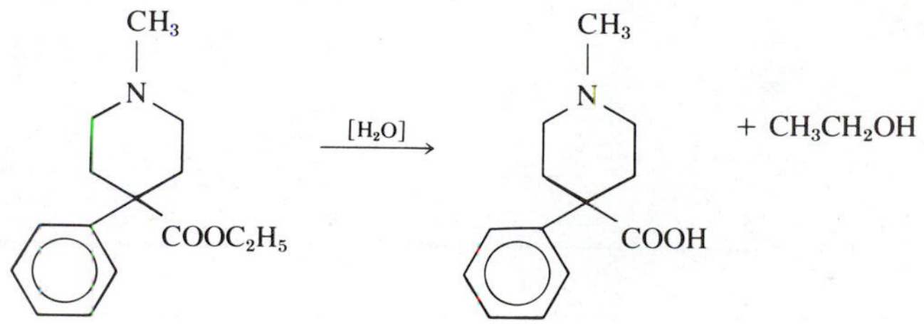

$RNHCOR' \rightarrow RNH_2 + R'COOH$
Amide hydrolysis

Meperidine: piperidine ring, N–CH_3, phenyl, $COOC_2H_5 \xrightarrow{[H_2O]}$ $COOH + CH_3CH_2OH$

Meperidine

Dehalogenation
Various reactions

$CF_3CHBrCl \xrightarrow{[O]} CF_3COOH$
Halothane

Continued.

Table 2-3. Phase I reactions—metabolic transformations—cont'd

Reaction	Example
Nonmicrosomal enzymes	
Oxidation	
$RCH_2OH \rightarrow RCHO$ **Alcohol dehydrogenation**	$CH_3CH_2OH \xrightarrow{[O]} CH_3CHO$ **Ethanol**
$RCHO \rightarrow RCOOH$ **Aldehyde oxidation**	
$RCH_2R' \rightarrow RCHR'$ with OH **Aliphatic hydroxylation**	Allopurinol $\xrightarrow{[O]}$ (hydroxylated product)
aromatic ring with R → aromatic ring with R and OH **Aromatic hydroxylation**	
$RCH_2NH_2 \rightarrow RCHO + NH_3$ **Deamination**	5-Hydroxytryptamine $CH_2CH_2NH_2 \xrightarrow{[O]} CH_2CHO + NH_3$

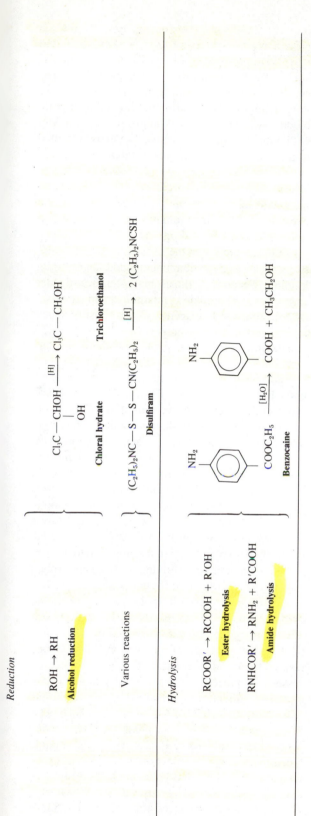

Reduction

ROH → RH
Alcohol reduction

$Cl_3C—CHOH \xrightarrow{[H]} Cl_3C—CH_2OH$
     |
    OH
Chloral hydrate   **Trichloroethanol**

Various reactions

$(C_2H_5)_2NC—S—S—CN(C_2H_5)_2 \xrightarrow{[H]} 2\ (C_2H_5)_2NCSH$
Disulfiram

Hydrolysis

RCOOR′ → RCOOH + R′OH
Ester hydrolysis

RNHCOR′ → RNH₂ + R′COOH
Amide hydrolysis

$COOC_2H_5 \xrightarrow{[H_2O]} COOH + CH_3CH_2OH$
Benzocaine

Glucuronide conjugation. The combination of compounds with glucuronic acid is the only phase II reaction catalyzed by microsomal enzymes (in this case, by a group of glucuronyl transferases). Originally derived from glucose, glucuronic acid is transferred from its donor, uridine diphosphate, to an appropriate reactive center on the drug molecule (Table 2-4). The glucuronide conjugate produced is then excreted, often by active secretion into the bile or urine. Although the liver is mainly responsible for glucuronide synthesis, other organs, especially the kidney, may also participate. Unlike many phase I reactions, conjugation with glucuronic acid almost invariably results in a total loss of pharmacologic activity. Some glucuronides excreted in the bile, however, are subject to hydrolysis by a bacterial enzyme, β-glucuronidase. If it has sufficient lipid solubility, the released drug may then be absorbed once again. Glucuronylation is a quantitatively significant metabolic pathway for many drugs and their metabolites; for agents like morphine, it represents the primary mode of inactivation.

Nonmicrosomal metabolism

The pattern of drug metabolism mediated by nonmicrosomal enzymes is considerably different from that of the microsomal system. Though important, the liver is not always predominant in nonmicrosomal biotransformations. The various major types of nonsynthetic reactions described above take place, but their relative frequencies of occurrence are dissimilar. In general, drugs must resemble natural substrates in order to be metabolized by most nonmicrosomal enzymes; certainly, the spectacular lack of specificity displayed in microsomal oxidation has no counterpart here.

Oxidation. Nonmicrosomal enzymes are responsible for the oxidation of a number of compounds. Selected alcohols and aldehydes are oxidized by dehydrogenases present in the cytosol of the liver. Other oxidation reactions include the oxidative deamination of drugs like tyramine and phenylephrine by mitochondrial enzymes found in the liver, kidneys, and other organs and the hydroxylation of, for example, the purine derivatives theophylline and allopurinol by xanthine oxidase.

Reduction. Nonmicrosomal enzymes promote the hydrogenation of double bonds and, through a reversal of the normal dehydrogenase pathway, the removal of oxygen atoms. The reduction of chloral hydrate to trichloroethanol by alcohol dehydrogenase is an often cited example of this latter type of reaction.

Hydrolysis. Most hydrolytic reactions of foreign substances are dependent on nonmicrosomal esterase and amidase enzymes. Nonspecific esterases are found throughout the body, but the two most important sites, by virtue of their hydrolytic capacity and availability to drugs, are the liver and plasma. Ester local anesthetics like procaine and benzocaine are hydrolyzed by these enzymes. Except for blood and other tissue peptidases responsible for the breakdown of pharmacologically active polypeptides, most amidase activities reside in the liver.

Conjugation reactions. A number of synthetic reactions are catalyzed by nonmicrosomal transferase enzymes. As with the microsomal synthesis of glucuronides, the body usually supplies an acidic moiety (e.g., sulfate, acetate, cysteine, glycine, glutamine, or riboside phosphate) attached to a particular cofactor or carrier molecule. The addition of methyl groups to phenols, mercaptans, and amines may lead to less polar compounds, but even here subsequent oxidation or conjugation reactions will decrease lipid solubility. With amines, methylation may even increase polarity, as in the formation of a quaternary ammonium cation. Phase II reactions can be expected whenever a drug carries one or more of the reactive centers listed in Table 2-4. Such conjugations generally result in the termination of drug effect, restriction in the apparent volume of distribution, and acceleration of drug excretion, often through active secretory processes.

Factors affecting drug metabolism

The rate of drug biotransformation is dependent on numerous variables. These include access to the site of metabolism, the concentration and phenotype of the enzyme present, and the effect of certain agents on enzymatic activity. Since most drugs are metabolized in the liver, attention will be centered on factors influencing hepatic drug biotransformation.

Entry into the liver. As stated previously, plasma protein binding can significantly reduce the rate of uptake and metabolism of drugs by the liver. Inverse correlations between the rate of biotransformation and the degree of protein binding have been reported for sulfonamides, warfarin, and phenytoin, among others.[14] A similar relationship should also hold for drugs bound to extravascular reservoirs. For some compounds, however, plasma protein binding does not hinder metabolism and may even enhance it. Lidocaine and propranolol are so effectively absorbed by hepatic tissues that, even with significant binding, the clearance of these drugs from the body is primarily limited by hepatic blood flow. Since protein binding retains extra drug within the vascular compartment, more is presented to the liver per unit time for metabolism.

Certain disease states and drug interactions can affect the accessibility of liver enzymes to pharmacologic agents. Uremia, by reducing the binding capacity of albumin, promotes the biotransformation of highly bound drugs. Hepatic damage can affect drug delivery to the liver in two ways. First, it may lead to hypoalbuminemia and altered drug binding. Second, cirrhosis may significantly decrease hepatic blood flow, retarding the metabolism of lidocaine and like agents. Cardiac insufficiency may also depress hepatic perfusion.

Enzyme inhibition. Drug metabolizing enzymes are subject to competitive and noncompetitive antagonism. Because so many drugs are acted upon by the cytochrome P-450 system, it is not surprising that competitive inhibition of microsomal oxidation is easily demonstrated in the laboratory. Fortunately, drug interactions of this type are usually not clinically important. In many instances, the rate of biotransformation is limited not by the cytochrome P-450 electron transport chain but by the movement of drugs into the smooth endoplasmic reticulum. some compounds, however, exhibit saturation kinetics and are restricted in metabolism by the rate of binding to cytochrome P-450. Competition involving these agents (phenytoin, dicumarol, etc.) is of practical significance.

A variety of metabolic poisons—carbon monoxide, cyanide, heavy metals—noncompetitively inhibit microsomal biotransformation. These actions are only of experimental interest, though, because effects on respiration and other vital processes take precedence in vivo. A much more specific inhibition of microsomal oxidation is achieved with proadifen (SKF 525A). This compound blocks the metabolism of a great number of agents dependent on cytochrome P-450; it can also inhibit glucuronylation. The effect on most drugs is a prolongation of action, but compounds requiring microsomal activation may suffer a loss of potency. The plethora of substances affected by SKF 525A prohibits its use in humans; however, similar compounds find application as potentiators of insecti-

Table 2-4. Phase II reactions—conjugations

Conjugation reaction (cofactor)	Substrates	Example
Glucuronide synthesis (uridine diphosphate)	Amines Carboxylic acids Alcohols Phenols Mercaptans	Salicylic acid → (UDP-glucuronide)
Acetylation (coenzyme A)	Amines Hydrazines	Sulfanilamide → (Acetyl-CoA)
Amino acid synthesis (coenzyme A)	Carboxylic acids	Salicylic acid → (CoA + Glycine)
Methylation (S-adenosyl-methionine)	Amines Phenols Mercaptans	Norepinephrine → (SAM)
Sulfate addition (3'-phosphoadenosine 5'-phosphosulfate)	Aromatic amines Alcohols Phenols	Acetaminophen → (PAPS)
Other reactions (various)	Purines Pyrimidines Epoxides	Naphthalene epoxide → (Glutathione)

cides that are inactivated by microsomal biotransformation.

Several drugs are employed clinically as inhibitors of selected nonmicrosomal enzymes. When the enzyme affected happens to be responsible for the inactivation of other therapeutic agents, drug interactions are likely to develop. Examples of such enzymes are monoamine oxidase, pseudocholinesterase, and xanthine oxidase. The inhibition of aldehyde dehydrogenase by disulfiram is exceptional because that drug's sole purpose is to interrupt the metabolism of another foreign compound, ethanol (see Chapter 41).

Enzyme induction. Microsomal drug metabolizing enzymes are inducible; under an appropriate chemical stimulus, catalytic activity will increase. Many chemicals, including therapeutic agents, "social" drugs, and environmental toxins, are capable of stimulating their own biotransformation and that of closely related compounds. In addition, some chemicals can augment the breakdown of a whole host of diverse substances. Phenobarbital illustrates this latter type of induction. Several hours after initiating phenobarbital treatment, an elevation in hepatic protein synthesis becomes apparent. Reductions in the metabolic half-lives of affected drugs then occur, which are paralleled by increases in microsomal weight and in the concentrations of NADPH-cytochrome P-450 reductase and cytochrome P-450. The liver eventually hypertrophies, and hepatic blood flow and bile secretion are likewise enhanced. By way of contrast, 3,4-benzpyrene exemplifies agents with a more restrictive form of induction. Although 3,4-benzpyrene requires new enzyme formation for its stimulation of metabolism (inhibitors of protein synthesis block its action), structural changes in the smooth endoplasmic reticulum are not prominent and may be undetectable.

No matter what the pattern of induction is, the rate of metabolism of affected compounds may be enhanced experimentally by as much as seven times the baseline. Stimulation is usually less pronounced clinically; nevertheless, enzyme induction has many important therapeutic ramifications. It is, for instance, a major cause of drug interactions. A classic example of this form of drug interaction is the stimulation by phenobarbital of the metabolism of the anticoagulant dicumarol, which causes standard doses of the anticoagulant to be ineffective.[9] Induction of microsomal enzymes may also lead to a gradual loss of pharmacologic responsiveness,

referred to as drug tolerance. Development of tolerance to the carcinogenic properties of 3,4-benzpyrene by self-enhancement of biotransformation may be vital to the avoidance of lung cancer in cigarette smokers.[21] Finally, enzyme induction may affect the function of endogenous chemicals metabolized microsomally. Acceleration of vitamin D oxidation to yield inactive products has become the leading cause of rickets and osteomalacia in epileptic patients receiving medications like phenytoin and phenobarbital.[17]

Genetic factors. Individuals vary in their ability to metabolize drugs. Although differences can result from the induction of microsomal enzymes (as seen in chemical factory workers, cigarette smokers, etc.), studies comparing identical and fraternal twins have conclusively established the preeminent influence of heredity on the rate of biotransformation.[35] For some drugs, the range in metabolic half-life may exceed an order of magnitude, but usually this figure is restricted to a value of two or three. The ability to metabolize a particular type of compound at an abnormal rate does not usually signify anything concerning the biotransformation of unrelated substances. A patient who oxidizes antipyrine quickly may, for instance, oxidize dicumarol more slowly than the general population. It is noteworthy, however, that normal individuals exhibiting the lowest microsomal metabolism rates are the most likely to undergo profound enzyme induction after phenobarbital treatment.[35]

Genetic influences on metabolism are most easily characterized when single genes are involved. A good example of this principle is provided by the plasma enzyme pseudocholinesterase. About 1 individual in 3000 is homozygous for an atypical gene whose enzyme product metabolizes esters very slowly. A conventional dose of the muscle relaxant succinylcholine will produce a prolonged apnea in these patients. Subjects with a combination of typical and atypical genes (heterozygotes) still have enough normal enzyme to hydrolyze the drug fast enough to avoid unusual clinical manifestations. Since the discovery of the atypical gene for pseudocholinesterase, other novel genotypes have been described, including one that is "silent" (its product has no enzymatic activity whatsoever)[2] and one that yields an enzyme so effective in catalysis that patients with it exhibit a remarkable innate resistance to the paralyzing effect of succinylcholine.[29]

Age. Neonates, especially premature infants, often lack certain functional drug metabolizing systems. The relative inability to conjugate bilirubin with glucuronic acid and the resultant development of hyperbilirubinemia is a commonly observed example of this deficiency in biotransformation. The failure to account for marked quantitative differences in neonatal metabolism is tragically highlighted by the gray syndrome and infant mortality associated with chloramphenicol.[36] Unlike newborn infants, children are often more adept at metabolizing drugs on a weight basis than are adults. In fact, biotransformation capacity appears to diminish with age; the elderly may often exhibit retarded rates of drug metabolism.

Pathology. Obviously, significant destruction of the hepatic parenchyma with loss of drug-metabolizing enzymes can directly depress the biotransformation of many agents. The clinical effect, however, may be quite small because of the liver's reserve metabolic capacity and because of enzyme induction in the unaffected tissue. (See Chapter 3 for further discussion of hepatic dysfunction and patient response.)

EXCRETION

Foreign substances, including therapeutic medications, are prevented from building up in the body by the combined action of metabolism and excretion. Drugs and their metabolites may be eliminated via a number of routes: urine, bile, sweat, saliva and other gastrointestinal secretions, pulmonary exhalation, tears, and milk. Quantitative considerations make the kidney the major organ of drug excretion.

Renal excretion

Three processes—glomerular filtration, tubular reabsorption, and active secretion—control the urinary elimination of drugs. Although all drugs are subject to filtration, the percentage filtered will vary inversely according to the degree of plasma protein binding and to the apparent volume of distribution. Once filtered, agents will tend to be resorbed in relation to their lipid/water partition coefficients. These considerations favor the renal excretion of highly polar compounds, but the exact rate of elimination will also depend on whether active transport into (or, rarely, out of) the tubular fluid also occurs.

Glomerular filtration. Each day the kidneys filter about 190 L of plasma. Arterial blood entering Bowman's capsule is routed through a tuft of capillaries collectively described as the glomerulus. These capillaries are uniquely modified for filtration, having large numbers of pores with an effective diameter of 80 Å penetrating through the endothelial membranes. About one fifth of the plasma entering the glomerular apparatus is actually filtered, the remainder exiting by way of efferent arterioles to supply other portions of the nephron. In general, molecules smaller than albumin (molecular weight 69,000) will appear in the tubular fluid. Because albumin is almost completely retained within the bloodstream, bound drugs are not subject to filtration.

Tubular reabsorption. Since only 1.5 L of urine is actually excreted every 24 hours (less than 1% of the daily filtered load), the kidney must have a very efficient reabsorption system. Indeed, were this not the case, the individual would lose valuable fluid and nutrients and quickly expire. About 80% of the glomerular filtrate is reclaimed by the proximal convoluted tubule. A high-capacity pump actively transports sodium back into the bloodstream, with anions (principally chloride) and water following passively. This process continues throughout the nephron (except in the ascending loop of Henle, where chloride is the actively absorbed ion). In addition, the reabsorption of sodium is aided by its active exchange with hydrogen and, in the distal convoluted tubule, potassium. The resultant concentration of the tubular fluid creates a chemical gradient for the diffusion of drugs back into the systemic circulation. Agents with a favorable lipid/water partition coefficient will then readily traverse the tubular epithelium and escape from the urine.

A major factor influencing the reabsorption of weak electrolytes from renal tubular fluid is the pH. Depending on the rate of hydrogen ion secretion, the urinary pH may vary from 4.5 to 8.0. Weak acids like aspirin and phenobarbital will be reabsorbed more effectively under acidic conditions; the reverse is true for weak bases like amphetamine and ephedrine. On occasion, the influence of pH on drug excretion is used to clinical advantage. Thus, a common strategy in the face of aspirin toxicity is to promote salicylate elimination through alkalinization of the urine by the systemic administration of sodium bicarbonate. For the sulfonamides (also weak acids), alkalinization of the urine may not only reduce the plasma half-life by 50% but may also prevent the development of crystalluria by increasing aqueous solubility.[14]

Of course, attempts to enhance renal excretion will be of little value for agents whose inactivation is largely dependent on biotransformation.

Active secretion. Numerous organic cations and anions are actively secreted by cells of the proximal convoluted tubule. The anionic transport system, responsible for the secretion of natural acids like uric acid, affects molecules containing carboxyl or sulfone groups. The cationic transport mechanism moves compounds with charged amino groups, like the endogenous substrates choline and histamine. Since each transport carrier is rather nonselective, competition for binding sites is sometimes observed. Probenecid, an acidic anion, has been used to block the active secretion of another acid, penicillin G. The inhibition of penicillin excretion was very beneficial at a time when the drug was in short supply and still finds use when it is necessary to maintain a high concentration of the antibiotic for prolonged periods of time.[33] Many of the conjugation products of drug metabolism are anions and subject to active transport by proximal tubular cells.

These carrier systems of the kidney can act bidirectionally. The most important active resorption of organic ions by this mechanism involves uric acid. Because probenecid can compete with urate ions as readily as it can with penicillin, probenecid finds application in gout as a promoter of uric acid excretion.

Active secretion of substances into the urine is not adversely affected by plasma protein binding. The transport is often so effective that drug dissociation takes place instantly, making available more drug for secretion, until all the drug has been cleared from the local blood supply. Binding to extravascular tissues, however, does reduce the rate of renal elimination, regardless of the mechanisms involved.

Clearance. The amount of drug removed by the kidney per unit time is often evaluated as a function of the plasma water "cleared" of drug. Mathematically, the volume of plasma cleared per minute (C) can be written as $C = UV/P$, where U is the urinary concentration of drug, V is the volume of urine produced per minute, and P is the plasma concentration. Agents that are filtered but not resorbed or secreted, such as inulin, yield a clearance of 130 ml per minute (assuming no plasma protein binding) and serve as a measure of the glomerular filtration rate. With a volume of distribution of 12 L, this clearance rate translates into a plasma half-

life for inulin of 64 minutes. Compounds actively secreted into the urine and not reabsorbed, such as penicillin and p-aminohippurate, may approach a clearance of 650 ml per minute, which is the rate of total plasma flow through the kidneys. Assuming a volume of distribution of 12 L, such a drug would have a plasma half-life of about 13 minutes. By way of contrast, drugs that are highly bound and subject to passive reabsorption may exhibit clearance rates approaching zero.

Biliary excretion

A number of cationic, anionic, and neutral molecules are selectively removed from the blood for excretion into the bile and eventually the feces. In general, these substances have molecular weights larger than 500. The transport process is an active one in which the dissolved substance is transferred from the plasma to the bile against a concentration gradient. As in all situations of this kind, special energy-requiring mechanisms of such transfer exist, in this instance one for each of the three categories of molecules. Competition for the transport mechanism may occur within each category. The ability to rapidly secrete the anionic dye sulfobromophthalein by the biliary route is the basis for a standard liver function test. The anionic transport mechanism is also involved in the transfer of acidic metabolites (e.g., glucuronides and sulfates) produced from neutral molecules by liver cells. Other carrier systems exist for quaternary ammonium compounds and for neutral substances (such as cardiac glycosides) that have both polar and nonpolar groups. Biliary excretion is responsible for all but a small portion of the fecal elimination of drugs. The remainder is due to direct transmucosal passage into the gastrointestinal tract from the bloodstream or represents compounds dissolved in one or more gastrointestinal tract secretions. Of course, the feces may also contain a variable amount of unabsorbed drug as well. Reabsorption of molecules excreted via the bile can occur, as for example with the laxative phenolphthalein. Such enterohepatic recycling can prolong the duration of action and may continue ad infinitum until the system is interrupted (by metabolism, curtailment of bile flow, ingestion of drug chelator, etc.).

Other routes of excretion

Pulmonary excretion is a primary route for the elimination of gases and some volatile compounds. Excepting the inhalation anesthetics, excretion of chemicals into the respiratory tree may be of more esthetic concern than pharmacokinetic interest. Halitosis produced by odoriferous agents (e.g., paraldehyde), however, may impair clinical suitability.

Elimination of drugs via milk is important, not because of any quantitative significance, but because it represents a potential danger to the nursing baby. Drugs to be particularly concerned about include lithium, various anticancer agents, and isoniazid, among others.[6] The primary variable influencing the passage of drugs into milk is lipid solubility.

Other minor routes of excretion include sweat, tears, saliva, and gastric, pancreatic, and intestinal secretions. In all cases, excretion is limited by the lipid/water partition coefficient. For saliva and related gastrointestinal fluids, drugs are deposited into the gastrointestinal tract after secretion and are available for reabsorption into the systemic circulation.

TIME COURSE OF DRUG ACTION

In previous sections of this text, the close correspondence between the plasma concentration of an agent and its magnitude of effect has been emphasized. Since drug administration usually encompasses the linear midrange of the log dose-response curve, the relationship between plasma titer and patient reaction is often straightforward. Thus, a temporal description of drug concentration based on pharmacokinetic principles is useful not only in illustrating how absorption, distribution, metabolism, and excretion influence drug effects in concert but also in providing guidance for adjusting dosage schedules to achieve therapeutic results with a minimum of drug toxicity.

Kinetics of absorption and elimination

Most biologic events involving the fate of drugs can be described in simple kinetic terms: zero-order, first-order, or capacity-limited (a combination of the two).

Zero-order kinetics. Zero-order kinetics define processes that occur at a constant rate per unit time. Mathematically this can be written as $dC/dt = k_o$, where dC/dt is the rate of change in concentration and k_o is a constant in units of amount/time. A good example of zero-order input of drugs is the continuous intravenous infusion in which the quantity of compound entering the bloodstream each minute is held constant (e.g., 5 mg/min). Another

example of zero-order absorption is provided by the intramuscular or subcutaneous injection of a depot form of drug. Poor aqueous solubility of the preparation permits a constant rate of drug release for several hours. With oral administration, essentially zero-order absorption is realized whenever the rate-limiting factor is the dissolution of the primary drug particles. Finally, topical therapy often results in zero-order uptake. So long as the agent is in great excess, a relatively fixed quantity of drug will permeate the skin per unit time.

First-order kinetics. First-order kinetics relate to events that occur at a constant fractional rate per unit time (e.g., 5%/min). Here $dC/dt = k_1C$, with k_1 depicting the fractional rate constant in units of time^{-1} and C representing the drug concentration. The absorption, distribution, and elimination of compounds commonly exhibit this type of kinetics because they generally rely on processes that are first-order in character: passive diffusion, filtration, blood flow, or drug transport or metabolism operating well below saturation. Since the fraction of drug affected per unit time is independent of concentration, it is often useful to refer to the reaction rate by its half-time (or half-life, $t_{1/2}$), the period required for the process to reach 50% of completion. The half-time is related to the fractional rate constant by the formula $t_{1/2} = 0.693/k_1$. Thus, the greater the rate constant, the shorter the half-life and the faster the reaction. It is easily shown that first-order processes are essentially complete (94%) after four half-times. Table 2-5 lists the elimination half-lives of representatives of some commonly used categories of drugs in dentistry.

Capacity-limited reactions. Capacity-limited reactions involve enzymes responsible for the metabolism of drugs and carrier molecules concerned with drug transport across membranes. This kind of process initially displays zero-order kinetics when the endogenous factor (enzyme or carrier) is saturated with drug; it gradually takes on the features of a first-order reaction as the plasma concentration falls. As stated above, doses employed clinically are usually below those required for saturation. There are some exceptions, however, in which saturation kinetics are evident. Alcohol, even in moderately intoxicating doses, is metabolized at a constant rate of about 8 gm per hour. Only when the concentration falls far below that producing any observable effect does alcohol dehydrogenation assume a first-order rate.

Another important instance of capacity-limited

Table 2-5. Approximate half-lives
of some common drugs

Drug	Elimination half-life (hours)
Antibiotics	
Ampicillin	1.3
Clindamycin	3
Erythromycin	1.4
Penicillin G	0.5
Tetracycline	10
Analgesics	
Acetaminophen	3
Aspirin (as salicylate)	3-20*
Codeine	3†
Meperidine	3
Morphine	3
Local anesthetics	
Bupivacaine	2.5
Lidocaine	1.5†
Procaine	0.13
Sedative agents	
Alcohol	1.4-20*
Diazepam	72†
Pentobarbital	45

*Capacity-limited metabolism.
†Converted to active metabolite(s).

biotransformation involves aspirin. Aspirin is quickly deacetylated to salicylate, the anion largely responsible for the drug's pharmacologic activity. The salicylate is then eliminated through several metabolic pathways and by renal excretion, yielding an overall elimination half-time of about 3 hours. Some of the inactivation routes, though, are easily saturated, so that when an overdose is ingested, the toxicity problem is compounded by a relative loss in elimination efficiency. Elimination half-lives can be calculated for drugs displaying capacity-limited kinetics, but the values obtained will vary continuously according to the drug concentration (Table 2-5). Thus, salicylate has a plasma half-life of 20 hours when a very high concentration is present in the bloodstream. As the salicylate titer falls into the therapeutic range, however, the elimination half-life will decrease to a constant of 3 hours.

Plasma concentration—single doses

Therapeutic agents are often administered in dental practice as single doses. Whether the drug is lidocaine injected for regional anesthesia, atropine to control salivation, or pentobarbital to provide preoperative sedation, the plasma concentration will rise to a peak during the absorptive phase and subsequently fall, eventually to zero, as the drug is eliminated from the bloodstream. The sojourn of many such agents can be described by a simple model system (Figure 2-9) in which the body is depicted as a single compartment whose size corresponds to the apparent volume of distribution.

Based on this model, it is possible to construct theoretical plasma concentration curves and observe how modifications of dosage, absorption, or elimination can alter drug concentrations and, presumably, drug effects. (Similar curves could also have been generated using zero-order absorption.) As shown in Figure 2-10, the plasma concentration is at all times directly proportional to the dose. (This relationship would, of course, not hold for agents that are capacity limited in absorption, binding, metabolism, or excretion.) So long as absorption is several times faster than elimination, changes in the rate of drug uptake have little effect other than to alter somewhat the peak concentration. The duration of action would be hardly influenced at all. A different pattern emerges, however, in those instances in which the rate of absorption approximates that of elimination (not shown in Figure 2-10). As exemplified by penicillin G (elimination half-time 30 minutes), the slow absorption achieved by oral ingestion results in a peak concentration that is, compared with intravenous injection, much reduced and considerably delayed. On the positive side, oral administration can result in a duration of effect that is significantly prolonged. Major differences in plasma concentration may be encountered with slowly absorbed preparations (e.g., timed-release formulations) or with compounds that are quickly metabolized or excreted. Variations in the elimination rate markedly affect the post-absorptive phase of drug action. As shown in Figure 2-10, a threefold decrease in elimination can be more effective than a similar increase in the dose in extending the duration of effect. Since the peak titer is generally not nearly as sensitive to changes in elimination as it is to alterations in dosage, retarding elimination may be the better approach to lengthening the effect duration of compounds with a low or moderate margin of safety. For penicillin G, retarding its elimination could be accomplished by inhibiting urinary excretion

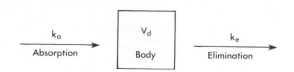

Figure 2-9. Single-compartment model of drug kinetics. Absorption into and elimination from the body are each assigned a single first-order rate constant. Distribution, assumed to be rapid with respect to both absorption and elimination, is not considered.

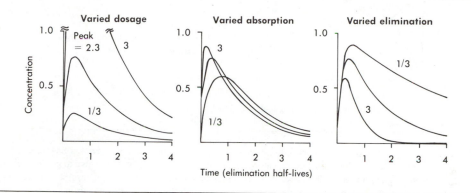

Figure 2-10. Time course of plasma concentration after single doses of drug. The various curves illustrate the influence of threefold increases (3) or decreases (⅓) of dosage, absorption, and elimination on drug titers. The standard curve reproduced in all three graphs represents an agent whose first-order absorption rate is 10 times faster than elimination. A concentration of 1.0 is the value that would result if the drug were absorbed instantaneously, as with an intravenous injection.

through the coadministration of probenecid. Once again, however, penicillin G is an exception to the rule. The antibiotic has such a low toxicity that it is also feasible to compensate for the drug's rapid elimination by simply multiplying the dose several times.

Plasma concentration—repeated doses

Whenever a drug is administered more than once every four elimination half-times, accumulation of the compound will occur within the body. Figure 2-11 demonstrates the result of continued use of a drug given either by intravenous infusion (a zero-order process) or by repetitive administration (first-order absorption in this case). Regardless of the administration format, a plateau concentration is reached in about four elimination half-lives. The periodic fluctuations obtained with intermittent administration are a function of the absorption rate and the dosage interval. Approaching 50% of the peak concentration when absorption is very rapid and the dosage period equals the elimination half-life, such variations can be minimized by increas-

ing the frequency of administration and retarding the rate of absorption.

The average plateau concentration relative to the peak value obtainable after an initial dose can be determined by multiplying the number of doses administered per elimination half-time by 1.44. Thus, the plateau concentration of a drug given once every half-life would equal 144% of the initial peak concentration. For diazepam ingested three times per day, the average equilibrium concentration would approximate, assuming a half-life of 3 days, 1.44 × 9 or 13 times the peak concentration after a single dose. Of course, it would take at least 12 days (four half-times) to reach this final drug titer.

The gradual approach to plateau concentrations associated with slowly eliminated drugs can either benefit or hinder therapy. On the positive side, a long half-time permits the clinician to administer the drug at convenient intervals, perhaps once a day, without having to be concerned with wide swings in plasma concentration. Should patient monitoring reveal an unusual buildup of drug be-

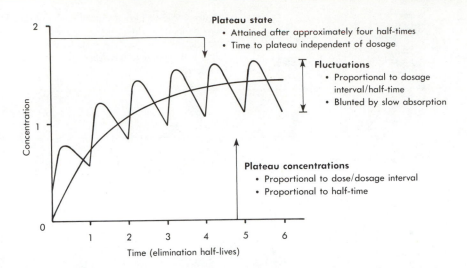

Figure 2-11. Time course of plasma concentration involving drug accumulation. The serrated line reflects the pattern of accumulation observed during the repeated administration of a drug at intervals equal to its elimination half-time, when drug absorption is 10 times as rapid as elimination. As the relative rate of absorption increases, the concentration maxima approach twice the minima during the plateau state. The smooth line depicts drug accumulation during the administration of an equivalent dosage by continuous intravenous infusion. (From Mayer, S.E., Melmon, K.L., and Gilman, A.G. Introduction; the dynamics of drug absorption, distribution, and elimination. In Gilman, A.G., Goodman, L.S., and Gilman, A., eds. Goodman and Gilman's The Pharmacological Basis of Therapeutics, ed. 6. New York, © 1980 Macmillan Publishing Co., Inc., 1980.)

cause of impaired metabolism or excretion or some other cause, time is available to adjust the dosage before toxic effects ensue. On the debit side, however, the attainment of a therapeutic effect will be delayed by the time required for drug accumulation to proceed. If an immediate pharmacologic effect is needed, it becomes necessary to administer a loading dose of the drug. A loading dose is a large, initial quantity of drug substituted for the normal amount to quickly produce a concentration approximating the plateau state. For an agent given once each half-time, the loading dose would equal twice the maintenance dose; for drugs given more frequently, the loading dose would have to be relatively larger. It is often wise, therefore, to divide a loading dose into several smaller fractions. The sacrifice of some speed in attaining a therapeutic concentration is usually more than compensated for by the ability to evaluate patient responses during the early phase of therapy. Indeed, the fact that elimination rates, which help regulate plateau concentrations, can vary greatly among individuals should dictate caution whenever cumulative drug effects are sought.

CITED REFERENCES

1. Adriani, J., and Campbell, D. Fatalities following topical application of local anesthetics to mucous membranes. Journal of the American Medical Association **162:**1527-1530, 1956.

2. Altland, K., and Goedde, H.W. Heterogeneity in the silent gene phenotype of pseudocholinesterase of human serum. Biochemical Genetics **4:**321-338, 1970.

3. Astwood, E.B. Occurrence in the sera of certain patients of large amounts of a newly isolated iodine compound. Transactions of the American Association of Physicians **70:**183-191, 1957.

4. Barchowsky, A., Stargel, W.W., Shand, D.G., and Routledge, P.A. Saliva concentrations of lidocaine and its metabolites in man. Therapeutic Drug Monitoring **4:**335-339, 1982.

5. Beckett, A.H., and Hossie, R.D. Buccal absorption of drugs. In Brodie, B.B., and Gillette, J.R., eds. Handbook of Experimental Pharmacology. Berlin, Springer-Verlag, 1971.

6. Berlin, C.M., Jr. Pharmacologic considerations of drug use in the lactating mother. Obstetrics and Gynecology **58**(Suppl.):17S-23S, 1981.

7. Collander, R. The permeability of plant protoplasts to small molecules. Physiologia Plantarum **2:**300-311, 1949.

8. Cooke, A.R., and Hunt, J.N. Absorption of acetylsalicylic acid from unbuffered and buffered gastric contents. American Journal of Digestive Diseases **15:**95-102, 1970.

9. Cucinell, S.A., Conney, A.H., Sansur, M., and Burns, J.J. Drug interactions in man. I. Lowering effect of phenobarbital on plasma levels of bishydroxycoumarin (Dicumarol) and diphenylhydantoin (Dilantin). Clinical Pharmacology and Therapeutics **6:**420-429, 1965.

10. Davson, H., and Danielli, J.F. The Permeability of Natural Membranes, ed. 2. Cambridge, Cambridge University Press, 1952.

11. Feller, K., and le Petit, G. On the distribution of drugs in saliva and blood plasma. International Journal of Clinical Pharmacology and Biopharmacy **15:**468-469, 1977.

12. Gangarosa, L.P. Iontophoresis for surface local anesthesia. Journal of the American Dental Association **88:**125-128, 1974.

13. Gangarosa, L.P., Park, N.H., and Hill, J.M. Iontophoretic assistance of 5-iodo-2′-deoxyuridine penetration into neonatal mouse skin and effects on DNA synthesis. Proceedings of the Society for Experimental Biology and Medicine **154:**439-443, 1977.

14. Gibaldi, M. Biopharmaceutics and Clinical Pharmacokinetics, ed. 2. Philadelphia, Lea & Febiger, 1977.

15. Goldstein, A., Aronow, L., and Kalman, S.M. Principles of Drug Action: The Basis of Pharmacology, ed. 2. New York, John Wiley & Sons, Inc., 1974.

16. Greenblatt, D.J., and Koch-Weser, J. Clinical toxicity of chlordiazepoxide and diazepam in relation to serum albumin concentrations: a report from the Boston Collaborative Drug Surveillance Program. European Journal of Clinical Pharmacology **7:**259-262, 1974.

17. Hahn, T.J., Hendin, B.A., Scharp, C.R., Boisseau, V.C., and Haddad, J.G., Jr. Serum 25-hydroxycalciferol levels and bone mass in children on chronic anticonvulsant therapy. New England Journal of Medicine **292:**550-553, 1975.

18. Hogben, C.A.M., Tocco, D.J., Brodie, B.B., and Schanker, L.S. On the mechanism of intestinal absorption of drugs. Journal of Pharmacology and Experimental Therapeutics **125:**275-282, 1959.

19. Inman, W.H.W., and Adelstein, A.M. Rise and fall of asthma mortality in England and Wales in relation to use of pressurized aerosols. Lancet **2:**279-285, 1969.

20. Lehner, T., and Lyne, C. Adrenal function during topical oral treatment with triamcinolone acetonide. British Dental Journal **129:**164-167, 1970.

21. Levine, R.R. Pharmacology: Drug Actions and Reactions, ed. 2. Boston, Little, Brown & Co., 1978.

22. Levy, G. Kinetics and implications of dissolution rate. Limited gastrointestinal absorption of drugs. In Ariëns, E.J., ed. Physio-Chemical Aspects of Drug Action, vol. 7. Proceedings of the Third International Pharmacology Meeting. Oxford, Pergamon Press, Inc., 1968.

23. Lovering, E.G., McGilveray, I.J., McMillan, I., Tostowaryk, W., Matula, T., and Marier, G. The bioavailability and dissolution behavior of nine brands of tetracycline tablets. Canadian Journal of Pharmaceutical Sciences **10:**36-39, 1975.

24. Magnussen, M.P. The effect of ethanol on the gastrointestinal absorption of drugs in the rat. Acta Pharmacologica et Toxicologica (Copenhagen) **26:**130-144, 1968.

25. Marier, J.R. Halogenated hydrocarbon environmental pollution: the special case of halogenated anesthetics. Environmental Research **28:**212-239, 1982.

26. Mark, L.C. Thiobarbiturates. In Papper, E.M., and Kitz, R.J., eds. Uptake and Distribution of Anesthetic Agents. New York, McGraw-Hill Book Co., 1963.

27. Melander, A. Influence of food on the bioavailability of drugs. In Gibaldi, M., and Prescott, L., eds. Handbook of Clinical Pharmacokinetics. Sydney, ADIS Health Science Press, 1983.

28. Murthy, K.S., Talim, S.T., and Singh, I. A comparative evaluation of topical application and iontophoresis of sodium fluoride for desensitization of hypersensitive dentin. Oral Surgery, Oral Medicine, Oral Pathology **36:**448-458, 1973.

29. Neitlich, H.W. Increased plasma cholinesterase activity and succinylcholine resistance: a genetic variant. Journal of Clinical Investigation **45:**380-387, 1966.

30. Ohki, S., Gravis, C., and Pant, H. Permeability of axon membranes to local anesthetics. Biochimica et Biophysica Acta **643:**495-507, 1981.

31. Rylance, G.W., and Moreland, T.A. Saliva carbamazepine and phenytoin level monitoring. Archives of Disease in Childhood **56:**637-652, 1981.

32. Singer, S.J., and Nicholson, G.L. The fluid mosaic model of the structure of cell membranes. Science **175:**720-731, 1972.

33. Treatment of syphilis and gonorrhea. Medical Letter on Drugs and Therapeutics **19:**105-107, 1977.

34. Van Der Reis, L., and Lazar, H.P. The Human Digestive System: Its Functions and Disorders. Basel, S. Karger AG, 1972.

35. Vesell, E.S. Advances in pharmacogenetics. Progress in Medical Genetics **9:**291-367, 1973.

36. Weiss, C.F., Glazko, A.J., and Weston, J.K. Chloramphenicol in the newborn infant: a physiological explanation of its toxicity when given in excessive dose. New England Journal of Medicine **262:**787-794, 1960.

37. Wilson, T.H. Intestinal Absorption. Philadelphia, W. B. Saunders Co., 1962.

GENERAL REFERENCES

Creasey, W.A. Drug Disposition in Humans. New York, Oxford University Press, 1979.

Curry, S.H. Drug Disposition and Pharmacokinetics, ed. 3. Oxford, Blackwell Scientific Publications, 1980.

Gibaldi, M. Biopharmaceutics and Clinical Pharmacokinetics, ed. 2. Philadelphia, Lea & Febiger, 1977.

Goldstein, A., Aronow, L., and Kalman, S.M. Principles of Drug Action: The Basis of Pharmacology, ed. 2. New York, John Wiley & Sons, Inc., 1974.

La Du, B.N., Mandel, H.G., and Way, E.L., eds. Fundamentals of Drug Metabolism and Drug Disposition. Baltimore, Williams & Wilkins Co., 1971.

Levine, R.R. Pharmacology: Drug Actions and Reactions, ed. 2. Boston, Little, Brown & Co., 1978.

Mayer, S.E., Melmon, K.L., and Gilman, A.G. Introduction; the dynamics of drug absorption, distribution, and elimination. In Gilman, A.G., Goodman, L.S., and Gilman, A., eds. Goodman and Gilman's The Pharmacological Basis of Therapeutics, ed. 6. New York, Macmillan, Inc., 1980.

3 Pharmacotherapeutics: the clinical use of drugs

John A. Yagiela

The primary goal of drug treatment is to achieve a desired pharmacologic effect without causing adverse reactions. Because no therapeutic regimen is without risk, the clinician must weigh the benefits expected from a drug against the dangers inherent in its use. If drugs are to be properly selected and administered, a number of factors should be considered that complicate both the attainment of therapeutic responses and the avoidance of unwanted effects.

As stated in Chapter 1, drugs are often selective in the effects they produce because they activate or inhibit specific drug receptors. However, even the most selective agents generally evoke a spectrum of reactions rather than a single pharmacologic outcome. Atropine in therapeutic concentrations, for example, specifically prevents the stimulation of muscarinic receptors by acetylcholine. Since these receptors are vital to the normal function of the entire parasympathetic nervous system, their blockade can result in a wide range of autonomic responses. Though specific in action, atropine is thus rather nonselective in effect. In addition, specificity of receptor binding is usually a matter of dose; in concentrations greater than therapeutic, atropine will block the nonmuscarinic effects of acetylcholine and may inhibit the actions of norepinephrine, histamine, and 5-hydroxytryptamine as well. Finally, nonspecific effects unrelated to receptor blockade may be observed. Large concentrations of atropine have local anesthetic activity and may directly affect the central nervous system and peripheral vasculature.

In addition to the fact that single agents can produce multiple effects, pharmacotherapeutics is complicated by variations in patient responsiveness. A therapeutic dose of drug for one individual may be ineffective for a second person and toxic to a third. Even highly inbred laboratory species display measurable biologic variations in drug sensitivity. Figure 3-1 is a quantal dose-effect graph illustrating the percentage of subjects responding to an agent as a logarithmic function of the dose. The graph is constructed by counting the number of animals or patients exhibiting a specified effect at various doses. With low amounts of drug, very few individuals react; as the dose is increased, however, more are affected, until a dose is reached at which the response is universal. Although similar in appearance, the *quantal* dose-effect relationship must not be confused with the *graded* dose-response curve described in Chapter 1 (see Figure 1-3). The quantal dose-response curve is sigmoidal in shape because of the log-normal distribution of drug sensitivities found in most populations (Figure 3-1). The ED50 (not ED_{50}) represents the median effective dose, the amount of drug required to produce a particular effect in 50% of the individuals treated. Although potency is represented in both quantal and graded relationships by the position of the curve on the abscissa, intrinsic activity (or efficacy) is apparent only in graded responses. On the other hand, biologic variation, which is inversely correlated with the slope of the quantal dose-effect curve, cannot be estimated from a single graded dose-response graph.

Patients who are unusually sensitive to a drug are said to be hyperreactive. Terms more or less synonymous with hyperreactivity include hypersusceptibility and drug intolerance. The term *hypersensitivity* is also employed on occasion, but this usage can be misleading as hypersensitivity is commonly employed to indicate drug allergy. Individuals unexpectedly resistant to conventional doses of drug are referred to as being hyporeactive. Tolerance, tachyphylaxis, and several additional

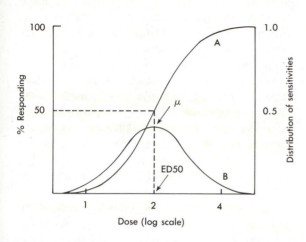

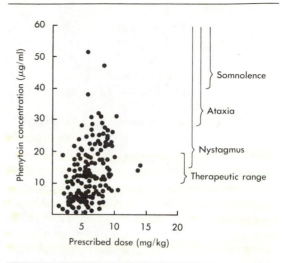

Figure 3-1. Quantal dose-response curves (log scale). Curve A represents the cumulative distribution and curve B the frequency distribution of patient responses in a normal population. As shown, the mean (μ) and median (50% responding) sensitivities fall on the same dose (median effective dose, ED50). (Adapted from Goldstein, A., Aronow, L., and Kalman, S.M. Principles of Drug Action: The Basis of Pharmacology, ed. 2. New York, John Wiley & Sons, Inc., 1974.)

Figure 3-2. Plasma phenytoin concentration as a function of the prescribed dose. Each dot represents a single patient (n = 294; data from Lund, L. Effects of phenytoin in patients with epilepsy in relation to its concentration in plasma. In Davies, D.S., and Prichard, B.N.C., eds. Biological Effects of Drugs in Relation to Their Plasma Concentrations. Baltimore, University Park Press, 1973.) Closed bracket indicates the accepted therapeutic concentration range for phenytoin in plasma; open-ended brackets denote concentrations at which the various toxic manifestations listed may occur (according to the data of Kutt, H., Winters, W., Kokenge, R., and McDowell, F. Archives of Neurology **11:**642-648, 1964.)

types of hyporeactivity will be discussed later. A great many variables influence the responsiveness of individuals to drugs. Some of these are readily apparent and under the control of the clinician; others are often hidden from view and not amenable to modification. Since it is impossible to predict how a given patient will respond to a particular agent, appropriate monitoring of drug effects is usually necessary to achieve optimal therapy.

FACTORS INFLUENCING DRUG EFFECTS

Differences between patients in reaction to a therapeutic agent may arise from disparities in drug concentration obtained with a standardized dose (pharmacokinetic differences) or from variations in individual responsiveness to a given drug concentration (pharmacodynamic differences) or from failure of patients to take their medication as prescribed (noncompliance). Figure 3-2 dramatizes the lack of correlation that can develop clinically between the prescribed dose of a drug, in this case

the anticonvulsant phenytoin, and the resultant plasma concentration and pharmacologic response. Even with the daily dose corrected for body weight, this study revealed that the steady-state concentration of phenytoin differed 20-fold or more.[24] It is apparent that, given a therapeutic concentration range of 10 to 20 μg/ml (the plasma concentration of phenytoin supposed to provide seizure protection with minimal adverse effects[13]), the majority of patients took either insufficient medication or an overdose. Although pharmacokinetic dissimilarities undoubtedly account for many differences in patient responsiveness, the fact that phenytoin has a "therapeutic range" rather than a single effective concentration indicates that there also exists some variation in pharmacodynamic sensitivity to the anticonvulsant. Indeed, a small percentage of individuals experience nystagmus, an early indication of drug toxicity, at plasma concentrations barely sufficient to control convulsions in other patients.[17] In view of these findings, the common practice of prescribing 300 mg of phenytoin per day for all patients cannot be condoned.[16]

Patient factors

Many factors that can influence drug effects clinically are highly variable with respect to individual patients. Although such attributes as size, age, and genetic make-up are not amenable to modification, they must be taken into account whenever drug therapy is planned.

Body weight and composition. Adults may differ three times or more in weight. Because the volume of distribution of a drug is a function of body mass, extremes in patient size may result in significant differences in plasma concentration when drugs are administered in the form of a "standard adult dose." Body composition is also an important variable here. Two equally heavy patients, one obese and the other muscular, may react quite differently to certain agents. Since adipose tissue contributes very little to body water, the obese individual will be more susceptible to a drug distributed essentially within one or more body fluid compartments. On the other hand, the same individual may demonstrate unusual resistance to a highly lipophilic agent like thiopental, especially when it is given in repeated doses.

Age. Pediatric patients generally cannot be given adult doses of drugs. The primary reason for this difference is body size, and various formulas (discussed in Chapter 49) have been devised to calculate pediatric fractions of the adult dose. For the following reasons, however, children must not be thought of as merely miniature adults. First, even with the size differential taken into account, neonates display an unusual hyperreactivity to drugs. Immature hepatic and renal systems during the first weeks of life tend to promote drug accumulation, and the relative inefficiency of drug binding by albumin (sometimes because of competition for binding sites by bilirubin[7]) may also lead to abnormal concentrations of drug in the vicinity of receptors. In addition, distribution of compounds into the central nervous system may be enhanced by an incomplete development of the blood-brain barrier. Second, in contrast to neonates, children and infants over 2 months of age often require large mg/kg doses of drugs during therapy. Part of this relative hyporeactivity may stem from a pediatric extracellular water space up to 75% greater in ml/kg than the adult volume, which tends to dilute absorbed drugs; the major reason, though, is an enhancement in the rate of elimination.[11] And last, children are especially vulnerable to the toxic effects of certain agents. Thus, sex steroids and other hormones may impair normal growth and development, atropine intoxication may readily cause hyperpyrexia, and salicylate overdose may quickly lead to acid-base and electrolyte disturbances.

Obviously, there is no method of pediatric dosage calculation suitable for all drugs and therapeutic situations. In older children, adjustments based on age, weight, or (preferably) surface area may be satisfactory, but no general guide is possible for the very young. Dosages for neonates and infants should be based on clinical trials; unfortunately, studies of this nature are often not done and dosage schedules for small children not provided.

Geriatric patients are frequently hyperreactive to drugs. Although increased sensitivity may result from organic pathology or from drug interactions, both more likely to occur in the elderly, age-related functional changes in drug disposition and cellular responsiveness are also involved. Because patients over the age of 65 are twice as likely to experience adverse reactions as are young adults, careful selection of dosage schedules is necessary, especially with drugs of low safety. The field of geriatric pharmacology is becoming increasingly important to the dentist as the general population ages and as a higher proportion of the elderly retain their teeth (thanks to improved oral hygiene and professional care); it is therefore covered in its entirety in Chapter 48.

Sex, pregnancy, and lactation. The sex of a patient is sometimes important with respect to drug effects. Because women tend to be smaller than men and have a higher percentage of body fat, dosage adjustments may be necessary for some agents. Hepatic disposition of drugs is affected by the ratio of female to male sex hormones. Women appear to be more susceptible to drug-induced blood dyscrasias, and those taking systemic contraceptives may be more prone to some drug interactions. For obvious reasons, side effects like hirsutism are less tolerable in women and gynecomastia more troublesome in men.

Pregnancy is a major concern in pharmacotherapeutics. Disturbances in liver and renal function are common and may delay the metabolism and excretion of numerous substances. The hepatic toxicity of tetracycline and certain other compounds is markedly accentuated by pregnancy. When present, toxemia may increase drug effects by reducing the binding capacity of albumin. Of primary importance are the actions of drugs on the unborn child. Spontaneous abortion, teratogenesis, mental retardation, drug dependence, and cancer have resulted from drug administration during pregnancy. Since few, if any, agents have been proved totally safe for the fetus, it is best to avoid all medications when possible. Drug administration should also be conservative in women of child-bearing age, as pregnancy is often undiagnosed during the first trimester (the most critical period of fetal development). Many drugs (e.g., methadone) are excreted in the milk. Since some of these agents may cause unwanted effects in the nursing infant, it is advisable to review carefully drug exposure during lactation as well.

Environmental factors. Probably the most important environmental factor influencing drug effects is the diet. The timing of meals and the types of food eaten can markedly affect drug absorption. Occasionally, individual substances in the diet can modify responses to selected agents. Patients receiving monoamine oxidase inhibitors, for example, risk severe hypertension and death should they eat foodstuffs containing tyramine (certain cheeses, beers, and wines, etc.). The therapeutic effects of levodopa in parkinsonism may be prevented by pyridoxine (vitamin B_6) present in foods and multivitamin supplements. Moreover, various chemicals that are ingested, inhaled, or absorbed through the skin can stimulate drug metabolism. Temperature, altitude, and probably other factors are also capable of influencing the disposition of drugs in the body.

The indigenous microflora represents a special kind of environmental variable. Several drugs given orally are metabolized by bacterial enzymes to such an extent that absorption may be significantly impaired. The dose of coumarin anticoagulants is partially governed by the amount of vitamin K produced by enteric bacteria. During antibiotic therapy, the type and number of microorganisms surviving play a large role in determining whether patients develop superinfection.

Physiologic variables. Numerous physiologic factors can modify clinical responses to drugs. Fluctuations in gastric, plasma, and urinary pH, for instance, may alter the pharmacokinetics of weak electrolytes. Salt and water balance, exercise, sleep, body temperature, circadian rhythms, and many other factors also influence patient reactions. The effects of blocking agents are particularly sensitive to variations in physiologic or biochemical events. Thus, isoproterenol, an adrenergic agonist, increases heart rate irrespective of autonomic nervous system tone, but atropine, an acetylcholine

antagonist, increases heart rate only in the face of tonic vagal activity.

Pathologic factors. Diseases may influence pharmacotherapeutics by modifying drug disposition or tissue responsiveness. Pathologic states most commonly associated with altered patient reactivity involve the organs of absorption, distribution, metabolism, and excretion. Diarrhea, malabsorption syndromes, and other disturbances of the gastrointestinal tract may depress the absorption of ingested agents. Although data are few, it is probable that actively absorbed substances are more likely to be affected by gastrointestinal disease than are drugs that reach the systemic circulation by passive diffusion.[29]

The distribution of drugs is sensitive to pathologic changes in the blood and circulatory system and to perturbations in anatomic barriers to diffusion. Disturbances in the concentration of plasma proteins (e.g., hypoalbuminemia) or in their function (as in uremia) may lead to drug toxicity or to a loss of therapeutic benefit. Congestive heart failure and arteriosclerosis may diminish tissue perfusion such that drug elimination is significantly retarded. Meningeal inflammation permits entry into the central nervous system of many drugs (e.g., penicillins) normally excluded by the blood-brain barrier.

Renal pathology is a common modifier of drug effects. The plasma half-lives of agents eliminated in the urine are often greatly prolonged by renal failure. Even for compounds completely destroyed in the liver, inadequate excretion of metabolites may increase the incidence of untoward reactions.[13] A good measure of renal status is provided by the endogenous creatinine clearance. By way of illustration, a 50% drop in creatinine clearance should theoretically indicate a twofold increase in the elimination half-time of a drug that is removed from the blood solely by renal excretion. For a drug partially eliminated in the urine, the increase in plasma half-life should be correspondingly less. The customary approach to avoiding excessive drug accumulation in patients with renal disease is to lengthen the dosage interval in accordance with the degree of elimination impairment. Table 3-1 lists, for several drugs commonly used in dentistry, the approximate dosage intervals indicated for patients with moderate or severe renal disability.[5] Hepatic dysfunction can markedly reduce the metabolism and biliary excretion of drugs. Unfortunately, standard liver function tests are of little

Table 3-1. Maintenance dose intervals in renal failure

Drug	Route of elimination	Dose interval (in hours) according to degree of renal failure*		
		Normal function	*Moderate impairment*	*Severe impairment*
Antibiotics				
Penicillin G	Mainly renal	8	8-12	12-16
Erythromycin	Hepatic	6	6	6
Cephalexin	Renal	6	6	6-12
Tetracycline†	Renal/hepatic	6	Avoid use	Avoid use
Analgesics				
Aspirin†	Renal/hepatic	4	4-6	Avoid use
Acetaminophen†	Hepatic	4	6	8
Phenacetin†	Hepatic	4	Avoid use	Avoid use
Ibuprofen	Renal	6	8	12
Codeine	Mainly hepatic	4	4	4
Meperidine	Mainly hepatic	4	4	4
CNS depressants				
Pentobarbital	Hepatic	8	8	8
Phenobarbital	Hepatic/renal	8	8	8-16
Diazepam	Hepatic	8	8	8
Chlordiazepoxide	Hepatic	8	8	12
Others				
Propranolol	Hepatic	8	8	8
Diphenhydramine	Mainly hepatic	6	6-9	9-12
Prednisone	Hepatic	12	12	12

Data from Bennett, W.M., Muther, R.S., Parker, R.A., Feig, P., Morrison, G., Golper, T.A., and Singer, I. Drug therapy in renal failure: dosing guidelines for adults. Annals of Internal Medicine **93:**62-89, 286-325, 1980.

*The degree of renal failure as defined by creatinine clearance: normal function, >80 ml/min: moderate impairment, 10 to 50 ml/min; severe impairment, <10 ml/min.

†Drugs that may accentuate renal damage.

prognostic value with respect to drug biotransformation. Some patients with demonstrable cirrhosis or hepatitis may show surprisingly little metabolic deficit while others may exhibit marked hyperreactivity to standard doses of drugs. Within the same individual, the metabolism of some drugs but not others may be impaired. The uncertainties of drug metabolism introduced by hepatic disease require that substances inactivated in the liver be used cautiously in affected patients and that careful monitoring of drug effects be performed in order to avoid serious adverse reactions. An insidious form of interaction between pathologic factors and drug effects occurs with agents potentially toxic to their primary organs of elimination. Acetaminophen accumulation permitted by liver disease may result in hepatic necrosis and further impairment of drug metabolism.[35] A similar "vicious cycle" involving the kidney has been observed with a variety of drugs.

Exaggeration of the systemic effects of epinephrine and reduction in the analgesic potency of morphine in uncontrolled hyperthyroidism are two examples of drug effects modified by disease states through nonpharmacokinetic means. While pathologic factors may influence drug-receptor interactions directly, as in myasthenia gravis (in which receptor reactivity to ACh agonists is reduced), most alterations of patient response occur indirectly through the augmentation of overt disease or the unmasking of latent physiologic deficits. Thus, agents that promote hyperuricemia may cause an acute exacerbation of gout, and propranolol may induce heart failure in patients with a severely compromised myocardium.

Genetic influences. Without question, genetic variables contribute greatly to the differences in drug responsiveness illustrated in Figure 3-1. Although the importance of heredity is underscored by the evolution of pharmacogenetics into a recognized field of study, the elucidation of multigenetic factors that lead to log-normal distributions in drug reactivity has proved difficult. In fact, the only variations in drug effects that have been shown unequivocally to be genetically linked are those that exhibit simple inheritance patterns and yield bimodal or otherwise discontinuous distribution curves and those that can be associated with certain groups of people on the basis of blood type, race, ethnic background, and so on. Genetic factors are responsible for idiosyncratic reactions and determine, in part, the relative likelihood of a patient experiencing an allergic response to an administered agent (see below). Genetic influences can alter drug effects quantitatively; they may also result in the appearance of novel pharmacologic outcomes.

Drug factors

In addition to individual variations in patient reactivity, certain drug factors, namely the formulation and dosage regimen of an agent and the development of tolerance, can markedly influence the success of drug therapy.

Variables in drug administration. Of all the factors influencing pharmacologic responses clinically, only those involved with drug selection and administration are totally under the control of the clinician. Some of these variables are discussed in detail in previous chapters: dose, drug formulation, route of administration, and drug accumulation. Two additional factors worthy of comment are the time of administration and the duration of therapy. Many disturbing side effects are minimized if an agent can be given shortly before sleep. These include the autonomic effects of the belladonna alkaloids, the vestibular component of nausea associated with narcotic analgesics, and the sedative properties of the antihistamines. Conversely, agents producing mild CNS stimulation are better tolerated in the daytime. The scheduling of doses with or between meals in order to limit gastrointestinal upset or to enhance absorption is mentioned in Chapter 2.

The duration of therapy has several important ramifications. Treatment must, of course, be sufficient in length to be effective. This is particularly true with antimicrobial agents, in which an inadequate duration of coverage can lead to reinfection. However, because adverse drug reactions are more likely to occur during extended courses of therapy, treatment should never be unduly prolonged. It is generally inappropriate, for example, to continue

a patient on medication after the condition requiring therapy has subsided. The duration of administration should be monitored especially carefully when drugs capable of producing physical or psychologic dependence are being used.

Drug tolerance. In pharmacology, tolerance to a drug refers to a state of decreased responsiveness that develops on repeated or continuous exposure to the agent or one of its congeners. Two major categories of tolerance are recognized: pharmacokinetic or drug-disposition tolerance, in which the effective concentration of the drug is diminished, and pharmacodynamic or cellular tolerance, in which the activity of a given concentration of the drug is reduced.

Most documented cases of drug-disposition tolerance involve agents that stimulate their own metabolism through induction of microsomal enzymes. Other mechanisms are possible, though, such as an "immune tolerance," in which circulating antibodies produced in response to an antigenic substance (e.g., bovine insulin) combine with the agent, thereby decreasing its effective concentration at the receptor site. When pharmacokinetic tolerance is encountered, clinical effectiveness can usually be restored through simple adjustment of the dose or administration interval.

Cellular tolerance is commonly observed with drugs that alter mood, perception, or thought: narcotic analgesics, barbiturates, benzodiazepines, alcohol, phenothiazines, tricyclic antidepressants, amphetamines, caffeine, cocaine, etc. Tolerance is usually acquired gradually, depending on the drug, its dose, and how often it is administered. Generally, cellular tolerance does not develop equally to all effects of a drug. Sometimes this is beneficial, as when undesirable side effects of an agent are lost but the therapeutic activity is retained (as with the phenothiazines). Unfortunately, differences in tolerance can also promote adverse reactions. Alcoholics, for example, become tolerant to the "therapeutic" effect of ethanol yet remain normally susceptible to the lethal effect. Continual use of ethanol leads to a potentially dangerous reduction in the drug's margin of safety as the user is forced to approach toxic concentrations in order to achieve the desired level of inebriety. A similar phenomenon occurs with other CNS depressants, such as the barbiturates. Clinical management of pharmacodynamic tolerance can often be accomplished by increasing the dose; however, this approach is occasionally ineffective in restoring drug activity and may result in serious toxicity or drug dependence. Normal sensitivity in a tolerant individual can be restored eventually through abstention from the drug.

Although the bases for most types of cellular tolerance are poorly understood, mechanisms have been established for certain drugs that evoke a rapidly developing form of tolerance known as tachyphylaxis. The sympathomimetic agent tyramine provides a classical example of tachyphylaxis. Administered intravenously to an animal whose vagal innervation of the heart has been interrupted, tyramine indirectly increases heart rate and blood pressure by causing the release of norepinephrine from adrenergic nerves. A subsequent dose given after the effects of the first have disappeared generates a smaller response, and, after a series of repetitions, the drug may lose essentially all activity. Acute tolerance to tyramine is produced by rapid depletion of the functional norepinephrine stores of the adrenergic nerve terminals. Two additional examples of tachyphylaxis are associated with histamine. Because endogenous stores of histamine can be quickly depleted but take a long time to be replenished, drugs that cause histamine release (e.g., morphine and tubocurarine) will generate tolerance in much the same manner as does tyramine. Tachyphylaxis may also occur to histamine itself. Repetition of increasing doses of intravenous histamine can produce in several hours a hyporeactivity a 100-fold less than normal. Other drugs capable of evoking acute tolerance include the barbiturates, nitrites, cholinergics, and anticholinergics.

Factors associated with the therapeutic regimen

Some factors influencing drug effects are related to the therapeutic context in which the agent is administered or prescribed. Attitudes, for example toward the drug regimen or practitioner, may determine whether an agent proves effective or even if it is taken. Concurrent use of other medicines may alter drug effects directly through pharmacologic mechanisms or indirectly by promoting errors in drug administration.

Placebo effects. A placebo effect is any effect attributable to a medication or procedure that is not related to its pharmacodynamic or specific properties.[48] The term *placebo* is derived from the Latin verb *placere,* meaning "to please." In pharmacotherapeutics, a placebo may be either "pure," in which the preparation is pharmacologically inert

(e.g., a lactose tablet), or "impure," in which the drug has pharmacologic activity but is given for a condition or in a manner such that no benefit can be obtained from its specific properties. A commonly held misconception is that placebos provide nothing more than a means of placating patients, that they may help in psychosomatic illness but are worthless when symptoms are organically based. Numerous studies have revealed, however, that placebo medication is effective in treating the subjective responses to a variety of "real" medical conditions (e.g., the pain of cancer, angina pectoris, headache, and surgical wounds).[4] Actually, the distinction between psychogenic and organic illness has become blurred by the realization that psychologic disturbances often produce physiologic or pathologic manifestations and that organic diseases, or at least their signs and symptoms, can be influenced by the central nervous system through regulation of hormonal secretion and peripheral nervous system activity. Placebo effects are not merely subjective in nature; the administration of pharmacologically inert substances has led to measurable changes in gastric acid secretion, in heart rate and blood pressure, in the number of circulating leukocytes, and in the plasma concentrations of various compounds, including adrenal steroids, catecholamines, electrolytes, and glucose.[4] Even so-called subjective responses to placebos may have a biochemical basis. It has been shown, for example, that placebo analgesia can be blocked by naloxone, a specific opioid antagonist.[20]

Placebo responses to drugs arise from expectations by the patient concerning their effects and from a wish to obtain benefit or relief. Expectations develop at the conscious and subconscious levels and are influenced by many factors. The patient, of course, must be aware that treatment is being rendered. It is the symbolic association of receiving medication in a therapeutic environment that generates placebo reactions. The patient must also be anxious about his problem and desirous of being cured. Placebo effects are unlikely if there is patient indifference to the condition or to the therapeutic regimen. Past experience is another important variable. Previous drug exposure informs a patient of what to expect from a drug; repeated administrations evoking prompt, noticeable effects may, in fact, produce conditioned reflexes. Because suggestion is involved, placebo effects are subject to modification by the practitioner's attitudes (to the patient, to the patient's illness, and to the drug or placebo) and how these feelings are communicated. In one study, a 45% reduction in placebo response occurred solely as a result of the administrators' negative bias toward the placebo medication.[3]

Several important similarities and differences between placebo and specific effects of drugs must be remembered if clinicians are to avoid being deceived by the preparations they employ. Therapeutic responses to placebos and to active agents may resemble each other in magnitude and duration. For example, the pain relief and cough suppression afforded by a placebo may parallel that of codeine. Toxicities can also overlap. Pure placebos cause many common side effects—nausea, drowsiness, sweating, xerostomia, etc.—and may occasionally induce such life-threatening emergencies as acute asthma, anaphylactic shock, and cardiac arrhythmia. By way of contrast, placebos suffer from a relative lack of predictability. Although some drugs can be relied on to produce a given effect in essentially all patients, only about one third of individuals receiving placebos usually react. Attempts to identify placebo responders on the basis of psychologic profile or other characteristics have been unfruitful; it appears that anyone may respond to placebos in the appropriate situation. Finally, there are many classes of drugs, such as the general anesthetics and the antibiotics, whose effects placebos cannot duplicate.

Placebo effects advantageous to therapy should be sought whenever a drug is administered. Sometimes, the effective communication of confidence and other positive attitudes by the practitioner can make the difference between therapeutic success and failure. The clinical application of placebos, though, should be restricted to those conditions for which no other agent is superior. Even then, the evolution of informed consent into a basic patient right complicates the administration of placebo medication. Clinicians, when using placebos, often favor the impure variety in order to reduce the chance of discovery and the possible loss of patient trust. This practice is questionable, however, because of the increased risk of toxicity associated with pharmacologically active compounds.

Medication errors, patient noncompliance. Drugs are often not administered in the manner intended by the prescriber. Occasionally, the clinician may miswrite the prescription, or the pharmacist may supply the wrong drug or incorrectly transcribe the instructions to the patient. The vast preponderance of medication errors, though, arise from the failure of patients to take their preparations as directed. Drug defaulting is a major problem in therapeutics; most studies document a noncompliance rate of 25% to 60%.[40] The reasons for noncompliance are varied: a lack of understanding of the drug, the purpose for which it was prescribed, or how it is to be administered; economic factors; negative feelings toward the drug or prescriber; development of adverse reactions; forgetfulness or carelessness; and resolution of the problem before the drug regimen is complete or, conversely, failure to notice any therapeutic benefit. Although infrequent omissions and minor mistakes in dosage or time of administration are often innocuous, complete failure to take the prescribed drug, premature discontinuance, or ingestion of excessive amounts can be disastrous. The possibility of noncompliance should be considered whenever a drug is seemingly without activity. Unfortunately, patients are notoriously inaccurate in reporting their own compliance, and physicians are not much better in estimating its occurrence.[38] When effective therapy is essential, direct assay of the patient's blood, urine, saliva, or feces for the drug or its metabolites may be necessary to detect noncompliance.

As with the placebo responder, attempts have been made to characterize the potential drug defaulter on the basis of such factors as age, sex, education, race, and socioeconomic status. While some correlations have been drawn (e.g., elderly patients are more apt to forget their medicine or to confuse one type of pill with another), many investigations have been either inconclusive or contradictory. The most important variables relate not to the patient but to the illness, the drug administered, the overall therapeutic regimen, and the doctor-patient relationship. Administration schedules are more faithfully followed by patients with life-threatening diseases than by those with minor ailments. However, even with serious illnesses like essential hypertension or chronic infection, compliance is generally poor (about 50%) when the benefits of therapy are not superficially apparent.[6] Other things being equal, drugs that produce unwanted side effects are more likely to be discontinued. Deviations in self-administration tend to increase progressively with drugs that are taken chronically. Also, the more complex the therapeutic regimen in terms of doses and drugs, the higher the incidence of drug default. The quality of the doctor-patient relationship is important in several respects. Patients who trust and respect their therapist are more likely to take prescribed medications. Effective communication further promotes compliance and reduces the possibility of a patient unilaterally terminating the drug should adverse effects occur. Measures that the clinician may employ to enhance patient compliance are discussed in Chapter 49.

Drug interactions. The effect of a drug may be increased, decreased, or otherwise altered by the concurrent administration of another compound. Because several agents routinely used in dental practice are implicated in drug interactions, the topic is of considerable interest to the clinician and is considered separately in Chapter 4.

ADVERSE DRUG REACTIONS

It has been estimated that 5% of all patients hospitalized in the United States each year are admitted because of adverse reactions to drugs.[28] Of these patients, 30% suffer an additional episode of drug toxicity while being treated for the initial problem. The introduction of new, highly efficacious compounds into pharmacotherapy during the past few decades has led to a disturbing increase in the incidence of adverse reactions; indeed, drug toxicity is now considered a major cause of iatrogenic disease. Recent reductions in mortality associated with certain drugs (e.g., aspirin) demonstrate, however, that toxic responses to therapeutic agents can be minimized through concerted efforts by the health professions, pharmaceutical industry, government, and lay public.

Classification of adverse drug reactions

Drug toxicity may come in many forms: acute versus chronic, mild versus severe, predictable versus unpredictable, local versus systemic. Therapeutic agents also differ widely in their tendency to elicit adverse reactions. Acetaminophen, for example, used to relieve headache rarely causes undesired responses, but methotrexate employed in cancer chemotherapy invariably produces some degree of toxicity. Agents quite safe for some individuals may be life-threatening to others. Thus, penicillin G, which normally enjoys an exceptionally high margin of safety, can, in small doses, initiate fatal anaphylaxis in allergic patients. Although no classification of adverse drug reactions is universally accepted, a taxonomy based on mechanism of toxicity is the most useful in promoting the recognition, management, and prevention of untoward responses to drugs.

Extension effects. Many drugs are employed clinically in doses that provide an intensity of effect that is less than maximal. The reason for this conservatism is simple: increasing drug effects beyond a certain point may be dangerous. The anticoagulant dicumarol provides a typical example of a drug whose therapeutic action must be held in check in order to avoid serious toxicity. For the treatment of peripheral vascular thrombosis, dicumarol is administered in doses sufficient to increase the one-stage prothrombin time by about 100%. Dicumarol could be given in larger amounts to further inhibit clotting, but the risk of spontaneous bleeding would be unacceptably high. Even with conventional therapy, hemorrhage, the toxic extension of dicumarol's anticoagulant effect, occurs in 2% to 4% of the patients treated. Inadvertent overmedication is, of course, one cause of dicumarol toxicity; however, many additional factors influencing drug effects may also be involved: diet, heredity, drug interactions, renal, hepatic, or cardiac insufficiency, gastrointestinal ulceration, and variable patient compliance. It is obvious that the "normal dose" has little meaning with respect to dicumarol because a therapeutic dose to one patient may represent an overdose to another.

Adverse responses arising from an extension of the therapeutic effect are dose-related and predictable. Theoretically, they are the only toxic reactions that can always be avoided without loss of therapeutic benefit by properly adjusting the dosage regimen. Additional examples of drugs that display this form of toxicity are provided in Table 3-2.

Side effects. Predictable, dose-dependent reactions unrelated to the goal of therapy are referred to as side effects. As illustrated in Table 3-3, drugs can produce an awesome array of deleterious side reactions. While many such effects are associated with only a single agent or class of drugs, others appear to be almost universal in occurrence. It is questionable, however, whether frequently noted side effects like nausea and drowsiness are always drug-related; similar symptoms are also commonly observed in patients after placebo administration and are even reported by individuals receiving no medication whatsoever.[36] Side effects are often produced by the same drug-receptor interaction responsible for the therapeutic effect, differing only in the tissue or organ affected. In these instances, the categorization of drug responses as toxic or therapeutic may depend on the purpose of treatment. Xerostomia induced by atropine is a side reaction during the management of gastrointestinal

Table 3-2. Examples of drug toxicity as an extension of the therapeutic effect

Drug	Medical indication	Therapeutic effect	Toxic extension of therapeutic effect
Amphetamine	Narcolepsy	Wakefulness	Insomnia
Furosemide	Edema	Diuresis	Water and electrolyte imbalance
Heparin	Thromboembolic disorders	Inhibition of coagulation	Spontaneous bleeding
Insulin	Diabetes mellitus	Reduction of blood glucose	Hypoglycemia
Pentobarbital	Insomnia	Hypnosis	Unconsciousness
Tubocurarine	Abdominal surgery	Skeletal muscle relaxation	Prolonged respiratory paralysis

Table 3-3. Some side effects of drugs

Drug	Effect	Drug	Effect
Oral cavity		**Neuromuscular system**	
Griseofulvin	Black hairy tongue	Theophylline	Tremors
Diphenhydramine	Xerostomia	Isoniazid	Convulsions
Phenytoin	Gingival hyperplasia	Chlorpromazine	Tardive dyskinesia
Tetracycline	Pigmentation, hypoplasia of the teeth		
		Central nervous system	
Skin and hair		Lithium	Anorexia
Methandrostenolone	Acne	Levodopa	Mania
Cyclophosphamide	Alopecia	Amphetamine	Hallucination
Ampicillin	Dermatitis	Diazepam	Confusion
Demeclocycline	Phototoxicity	Reserpine	Suicidal depression
		Clonidine	Drowsiness and lethargy
Bone			
Prednisolone	Osteoporosis	**Cardiovascular system**	
Fluoride	Osteosclerosis	Nifedipine	Hypotension
Phenobarbital	Osteomalacia	Pargyline	Hypertensive crisis
		Propranolol	Cardiac failure
Sensory apparatus			
Fluphenazine	Blurred vision	**Respiratory system**	
Digitalis	Yellow vision	Ibuprofen	Bronchospasm
Thioridazine	Pigmentary retinopathy	Meperidine	Respiratory depression
Streptomycin	Ototoxicity	Ketamine	Laryngospasm
Blood		**Gastrointestinal tract**	
Phenacetin	Anemia	Indomethacin	Ulcer formation
Phenylbutazone	Agranulocytosis	Aspirin	Melena
Cytarabine	Pancytopenia	Erythromycin	Diarrhea
Mithramycin	Thrombocytopenia	Morphine	Constipation
Prilocaine	Methemoglobinemia		
		Genitourinary system	
Metabolic effects		Mecamylamine	Impotence
Phenformin	Lactic acidosis	Sulfadiazine	Crystalluria
Dextrothyroxine	Hyperglycemia	Testosterone	Priapism
Rifampin	Jaundice	Ergonovine	Abortion

hypermotility but is a desired effect when the drug is used to control excessive salivation. Side effects unrelated pharmacodynamically to the therapeutic action are also quite common, and they too may occasionally be useful. Table 3-4 lists some drugs whose side effects were found sufficiently note-worthy to provide new and unanticipated indications for therapeutic use.

Many side effects, particularly the more dangerous forms, develop only during drug overdose. Careful alteration of the administration regimen will usually resolve these problems while main-

Table 3-4. Useful side effects of some drugs

Drug	Original use	Subsequent use
Diphenhydramine	Antihistaminic	Sedative
Probenecid	Inhibition of penicillin excretion	Uricosuric
Iproniazid	Tuberculostatic	Antidepressant
Amphetamine	CNS stimulant	Management of hyperkinetic children
Lidocaine	Local anesthetic	Antiarrhythmic
Methadone	Analgesic	Heroin substitute
Quinidine	Antimalarial	Antiarrhythmic
Diazoxide	Antihypertensive	Antihyperglycemic
Chlorothiazide	Diuretic	Antihypertensive
Phenytoin	Anticonvulsant	Antiarrhythmic

taining effective treatment. Many other side effects, however, appear at therapeutic or even subtherapeutic concentrations and cannot be avoided by dosage adjustment without loss of drug benefit. Such reactions can be tolerated, though, if they are mild, brief in duration, reversible, and compatible with therapy. Occasionally, even disturbing side effects will be accepted if the need for medication is great. Drugs used in the treatment of various cancers, for example, produce severe toxicities that must be tolerated since no therapeutic alternative is available.

When two drugs share a common desired effect but cause different side reactions, it is sometimes possible to limit toxic responses by using reduced doses of the agents in combination. Another pharmacologic approach to avoiding side effects is to add a secondary agent that is capable of blocking or otherwise compensating for the unwanted activity of the principal drug. These strategies presuppose that no additional toxicity will be generated by the combination over that produced by a single effective drug. The association of renal papillary necrosis with chronic abuse of analgesic mixtures that contained aspirin, phenacetin, and caffeine is highly instructive regarding the noncritical acceptance of this assumption.[39] Undoubtedly, the most fruitful pharmacologic approach to eliminating undesired side effects is through the development of more selective drugs. Studies of structure-activity relationships have proved invaluable in removing side effects unrelated to therapeutic actions and in reducing side effects that are related.

Idiosyncratic reactions. An idiosyncratic reaction is a "genetically determined abnormal response to a drug."[14] Although dose-dependent, such reactions are unpredictable in most instances because exceedingly few patients given an agent respond idiosyncratically and because the genetic trait responsible for an atypical reaction may be completely "silent" in the absence of drug challenge. When confronted with an unexpected response to a drug, it is a common, though erroneous, practice to describe the event as an idiosyncrasy. This habit may explain why the idiosyncratic reaction is jocularly defined as a reaction the "idiots can't explain." Most responses lying outside the normal range of drug reactivity are not truly idiosyncratic in nature but represent allergic manifestations or reflect extension or side effects in patients intolerant to the drug by virtue of age, weight, existing pathology, and the like. In dentistry, the majority of "idiosyncratic reactions" to local anesthetics are actually the result of accidental intravascular injections or anxiety reactions to the process of injection.

Often, an idiosyncratic reaction is manifested as an abnormal drug sensitivity in which the agent produces its characteristic effect at an unconventional dose. Drug effects may be unusually strong or weak in intensity or brief or prolonged in duration. In most such instances (e.g., involving succinylcholine, isoniazid, vitamin D, or phenytoin), altered drug metabolism is responsible for the abnormal responses; however, additional mechanisms have also been identified, such as abnormal distribution (iron, thyroxine) and unusual receptor affinity (phenylthiourea, coumarin anticoagulants). In addition to perturbing characteristic drug responses, genetic singularities can produce novel drug effects that regardless of dose may never occur in normal individuals. One example of a novel drug effect is the hemolytic anemia caused by the antimalarial drug primaquine. Red blood cells of sensitive individuals are deficient in glucose-6-phosphate dehydrogenase, an enzyme in-

Table 3-5. Idiosyncratic reactions to drugs used in dentistry

Genetic abnormality	Drugs affected	Idiosyncratic response
NADH methemoglobin reductase deficiency	Phenacetin, prilocaine, sulfonamides	Methemoglobinemia
Abnormal hemoglobin	Phenacetin, prilocaine, sulfonamides	Methemoglobinemia, hemolytic anemia
Erythrocyte glucose-6-phosphate dehydrogenase deficiency	Aspirin, phenacetin, sulfonamides	Hemolytic anemia
Abnormal induction of heme synthesis	Barbiturates and other CNS depressants, sulfonamides	Porphyria
Low plasma cholinesterase activity	Procaine and other ester local anesthetics	Local anesthetic toxicity

volved in the intermediary metabolism of glucose. Lacking the ability to produce normal amounts of reducing equivalents, these erythrocytes are susceptible to oxidative destruction by primaquine and several dozen other compounds. The genetic basis of primaquine hemolysis is clear: the reaction occurs almost exclusively in males of certain racial and ethnic groups (blacks, Sardinians, Sephardic Jews, Iranians, Filipinos, etc.).[27]

Several idiosyncrasies are known to be associated with drugs used in general dental practice (Table 3-5). If an adverse response is suspected of having a genetic basis, it becomes important to determine whether the patient has a personal or familial history of atypical reactivity to the drug. Since idiosyncratic reactions are quite reproducible within any individual, a single episode of serious toxicity should preclude future use of the inciting compound. Examination of the patient's family is helpful not only in establishing the hereditary nature of the reaction but also in identifying other individuals at risk.

Drug allergy. Adverse responses of immunologic origin account for approximately 10% of all untoward reactions to drugs. Allergy can be distinguished from other forms of drug toxicity in several respects. First, prior exposure to the drug or a closely related compound is necessary to elicit the reaction. Second, the severity of response is frequently dose-independent. Third, the nature of the unfavorable effect is a function not of the offending drug but of the immune mechanism involved. And last, the reaction is unpredictable; it usually occurs in a small portion of the population, sometimes in patients who had been previously treated on numerous occasions without mishap.

Drugs differ enormously in antigenic potential. Certain compounds (e.g., caffeine and epineph-

rine) never cause drug allergy; others (e.g., phenylethylhydantoin) have proved too allergenic for human use. With drugs commonly implicated clinically in allergic reactions (penicillins, sulfonamides, quinidine, etc.), the incidence of such responses is about 5%. On occasion, it is not the drug itself that causes the reaction but some other substance in the preparation, such as a preservative or coloring agent.

Aside from agents of high molecular weight (insulin, dextran, polypeptides), drugs are not antigenic in the free state but must be covalently linked to endogenous carrier molecules, normally proteins such as albumin, in order to generate immunologic responses. Because these therapeutic agents are often chemically inert, they generally require activation by metabolism or by sunlight (photoallergy) before serving as haptens in the formation of antigen. Penicillins, which are responsible for most fulminating reactions, are exceptional in that they spontaneously convert to highly reactive derivatives.

Four types of drug allergy can be differentiated on the basis of the immune elements that cause them and the loci of their actions.[9] Type I, or anaphylactic, responses include the immediate forms of drug allergy, in which disturbances appear within minutes or hours of taking the drug. The underlying immune reaction is initiated by the attachment of antigen to IgE antibodies bound to the surface of mast cells and basophils. Subsequent cellular degranulation and release of histamine and other vasoactive substances is responsible for the undesired effects. Major signs and symptoms of type I allergy involve the gastrointestinal tract (cramps and diarrhea), skin and mucous membranes (erythema, urticaria, angioneurotic edema), lungs (bronchoconstriction), and blood vessels (vasodilatation, increased permeability). In its severest form, anaphylaxis can cause death by airway obstruction or cardiovascular collapse within a few minutes after drug exposure. Parenteral injection of the drug is more likely to produce life-threatening reactions than is oral or topical use. Nevertheless, patients have died from topical application of less than 1 μg of penicillin.[14] It is believed that patients with allergic diathesis (noted by a history of hay fever or bronchial asthma) are more prone to develop serious type I reactions. The immediate anaphylactic response is the only type of drug allergy that the dentist may be forced to treat without the benefit of medical back-up. Epinephrine is the drug of choice to reverse the manifestations of a severe response; antihistamines and adrenal corticosteroids are useful as adjunctive medications.

Type II, or cytotoxic, reactions are caused by circulating antibodies such as IgG. When a plasma membrane constituent serves as the hapten carrier, the binding of immunoglobulin is followed by complement fixation and lysis of the cell. Many drug-induced hemolytic anemias, leukopenias, and thrombocytopenias are the result of immunologic destruction. Type II responses are usually delayed, being manifest from several hours to days after drug administration.

Type III, or immune-complex, reactions occur when insoluble antigen-antibody complexes form in intravascular or interstitial spaces. Deposition of the complexes on the walls of small blood vessels and activation of complement attracts neutrophils to the area. These cells degranulate in attempts to remove the complexes, releasing lysosomal enzymes which cause local tissue damage and promote thrombosis of affected vessels. Type III reactions can induce a number of unpleasant sequelae, some of which can be quite serious (neuropathy, glomerulonephritis, serum sickness). Reactions indistinguishable from disease states like lupus erythematosus and erythema multiforme are also observed.

Type IV reactions are synonymous with cell-mediated immunity. Sensitized T lymphocytes exposed to the drug hapten or its conjugate release soluble mediators, called lymphokines, that attract additional cells (lymphocytes, macrophages) to the antigenic site. Lysozymes and other substances (including toxic lymphokines) elaborated by the recruited cells produce local tissue necrosis. Type IV reactions are usually delayed because of the time required for effector cells to concentrate in the area

involved. For dentists, an important cellular immune reaction is the contact dermatitis acquired from repeated exposure of the hands to ester local anesthetics like procaine. Before the availability of amide anesthetic drugs, allergy to procaine markedly complicated clinical practice. Even today, allergy to ester-based local anesthetics presents a considerable problem because of the variety of substances that may cross-react to elicit an eczematoid rash: methylparaben, a pharmaceutical preservative in widespread use; *p*-phenylenediamine, a component of hair dyes; and dichlorophene, a germicide in soaps.[1]

While drug allergies cannot always be prevented, their frequency of occurrence can be minimized by observing the following precautions.

1. *Take an adequate medical history*. If a patient has a presumptive history of drug allergy, it is important to discover the identity of the inciting preparation and to determine whether the reaction is, in fact, consistent with an immunologic etiology.

2. *Avoid the offending drug and likely cross-reactors*. A patient truly allergic to a drug should not receive the agent or congener again, unless need for the particular medication is great.

3. *Avoid inappropriate drug administration*. In one study, a review of 30 fatalities to penicillin revealed that the antibiotic was not even indicated in over 50% of the cases examined.[37]

4. *Promote oral use and limit topical exposure.* On a quantitative basis, the oral and topical routes are, respectively, the least and most allergenic avenues of drug administration.

5. *Request allergy testing, when appropriate*. Although such methods are generally unreliable and can be dangerous, skin tests for penicillin allergy have proved highly predictive,[34] and success has also been claimed regarding local anesthetics.[2] Allergy testing may be necessary when suitable alternatives to the drug in question are not available.

Adherence to these recommendations will reduce the incidence of allergic reactions to drugs. It is encouraging to note that a more prudent use of penicillin in recent years may have led to a decline in the drug's mortality, once estimated to be as high as 500 per year.[33]

Carcinogenesis. One aspect of drug toxicity that has had a strong impact on public awareness is carcinogenesis. Although most attention is currently focused on environmental pollutants, especially those chemicals that pose an occupational hazard, the association of reserpine with breast cancer and diethylstilbestrol with uterine neoplasia underscores the tumorigenic potential of certain drugs. Of course, the most pervasive cancer-producing substances in our society are derived from a "social" drug—the cigarette.

A peculiar feature of chemical carcinogenesis is that it occurs as two-stage phenomenon. Certain compounds cause tumors only after prior treatment with another agent. The first chemical appears to initiate neoplastic transformation while the second is required to promote tumor growth. Neither chemical acting alone is carcinogenic, and reversal of the order of administration also prevents activity. Drugs can thus be classified as *initiators* or *promoters,* depending on their particular effect. (Many agents, however, have both capabilities.) The dual roles of initiation and promotion are consistent with the view that chemical carcinogenesis is a manifestation of somatic mutation, an alteration in the genetic make-up of a nongerminal cell of the body. The initiator may be responsible for triggering mutability in the genetic apparatus of the cell, a change that permits the promoter to remove the control of growth that distinguishes normal from cancerous cells.

Virtually any agent capable of altering the structure of DNA is a potential carcinogen. Agents known to be carcinogenic include radioactive substances, alkylating agents, nitrosamines, and various aromatic amines and polycyclic hydrocarbons. Immunosuppressive drugs, though not inherently carcinogenic, may nevertheless promote cancer development by interfering with immunologic surveillance mechanisms responsible for the elimination of transformed neoplastic cells.

Major difficulties are encountered in assessing the carcinogenicity of agents intended for human use. First, the latency period between the initiation and clinical appearance of neoplasia may extend for years to decades. Second, although the incidence of tumor induction is dose-dependent, it is not established whether a dose or duration of exposure below which tumors will not be produced can be found for any drug. Third, an administered agent that is not carcinogenic may be converted by metabolism into a chemical that is. Interspecies differences in biotransformation severely limit the utility of animal testing in such instances. Without a foolproof method of screening drugs, continued appraisal of cancer rates with respect to drug intake

is a necessary, if not ideal, approach to identifying carcinogenic compounds. In view of the prolonged latency of cancer development and the flood of agents introduced into pharmacology since World War II, it would be surprising not to witness the discovery of new carcinogens among therapeutic agents now in use.

Special problems

Hazards of medication pertaining to abuse, poisoning, and effects on the unborn child deserve special comment inasmuch as the persons affected are generally not exposed to the agent for therapeutic purposes. In these situations, the prevention and the management of adverse reactions can be complicated by such matters as the intent of the individual taking the drug, an inability to identify the offending agent, and the unique susceptibility of the embryo to drug toxicity.

Drug abuse. Typified by persistent and excessive self-administration, drug abuse refers to the inappropriate and deviant use of any drug. Drug abuse presents a special problem in toxicology because, in addition to the hazards of taking pharmacologically active agents without proper medical supervision (drug toxicity, infection from inadequate antisepsis), adverse consequences may arise from the acts involved in procuring and using such compounds. Compulsive behavior is especially strong with drugs that act on the central nervous system, and, except for substances to which little stigma is attached (e.g., coffee and tobacco products), the attendant social, economic, and legal costs of the abuse of these agents can be enormous. Moreover, abstinence from drugs producing physical dependence results in the appearance of withdrawal symptoms characteristic of the substance involved and the intensity of previous use. A thorough discussion of drug abuse involving centrally acting agents is presented in Chapter 46.

Drug poisoning. It is estimated that each year over 1.5 million people in the United States suffer from accidental or intentional poisoning.[21] Of the 5000 poisoning deaths recorded annually, more than half are the result of suicide, with CNS depressants most frequently implicated. Tabulations over a 15-year period beginning in 1959 revealed that accidental deaths due to poisoning by solid and liquid substances increased by 150%.[45] As medicinal compounds are responsible for two thirds of such fatalities, drug poisoning is obviously a major concern for health professionals and lay persons alike.

One of the more tragic aspects of accidental ingestion is that children under the age of 5 account for the majority of poisonings and for about 2% of the deaths. Against this backdrop of statistics, however, it is pleasing to note that fatal poisonings of small children have actually decreased by over 70% since 1959.[46] Aspirin, historically the leading cause of drug toxicity in the very young, provides a noteworthy example of how unintentional poisoning can be controlled. Recognizing the special hazard of flavored baby aspirin, the pharmaceutical industry voluntarily limited the number of aspirin tablets per bottle to a (normally) sublethal total of 36. Safety packaging, which became mandatory after the passage of the Poison-Prevention Packaging Act of 1970, further reduced the incidence of fatal ingestion. Finally, increased public awareness of the danger of aspirin overdose, engendered in part by the proliferation of Poison Control Centers throughout the country, led to a safer storage of aspirin in the home. In combination, these events reduced aspirin fatalities by 83% between 1959 and 1974. Further decrements in aspirin mortality have occurred, if only because of the increased reliance on liquid acetaminophen preparations for analgesia and antipyresis. As one might predict, however, acetaminophen poisoning, once quite rare, is now relatively common. The principles of toxicology and the prevention and management of drug poisoning are covered in Chapter 47.

Drugs and pregnancy. The hazard to the unborn child of administering drugs during pregnancy has received considerable attention in the lay and professional literature. Over the years, certain compounds have become implicated in the development of congenital abnormalities. These teratogens disturb organogenesis in the developing embryo such that defects in one or more structures are produced. If the defects are incompatible with life, fetal death and either resorption or spontaneous abortion ensues; if they are less severe, the result is a malformed child.

Very little is known about the teratogenic potential of most drugs in humans, but the thalidomide disaster of 1960 to 1962 proved that an ordinary drug, extremely safe in adults, could induce extensive malformation of the human fetus. Thalidomide is a sedative-hypnotic that was released for clinical use in Europe and elsewhere in the late 1950s. The drug quickly gained wide acceptance

and was commonly used by women to relieve the nausea of "morning sickness." Shortly after its introduction, however, there occurred an epidemic of infants born with phocomelia, "seal limb" malformation of the arms and legs. Retrospective studies determined that phocomelia was caused by thalidomide when the agent was taken on or about the twenty-fifth day of gestation.[19] Other defects were also produced by thalidomide (absence of external ears, anorectal stenosis, etc.), depending on the time of administration.

Laboratory experiments in animals and investigations of accidental teratogenesis in humans have found that drug-induced malformation is governed by the sequential pattern of embryonic and fetal development. From fertilization to about 20 days, an embryo will either survive or succumb to a chemical insult. No malformations will occur, though, because the cells remain undifferentiated during this period. Beginning at day 21 (when the embryo divides into somites) and continuing until the end of the first trimester (when differentiation and organogenesis are well established), malformations are possible when the embryo is exposed to a teratogen. The defects produced will vary with the toxic action of the agent and with the time of administration. Certain malformations, such as cleft palate, may be produced by a variety of substances; some teratogens, for example antifolate drugs, can evoke a wide spectrum of structural defects.[43] Selective toxicity of drugs to the unborn child does not end after 3 months' gestation. Although gross malformation may not occur, normal development may be retarded or otherwise affected throughout pregnancy. Immaturities in physiology and biochemistry may promote adverse reactions in the fetus at doses quite safe to the mother. The administration of drugs at time of delivery is commonly associated with exaggerated effects in the neonate. Table 3-6 lists several agents known to elicit toxic effects during pregnancy and indicates when their administration is most dangerous to the fetus.

Despite uncertainties concerning the effects of most drugs on fetal development and health, pharmacologic agents are extensively used by pregnant women. In one survey, 82% of the women questioned received prescription drugs and 65% took over-the-counter medications.[12] The major drug categories included (in decreasing order of usage) iron supplements, analgesics, vitamins, barbiturates, diuretics, antiemetics, antibiotics, sulfon-

Table 3-6. Toxic effects of selected drugs during pregnancy

Drug	Toxic effect to the fetus	1st	2nd	3rd	Term
Anticancer drugs	Cleft palate, extremity defects, severe stunting, death	✔			
Chloramphenicol	Gray syndrome and death				✔
Cortisone	Cleft palate	✔			
Coumarin anticoagulants	Hemorrhage, death	✔	✔	✔	✔
Diazepam	Cleft palate, respiratory depression	✔			✔
Local anesthetics	Bradycardia, respiratory depression				✔
Lysergic acid diethylamide	Chromosomal damage, stunted growth	✔			
Narcotic analgesics	Respiratory depression, neonatal death				✔
Nicotine (smoking)	Decreased size at birth	✔	✔	✔	✔
Potassium iodide	Goiter, mental retardation	✔	✔	✔	✔
Quinine	Deafness, thrombocytopenia			✔	✔
Reserpine	Nasal block				✔
Sex steroids	Masculinization, vaginal carcinoma (delayed)	✔	✔	✔	✔
Streptomycin	Eighth nerve damage, micromelia, multiple skeletal anomalies	✔	✔	✔	✔
Tetracyclines	Inhibition of bone growth; tooth discoloration, micromelia, syndactyly	✔	✔	✔	✔
Thalidomide	Phocomelia, multiple defects	✔			
Thiazide diuretics	Thrombocytopenia, neonatal death			✔	✔

Adapted from Underwood, T., Iturrian, W.B., and Cadwallader, D.E. Some aspects of chemical teratogenesis. American Journal of Hospital Pharmacy **27:**115-122, 1970.

amides, cough medicines, antihistamines, hormones, tranquilizers, bronchodilators, hypnotics, and appetite suppressants. More than half of the women smoked, and over 85% used alcohol. Even though most pregnancies end in the birth of a normal infant regardless of drug consumption, the admonition to restrict usage of therapeutic agents, especially during the first trimester, bears reiteration. In general, only emergency dental treatment should be rendered during the critical period of fetal development. Regular dental care need not be postponed, however, during the second and most of the third trimester, so long as reasonable attention and care are given to avoiding undue physical and emotional stress in the patient.

DEVELOPMENT OF NEW DRUGS

Advances in pharmacotherapy are ultimately dependent on the discovery, evaluation, and marketing of new drugs. The past several decades have witnessed an unprecedented proliferation of medicinal agents. Although the discovery of fundamentally different drugs has slowed somewhat in recent years, major revisions in how drugs intended for human use are evaluated have contributed to the manufacture of safer as well as more effective compounds. As an employer of drugs, the practitioner should be aware of the attendant problems

and costs of developing therapeutic agents and of the unavoidable limitations in assessing drug safety before widespread use. Only with this knowledge can the clinician arrive at a balanced attitude toward new drugs and claims made for them.

Sources of new drugs

Most major categories of drugs have their origins in prescientific or folklore medicine. For many years, considerable effort in pharmacology was devoted to the purification of active constituents from natural plant and animal products previously used for medicinal purposes. Although new agents may still emerge from home remedies or apothecary formulations, these traditional sources of drugs are, for the most part, depleted.

Many new therapeutic agents are discovered by empirical screening. In screening tests, thousands of compounds from natural materials or synthetic chemistry are examined for a particular pharmacologic activity. Though inefficient, time-consuming, laborious, and costly, screening is a very important method of finding new drugs capable of producing a defined drug effect. With the exception of penicillin, all of the antibiotics have been isolated by the screening of soils and other materials for antimicrobial activity. It appears, however, that the likelihood of finding new antibiotics of therapeutic utility is diminishing with time. Indeed, much effort is currently wasted on screening promising soil samples, only to rediscover old agents like streptomycin as the source of antimicrobial activity. Screening of synthetic chemicals, though, will probably be fruitful for many years to come.

One of the more interesting techniques of finding new drugs is to alter the molecular structure of an existing agent. Obviously, structure-activity relationship studies are intimately involved in this approach. When successful derivatives are produced, they are frequently little more than "me too" drugs, agents that, though similar in activity to the parent compound, offer no therapeutic advantage but are marketed anyway for economic reasons. Less often, a drug is synthesized that differs substantially from its predecessor in pharmacokinetic properties. Penicillin V, which is nearly identical to its precursor, penicillin G, in antimicrobial activity, is nevertheless preferred for oral use because its absorption is two to five times better. Pharmacokinetic differences are especially prominent among the congeners of barbital. Some barbiturates are useful as ultra-short-acting intravenous anesthetics, while others can provide sedation for hours following a single administration. The least common but usually most desirable outcome of molecular modification is the synthesis of a derivative that differs qualitatively from the parent drug in pharmacodynamic effect. Such discoveries are generally the result of attempts to enhance one aspect of an agent's spectrum of activity over all others. Thus, the observations that sulfonamides used in chemotherapy of bacterial infections could lower blood glucose and promote urine flow under appropriate conditions eventually led to the manufacture of several new classes of drugs: carbonic anhydrase inhibitors, thiazide diuretics, and sulfonylurea hypoglycemic agents.

Increasingly, discoveries of new drugs are evolving from advances in our understanding of basic physiology and biochemistry. The extraction of some natural effectors (e.g., insulin, calcitonin, and adrenocorticotropin) and the synthesis of others (e.g., adrenal and sex steroids, epinephrine, vitamin D derivatives, and prostaglandins) have provided a host of new therapeutic agents. Recombinant DNA technology, through which bacteria can be altered genetically to synthesize foreign proteins, promises to provide a means for the large-scale production of human biologicals (e.g., interferon, insulin, calcitonin, and growth hor-

mone) that are currently obtainable only in small amounts.[26] Occasionally, it has also been possible to tailor compounds for a specific purpose. Nowhere is this approach more apparent than in the synthesis of antimetabolites for cancer chemotherapy.

A burgeoning source of new pharmaceutical products consists of the development of novel delivery systems for existing drugs. Monoclonal antibodies, whose production is outlined in Chapter 39, are being studied in cancer patients as vehicles for cytotoxic substances (e.g., diphtheria toxin) and various anticancer drugs and radioactive isotopes.[32] The antibody attaches to tumor-associated surface antigens; the active ligand provides the tumoricidal effect. Similar drug-carrying monoclonal antibodies directed against discrete cellular elements of the immune system may find use in preventing transplant rejection and in the treatment of autoimmune diseases.[25] Attaching drugs, often covalently, to polymeric carriers is proving effective in localizing and prolonging drug effects, either because the controlled release of free drug from the immobilized matrix permits only local effects or because the drug is active in the bound state.[44] In either case, the distribution of drug action is determined by the properties of the carrier. There are many potential applications for such systems; in dentistry, the controlled release of fluoride and antibiotics may be useful, respectively, in preventing dental caries[31] and in treating advanced periodontitis.[15]

The last major source of new drugs is serendipity. Probably the greatest single breakthrough in pharmacotherapeutics in the twentieth century was the isolation of penicillin, made possible by the chance but astute observation by Fleming that bacteria in a culture dish were lysed by a mold contaminant of the genus *Penicillium*. Other classes of agents that originated by accident include the antiarrhythmic drugs (quinine) and the oral anticoagulants (dicumarol). Table 3-4 lists several drugs for which new therapeutic applications were fortuitously discovered after marketing.

Evaluation of new drugs

Before a drug can be released for general use, it must pass a rigorous evaluation program established by the Food and Drug Administration (FDA). This program, though subject to some modification depending on the drug's intended use, invariably includes a series of animal and human

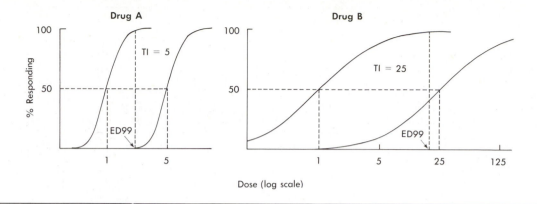

Figure 3-3. Quantal dose-response relationships (log scale) of two drugs, A and B. For each drug, the curve on the left reflects therapeutic responses, while the curve on the right represents toxic reactions. TI = therapeutic index; ED99 = dose effective in 99% of the population.

investigations to ensure the product's safety and efficacy. (See Chapter 49 for a review of drug regulations pertaining to the FDA and the development of new drugs.)

Preclinical testing. The first step in evaluating a newly discovered compound is to ascertain its pharmacologic activity in animals. Initially, a few rats may be given several different doses of the chemical and observed for any disturbances that may occur in physiology or behavior. If the drug was developed for a given purpose (e.g., to lower blood pressure), it would be tested for that particular effect as well. Agents that appear to have a useful action are then enrolled in more extensive examinations. Graded dose-response curves are constructed to determine the potency and maximal efficacy obtainable with the compound. When a specific therapeutic effect is identified, quantal dose-effect relationships are drawn to estimate the compound's relative safety. As shown in Figure 3-3, quantal dose-effect curves can be prepared for both desired and toxic responses.

When one is working with laboratory animals, one of the most convenient toxic effects to monitor is lethality. Death is universal, all drugs are capable of producing it, and it represents a definite endpoint that can be quickly and unequivocally recognized. The dose causing death in 50% of the test animals in a given period of time is designated as the median lethal dose (LD50). The ratio of this dose to the median effective dose (LD50/ED50) defines the therapeutic index, a crude but useful measure of drug safety. Other things being equal, a drug with a large therapeutic index is safer than an agent with

a smaller value. Indeed, when many congeners are being tested concurrently, those with the most favorable therapeutic indexes are given preference in further investigations, being considered the most promising candidates for clinical application. Unfortunately, the LD50/ED50 ratio is not fully predictive of relative safety. Drugs produce many toxic effects besides death that can prevent their use in humans. An agent that enjoys a large therapeutic index with respect to one adverse reaction may fare poorly in regard to another type of toxicity.

Table 3-7 compares a group of local anesthetics in their propensity to elicit two separate toxic effects—death and local tissue irritation—as a function of the anesthetic concentration.[23] Each test was performed in a different species: lethality in mice, irritancy in rabbits, and anesthesia in guinea pigs. Procaine being used as a standard, propoxycaine was 4.6 times safer with respect to tissue irritation but essentially equivalent in relation to lethality. From these data, cocaine would appear to be the safest local anesthetic for human administration; however, cocaine has some additional liabilities (CNS stimulation, abuse potential) not shared by the other agents, which severely restrict its medical usefulness.

A second limitation of the therapeutic index is that biologic variability is not taken into account. In Figure 3-3, drug B has a larger therapeutic index than drug A but is nevertheless inferior clinically. The goal of pharmacotherapy is to achieve a desired effect in virtually all patients without producing toxicity in any. Because the slopes of the quantal dose-effect curves of drug A are steep (indicating

Table 3-7. Comparison of potency, irritancy, and lethality of several local anesthetics

Drug	Anesthesia* ED50 (mM)	Local irritancy†		Lethality‡	
		TD50 (mM)	Relative safety	TD50 (mM)	Relative safety
Procaine	8.8	176	1.0	220	1.0
Tetracaine	0.69	12	0.9	27	1.6
Propoxycaine	0.81	75	4.6	22	1.1
Lidocaine	2.69	62	1.2	85	1.3
Cocaine	1.16	79	3.4	62	2.1

Data from Luduena, F.P., and Hoppe, J.O. 2-Alkoxy benzoate and thiolbenzoate derivatives as local anesthetics. Journal of Pharmacology and Experimental Therapeutics **117:**89-96, 1956.
*Intracutaneous wheal test in guinea pigs.
†Trypan blue test in rabbits.
‡Intravenous injection in mice.

little variation in responsiveness to the drug), a dose effective in 99% of the population (ED99) can be administered with essentially no risk to the recipients. Although drug B exhibits a therapeutic index five times greater than drug A, the biologic variability to it is so great that an ED99 would produce toxicity in a significant fraction of the population.

To thoroughly evaluate drug safety in animals, acute, subacute, and chronic toxicity testing must be carried out in several different species and by several different routes of administration. Special studies are performed in order to detect carcinogenic and teratogenic activity, and adjuvants (e.g., Freund's) are used to test new products for their propensity to cause contact dermatitis. In addition to toxicity evaluations, pharmacokinetic investigations are run to determine the rate and extent of drug absorption, pattern of distribution, plasma half-life, and routes of elimination. Correlation of pharmacologic effect with plasma titer has some predictive value for the therapeutic concentration in humans and can indicate if the parent drug or a metabolite is the active moiety. Some of the more protracted and costly investigations may be run concurrently with human studies to save time and expense (should the drug prove unsuitable during initial clinical trials).

Regardless of the number, size, or sophistication of animal tests employed, studies in humans are necessary to establish the clinical worth of any drug. Primarily because of unpredictable differences in biotransformation, pharmacokinetic studies in animals cannot be relied on to determine the correct dose or the duration of action of a drug in humans. Of even greater importance is the inability of preclinical studies to detect many forms of drug

toxicity that occur in humans. Most revealing in this regard was a retrospective compilation of adverse reactions to six unrelated drugs, each used in humans, rats, and dogs.[22] Considering only toxic signs that are observable in animals as well as humans, 43% of the various kinds of human toxicity caused by the drugs were not found in either of the test species. When subjective responses (e.g., depression and giddiness) and other effects (urticaria, nausea, headache, etc.) not detectable in animals are taken into account, it becomes apparent that at least half of untoward responses frequently caused by drugs cannot be ascertained preclinically. Thus, the need for human experimentation in drug development is unassailable.

Clinical trials. If an agent appears sufficiently promising on the basis of its preclinical evaluation to warrant testing in humans, the drug sponsor (generally a large pharmaceutical company) must first submit an application to the FDA in the form of a *Notice of Claimed Investigational Exemption for a New Drug* (IND) detailing, among other things, (1) the identity of the drug and how it is prepared, (2) all results of preclinical investigations to date, (3) the intended use of the agent, dosage form, and route of administration, and (4) the procedures to be followed in assessing the drug's safety and effectiveness in humans. On FDA approval of the IND, the first phase of clinical evaluation can begin.

Phase 1 trials represent an intensive study of the drug in a few, usually healthy volunteers. The safe or tolerable human dose is arrived at by cautiously administering increasing increments of the drug to subjects until the desired response is obtained or a toxic side effect intervenes. Pharmacokinetic data from single as well as repeated administrations are collected to determine the bioavailability of the compound, its time course of action, and how it is eliminated from the body. Careful attention is given to any adverse effects that may appear. As with subsequent clinical studies, informed consent must be obtained from all subjects involved in phase 1 trials. Regulations by the FDA involving human experimentation conform to the principles incorporated in the Declaration of Helsinki of the World Medical Association.[10]

The second phase of clinical evaluation involves administration of the drug to a small number of "target" patients. Phase 2 trials are the first real attempt to establish efficacy, and many drugs are withdrawn from further investigation at this point. The exact studies made during phase 2 are determined in large measure by the drug. However, the major goals of investigation are constant: to establish efficacy and safety in patients and to arrive at the therapeutic dose. These first two phases are conducted exclusively by individuals trained and experienced in clinical pharmacology.

The decision to proceed to phase 3 trials commits the drug sponsor to a large-scale, controlled study of the drug. In phase 3, the agent must be proved to be relatively safe and effective in a clinical setting. Such proof may require the combined efforts of over a hundred practitioners administering the drug to several thousand patients. It is most important that these trials be designed and organized to provide a scientifically sound appraisal of the drug's therapeutic value. There must, for example, be a clearly defined endpoint of treatment so that drug effectiveness can be accurately determined. Proper controls (placebos when appropriate, active drugs when available) must be run concurrently to provide the necessary comparisons of drugs, and sufficient numbers of subjects must be used in the study to make such comparisons meaningful. The assignment of subjects to control and test categories must be unbiased. This generally requires either a randomized allotment of patients, in which each volunteer has an equal chance of being in any treatment group, or a crossover design, in which every subject receives each drug in a balanced order. Bias in reporting drug effects must also be avoided. Many times, this can only be accomplished by performing the trial under "blind" conditions. In a single-blind study, patients are not informed of which drug they receive; in a double-blind investigation, the identity of the medication is concealed from all individuals directly engaged in the study.

Finally, appropriate statistical methodology must be employed to verify any conclusions reached about the drug.

Drug approval, continued surveillance. At the conclusion of phase 3, a considerable body of information will have been gathered about the drug. These data are submitted to the FDA in the form of a *New Drug Application* (NDA). If accepted as "complete," the drug will be approved for marketing as a prescription drug or as an over-the-counter item, depending on the need for professional supervision to ensure user safety. More often than not, however, the application is labeled "incomplete," and the sponsor is advised of additional evaluations that must be performed in order for the drug application to be accepted. Even with approval of the agent, the sponsor must continue to submit reports to the FDA at regular intervals describing the quantity of drug distributed and detailing any unusual responses to the preparation, such as allergic reactions, idiosyncratic responses, or unanticipated drug interactions. This review constitutes the fourth phase of clinical investigation. Continued surveillance of the drug after general release is often the only method available for identifying uncommon or delayed toxic effects. For instance, chloramphenicol was extensively employed for 2 years before it was discovered to be capable of inducing severe blood dyscrasias (in about 0.002% of treated patients)[30] and for 17 years before it was recognized to be capable of causing visual impairment.[8] It seems an ever-repeating cycle that a new drug is initially hailed as being essentially nontoxic, only to have enthusiasm dampened several years later by the realization that adverse effects are, in fact, an integral part of the agent's pharmacologic profile.

Impact of FDA regulations on the development of new drugs. Regulations by the FDA governing the development and marketing of therapeutic agents exist largely as a result of public concern over the toxic liabilities of drugs. Indeed, had similar regulations been in force in Europe before 1959, the thalidomide disaster affecting some 10,000 children could probably have been averted. There are, however, several disadvantages to the present evaluation system employed in the United States. For a drug to successfully negotiate the obstacle course of preclinical and clinical testing takes on the average about 8 years. For every 20 drugs that look sufficiently promising in animal studies for their sponsors to request permission of the FDA to begin phase 1 trials, only one agent ever receives final approval for general release.[21] Including the development costs associated with unfruitful compounds, it is estimated that $70 million is spent on the average to bring a new drug to market in the United States.[18]

The uncertainty and expense of drug development in recent years have had a marked influence on the pharmaceutical industry. Only the largest drug manufacturers have the resources to meet FDA guidelines. Since pharmaceutical companies are profit-oriented enterprises, the multimillion dollar cost of developing a drug will be incurred only if a reasonable return on the investment can be anticipated. Thus, without some additional incentive, the development of drugs for rare diseases has been priced out of consideration. It is also to be expected that agents under patent protection will be highly priced and heavily promoted.

The delay in introducing new drugs into pharmacotherapeutics has opened up a "drug lag" between the United States and other countries, for example, Great Britain.[47] Although the British people may be exposed to some increased risk of toxicity from new drugs, this danger is counterbalanced by the greater therapeutic benefits afforded by these agents. The FDA has reduced the drug lag somewhat by expediting approval of a few drugs, such as the anticonvulsant valproic acid; nevertheless, the debate over the benefits of the present regulations as opposed to their liabilities continues.

Recent legislation by Congress allows the FDA to contract with nongovernmental enterprises for the development and approval of drugs that have limited use or cannot be patented. These "orphan" drugs have, until this change, been ignored for economic reasons in spite of promising success for the treatment of specific but rather rare diseases.

Drug nomenclature

During the course of development and marketing, a drug will acquire a variety of names or designations (Figure 3-4). The first identification of a drug is the formal chemical name. Though descriptive of the molecular structure of the compound, the chemical name is usually too unwieldy for practical purposes. Often, therefore, a newly synthesized drug is given a simple code name by the parent pharmaceutical firm to denote the agent during the various stages of drug evaluation. Should the drug manufacturer intend to request approval by the FDA for distributing the agent, a nonpro-

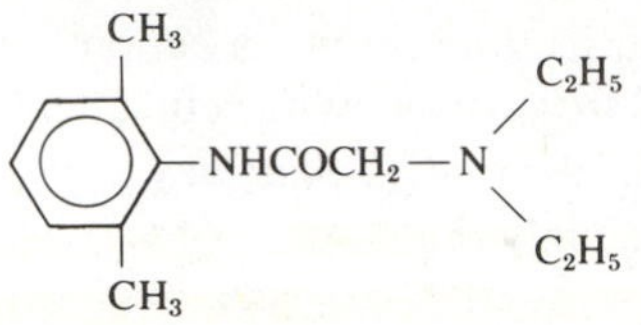

Chemical name:	Diethylaminoaceto-2,6-xylidide
Code name:	LL 30
Nonproprietary name:	Lidocaine
Official name:	Lidocaine
Trade names:	Xylocaine, Alphacaine, Codescaine, Dilocaine, Dolicaine, L-Caine, Nervocaine, Nulicaine, Octocaine, Ultracaine

Figure 3-4. Full nomenclature of a local anesthetic.

prietary name, or United States Adopted Name (USAN), will be assigned to the drug by the USAN Council, an organization jointly sponsored by the United States Pharmacopeial Convention, the American Medical Association, and the American Pharmaceutical Association. The nonproprietary name is commonly referred to as the "generic" name, but, by definition, the generic designation should be reserved to indicate a family of compounds (e.g., penicillins) rather than a single entity (e.g., ampicillin). If the drug is eventually admitted to the United States Pharmacopeia, its nonproprietary name then becomes the official name.

Much confusion over drug nomenclature arises because a single drug may be marketed under many different trade names. A trade, or proprietary, name is given to a drug by the manufacturer when the agent is approved for general release. Unlike the nonproprietary name, which is publicly owned, a trade name receives copyright protection and is the sole property of the drug company. On occasion, a manufacturer may distribute the agent under several different trade names to promote separate uses of the drug. In addition, it may arrange with other pharmaceutical firms to sell the drug, each employing their own trade name. A profusion of trade names may develop when the drug patent expires at the end of 17 years and all companies are permitted by law to produce the agent. Assignment of trade names to drug combination products contributes yet another "voice" to the "babel" of drug names.

Throughout this book, nonproprietary names will be emphasized in discussions of the various drugs. This practice will reduce confusion and equip the reader to use other sources of drug information to best advantage. The benefits and debits of employing nonproprietary designations in prescription writing are presented in Chapter 49.

SOURCES OF DRUG INFORMATION

The continued development of new drugs and the acquisition of new information about existing agents make pharmacology a discipline requiring continual study. A variety of resources are available to aid the clinician in keeping abreast of advances in pharmacotherapeutics.

Official compendia

The United States Pharmacopeia (USP) and *The National Formulary* (NF) were designated as official compendia of drugs in the United States by the Pure Food and Drugs Act of 1906. First published in 1820, the USP is revised every 5 years, with interim supplementation as needed, by a Committee on Revision of the United States Pharmacopeial Convention, Inc. Members of the Council on Dental Therapeutics of the American Dental Association serve in an advisory capacity to the Committee on Revision. Prior to 1975, only single-entity drugs (preparations with a single active ingredient) of proven therapeutic value were considered for inclusion in the USP. The NF, first released in 1888, was a publication of the American Pharmaceutical Association. In addition to single-entity agents of therapeutic value, the NF admitted combination products "for which there is a therapeutic advantage to the patient as contrasted with administration of the separate individual therapeutically-active ingredients."[41] After publication of the fourteenth edition in 1975, the NF was consolidated with the USP under the management of the USP organization. With this consolidation, the USP was expanded to include "all drugs having proven efficiency as therapeutic agents," including selected combination products, whereas the NF was restricted to describing pharmaceutical ingredients used in the formulation of marketed products.[42] The USP-NF is not a good source of information about the clinical use of drugs. However, it provides an invaluable service to the practitioner by defining criteria for the manufacture of pharmaceutical preparations. It ensures that when a prescription is written for an official drug, the medication supplied to the patient will meet certain standards of strength, purity, and chemical and physical properties.

A number of other nations have their own official compendia. In Great Britain and Canada, for example, the *British Pharmacopoeia* and the *Pharmaceutical Codex* are equivalent to the USP and the NF, respectively. The *Pharmacopoeia Internationalis* (PI) is issued by the World Health Organization. Although not "official" in the sense of the United States or British pharmacopeias, the PI is instrumental in promoting the standardization and unification of the various national compendia.

Unofficial compendia

The *Physicians' Desk Reference* (PDR) is perhaps the most widely distributed source of prescribing information available to health professionals. The PDR is published annually (with interim revisions as necessary) by the Medical Economics Company in cooperation with over 200 pharmaceutical manufacturing and distributing concerns. Approximately 2000 preparations are listed by proprietary name in an alphabetical arrangement according to drug distributor. (The cost of including a drug deters many companies from listing all of their products.) Although the PDR is well indexed, its organization makes difficult the comparison of similar agents. The product information, which is largely derived from phase 3 trials and must legally conform to FDA regulations, contains concise summaries of the uses, dosage forms and schedules, contraindications, and adverse effects of the drugs listed. Nevertheless, the lack of critical appraisals of, or relative comparisons between, the various preparations included in the PDR prohibits its use as a reliable guide for the rational selection of drugs in therapy.

A very suitable alternative to the PDR is *Facts and Comparisons*. Published independently of the pharmaceutical industry, *Facts and Comparisons* contains monographs on over 8000 preparations arranged in a format designed to facilitate comparisons between drugs. Constructed as a loose-leaf binder, the compendium readily incorporates page revisions, which are distributed monthly to keep the drug information up to date. An interesting feature of the book is the inclusion of a "relative cost index," which is useful in comparing the costs of chemically ("generically") equivalent agents.

In 1975, the USP organization decided "to directly assist and benefit practitioners of medicine and pharmacy in the use of drugs."[42] Publication of the *USP Dispensing Information* (USPDI) was a major outcome of that decision. In its current form, the USPDI comprises two separate volumes, one detailing for the health care provider the prescribing information for numerous drugs, the second providing advice to the patient regarding the proper use of these medications, precautions to consider, and adverse effects that may occur. Drug monographs from the latter volume may be reproduced and distributed without prior authorization by the USP Convention, Inc., to patients receiving the medications. The USPDI has some highly desirable features. For example, it is arranged in a uniform outline format, and adverse effects are listed according to frequency of occurrence. One limitation for many clinicians is that the USPDI is currently incomplete in its coverage of drug products.

Books on pharmacology and therapeutics

Textbooks of general pharmacology usually present basic principles of drug action and pharmacologic profiles of the various classes of therapeutic agents. Relationships between pathophysiology and drug effects described in textbooks contribute significantly to the understanding of pharmacotherapeutics. Although textbooks can provide perhaps the best overview of pharmacology, for clarity of presentation and because of limitations of space, detailed coverage of individual agents in each drug category is generally restricted to a few prototypical compounds. Thus, epinephrine may be discussed in depth while other sympathomimetic amines commonly employed by practitioners (e.g., levonordefrin used as a vasoconstrictor in local anesthetic solutions) or patients (e.g., phenylpropanolamine used as a vasoconstrictor in cold remedies) are only briefly mentioned, if at all. Textbooks are also limited in that they cannot include information on the most recent advances in pharmacotherapeutics, such as the introduction of new drugs.

AMA Drug Evaluations is a product of the Department of Drugs of the American Medical Association in cooperation with the American Society for Pharmacology and Experimental Therapeutics. Released every few years, the book provides an unbiased review of most of the prescribed drugs in the United States, including agents listed in the USP-NF and other drugs judged to be of importance. Dosages, routes of administration, and therapeutic indications for the various drugs are based on clinical effectiveness and are not necessarily identical with those approved by the FDA or listed in the package insert.

The *Handbook of Nonprescription Drugs,* published by the American Pharmaceutical Association, is one of the very few sources of information concerning over-the-counter drugs. The handbook presents critical evaluations of the various preparations available to the lay public. Of special interest to dentists are the chapters on analgesics, vitamins, and dental products.

Periodicals

A number of journals and reviews are expressly devoted to pharmacology and therapeutics. Although some of these are primarily concerned with experimental aspects of pharmacodynamics, the following regularly feature articles dealing with drug effects in humans: *Clinical Pharmacology and Therapeutics, Journal of Pharmacy and Pharmacology,* and *Journal of Pharmaceutical Sciences.* A particularly good source of basic pharmacologic information, often with direct clinical relevance, is provided by *Annual Review of Pharmacology and Toxicology.* Though not restricted in scope to drugs, the *New England Journal of Medicine* is noteworthy for its excellent coverage of pharmacotherapeutics. Specialty journals of significance to dentistry include the *Journal of Anesthesiology* and *Anesthesia and Analgesia.*

The *Medical Letter on Drugs and Therapeutics* provides a unique service to practitioners in this country. Published biweekly, *The Medical Letter* offers current, concise, and critical reviews of new drugs and pharmaceutical preparations. Expert opinion is also provided regarding the therapeutic efficacies and toxicities of established drugs. In this respect, the periodic updates on drug interactions and on clinical selection of antimicrobial agents are especially helpful.

Dental sources of information

Accepted Dental Therapeutics (ADT) is published biannually by the Council on Dental Therapeutics of the American Dental Association. Before a drug is accepted by the Council for inclusion in ADT, it must be safe and effective and meet certain advertising and labeling standards. Some drugs are also listed that have not been submitted by the manufacturer for consideration but are potentially useful in dental practice (e.g., dicloxacillin). ADT is an excellent reference for the therapeutic application of drugs in dentistry. In addition to providing information on pharmacology and drug administration, ADT offers guidance for the treatment of various intraoral maladies and for the prevention and management of medical emergencies.

Although there is currently no dental periodical solely concerned with pharmacology, a number of journals feature articles dealing with drugs in dental practice. *Anesthesia Progress* is the official journal of the American Dental Society of Anesthesiology. It publishes papers on drugs useful in pain and anxiety control and prints abstracts from other periodicals of related papers of interest. The *Journal of the American Dental Association* (JADA) is also a good source of information about dental pharmacotherapeutics. In addition to publishing original contributions and review articles, JADA provides evaluations from the Council on Dental Therapeutics of pharmaceutical preparations submitted for its review. Specialty journals, such as the *Journal of Oral and Maxillofacial Surgery, Journal of Periodontology,* and *Oral Surgery, Oral Medicine, and Oral Pathology,* occasionally publish papers on dental pharmacotherapeutics. Often the easiest and most economical method of identifying these items of interest is to use an abstract service, for example, *Dental Abstracts.*

CITED REFERENCES

1. Adams, R.M. Occupational Contact Dermatitis. Philadelphia, J.B. Lippincott Co., 1969.
2. Arora, S., and Aldrete, J.A. Investigation of possible allergy to local anesthetic drugs: correlation of intradermal with intramuscular injections. Anesthesia Review **3**:13-16, 1976.
3. Beck, F.M. Placebos in dentistry: their profound potential effects. Journal of the American Dental Association **95**:1122-1126, 1977.
4. Beecher, H.K. The powerful placebo. Journal of the American Medical Association **159**:1602-1606, 1955.
5. Bennett, W.M., Muther, R.S., Parker, R.A., Feig, P., Morrison, G., Golper, T.A., and Singer, I. Drug therapy in renal failure: dosing guidelines for adults. Annals of Internal Medicine **93**:62-89, 286-325, 1980.
6. Bourne, H.R. The placebo—a poorly understood and neglected therapeutic agent. Rational Drug Therapy **5**:1-6, 1971.
7. Chignell, C.F., Vesell, E.S., Starkweather, D.K., and Berlin, C.M. The binding of sulfaphenazole to fetal, neonatal, and adult human plasma albumin. Clinical Pharmacology and Therapeutics **12**:897-901, 1971.
8. Cocke, J.G., Jr., Brown, R.E., and Geppert, L.J. Optic neuritis with prolonged use of chloramphenicol. Journal of Pediatrics **68**:27-31, 1966.
9. Coombs, R.R.A., and Gell, P.G.H. Classification of allergic reactions responsible for clinical hypersensitivity and disease. In Gell, P.G.H., Coombs, R.R.A., and Lachmann, P.J., eds. Clinical Aspects of Immunology, ed. 3. Oxford, Blackwell Scientific Publications, 1975.
10. Declaration of Helsinki. Recommendations guiding doctors in clinical research. World Medical Journal **11**:281, 1964.
11. Done, A.K., Cohen, S.N., and Strebel, L. Pediatric clinical pharmacology and the "therapeutic orphan." Annual Review of Pharmacology and Toxicology **17**:561-573, 1977.
12. Forfar, J.O., and Nelson, M.M. Epidemiology of drugs taken by pregnant women: drugs that may affect the fetus adversely. Clinical Pharmacology and Therapeutics **14**:632-642, 1973.
13. Gibaldi, M. Biopharmaceutics and Clinical Pharmacokinetics, ed. 2. Philadelphia, Lea & Febiger, 1977.
14. Goldstein, A., Aronow, L., and Kalman, S.M. Principles of Drug Action: The Basis of Pharmacology, ed. 2. New York, John Wiley & Sons, Inc., 1974.
15. Goodson, J.M., Holborow, D., Hogan, P., and Dunham, S. Characteristics of monolithic tetracycline containing fibers for periodontal therapy. Journal of Dental Research **61**:274, 1983.
16. Koch-Weser, J. The serum level approach to individualization of drug dosage. European Journal of Clinical Pharmacology **9**:1-8, 1975.
17. Kutt, H., Winters, W., Kokenge, R., and McDowell, F. Diphenylhydantoin metabolism, blood levels, and toxicity. Archives of Neurology **11**:642-648, 1964.
18. Lasagna, L. Will all new drugs become orphans? Clinical Pharmacology and Therapeutics **31**:285-289, 1982.
19. Lenz, W. Epidemiology of congenital malformations. Annals of the New York Academy of Sciences **123**:228-236, 1965.
20. Levine, J.D., Gordon, N.C., and Fields, H.L. The mechanism of placebo analgesia. Lancet **2**:654-657, 1978.
21. Levine, R.R. Pharmacology: Drug Actions and Reactions, ed. 3. Boston, Little, Brown & Co., 1983.
22. Litchfield, J.T., Jr. Evaluation of the safety of new drugs by means of tests in animals. Clinical Pharmacology and Therapeutics **3**:665-672, 1962.
23. Luduena, F.P., and Hoppe, J.O. 2-Alkoxy benzoate and thiolbenzoate derivatives as local anesthetics. Journal of Pharmacology and Experimental Therapeutics **117**:89-96, 1956.
24. Lund, L. Effects of phenytoin in patients with epilepsy in relation to its concentration in plasma. In Davies, D.S., and Prichard, B.N.C., eds. Biological Effects of Drugs in Relation to Their Plasma Concentrations. Baltimore, University Park Press, 1973.
25. Macek, C. Monoclonal antibodies: key to a revolution in clinical medicine. Journal of the American Medical Association **247**:2463-2470, 1982.
26. Malik, V.S. Recombinant DNA technology. Advances in Applied Microbiology **27**:1-84, 1981.
27. Marks, P.A., and Banks, J. Drug-induced hemolytic anemias associated with glucose-6-phosphate dehydrogenase deficiency: a genetically heterogeneous trait. Annals of the New York Academy of Sciences **123**:198-206, 1965.
28. Martin, E.W. Hazards of Medication, ed. 2. Philadelphia, J.B. Lippincott Co., 1978.

29. Mattila, M.J., Jussila, J., and Takki, S. Drug absorption in patients with intestinal villous atrophy. Arzneimittel-Forschung **23**:583-585, 1973.

30. McCurdy, P.R. Chloramphenicol bone marrow toxicity. Journal of the American Medical Association **176**:588-593, 1961.

31. Mirth, D.B., Adderly, D.D., Amsbaugh, S.M., Monell-Torrens, E., Li, S.-H., and Bowen, W.H. Inhibition of experimental dental caries using an intraoral flouride-releasing device. Journal of the American Dental Association **107**:55-58, 1983.

32. Moolten, F.L., Schreiber, B.M., and Zajdel, S.H. Antibodies conjugated to potent cytotoxins as specific antitumor agents. Immunological Reviews **62**:47-73, 1982.

33. Parker, C.W. Drug allergy (first of three parts). New England Journal of Medicine **292**:511-514, 1975.

34. Parker, C.W. Drug allergy (third of three parts). New England Journal of Medicine **292**:957-960, 1975.

35. Prescott, L.F., Wright, N., Roscoe, P., and Brown, S.S. Plasma-paracetamol half-life and hepatic necrosis in patients with paracetamol overdosage. Lancet **1**:519-522, 1971.

36. Reidenberg, M.M., and Lowenthal, D.T. Adverse nondrug reactions. New England Journal of Medicine **279**:678-679, 1968.

37. Rosenthal, A. Follow-up study of fatal penicillin reactions. Journal of the American Medical Association **167**:1118-1121, 1958.

38. Roth, H.P., and Caron, H.S. Accuracy of doctors' estimates and patients' statements on adherence to a drug regimen. Clinical Pharmacology and Therapeutics **23**:361-370, 1978.

39. Shelley, J.H. Phenacetin, through the looking glass. Clinical Pharmacology and Therapeutics **8**:427-471, 1967.

40. Stewart, R.B., and Cluff, L.E. A review of medication errors and compliance in ambulant patients. Clinical Pharmacology and Therapeutics **13**:463-468, 1972.

41. The National Formulary, ed. 14. Washington, D.C., American Pharmaceutical Association, 1975.

42. The United States Pharmacopeia, rev. 20. Rockville, Maryland, The United States Pharmacopeial Convention, Inc., 1979.

43. Underwood, T., Iturrian, W.B., and Cadwallader, D.E. Some aspects of chemical teratogenesis. American Journal of Hospital Pharmacy **27**:115-122, 1970.

44. Venter, J.C. Immobilized and insolubilized drugs, hormones, and neurotransmitters: properties, mechanisms of action and applications. Pharmacological Reviews **34**:153-187, 1982.

45. Vital Statistics—Special Reports, National Summaries. Washington, D.C., National Office of Vital Statistics, U.S. Department of Health, Education, and Welfare, 1959-1974.

46. Walton, W.W. An evaluation of the Poison Prevention Packaging Act. Pediatrics **69**:363-370, 1982.

47. Wardell, W.M. Therapeutic implications of the drug lag. Clinical Pharmacology and Therapeutics **15**:73-96, 1974.

48. Wolf, S. The pharmacology of placebos. Pharmacological Reviews **11**:689-704, 1959.

GENERAL REFERENCES

Gibaldi, M., and Prescott, L. Handbook of Clinical Pharmacokinetics. Balgowlah, Australia, ADIS Health Science Press, 1983.

Goldstein, A., Aronow, L., and Kalman, S.M. Principles of Drug Action: The Basis of Pharmacology, ed. 2. New York, John Wiley & Sons, Inc., 1974.

Levine, R.R. Pharmacology: Drug Actions and Reactions, ed. 3. Boston, Little, Brown & Co., 1983.

Martin, E.W. Hazards of Medication, ed. 2. Philadelphia, J.B. Lippincott Co., 1978.

Melmon, K.L., Gilman, A.G., and Mayer, S.E. Principles of therapeutics. In Gilman, A.G., Goodman, L.S., and Gilman, A., eds. Goodman and Gilman's The Pharmacological Basis of Therapeutics, ed. 6. New York, Macmillan, Inc., 1980.

4 General mechanisms of drug interactions

Norton M. Ross
Anthony Picozzi

Numerous studies have documented that drugs are rarely taken in isolation. It is well known, for example, that adults in contemporary society may take an average of four to five drugs daily and that hospitalized patients may receive from 9 to 13 different agents every 24 hours, depending on the institution, the patient's status, and the intercommunication among attending physicians.[1] As the number of administered drugs increases arithmetically, the risk of an adverse drug reaction increases geometrically (Figure 4-1).[2] Drug interactions, in fact, may be responsible for extending the hospital stay of approximately 15% of admitted patients. However, not all drug interactions are clinically significant or undesired, and some are actively sought in pharmacotherapeutics to increase drug effectiveness, decrease toxicity, or both. The purpose of this chapter is to review the basic principles and general mechanisms of drug interactions and to illustrate these interactions with selected examples. Some interactions will not be included here, for example, medication interference with laboratory tests and metabolic interactions with environmental chemicals, such as pesticides that alter in vivo enzyme activity. In addition, it will be assumed for the sake of simplicity that only two agents are interacting concurrently.

Basically, there are three types of drug action: (1) that between the drug and the disease state of the patient, which is, of course, the objective of therapy, (2) that between the drug and the patient, which is unrelated to the disease state (known as an undesired patient reaction), and (3) that between two or more drugs being concurrently administered to the patient, thus, a drug interaction that can alter either the therapeutic effect or other drug reactions. The sources of drugs that may be involved in drug

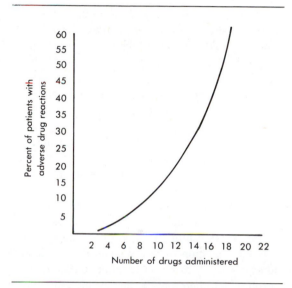

Figure 4-1. Relationship of rate of adverse reactions to number of drugs administered. The exponential curve indicates that drug interactions account for many episodes of toxicity during multiple drug therapy. (From Smith, J.W., Seidl, L.G., and Cluff, L.E. Annals of Internal Medicine **65:**629-640, 1966.)

interactions are varied. They may be prescribed or administered by a single physician or dentist or by several practitioners. Patients may also medicate themselves with over-the-counter (OTC) preparations, with drugs provided by relatives or friends, or with medication remaining from a previous prescription. Finally, certain substances in foods may interact with administered drugs. Potential interactions between concurrently administered drugs are both dose and duration dependent; nevertheless, the degree or severity of an adverse interaction is seldom predictable.

CLASSIFICATION OF DRUG INTERACTIONS

Historically, complex systems of nomenclature were developed in an attempt to explain the many combined effects of two or more drugs. These classification schemes attempted to scale the total drug response in mathematical terms. With a better understanding of the mechanisms of action of drugs, the usefulness and need of such schemes have diminished, so that today only three terms remain in common use: *antagonism, summation,* and *potentiation.*

Antagonism

Antagonism implies that the biologic or clinical response to a drug is reduced by the administration of a second agent. In some cases, the action of one or both of the drugs might be diminished or completely lost. An example of this type of interaction is seen in antibiotic therapy, where the combined use of a drug that acts by inhibiting the synthesis of bacterial cell walls, such as penicillin, and one that acts by inhibiting bacterial protein synthesis, such as erythromycin or tetracycline, results in less antimicrobial activity than might have been obtained by adequate doses of either antibiotic used alone.

Antagonism can occur when an antagonist produces a physical or chemical change in the agonist, reducing or abolishing its activity. An example of this is the chelation of heavy metal ions in dairy products or antacids by tetracycline, reducing the absorption and therefore the therapeutic effectiveness of that antibiotic. A second form of antagonism may develop when one drug modifies the disposition of a second agent. Most commonly, an antagonism of this nature is caused by a compound that stimulates drug metabolism and shortens the biologic half-life of the agonist; in a few instances, however, drugs may inhibit the enzymatic activation of other agents. Third, competition can develop between drugs for the same receptor site, diminishing or even abolishing the effectiveness of the active drug. Such pharmacologic antagonisms occur frequently with drugs that act on the autonomic nervous system, such as the blockade of sympathomimetic amines by α- and β-adrenergic antagonists. Finally, drugs having opposing actions at different receptor sites may partially or completely antagonize the effects of either or both drugs. Examples of this type of antagonism are the opposing effects of simultaneous administration of

CNS stimulants and depressants or the physiologic antagonism of corticosteroids and insulin.

Summation

Summation refers to the combined activities of two drugs that elicit common pharmacologic effects. If the two drugs act at the same site and produce simple mathematical summation of effects in the linear range of the dose-response curve, they are said to be additive. Examples of drugs that summate by acting at different and identical receptor sites include trimethoprim and sulfamethoxazole, and morphine and meperidine, respectively.

Potentiation

Potentiation is said to occur when a combination of two drugs that do not share similar pharmacologic activities results in an effect of one of the drugs that is greater than expected. Although not active in producing the effect by itself, the potentiator ''sensitizes'' the individual to the active agent. For instance, a patient receiving a monoamine oxidase inhibitor is rendered unusually susceptible to meperidine because the metabolism of the analgesic is altered.

MECHANISMS OF DRUG INTERACTIONS

Any of the classes of drug interactions described above can occur at any point along the pharmacologic pathway of the agonist, from even before the drug is administered to a patient, to the period when it is in contact with its site of action, to the point at which it is eliminated. The various mechanisms involved in drug interactions can be grouped taxonomically into three broad categories: pharmaceutical, pharmacokinetic, and pharmacodynamic interactions.

Pharmaceutical interactions

Pharmaceutical interactions represent drug incompatibilities of a physical or chemical nature (Table 4-1). In general, pharmaceutical interactions can be anticipated between organic acids and bases, resulting in precipitation of one or both drugs. Chemical reactions between drugs may also occur, but these are less common. Most pharmaceutical interactions of importance to dentistry involve drugs that are given parenterally for intravenous sedation. As a general rule, it is best to avoid mixing drugs within the same syringe.

Table 4-1. Examples of pharmaceutical drug interactions*

·Drug A	with	Drug B
Kanamycin		Methicillin
Diazepam		Intravenous fluids
Barbiturates		Narcotic analgesics
Norepinephrine		Sodium bicarbonate
Hydroxyzine		Amobarbital
Metaraminol		Hydrocortisone

*Mixing of any of the above pairs of drugs in the same bottle, tubing, syringe, or intravenous drip may result in the precipitation or destruction of the constituents.

Pharmacokinetic interactions

Pharmacokinetic interactions derive from the influence of one drug on the absorption, distribution, biotransformation, or excretion of another (Table 4-2).

Absorption. Many times an interaction will affect the rate or extent of effective absorption of the principal drug into the systemic circulation, causing a decrease or increase in that drug's effect. Factors influencing absorption include the pH of lumen fluids, enzyme activity, and intestinal motility. Familiar examples of interactions that decrease drug absorption include the previously mentioned chelation by tetracycline of multivalent heavy metal cations (Ca^{++}, Mg^{++}, Fe^{+++}, and Al^{+++}) in dairy products, antacids, or ferrous salts and the hydrolysis of penicillin G by fruit juice acids, resulting in a decrease in the amount of antibiotic available for absorption and therefore a decrease in the therapeutic effects of these antibiotics. Dentists are familiar with combining vasoconstrictors with local anesthetic preparations to retard absorption of the anesthetic from the site of administration.

A well-known example of an interaction that facilitates or increases absorption occurs in patients taking monoamine oxidase inhibitors. Tyramine in beer, ripened cheese, red wine, and many other fermented foods is normally not absorbed because it is enzymatically inactivated by monoamine oxidases in the intestinal mucosa and liver. When monoamine oxidase inhibitors suppress these enzymes, tyramine, a sympathomimetic amine, is absorbed in excessive amounts, releasing norepinephrine and epinephrine from sympathetic nerve endings and adrenal glands. The effect frequently results in drug toxicity, including severe headache and, occasionally, hypertensive crisis and death.

Distribution. Once the principal drug is absorbed, an interaction may modify its distribution or the rate of transfer of the drug from one location to another. Drugs may be free in the bloodstream or become reversibly bound to plasma or tissue components. Plasma proteins, usually albumin but sometimes globulins, act as acceptor or storage sites for many drugs. Protein-bound drugs are inactive, being unavailable for active combination with a receptor site, for biotransformation, or for glomerular filtration. Since a bound drug is in equilibrium with the free drug in plasma and tissue fluids, an interacting drug that displaces an agonist from its protein-binding sites raises the plasma concentration of the pharmacologically active, unbound agonist. This increases its pharmacologic activity; it also increases the amount available for metabolism and excretion, thus shortening its duration of action. Because some drugs are highly protein bound, displacement of even a small percentage of these drugs from their binding sites can result in a relatively large increase in pharmacologic activity.

Oral anticoagulants, which are highly protein bound, are displaced from their plasma protein-binding sites by certain antibiotics, barbiturates, and antiinflammatory agents, thus potentiating the anticoagulant effect and resulting in an increased prothrombin time and an increased tendency for bleeding or spontaneous hemorrhage. Although many interactions are due to displacement of drugs from their binding sites, the reverse is rare.

Metabolism. The degree and duration of activity of a drug is often a function of its metabolism; therefore, an interacting drug could modify the effect of an agonist by altering its rate of biotransformation. For example, phenobarbital and many other CNS depressants are known to induce the production of hepatic microsomal enzymes that are responsible for their biotransformation. These same microsomal enzymes, however, may also metabolize other drugs, such as oral anticoagulants, resulting in an increase in the rate of biotransformation of the anticoagulant and a consequent decrease in the active free form, with a resultant loss of therapeutic effectiveness. Care must be taken to reassess the anticoagulant dosage when an enzyme-inducing agent is withdrawn, since removal of enzyme induction may then result in an increase in anticoagulant activity and spontaneous hemorrhage. Corticosteroids also cause enzyme induction, resulting in a decreased efficiency of hydro-

Table 4-2. Some examples of pharmacokinetic drug interactions

Mechanism of drug interaction	Drug A given with	Drug B or dietary constituent	Produces	Net effect
Inhibition of drug absorption	Penicillin G	Acidic fruit juice	Hydrolysis of penicillin	Less antibiotic is absorbed and blood concentrations are reduced
	Digitalis	Cholestyramine	Adsorption of digitalis by the anion exchange resin	More digitalis is excreted and less is absorbed from the gastrointestinal tract; lower blood concentrations
	Local anesthetic (lidocaine, etc.)	Vasoconstrictor (epinephrine, etc.)	Vasoconstriction in the area of injection	Decreased absorption of anesthetic with prolongation of anesthesia
	Many oral medications	Cathartics	Increased gastrointestinal motility	Decreased absorption of oral medication; decreased blood concentrations
	Tetracyclines	Milk, antacids, drugs containing multivalent metallic ions	Chelation by tetracycline	Formation of insoluble tetracycline complex that is poorly absorbed
	Vitamins A, D, K	Mineral oil	Vitamins are sequestered in the oil; inadequate contact with intestinal epithelium	Decreased absorption of vitamins
	Cimetidine	Antacids	Complexation of Mg^{++} and Al^{+++} to cimetidine	Decreased cimetidine blood concentrations
Increased drug absorption	Monoamine oxidase inhibitors	Tyramine-containing foods (wine, beer, aged cheese, etc.)	Increased absorption of tyramine and release of norepinephrine from neuron terminals	Severe headache, hypertensive crisis
	Many oral medications	Narcotic analgesics, antimuscarinics	Delay in gastric emptying	Increased absorption of drugs normally absorbed in stomach; increased blood concentrations
Alteration of drug binding	Dicumarol	Chloral hydrate, phenylbutazone	Displacement of oral anticoagulant from protein-binding site	Activity of anticoagulant increased significantly; increased bleeding
	Nonsteroidal antiinflammatory agents (indomethacin, etc.)	Endogenous corticosteroids	Displacement of corticosteroids from secondary binding sites	Beneficial antiinflammatory effects
	Digoxin	Quinidine	Displacement of digoxin from tissue binding sites	Increased risk of digitalis intoxication
Induction of drug-metabolizing enzymes	Warfarin	Barbiturates	Induction of hepatic microsomal enzymes for destruction of warfarin	Decreased blood concentrations of warfarin
	Phenytoin	Barbiturates	Hepatic microsomal induction of enzymes for phenytoin	Decreased blood concentrations of phenytoin
	Barbiturates	Alcohol	Induction of enzymes for inactivation of barbiturates	Decreased blood concentrations of barbiturates

	Drug	Interacting drug	Mechanism	Result
Inhibition of biotransformation	Levodopa	Decarboxylase inhibitor	Destruction of levodopa prevented before it reaches the brain	Allows a reduction in dosage of levodopa and decreased toxicity
	Tolbutamide	Dicumarol, phenylbutazone	Inhibition of microsomal enzymes for metabolism of tolbutamide	Increased blood concentrations of tolbutamide; hypoglycemia
	Phenytoin	Aminosalicylic acid, methylphenidate	Inhibition of microsomal enzymes for metabolism of phenytoin	Increased blood concentrations of phenytoin; increased toxicity
	Meperidine	MAO inhibitors	Decrease in rate of biotransformation of meperidine	Retention of toxic intermediary metabolite; potentially fatal
	Alcohol	Disulfiram	Inhibition of acetaldehyde dehydrogenase	Increased blood concentration of acetaldehyde; unpleasant side effects
	Methotrexate	Antibiotics	Methotrexate is normally excreted via the enterohepatic route and metabolized by microflora of the gastrointestinal tract; microflora are killed by the antibiotics	Decreased rate of biotransformation of methotrexate and lower dose required or increased toxicity
	Diazepam	Cimetidine	Inhibition of microsomal enzymes for metabolism of diazepam	Excessive accumulation of diazepam; increased toxicity
Alteration of excretion	Aspirin, long-acting barbiturates	NaHCO₃	Urine is alkalinized	Acidic drugs are less readily reabsorbed by kidneys; excretion enhanced
	Penicillin	Probenecid	Competition with penicillin for renal tubular secretory pathway	Half-life of penicillin is increased

cortisone used in the treatment of acute asthma. Conversely, the monoamine oxidase inhibitors, by inhibiting the oxidative enzymes that metabolize drugs such as phenylephrine, pentobarbital, and chlorpromazine, increase the available active forms of these agonists and potentiate their activity.

Excretion. Increasing or decreasing the rate of excretion, or renal or biliary clearance, of a drug also alters its elimination rate constant and therefore the amount of drug available in the circulating plasma, thus affecting the duration as well as the degree of activity of the drug. Renal excretion is affected by urinary pH and tubular reabsorption, as well as by inhibition of active transport. For example, weak acids, such as aspirin, are more rapidly excreted in an alkaline urine produced by sodium bicarbonate, whereas weak bases, such as amphetamine, are more readily excreted in a urine acidified by ammonium chloride. Tubular secretion of a principal drug might also be decreased by an interacting drug. A common example is that of probenecid, which, by competing for the same renal transport system as penicillin, increases the serum concentration and the duration of action of penicillin.

Pharmacodynamic interactions

Pharmacodynamic interactions represent modifications in the pharmacologic effects of a drug independent of any change in the quantitative disposition of that drug (Table 4-3). Such interactions may increase, diminish, or alter qualitatively the therapeutic effect of drug administration.

There are many interactions that take place at or near receptor sites. The mechanisms involved can include competition for the receptor or alterations of either the transmitter or receptor. This type of interaction is especially common among autonomic drugs. For instance, a drug such as reserpine affects the synthesis, storage, release, and reuptake of the neuromediator norepinephrine, resulting in depletion of norepinephrine in the neuronal vesicles. Subsequent administration of an agent that acts by evoking the release of norepinephrine (e.g., ephedrine, amphetamine) will then be ineffective. An example of the opposite effect is that of the monoamine oxidase inhibitors, such as pargyline, which permit the accumulation of norepinephrine by forming complexes with the enzyme that metabolizes the neuromediator within the nerve terminals. In this instance, ephedrine or amphetamine will produce markedly exaggerated effects. Other drugs

Table 4-3. Some examples of pharmacodynamic interactions

Mechanism of drug interaction	Drug A given with	Drug B or dietary constituent	Produces	Net effect
Competition for same receptor	Acetylcholine, pilocarpine	Atropine	Competition for the muscarinic receptor	Responses to muscarinic drugs and parasympathetic nerve stimulation are blocked
	Histamine	Tripelennamine, diphenhydramine, etc.	Competition for the histamine receptor	Responses of the H_1 receptor are blocked; many manifestations of allergy are prevented
	Epinephrine	Propranolol	Competition for the β receptors	Responses to epinephrine are blocked; epinephrine therapy for bronchospasm would be ineffective
	Indomethacin	Aspirin	Competition for same receptor site	Decreased indomethacin response
Inactivation of an enzyme	Physostigmine	Atropine	Reversible inactivation of acetylcholinesterase; excess ACh is denied access to the muscarinic receptor	Atropine is a specific antidote for overdose of physostigmine
	Neostigmine	Tubocurarine	Inhibition of AChE and build-up of ACh at the motor endplate	Neuromuscular blockade produced by tubocurarine is terminated
Opposite pharmacologic effects on different receptors	Histamine	Epinephrine	Effects of histamine on blood vessels, bronchial muscle, etc. are counteracted by opposite effects, on different receptors, of epinephrine	Epinephrine is an effective physiologic antidote to histamine overdose
	Barbiturates, other CNS depressants	Amphetamines, caffeine, other CNS stimulants	Depression produced by the depressants is counteracted by an effect, on different sites, of the stimulants	(In practice, the stimulants are rarely used to treat depression produced by overdose of depressants)
Additive pharmacologic effects at same or different sites	Alcohol	Phenothiazines	Sedative effects of alcohol are increased	Severe depression may result; coma and death
	Alcohol	Diazepam	Additive effects of hypotensive and other CNS depressant effects	Severe CNS depression
	Alcohol	Aspirin	Potentiation of aspirin-induced prolongation of bleeding time	Possible increased postoperative bleeding
	Neuromuscular blocking agents (nondepolarizing)	General anesthetics (ether, halothane, etc.)	Potentiation of the action of the blocking agent	More profound paralysis necessitating a reduction in dosage of blocking agent
	Neuromuscular blocking agents (depolarizing and nondepolarizing)	Propranolol	Intensification and prolongation of blockade because propranolol stabilizes the postjunctional membrane	Intensification and prolongation of blockade
	Neuromuscular blocking agents (depolarizing)	Neostigmine	Accumulation of ACh at the endplate	Potentiation of the effects of the neuromuscular blocking agent
	Ether	Aminoglycoside antibiotics (e.g., kanamycin)	Potentiation of neuromuscular blocking effects of ether	Apnea, respiratory depression, respiratory paralysis
	Halothane	Epinephrine	Sensitization of the myocardium to epinephrine	Cardiac arrhythmias
	Halothane	Succinylcholine	Increased muscle catabolism	Malignant hyperthermia
	Pancuronium	Aminophylline	Enhanced adrenergic effects	Paroxysmal atrial tachycardia

may increase (dextrothyroxine) or decrease (propranolol, phenoxybenzamine) the affinity of the drug for the receptor site.

Interacting drugs may also have their effects at sites of action in different locations. A previously cited example of this phenomenon is the physiologic antagonism of the CNS stimulants, such as caffeine or amphetamine, by the CNS depressants, such as the barbiturates or the anticonvulsants. When the agents are administered simultaneously, these drug groups produce opposing actions that partially or completely cancel each other. Probably the most common interactions involve drugs that evoke similar pharmacologic effects. Combinations of alcohol, barbiturates, benzodiazepines, phenothiazines, antihistamines, bromides, or other drugs capable of producing CNS depression are often unwittingly consumed by individuals, resulting in somnolence, unconsciousness, or even death.

FACTORS INFLUENCING DRUG INTERACTIONS

Several variables can affect the occurrence and intensity of potential interactions. Prime among these are individual or biologic variations in the handling of and reaction to administered drugs, including genetic differences that affect metabolism. As previously mentioned, drug interactions, as well as drug effects, are both dose-dependent and duration-dependent; thus, an interaction may not be clinically discernible each time interacting drugs are administered. The higher the dosage and the longer the administration, the greater the chance that an interaction may occur. Individual tolerance or sensitivity, previous exposure affecting drug metabolism, and the degree of protein binding of the drugs may alter the potential for interaction. In addition, many drugs have a long biologic half-life, and effective concentrations may be present in the blood or tissue for many days after the cessation of therapy; interactions may occur, therefore, days and occasionally weeks after discontinuation of therapy with one of the interacting drugs.

DRUG INTERACTIONS USED IN PHARMACOTHERAPEUTICS

Combinations of drugs are employed in therapy to provide enhanced effects and to prevent adverse reactions. Purposeful drug interactions are especially common in the treatment of certain diseases, such as essential hypertension, tuberculosis, and cancer, in which the concurrent administration of two or more drugs is routine. Drugs may also be given sequentially in order for the second agent to abruptly terminate the action of the first. Thus, edrophonium, a cholinesterase inhibitor, is administered to reverse the neuromuscular blockade of tubocurarine, and leucovorin (folinic acid) is administered to "rescue" patients given potentially lethal doses of methotrexate, a folic acid analogue used in cancer chemotherapy. Agents useful as specific antidotes in accidental drug overdosage include protamine for heparin, naloxone for narcotic analgesics, and atropine for anticholinesterases.

Particular mention should be made of fixed-dose combination products. Such preparations make up the majority of all drugs sold in the United States, from OTC remedies to prescription items to agents administered by practitioners. The fixed combination of a local anesthetic with epinephrine to provide safer, more prolonged anesthesia is a notable example. In general, drug mixtures include a principal ingredient for the main therapeutic effect, adjuvants that summate with, potentiate, or otherwise complement the first drug, and correctives that antagonize or minimize undesired side effects.

The major criticisms of fixed-dose combinations are (1) the inability to adjust the dosages of the individual ingredients to the needs of a particular patient, (2) discrepancies in half-lives of individual agents leading to the accumulation of some but not other constituents during repeated administration, (3) the likelihood of taking unnecessary drugs, (4) the possibility of increased toxicity or allergenicity without correspondingly increased therapeutic efficacy, and (5) the possibility of a higher cost from the manufacturer. There are, however, certain potential advantages to fixed-dose combinations. Certain mixtures offer therapeutic gains in effectiveness and safety (e.g., aspirin with codeine combinations and local anesthetic-vasoconstrictor solutions). In addition, drug combinations may improve patient compliance by reducing the number of medications the patient must take. Finally, the reduced number of individual prescriptions can be less expensive to the patient.

Although certain fixed-dose combinations are useful, such preparations should be avoided as a general rule, and only those mixtures that have been demonstrated to be therapeutically advantageous to the patient should be employed.

CITED REFERENCES

1. Ross, N.M. General mechanisms of drug interactions. In Bourgault, P.C., and Ross, N.M., eds. Drug Interactions, vol. 3. The Third Symposium of the Pharmacology, Therapeutics, and Toxicology Group. International Association for Dental Research, 1976.
2. Smith, J.W., Seidl, L.G., and Cluff, L.E. Studies on the epidemiology of adverse drug reactions. V. Clinical factors influencing susceptibility. Annals of Internal Medicine **65:**629-640, 1966.

GENERAL REFERENCES

Adverse interactions of drugs. Medical Letter on Drugs and Therapeutics **23:**17-28, 1981.

AMA Drug Evaluations, ed. 5. Chicago, American Medical Association, 1983.

Bourgault, P.C., and Ross, N.M., eds. Drug Interactions, vol. 3. The Third Symposium of the Pharmacology, Therapeutics, and Toxicology Group. International Association for Dental Research, 1976.

Cohen, S.N., and Armstrong, M.F. Drug Interactions: A Handbook for Clinical Use. Baltimore, The Williams & Wilkins Co., 1974.

Cooper, J.W., Jr., Wellins, I., Fish, K.H., Jr., and Loomis, M.E. A seven-nursing home study: frequency of potential drug-drug interactions. Journal of the American Pharmaceutical Association **15:**24-27, 1975.

Evaluation of Drug Interactions. Washington, D.C., American Pharmaceutical Association, 1973.

Gage, T.W., and Radman, W.P. Drug interactions: a professional responsibility. Journal of the American Dental Association **84:**848-853, 1972.

Gilman, A.G., Goodman, L.S., and Gilman, A., eds. Goodman and Gilman's The Pharmacological Basis of Therapeutics, ed. 6. New York, Macmillan, Inc., 1980.

Hansten, P.D. Drug Interactions, ed. 4. Philadelphia, Lea & Febiger, 1979.

Hussar, D.A. Mechanisms of drug interactions. Journal of the American Pharmaceutical Association **9:**208-209, 1969.

Martin, E.W. Hazards of Medication, ed. 2. Philadelphia, J.B. Lippincott Co., 1978.

Melmon, K.L., and Morelli, H.F. Drug reactions. In Melmon, K.L., and Morelli, H.F., eds. Clinical Pharmacology: Basic Principles in Therapeutics, ed. 2. New York, Macmillan, Inc., 1978.

Morselli, P.L., Cohen, S.N., and Garattini, S., eds. Drug Interactions. New York, Raven Press, 1974.

Yaffee, S.J. Drug Interactions. I. Pediatrics **49:**452-453, 1972.

PHARMACOLOGY OF SPECIFIC DRUG GROUPS

5 Introduction to autonomic nervous system drugs

Enid A. Neidle

The term *autonomic nervous system drugs* is an umbrella that covers a vast number of agents possessing a variety of mechanisms and sites of action and pharmacologic activity. Some of these drugs act on postjunctional receptor sites, and some act on the nerve terminals. Some mimic the action of naturally occurring mediators; some interfere with the action of these mediators; and still others owe their activity to complex effects on mediator formation, destruction, or release. An understanding of this large class of drugs rests on two foundations: a knowledge of the organization and function of the autonomic nervous system and an understanding of how certain endogenous chemical entities, called transmitters or mediators or neurohumors, affect cellular function.

AUTONOMIC NERVOUS SYSTEM

The autonomic nervous system, also referred to as the visceral, vegetative, or involuntary nervous system, regulates the function of involuntary structures: smooth muscle, secretory glands, and cardiac muscle. These structures possess intrinsic mechanisms that make it possible for them to function entirely in the absence of innervation, but the autonomic nervous system contributes a regulatory and coordinating function. Essentially, it is an efferent system. At the present time little is known about the afferent limb other than that sensory nerves carry impulses that are received and organized centrally, often at an unconscious level. Thus, a person is not aware of impulses generated at the baroreceptors, although these impulses may trigger a generalized body response, such as a reflex fall in blood pressure, that the individual would indeed recognize.

The structural organization of the efferent arm of the autonomic nervous system differs from that of the somatic nervous system in that autonomic fibers leaving the brainstem and spinal cord synapse once outside the central nervous system. This means that the autonomic nervous system consists of a two-neuron outflow, one neuron being located within the central nervous system and the other lying outside. This two-neuron arrangement gives rise to the terms *preganglionic* for the cell body and fiber that originate in the cerebrospinal axis and *postganglionic* for the neuron that originates in ganglia outside the central nervous system (Figure 5-1).

The autonomic nervous system is divided into two parts, the parasympathetic (craniosacral) and sympathetic (thoracolumbar), a division based on anatomical, functional, and chemical characteristics of each division.

Anatomy

The anatomy of the two divisions of the autonomic nervous system is shown in Figure 5-1. The sympathetic nervous system, or thoracolumbar division, originates from cells located in the intermediolateral columns of the spinal cord, extending from the first thoracic to the second or third lumbar segments. As shown in Figure 5-2, the myelinated preganglionic fibers emerge with the ventral root of the spinal nerve and synapse with the second neuron in one of three possible types of ganglia: the vertebral (paravertebral or lateral), the prevertebral, or the terminal. The vertebral chains consist of 22 pairs of ganglia lying on either side of the spinal cord and connected to each other by nerve fibers. The prevertebral ganglia are located in the abdomen and pelvis and include the celiac, inferior mesenteric, and superior mesenteric. The few terminal ganglia lie near the organs they innervate, principally the urinary bladder and rectum.

Preganglionic fibers emerging from the spinal

89

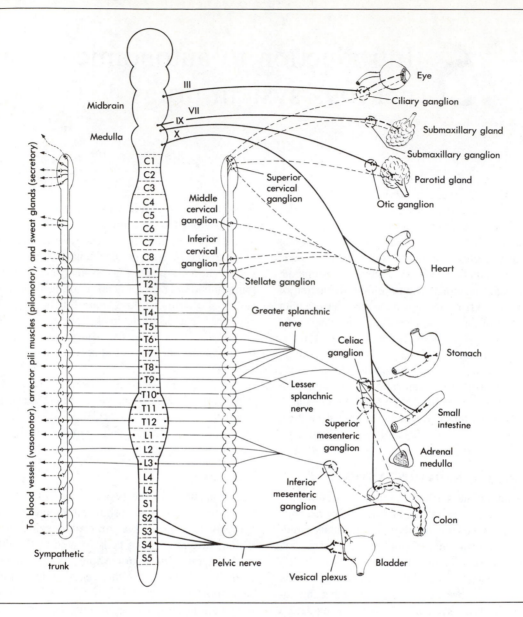

Figure 5-1. General arrangement of the autonomic nervous system showing one side of bilateral outflow. The brain and spinal cord are represented at left. Preganglionic fibers of the sympathetic nervous system are indicated by light solid lines; postganglionic fibers of the sympathetic nervous system are indicated by light dashed lines. Preganglionic fibers of the parasympathetic system are shown by bold solid lines; postganglionic fibers of the parasympathetic system are shown by bold dashed lines. (From Copenhaver, W.M., ed. Bailey's Textbook of Histology, ed. 15. © 1964, The Williams & Wilkins Co., Baltimore.)

cord enter the chain of vertebral ganglia via the white rami and then follow one of three anatomical courses. First, the fibers may synapse with neurons lying in the segment or, by passing up or down in the chain, synapse in superior or inferior segments. In this way, ganglia of spinal cord segments that do not give rise to sympathetic outflow (e.g., the superior cervical ganglion) receive input from the sympathetic nervous system, and it is these fibers that make up the nervous interconnections between the vertebral ganglia. Postganglionic fibers exit by way of the gray rami, so called because they are made up of nonmyelinated nerves, and are then conveyed via segmental spinal nerves to blood vessels, secretory glands, and other smooth muscle. The sympathetic innervation to the head and neck,

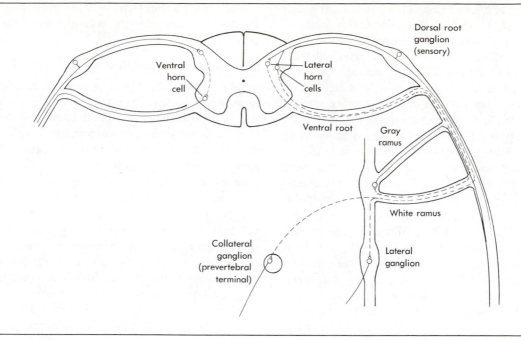

Figure 5-2. Different arrangements of neurons in the somatic and autonomic nervous systems. A single poly-synaptic reflex is shown on the left; a reflex involving the sympathetic nervous system is shown on the right. Preganglionic fibers are represented by dashed lines and postganglionic fibers by solid lines. Note that pre-ganglionic fibers emerging from the white ramus make synaptic connection in more than one lateral chain ganglion or a collateral ganglion. (From Koizumi, K., and Brooks, C.M. The autonomic nervous system and its role in controlling body functions. In Mountcastle, V.B., ed. Medical Physiology, ed. 14. St. Louis, The C. V. Mosby Co., 1980.)

including the vascular smooth muscle, the salivary glands and other secretory organs, the iris, and the pilomotor apparatus, receives fibers that originate from cell bodies located in the cervical sympathetic chain, which consists of the superior, middle, and inferior cervical ganglia.

Second, preganglionic fibers may pass directly through the chain of vertebral ganglia without synapsing and eventually enter the prevertebral or terminal ganglia where they synapse. For example, it will be noted from Figure 5-1 that preganglionic fibers from T5 through T10 are gathered together to form the greater splanchnic nerve, which synapses in the celiac ganglion and gives rise to fibers that travel with major arteries and with other postganglionics to supply the smooth muscle of the viscera, the glands of the gastrointestinal tract, and the blood vessels of this area.

A third route for preganglionics is to pass via the greater splanchnic nerve and terminate in the adrenal medulla, without any further synapse. Since the adrenal medulla is embryologically and anatomically analogous to other sympathetic gan-

glia, it is not surprising that its innervation is pre-ganglionic.

One of the striking anatomical aspects of the sympathetic nervous system, and one that has great functional significance, is that a single preganglion-ic fiber may contact as many as 20 or more post-ganglionic neurons. This means that impulses aris-ing in one neuron of the sympathetic nervous sys-tem may ultimately affect many postganglionic neurons, and it goes far to explain the diffuse and widespread character of sympathetic nervous sys-tem responses. The involvement of the adrenal me-dulla in sympathetic activity and its capability of releasing, on preganglionic stimulation, a mixture of epinephrine and norepinephrine provide yet an-other explanation for the nonselective character-istics of sympathetic activity. These factors make logical the use of the term *sympathoadrenal system.*

The parasympathetic nervous system, or cra-niosacral division, has its origin in cell bodies located in the brainstem nuclei of four cranial nerves—the oculomotor (3), facial (7), glossopharyngeal (9), and vagus (10)—and in cell bodies located in the second, third, and fourth segments of the sacral spinal cord. The preganglionic fibers form part of the cranial nerves and travel with them to synapse with postganglionic neurons located in ganglia near or actually within the structures innervated. The midbrain outflow from the nucleus of the third cranial nerve synapses in the ciliary ganglion located in the orbit. The ganglion gives rise to fibers that supply the ciliary muscle and the sphincter muscle of the iris. Fibers of the facial nerve that synapse in the sublingual and submaxillary ganglia form the chorda tympani. Other neurons of the facial nerve synapse in the sphenopalatine ganglion. Fibers from the glossopharyngeal nuclei synapse in the otic ganglion; its postganglionic fibers innervate the parotid gland. A major component of the cranial outflow is the vagus nerve, which originates from vagal nuclei in the medulla. Preganglionic fibers pass to ganglia located within the heart and the viscera of the thorax and abdomen. Postganglionic fibers, very short in length, arise from these neurons to terminate in the aforementioned structures. Fibers originating from sacral segments form the pelvic nerves, or nervi erigentes, which synapse in terminal ganglia lying near or within the uterus, bladder, rectum, and sexual organs.

From the foregoing, it should be clear that, unlike the arrangement in the sympathetic nervous system, there is very little overlap or divergence in the parasympathetic nervous system. With few exceptions (for instance in Auerbach's plexus, where one preganglionic fiber exists for every 8,000 postganglionic cells), there is a one-to-one relationship between pre- and postganglionic fibers, which makes possible very discrete and limited responses in the parasympathetic nervous system. It should also be clear that the parasympathetic nervous system is characterized by relatively long preganglionic and very short postganglionic fibers and that the well-defined, anatomically distinct ganglia of the sympathetic nervous system are not, with only a few exceptions, major features of the parasympathetic. Finally, as shown in Figure 5-1 and Table 5-1, some organs are dually innervated, for example, the salivary glands, heart, lungs (bronchial muscle), and abdominal and pelvic viscera, whereas other organs receive innervation from only one division. The sweat glands, adrenal medulla, piloerectors, and most of the blood vessels receive innervation from only the sympathetic nervous system. On the other hand, the paren-chyma of the parotid, lacrimal, and nasopharyngeal glands are supplied only with parasympathetic fibers.

Functional characteristics

Table 5-1 lists the organs to which fibers of the parasympathetic and sympathetic nervous systems are distributed, the effects of stimulation of these fibers, and the kinds of receptors that have been identified. In order to understand or predict the effects of autonomic drugs on a specific organ, it is necessary to know not only how each division of the autonomic nervous system affects that organ but also whether the organ is singly or dually innervated and, if dually, which of the two systems is dominant in the organ. In certain circumstances, one or the other of the two divisions may provide the dominant influence, but it should be noted that a fine push-pull adjustment exists between the two divisions in many of the dually innervated organs. The role of the two divisions in modulating intrinsic activity of the various tissues cannot be overemphasized.

The anatomical and functional characteristics of the two divisions should make it clear that there are striking differences between the sympathetic and parasympathetic nervous systems. Cannon was the first to recognize that the sympathetic nervous system is capable of producing the kind of widespread and massive response that would enable an organism confronted with a sudden emergency (such as pain, asphyxia, or strong emotions) to mount an appropriate response (i.e., either "fright, fight, or flight").[12] On the other hand, the parasympathetic division is primarily concerned with the protection, conservation, and restoration of bodily resources. These differences in function are subserved by some of the anatomical characteristics that have already been mentioned, that is, the involvement of the adrenal medulla and the high ratio of postganglionic to preganglionic fibers in the sympathetic nervous system, but they are also subserved by the characteristics of the chemical mediators for the two systems.

NEUROTRANSMITTERS OF THE SYMPATHETIC AND PARASYMPATHETIC NERVOUS SYSTEMS

The concept that transmission in the autonomic nervous system is accompanied by the release of chemical mediators emerged at the end of the nineteenth and the beginning of the twentieth century.

Table 5-1. Responses of various effectors to stimulation by autonomic nerves

Effector	Sympathetic Response	Receptor	Parasympathetic response
Eye			
Radial muscle of the iris	Contraction (mydriasis)	α	—
Sphincter of the iris	—		Contraction (miosis)
Ciliary muscle	Slight relaxation (far vision)	β_2	Contraction (near vision)
Heart			
S-A node	Increase in rate	β_1	Decrease in rate
Atria	Increased contractility and conduction velocity	β_1	Decreased contractility, usually increased conduction velocity
A-V node	Increase in automaticity and conduction velocity	β_1	Decrease in conduction velocity
Ventricles	Increased contractility, conduction velocity, and automaticity	β_1	—
Blood vessels			
Coronary	Functional significance is doubtful	α, β_2	Same as sympathetic
Skin and mucosa	Constriction	α	Dilation, but of questionable significance
Skeletal muscle	Constriction, dilation	α, β_2	*
Abdominal viscera	Constriction, dilation	α, β_2	—
Salivary glands	Constriction	α	Dilation
Erectile tissue	Constriction	α	Dilation
Lungs			
Bronchial smooth muscle	Relaxation	β_2	Constriction
Bronchial glands	—		Stimulation of secretion
Gastrointestinal tract			
Smooth muscle	Decreased motility and tone	β_2, α	Increased motility and tone
Sphincters	Contraction	α	Relaxation
Secretion	—		Stimulation
Salivary glands	Vicous secretion, amylase secretion†	α, β	Profuse, watery secretion
Spleen capsule	Contraction, mild relaxation	α, β_2	
Urinary bladder			
Detrusor	Relaxation	β	Contraction
Trigone and sphincter	Contraction	α	Relaxation
Ureter			
Motility and tone	Increased	α	Increased (?)
Uterus	Variable, depending on species, endocrine status, etc.	α, β_2	Variable
Skin			
Pilomotor muscles	Contraction	α	—
Sweat glands‡	Secretion		—
Liver	Glycogenolysis, gluconeogenesis, etc.	α, β_2	Glycogen synthesis
Adipose tissue	Lipolysis	α, β_1	

*Skeletal muscle receives some cholinergic fibers of sympathetic origin that cause vasodilation.
†The parotid glands do not receive adrenergic fibers.
‡The sweat glands are supplied with postganglionic fibers of the sympathetic nervous system, but the transmitter is acetylcholine and the receptors are classified as muscarinic.

Of particular note was the observation by Elliott in 1905 that an injection of adrenal medullary extract produced effects very similar to those obtained by stimulation of sympathetic nerves.[24] Elliott suggested that minute quantities of a substance related to adrenal medullary extract might be released during sympathetic nerve stimulation. Other investigators, studying the properties of acetylcholine, the alkaloid muscarine, and some congeners of acetylcholine, noted a correspondence between parasympathetic stimulation and drugs resembling acetylcholine.[17,21,37] In 1921, Loewi demonstrated in a brilliant yet basically simple experiment that the slowing produced by vagal stimulation in a perfused frog heart could be produced in a recipient frog heart by exposing it to the perfusate from the donor heart.[44] Loewi deduced from this that a substance, which he called *Vagusstoff*, was released from vagal nerve endings during stimulation. This "vagus substance" was subsequently identified as acetylcholine by Loewi and Navratil.[45] In Loewi's earlier experiment, he also demonstrated in the same preparation the release of an accelerator substance when the cardiac accelerator or sympathetic nerves were stimulated. While the mediator for the parasympathetic nervous system was clearly identified as acetylcholine by 1926, the mediators for the sympathetic nervous system were characterized only as sympathin E and sympathin I, compounds that were thought to be very similar to epinephrine but not necessarily identical with it.[13] In 1947, von Euler presented evidence that the substance in the adrenergic nerve terminal is norepinephrine,[26] and subsequently he, as well as others, showed that epinephrine is the chief mediator released from the adrenal medulla.[27] Thus, over this half century the basic concept of neurohumoral transmission was developed. At its simplest, the theory holds that conduction in any part of the nervous system, whether from one nerve to another or from a nerve to an effector organ, is accompanied by the release of a specific molecule that can, by attaching to the receptor site, alter the permeability of the nerve cell or effector membrane. This concept applies to the effectors of the autonomic nervous system, to the adrenal medulla, to ganglia, to skeletal muscle, and even to the central nervous system, where evidence has been accumulating that a variety of transmitters are involved not only in normal CNS function but in disorders of the central nervous system such as Parkinson's disease,[34] schizophrenia, and depressive psychoses.[51]

While acetylcholine, norepinephrine, epinephrine, and more recently dopamine[54] have come to be recognized as the principal mediators of autonomic nervous activity and are ubiquitous throughout the central nervous system, considerable evidence exists that other molecules serve as chemical transmitters for specific neuronal circuits. Among these are bradykinin, histamine, 5-hydroxytryptamine (serotonin, 5-HT), γ-aminobutyric acid (GABA), prostaglandins, aspartate, adenosine triphosphate (ATP), glutamate, and glycine.[16,23,60] The criteria for establishing that a particular molecule is a transmitter at a given synapse have been described as follows:[22]

1. The specific molecule must be liberated from activated terminals.
2. The neuron must contain both the substance and the enzymes necessary for its synthesis.

3. It must be possible to demonstrate the presence in the axon terminal of synaptic vesicles in close relationship to the synaptic membrane.
4. There must be a mechanism for inactivation of the transmitter; this may involve an enzyme, a reuptake mechanism, or both.
5. Exogenous application of the substance to a receptor should produce the same effects as the transmitter does when it is released by nerve stimulation.
6. Drugs that decrease or increase nerve-mediated responses should have a similar effect on responses to exogenously applied transmitter.

GENERAL SCHEME OF CHEMICAL MEDIATION

The present concept of neurohumoral transmission arises out of the work of Hodgkin and Huxley[33] and is shown in a schematic representation adapted from the work of Hubbard[35] (Figure 5-3). In this scheme, when an action potential reaches the nerve axon terminal, it causes a massive depolarization of the membrane, and stored transmitter is released into the synaptic cleft. The transmitter crosses the synaptic cleft, a distance usually of 20 to 40 nm (200 to 400 Å), and attaches to a specific site on the postsynaptic membrane, which could be located on a ganglion cell, a striated muscle fiber, an autonomic effector, or a cell in the central nervous system. To this basic conception of the manner in which the neurotransmitter leaves the neuron terminal, traverses the synaptic membranes, and attaches to the postsynaptic receptor site various refinements have been added over the years. Katz and Miledi,[41] for instance, proposed the calcium hypothesis, in which the depolarization of the terminal brings about an increase in the permeability of the plasma membrane to calcium. Entry of calcium into the terminal causes a rise in the intraneuronal concentration of Ca^{++}, and this triggers the release of the transmitter. More recently, the identification of calmodulin, a major Ca^{++}-receptor protein (capable of combining with four calcium ions) has led to the proposal that it plays an important role in neurotransmitter release. This has been strengthened by experiments that have shown that calmodulin is present in the nerve terminal, is bound to synaptic vesicles, and therefore exists in very close proximity to the presynaptic membrane.[19] At the present time, it is postulated

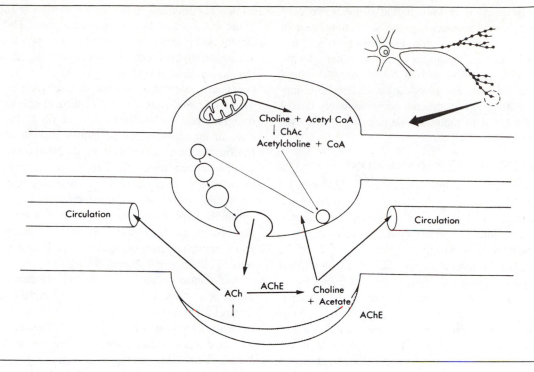

Figure 5-3. Autonomic cholinergic nerve terminal and its effector, in which are shown the intraneuronal synthesis of ACh, the vesicles containing ACh, the discharge of ACh into the synaptic cleft, and the removal of ACh from the receptor by the action of AChE and by diffusion. ACh = acetylcholine, CoA = coenzyme A, ChAc = choline acetylase (sometimes choline acetyltransferase), AChE = acetylcholinesterase. (Adapted from Hubbard, J.I. Annals of the New York Academy of Sciences **183**:131-146, 1971.)

that after depolarization, Ca^{++} enters the nerve terminal and is immediately bound to calmodulin near the membrane. Calmodulin then activates a vesicle-bound protein kinase system that phosphorylates several synaptic vesicle proteins and modulates the Ca^{++}-stimulated release of norepinephrine and ACh from isolated vesicles.

The combination of mediator with receptor is a reversible one and may either increase permeability of the membrane to all ions or selectively increase permeability only to smaller ions. In the first case, the result will be an excitatory postsynaptic potential (EPSP), and in the second case, an inhibitory postsynaptic potential (IPSP). Eccles has demonstrated that the mediator may also cause a prolonged depolarization of the presynaptic membrane, thereby bringing about a decrease in the amount of transmitter released by the terminal and an apparent inhibition.[23] An EPSP will initiate activity in the effector, whether it be a ganglion cell, a smooth muscle, or a secretory cell. An IPSP will tend to inhibit excitatory impulses arriving at the same site. In a very short time the mediator is

removed from the receptor site by a variety of mechanisms: metabolism by specific enzymes, diffusion from the synaptic area into the systemic circulation, uptake and binding by postjunctional tissues, and active reuptake by the nerve terminal. In order for the axon terminal to respond to repetitive stimulation by the rapid release of stored mediator, mechanisms must exist by which the transmitter is continuously resynthesized and stored.

Recently attention has been focused on the fact that certain neurons release more than one transmitter, as, for instance, serotonin with dopamine, norepinephrine with ACh, and dopamine with transmitter-like peptides. When this occurs, it is possible that the two transmitters have different functions, one functioning as a transmitter and the other as a modulator, or that they act cooperatively as transmitters to elicit some physiologic response. The nature and location of the receptors on which they act are still undetermined; they could be on different postsynaptic sites, on the same site, or on the presynaptic receptor of one cell and the postsynaptic receptor of another.[49] Finally, in another arrangement, it is known that some nerve cells release two substances at the same time, one of them being a transmitter and the other not. Examples are catecholamines with ATP, norepinephrine with peptides, and ACh with acetylcholinesterase (AChE). The physiologic role of these nontransmitters is not understood; presumably one of their roles is to maintain the integrity of the synapse.[14]

ADRENERGIC TRANSMISSION*

In the three quarters of a century that has elapsed since Elliott first suggested that a substance related to adrenal medullary secretions might be released on sympathetic nerve stimulation, an enormous amount of information has been amassed on the nature of the adrenergic terminal, its mediator, and the postjunctional receptors. As mentioned previously, von Euler first recognized that norepinephrine is the transmitter for the sympathetic nervous system; but much earlier a pathway had been proposed for the synthesis of norepinephrine in the nerve terminal.[6,7] This synthetic process, shown in Figure 5-4, involves a number of enzymes that are synthesized in the perikaryon and carried by tubular transport mechanisms to the nerve endings. The enzyme tyrosine hydroxylase, which catalyzes the conversion of tyrosine to dihydroxyphenylalanine (dopa), is the rate-limiting enzyme in this process; any drugs that affect the function of tyrosine hydroxylase will affect the rate at which norepinephrine is produced in the nerve terminal. It appears too that the concentration of norepinephrine in the axoplasm is one of the factors that regulates its own formation, principally through an inhibitory effect on tyrosine hydroxylase activity and, as shall be described, probably mediated by a presynaptically located adrenergic receptor.[47] The enzyme phenylethanolamine-N-methyltransferase (PNMT), which catalyzes the conversion of norepinephrine to epinephrine, occurs almost exclusively in the chromaffin cells of the adrenal medulla and is therefore missing in peripheral nerve terminals.[4] Hence, norepinephrine is the final step in the synthetic process in most adrenergic nerves.

The evidence at present suggests that 90% to 95% of the neurotransmitter is sequestered in small granulated vesicles, where it is protected from intracellular enzymatic destruction until it is released

on neural command, whereas 5% to 10% is found in the axoplasm or presynaptic membrane. The vesicular norepinephrine is stored in a complex with adenosine triphosphate, chromogranin, the enzyme dopamine β-hydroxylase, and Mg^{++}-, Ca^{++}-dependent adenosine triphosphatase (ATPase).[53] There are two different norepinephrine pools inside the granule: a mobile and a reserve pool. The arrival of an action potential causes release of the transmitter from the mobile pool. Newly synthesized norepinephrine would appear to compose the mobile pool, because it is preferentially released on neural command.[59] The function of the small cytoplasmic pool, and its relationship to vesicular norepinephrine, is not well understood. A diagrammatic representation of the adrenergic nerve terminal is shown in Figure 5-5.

Autonomic nerve terminals and effector junctions are less structurally organized than the classic myoneuronal junction. The axon resembles a string of beads as it passes among smooth muscle fibers in blood vessels and intestines (see top right of Figure 5-5). The beaded varicosities release the transmitter near relatively few directly innervated smooth muscle or glandular cells. Most of the effector cells are either directly or indirectly coupled to those cells that are innervated. As the nerve impulse passes down the axon and depolarization successively involves each varicosity, extracellular Ca^{++} is taken into the terminals, and norepinephrine is released into the synaptic cleft by a process of exocytosis. The cleft distances in both the sympathetic and parasympathetic nervous systems are quite variable, ranging from 15 nm (150Å) up to many hundreds, depending on the relative development of the junction.[5,53] The transmitter then crosses the synaptic cleft and becomes attached to receptor sites on the effector organ. The nature of these receptor sites and the way in which the receptor-agonist combination is translated into a response will be described in some detail below.

The fate of the released transmitter, and the resultant termination of its action on the effector organ, is quite different from that which occurs at cholinergic nerve synapses. At adrenergic synapses, enzymatic destruction of the transmitter normally plays a relatively minor role. Uptake of the transmitter accounts for the greatest proportion of the transmitter, with enzymatic transformation and diffusion away from the synapse responsible for only a small percentage of the total. Uptake can be neuronal (uptake 1) or extraneuronal (uptake

---

*This section was written by Enid A. Neidle and Donald C. Kroeger.

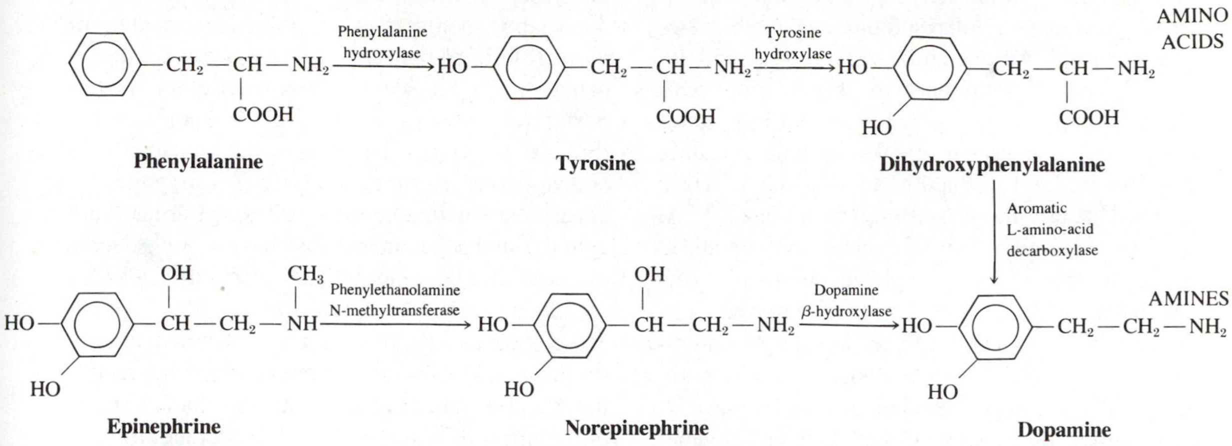

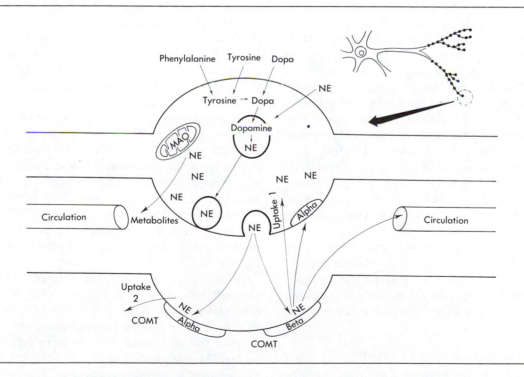

Figure 5-4. Biosynthesis of adrenergic transmitters in the neuron terminal. The amino acids in the top row can penetrate the blood-brain barrier, while the compounds shown in the bottom row cannot. Conversion of dopamine to norepinephrine takes place in the granules, while conversion of norepinephrine to epinephrine occurs only in the adrenal medulla and in some neurons of the central nervous system.

Figure 5-5. Adrenergic nerve terminal and its effector. The diagram shows the precursors of norepinephrine, the sites of synthesis and storage of dopamine and norepinephrine, the enzymes principally responsible for biotransformation of norepinephrine, and the location and variety of adrenergic receptors. It also shows the mechanisms by which the action of norepinephrine is terminated. Dopa = dihydroxyphenylalanine, NE = norepinephrine, MAO = monoamine oxidase, COMT = catechol-O-methyltransferase.

2).[38] Uptake 1 is an active process that requires energy and extracellular sodium and exhibits stereospecificity. Amphetamines, tyramine, and levonordefrin (α-methylnorepinephrine) are examples of chemicals that are taken up by this system. Inhibitors of neuronal uptake include cocaine, imipramine, and guanethidine. Uptake 2 has a greater capacity but less affinity than uptake 1. At high concentrations of norepinephrine, uptake 2 results in the relatively rapid metabolism of the transmitter. Uptake 2 is sometimes referred to as the cocaine-insensitive uptake. Uptake of norepinephrine into the membrane-bound storage granules within the nerve terminal also takes place. It is an active process, requiring ATP and magnesium, and it is by this mechanism that norepinephrine and structurally related compounds (such as the vasoconstrictors that are added to local anesthetic solutions) are returned to the membrane-bound vesicles. The drug best known for its ability to inhibit this transfer of norepinephrine and related compounds from the cytoplasm to storage vesicles is reserpine.

In the cytoplasmic pool, the transmitter is susceptible to the enzymatic action of a mitochondrial enzyme, monoamine oxidase (MAO), that is capable of deaminating the molecule. While MAO is widely distributed through the body, especially in the liver, kidney, and brain, it is chiefly associated with the mitochondria of the adrenergic nerve terminals and is viewed as the principal intraneuronal enzyme concerned with the transformation of norepinephrine. Certain drugs are capable of inhibiting MAO, leading to an accumulation of the transmitter in the nerve terminal, an effect that has both physiologic and therapeutic implications. A second enzyme concerned with the transformation of norepinephrine is catechol-O-methyltransferase (COMT). It is widely distributed in the tissues, again particularly in the liver and kidney, and is believed to be closely associated with the receptor. COMT is regarded as the principal extraneuronal enzyme involved with the metabolism of norepinephrine. Inhibition of COMT has no current therapeutic importance.

The nature of adrenergic receptors

In 1948, Ahlquist proposed that there might be two kinds of adrenergic receptors. He called these alpha (α) and beta (β).[1] Two subtypes of the β receptor, called β_1 and β_2, were identified by Lands and others[42] in 1967, and evidence has mounted for two different α receptors, one located on the postsynaptic membrane (α_1) and the other on the presynaptic membrane (α_2).[55] The identification of these different adrenergic receptors provides an explanation for the seemingly contradictory (or opposing) actions of the adrenergic transmitters (as, for instance, vasodilation in some vascular beds and vasoconstriction in others) and is supported by experiments with recently synthesized drugs (both agonists and antagonists) that have a high degree of specificity for one but not necessarily all four of the currently accepted adrenergic receptors. More recently, studies with radiolabeled ligands (radioactively labeled compounds that interact at the receptor site and demonstrate the characteristics of the drug- or hormone-receptor interaction) have proved to be valuable tools in the characterization and classification of receptors. Such studies have employed relatively purified cell membranes from mammalian and nonmammalian tissues (e.g., human platelets, rat heart, turkey erythrocytes) that obviate problems associated with diffusion of drugs to receptors and loss due to metabolism or cellular uptake. In this way accurate data on the affinities of receptors for agonists and antagonists have been acquired for all four receptor subtypes.

It has been possible, using recently developed techniques, to describe the fine structure of some receptors. Thus a proposed model for the β_2 receptor consists of a dimer with each identical subunit containing a catecholamine binding site and having a molecular weight of 58,000. A model for the β_1 receptor of the dog heart gives it a molecular weight of 65,000 to 70,000 and visualizes it as a monomer with a single binding site. Preliminary data on the α_1 receptor indicate a dimeric structure, each subunit having a molecular weight of 85,000. Similar data regarding the muscarinic receptor (mChR) suggest that the α_1 receptor and mChR are structurally related and, in fact, that neurotransmitter receptors may have evolved from a common ancestor.[57]

As can be seen in Table 5-1, some organs are provided with one kind of receptor, while others have several kinds. Receptors of the subtype α_2 have been located on the axon terminal, and it is believed that previously released norepinephrine acts on the presynaptic receptors to inhibit transmitter release by subsequent impulses. This theory is supported, for instance, by the observation that drugs that block these α_2 receptors (e.g., phenoxybenzamine) cause an increase in the efflux of transmitter in response to nerve stimulation.[55] It is worth noting, however, that evidence has been presented

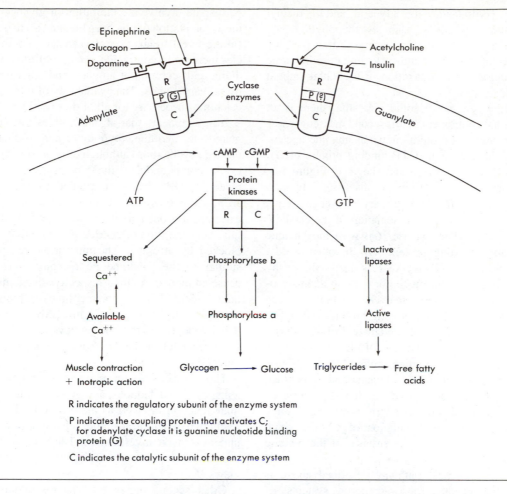

Figure 5-6. Sites of action of primary messengers, such as epinephrine, glucagon, and ACh, and their role in regulating the formation of second messengers in target cells. The agonist plus the receptor (R) causes cyclase enzymes (C), activated by a binding protein (P), to catalyze the conversion of ATP to cAMP. cAMP stimulates the protein kinases to regulate cytoplasmic Ca^{++}, phosphorylase a (via another enzyme, phosphorylase kinase), and lipase activities (vertical arrows on the left). cGMP, produced in a cascade of reactions similar to that described for cAMP and involving a different binding protein, has opposite effects (vertical arrows on the right).

recently to cast doubt on this hypothesis.[39]

The α_1-receptor response is characterized by a fairly rapid depolarization of the postjunctional membrane and a change in permeability to ions, but the course of the reaction is not as rapid as that seen at the myoneural junction. Responses to β-receptor activation are relatively small in amplitude but of a much longer course than that for α_1 receptors.[46]

Second messengers

The identification of the adrenergic neurotransmitter and the receptors with which it interacts did not answer the question of how the receptor-agonist interaction triggers an intracellular response.

Transmitters, or primary messengers such as acetylcholine and norepinephrine, histamine, and a variety of hormones have been known for a long time, but it was not until Sutherland and his coworkers isolated an enzyme system activated by epinephrine that the concept of second messengers became established. As shown in Figure 5-6, the second messenger theory holds that the combination of epinephrine with the receptor activates an enzyme, adenylate cyclase, located in the membrane, and that the enzyme in turn converts ATP into 3′-5′ adenosine monophosphate (cAMP).[56] Once formed, cAMP is subject to breakdown by a second enzyme, phosphodiesterase. Inhibition of this enzyme preserves and prolongs the life of cAMP. Hydralazine, nitroglycerin, and the methyl xanthine derivatives such as theophylline are known to inhibit phosphodiesterase,[2] thus possibly accounting for their ability to imitate adrenergic stimulation, as in relaxation of bronchial smooth muscle.

Recently it has become clear that there is an additional component in this second messenger system, a coupling protein known as guanine nucleotide binding protein (GTP binding protein or *G*). As currently visualized and shown in Figure 5-6, adenylate cyclase activity results from activation of a receptor *(R)* by a primary messenger (e.g., epinephrine) and from association of the catalytic moiety, adenylate cyclase *(C)*, with the guanine nucleotide binding protein *(G)*. In other words, conversion of ATP to cAMP is accomplished by the combination of a receptor with an agonist, together acting on adenylate cyclase, which has been activated by the GTP binding protein. Adenylate cyclase activity is terminated by hydrolysis of GTP to guanosine diphosphate (GDP) by a GTPase. A deficiency in GTP binding protein has been found in 45% of patients with a clinical condition known as type I hypoparathyroidism. It is hypothesized that parathyroid hormone exerts its effect on kidney and bone through stimulation of cAMP, which would be deficient in the absence of the binding protein.[28]

The biochemical pathway described above is generally accepted for β-adrenergic systems; α-adrenergic receptors are not as well understood. It is known that $α_2$-adrenergic receptor activation leads to inhibition of adenylate cyclase experimentally and therefore to decreased cAMP concentrations.[43] This effect is probably mediated by a GTP inhibitory protein that presumably inhibits the association of adenylate cyclase and GTP binding protein.

The manner in which cAMP acts is still under investigation, but it is known to participate in the activation of a group of enzymes, the protein kinases. These kinases catalyze the phosphorylation of other enzymes, using ATP as the energy source. Protein kinases, like the cyclase enzymes, occur as an association of regulatory and catalytic subunits. It is conjectured that the combination of cAMP with the regulatory subunit of a protein kinase allows activation of its catalytic subunit or, in certain situations, association with the catalytic subunit to form an inactive enzyme complex.

Some of the roles in which cAMP is known to participate involve the inhibition of glycogen synthesis, activation of glycogen breakdown to glucose (in the liver), relaxation of vascular smooth muscle, increase in contractile strength of the myocardium, and secretion of amylase and other proteins by salivary glands. The availability of intracellular calcium is necessary for all of these actions.[3,11,25,52]

It now appears that all nucleotides (adenosine, guanosine, cytidine, thymidine, and uridine) can undergo cyclization, although only one other of the cyclic compounds, cyclic guanosine monophosphate (cGMP), has been studied to any extent. ACh, acting on cortical brain slices or on the myocardium, has been shown to increase the intracellular concentration of cGMP, an action that can be blocked by atropine. The muscarinic receptor is similar to the β-adrenergic receptor since both cause an increase in their respective cyclic nucleotides.[32] (Stimulation of the nicotinic receptors does not cause any such changes in cGMP or cAMP.) It is hypothesized that the two cyclic nucleotides, cAMP and cGMP, have opposing actions on some intracellular functions.

The roles of calcium, calmodulin, binding proteins, cyclic nucleotides, and prostaglandins in cellular function, as well as more specifically in the regulation of neurotransmitter release, are currently under extensive investigation. The interested reader is advised to consult one of many available reviews.[58]

Other second messenger systems undoubtedly exist besides the cyclic nucleotides, such as calcium and the prostaglandins. Further studies are needed to understand this interesting new field of cell physiology.

DOPAMINERGIC TRANSMISSION

It is now known that dopaminergic receptors exist outside the central nervous system, almost certainly in the kidney (where their activation leads to vasodilation) and possibly in the mesenteric bed, the coronary vessels, and other vascular and nonvascular smooth muscle. Identification of these dopamine receptors has been made possible in recent years through the discovery that a number of psychoactive drugs (e.g., haloperidol and chlorpromazine) are dopamine antagonists. The discovery of dopamine receptors in the periphery has led to the application of dopamine to a number of clinical situations, as for instance in the treatment of cardiogenic shock and renal failure, where it has the capacity to increase renal blood flow without causing vasodepressor effects.[31] The existence of dopaminergic nerves in the periphery is less settled; one location where dopamine may be a transmitter is the gastrointestinal tract. Most of the evidence to date indicates that dopamine is synthesized, stored, released, and taken up in a manner similar to, if not identical with, that involving norepinephrine.[30] The response to dopamine in brain studies indicates that cAMP is involved; however, the adenylate cyclase receptor for dopamine is different from the conventional β receptor in that it does not bind epinephrine.

CHOLINERGIC TRANSMISSION

The general scheme of chemical mediation presented previously applies in all its particulars to the cholinergic synapse of the autonomic nervous system. As shown in Figure 5-3, the conversion of choline to ACh in the neuron terminal is accomplished by the enzyme choline acetyltransferase (or choline acetylase).[48] The mitochondrial cofactor acetyl coenzyme A serves as the acetyl group donor for the reaction. The newly synthesized ACh is then stored in vesicles[20,36] that carry a charge and are enveloped by a ring of water molecules. The vesicles move toward the membrane, eventually making contact with it; on the arrival of a nerve action potential, the contents of the vesicles are released by a process of exocytosis and cross the synaptic gap.[35] The transmitter ACh attaches reversibly to the protein receptor,[50] which exists in very close proximity to a highly specific enzyme, AChE.[15] ACh becomes closely associated with the enzyme at two possible sites (see Figure 8-3) and is hydrolyzed into choline and acetate at such a rapid rate that the nerve can respond to another stimulus milliseconds later. AChE is believed to be located on or within the folds of the postsynaptic membrane[35] or highly concentrated in the endplate region.[18] But, even in the total absence or inactivity of this highly specific enzyme, the action of ACh can be terminated very quickly by a nonspecific plasma enzyme, pseudocholinesterase, also known as butyrocholinesterase (BuChE), which is found in many tissues, including blood. ACh is also removed by the simple process of diffusion. The choline produced by the action of AChE is then returned to the nerve terminal by means of a carrier mechanism and is once more used in the synthesis of ACh.

Each vesicle is considered to contain a uniform packet or quantum of ACh corresponding to several thousand molecules.[29] Under resting conditions, a single quantum may be released, leading to the appearance of a miniature endplate potential (MEPP). When a nerve action potential arrives at the terminal, many quanta (100 to 200) are released, leading to an endplate potential (EPP).[40]

PURINERGIC TRANSMISSION

Evidence has accumulated that there are noncholinergic, nonadrenergic nerves, designated as purinergic, that are found in the gastrointestinal tract of all vertebrates as well as in certain areas of the central nervous system, the vascular system, and the lungs, trachea, and bladder.[10] It was visualized that ATP is stored in vesicles in the nerve terminal and when released engages purinergic receptors, prior to being broken down to adenosine. In 1978 Burnstock proposed two purinergic receptors in the periphery, P_1 purine receptors, which are sensitive to adenosine and would constitute presynaptic receptors, and P_2 purine receptors, which are responsive to ATP and constitute the postsynaptic receptors.[9] It was further postulated that adenosine, by reducing the available Ca^{++}, suppresses the release of transmitter from nerve terminals. Other purine and pyrimidine nucleotides are able to activate the postsynaptic receptor in the guinea pig ileum, thus producing relaxation,[8] but these compounds are considerably less potent than ATP.

LOCATION OF ADRENERGIC AND CHOLINERGIC SYNAPSES

Figure 5-7 shows the sites at which ACh and norepinephrine are mediators. (Dopaminergic and purinergic receptors are not shown.) It should be clear from this diagram that, with the exception of effectors that receive postganglionic fibers of the sympathetic nervous system where the mediator is norepinephrine, all other sites are cholinergic, including the ganglia of the autonomic nervous system, the adrenal medulla, certain effectors of the sympathetic nervous system, and all the effectors of the parasympathetic nervous system. That these ubiquitous cholinergic receptors are not identical has become increasingly evident, beginning with the observation that administration of the alkaloid muscarine could duplicate the effects of vagal stimulation. Subsequently, it was found that muscarine mimics the activation of postganglionic parasympathetic and cholinergic sympathetic fibers and most cholinergic neurons in the central nervous sys-

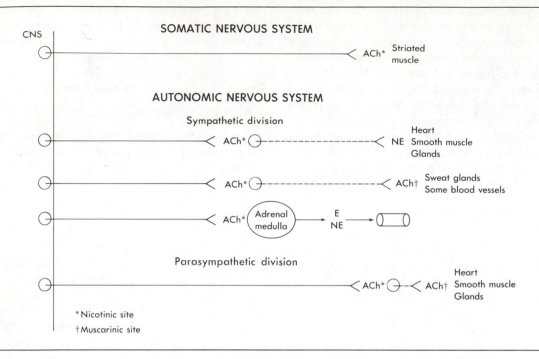

Figure 5-7. Fibers of the somatic and autonomic nervous systems, with the structures innervated by the different fibers and the chemical mediators responsible for transmission at the various loci. Dashed lines indicate postganglionic autonomic fibers. (ACh = acetylcholine, E = epinephrine, NE = norepinephrine.)

Table 5-2. Cholinergic agonists and antagonists and their sites of action

	Transmitter	Antagonist(s)	Other agonists
Muscarinic sites			
Parasympathetic effectors	ACh	Atropine	Muscarine, bethanechol
Some sympathetic effectors	ACh	Atropine	Muscarine, bethanechol
Most CNS neurons	ACh	Atropine	Muscarine, oxotremorine
Nicotinic sites			
All autonomic ganglia, including adrenal medulla	ACh	Hexamethonium (C-6), tubocurarine*	Nicotine, dimethylphenylpiperazinium
Skeletal muscle	ACh	Tubocurarine, decamethonium (C-10)	Nicotine, phenyltrimethylammonium
Some CNS neurons	ACh	Tubocurarine	Carbachol

*At higher than normal doses.

tem, effects that can be antagonized by atropine. The alkaloid nicotine mimics the effects of ACh at a larger number of loci, including autonomic ganglia, the adrenal medulla, skeletal muscle, and some neurons in the central nervous system. Dale introduced the term *muscarinic* to describe the action of ACh or related compounds at postganglionic sites and the term *nicotinic* to describe its actions at other sites.[17] The differences in these receptors have been further substantiated by the discovery that there are agonists that have an affinity for muscarinic but not nicotinic sites and that there are blocking agents or antagonists that are similarly effective at one but not the other site. In fact, certain agonists and antagonists are specific for only one kind of nicotinic receptor, as is shown in Table 5-2.

Table 5-3. Some autonomic drugs listed according to mechanism and site of action

Mechanism of action	Site of action	
	Cholinergic synapses	Adrenergic synapses
Interfere with synthesis of transmitter	Hemicholinium	Metyrosine
Cause formation of "false" transmitter	—	Methyldopa
Prevent release of transmitter	Botulinus toxin	Bretylium
Prevent reuptake of transmitter from synapse	—	Imipramine, amitriptyline, cocaine
Prevent reincorporation of transmitter in storage vesicles	—	Reserpine
Cause rapid release of transmitter	Carbachol	Tyramine, amphetamine
Cause slow release of transmitter	—	Guanethidine
Occupy postsynaptic receptor site	Muscarinic: choline esters, cholinomimetic alkaloids Nicotinic: nicotine	α_1 receptor: phenylephrine; α_2 receptor: clonidine; β_1 and β_2 receptors: isoproterenol; β_2 receptor: metaproterenol
Block access of transmitter to receptor site	Muscarinic: atropine Nicotinic: tubocurarine, hexamethonium	α_1 and α_2 receptors: phenoxybenzamine; α_1 receptor: prazosin; α_2 receptor: yohimbine; β_1 and β_2 receptors: propranolol; β_1 receptor: metoprolol
Inhibit enzymatic breakdown of transmitter	Physostigmine, isoflurophate	MAO inhibitors (tranylcypromine, pargyline)

CENTRAL CONTROL OF AUTONOMIC FUNCTION

Virtually all levels of the central nervous system contribute significantly to the regulation of the autonomic nervous system—from the spinal cord and brainstem, where reflexes regulating blood pressure are integrated, to the higher centers in the hypothalamus, limbic system, and cerebral cortex, which integrate very complex autonomic responses involved in behavior, reproduction, and emotional states. While the precise location of "centers" that regulate such functions as blood pressure, respiration, micturition, and sweating are the province of a physiology textbook, it is appropriate to point out that the hypothalamus plays a very important role in the integration of responses to changes in temperature, emotional states, and patterns of sexual and reproductive activity, all of which involve integration of the endocrine, autonomic, and somatic nervous systems. Furthermore, the limbic system has been shown, through stimulation experiments, to cause changes in blood pressure, sexual activity, rage-like responses, and a host of other reactions characteristic of autonomic nervous system stimulation. Thus, it is currently believed that the limbic system plays an important role in patterns of sexual activity and states of rage and fear and that its effects may be superimposed on those exerted by the hypothalamus. The cerebellum and the cerebral cortex also make contributions to patterns of autonomic activity, but their importance is less than that of the hypothalamus.

SPECIFIC SITES AND MECHANISMS OF ACTION OF AUTONOMIC DRUGS

The foregoing sections of this chapter have shown that transmission in the autonomic nervous system, and therefore normal function of the two autonomic divisions, depends on a number of integrated steps, including synthesis of mediator, release of mediator, combination of the transmitter with the receptor, destruction by highly specific enzymes, or reuptake and reincorporation of mediator in the nerve terminal. The explosion of knowledge about the function of the autonomic nervous system at the neuronal level has been accompanied by the discovery and development of drugs that interfere with one or several steps in the complex processes described in the earlier sections on cholinergic and adrenergic transmission.

Some of these drugs, and their specific mechanisms and sites of action, are listed in Table 5-3. Their pharmacology is described in the appropriate sections of the text. But, with a working knowledge of the autonomic nervous system and the role it plays in the normal function of the various organs, it is possible to predict what effects a drug with a known mechanism of action would have. A single example will perhaps make this point clear. If a drug (in this instance reserpine) prevents norepinephrine from being transferred from the cytoplasm of the neuron terminal to the storage granules, it is reasonable to expect that the norepinephrine that has been taken back from the synaptic cleft will remain in the cytoplasm. Here it will be subject to the destructive action of MAO, and in time (a remarkably short time, in fact) the stores of norepinephrine will be degraded, leaving adrenergic terminals throughout the body depleted of norepinephrine. It is finally possible to predict that the depletion of norepinephrine throughout the sympathetic nervous system will place the animal under the control of the parasympathetic system, entirely unopposed by the sympathetic. Thus, the pupils will be constricted, there will be copious secretion of watery saliva, and gastrointestinal motility and secretion will be increased.

CITED REFERENCES

1. Ahlquist, R.P. A study of adrenotropic receptors. American Journal of Physiology **153**:586-600, 1948.
2. Andersson, R. Cyclic AMP as a mediator of the relaxing action of papaverine, nitroglycerine, diazoxide, and hydralazine in intestinal and vascular smooth muscle. Acta Pharmacologica et Toxicologica **32**:321-336, 1973.
3. Andersson, R., and Nilsson, K. Cyclic AMP and calcium in relaxation in intestinal smooth muscle. Nature **238**:119-120, 1972.
4. Axelrod, J. Purification and properties of phenylethanol-amine-N-methyl-transferase. Journal of Biological Chemistry **237**:1657-1660, 1962.
5. Bevan, J.A. Some functional consequences of variation in adrenergic synaptic cleft width and on nerve density and distribution. Federation Proceedings **36**:2439-2443, 1978.
6. Blaschko, H. The specific action of *l*-dopa decarboxylase. Journal of Physiology **96**:50P, 1939.
7. Blaschko, H. Catecholamine biosynthesis. British Medical Bulletin **29**:105-109, 1973.
8. Brown, C.M., and Burnstock, G. The structural conformation of the polyphosphate chain of the ATP molecule is critical for its promotion of prostaglandin biosynthesis. European Journal of Pharmacology **69**:81-86, 1981.
9. Burnstock, G. A basis for distinguishing two types of purinergic receptor. In Straub, R.W., and Bolis, L. eds. Cell Membrane Receptors for Drugs and Hormones: a Multi-Disciplinary Approach. New York, Raven Press, 1978.
10. Burnstock, G., Campbell, G., Satchell, D., and Smythe, A. Evidence that adenosine triphosphate or a related nucleotide is the transmitter substance released by non-adrenergic inhibitory nerves in the gut. British Journal of Pharmacology and Chemotherapy **40**:668-688, 1970.
11. Butcher, F.R. The role of calcium and cyclic nucleotides in α-amylase release from slices of rat parotid: studies with the divalent cation ionophore A-23187. Metabolism **24**:409-418, 1975.
12. Cannon, W.B. Bodily Changes in Pain, Hunger, Fear, and Rage, ed. 2. New York, D. Appleton-Century Co., 1929.
13. Cannon, W.B., and Rosenblueth, A. A comparison of the effects of sympathin and adrenin on the iris. American Journal of Physiology **113**:251-258, 1935.
14. Chubb, I.W., and Hodgson, A.J. Release of non-transmitter substances: especially acetylcholinesterase. In Kalsner, S., ed. Trends in Autonomic Pharmacology, vol. 2. Baltimore, Urban & Schwarzenberg, 1982.
15. Cohen, J.B., and Changeux, J.P. The cholinergic receptor protein in its membrane environment. Annual Review of Pharmacology **15**:83-103, 1975.
16. Curtis, D.R., Hösli, L., Johnson, G.A.R., and Johnston, I.H. Glycine and spinal inhibition. Brain Research **5**:112-114, 1967.
17. Dale, H.H. The action of certain esters of choline and their relation to muscarine. Journal of Pharmacology and Experimental Therapeutics **6**:147-190, 1914.
18. David, R., and Koelle, G.B. Electron microscopic localization of acetylcholinesterase and nonspecific cholinesterase at the neuromuscular junction by the gold-thiocholine and gold-thiolacetic acid methods. Journal of Cell Biology **34**:157-171, 1967.
19. DeLorenzo, R.J., Freedman, S.D., Yohe, W.B., and Maurer, S.C. Stimulation of Ca^{2+}-dependent neurotransmitter release and presynaptic nerve terminal protein phosphorylation by calmodulin and a calmodulin-like protein isolated from synaptic vesicles. Proceedings of the National Academy of Sciences of the United States of America **76**:1838-1842, 1979.
20. DeRobertis, E.D.P., and Bennett, H.S. Some features of the submicroscopic morphology of synapses in frog and earthworm. Journal of Biophysical and Biochemical Cytology **1**:47-58, 1955.
21. Dixon, W.E. Vagus inhibition. British Medical Journal **2**:1807, 1906.
22. Eccles, J.C. The Physiology of Synapses. New York, Academic Press, Inc., 1964.
23. Eccles, J.C. The Inhibitory Pathways of the Central Nervous System. Springfield, Ill., Charles C Thomas, Publisher, 1969.
24. Elliott, T.R. The action of adrenalin. Journal of Physiology **32**:401-467, 1905.
25. Entman, M.L., Levey, G.S., and Epstein, S.E. Mechanism of action of epinephrine and glucagon on the canine heart: evidence for increase in sarcotubular calcium stores mediated by cyclic $3',5'$-AMP. Circulation Research **25**:429-438, 1969.
26. Euler, U.S. von. A specific sympathomimetic ergone in adrenergic nerve fibers (sympathin) and its relation to adrenaline and nor-adrenaline. Acta Physiologica Scandinavica **12**:73-97, 1947.
27. Euler, U.S. von, Franksson, C., and Hellström, J. Adrenaline and noradrenaline content of surgically removed human suprarenal glands. Acta Physiologica Scandinavica **31**:6-8, 1954.
28. Farfel, Z., Brickman, A.S., Kaslow, H.R., Brothers, V.M., and Bourne, H.R. Defect of receptor-cyclase coupling protein in pseudohypoparathyroidism. New England Journal of Medicine **303**:237-242, 1980.
29. Fatt, P., and Katz, B. Some observations on biological noise. Nature **166**:597-598, 1950.
30. Goldberg, L.I. Cardiovascular and renal actions of dopamine: potential clinical applications. Pharmacological Reviews **241**:1-29, 1972.

31. Goldberg, L.I., Hsieh, Y-Y., and Resnekof, L. Newer catecholamines for treatment of heart failure and shock: an update on dopamine and a first look at dobutamine. Progress in Cardiovascular Diseases **19:**327-340, 1977.

32. Goldberg, N.D., Haddox, M.K., Nicol, S.E., Glass, D.B., Stanford, C.H., Kuehl, F.A., and Estensen, R. Biologic regulation through opposing influences of cyclic GMP and cyclic AMP: the yin yang hypothesis. Advances in Cyclic Nucleotide Research **5:**307-330, 1975.

33. Hodgkin, A.L., and Huxley, A.F. A quantitative description of membrane current and its application to conduction and excitation in nerve. Journal of Physiology **117:**500-544, 1952.

34. Hornykiewicz, O. Die topische Lokalisation und das Verhalten von Noradrenalin und Dopamin (3-hydroxytyramin) in der Substantia Nigra des normalen und Parkinson-kranken Menschen. Wiener Klinische Wochenschrift **75:**309-312, 1963.

35. Hubbard, J.I. Mechanism of transmitter release from nerve terminals. Annals of the New York Academy of Sciences **183:**131-146, 1971.

36. Hubbard, J.I., and Kwanbumbumpen, S. Evidence for the vesicle hypothesis. Journal of Physiology **194:**407-420, 1968.

37. Hunt, R., and Taveau, R. deM. The effects of a number of derivatives of choline and analogous compounds on the blood pressure. Treasury Department Public Health and Marine Hospital Service. United States Hygiene Laboratory Bulletin, No. 73, Washington, D.C., 1911.

38. Iversen, L.L. Catecholamine uptake processes. British Medical Bulletin **29:**130-135, 1973.

39. Kalsner, S. Feedback regulation of neurotransmitter release through adrenergic presynaptic receptors: time for a reassessment. In Kalsner, S., ed. Trends in Autonomic Pharmacology, vol. 2. Baltimore, Urban & Schwarzenberg, 1982.

40. Katz, B. Microphysiology of the neuromuscular junction. Bulletin of the Johns Hopkins Hospital **102:**275-312, 1958.

41. Katz, B., and Miledi, R. The measurement of synaptic delay, and the time course of acetylcholine release at the neuromuscular junction. Proceedings of the Royal Society of London; B: Biological Sciences **161:**483-495, 1965.

42. Lands, A.M., Arnold, A., McAuliff, J.P., Luduena, F.P., and Brown, T.G., Jr. Differentiation of receptor systems activated by sympathomimetic amines. Nature **214:**597-598, 1967.

43. Limbird, L.E. α_2-Adrenergic systems: models for exploring hormonal inhibition of adenylate cyclase. Trends in Pharmacological Sciences **4:**135-138, 1983.

44. Loewi, O. Über humorale Übertragbarkeit der Herznervenwirkung. Pfluegers Archiv für die Gesamte Physiologie **189:**239-242, 1921.

45. Loewi, O., and Navratil, E. Über humorale Übertragkeit der Herznervenwirkung. X. Über das Schicksal des Vagusstoffes. Pfluegers Archiv für die Gesamte Physiologie **214:**678-688, 1926.

46. Marshall, J.M. Modulation of smooth muscle activity by catecholamines. Federation Proceedings **36:**2450-2455, 1977.

47. Mueller, R.A., Thoenen, H., and Axelrod, J. Increase in tyrosine hydroxylase activity after reserpine administration. Journal of Pharmacology and Experimental Therapeutics **169:**74-79, 1969.

48. Nachmansohn, D., and Machado, A.L. The formation of acetylcholine. A new enzyme: "choline acetylase." Journal of Neurophysiology **6:**397-403, 1943.

49. Osborne, N.N. Do some nerves use more than one neurotransmitter? A look at the evidence. In Kalsner, S., ed. Trends in Autonomic Pharmacology, vol. 2. Baltimore, Urban & Schwarzenberg, 1982.

50. Raftery, M.A., Vandlen, R.L., Reed, K.L., and Lee, T. Characterization of *Torpedo californica* acetylcholine receptor: its subunit composition and ligand-binding properties. Cold Spring Harbor Symposia on Quantitative Biology **40:**193-202, 1975.

51. Schildkraut, J.J., and Kety, S.S. Biogenic amines and emotion. Science **156:**21-30, 1967.

52. Schramm, M., and Selinger, Z. The functions of cyclic AMP and calcium as alternative second messengers in parotid gland and pancreas. Journal of Cyclic Nucleotide Research **1:**181-192, 1975.

53. Smith, A.D. Mechanisms involved in the release of noradrenaline from sympathetic nerves. British Medical Bulletin **29:**123-129, 1973.

54. Sporrong, B., Clase, L., Owman, Ch., and Sjöberg, N.-O. Electron microscopy of adrenergic, cholinergic, and "P-type" nerves in the myometrium, and a special kind of synaptic contact with the smooth muscle cells. Acta Physiologica Scandinavica Supplement **452:**93-96, 1977.

55. Starke, K. Regulation of noradrenaline release by presynaptic receptor systems. Reviews of Physiology, Biochemistry, and Pharmacology (Berlin) **77:**1-24, 1977.

56. Sutherland, E.W., Robison, G.A., and Butcher, R.W. Some aspects of the biological role of adenosine 3',5'-monophosphate (cyclic AMP). Circulation **37:**279-306, 1968.

57. Venter, J.C., and Fraser, C.M. The structure of α- and β-adrenergic receptors. Trends in Pharmacological Sciences **4:**256-258, 1983.

58. Watterson, D.M., and Vincenzi, F.F., eds. Calmodulin and Cell Functions. Annals of the New York Academy of Sciences **356:**1-446, 1980.

59. Weiner, N., Cloutier, G., Bjur, R., and Pfeffer, R.I. Modification of norepinephrine synthesis in intact tissue by drugs and during short-term adrenergic nerve stimulation. Pharmacological Reviews **24:**203-221, 1972.

60. Werman, R., Davidoff, R.A., and Aprison, M.H. Inhibition of motoneurones by iontophoresis of glycine. Nature **214:**681-683, 1967.

GENERAL REFERENCES

Burnstock, G. Purinergic nerves. Pharmacological Reviews **24:**509-581, 1972.

Burnstock, G. Cholinergic, adrenergic, and purinergic neuromuscular transmission. Federation Proceedings **36:**2434-2438, 1977.

Calmodulin-regulated enzymes: modification by drugs and disease. Symposium. Federation Proceedings **41:**2251-2299, 1982.

DeRobertis, E. Molecular biology of synaptic receptors. Science **171:**963-971, 1971.

Euler, U.S. von. The nature of adrenergic nerve mediators. Pharmacological Reviews **3:**247-277, 1951.

Hebb, C. Biosynthesis of acetylcholine in nervous tissue. Physiological Reviews **52:**918-957, 1972.

Hornykiewicz, O. Psychopharmacological implications of dopamine and dopamine antagonists: a critical evaluation of current evidence. Annual Review of Pharmacology and Toxicology **17:**545-549, 1977.

Kalsner, S., ed. Trends in Autonomic Pharmacology, vol. 2. Baltimore, Urban & Schwarzenberg, 1982.

Otsuka, M., and Takahashi, T. Putative peptide neurotransmitters. Annual Review of Pharmacology and Toxicology **17:**425-439, 1977.

Robison, G.A., Butcher, R.W., and Sutherland, E.W. Cyclic AMP. New York, Academic Press, Inc., 1971.

Scriabine, A., Clineschmidt, B.V., and Sweet, C.S. Central noradrenergic control of blood pressure. Annual Review of Pharmacology **16:**113-123, 1976.

Shore, P.A. Release of serotonin and catecholamines by drugs. Pharmacological Reviews **14:**531-550, 1962.

Triggle, D.J. Neurotransmitter-Receptor Interactions. London, Academic Press, Inc., 1971.

Triggle, D.J., and Triggle, C.R. Chemical Pharmacology of the Synapse. London, Academic Press, Inc., 1976.

6 Adrenergic drugs

Donald C. Kroeger

Agents that bring about tissue responses resembling those produced by stimulation of the sympathetic nervous system represent an important group of drugs. The therapeutic uses of these compounds are several. In dentistry, they are used as vasoconstrictors for local anesthetic solutions and for hemostasis, and, in medicine, as vasoconstrictors for ophthalmic and nasal preparations, as pressor agents to maintain blood pressure in vascular shock states, and as bronchodilators for asthmatic attacks and for allergic states, including anaphylactic shock. Several CNS stimulants are also useful in treating narcolepsy and hyperkinetic syndrome.

Many terms have been used to describe these agents, and this variety of terminology is often confusing. The terms *adrenergic drugs, sympathomimetics,* and *sympathetic amines* are almost always synonymous. The term *catecholamine* is often used in reference to these agents as a class, but it is properly reserved for those sympathomimetic amines that are actually derivatives of catechol. Many hundreds of chemicals have been synthesized and tested for their adrenergic activity, and an extensive structure-activity relationship profile can be described for these agents.

HISTORY

As is true for many other drugs, adrenergic agents have been known to humans in folk medicine. With the development of chemistry in the nineteenth century, attempts were made to isolate and identify the active ingredients in these folk remedies. The first recorded study of an adrenergic agent resulted in the isolation in 1887 of ephedrine from the herb ma huang, which had been grown and used in China for centuries. Thus, the first sympathomimetic agent to be identified was derived from a plant, not an animal, source.

At the same time, investigators were making extracts of all the organs of the body in an attempt to discover new hormones. Studies by Oliver and Schäfer in the early 1890s demonstrated a potent pressor substance in extracts of the adrenal gland. The active agent, epinephrine, was soon isolated, prepared commercially, and marketed under the name Adrenalin(e). By 1905, it had been synthesized and was being incorporated with local anesthetics. In fact, in that year an account was published of the results of mixing procaine with epinephrine to obtain dental anesthesia.[6]

CHEMISTRY AND STRUCTURE-ACTIVITY RELATIONSHIPS

Sympathomimetic drugs may act as agonists, combining with adrenergic receptors; in this case, they are called direct-acting drugs. Sympathomimetic drugs may also cause the release of the adrenergic mediator from the nerve terminal, in which case they are known as indirect-acting drugs. Finally, adrenergic agents may exert a combination of these actions (mixed-acting drugs). The actions of other drugs that influence sympathetic nervous system activity result from interference with or activation of any one or more of the receptors described in Chapter 5 or the physiologic processes outlined in Table 5-4.

Of the countless number of compounds that have been isolated or synthesized, only a few will be discussed. The three naturally occurring adrenergic amines known to play roles in the sympathetic nervous system are dopamine, norepinephrine, and epinephrine. The chemical structures of these adrenergic amines are illustrated in Figure 6-1. It should be noted that these compounds are synthesized sequentially in nerve terminals and specialized cells. All three metabolites are derived from tyrosine. Although they are catechol derivatives,

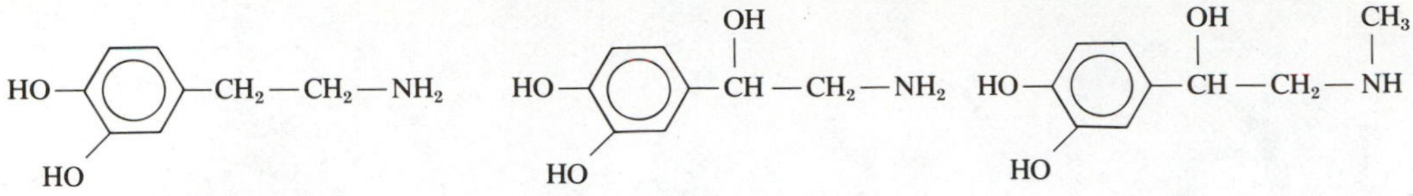

Figure 6-1. Chemical structures of three naturally occurring adrenergic amines.

Table 6-1. Structure-activity relationships of selected adrenergic agonists

Agonist	Receptor preference	Structure (phenylethylamine nucleus)			
		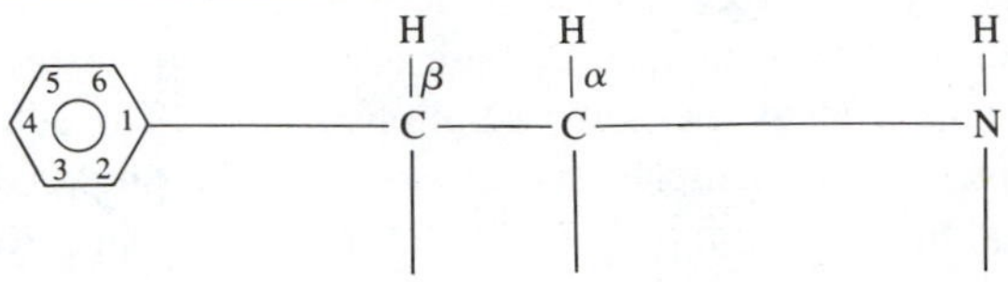 (ring)	H β C	H α C	H N
Direct action					
Dopamine	DA, α, β_1	3 — OH, 4 — OH	H	H	H
Dobutamine	β_1	3 — OH, 4 — OH	H	H	CH — (CH$_2$)$_2$—(ring)— OH / CH$_3$
Norepinephrine	α, β_1	3 — OH, 4 — OH	OH	H	H
Levonordefrin	α, β	3 — OH, 4 — OH	OH	CH$_3$	H
Epinephrine	α, β	3 — OH, 4 — OH	OH	H	CH$_3$
Isoproterenol	β	3 — OH, 4 — OH	OH	H	CH(CH$_3$)$_2$
Metaproterenol	β_2	3 — OH, 5 — OH	OH	H	CH(CH$_3$)$_2$
Terbutaline	β_2	3 — OH, 5 — OH	OH	H	C(CH$_3$)$_3$
Albuterol	β_2	3 — CH$_2$OH, 4 — OH	OH	H	C(CH$_3$)$_3$
Ritodrine	β_2	4 — OH	OH	CH$_3$	CH$_2$ — CH$_2$—(ring)— OH
Isoxsuprine	β_2	4 — OH	OH	CH$_3$	CH — CH$_2$ — O—(ring) / CH$_3$ 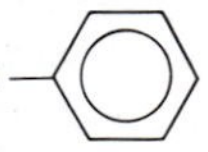
Isoetharine	β_2	3 — OH, 4 — OH	OH	CH$_2$CH$_3$	CH(CH$_3$)$_2$
Mainly direct action					
Methoxamine	α	2 — OCH$_3$, 5 — OCH$_3$	OH	CH$_3$	H
Phenylephrine	α	3 — OH —	OH	H	CH$_3$
Mixed action					
Ephedrine	α, α(CNS), β	— —	OH	CH$_3$	CH$_3$
Metaraminol	α, β_1	3 — OH —	OH	CH$_3$	H
Mainly indirect action					
Tyramine	α, β_1	4 — OH —	H	H	H
Hydroxyamphetamine	α, β_1	4 — OH —	H	CH$_3$	H
Amphetamine	α(CNS)	— —	H	CH$_3$	H
Methamphetamine	α(CNS)	— —	H	CH$_3$	CH$_3$

it is advantageous to consider all adrenergic amines as derivatives of phenylethylamine.

Table 6-1 lists some of the adrenergic amines currently in use and illustrates certain major alterations in biologic activity that occur with structural modifications. The following conclusions about the relationship between structure and activity can be drawn:

1. Direct-acting sympathetic amines (those that interact with the receptor) require a metahydroxyl group on the ring plus a hydroxyl group on the β-carbon atom of the side chain to stimulate the classic α- or β-adrenergic receptors.

2. Indirect-acting compounds have no β-hydroxyl group and either no or one hydroxyl group on the ring. Those agents lacking an aromatic hydroxyl substitution can penetrate the blood-brain barrier and exert prominent CNS effects. Some indirect-acting compounds (such as tyramine) occur naturally in food and beverages.

3. Mixed agents (those having both actions described above) generally have a β-hydroxyl group and a single ring hydroxyl group.

4. Dopamine, which lacks the β-carbon hydroxyl moiety present in other endogenous catecholamines, appears to activate a particular set of receptors, in addition to those also responsive to norepinephrine.

5. Repeated doses of either mixed or indirect-acting adrenergic amines may lead to a depletion of available pools of the neurotransmitter, resulting in a reduction or loss of activity of the exogenous amine. This is one of the mechanisms for the relatively rapid decrease in drug effect known as tachyphylaxis.

6. Slight structural modifications in the chemical structure confer specificity for certain receptors. Therapeutic agents can be designed to provide selective responses. For example, methyl substitution on the α carbon yields orally active compounds able to resist enzymatic destruction in the stomach and small intestine.

7. As the alkyl substitution on the amine nitrogen is increased in molecular weight, a shift in receptor affinity-efficacy toward the β receptor is observed. The affinity of norepinephrine with hydrogens is almost entirely toward α receptors, the affinity of epinephrine with a methyl group is mixed, and that of isoproterenol with an isopropyl group is toward β receptors. Further increases in molecular weight and changes in the position of ring hydroxyl groups (to the 3 and 5 positions, or

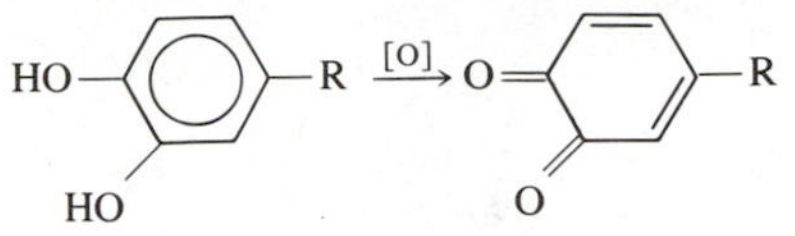

Figure 6-2. Oxidation of the catecholamine nucleus.

a single hydroxyl group in the 4 position) lead to compounds with greater affinities for the β_2 receptors of bronchioles (terbutaline) or skeletal muscle arterioles (isoxsuprine).

8. Besides structural modifications, many of the above compounds exist as optical isomers. Substitutions on either the α or β carbon atom of the side chain produce stereoisomeric pairs. Levorotatory substitution on the carbon chain enhances the peripheral α-receptor effects. Dextrorotatory substitution on the α carbon increases the CNS stimulant activity (e.g., *d*-amphetamine).

9. The catecholamine nucleus is extremely sensitive to oxidation. This chemical reaction results in the formation of a quinone, adrenochrome (Figure 6-2), which accounts for color changes that may occur in solution of catecholamines, as for example in dental anesthetic cartridges. Sodium bisulfite is incorporated in such solutions as an antioxidant to prevent catecholamine degradation.

10. All of the commercially available adrenergic amines are marketed as water-soluble salts (i.e., hydrochlorides, sulfates, and bitartrates). The sulfates are quite frequently used for the orally effective forms.

PHARMACOLOGIC EFFECTS

Sympathomimetic drugs can elicit a wide variety of responses depending on their mode of action, the receptors they activate, and their ability to enter the central nervous system. In this section, the pharmacologic effects of some important and representative catecholamines are described. Meaningful differences between these drugs and other adrenergic amines will be reviewed in the section on general therapeutic uses.

Norepinephrine and epinephrine

Vascular effects. The net action of norepinephrine and epinephrine on the human cardiovascular system is dependent on the route of administration

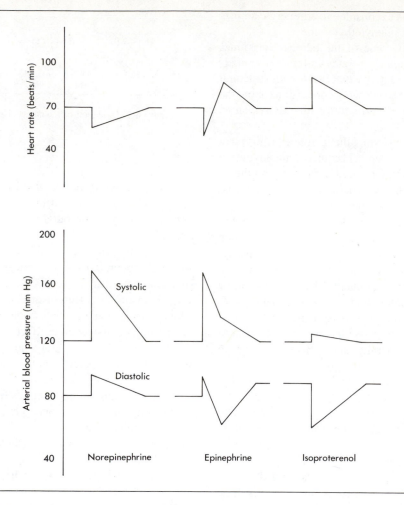

Figure 6-3. Schematic representation of the effects of three catecholamines on heart rate and arterial blood pressure in the dog. The drugs were administered intravenously by bolus injection at a dose of 1 μg/kg. Note the biphasic effect of epinephrine. Initially the drug resembles norepinephrine by causing an increased blood pressure and cardiac slowing. As the concentration of epinephrine falls into the physiologic range, however, β-receptor activation predominates. There is a fall in diastolic pressure, and direct cardiac effects are unmasked. The decreased heart rates seen with norepinephrine and at the beginning of the epinephrine response are indirectly produced by an active carotid sinus reflex. The drug effects last for approximately 5 minutes.

and the dose. When injected locally, both mediators cause vasoconstriction, irrespective of the vascular bed to which they are applied. When administered intravascularly, the net response is dependent on the dose and the rate of administration. With intravenous infusion of physiologic amounts (0.5 μg/min or less) a predictable effect, based on the theory of α and β receptors, is obtained. Norepinephrine elicits primarily the α-receptor response: increased systolic and diastolic pressure, with a reflex bradycardia brought on by carotid sinus and other cardiodeaccelerator reflexes. On the other hand, epinephrine in moderate to large doses

will stimulate both receptors, but the α-receptor pressor response initially masks the response to the β receptor. As epinephrine is metabolized, the more sensitive β-receptor depressor response is observed (Figure 6-3). The slow administration of epinephrine in dilute concentrations, less than 0.1 μg/kg/min, will elicit only the β-receptor response. If pressure elevations are mild, a direct chronotropic effect of epinephrine on the myocardium may be observed. Increased doses or faster rates of administration may elicit greater degrees of the less sensitive α-receptor responses (vasoconstriction), as well as compensatory vascular re-

Table 6-2. Relative activity of certain adrenergic amines on peripheral sympathetic receptors

Drug	Potency ratio (epinephrine = 1)	Receptor ratio (α/β)
Phenylephrine	0.05	95/5
Norepinephrine	0.7	90/10
Levonordefrin	0.2	75/25
Epinephrine	1.0	50/50
Ethylnorepinephrine	0.1	25/75
Isoproterenol	0.9	5/95

flexes. At higher pharmacologic doses, there are few differences between the two mediators.

Cardiac effects. Norepinephrine and epinephrine produce excitation of the β_1 receptors located in the myocardium, pacemaker, and conducting tissues of the heart. Not only is the strength of contraction increased, but the rate of force development is accentuated. (This is known as the positive inotropic effect). The spread of the excitation through the conductile tissues is also increased (positive dromotropic action). Pacemaker tissues increase their rate (positive chronotropic effect), and automaticity is enhanced in normally quiescent muscle (latent pacemakers are activated). Almost all of the effects described above are effectively antagonized by β blockade, although α blockade with phenoxybenzamine is useful in preventing epinephrine-induced arrhythmias that may occur during general anesthesia with certain agents.

β-Receptor stimulation also increases oxygen consumption of the heart, but efficiency is diminished. The oxygen supply via the coronary arteries will be variably affected by the relative amount of α- or β-receptor activation produced by each adrenergic amine (Table 6-2), as well as by metabolic regulators of local blood flow.

Effects on smooth muscle. The effect of adrenergic amines on smooth muscle in the hollow organs of the thoracic and abdominal cavities is, with few exceptions, relaxation. The gastrointestinal tract is relaxed and shows decreased motility, but the sphincters are usually constricted, particularly if they were relaxed before drug administration. A similar situation exists for the urinary bladder and its sphincters. The uterine smooth muscle response varies with the species, the stage of the sex cycle, and pregnancy. Ritodrine, a selective β_2-receptor agonist, is approved for use to relax the smooth muscle of the uterus and delay pre-

mature labor. In any case, these activities are not usually affected by doses of epinephrine administered for other therapeutic purposes.

Bronchial dilation is an example of smooth muscle relaxation that is of major therapeutic importance. The β_2 receptors of this tissue are intensely affected by epinephrine, isoproterenol, and the newer β_2-receptor stimulants terbutaline, metaproterenol, albuterol, and isoetharine.[1] These compounds produce bronchodilation with less of the concomitant β_1-receptor stimulation of the myocardium than is caused by isoproterenol. This reduced positive inotropic effect on the heart is useful in asthmatic patients, who often have accompanying cardiac problems.

In contrast to the above, adrenergic amines cause the splenic capsule to contract, although in humans this does not appear to play an important role in increasing the hematocrit. The pilomotor muscles and the radial muscle of the iris also contract in response to norepinephrine and epinephrine.

Effects on salivary glands. Sympathetic nerve stimulation of mucus-secreting cells of the submaxillary and sublingual glands causes an increase in the secretion of viscous saliva. Serous secretion by the parotid gland does not appear to be directly influenced by adrenergic drugs, but it is indirectly affected through vasomotor responses in the gland and contraction of the myoepithelial elements in the ducts. After an initial expression of serous saliva from the ducts, mucous secretion from the other glands predominates. Adrenergic agents acting on the salivary glands have no therapeutic importance.

Metabolic responses. The major metabolic effect produced by adrenergic drug stimulation is related to the second-messenger response discussed in Chapter 5. Metabolic responses result from β-receptor stimulation and occur primarily in the liver and in adipose tissue. Injections of adrenergic agents with β-receptor activity bring about a transitory increase in circulating blood glucose as a result of liver glycogenolysis.[3] In a similar enzymatic action, cAMP is involved in the hydrolysis of triglycerides, causing an increase in circulating free fatty acids. Other effects that occur are a decreased synthesis of cholesterol, a numerical reduction in circulating eosinophils, and an increase in oxygen consumption. These last effects are thought to be indirect actions involving a variety of responses. To date no therapeutic use has been made of the metabolic effects.

Central nervous system effects. Although the catecholamines are extensively involved with neuronal transmission in the central nervous system, peripherally administered adrenergic agents of the catecholamine variety do not gain access to the central nervous system because hydroxyl groups on the aromatic ring deter passage across the blood-brain barrier.

Intravenous injection of epinephrine does, however, produce a variety of apparently central effects—feelings of anxiety, jitteriness, and apprehension. Most, if not all, of these effects, though, are indirect, resulting from sensory input from the periphery. Reflex respiratory apnea is induced by increased blood pressure and can be diminished by desensitization of the carotid sinus and aortic arch receptors by topical application or intravenous injection of a local anesthetic.[32]

Isoproterenol

Although there have been suggestions that isoproterenol (isopropylarterenol) is a natural transmitter, this claim has not been substantiated. Even so, isoproterenol is important because it is an almost pure β-receptor agonist, affecting both β_1 and β_2 receptors. It is used clinically in bronchoconstrictive diseases, and its pharmacologic actions can induce serious side effects on other bodily systems.

Cardiac and vascular effects. The actions of isoproterenol on the cardiovascular system are based on its being essentially a pure β-receptor agonist. It causes a marked fall in diastolic blood pressure but little or no change in systolic pressure because of increased cardiac output due to its positive inotropic action on the myocardium. The principal vasculature affected is that supplying skeletal muscle, with some additional vasodilation in the renal and mesenteric beds. The powerful inotropic action may increase myocardial oxygen demand sufficiently to cause ischemia and heart damage. Its action on the excitability of the myocardium may induce palpitations and arrhythmias.

Effects on bronchial smooth muscle. The β_2-receptor action of isoproterenol causes dilation of the bronchioles without the vasoconstriction and drying effect (cessation of mucous membrane activity) associated with epinephrine (α-receptor effect). Tolerance to the bronchorelaxing effect of isoproterenol may develop with extended use.[26]

Effects on salivary glands. Isoproterenol stimulates the secretion of a mucous saliva rich in amylase activity. The effect is minor, however, and of little clinical significance.

Metabolic effects. The β-receptor agonist activity of isoproterenol does bring about changes in liver function. Although not as potent as epinephrine in stimulating glycogenolysis, isoproterenol is more active in producing lipolysis and release of free fatty acids.

Dopamine

Dopamine, first synthesized in 1910, was not recognized as a neural transmitter in the central nervous system until the late 1950s.[5,10] Dopamine has effects in the periphery, and specific receptors to dopamine have been identified in many peripheral tissues. Peripheral dopaminergic neurons have so far been demonstrated in the small intensely fluorescent (SIF) cells in autonomic ganglia, kidney glomeruli, and the foot pads of dogs.[21] Evidence is suggestive that dopaminergic neurons play a role in the function of the peripheral autonomic nervous system, especially in some vascular beds.

Vascular effects. Dopamine has both direct and indirect actions at effector sites. In high doses, it excites both α and β receptors, effects that can be abolished by the appropriate blocking agents. In low doses, it produces responses that are unique to dopamine. The renal, celiac, hepatic, and mesenteric vasculatures are dilated, resulting in increased blood flow in these regions. These responses can be briefly blocked by the simultaneous administration of a dopamine antagonist such as a butyrophenone (e.g., haloperidol) or a phenothiazine (e.g., chlorpromazine).[18]

Other effects. Dopamine has also been shown to be involved with the sensory division of the autonomic nervous system. The high concentration of dopamine in the glomus cells of the carotid body and the effects of hypoxia on these suggest that dopamine is an inhibitory transmitter that modulates the frequency of discharge of the sensory fibers from that structure.[20] It is theorized that via this mechanism dopamine may affect cardiovascular and respiratory responses.

Levodopa, when administered for Parkinson's disease (Chapter 16), has peripheral side effects attributable to dopamine, because approximately 95% of an oral dose of levodopa is decarboxylated in the periphery to dopamine.[2] Dopamine itself does not penetrate the blood-brain barrier, but it does produce nausea and vomiting due to excitation of the medullary chemoreceptor trigger zone (CTZ), which is outside the barrier.

Dobutamine

The synthesis of dobutamine, a synthetic catecholamine analogue of dopamine (Table 6-1), was the result of a search for a drug that would provide inotropic support for the heart with little effect on cardiac rate and rhythm and blood pressure. While isoproterenol has marked inotropic effects and does not elevate blood pressure, it has a tendency to cause arrhythmias, to lower peripheral resistance, and thereby to diminish coronary perfusion pressure. Norepinephrine and dopamine, on the other hand, are capable of stimulating β_1 receptors in the heart but have considerable vasoconstrictor activity that results in increased cardiac work. Dobutamine appears to be highly cardioselective, acting directly on β_1 receptors to increase the force of contraction but having little effect on cardiac rate, rhythm, or β_2 receptors. It increases cardiac output without the peripheral vasoconstriction that would be associated with norepinephrine and dopamine. Dobutamine is used for short-term treatment of acute myocardial insufficiency resulting from organic heart damage or cardiac surgery.[29] It may also have a beneficial hemodynamic effect in some forms of shock.

ABSORPTION, FATE, AND EXCRETION

As noted in the section on the chemistry and structure-activity relationships of these compounds, the route for administering adrenergic amines is determined by the chemical structure. All catecholamines and certain other drugs, unless specifically modified at the α carbon of the side chain, are subject to enzymatic destruction in the gastrointestinal tract. Catecholamines are usually administered systemically by inhalation, by injection, or by the sublingual route; absorption is rapid with all of these techniques.

The inactivation and metabolic disposal of catecholamines can involve many processes (Figure 6-4), as illustrated by the fate of endogenous norepinephrine. After neuronal release, most of the adrenergic transmitter is returned to the nerve terminal by an active uptake process. What remains in the cleft, approximately 20%, is subjected to O-methylation by COMT after uptake by postsynaptic tissues. Once the transmitter is O-methylated to normetanephrine, it can no longer be returned to the adrenergic neuron but is instead carried by the blood to the liver, where it is largely deaminated by that organ's MAO.[13] Some portion of the released transmitter also diffuses away from the cleft to enter the circulation intact.

Of the norepinephrine that is actively pumped back into the neuron, the greater part enters the granulated vesicle where it can again be released on neural command. A smaller portion is deaminated by MAO located in mitochondria to form

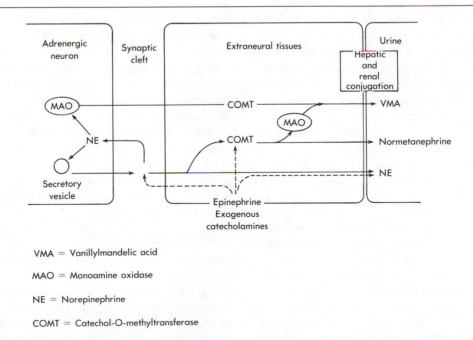

VMA = Vanillylmandelic acid

MAO = Monoamine oxidase

NE = Norepinephrine

COMT = Catechol-O-methyltransferase

Figure 6-4. Biotransformation and excretion of catecholamines.

3,4-dihydroxymandelic aldehyde. Most of the aldehyde is converted to an acid, the remainder to an alcohol. Both metabolites enter the circulation and are eventually O-methylated by COMT. The major metabolic product of norepinephrine resulting from the combined action of MAO and COMT is 3-methoxy-4-hydroxymandelic acid, also referred to as vanillylmandelic acid (VMA). Indeed, about 90% of the total endogenous catecholamine load excreted in the urine is VMA, with the remainder consisting of the O-methylated compounds and lesser quantities of other derivatives and unmetabolized transmitters.[25] Variable amounts of these products may be conjugated as the glucuronide or sulfate before being excreted by the kidney.

Exogenously administered catecholamines and endogenous dopamine and epinephrine are metabolized in much the same manner as norepinephrine. Nevertheless, there are some differences of note. Dopamine, for example, may be converted to norepinephrine by β-hydroxylation. The metabolism of epinephrine and injected catecholamines (including norepinephrine) is modified because these compounds gain access to the bloodstream without having been exposed to intraneuronal MAO. Because of its widespread distribution through the body, COMT is primarily responsible for the inactivation of these substances. The relative shift toward COMT for the initial enzymatic attack is reflected in a considerable increase in the recovery of O-methylated derivatives in the urine. It is noteworthy, however, that a small percentage of epinephrine injected as a vasoconstrictor during local anesthesia will ultimately reside in the patient's nerve terminals and will be released during sympathetic nervous system activity.[15]

Recently, attention has been drawn to a different pathway of metabolism, one similar to that which accounts for the discoloration that can occur in local anesthetic cartridges.[11] The quinoid radical may combine covalently with macromolecules of the liver cells, resulting in a toxic reaction and tissue necrosis. Such a reaction is thought to explain the extremely serious drug toxicity occurring in some patients receiving methyldopa for the treatment of high blood pressure (see Chapter 7).

The indirect-acting adrenergic amines that act by displacing the transmitter from the labile pool must enter the neuron to cause this release. While in the cytoplasm, these compounds may be subjected to deamination by MAO and other enzymes. A small amount of tyramine is β-oxidized in the neuron to form octopamine, which can enter the labile pool in the vesicles.[24] Only compounds with a β-hydroxyl group can be taken into the vesicle. Other avenues for the metabolism of noncatecholamines include *p*-hydroxylation, N-demethylation, deamination, or conjugation in the liver and kidney, or a combination of all these. Amphetamine and ephedrine, being resistant to the actions of MAO, can be administered orally.

GENERAL THERAPEUTIC USES

Clinical applications of the adrenergic amines can be divided into seven major categories: ophthalmic uses, local vasoconstriction, vasoconstriction in hypotension and shock, relief of allergic states (including anaphylaxis), bronchodilation, CNS stimulation and, surprisingly, control of hypertension. The choice of specific drugs for each of these uses depends on the relative amounts of α-receptor, β-receptor, or dopaminergic receptor activity; whether the drug action is direct, indirect, or mixed; and other factors involving absorption, duration of action, metabolic fate, and the like. The following section will examine each of the uses, indicating in each case one or more preferred drugs.

Ophthalmic uses

The two major ocular applications of adrenergic amines are for the production of mild mydriasis and the reduction of intraocular pressure. Although cholinergic blocking agents such as atropine produce a much stronger pupillary dilation, adrenergic amines are useful because they cause mydriasis without paralysis of ciliary muscle (cycloplegia). Even greater mydriasis can be obtained if a combination of a cholinergic blocking drug and a sympathomimetic drug is used. Phenylephrine, epinephrine, ephedrine, and hydroxyamphetamine are frequently used for this purpose. Because they restrict ocular blood flow and, hence, the formation of aqueous humor, some adrenergic drugs like epinephrine are useful adjuncts in the treatment of wide-angle glaucoma.

Local vasoconstriction

To provide temporary symptomatic relief of nasal congestion associated with a variety of causes, drops, sprays, aerosols, and even oral dosage forms of several adrenergic amines have proved useful. In these situations, drugs with primarily an α-receptor response and a prolonged duration of action are preferred. Most of the compounds in current use have a mixture of direct and indirect actions, and many are not derivatives of phenylethylamine but are straight-chain or other ring structures that possess potent α-adrenergic activity and have minimal CNS stimulant action.

An adverse effect associated with the use of nasal decongestants is rebound congestion, a chronic swelling of the nasal mucous membranes. Overdosage, with systemic effects, is frequently manifested by the appearance of symptoms of excessive adrenergic stimulation. Imidazoline derivatives, such as tetrahydrozoline and oxymetazoline, paradoxically can produce drowsiness, comatose sleep with hypotension, and bradycardia. Children and infants are especially prone to these adverse effects.

Decongestants have also been used to relieve itching in hyperemic (bloodshot) eyes by causing vasoconstriction. Such agents include ephedrine, phenylephrine, and tetrahydrozoline. Sometimes these drugs are mixed with other agents used to treat disorders of the conjunctiva or corneal epithelium.

Adrenergic drugs are often used to produce hemostasis for surgery and for local anesthesia. Whether applied topically or administered by injection with or without a local anesthetic, α agonists can in certain situations significantly improve visibility of the operative field. As vasoconstriction is temporary, however, the use of these drugs is no substitute for the adequate surgical control of bleeding. Furthermore, sympathomimetic amines must often be used with special caution during general anesthesia, because certain inhalation anesthetics (e.g., halothane) predispose the heart to arrhythmias.[14,22] Finally, the injection of vasoconstrictors into appendages supplied by end-arteries is absolutely contraindicated. Failure to heed this admonition has been the cause of tissue necrosis and gangrene of the fingers, toes, ears, and penis. Employment of vasoconstrictors for surgical hemostasis and as adjuvants for local anesthetics is discussed in the section on dental uses.

Vasoconstriction in hypotension and shock

Shock is a condition in which the mean arterial pressure falls, and signs of inadequate tissue perfusion result. In cases of hypotension unrelated to sympathetic nervous system failure, increased adrenergic activity occurs, as manifested by excessive sweating, tachycardia, dyspnea, and mental disturbances. If shock is the result of blood loss (hypovolemia), blood volume is usually restored with blood, plasma, or plasma expanders. When shock develops under normovolemic conditions, adrenergic amines can prove useful in restoring blood pressure and in correcting distribution of blood flow, especially to the vital organs.

There are three goals in the treatment of shock: (1) constriction of capacitance vessels to reduce venous pooling, (2) dilation of resistance vessels to increase arteriolar perfusion of vital organs, and (3) improvement of myocardial contractility to increase cardiac output. Both natural and synthetic amines are used to treat various shock conditions. Strong α-receptor agonists (e.g., methoxamine and phenylephrine), which improve blood pressure by inducing vasoconstriction, are most useful during episodes of inadequate sympathetic nervous system function as may result from spinal anesthesia or hypotensive drug overdose. Drugs with purely α-receptor activity are less beneficial in other shock states and may impair blood flow to the kidneys and mesenteric organs. Strong β₁-receptor agonists have been advocated for cardiogenic shock. Through stimulating cardiac output, isoproterenol may enhance tissue perfusion and coronary blood flow. Unfortunately, by markedly increasing myocardial oxygen demand, isoproterenol may actually worsen cardiac ischemia. Drugs with mixed α- and β₁-receptor effects (e.g., norepinephrine and metaraminol) appear more effective in lessening myocardial hypoxia while increasing blood pressure. All drugs with β₁-receptor activity, however, may impair cardiac perfusion as well as cause tachycardia and predispose the heart to other dysrhythmias. Dopamine is used in the treatment of shock due to myocardial infarction, trauma, cardiac surgery, renal failure, and chronic cardiac decompensation. In small doses, it has only mild α- and β-stimulating properties, but through stimulation of the dopamine receptors it improves renal and mesenteric perfusion.[17]

Treatment of shock may involve other kinds of medication, including glucocorticoids, antibiotics for bacteremic states, or adrenergic blocking agents to lessen vasoconstriction induced by α agonists. Volume replacement is primary in those cases where true or relative hypovolemia is involved.

Relief of allergic states

Adrenergic amines such as ephedrine and epinephrine are especially useful in reversing the actions of histamine and other mediators associated with allergic phenomena. Unlike the antihistamines, adrenergic amines are physiologic antagonists, producing responses opposite to the acute effects produced by histamine and associated autacoids. Ephedrine has the advantage of being well absorbed orally and of providing activity for an hour or more. It is useful for mild rashes and other symptoms caused by food, drugs, or insect bites. Epinephrine solutions, which must be given parenterally, provide the same relief and protection but much more effectively and rapidly. For acute allergic reactions involving urticaria and angioneurotic edema, subcutaneous injection of 0.3 to 0.5 ml of 1:1000 epinephrine should be adequate. Fulminating disturbances such as anaphylactic shock require a faster absorption of epinephrine than provided by subcutaneous injection, especially if circulation is impaired. Intramuscular (intralingual) injection of 0.4 to 0.6 ml 1:1000 epinephrine or, if the patient has previously been prepared for intravenous injections, slow intravenous administration of 1:10,000 epinephrine is recommended. With this latter route of administration, there is a considerable risk of precipitating serious cardiac arrhythmias and ventricular fibrillation.

Bronchodilation

Acute and chronic obstructive pulmonary diseases are marked by increased inspiratory and expiratory resistance. Ephedrine given orally or epinephrine administered by spray or aerosol is usually promptly effective in relaxing constricted bronchial passageways. However, the resultant vasoconstriction in the pulmonary vasculature is associated with a drying effect due to decreased secretions. Isoproterenol in aerosols or sublingual tablets gives prompt relief without eliciting detrimental α-receptor effects, but the strong β_1-receptor effect can produce cardiac arrhythmias and palpitations.

As mentioned earlier, drugs selective for β_2 receptors have become available; these drugs (e.g., terbutaline, metaproterenol, and albuterol) produce marked bronchodilation with little effect on the heart or blood pressure. Durations of action up to 4 hours are partly explained by the failure of these compounds to be metabolized by COMT. Many of the compounds are excreted in the urine as conjugates, the percentage varying with the route of administration. Side effects include reactions commonly seen with epinephrine—nervousness, trem-

or, and other CNS effects.[1] (See Chapter 32 for a discussion of the use of these agents in bronchial asthma.)

CNS stimulation

For many years certain adrenergic amines have been employed clinically because of their ability to produce stimulation of certain functions of the central nervous system that results in increased alertness, decreased sense of fatigue, and euphoria. Other actions of these agents include stimulation of hypothalamic centers involved with satiation of the food drive and an increase in the concentration and initiative powers of the brain to prevent drowsiness and even narcolepsy.

The principal drugs in this group are dextroamphetamine, methamphetamine, and methylphenidate. Because of the history of abuse of these and related drugs, their procurement and use are strictly controlled by various state and federal statutes. The principal therapeutic indications for these agents are for the treatment of narcolepsy, a disorder characterized by uncontrollable attacks of sleep in the daytime, and for the management of children with hyperkinetic child syndrome (minimal brain dysfunction [MBD] syndrome). Another use, which has drawn considerable criticism, is as adjuvant therapy in weight loss programs. While the amphetamines and related CNS stimulants do produce anorexia, their use is accompanied by amphetamine-like effects, including the development of psychic dependence. At best, their effect is marginal, not all patients respond, and drug therapy should not be continued for more than 4 to 6 weeks.

Although these drugs were developed for their ability to cross the blood-brain barrier and produce central effects, most of the agents have some slight to moderate action on the peripheral cardiovascular system. Thus, they are contraindicated in patients with hypertension, cardiac arrhythmias, or thyrotoxicosis. The contraindication for anorexiants is especially applicable to patients who are taking MAO inhibitors and antihypertensives such as guanethidine or methyldopa. Fenfluramine, a relatively new anorexiant, is contraindicated only in those patients with severe cardiovascular disease or who are taking MAO inhibitors.

Control of hypertension

The α_2-receptor agonists are discussed in detail in Chapter 7 because their major therapeutic effect is to reduce sympathetic outflow from the central nervous system. The three drugs in this category that are currently approved in the United States for the treatment of hypertension are methyldopa, clonidine, and guanabenz. A fourth drug, guanfacine, is under investigation. These drugs are partial agonists of the α_2 receptor and as such cause effects quite different from those elicited by the α_1 agonists. While the precise locations of the α_2 receptors are still under investigation, they are known to exist in the presynaptic membranes of adrenergic neurons in both the peripheral and the central nervous systems. Certain central neuronal tracts (e.g., the pontoreticular) and some innervated peripheral tissues are known to possess these receptors, as do also blood platelets. The term *presynaptic* α *receptor* once used to denote these receptors has fallen into disfavor because of the additional sites of activity that have been identified.

In most of the tissues studied to date, stimulation of the α_2 receptor inhibits adenylate cyclase activity, which in turn causes a reduction or depression of tissue activity. The tissues considered to be most influenced by these agonists are central neurons involved in the regulation of the cardiovascular system. Activation of inhibitory neurons brings about peripheral vasodilation via inhibition of the sympathetic system and a decrease in cardiac output via enhanced vagal tone.

THERAPEUTIC USES IN DENTISTRY

Vasoconstrictors are widely used in conjunction with local anesthetic solutions. Three adrenergic amines are currently being used for this purpose: norepinephrine, epinephrine, and levonordefrin. All three compounds are direct-acting catecholamines.

Table 6-3 lists the concentrations and amounts of adrenergic vasoconstrictors contained in commercially available dental local anesthetic cartridges. The concentrations listed for norepinephrine and levonordefrin are considered equivalent in efficacy to 1:100,000 epinephrine as judged by prolongation of dental anesthesia. The recommended dilution of the vasoconstrictor is 1:100,000 epinephrine equivalency for routine nerve-block anesthesia. The periodontist who wishes to obtain local tissue hemostasis may additionally choose to infiltrate the area with local anesthetic solution containing 1:50,000 epinephrine, but repeated injections of 2% lidocaine with 1:50,000 epinephrine may cause muscle cell necrosis and microscarring of the tissue.[4] The total

Table 6-3. Concentrations and amounts of adrenergic vasoconstrictors in dental local anesthetic cartridges

Vasoconstrictor	Dilution	Amount per dental cartridge ($\mu g/1.8$ ml)
Epinephrine hydrochloride	1:200,000	9
Epinephrine hydrochloride	1:100,000	18
Epinephrine hydrochloride	1:50,000	36
Norepinephrine hydrochloride	1:30,000	60
Levonordefrin hydrochloride	1:20,000	90

Table 6-4. Effect of epinephrine on the duration of local anesthesia*

Local anesthetic	Vasoconstrictor	Duration Mean (min)	Maximum (min)
Lidocaine 2%	None	44	100
Lidocaine 2%	Epinephrine 1:1,000,000	57	130
Lidocaine 2%	Epinephrine 1:750,000	67	145
Lidocaine 2%	Epinephrine 1:250,000	90	175
Lidocaine 2%	Epinephrine 1:50,000	88	210

Adapted from Keesling, G.G., and Hinds, E.C. Optimal concentration of epinephrine in lidocaine solutions. Journal of the American Dental Association **66**:337-340, 1963.

*These data were obtained by oral surgeons from patients undergoing exodontia. The mean and maximum duration of anesthesia was judged by luxation of the tooth and by the use of probes for soft-tissue effects. All injections were inferior alveolar nerve blocks; 24 patients were included in each group.

amount of epinephrine administered to an adult at one appointment should not exceed that amount equivalent to 10 cartridges of local anesthesia with 1:100,000 epinephrine, or 180 μg. Many clinicians and schools of dentistry limit injections to five cartridges, which may be safer.

The vasoconstrictor most commonly employed in commercial cartridges of local anesthetics is *l*-epinephrine, with levonordefrin (the *l* isomer of nordefrin) being employed somewhat less frequently, usually with mepivacaine. Norepinephrine is only occasionally used by manufacturers.

Vasoconstrictors serve several useful purposes when employed with local anesthetic solutions. First, they prolong the duration of local anesthesia severalfold and may improve the frequency of successful nerve block.[23] Second, toxicity may be minimized by delaying and reducing the peak blood concentration of the anesthetic agent.[9] Third, when anesthetic solutions are given by infiltration, vasoconstrictors reduce blood loss associated with surgical procedures. Tables 6-4 and 17-2 illustrate the effect of vasoconstrictors on duration of local anesthesia.

Local anesthesia with vasoconstrictors has been implicated, however, with ischemic conditions of the pulp and alveolar bone, the latter being associated with an increased incidence of osteitis following extractions.[7,28] Furthermore, local tissue damage at the site of injection is related to or accentuated by the presence of adrenergic amines.

The question often faced by the dentist is whether to administer a vasoconstrictor-containing local anesthetic solution to a known cardiac or cardiovascular patient. A joint report of the American Heart Association and the Council on Dental Therapeutics of the American Dental Association[27] recommends that the cardiac patient be given adequate anesthesia, because the benefits of satisfactory anesthesia far outweigh the risks of the small amount of vasoconstrictor. In spite of these recommendations, many physicians will specifically advise against using a mixture of a vasoconstrictor and local anesthetic for their cardiovascular patients undergoing dental treatment. It is often useful to remind the physician that the normal adrenal medulla may release much more catecholamine per minute in an acutely stressful period than the 18 μg of epinephrine contained in a typical dental cartridge.[19] Reviews of the literature indicate that adverse reactions attributable to vasoconstrictors used with local anesthetics in dentistry are extremely rare.[8,31]

Frequently, it is necessary to produce gingival retraction for the preparation of cavities and for making impressions. Besides astringents such as zinc and aluminum salts, cotton cord impregnated with racemic epinephrine, containing up to 1.0 mg drug per inch of cord, is commercially available. Racemic epinephrine has about only half the potency of the levorotary epinephrine, *d*-epinephrine having only one fifteenth the activity of *l*-epinephrine.

Whether these large amounts of epinephrine present a hazard to the normal as well as to the cardiovascular patient depends on the status of the oral epithelium. Both experimental and clinical studies indicate a relatively high absorption of the vasoconstrictor if the epithelium is abraded or the vasculature is exposed, which is common in extensive restorative procedures.[16] Systemic absorption is marked by signs of anxiety, elevated blood pressure, increased heart rate, and occasional arrhythmias. These effects can be extremely serious in a patient with cardiovascular disease or in one who is taking medication that affects the disposition of the adrenergic amines.[30]

Various products are available to control capillary bleeding occurring with surgical procedures on gingival tissues. Epinephrine hydrochloride (1:1000) or phenylephrine (1:100) is recommended. Stronger concentrations have occasionally been advocated, but their use can only heighten the risk of cardiovascular problems without producing any signficant increased efficacy in reducing hemorrhage.

TOXIC REACTIONS AND SIDE EFFECTS

Almost all toxic effects of the adrenergic amines are due to overdosage. These can result from the administration of too large a dose, impaired uptake or metabolic degradation, accidental intravascular injection, or therapeutic doses given to an exquisitely sensitive individual. Serious complications may be expected with doses of epinephrine above 0.5 mg; fatalities are likely to occur with doses of 4 mg or more, although one patient is reported to have survived an injection of 30 mg.[31] Correct calculations, careful reading of labels, and a complete medical history can help reduce accidents.

Most serious of the toxic effects are cardiac disturbances, such as increased excitability of the myocardium leading to arrhythmias including ventricular fibrillation. Patients with a history of hyperthyroidism, hypertension, or angina pectoris are particularly susceptible, as are patients who are taking β_2-adrenoceptor blocking agents (see Chapter 7). In the latter situation, unopposed α-receptor stimulation causes excessive vasoconstriction. The increase in blood pressure can be so severe as to result in hypertensive crisis, which can cause cardiac disturbances or cerebrovascular accidents in patients with weakened vessel walls.[12]

CNS reactions include nervousness, excitability, insomnia, dizziness, and tremors. With long-acting compounds such as ephedrine, a sedative may be needed to counteract these effects. The paradoxical CNS depression produced by imidazoline derivatives in the young and elderly has been mentioned.

Adrenergic drugs

Nonproprietary name	Proprietary name

Ophthalmic products
Mydriatics

epinephrine	Adrenalin Chloride
hydroxyamphetamine	Paredrine
phenylephrine	Neo-Synephrine

Decongestants

naphazoline	Naphcon Forte
phenylephrine	Neo-Synephrine
tetrahydrozoline	Visine, Murine

Antiglaucoma agents

dipivefrin	Propine
epinephrine	Epifrin, Epitrate, Eppy/N

Respiratory tract products
Nasal decongestants

ephedrine	Vatronol
epinephrine	Adrenalin Chloride
naphazoline	Privine
oxymetazoline	Afrin
phenylephrine	Neo-Synephrine
phenylpropanolamine	Propadrine
pseudoephedrine	Sudafed
tetrahydrozoline	Tyzine
xylometazoline	Neo-Synephrine II

Cold remedies

These preparations consist of a mild analgesic, usually aspirin, one or two antihistamines, an antimuscarinic drug, and one of the following adrenergic agents:

phenylephrine	Neo-Synephrine
phenylpropanolamine	Propadrine
pseudoephedrine	Sudafed

Bronchodilators

albuterol	Proventil, Ventolin
ephedrine	—
epinephrine	Adrenalin Chloride
ethylnorepinephrine	Bronkephrine
isoetharine	Bronkosol
isoproterenol	Isuprel
isoproterenol and phenylephrine	Duo-Medihaler
metaproterenol	Alupent, Metaprel
terbutaline	Brethine, Bricanyl

Products used for treatment of shock and hypotension

dobutamine	Dobutrex
dopamine	Intropin
ephedrine	—
epinephrine	Adrenalin Chloride
isoproterenol	Isuprel
mephentermine	Wyamine Sulfate
metaraminol	Aramine
methoxamine	Vasoxyl
norepinephrine (levarterenol)	Levophed
phenylephrine	Neo-Synephrine

Miscellaneous products

ritodrine	Yutopar
isoxsuprine	Vasodilan

CITED REFERENCES

1. Alexander, M.R., Hendeles, L., and Guernsey, B. The beta-2 agonist bronchodilators. Drug Intelligence and Clinical Pharmacology **11**:526-532, 1977.
2. AMA Drug Evaluations, ed. 5. Chicago, American Medical Association, 1983.
3. Arnold, A., McAuliff, J.P., Colella, D.F., O'Connor, W.V., and Brown, Th. G., Jr. The β-2 receptor mediated glycogenolytic responses to catecholamines in the dog. Archives Internationales de Pharmacodynamie et de Therapie **176**:451-457, 1968.
4. Benoit, P.W. Microscarring in skeletal muscle after repeated exposures to lidocaine with epinephrine. Journal of Oral Surgery **36**:530-533, 1978.
5. Blaschko, H. Metabolism and storage of biogenic amines. Experientia **13**:9-12, 1957.
6. Braun, H. Über einige neue örtliche Änasthetica (Stovain, Alypin, Novocain). Deutsche Medizinische Wochenschrift **31**:1667-1671, 1905.
7. Calhoun, N.R. Dry socket and other postoperative complications. Dental Clinics of North America **15**(2):337-348, 1971.
8. Campbell, R.L. Cardiovascular effects of epinephrine overdose: case report. Anesthesia Progress **24**:190-193, 1977.
9. Cannell, H., Beckett, A.H., Walters, H., and Saunders, A. Circulating levels of lignocaine after peri-oral injections. British Dental Journal **138**:87-93, 1975.
10. Carlsson, A. The occurrence, distribution, and physiological role of catecholamines in the nervous system. Pharmacological Reviews **11**:490-493, 1959.
11. Dybing, E., Nelson, S.D., Mitchell, J.R., Sasame, H.A., and Gillette, J.R. Oxidation of α-methyldopa and other catechols by cytochrome P-450–generated superoxide anion: possible mechanism of methyldopa hepatitis. Molecular Pharmacology **12**:911-920, 1976.
12. Foster, C.A., and Aston, S.J. Propranolol-epinephrine interaction: a potential disaster. Plastic and Reconstructive Surgery **72**:74-78, 1983.
13. Fuller, R.W., and Roush, B.W. Substrate-selective and tissue-selective inhibition of monoamine oxidase. Archives Internationales de Pharmacodynamie et de Therapie **198**:270-276, 1972.
14. Funakoshi, Y., Iwai, S., Kaneda, H., and Iuchi, Y. Hemodynamic effects of locally applied epinephrine used with various general anesthetic techniques. Journal of Oral Surgery **35**:713-718, 1977.
15. Gerke, D.C., Ahrns, B., Frewin, D.B., and Frost, B.R. The effect of local anaesthetics on the neural uptake of catecholamines in isolated arteries—a histochemical study. Australian Journal of Experimental Biology and Medical Science **54**:601-604, 1976.
16. Gogerty, J.H., Strand, H.A., Ogilvie, A.L., and Dille, J.M. Vasopressor effects of topical epinephrine in certain dental procedures. Oral Surgery, Oral Medicine, and Oral Pathology **10**:614-622, 1957.
17. Goldberg, L.I. Dopamine—clinical uses of an endogenous catecholamine. New England Journal of Medicine **291**:707-710, 1974.
18. Goldberg, L.I., Volkman, P.H., Kohli, J.D., and Kotake, A.N. Similarities and differences of dopamine receptors in the renal vascular bed and elsewhere. Advances in Biochemical Psychopharmacology **16**:251-256, 1977.

19. Guyton, A.C. Textbook of Medical Physiology, ed. 5. Philadelphia, W.B. Saunders Co., 1976.
20. Hanbauer, I. Regulation of tyrosine hydroxylase in carotid body. Advances in Biochemical Psychopharmacology **16:**275-280, 1977.
21. Is dopamine a peripheral transmitter? Symposium. Federation Proceedings **42:**2998-3021, 1983.
22. Katz, R.L., and Epstein, R.A. The interaction of anesthetic agents and adrenergic drugs to produce cardiac arrhythmias. Anesthesiology **29:**763-784, 1968.
23. Keesling, G.R., and Hinds, E.C. Optimal concentration of epinephrine in lidocaine solutions. Journal of the American Dental Association **66:**337-340, 1963.
24. Kopin, I.J., Fischer, J.E., Musacchio, J.M., Horst, W.D., and Weise, V.K. "False neurochemical transmitters" and the mechanism of sympathetic blockade by monoamine oxidase inhibitors. Journal of Pharmacology and Experimental Therapeutics **147:**186-193, 1965.
25. Labosse, E.H., Axelrod, J., Kopin, I.J., and Kety, S.S. Metabolism of 7-H^3-epinephrine-*d*-bitartrate in normal young men. Journal of Clinical Investigation **40:**253-260, 1961.
26. Lin, C.-S., Hurwitz, L., Jenne, J., and Avner, B.P. Mechanism of isoproterenol-induced desensitization of tracheal smooth muscle. Journal of Pharmacology and Experimental Therapeutics **203:**12-22, 1977.
27. Management of dental problems in patients with cardiovascular disease. Council on Dental Therapeutics, American Dental Association and American Heart Association Joint Report. Journal of the American Dental Association **68:**333-342, 1964.
28. Nilsson, E., and Wendeberg, B. Effect of local anaesthetics on wound healing. Acta Anaesthesiologica Scandinavica **1:**87-99, 1957.
29. Stoner, J.D., III, Bolen, J.L., and Harrison, D.C. Comparison of dobutamine and dopamine in treatment of severe heart failure. British Heart Journal **39:**536-539, 1977.
30. Vernale, C.A. Cardiovascular responses to local dental anesthesia with epinephrine in normotensive and hypertensive subjects. Oral Surgery, Oral Medicine, and Oral Pathology **13:**942-952, 1960.
31. Verrill, P.J. Adverse reactions to local anaesthetics and vasoconstrictor drugs. The Practitioner **214:**380-387, 1975.
32. Weatherred, J., Kroeger, D.C., and Smith, E.L. Some cardiovascular effects of intravascular local anesthesia. Federation Proceedings **17:**358, 1958.

GENERAL REFERENCES

Goldberg, L.I. Cardiovascular and renal actions of dopamine: potential clinical applications. Pharmacological Reviews **24:**1-30, 1972.
Guldberg, H.C., and Marsden, C.A. Catechol-O-methyl transferase: pharmacological aspects and physiological role. Pharmacological Reviews **27:**135-206, 1975.
Jastak, J.T., and Yagiela, J.A. Vasoconstrictors and local anesthesia: a review and rationale for use. Journal of the American Dental Association **107:**623-630, 1983.
Patil, P.N., Miller, D.D., and Trendelenberg, U. Molecular geometry and adrenergic drug activity. Pharmacological Reviews **26:**323-392, 1974.
Persson, G. General side effects of local dental anesthesia with special reference to catecholamines as vasoconstrictors and to the effect of some premedicants. Acta Odontologica Scandinavica Supplement **53:**1-60, 1969.
Vandam, L.D. Symposium on the autonomic nervous system. Anesthesiology **29:**621-827, 1968.

7 Adrenergic blocking drugs

Donald C. Kroeger

An explosion of research in the past several decades has led to an increasingly precise understanding of the mechanisms of transmission in the sympathetic nervous system. Some of the impetus for this research has come both from an understanding of the action of drugs on the central nervous system and from extensive research on an economically important disease, essential hypertension (see Chapters 12 and 28). The result of this research has been the development of a large number of new pharmacologic agents with such diverse mechanisms as to make a simple nomenclature difficult.

In Chapter 5 (see Table 5-3), there was a discussion of the theoretical mechanisms by which drugs could produce effects on the autonomic nervous system. The drugs to be presented in this chapter all interfere with the function of the adrenergic components of the autonomic nervous system; that is, they have the effect of blocking transmission in those parts of the autonomic nervous system in which norepinephrine is a transmitter. Because of their varied mechanisms of action, these drugs can be classified according to the site of action. Some of these drugs act on the postjunctional, or receptor, site. Among these are the α- and β-adrenergic receptor blocking agents. The α-adrenergic receptor blocking agents can be divided for discussion into reversible, competitive agents and irreversible agents. In addition, there are several drugs that act on the prejunctional, or neuronal, sites (i.e., the neuron terminal blocking agents). Finally, there are drugs that act on synapses in the central nervous system.

HISTORY

In 1906, shortly after the isolation and synthesis of epinephrine, Dale and his co-workers noticed that certain alkaloids of ergot, produced by a fungus disease of rye grain, blocked the pressor response to epinephrine. Whereas the usual reaction to an injection of epinephrine into an experimental animal is a marked rise in blood pressure, after an injection of ergotoxine (a mixture of ergot alkaloids), a depressor response was observed, and it was aptly named by Dale the "epinephrine reversal" response. Subsequent investigations by others soon showed that while certain ergot alkaloids were capable of blocking some of the actions of epinephrine, they did not block all the effects of sympathetic nerve stimulation.

In 1947, Nickerson and Goodman reported the development of a drug, dibenamine, that not only inhibited the responses to exogenous epinephrine but could also prevent some of the responses to nerve stimulation. Dibenamine and other drugs that followed were capable of blocking the pressor effects of norepinephrine and were labeled α-adrenergic receptor blocking agents. With the studies of Lands and Tainter came the development of isoproterenol, with potent β-receptor stimulant properties.[26] Shortly thereafter, it was shown that dichloroisoproterenol, the dichloro derivative of isoproterenol, blocked the vasodepressor and cardiac-stimulating properties of epinephrine. This drug was the first β-adrenergic receptor blocking agent to be isolated. During this same period, it was discovered that the drug bretylium interferes with the release of norepinephrine in response to nerve stimulation, and in a short time other studies of indirect- and direct-acting amines, depletion of transmitter by reserpine, blockade of the reuptake mechanism by cocaine, and transmitter metabolism began a second era of drug development, that of the neuronal blocking agents. Many authors refer to these latter agents as sympatholytics, because they block actions of the sympathetic nervous system by decreasing or preventing transmitter release.

Before the specific drugs used to reduce sympathetic activity are discussed, it is important to emphasize the complexity of the mechanisms involved with the release of transmitter. One of these, autoregulation via presynaptic receptors, plays a clinically significant role.[27] Also, it has been shown that receptors are extremely labile and that their number is a net result of formation and destruction and is subject to disease states and aging. The unusually rapid loss of receptor activity called ''down regulation'' has been confused with receptor blockade and is now understood to be due to a disappearance of the receptor.[32]

Besides down regulation or a decrease in the receptor population, other mechanisms for reduction of agonist-receptor activity have been shown to exist, such as decreases in receptor sensitivity or increases in phosphodiesterase activity.[17] The drop in responsiveness to exogenously administered agonists known as tachyphylaxis may be the result of all of these activities, as well as the depletion of endogenously released neurotransmitter.

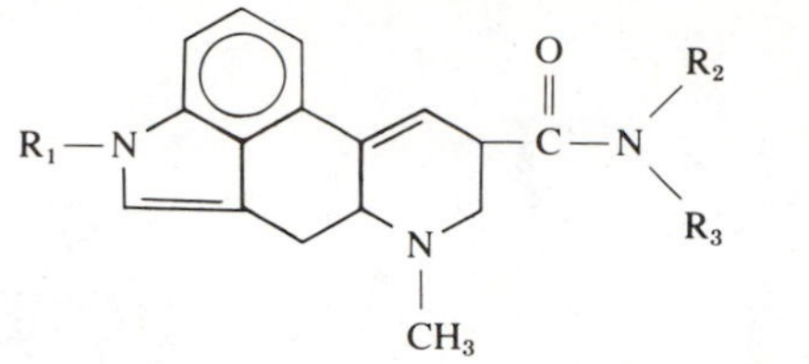

α-ADRENERGIC RECEPTOR BLOCKING AGENTS

Those agents that combine with and prevent the action of the adrenergic transmitters on the α receptors are known as the α-adrenergic receptor (adrenoceptor) blocking agents. As is explained in Chapters 5 and 6, two types of α receptor have now been identified, the α_1, which is located on the postsynaptic membrane, and the α_2, which is found on the presynaptic membrane where it is believed to play a role in the regulation of norepinephrine release and on the postsynaptic membrane where its function is not well known.[19,28] Also, α_2 receptors are found in the central nervous system; their function and the drugs that affect them are mentioned in Chapter 6 and in this chapter under the heading of ''centrally active agonists.''

Because of the differences in affinity and binding characteristics, the α-adrenergic blocking drugs are best subdivided into several groups.

Reversible α-adrenoceptor blockers

There are three classes of α-adrenergic receptor blocking agents that exert reversible and competitive effects: those derived from the ergot fungus, analogues of the imidazoline adrenergic amines, and a group of agents that act solely on the postjunctional site.

Ergot alkaloids. The ergot alkaloids compose an interesting group of drugs, both historically and

	R_1	R_2	R_3
Ergonovine	H	H	—CH (CH$_2$OH / CH$_3$)
Lysergic acid diethylamide (LSD-25)	H	—C$_2$H$_5$	—C$_2$H$_5$

Figure 7-1. Lysergic acid amide nucleus of the ergot alkaloids. Also shown are the substitutions at R_1, R_2, and R_3 which specifically characterize ergonovine and lysergic acid diethylamide.

pharmacologically. Rye infected with the ergot fungus *Claviceps purpurea* has for centuries caused outbreaks of severe poisoning, particularly in Eastern Europe. Even today, small outbreaks of ergotism occur after bread and other foodstuffs made from infected grain are eaten. Saint Anthony's fire is an early name given to describe the symptoms of poisoning, which include hallucinations, delirium, and a burning feeling in the legs caused by developing gangrene.

Two major groups of alkaloids have been isolated from ergot. One group has adrenergic blocking actions, whereas the other includes smooth muscle stimulants used therapeutically as oxytocics to reduce postpartum hemorrhage of the uterus and as vasoconstrictors in the treatment of migraine headaches. A few hydrogenated, alcohol-soluble alkaloids are used as vasodilators.

It is interesting to note that the chemical nucleus of the ergot alkaloids is lysergic acid and that some of the symptoms of ergot poisoning resemble the more classic hallucinatory events seen with lysergic acid diethylamide or LSD (Figure 7-1).

Imidazoline derivatives. Analogues of the imidazoline adrenergic amines (Chapter 6) were among the first synthetic adrenergic blocking agents to be identified. They possess a high affinity for the adrenergic receptor but little intrinsic activity. Through a loose binding to the receptor (competitive blocking), they can reduce or block the

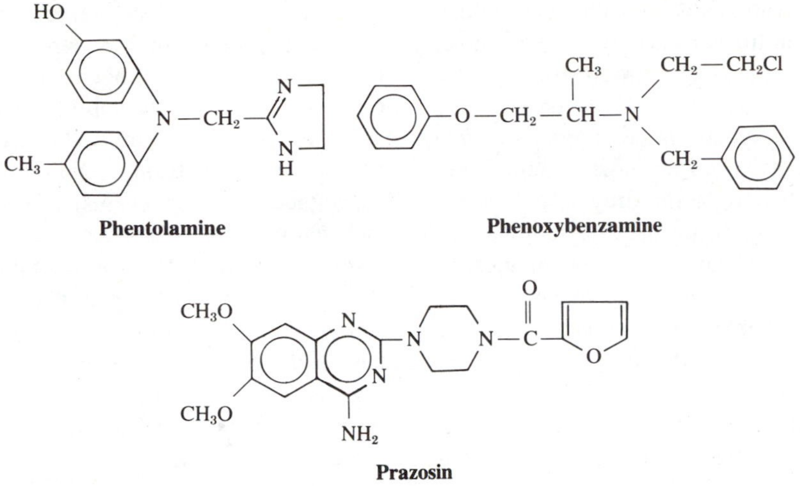

Figure 7-2. Structural formulas of three α-receptor blocking agents, one of which, prazosin, is specific for α_1 receptors.

action of exogenous epinephrine. Their action, however, can be readily reversed by the administration of more agonist.[44]

Two substituted imidazoline derivatives, tolazoline and phentolamine (Figure 7-2), and a dibenzazepine derivative, azapetine, are capable of producing a moderate degree of α-receptor blockade lasting for several hours. This blockade is more effective against circulating epinephrine than it is against neurally released transmitter. Phentolamine is considered more active than tolazoline and azapetine. Because these compounds are partial agonists, it is not surprising that they have sympathomimetic activity; they also have actions similar to acetylcholine and histamine. Therapeutically, doses sufficient to achieve adrenergic blockade produce side effects attributable to these other actions.

A complication arises from the use of these compounds; that is, by blocking the prejunctional α_2 as well as the postjunctional α_1 receptors, they interfere with the negative feedback mechanism (autoregulation) that normally limits the amount of norepinephrine released. The neuron fails to shut itself off, and the excess transmitter may produce many sympathetic side effects via unblocked β receptors.[43]

Although the use of all these agents was at one time promoted for the treatment of essential hypertension, none proved successful or remains in current use for that purpose. Phentolamine is used,

however, to diagnose pheochromocytoma, a chromaffin cell tumor of the adrenal medulla that releases norepinephrine and epinephrine into the circulatory system, producing a form of secondary hypertension.

A number of other compounds have mixed competitive α-adrenergic blocking properties, including the benzodioxans, butyrophenones, and phenothiazines.

Agents acting only postjunctionally. Prazosin is an example of a different kind of α-adrenergic blocking agent (Figure 7-2). It differs from older blocking agents in possessing an affinity only for the α_1 receptor and not the α_2 receptor involved in autoregulation.[31] Prazosin produces hypotension by reducing peripheral resistance, mainly by the relaxation of small arterioles. Like phentolamine, it causes the epinephrine-reversal reaction, an effect usually regarded as evidence for α-receptor blocking activity. Unlike conventional α-receptor blocking agents, prazosin does not cause tachycardia or renin release. Reduction in mean blood pressure occurs in patients in the supine position, at rest, and during exercise. Unlike other antihypertensive agents, prazosin causes only insignificant changes in cardiac rate and cardiac output.[4]

Irreversible α-adrenoceptor blockers

The β-haloalkylamines have the ability to form a stable covalent bond with α receptors. Dibenamine and phenoxybenzamine (Figure 7-2) are examples of such compounds. Phenoxybenzamine, which is six to ten times as active as dibenamine, is the only compound of this group still available for therapeutic use. The half-life of the blockade produced by phenoxybenzamine is approximately 24 hours; thus, daily doses have a cumulative effect. The full action of the drug is not immediate, even though the drug may be administered intravenously. This delay, up to 60 minutes, is the time required to convert a reversible blockade to an irreversible (noncompetitive) block through rearrangement of the drug molecule. Because these agents can block both the α_1 and α_2 receptors, they produce many of the same side effects as do the reversible agents such as phentolamine.

General therapeutic uses

Initially, the α-receptor blocking agents were developed and promoted for the treatment of essential hypertension, but the many side effects related to blockade of the sympathetic nervous system eventually led to their discontinuance. The major problems resulted from the difficulty of maintaining adequate pressure and blood flow to the head region while standing (i.e., orthostatic hypotension). Prazosin produces less postural hemodynamic deficit and remains a useful drug for essential hypertension.

At present, the nonselective α-blocking agents are relegated to the treatment of acute cardiac arrhythmic conditions occurring in the hospitalized patient and hypertensive crises. Circulatory shock is a condition in which there is a lowering of blood pressure and inadequate perfusion of vital organs. Phenoxybenzamine has been investigated for its ability to restore circulation in such affected vascular beds as the mesenteric and renal. The administration of α-blocking agents is considered an adjuvant therapy to other recognized modes of treatment.[33]

Phentolamine, a short-acting agent, is useful in diagnosing unexplained hypertensive crisis and hypertension. The intravenous administration of phentolamine will bring about a prompt reduction of elevated blood pressure if the condition is due to catecholamines. Phentolamine not only is used to diagnose pheochromocytoma but also is administered along with a β-blocking agent during the surgical procedure to remove the tumor.

Toxic reactions and side effects

The lowering of blood pressure caused by blockade, both prejunctional and postjunctional, of α receptors results in compensatory reflex activity, especially increased excitability, contractility, rate, and output of the heart. Orthostatic hypotension commonly results from the loss of control over the capacitance vessels (veins). The symptoms of tachycardia, dizziness, headache, and syncope are disturbing to the patient. Abdominal distress and diarrhea due to uncompensated parasympathetic activity are added problems. In addition, impotence has made compliance among male patients extremely poor. It is not surprising that the symptoms of therapy with these drugs often seem worse than those of the disease.

β-ADRENERGIC RECEPTOR BLOCKING AGENTS

Dichloroisoproterenol (DCI), the first synthetic β-blocking agent, did not prove suitable for therapeutic use, but it did lead to the development of other agents that have gained wide clinical acceptance. The β-receptor blocking drugs represent an important class of therapeutic agents for cardiovascular problems and for a number of other disease states. In fact, one of these drugs, propranolol, is among the most widely prescribed medicines in the United States. At the present time, there exist drugs that are nonselective β-receptor antagonists, meaning that they block both β_1 and β_2 receptors, and selective antagonists that are specific for either β_1 or β_2 receptors. No therapeutic application is currently recognized for agents specific for β_2 receptors.

Chemistry

As exemplified by the first β blocker, DCI, halogen substitution of the catechol hydroxyl groups results in a partial agonist/antagonist of the receptor. As illustrated in Figure 7-3, the currently available β-adrenoceptor blocking agents all possess one of two similar side chains attached to a variant ring structure. Two compounds, atenolol and nadolol, have low lipid solubility due either to the saturated ring hydroxyl groups (nadolol) or to an amide structure (atenolol). It should be noted that the suffix *olol* has been authorized by the USAN Council as denoting β-blocking activity. Several other drugs that have enjoyed popularity for some years in Europe have not been approved for use in the United States.

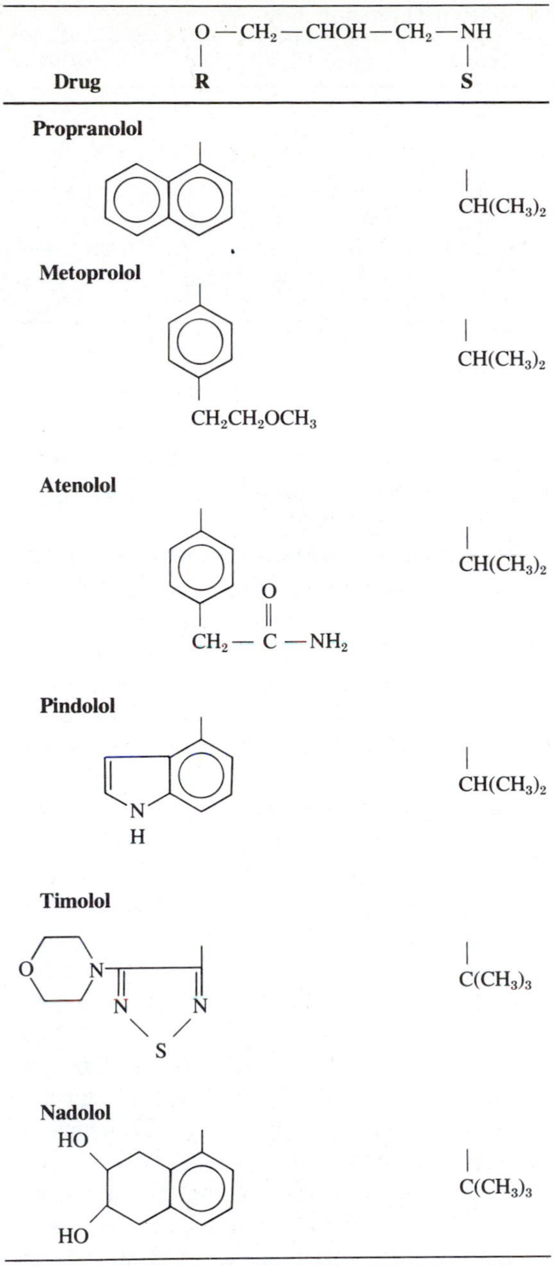

$$O - CH_2 - CHOH - CH_2 - NH$$

Drug	R	S

Propranolol — $CH(CH_3)_2$

Metoprolol — $CH_2CH_2OCH_3$ — $CH(CH_3)_2$

Atenolol — $CH_2 - \overset{O}{\overset{\|}{C}} - NH_2$ — $CH(CH_3)_2$

Pindolol — $CH(CH_3)_2$

Timolol — $C(CH_3)_3$

Nadolol — $C(CH_3)_3$

Figure 7-3. Structural formulas of β-adrenoceptor blocking agents currently approved in the United States. All the drugs share a similar side chain differing only in the terminal hydrocarbon group (S). Considerable variation exists in the ring structures (R).

Mechanism of action

Current theories on the mechanism of action of β-adrenergic agonists are discussed in Chapters 5 and 6. With respect to the antagonists, it is believed that combination of the receptor with an antagonist causes a failure of the GTP binding protein to accept GTP. As a result, the adenylate cyclase is not activated, and cAMP synthesis is retarded.

Pharmacologic effects

Since propranolol was the first β-adrenoceptor blocking agent to be approved in the United States, much of this discussion will be concerned with that drug. However, some of the newer agents have different pharmacodynamic and pharmacokinetic properties; Table 7-1 presents a comparison of propranolol with the other currently approved β blockers.

Propranolol is capable of blocking both β_1 and β_2 receptors; thus, its pharmacologic effects are quite predictable. Several compounds, for instance pindolol, have agonist properties, referred to as intrinsic sympathomimetic activity (ISA). Clinically, such activity should lessen the resultant β-blockade, and indeed pindolol does not depress resting cardiac output or plasma renin activity as do the other drugs listed in Table 7-1. Several of these drugs have a local anesthetic action, sometimes referred to as quinidine-like (in Table 7-1 this is indicated as membrane-stabilizing activity), but this action requires higher blood concentrations than those necessary for β blockade. Propranolol and other compounds with lipophilic properties also penetrate the blood-brain barrier and may act on central adrenergic receptors that are involved with renin release and other functions related to blood pressure regulation.

Cardiac effects. By blocking β_1 receptors in the heart, propranolol causes a reduction in most aspects of cardiac activity, a decreased rate of firing by the sinoatrial (S-A) node, slowed conduction through the atrioventricular (A-V) node and conducting tissue, and reduced contractile strength and automaticity. Collectively, these bring about a decrease in cardiac output. As mentioned before, compounds that have intrinsic agonistic activity produce less of an effect on the heart.

At much higher doses, propranolol can exert a nonspecific action on myocardial muscle membranes similar to that caused by lidocaine.[9] The effects are a shortening of the upstroke of the action potential (phase 1) and a prolongation of the refractory period of the A-V node. These reactions occur at concentrations of propranolol that are about 100 times as great as those required to produce substantial and therapeutically useful β-receptor blockade.[8]

Clinical studies have shown that the *d*-isomer

Table 7-1. Comparison of β-adrenoceptor blocking agents with propranolol

Property	Propranolol	Metoprolol	Timolol	Nadolol	Atenolol	Pindolol
ISA*	—	—	—	—	—	Yes
Membrane-stabilizing activity	High	Low	—	—	—	Low
β₁ selectivity	—	Yes	—	—	Yes	—
Relative potency	1	1	6-8	0.5	1	6
Half-life (hours)	3-5	3-4	4	20-24	6-9	3-4
Route of elimination	Hepatic	Hepatic	Hepatic/renal	Renal	Renal	Hepatic/renal
Lipophilicity	High	Moderate	Moderate	Low	Low	Moderate
Absorption† (%)	90	95	90	30	50	90

*Intrinsic sympathomimetic activity.

†After oral administration. Bioavailability of propranolol and metoprolol is reduced by first-pass metabolism in the liver.

fails to correct arrhythmias even at doses three to four times those of the racemic mixture. The *d*-isomer has the same potency as the *l*-isomer with respect to the nonspecific actions, but the *d*-isomer has very little β-receptor blocking ability. The therapeutic actions of propranolol in treating cardiac arrhythmias appear to be mainly due to the β-blocking effects.

In recent years the use of β blockers in the treatment of postmyocardial infarction patients has produced significant reductions of mortality and reinfarction.[30] The actions presumed to account for the results of these studies are a reduction in heart rate, reduced cardiac output at rest and during exercise, an antiarrhythmic action, and protection of the ischemic heart by a reduction in oxygen demand.

Vascular system effects. Propranolol lowers blood pressure equally in both the supine and standing positions, with no orthostatic hypotension. This attribute was discovered serendipitously while propranolol was being used to treat angina pectoris. Since that time, propranolol, alone or in combination with other antihypertensive drugs, has gained status as a major antihypertensive agent. Although the mechanism by which it accomplishes a lowering of blood pressure is not well understood, certain facts are known. The reduction in blood pressure is associated only with the *l*-isomer, which has the β-receptor blocking activity. When the drug is first administered to a patient, cardiac output decreases and peripheral resistance increases. However, with continued therapy, peripheral resistance also decreases. Propranolol also causes a lowering of plasma renin in most patients, even though the dose may have to be considerably increased. The exact relationship of plasma renin activity to hypertension, as well as to the effects of propranolol, is still quite controversial. Finally, recent studies have revealed that some of the antihypertensive effects of propranolol may be central in origin, especially at high doses.[16]

Effects on bronchial smooth muscle. By blocking the sympathetic innervation of the bronchiolar smooth muscle, propranolol causes a preponderance of parasympathetic activity, resulting in marked constriction. This important side effect of propranolol has been the major impetus for development of blocking agents with only β₁-receptor blocking properties.

Gastrointestinal tract effects. Like other adrenergic blocking agents, propranolol produces an excess of parasympathetic activity in the gastrointestinal tract. The net effect is related to the amount of sympathetic activity that is blocked.

Metabolic effects. Propranolol can block the receptors in the liver that are responsible for initiating glycogenolysis. Hypoglycemia resulting from this blockade is rare in the nondiabetic individual. In the diabetic patient taking hypoglycemic agents, however, compensatory autonomic adjustments to a lowered blood sugar may be blocked.[39]

Ocular effects. While studying the antihypertensive effects of the β-adrenoceptor blockers it was noticed that intraocular pressure in patients with open-angle glaucoma was reduced. The mechanism is presumed to be a decrease in production of aqueous humor, not an increase in outflow.[45]

CNS effects. Those compounds with high lipid solubility can cross the blood-brain barrier and have been used to treat a variety of conditions: migraine headaches, tremors associated with anxiety (stage fright), thyrotoxicosis, Parkinson's disease, benign essential tremor, and drug withdrawal (e.g., from lithium, benzodiazepines, opioids, and alcohol).[15]

Absorption, fate, and excretion

All β-adrenoceptor blockers, except nadolol and atenolol which have low lipid solubility, are readily absorbed after oral administration. Propranolol is subject to an approximately 50% first-pass removal from the portal circulation by the liver.

The first-pass extraction can vary widely among patients, thus necessitating individualized dose regimens. Peak plasma concentrations occur in about 90 minutes, with as much as 90% of the drug being bound to plasma protein. The half-life after oral administration is 3 to 5 hours; intravenous administration results in a half-life of 1½ to 2 hours. The extensive metabolism of propranolol explains why more than 400 to 600 mg daily may be needed in some patients.[34] The bioavailability of propranolol and metoprolol may be significantly improved if the drugs are taken after a high-protein meal, presumably because the protein reduces the first-pass metabolism of the drugs. To mimimize variation in the drug effects, the daily regimen should be consistent with regard to meals.

Metabolism of propranolol occurs almost exclusively in the liver, with oxidative reactions involving both the ring and the side chain. One metabolite, 4-hydroxy propranolol, is as active as the parent compound.[7] Only about 5% of the administered drug is excreted intact in the urine. As noted in Table 7-1, most of the other blocking agents are excreted more extensively by the kidney.

General therapeutic uses

At the present time, propranolol is approved for six major conditions: arrhythmias, angina pectoris, hypertension, myocardial infarction, migraine headache (prophylaxis only[29]), and hypertrophic subaortic stenosis. It is also employed to block the reflex tachycardia occurring in patients receiving hydralazine and minoxidil for hypertension. Propranolol and an α-adrenergic blocking agent are sometimes used both before and during an operation for the control of blood pressure in patients with pheochromocytoma. Other conditions for which propranolol is under consideration are hyperthyroidism and recurrent gastrointestinal bleeding in cirrhotic patients. Noncardiovascular uses being investigated include the treatment of various tremors, stage fright, and drug dependence.[15,20]

Timolol, a nonspecific β-receptor blocking agent without local anesthetic, cardiac depressant, or sympathomimetic actions, has been used topically in the treatment of open-angle glaucoma.[45] Its effectiveness in reducing intraocular pressure is equivalent to or greater than that of pilocarpine and epinephrine, and its use as an ophthalmic solution is attended by fewer side effects (miosis, spasm of accommodation, and irritation). Timolol was also the first β blocker to be approved for use in myocardial infarction patients to reduce the incidence of reinfarction.

Because of limited clinical experience in their use, the other β-receptor blocking drugs are approved currently only for treatment of hypertension (except nadolol, which is also classified as an antianginal drug). It is expected that with time more indications will be added.

Toxic reactions and side effects

The toxic effects of propranolol (Table 7-2) are logical extensions of its principal pharmacologic action—the blockade of β-adrenergic receptors. These effects are seen most prominently in the heart, bronchial smooth muscle, and organs that mediate metabolic responses.[42] The effects of propranolol, a competitive antagonist, can be reversed by giving a β-receptor agonist such as isoproterenol. However, this treatment is reserved for emergency situations, since reversal of the blockade may quickly precipitate dangerous cardiovascular responses. The abrupt withdrawal of propranolol has been linked with myocardial infarction and sudden death;[1] for this reason withdrawal from β-blocking drugs must be done slowly, over a period of 1 to 2 weeks.

Effects on the heart. Patients with congestive heart failure compensate for the diminished myocardial contractile ability by increasing the sympathetic reserve activity. Blockade of this sympathetic reserve can precipitate rapid decompensation, bradyarrhythmias, and cardiac failure. Most often such effects from propranolol are observed during the early phase of therapy and can be largely prevented by careful adjustment of the dose.

Effects on bronchioles. The term *asthmagenic* has been used to describe the effects of β2-receptor blockade on the bronchioles. Acute bronchospasm is apt to occur in patients with chronic pulmonary constrictive disease and bronchitis. Metoprolol and atenolol, agents selective for β1 receptors, are said to spare the β2 receptors of the bronchial smooth muscle.

Metabolic effects. Propranolol can block compensatory metabolic reflexes in patients receiving hypoglycemic medication. Lactic acid release from

Table 7-2. Major side effects of drugs that suppress the activity of the sympathetic nervous system

Side effect	Postsynaptic blocking agents			Presynaptic blocking agents		MAO inhibitors	Agents acting on the central nervous system	
	Nonselective α-receptor blocking agents	Selective α₁-receptor blocking agents (prazosin)	β-Receptor blocking agents	Reserpine	Guanethidine	MAO inhibitors	Methyldopa	Clonidine
CNS effects								
Depression			+	+++	+		+	+
Drowsiness			++	+++		++	++	+++
Dreams/insomnia			++	++		++		
Cardiovascular effects								
Orthostatic hypotension	+++	++ (1st dose)		+	+++	+++	+	+
Heart rate	↑		↓		∿	↑	↓	↓
General autonomic effects								
Diarrhea	++	+		+++	+++		++	Constipation
Nasal stuffiness	++	+		+++			++	
Xerostomia		+		+++			+	+++
Asthma			++					
Fluid retention				++	+++		+	++
Special reactions			Heart failure, withdrawal reaction		Enhanced adrenergic amine response	Hypertensive crisis	Positive Coombs' test, hemolytic anemia, hepatitis	Withdrawal reaction

Key: + = rare, + + = occasional, + + + = common, ↑ = increase, ↓ = decrease, ∿ = arrhythmia.

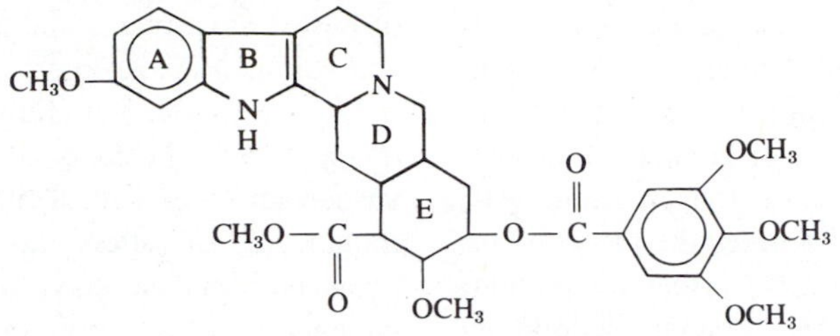

Figure 7-4. Structural formula of reserpine.

skeletal muscle and its conversion to glucose by the liver may be prevented, and this may cause further hypoglycemia. Diagnosis of insulin shock is made difficult by the prevention of tachycardia. Interestingly, a depressed formation of ketone bodies may also mask typical symptoms of diabetes mellitus.

NEURONAL BLOCKING AGENTS

The category of neuronal blocking agents encompasses a wide variety of drugs having different mechanisms of action. Whatever their specific mechanism, the result is usually the same—a depletion of mediator in the neuron terminal or an inability of the mediator to be released from the terminal.

Drugs affecting synthesis of neurotransmitter

Metyrosine and 6-hydroxydopamine are agents that affect synthesis of the neurotransmitter. The former is used in the management of pheochromocytoma; the latter is used as an investigational tool only. Metyrosine inhibits tyrosine hydroxylase, the rate-limiting enzyme in the synthesis of norepinephrine, preventing the formation of dopa from tyrosine and ultimately the synthesis of norepinephrine.[13] 6-Hydroxydopamine causes lysis of the adrenergic nerve terminal, and only after regeneration of the nerve is there a restoration of neuronal activity.[24]

Drugs causing depletion of catecholamines

The most important example of drugs that cause depletion of catecholamines is reserpine, although guanethidine, as will be pointed out later, has some reserpine-like properties. In the early 1950s, much attention was given to several groups of drugs that

could produce tranquilization in both humans and animals without serious impairment of motor reflexes and responses. One group of these drugs was the alkaloids obtained from the root of a shrub, *Rauwolfia serpentina (Benth)*, grown in India and nearby countries. Among the alkaloids extracted, reserpine is predominant and has activity typical of the some 20 other alkaloids present in the crude drug. Reserpine and similar alkaloids briefly gained major status in the treatment of psychotic states. However, serious mental depression and other side effects, as well as the discovery of the phenothiazines, soon brought them into disfavor. An antihypertensive action now accounts for the wide therapeutic use of reserpine. Its ability to deplete neuronal stores of both catecholamines and indoleamines has also made it an important investigational tool.

Chemistry. Initially, the whole ground root or a semipurified fraction containing many alkaloids was used. More recently, purified reserpine or synthetic modifications of this alkaloid have largely replaced the other forms. The structure of reserpine includes an indole moiety, rings A and B (Figure 7-4), which is thought to account for some of its action. Other compounds derived from reserpine are deserpidine, rescinnamine, and syrosingopine. These derivatives of reserpine are produced by modifications of side groups on rings A and E.

Mechanism of action. Reserpine induces the release of monoamines from intracellular vesicles, both in the periphery and in the central nervous system. It causes depletion of dopamine, norepinephrine, epinephrine, and 5-hydroxytryptamine (serotonin, 5-HT) from their respective nerve terminals. Besides releasing stored monoamines into the neuronal cytoplasm, it also blocks their uptake by the vesicles, thus indirectly preventing synthesis of norepinephrine and epinephrine.[6] The binding of reserpine with the vesicular amine-concentrating mechanism is quite permanent, and the effect of reserpine lasts considerably longer than its plasma half-life would indicate. Clinically, a reduction in stored catecholamine of 70% or greater is required to impair sympathetic nerve transmission. Although reserpine easily penetrates the blood-brain barrier to exert prominent CNS effects, depletion of catecholamines from the adrenal medulla is slower and less complete than for nerve terminals. Reserpine differs from guanethidine in not possessing a tyramine-like action; that is, it does not release the transmitter through the neuronal membrane. The release of the transmitter occurs intraneuronally, and unless MAO is inactivated, adrenergic effects on blood pressure and cardiac activity are not observed.[21]

Pharmacologic effects. The tranquilizing, antihypertensive, and adverse side effects of reserpine are caused by depletion of monoamines. Centrally, the loss of dopamine and serotonin disrupts many neural circuits known to be involved with emotional and behavioral states. The depletion of biogenic amines also alters the sleep state, affecting the patterns of both REM (rapid eye movement) and non-REM sleep.

Similarly, depletion of both central and peripheral stores of transmitters brings about a mild reduction of blood pressure. This effect is the result of a reduction in the contractile strength of the myocardium and a decrease in peripheral resistance through vasodilation of the arterioles. In high doses, reserpine has a direct vasodilator action thought to be due to its phosphodiesterase inhibitor activity.[37]

General therapeutic uses. The use of reserpine in the treatment of hypertension has generally been relegated to the mild forms, and it is usually prescribed as a supplement to diuretic therapy. With the advent of newer antihypertensives, the use of reserpine has decreased. Chapter 28 contains further information on reserpine.

Toxic reactions and side effects. Most, if not all, of the side effects of reserpine are attributable to a reduction of sympathetic activity and the resultant relative increase in parasympathetic tone. An important central effect, mental depression, occasionally results in suicide. Disturbed sleep patterns, including insomnia and nightmares, are frequently noted.[40] Common manifestations of reserpine's peripheral actions are nasal stuffiness, increased secretion of gastric acid associated with

ulcers and hemorrhaging, and increased frequency of bowel movements and diarrhea. Paradoxically, xerostomia is also a commonly reported side effect.

Recovery after withdrawal of the drug is slow, taking several weeks or longer. Use of adrenergic vasoconstrictors with local anesthesia is not contraindicated in patients taking only reserpine. Hypotensive episodes have occurred in reserpinized patients given general anesthesia. Adverse responses have been treated with those adrenergic amines typically used for hypotensive states, (e.g., epinephrine, mephentermine, and metaraminol).

Drugs preventing release and causing depletion of catecholamines

Guanethidine, bretylium, and guanadrel are currently approved for use in the United States. Chemically, bretylium is unrelated to guanethidine and guanadrel, but all show enough structural similarity to norepinephrine to account for their activity (Figure 7-5). Two other agents, bethanidine and debrisoquin, not yet approved for use in the United States, have actions that are similar but of shorter duration.

Pharmacologic effects. These compounds diminish the activity of sympathetic postganglionic nerve fibers. They do not block the effects of exogenous direct-acting adrenergic amines, but they do block the action of indirect-acting amines such as tyramine and amphetamine. They are taken up by the nerve terminals (uptake 1) by the same mechanism as norepinephrine, are stored in the vesicles, and are released by action potentials.[5] However, failure of functional transmission can occur before nerve-terminal concentrations of norepinephrine have been reduced to any degree. In the case of bretylium, there is an alteration of the excitation-release mechanism, which blocks the release of the transmitter by the nerve action potential.

Guanethidine is considered to have four mechanisms of action: bretylium-like, tyramine-like, reserpine-like, and cocaine-like. These actions of guanethidine are time-related. With acute administration, inhibition of transmitter release occurs before there is any measurable depletion in norepinephrine stores. This action is similar to that of bretylium. Guanethidine's tyramine-like action causes a transitory stimulation of sympathetic nervous activity, manifested by piloerection, hypertension, and some myocardial stimulation. If the stores of norepinephrine are increased, as will oc-

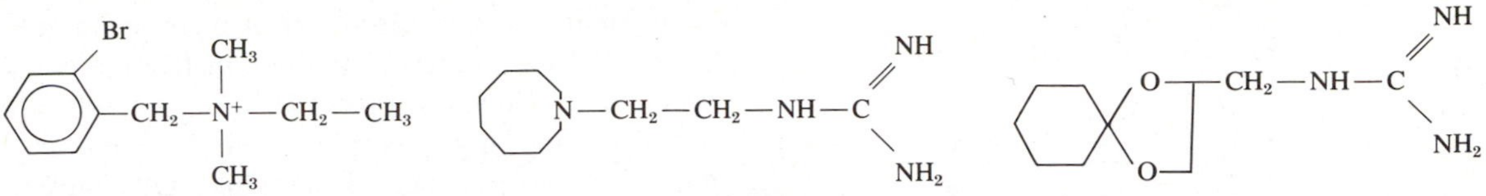

Figure 7-5. Structural formulas of bretylium, guanethidine, and guanadrel.

cur with pretreatment with MAO inhibitors, oral administration of guanethidine may cause a release of stored norepinephrine, resulting in an elevation of blood pressure similar to that seen when the drug is given intravenously to normal patients. Continued administration of guanethidine allows for its accumulation in the vesicles, where it replaces norepinephrine to a considerable extent. After the initial bretylium-like effect, nerve stimulation can now cause a parallel release of both guanethidine and norepinephrine. In this instance, guanethidine is acting as a false transmitter. Finally, guanethidine, like cocaine, inhibits the uptake-1 mechanism, especially that for the true transmitter.[41]

Absorption, fate, and excretion. The absorption of guanethidine from the intestinal tract is quite variable, with as little as 3% of the drug reaching the systemic circulation. The drug is rapidly removed from the blood by being sequestered in the various storage sites in tissues. The elimination of the drug from these various extravascular compartments is prolonged, leading to a half-life of 5 days. This "cumulative" effect of guanethidine allows for a maintenance dose to be given daily once the steady state drug concentration has been achieved, usually in about 2 weeks.

Guanadrel is rapidly absorbed after oral administration, reaching peak blood concentrations after 1.5 to 2 hours. With a mean plasma half-life of 10 hours, twice daily dosing is usually necessary. Bretylium is so poorly absorbed that parenteral administration is required.

General therapeutic uses. As is discussed in Chapter 28, the major indication for guanethidine and guanadrel is in the treatment of moderate to severe hypertension. Because of their side effects, these agents are not considered to be primary drugs and are reserved for patients whose hypertension is not adequately controlled by safer or better tolerated drugs. Bretylium finds use in the treatment

of ventricular arrhythmias not amenable to lidocaine therapy (see Chapter 24).

Toxic reactions and side effects. These drugs belong to a group of agents that are often referred to as orthostatic antihypertensives, because the reflex adjustment of blood pressure in response to postural changes and exertion is affected. In common with other drugs affecting adrenergic neurons, an increase in parasympathetic activity is noted, mainly because there is little or no compensatory response from the sympathetic division. Salt and water retention occurs and may require therapy with a thiazide diuretic. Other side effects, such as diarrhea, failure to ejaculate, and a feeling of weakness, are also quite common.

Drug interactions. Because the actions of guanethidine are dependent on uptake into the nerve ending, its actions are blocked or reversed by the tricyclic antidepressants and the phenothiazines. In a similar manner, amphetamines and other indirect-acting amines may displace guanethidine from the vesicles. Prolonged reduction in the amount of neurotransmitter caused by guanethidine may bring about an increased reactivity to adrenergic amines that resembles denervation supersensitivity. This effect and the cocaine-like action of guanethidine may cause an exaggeration of the effect of the direct-acting amines such as norepinephrine, epinephrine, and some of the sympathomimetics present in cold remedies.

Monoamine oxidase inhibitors

Paradoxical as it may seem, MAO inhibitors, drugs capable of inhibiting the intracellular enzyme responsible for the inactivation of norepinephrine, cause a lowering of blood pressure. One such drug, pargyline (Figure 7-6), was specifically marketed for the treatment of essential hypertension. (See Chapter 12 for the antidepressant uses of these drugs.) Although the exact mechanism of action is not understood, evidence suggests that autoregu-

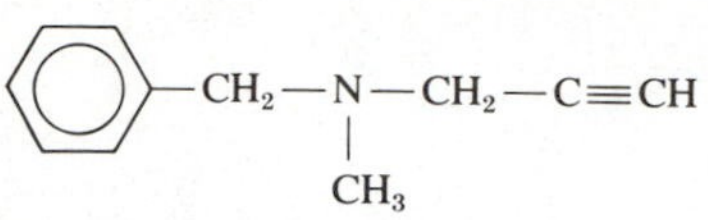

$$\langle\!\!\bigcirc\!\!\rangle - CH_2 - N - CH_2 - C \equiv CH$$
$$\hspace{3.2cm} | $$
$$\hspace{3.2cm} CH_3$$

Figure 7-6. Structural formula of the MAO inhibitor pargyline.

lation may play a role. By preventing inactivation of the transmitter, pargyline allows it to accumulate in nerve terminals. Such an accumulation, via a negative feedback loop, prevents the release of norepinephrine. Another theory to explain the antihypertensive actions of MAO inhibitors involves the accumulation of a false transmitter in vesicles. With the inhibition of MAO, tyramine is hydroxylated to form octopamine, a false transmitter with about 1% of the activity of norepinephrine. This theory presumes a daily consumption of small amounts of tyramine from ordinary foods (other than those mentioned in the following section).[23]

Toxic reactions and side effects. The risks of pargyline therapy for hypertension appear to outweigh the benefits, and its use as an antihypertensive has declined. The most frequent adverse effects are those associated with other adrenergic and ganglionic blocking agents: orthostatic hypotension, dizziness, weakness, and syncope. Difficulties in micturition and ejaculation are also experienced. Most serious is the hypertensive crisis that can occur after eating or drinking foodstuffs containing substantial amounts of tyramine. Aged cheese, liver, beer, and wines are among the most common of these tyramine-containing foods. The hypertension is the result of three factors: (1) the metabolism of tyramine by MAO, which would normally take place in the gastrointestinal tract, is blocked by MAO inhibitors, (2) tyramine is an indirect-acting amine and causes release of neurotransmitter from the vesicles, and (3) large amounts of the transmitter accumulate as a result of the inhibition of MAO. Besides the typical symptoms of acute hypertension, such effects as throbbing headaches, flushing and hyperpyrexia, cerebral vascular accidents, and occasionally death have occurred.[38]

Drug interactions. Pargyline can inhibit other oxidative enzymes throughout the body, including those in the liver. The use of the analgesic meperidine is contraindicated in patients taking pargyline

because the oxidative reactions primarily responsible for the biotransformation of meperidine are blocked. As a result, a convulsant metabolite may accumulate. However, opioid analgesics unrelated to meperidine (e.g., morphine) are not contraindicated in the presence of pargyline. Other drug interactions of importance are detailed in Chapter 12.

CENTRALLY ACTING AGENTS

Three centrally acting agents, methyldopa, clonidine, and guanabenz, are currently approved for use in the treatment of hypertension. A fourth drug, guanfacine, is at present in the clinical trial phase for the same condition. It should be noted that clonidine, guanabenz, and guanfacine are guanidine derivatives similar in some respects to the neuronal depleters guanethidine and guanadrel. Their structures are shown in Figure 7-7.

Methyldopa, originally studied as an inhibitor of histamine synthesis, was found to cause a marked lowering of blood pressure in hypertensive rats.[36] While the compound does block the decarboxylase responsible for converting dopa to dopamine, this action does not appear to account for its antihypertensive activity. The drug is a methyl derivative of dopa, an important intermediate in the synthesis of norepinephrine. An amino acid, methyldopa readily crosses the blood-brain barrier, and once it passes into the nerve terminal it is subjected to biotransformation just like its nonmethylated analogue, dopa. Thus, methyldopa is converted to methyldopamine and then to α-methylnorepinephrine.

Initially, it was thought that α-methylnorepinephrine was a false transmitter, an inactive metabolite replacing norepinephrine in the nerve terminals. While it does exist in the vesicles, research has shown that the compound is nearly equipotent to norepinephrine in humans.[2] Indeed, the agent has been assigned the nonproprietary name of levonordefrin and is commonly used as a vasoconstrictor in local anesthetic solutions. Since it is not metabolized by MAO, it has a longer action than norepinephrine in inhibiting transmitter release by a negative feedback mechanism.

Clonidine was first used as a nasal decongestant, but it was soon found to produce a lowering of blood pressure. An imidazoline, clonidine is an α_2-receptor agonist with relatively weak peripheral effects.[10]

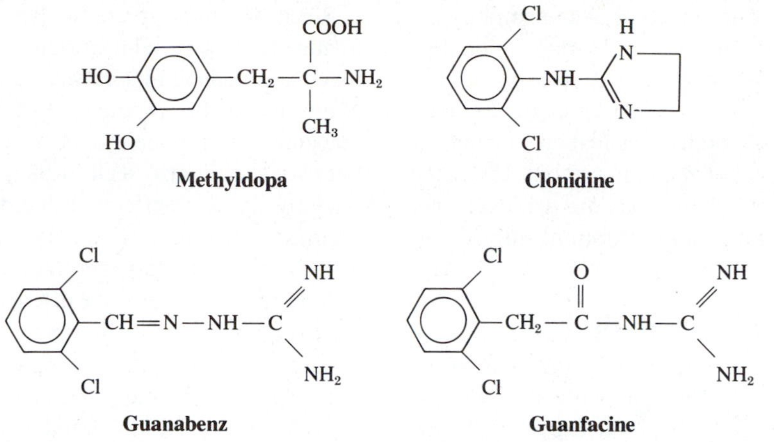

Figure 7-7. Structural formulas of the centrally acting α_2-adrenoceptor agonists.

Pharmacologic effects

While the central mechanisms regulating cardiovascular activity are not yet fully understood, the nucleus tractus solatarius (NTS) in the brainstem is known to be the primary recipient of impulses from the peripheral baroreceptors and chemoreceptors and acts as an important relay station for the distribution of this input to all levels of the central nervous system. The nucleus also receives processed information from some of the major brain areas involved with cardiovascular reflexes. Recent experiments have shown that administration by stereotactic techniques of the α agonists norepinephrine, dopamine, α-methylnorepinephrine, and clonidine into the NTS causes a reduction in blood pressure and a slowing of the heart attributable to increases in vagal tone and decreases in sympathetic activity.[14] These effects can be prevented by administration into the cerebrospinal fluid of α-receptor blocking agents[22] or, in the case of α-methylnorepinephrine, by pharmacologically preventing its synthesis from methyldopa.[18] Other studies indicate that stimulation of the NTS with α agonists activates second-order neurons,[35] those going to the nucleus ambiguus facilitating vagally induced bradycardia and those going to the vasomotor centers causing inhibition of sympathetic activity to the vascular beds.

The administration of these centrally acting drugs in humans results in a moderate decrease in the systemic mean blood pressure, not from a decrease in peripheral resistance but through a decreased cardiac output by a combination of slowing the heart rate and reducing venous return.

Serendipity has played a role in the use of clonidine in treating the withdrawal symptoms of opioid addiction.[25] Clonidine, when given to addicts undergoing withdrawal treatment, blocks the nausea, vomiting, sweating, diarrhea, and other symptoms of excessive autonomic discharge (see Chapter 46). Although precise evidence is not yet available, it appears that the neurons of the locus ceruleus of the dorsolateral pons are inhibited by opioids. When the opioids are withdrawn, the neurons are disinhibited and release excessive norepinephrine, which gives rise to the many symptoms of withdrawal. Clonidine, by activating the α_2 receptors on these same neurons, likewise causes inhibition and a reduction of neurotransmitter release. The current clinical practice is to follow abrupt withdrawal of the opioid with oral administration of clonidine for 2 weeks or until the absence of withdrawal symptoms to a naloxone challenge indicates opioid detoxification is complete. Clonidine is then discontinued and more conventional therapy instituted. Similarly, patients with alcohol-abuse problems, certain neurologic diseases, or some forms of psychotic illness show therapeutic results with clonidine.

Metabolism, fate, and excretion

Methyldopa is incompletely absorbed when taken orally. It reaches its maximal effect in about 6 hours, the effect lasting over 24 hours. The drug is excreted either unchanged or as the sulfate conjugate. Better absorbed than methyldopa, clonidine is excreted largely unchanged in the urine. The half-life of clonidine is approximately 8 hours when administered orally. Guanabenz is rapidly absorbed and metabolized, only about 1% being excreted unchanged. Its actions are apparent after 1 hour. Twice daily administration suffices for many patients.

Toxic reactions and side effects

Although the exact mechanism and sites of action of these drugs differ, clinically methyldopa, clonidine, and guanabenz produce essentially the same reactions. Orthostatic hypotension with the centrally acting drugs is rare. Cardiac output and blood flow to the kidneys are well maintained. Sleepiness and drowsiness are seen during therapy with all three drugs. One distinctive difference is that xerostomia is commonly seen with clonidine and guanabenz and rarely with methyldopa. Occasionally, the centrally acting α_2-receptor agonists cause impotence.

Unique to methyldopa is the occurrence of drug-induced hepatitis, with a fever that may reach alarming levels (105 F). Withdrawal of the drug usually allows liver function to return to normal. This reaction has been shown to be related to the transformation of methyldopa to reactive compounds that combine covalently with cellular macromolecules.[11]

Clonidine and guanabenz when withdrawn may cause an alarming increase in blood pressure within a few hours. Patients should be warned not to terminate medication abruptly, and when a patient is being considered for hospitalization and surgery, attention should be given to the continuation of antihypertensive therapy.[3]

IMPLICATIONS FOR DENTISTRY

Agents that suppress functions of the sympathetic nervous system as well as those that block the actions of exogenous adrenergic amines have a number of important implications for the practice of dentistry. Almost without exception, these drugs are used to treat serious cardiovascular problems. Drug therapy with any of these blocking agents results in a patient whose autonomic reflexes for maintaining homeostasis have been compromised.

Physical implications

Since the greatest use of these drugs is for the treatment of essential hypertension, the mention of them in a medical history should immediately alert clinicians to this problem. Not only should they recognize the probable existence of hypertension, but they should also seek further information, particularly any side effects to the drug and the dose regimen. This information should allow the clinician to schedule the patient at a time of day when sedation and lethargy, side effects common to most antihypertensives, are minimal.

A second consideration for patients being treated with these drugs is the patient's position during and after dental procedures. Suddenly standing upright after being in a supine position in the dental chair is very apt to cause syncope. This is particularly true for the orthostatic hypotensive drugs (e.g., α-adrenergic blocking agents and guanethidine). Accidents ranging from broken teeth and restorations to fractured mandibles and worse have resulted from such falls. Contemporary practice standards require the monitoring of blood pressure of such patients during the course of dental therapy.

Drug implications

For many people, the dentist represents still another practitioner from whom they receive therapy. Increasingly, incidents are reported of patients who are receiving medication from one practitioner failing to inform the dentist of a change in drug therapy or dosage. With the sympathetic inhibitors this can be a very serious problem. Patients taking MAO inhibitors, neuronal depleters, and β blockers have an impaired ability to metabolize, sequester, or counteract the influences of the adrenergic agonists. Hypertensive crises have occurred in the office as a result of these impairments. With patients taking propranolol for hypertension, blood pressures have risen precipitously as the result of infiltrating tissues about the face with a local anesthetic containing epinephrine. Hemostatic preparations containing high concentrations of epinephrine are absolutely contraindicated. However, the requirement for adequate control of anxiety and pain is still valid since the adrenal gland represents a sizeable store of catecholamines (except when reserpine has been given).

In the case of guanethidine, a condition resembling denervation supersensitivity may be clinically significant: the intensity of the response to exogenous amines may be increased severalfold as the result.[12] Agents acting centrally or on the postganglionic fibers have little tendency to produce this effect, but they do cause a rebound hypertension when the patient is removed from therapy even for a short period of time (8 to 12 hours).

Adrenergic blocking drugs

Nonproprietary name	Proprietary name
α-Adrenergic blocking agents	
azapetine	Ilidar
dihydrogenated ergot alkaloids	Hydergine
phenoxybenzamine	Dibenzyline
phentolamine	Regitine
prazosin	Minipress
tolazoline	Priscoline
β-Adrenergic blocking agents	
atenolol	Tenormin
metoprolol	Lopressor
nadolol	Corgard
oxprenolol	Trasicor, Iset
pindolol	Visken
propranolol	Inderal
timolol	Timoptic, Blocadren
α- and β-adrenergic blocking agents	
labetalol*	Trandate, Vescal
Neuronal blocking agents	
alseroxylon	Rauwiloid
bretylium	Bretylol
deserpidine	Harmonyl
guanadrel	Hylorel
guanethidine	Ismelin
metyrosine	Demser
pargyline	Eutonyl
rauwolfia, crude root	Raudixin
rescinnamine	Moderil
reserpine	Serpasil
Centrally acting agents	
clonidine	Catapres
guanabenz	Wytensin
guanfacine*	—
methyldopa	Aldomet

*Not currently available in the United States.

CITED REFERENCES

1. Alderman, E.L., Coltart, D.J., Wettach, G.E., and Harrison, D.C. Coronary artery syndromes after sudden propranolol withdrawal. Annals of Internal Medicine **81**:625-627, 1974.
2. Altura, B.M. Pharmacological effects of alpha-methyldopa, alpha-methylnorepinephrine, and octopamine on rat arteriolar, arterial, and terminal vascular smooth muscle. Circulation Research **36**(suppl. 6, part I):233-240, 1975.
3. Brodsky, J.B., and Bravo, J.J. Acute postoperative clonidine withdrawal syndrome. Anesthesiology **44**:519-520, 1976.
4. Brogden, R.N., Heel, R.C., Speight, T.M., and Avery, G.S. Prazosin: a review of its pharmacological properties and therapeutic efficacy in hypertension. Drugs **14**:163-197, 1977.
5. Cass, R., and Spriggs, T.L.B. Tissue amine levels and sympathetic blockade after guanethidine and bretylium. British Journal of Pharmacology **17**:442-450, 1961.
6. Chidsey, C.A., Braunwald, E., Morrow, A.G., and Mason, D.T. Myocardial norepinephrine concentration in man: effects of reserpine and of congestive heart failure. New England Journal of Medicine **269**:653-658, 1963.
7. Cleaveland, C.R., and Shand, D.G. Effect of route of administration on the relationship between β-adrenergic blockade and plasma propranolol level. Clinical Pharmacology and Therapeutics **13**:181-195, 1972.
8. Coltart, D.J., Gibson, D.G., and Shand, D.G. Plasma propranolol levels associated with the suppression of ventricular ectopic beats. British Medical Journal **1**:490-491, 1971.
9. Davis, L.D., and Tempte, J.V. Effects of propranolol on the transmembrane potentials of ventricular muscle and Purkinje fibers of the dog. Circulation Research **22**:661-677, 1968.
10. Dollery, C.T., Davies, D.S., Draffan, G.H., Dargie, H.J., Dean, C.R., Reid, J.L., Clare, R.A., and Murray, S. Clinical pharmacology and pharmacokinetics of clonidine. Clinical Pharmacology and Therapeutics **19**:11-17, 1976.
11. Dybing, E., Nelson, E.D., Mitchell, J.R., Sasame, H.A., and Gillette, J.R. Oxidation of α-methyldopa and other catechols by cytochrome P-450–generated superoxide anion: possible mechanism of methyldopa hepatitis. Molecular Pharmacology **12**:911-920, 1976.
12. Emmelin, N., and Engström, J. Supersensitivity of salivary glands following treatment with bretylium or guanethidine. British Journal of Pharmacology **16**:315-319, 1961.
13. Engelman, K., Horwitz, D., Jéquier, E., and Sjoerdsma, A. Biochemical and pharmacologic effects of α-methyltyrosine in man. Journal of Clinical Investigation **47**:577-594, 1968.
14. Finch, L., and Haeusler, G. Further evidence for a central hypotensive action of α-methyldopa in both the rat and cat. British Journal of Pharmacology **47**:217-228, 1973.
15. Fisher, R.G., and Byrd, H.J. Beta-adrenergic blocking agents. U.S. Pharmacist **7**:46-60, 1982.
16. Garvey, H.L., and Ram, N. Comparative antihypertensive effects and tissue distribution of *beta* adrenergic blocking drugs. Journal of Pharmacology and Experimental Therapeutics **194**:220-233, 1975.
17. Harden, T.K. Agonist-induced desensitization of the β-adrenergic receptor-linked adenylate cyclase. Pharmacological Reviews **35**:5-32, 1983.

18. Heise, A., and Kroneberg, G. Central nervous alpha-adrenergic receptors and mode of action of alpha-methyldopa. Naunyn-Schmiedeberg's Archives of Pharmacology **279**:285-300, 1973.

19. Hoffman, B.B., and Lefkowitz, R.J. Alpha-adrenergic receptor subtypes. New England Journal of Medicine **302**:1390-1396, 1980.

20. Hollister, L.E., and Prusmack, J.J. Propranolol in withdrawal from opiates. Archives of General Psychiatry **31**:695-698, 1974.

21. Iverson, L.L. Catecholamine uptake processes. British Medical Bulletin **29**:130-135, 1973.

22. Kobinger, W., and Walland, A. Facilitation of vagal reflex bradycardia by an action of clonidine on central α-receptors. European Journal of Pharmacology **19**:210-217, 1972.

23. Kopin, I.J., Fischer, J.E., Musacchio, J.M., Horst, W.D., and Wiese, V.K. "False neurochemical transmitters" and the mechanism of sympathetic blockade by monoamine oxidase inhibitors. Journal of Pharmacology and Experimental Therapeutics **147**:186-193, 1965.

24. Kostrzewa, R.M., and Jacobwitz, D.M. Pharmacological actions of 6-hydroxydopamine. Pharmacological Reviews **26**:199-288, 1974.

25. Lal, H., and Fielding, S. Clonidine in the treatment of narcotic addiction. Trends in Pharmacological Sciences **4**:70-71, 1983.

26. Lands, A.M., Arnold, A., McAuliff, J.P., Luduena, F.P., and Brown, T.G., Jr. Differentiation of receptor systems activated by sympathomimetic amines. Nature **214**:597-598, 1967.

27. Langer, S.Z. The role of α and β presynaptic receptors in the regulation of noradrenaline release elicited by nerve stimulation. Clinical Science and Molecular Medicine **51**:423S-426S, 1976.

28. Leclerc, G., Rouot, B., Velly, J., and Schwartz, J. β-adrenergic receptor subtypes. Trends in Pharmacological Sciences **2**:18-20, 1981.

29. Ludvigsson, J. Propranolol used in prophylaxis of migraine in children. Acta Neurologica Scandinavica **50**:109-115, 1974.

30. Lund-Johansen, L. Beta-blockers in post-myocardial infarction patients: the Norwegian timolol trial. Trends in Pharmacological Sciences **4**:36-40, 1983.

31. Massingham, R., and Hayden, M.L. A comparison of the effects of prazosin and hydrallazine on blood pressure, heart rate, and plasma renin activity in conscious renal hypertensive dogs. European Journal of Pharmacology **30**:121-124, 1975.

32. Mickey, J., Tate, R., and Lefkowitz, R.J. Subsensitivity of adenylate cyclase and decreased β-adrenergic receptor binding after chronic exposure to (−)-isoproterenol in vitro. Journal of Biological Chemistry **250**:5727-5729, 1975.

33. Nickerson, M., and Gourzis, J.T. Blockade of sympathetic vasoconstriction in the treatment of shock. Journal of Trauma **2**:399-411, 1962.

34. Nies, A.S., and Shand, D.G. Clinical pharmacology of propranolol. Circulation **52**:6-15, 1975.

35. Nijkamp, F.P., and DeJong, W. α-Methylnoradrenaline induced hypotension and bradycardia after administration into the area of the nucleus tractus solitarii. European Journal of Pharmacology **32**:361-364, 1975.

36. Oates, J.A., Gillespie, L., Udenfriend, S., and Sjoerdsma, A. Decarboxylase inhibition and blood pressure reduction by α-methyl-3,4-dihydroxy-D,L-phenylalanine. Science **131**:1890-1891, 1960.

37. Parks, V.J., Sandison, A.G., Skinner, S.L., and Whelan, R.F. The mechanism of the vasodilator action of reserpine in man. Clinical Science and Molecular Medicine **20**:289-295, 1961.

38. Pettinger, W.A., and Oates, J.A. Supersensitivity to tyramine during monoamine oxidase inhibition in man: mechanism at the level of the adrenergic neuron. Clinical Pharmacology and Therapeutics **9**:341-344, 1968.

39. Podolsky, S., and Pattavina, C.G. Hyperosmolar nonketotic diabetic coma: a complication of propranolol therapy. Metabolism **22**:685-693, 1973.

40. Quetsch, R.M., Achor, R.W.P., Litin, E.M., and Faucet, R.L. Depressive reactions in hypertensive patients: a comparison of those treated with rauwolfia and those receiving no specific antihypertensive treatment. Circulation **19**:366-375, 1959.

41. Shand, D.G., Morgan, D.H., and Oates, J.A. The release of guanethidine and bethanidine by splenic nerve stimulation: a quantitative evaluation showing dissociation from adrenergic blockade. Journal of Pharmacology and Experimental Therapeutics **184**:73-80, 1973.

42. Stephen, S.A. Unwanted effects of propranolol. American Journal of Cardiology **18**:463-468, 1966.

43. Stokes, G.S., and Oates, H.F. Prazosin: new alpha-adrenergic blocking agent in the treatment of hypertension. Cardiovascular Medicine **3**:41-57, 1978.

44. Struyker Boudier, J., Smeets, G., Brouwer, G., and van Rossum, J. Central and peripheral alpha-adrenergic activity of imidazoline derivatives. Life Sciences **15**:887-899, 1974.

45. Zimmerman, T.J., and Kaufman, H.E. Timolol: a β-adrenergic blocking agent for the treatment of glaucoma. Archives of Ophthalmology **95**:601-604, 1977.

GENERAL REFERENCES

Antonaccio, M.J. Neuropharmacology of central mechanisms governing the circulation. In Antonaccio, M., ed. Cardiovascular Pharmacology. New York, Raven Press, 1977.

Kellaway, G.S.M. Adverse drug reactions during treatment of hypertension. Drugs **11**(suppl. 1):91-99, 1976.

Moore, K.E., and Dominic, J.A. Tyrosine hydroxylase inhibitors. Federation Proceedings **30**:859-870, 1971.

Orme, M.L. Clinical pharmacology and therapeutic uses of beta adrenergic blocking drugs. Hospital Formulary **13**:366-383, 1978.

Potter, D.K. Adrenergic pharmacology of aqueous humor dynamics. Pharmacological Reviews **33**:133-153, 1981.

Taylor, S.H., Silke, B., and Lee, P.S. Intravenous beta-blockade in coronary heart disease. New England Journal of Medicine **306**:631-635, 1982.

Vedin, J.A., and Wilhelmsson, C.E. Beta receptor blocking agents in the secondary prevention of coronary heart disease. Annual Review of Pharmacology and Toxicology **23**:29-44, 1983.

8 Cholinergic drugs

Enid A. Neidle

Cholinergic drugs are compounds that mimic the actions of the endogenous neurotransmitter ACh. Direct-acting, or *cholinomimetic,* agents combine with cholinergic receptors, muscarinic or nicotinic or both, to cause a response in an effector. These drugs include ACh, various choline-ester congeners of ACh, and some alkaloids. With few exceptions (i.e., nicotine and other ganglionic stimulants), these agents exert prominent muscarinic or *parasympathomimetic* effects. The indirect-acting cholinergic drugs discussed herein are those substances that are capable of inhibiting the esterases responsible for the inactivation of ACh. These *anticholinesterases* derive their effects from their ability to prolong the life of ACh at receptor sites.

ACETYLCHOLINE AND CHOLINE ESTERS

The history of the discovery of ACh and its identification was covered in Chapter 5. In 1909, Hunt synthesized the acetyl ester of choline, and earlier Hunt and Taveau reported on the pharmacology of a number of synthetic congeners of ACh.[12] Interest in the choline esters arose, in part, out of the hope that some of these compounds would have a longer duration of action than ACh and, at the same time, a greater degree of selectivity. This goal has only partially been realized, and in general ACh and related drugs are either not used therapeutically or used only in very rare instances. The structure of ACh and the three principal esters of choline are shown in Figure 8-1.

PILOCARPINE AND MUSCARINE

Several alkaloids including pilocarpine, which is derived from the leaves of *Pilocarpus jaborandi,* a tropical South American shrub, and muscarine, found in such poisonous mushrooms as *Amanita muscaria,* have been known for some time to mimic the actions of ACh and to have the property of combining with cholinergic receptors, particularly of the muscarinic variety. In fact, as was pointed out in Chapter 5, the term *muscarinic* derives from the observation that muscarine has a very selective effect on certain cholinergic receptors, such as those found in the sweat glands, secretory glands, heart, and bronchial muscle. As can be seen in Figure 8-2, pilocarpine is a tertiary amine and muscarine is a quaternary ammonium compound. There are no therapeutic indications for muscarine because it is highly toxic; pilocarpine remains in the armamentarium for a few specific uses.

ANTICHOLINESTERASES

Physostigmine, or eserine, the earliest and best known anticholinesterase, has a colorful history. An alkaloid, it is derived from a bean, or nut, known as the Calabar, ordeal, or Esére bean, and was used in witchcraft trials by certain native tribes in West Africa. The bean was brought to England by a British medical officer stationed in Calabar in the mid-1800s, and its pharmacologic properties were investigated in a number of laboratories, including those of Fraser, who studied its toxicity in the 1860s and noted that its actions were antagonized by atropine.[19] As early as 1877, eserine, or physostigmine, was used for the treatment of glaucoma, which remains one of its principal uses today. In 1914, noting the extreme brevity of the action of ACh, Dale[5] suggested that an enzyme capable of destroying ACh must exist in the body, and in 1930 it was found that physostigmine could prevent the rapid destruction of ACh.[9] By the 1930s, the chemical structure of physostigmine had been elucidated,[1,26] a series of synthetic analogues had been synthesized, and several researchers had

137

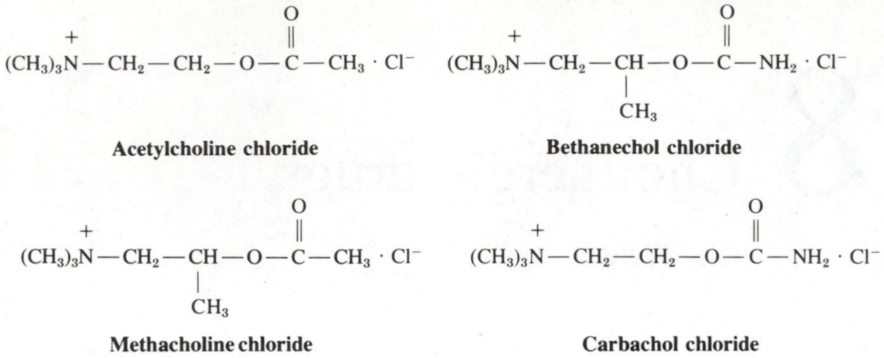

$$(CH_3)_3 \overset{+}{N} - CH_2 - CH_2 - O - \overset{\overset{O}{\|}}{C} - CH_3 \cdot Cl^-$$

Acetylcholine chloride

$$(CH_3)_3 \overset{+}{N} - CH_2 - \underset{\underset{CH_3}{|}}{CH} - O - \overset{\overset{O}{\|}}{C} - NH_2 \cdot Cl^-$$

Bethanechol chloride

$$(CH_3)_3 \overset{+}{N} - CH_2 - \underset{\underset{CH_3}{|}}{CH} - O - \overset{\overset{O}{\|}}{C} - CH_3 \cdot Cl^-$$

Methacholine chloride

$$(CH_3)_3 \overset{+}{N} - CH_2 - CH_2 - O - \overset{\overset{O}{\|}}{C} - NH_2 \cdot Cl^-$$

Carbachol chloride

Figure 8-1. Structural formulas of ACh and three congeners.

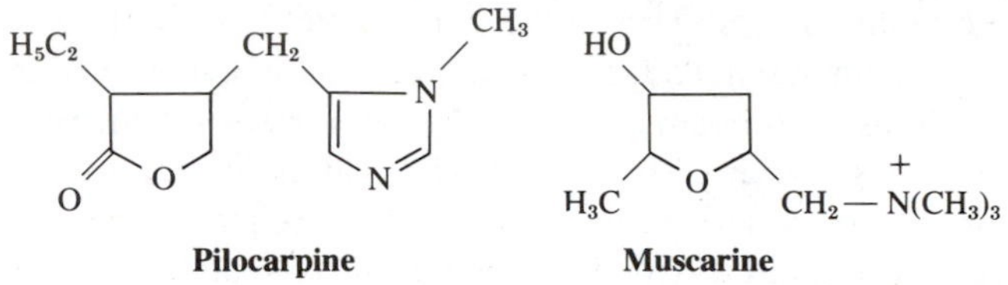

Pilocarpine

Muscarine

Figure 8-2. Structural formulas of pilocarpine and muscarine.

reported independently that the derivative neostigmine was effective in the treatment of myasthenia gravis.[21,29] Until the basic mechanism of neurohumoral transmission was elucidated, however, it was not understood that these drugs acted as anticholinesterases.

The first organophosphate anticholinesterase was actually synthesized in 1854, before physostigmine was known, by de Clermont, who made and tasted tetraethyl pyrophosphate (and survived to record the fact). Modern interest in these compounds did not begin, though, until 1932 when Lange and Krueger synthesized some compounds with a P-F (phosphorofluoride) linkage and gave a remarkable description of the pharmacologic properties of this group of chemicals.[14] Lange believed that these compounds would prove useful as insecticides, and he offered them to the I.G. Farben Company in Germany. It was some years before this company took an active interest, but they soon realized the potential of these compounds as chemical warfare agents. The manufacture of nerve gas began in Germany in 1940. Related investigations were being carried out in England at the same time,

and in the United States diisopropyl fluorophosphate (DFP) was being studied during World War II. (This agent has been given the official name of isoflurophate.) Two compounds developed by the Germans, tabun and sarin, are among the most toxic nerve gases known. Of the thousands of organophosphates that have been tested, several dozen are widely available as insecticides and a number of others find military application as lethal nerve gases.[10]

MECHANISMS OF ACTION

ACh and its congeners act by reversibly combining with the cholinergic receptors (AChRs) at muscarinic and nicotinic sites. Pilocarpine and muscarine act principally on muscarinic receptors.

In Chapter 5 it was pointed out that acetylcholinesterase hydrolyzes ACh with great rapidity, that it is localized in the region of the receptor, and that it acts most efficiently when ACh is present in low concentrations. There is also a nonspecific cholinesterase, or pseudocholinesterase (butyrocholinesterase, BuChE), which has a greater affinity for butyric esters than for acetyl esters and is more

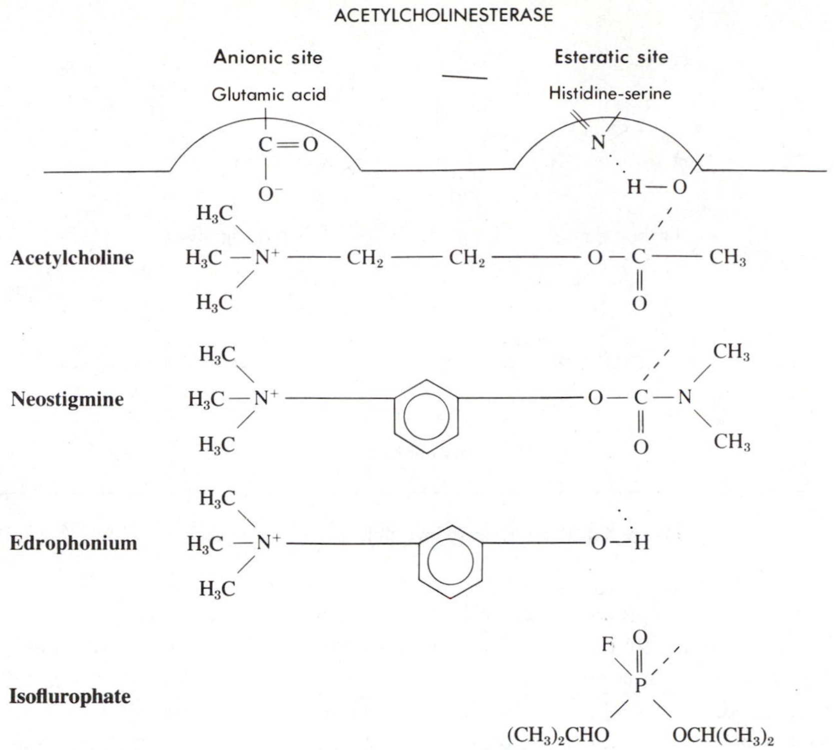

Figure 8-3. Interaction between ACh and acetylcholinesterase shown occurring at both anionic and esteratic sites. As a result, choline is split off, and the enzyme is acetylated. Neostigmine is shown bonding to the anionic and esteratic sites, whereas the organophosphate isoflurophate reacts only at the esteratic site. Edrophonium binds primarily to the anionic site but also participates in a hydrogen bond with the nitrogen of the esteratic site.

effective when the concentration of the agonist is high.[19] Acetylcholinesterase has been isolated from the receptor protein of the eel, *Electrophorus electricus*. It is calculated to have a molecular weight of 10^6 and is composed of protein units having individual weights of 80,000.[6,15]

The ACh molecule is believed to react with the enzyme at at least two sites[33]; these sites are shown, with ACh and a number of anticholinesterases, in Figure 8-3. The enzyme is depicted as having a negatively charged anionic site, to which the quaternary ammonium portion of the ACh molecule is attracted, and an esteratic site, with an affinity for the ester portion of the molecule. It is at the esteratic site that the ACh molecule is split, leaving the acetylated enzyme, which is rapidly regenerated after it combines with water. The simplest quaternary anticholinesterases such as edrophonium combine reversibly with the enzyme largely at the anionic site and therefore compete with ACh

for the receptor site on the enzyme. The organophosphate anticholinesterases have an affinity chiefly for the esteratic site of the enzyme molecule. They produce a very stable covalent attachment; indeed, there is virtually no hydrolysis, and cholinesterase activity remains depressed until new enzyme is synthesized. Since enzyme turnover may take from several days to months, the organophosphates are referred to as *irreversible* in action. The anticholinesterase agents that enjoy the greatest therapeutic use are those drugs, like neostigmine and physostigmine, which interact strongly with both binding sites of the receptor. As with the organophosphates, attachment of such drugs to the serine residue at the esteratic site is achieved by means of a covalent linkage. This bond is subject to hydrolysis, however, and these drugs are categorized along with edrophonium as *reversible* cholinesterase inhibitors.

The anticholinesterases, whether reversible or ir-

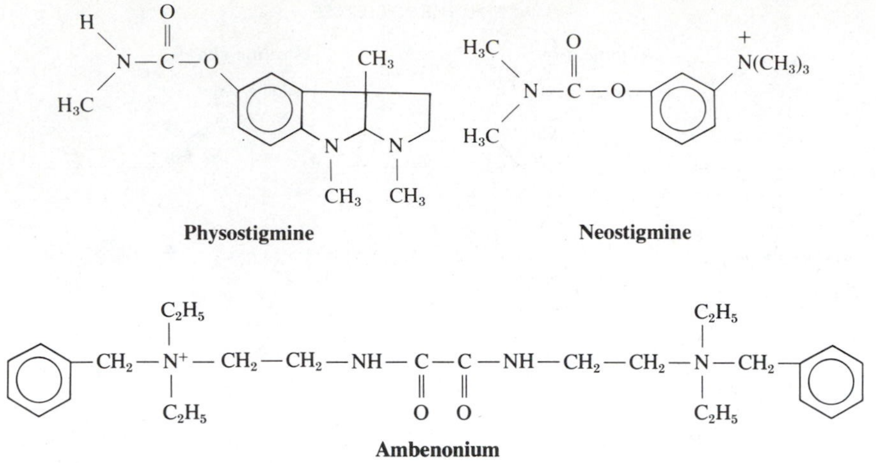

Figure 8-4. Representative reversible anticholinesterases.

reversible, owe their pharmacologic effects chiefly to the fact that they prolong the life of ACh at sites where it is a mediator. Thus, their actions are often identical with those of ACh, although much more prolonged and in most cases dependent on the presence of endogenous ACh in the area of the effector. For this reason most of the anticholinesterases are ineffective in denervated organs. In exception to this effect, quaternary ammonium compounds like neostigmine and pyridostigmine and the *bis*-quaternary amine ambenonium have direct actions on cholinergic sites, either stimulating the effectors or blocking transmission. Neostigmine, for example, is capable of direct stimulation of the neuromuscular junction and is effective on denervated skeletal muscle. Its pharmacology, therefore, is the result of a combination of anticholinesterase and cholinomimetic properties.

CLASSIFICATION OF ANTICHOLINESTERASES

Reversible anticholinesterases include the truly reversible nonester quaternary ammonium compounds and the esters of carbamic acid that react with the enzyme surfaces. The enzyme is regenerated by hydrolysis over a period of hours. The reversible anticholinesterases may be classified as simple quaternary ammonium compounds (edrophonium) or carbamate ester derivatives, including tertiary amines (physostigmine), quaternary amines (neostigmine), and bisquaternary amines (ambenonium). Three representative reversible an-

ticholinesterases are shown in Figure 8-4.

Irreversible anticholinesterases are organophosphates that react only at the esteratic site and are not significantly regenerated by hydrolysis. They have relatively little therapeutic value but are of great toxicologic significance. Four examples include (1) isoflurophate (DFP), the best known and studied compound of this class, (2) malathion, a widely used insecticide, (3) echothiophate, one of the first compounds in this class to have a therapeutic application, and (4) tabun, one of the most potent and toxic nerve gases. Structures of several irreversible anticholinesterases are given in Figure 8-5. The anticholinesterases are classified according to their use in Table 8-1.

PHARMACOLOGIC EFFECTS

The effects of stimulation of cholinergic nerves are shown in Table 5-1. As is documented in Chapter 5, ACh is the transmitter at a variety of sites in the autonomic, peripheral, and central nervous systems. These sites are designated muscarinic or nicotinic, and it is clear that there are at least two kinds of nicotinic receptors.

The cholinergic drugs—whether they are ACh and the choline esters, the alkaloids muscarine and pilocarpine, or the anticholinesterases—all have basically similar actions, even though the mechanism, extent, and duration of action may be significantly different. ACh and its congeners act directly on the receptor, but their duration of action is determined by their susceptibility to the action

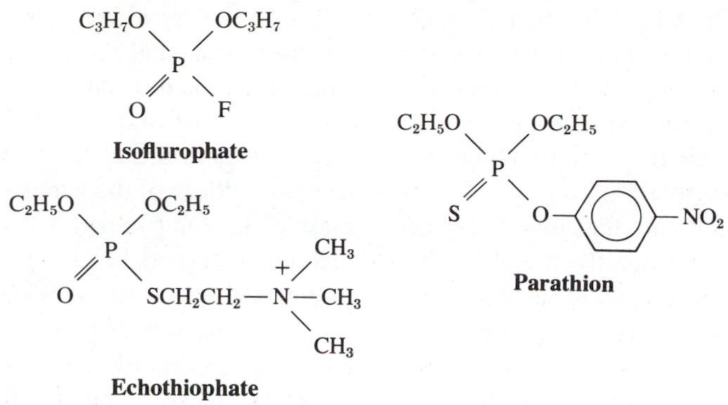

Figure 8-5. Representative irreversible anticholinesterases.

Table 8-1. Some anticholinesterases and their uses

For treatment of glaucoma	For treatment of myasthenia gravis	As nerve gas	As insecticide
Demecarium	Ambenonium	Soman	Malathion
Echothiophate	Edrophonium	Sarin	Octamethyl pyrophosphoramide (OMPA)
Isoflurophate	Neostigmine	Tabun	Paraoxon
Physostigmine			Parathion
			Tetraethyl pyrophosphate (TEPP)

of acetylcholinesterase and pseudocholinesterase. Thus methacholine, with a susceptibility only to acetylcholinesterase, has a longer duration of action than ACh, and bethanechol and carbachol, which are not affected by the cholinesterases, have an even longer duration. There is evidence that carbachol not only occupies the cholinergic receptor but also causes the release of ACh from nerve terminals in certain locations, specifically certain vascular smooth muscle and autonomic ganglia.[22,28]

The cholinomimetic alkaloids also act directly on the receptor, but they are not at all affected by the cholinesterases and therefore have a much more prolonged action than ACh. It should be noted too that the esters of ACh, as well as the cholinomimetic alkaloids, have a different affinity for muscarinic and nicotinic sites, so that carbachol has much more pronounced nicotinic effects than ACh, and bethanechol has no nicotinic properties whatever. Also, they have different intensities of effect on different effectors. Thus, carbachol is a very effective stimulant of the urinary tract, whereas ACh and methacholine are not. The activity of the

anticholinesterases is greatest for those organs that receive more or less continuous cholinergic nerve stimulation. As a result, their effects are seen first in the smooth muscles of various ocular structures, the gastrointestinal tract, and the urinary bladder. Finally, as has been pointed out, quaternary ammonium compounds penetrate biologic membranes poorly, so anticholinesterases that contain a quaternary ammonium group, such as neostigmine or edrophonium, are poorly absorbed after oral administration and do not readily pass through the blood-brain barrier. Predictably they are quite effective at skeletal neuromuscular junctions but have no central effects.

The following listing of the specific pharmacologic effects of the cholinergic drugs will be limited to those actions that have some therapeutic or practical application, and it is emphasized once more that not all cholinergic drugs possess all of these actions.

Muscarinic effects

Eye. Cholinergic drugs in general produce constriction of the pupil (miosis), which is very pronounced with some of the anticholinesterases and less prominent with ACh and its congeners. At the same time there is contraction of the ciliary muscles so that the eye is fixed for near vision. Intraocular pressure is decreased, particularly if the tension was elevated initially. There may also be a transient hyperemia of the conjunctiva.

Secretory glands. All glands that are innervated by cholinergic fibers are potentially stimulated by cholinergic drugs. This includes the salivary, lacrimal, bronchial, sweat, gastric, intestinal, and pancreatic glands.

Heart. Cardiac effects are similar to those associated with vagal stimulation. The heart rate is slowed (negative chronotropic effect), unless the dose of cholinergic drug is great enough to cause the release of catecholamines. There is also a decrease in the force of contraction (negative inotropic effect). While the effective refractory period is shortened in atrial muscle, the refractory period in the A-V node and conducting system of the heart is increased at the same time that conduction is slowed.

Vascular smooth muscle. Many of the cholinomimetic drugs produce a generalized vasodilation that, with the negative chronotropic and inotropic effects, is the cause of the fall in blood pressure associated with administration of these drugs. All vascular beds are affected by this class of drugs, and there is ample pharmacologic evidence that all parts of the vasculature, including the coronary vessels, are supplied with cholinergic receptors. The functional significance of these receptors is still very much in doubt. It is likely that vasodilation in vascular beds occurs most often in response not to stimulation of cholinergic nerves but to autoregulatory factors such as carbon dioxide, oxygen, and pH.

Bronchial smooth muscle. The smooth muscle of the bronchioles is constricted by cholinergic drugs.

Gastrointestinal smooth muscle. Motility, peristaltic contractions, amplitude of contraction, and tone are all increased by cholinomimetic drugs.

Urinary tract. Cholinergic drugs are potentially capable of stimulating the detrusor muscle of the bladder to contract and of decreasing the capacity of the bladder, but in actual fact some drugs in this class (anticholinesterases) are very active in this respect and others are not. Peristaltic activity in ureteral smooth muscle may also be stimulated.

Nicotinic effects

The cholinergic drugs have varying effects at nicotinic sites, and these effects are related to the structure of the molecule,[2,4] the dosage of the drug, and the location of the nicotinic receptor. It is probable that there are at least two kinds of nicotinic receptors, those of the ganglia and those in skeletal muscle. It is not known to which group the CNS nicotinic receptors belong or whether ACh, except in the case of the Renshaw cells, can be regarded as a true transmitter in the central nervous system. Exogenous ACh at low doses activates muscarinic receptors, in substantially higher doses activates ganglia, and by close intraarterial injection of high doses activates skeletal muscle. Several ACh congeners, such as methacholine and to an even greater extent carbachol, have nicotinic properties at therapeutic doses. The cholinomimetic alkaloids are primarily muscarinic in action, although pilocarpine has been reported to produce ganglionic stimulation at relatively high doses.

ABSORPTION, FATE, AND EXCRETION
Acetylcholine and choline esters

All of these drugs are absorbed after administration by both oral and parenteral routes, although the absorption of quaternary ammonium compounds from the gastrointestinal tract is likely to be unpredictable. Parenteral administration of the choline esters must be carried out with extreme caution because of the profound effects they may have on blood pressure, bronchial smooth muscle, and other cholinergic effectors. ACh is destroyed by acetylcholinesterase and pseudocholinesterase, whereas methacholine is susceptible to acetylcholinesterase only. Its duration of action is therefore longer than that of ACh. Carbachol and bethanechol are, for all practical purposes, not affected by the cholinesterases, so they have a very long duration of action and the potential for producing widespread and prolonged cholinergic effects.

Cholinomimetic alkaloids

Pilocarpine is well absorbed after oral, subcutaneous, or topical administration. It also gains ready access to the central nervous system; thus, it is well distributed through the tissues and organs of the body. A large part is excreted unchanged by the kidney.

Anticholinesterases

Physostigmine is readily absorbed after oral, subcutaneous, and topical administration, and it is rapidly destroyed, principally through hydrolysis at the ester linkage, by cholinesterases. The other reversible cholinesterases listed in this chapter, neostigmine and pyridostigmine for instance, are quaternary ammonium compounds, which means that they pass through biologic membranes with difficulty. Some of these compounds are broken down by cholinesterases or by hepatic microsomal enzymes, and they appear in the urine in both changed and unchanged forms.

The organophosphate anticholinesterases, with the exception of echothiophate, are highly lipid soluble, and they are rapidly absorbed from the gastrointestinal tract, the skin and mucous membranes, and the lungs. These characteristics explain their potential toxicity when used as aerosols, dusts, vapors, or liquids. Most of the organophosphates are inactivated by hydrolysis and oxidation; but in some instances the enzymatic transformation of these compounds results in a more toxic product than the original compound.[18] In the case of DFP, about 80% of the drug is metabolized and excreted in the urine and feces in changed forms, and about 20% remains protein-bound in the tissues for a prolonged period.

GENERAL THERAPEUTIC USES

ACh itself has had very little therapeutic application because of the extreme brevity of its action. The synthesis of congeners to some extent solved this problem, because compounds were produced that not only were more potent than ACh but also were relatively unaffected by the cholinesterases. Nevertheless, in contemporary therapeutics these compounds enjoy very limited use. The alkaloid pilocarpine is still widely used for several purposes, as are the reversible anticholinesterases. The irreversible anticholinesterases are principally used as laboratory tools, as insecticides, in nerve gases, and therapeutically for ophthalmologic purposes.

Glaucoma

Miotics are the initial and principal drugs used in the treatment of chronic open-angle glaucoma, even though their mechanism of action is not clearly understood. Pilocarpine is the miotic most commonly used for chronic glaucomas. It is available for topical administration in various solutions, combined with physostigmine or epinephrine, or in a new drug delivery system that is placed in the cul-de-sac of the eye and provides sustained delivery of the drug over a period of about 7 days. Carbachol is also used in chronic open-angle glaucoma, especially when intolerance or resistance to pilocarpine has developed. It is applied topically as a solution. The anticholinesterases are generally employed in emergencies and when other agents have proved to be inadequate. Physostigmine, usually in solution with pilocarpine, is very effective in the acute and long-term management of chronic simple glaucoma, secondary glaucoma, and acute congestive glaucoma. Its effects last from 12 to 36 hours, and it is therefore classified as a short-acting miotic. Longer acting anticholinesterases include the reversible anticholinesterase demecarium and the so-called irreversible organophosphates echothiophate and isoflurophate. They are very potent and are administered in the lowest possible concentrations. Long-term administration (6 months or more) of these potent and long-acting anticholinesterases has been associated with the development of cataracts, and this clearly limits their usefulness in the therapy of glaucoma.

Paralytic ileus and bladder atony

After abdominal and pelvic surgery there is often a failure of normal peristalsis that leads to postoperative abdominal distension and discomfort. Neostigmine has been used to advantage in the treatment of this condition, as has bethanechol, which is preferred to other choline esters because of its lack of effect on the heart.

Bladder atony also follows surgery and sometimes parturition. It leads to urinary retention and is treated with bethanechol, neostigmine, or sometimes pilocarpine.

Paroxysmal atrial tachycardia

Methacholine (which is no longer available) was occasionally used for this particular disorder of cardiac rhythm, especially when other drugs had failed. The very short-acting reversible anticholinesterase edrophonium, vagal stimulation via massage of the carotid sinus, and digitalis have also been successfully used in this form of supraventricular arrhythmia.

Xerostomia

A dry mouth may result from a number of causes, including radiation to the salivary glands, therapy with antineoplastic agents, aging, and treatment with a variety of drugs. Xerostomia can be unsupportably uncomfortable as well as threatening to the health of oral tissues. Pilocarpine and neostigmine have been used to relieve xerostomia, but they produce many undesirable side effects, which make the use of masticatory stimulants and oral fluids preferable to the use of cholinomimetic drugs for the relief of xerostomia.

Vasospastic disorders

Methacholine was used in the past for the treatment of certain kinds of peripheral vascular disease, but its use has been supplanted by other drugs.

Antidote for atropine poisoning

All of the cholinergic drugs should theoretically be useful in antagonizing the effects of atropine, but the most effective drugs for this purpose are the anticholinesterases, and the drug of choice is physostigmine. When the diagnosis of atropine poisoning is confirmed, physostigmine is administered intravenously, and it rapidly relieves the delirium and coma.[23] Neostigmine and other quaternary ammonium compounds are of limited use because they are incapable of counteracting the CNS effects of atropine.

A number of psychotropic agents (e.g., tricyclic antidepressants, phenothiazines, and antihistamines) share to varying degree the antimuscarinic effects of atropine. Particularly when used in combination (for intravenous sedation or for other reasons), these agents may induce a central anticholinergic syndrome consisting of confusion, delirium, hallucination, and psychotic behavior. Intravenous physostigmine in doses of 0.5 to 2 mg is effective in reversing this syndrome, and it may also be useful in treating various adverse reactions to the benzodiazepines.[3] Inasmuch as the duration of action of parenteral physostigmine is 1 to 2 hours, several administrations may be necessary to avoid recurrence of the syndrome.

Reversal of neuromuscular block

The use of reversible anticholinesterases to terminate the neuromuscular block of curare-like drugs in general anesthesia is covered in Chapter 11.

Myasthenia gravis

Myasthenia gravis (MG) is a disease characterized by weakness and easy fatigability of the skel-etal muscles, particularly the ocular and oropharyngeal, and by marked variations in severity of symptoms even in the course of a single day. It is thought that there are approximately 30,000 cases in the United States, with two peaks of age incidence: in the twenties for women and in the fifties for men. About 10% of patients die from the disease. There is also a neonatal form of myasthenia which tends to be transient.[11] Although the disease was described over 300 years ago, the underlying mechanisms and suitable treatment were unclear until two investigators, Remen in 1932[21] and Walker in 1934,[29] unknown to each other, administered neostigmine to patients suffering from myasthenia and reported relief of symptoms.

The typical myasthenic initially has ocular complaints—double vision or ptosis—and difficulty in chewing and swallowing. Later, dyspnea and other respiratory problems may arise. About 10% of myasthenic patients have a tumor of the thymus, and approximately 75% have some abnormality of the thymus. At least 30% of patients with an enlarged thymus experience a remission of myasthenic symptoms after thymectomy. Since the work of Remen and Walker, it has been accepted that the defect in MG is probably at the neuromuscular junction, and one of the early findings was that the synaptic vesicles of the myasthenic patient appeared to contain less than normal amounts of ACh.[7] Other investigators showed that while synaptic vesicle diameter is unaltered, the mean nerve terminal area and the postsynaptic membrane are abnormally simple with clefts that are sparse, shallow, wide, or absent.[24] The favorable response of some patients to thymectomy and certain features of the muscle response in myasthenia have led to the hypothesis that the condition might be the result of an autoimmune phenomenon, an idea that was given a solid basis by the demonstration in rabbits that injection of highly purified receptor protein from the electric eel results in the production of a precipitating antibody specific for the ACh receptor (AChR).[20] Later it was shown that rats immunized with eel electroplax AChR protein develop a myasthenia-like syndrome[8] and that, as a result of such immunization, AChRs degenerate.[13] A similar alteration of AChRs was induced in mice by the injection of immunoglobulin from myasthenic patients,[25,27] whose blood had been shown to contain receptor-binding antibodies.[17] Experimental autoimmune myasthenia gravis (EAMG) is characterized, then, by simplified postsynaptic membrane structures, high concentrations of anti-AChR antibodies in the serum, binding of antibodies to most AChR in the muscle, and reduction of the AChR content to about 30% of normal. The primary factor in impaired neuromuscular transmission in both EAMG and human MG is loss of AChR, through accelerated destruction of receptors without concomitant increase in rate of synthesis, and by complement-mediated focal lysis of the postsynaptic membrane.[16]

Even if the precise mechanism is not thoroughly understood, treatment for MG is now fairly standardized. Diagnosis is usually made after the intravenous or intramuscular injection of edrophonium, a short-acting anticholinesterase that will briefly improve muscle strength in the MG patient while the injection of a placebo will not. For treatment of the diagnosed myasthenic patient, one of three reversible anticholinesterases with weak cholinergic activity at the neuromuscular junction is used: neostigmine, pyridostigmine, or ambenonium. These drugs are given orally, unless the patient is desperately ill and does not respond to oral medications. Some patients are helped by the addition of ephedrine and potassium and calcium salts to their drug regimen, and occasionally patients are given adrenocorticosteroids (e.g., prednisone) or, if hospitalized, adrenocorticotropic hormone (ACTH). The immunosuppressive drugs azathioprine and mercaptopurine have been reported to be useful in some cases.

Therapy with an anticholinesterase is likely to be complicated by side effects resulting from the accumulation of ACh at cholinergic receptor sites. Some of these effects will be characteristically muscarinic—abdominal cramps, diarrhea, sweating, salivation, lacrimation—and can be well controlled by administration of atropine and related drugs. Other side effects, such as muscle fasciculations and CNS symptoms, will not be controlled by the muscarinic blocking drugs and may be warning signs of an impending cholinergic crisis, which results from overdosage with the anticholinesterases. Cholinergic crisis is characterized by muscle weakness, particularly of the respiratory muscles, resulting from persistent depolarization of the neuromuscular junction. Cholinergic crisis very closely resembles myasthenic crisis, which may come about because of inadequate medication, and it is urgently necessary in such patients to determine quickly which of the two conditions exists. This can be done by giving, with great caution and

with resuscitation apparatus available, a very low dose of edrophonium. If the symptoms are relieved, the problem is myasthenic weakness; if muscle strength decreases, cholinergic crisis is established.

TOXIC REACTIONS AND SIDE EFFECTS

The mushrooms *Amanita muscaria* and *Amanita pantherina* contain muscarine but in amounts that are probably too small to account for the symptoms of poisoning that result from their ingestion. On the other hand, the mushroom *Inocybe lateraria,* with a much higher muscarine content, produces symptoms of intoxication that resemble those produced by muscarine and include profuse salivation and sweating, miosis, bradycardia, severe abdominal pain with vomiting, cramps, and diarrhea, and respiratory difficulties arising from the constriction of bronchial muscle and increased secretion in the respiratory tract.[30] The onset of poisoning is rapid, and treatment consists of the administration of atropine in large quantities, gastric lavage, and appropriate supportive measures. Recovery usually takes place in 1 or 2 days. In many cases of mushroom poisoning there are delayed symptoms, including violent emesis and diarrhea and damage to parenchymatous organs, principally the liver, that are not amenable to atropine treatment and are presumably produced by toxins that may be unusual cyclopeptides.[31]

In humans, intoxication from anticholinesterases has resulted from overdosage with drugs used in the treatment of myasthenia gravis, as described earlier, and from exposure to toxic amounts of organophosphates in insecticides or chemical warfare agents.[10] Organophosphate insecticides have gained wide use in many countries, and thousands of cases of poisoning are attributable to these compounds, especially parathion. Most of the organophosphates are volatile liquids at ordinary temperatures and are highly lipid soluble. They are readily absorbed through the skin, the respiratory tract, the gastrointestinal tract, and the eyes. The symptomatology of anticholinesterase poisoning reflects ACh's role as a neuromediator at muscarinic, nicotinic, and CNS sites. In high doses the reversible anticholinesterases can produce the same symptoms as the irreversible anticholinesterases; the chief difference between these two groups lies in the wide public use of the latter compounds, their ready access to the circulation, and their longer duration of action.

Table 8-2. Some manifestations of overdosage with anticholinesterases

Muscarinic effects	*Nicotinic effects*	*Central effects*
Miosis, frontal headache (brow ache), conjunctival hyperemia, blurred vision	Muscular weakness, twitching, fasciculations	Restlessness, giddiness, tension, anxiety, insomnia
Rhinorrhea, nasal hyperemia	Tachycardia	Tremors, EEG changes
Lacrimation, salivation, sweating	Elevation of blood pressure	Confusion, ataxia, convulsions
Increased bronchial secretions, tightness of chest, bronchoconstriction, wheezing	**Death from respiratory failure**	Depression of respiratory and circulatory centers, cyanosis, coma, respiratory and circulatory collapse
Anorexia, nausea, vomiting, cramps, diarrhea, involuntary defecation		**Death from respiratory failure**
Urinary urgency, involuntary micturition		
Bradycardia, hypotension		

The first symptoms to appear, especially after local exposure through aerosols, vapor, or dust, are an intense miosis, an inability to accommodate for far vision, severe rhinorrhea, and a frontal headache attributable to ciliary muscle spasm. The respiratory tract is also affected very soon after exposure. In addition to the watery nasal discharge, there is nasal hyperemia, a sensation of tightness in the chest, probably because of bronchoconstriction, and increased bronchial secretion. Audible wheezing may follow, related to both the bronchoconstriction and the hypersecretion. Laryngospasm may occur because of the secretory activity, which triggers a reflex spasm of laryngeal muscle. In fact, respiration can be severely compromised very rapidly. There are other manifestations of muscarinic stimulation, including such gastrointestinal effects as anorexia, nausea, vomiting, severe cramps, diarrhea, and even involuntary defecation. There is also sweating, lacrimation, bradycardia, urinary frequency, and involuntary micturition. With the onset of muscarinic effects, various nicotinic effects also become apparent. The subject shows easy fatigability and generalized weakness, especially on exertion. Involuntary muscle twitching, fasciculations, and muscle cramps follow; then generalized muscle weakness, including the muscles of respiration, increases in severity. Respiratory movements become more shallow and rapid, and respiratory failure may take place in a matter of minutes unless artificial respiration is instituted. It should be remembered that respiration is also greatly hampered by the constriction of the airway and the intense secretory activity in the respiratory tract. Sympathetic ganglia may be stimulated in moderate to severe intoxication, but this does not pose a life-threatening problem. Finally, there are outstanding CNS manifestations that start with tension, restlessness, and jitteriness and progress to confusion and ataxia, coma, disappearance of reflexes, Cheyne-Stokes respiration, and finally generalized convulsions. The cause of death is respiratory failure resulting from paralysis of the muscles of respiration, central depression of respiration, and airway obstruction. Table 8-2 summarizes the signs of poisoning with the anticholinesterases according to muscarinic and nicotinic effects.

The treatment of acute intoxication with the organophosphates includes the following actions:

1. Remove the victim from the source of contamination, or remove the organophosphate-containing contaminant.
2. Administer atropine in very large doses. Atropine will not relieve the neuromuscular blockade produced by these agents, but it will alleviate the muscarinic and central manifestations of poisoning. Repeated, often heroic doses may be required.
3. Maintain the airway and administer artificial respiration.
4. Inject diazepam, if atropine fails to relieve the convulsions.
5. Administer pralidoxime (PAM). This molecule, an oxime, is one of several that were synthesized in the 1950s as ideal cholinesterase *reactivators*.

Once the mechanism of organophosphate poisoning was fully understood, it became possible to conceptualize a molecule that could reverse the inhibition of the enzymes. It was reasoned that by attaching a nucleophilic group to a cationic qua-

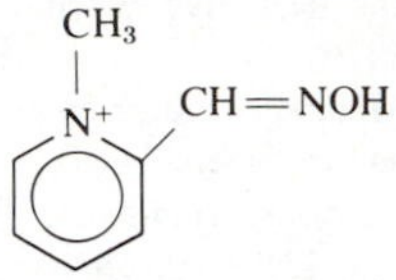

$$CH_3$$
$$N^+ \quad CH=NOH$$

Figure 8-6. Structural formula of pralidoxime.

ternary nitrogen group at a proper atomic distance, the phosphorus group of the alkyl phosphate would be attacked and would be removed from acetylcholinesterase in a displacement reaction. It was further reasoned that the cationic group of this ideal molecule would be attracted to the anionic site and the nucleophilic atom would be directed toward the phosphorus atom.[32] A number of compounds were synthesized, and one of the most potent was pralidoxime,[34] the structure of which is shown in Figure 8-6. Intravenous administration of the oximes produces a remarkably rapid reactivation of the acetylcholinesterase at neuromuscular junctions in which transmission has failed as a result of poisoning with irreversible anticholinesterases. The reactivation occurs within minutes, but the effect of the oximes is much less dramatic at muscarinic sites and negligible in the central nervous system, because many of the reactivators are quaternary compounds and cannot pass the blood-brain barrier. Also, the oximes are most effective when given immediately after exposure to organophosphates. Therapeutic use of pralidoxime and its congeners is reserved for cases of intoxication with the irreversible anticholinesterases.

THERAPEUTIC USES IN DENTISTRY

All of the cholinomimetic drugs that have an affinity for muscarinic sites are capable of stimulating salivation. Xerostomia is a common problem encountered by dentists in patients who are elderly or are undergoing treatment with certain drugs or radiation. While pilocarpine is of questionable value in stimulating salivary flow, it is useful for diagnosing functional salivary activity.

As mentioned previously, physostigmine may be of value in treating certain adverse reactions to drugs used for intravenous sedation.

Cholinergic drugs

Nonproprietary name	Proprietary name
Cholinomimetics	
acetylcholine	in Miochol Intraocular
bethanechol	Urecholine
carbachol	Carbacel, Isopto Carbachol
methacholine*	—
pilocarpine hydrochloride	Isopto Carpine, Pilocar, Pilocel
pilocarpine nitrate	P.V. Carpine Liquifilm
pilocarpine ocular therapeutic system	Ocusert Pilo-20, Ocusert Pilo 40
pilocarpine and epinephrine	E-Pilo-1
pilocarpine and physostigmine	Isopto P-ES, Miocel
Anticholinesterases	
ambenonium	Mytelase Caplets
demecarium	Humorsol
echothiophate	Phospholine Iodide
edrophonium	Tensilon
isoflurophate (diisopropyl fluorophosphate)	Floropryl
neostigmine	Prostigmin Bromide
physostigmine	Eserine Sulfate, Isopto Eserine
physostigmine salicylate	Antilirium
pyridostigmine	Mestinon Bromide, Regonol
Cholinesterase reactivator	
pralidoxime	Protopam Chloride

*No longer available in the United States for clinical use.

CITED REFERENCES

1. Aeschlimann, J.A., and Reinert, M. Pharmacological action of some analogues of physostigmine. Journal of Pharmacology and Experimental Therapeutics **43**:413-444, 1931.

2. Beers, W.H., and Reich, E. Structure and activity of acetylcholine. Nature **228**:917-922, 1970.

3. Caldwell, C.B., and Gross, J.B. Physostigmine reversal of midazolam-induced sedation. Anesthesiology **57**:125-127, 1982.

4. Chothia, C. Interaction of acetylcholine with different cholinergic nerve receptors. Nature **225**:36-38, 1970.

5. Dale, H.H. The action of certain esters of choline and their relation to muscarine. Journal of Pharmacology and Experimental Therapeutics **6**:147-190, 1914.

6. Dudai, Y., Herzberg, M., and Silman, I. Molecular structures of acetylcholinesterase from electric organ tissue of the electric eel. Proceedings of the National Academy of Sciences of the United States of America **70**:2473-2476, 1973.

7. Elmqvist, D., Hofmann, W.W., Kugelberg, J., and Quastel, M.J. An electrophysiological investigation of neuromuscular transmission in myasthenia gravis. Journal of Physiology (London) **174**:417-434, 1964.

8. Engel, A.G., Tsujihata, M., Lambert, E.H., Lindstrom, J.M., and Lennon, V.A. Neuromuscular junction ultrastructure in experimental autoimmune myasthenia (EAM). Journal of Neuropathology and Experimental Neurology **35**:113, 1976.

9. Engelhardt, E., and Loewi, O. Fermentative Azetylcholinspaltung im Blut und ihre Hemmung durch Physostigmine. Naunyn-Schmiedebergs Archiv für Pharmakologie **150**:1-13, 1930.

10. Grob, D. Anticholinesterase intoxication in man and its treatment. In Koelle, G.B., ed. Cholinesterases and Anticholinesterases. Handbuch der Experimentellen Pharmakologie, vol 15. Berlin, Springer-Verlag, 1963.

11. Grob, D. Cause of weakness in myasthenia gravis. New England Journal of Medicine **294**:722-723, 1976.

12. Hunt, R., and Taveau, R. deM. On the physiological action of certain choline derivatives and new methods for detecting choline. British Medical Journal **2**:1788-1791, 1906.

13. Kao, I., and Drachman, D.B. Myasthenic immunoglobulin accelerates acetylcholine receptor degradation. Science **196**:527-529, 1977.

14. Lange, W., and von Krueger, G. Über Ester der Monofluorphosphorsäure. Bericht der Deutschen Keramischen Gesellschaft **65**:1598-1601, 1932.

15. Leuzinger, W., Baker, A.L., and Cauvin, E. Acetylcholinesterase. II. Crystallization, absorption, spectra, isoionic point. Proceedings of the National Academy of Sciences of the United States of America **59**:620-623, 1968.

16. Lindstrom, J., and Dau, P. Biology of myasthenia gravis. Annual Review of Pharmacology and Toxicology **20**:337-362, 1980.

17. Lindstrom, J.M., Seybold, M.E., Lennon, V.A., Whittingham, S., and Duane, D.D. Antibody to acetylcholine receptor in myasthenia gravis: prevalence, clinical correlates, and diagnostic value. Neurology (Minneapolis) **26**:1054-1059, 1976.

18. Mounter, L.A. Metabolism of organophosphorus anticholinesterase agents. In Koelle, G.B., ed. Cholinesterases and Anticholinesterases. Handbuch der Experimentellen Pharmakologie, vol 15. Berlin, Springer-Verlag, 1963.

19. Paton, W.D.M. Anticholinesterases. In Lectures on the Scientific Basis of Medicine, vol 3. London, The Athlone Press, University of London, 1955.

20. Patrick, J., and Lindstrom, J. Autoimmune response to acetylcholine response. Science **180**:871-872, 1973.

21. Remen, L. Zur Pathogenese und Therapie der Myasthenia gravis pseudoparalytic. Deutsche Zeitschrift für Nervenheilkunde **128**:66-78, 1932.

22. Renshaw, R.R., Green, D., and Ziff, M. A basis for the acetylcholine action of choline derivatives. Journal of Pharmacology and Experimental Therapeutics **62**:430-448, 1938.

23. Rumack, B.H. Anticholinergic poisoning: treatment with physostigmine. Pediatrics **52**:449-451, 1973.

24. Santa, T., Engel, A.G., and Lambert, E.H. Histometric study of neuromuscular junction ultrastructure. Neurology **22**:71-82, 1972.

25. Stanley, E.F., and Drachman, D.B. Effect of myasthenic immunoglobulin on acetylcholine receptors of intact mammalian neuromuscular junction. Science **200**:1285-1287, 1978.

26. Stedman, E., and Barger, G. Physostigmine (eserine). Part III. Journal of the Chemical Society; Perkin Transactions I: Organic and Bio-organic Chemistry **127**:247-258, 1925.

27. Toyka, K.V., Drachman, D.B., Griffin, D.E., Pestronk, A., Winkelstein, J.A., Fischbeck, K.H., Jr., and Kao, I. Myasthenia gravis: study of humoral immune mechanisms by passive transfer from man to mouse. New England Journal of Medicine **296**:125-131, 1977.

28. Volle, R.L., and Koelle, G.B. The physiological role of acetylcholinesterase (AChE) in sympathetic ganglia. Journal of Pharmacology and Experimental Therapeutics **133**:223-240, 1961.

29. Walker, M.B. Case showing the effect of prostigmine on myasthenia gravis. Proceedings of the Royal Society of London; B: Biological Sciences **28**:759-761, 1935.

30. Waser, P.G. Chemistry and pharmacology of muscarine, muscarone, and some related compounds. Pharmacological Reviews **13**:465-515, 1961.

31. Wieland, T., and Wieland, O. Chemistry and toxicology of the toxins of *Amanita phalloides*. Pharmacological Reviews **11**:87-107, 1956.

32. Wilson, I.B. Acetylcholinesterase. XI. Reversibility of tetraethyl pyrophosphate inhibition. Journal of Biological Chemistry **190**:111-117, 1951.

33. Wilson, I.B., and Bergmann, F. Acetylcholinesterase. VII. Dissociation constants of the active groups. Journal of Biological Chemistry **186**:683-692, 1950.

34. Wilson, I.B., and Ginsburg, S. A powerful reactivator of alkylphosphate-inhibited acetylcholinesterase. Biochimica et Biophysica Acta **18**:168-170, 1955.

GENERAL REFERENCES

Cohen, J.A., and Warringa, G.P.J. The fate of P^{32} labelled diisopropyl flurophosphonate in the human body and its use as a labelling agent in the study of turnover of blood plasma and red cells. Journal of Clinical Investigation **33**:459-467, 1954.

Drachman, D.B. Myasthenia gravis. The New England Journal of Medicine **298**:136-142, 186-193, 1978.

Engel, A.G., and Santa, T. Histometric analysis of the ultrastructure of the neuromuscular junction in myasthenia gravis and in the myasthenic syndrome. Annals of the New York Academy of Sciences **183**:46-63, 1971.

Fambrough, D.M., Drachman, D.B., and Satyamurti, S. Neuromuscular junction in myasthenia gravis: decreased acetylcholine receptors. Science **182**:293-295, 1973.

Kao, I., and Drachman, D.B. Thymic cells bear acetylcholine receptors: possible relation to myasthenia gravis. Science **195**:74-75, 1977.

Koelle, G.B. Acetylcholine—current status in physiology, pharmacology, and medicine. New England Journal of Medicine **286**:1086-1090, 1972.

Lambert, E.H., and Elmqvist, D. Quantal components of endplate potentials in the myasthenic syndrome. Annals of the New York Academy of Sciences **183**:183-199, 1971.

Mittag, T., Kornfeld, P., Tormay, A., and Woo, C. Detection of antiacetylcholine receptor factors in serum and thymus from patients with myasthenia gravis. New England Journal of Medicine **294**:691-694, 1976.

Nachmansohn, D. Actions on axons and evidence for the role of acetylcholine in axonal conduction. In Koelle, G.B., ed. Cholinesterases and Anticholinesterases. Handbuch der Experimentellen Pharmakologie, vol. 15. Berlin, Springer-Verlag, 1963.

Stedman, E., Stedman, E., and Easson, L.H. Cholinesterase: an enzyme present in the blood serum of the horse. Biochemical Journal **26**:2056-2066, 1932.

Wilson, I.B. Acid-transferring inhibitors of acetylcholinesterase. In Burger, A., ed. Drugs Affecting the Peripheral Nervous System. New York, Marcel Dekker, Inc., 1967.

9 Antimuscarinic drugs

Enid A. Neidle

There is a variety of drugs that interfere with transmission of nerve impulses at cholinergic junctions. As shown in Table 5-3, there are drugs that prevent the uptake of choline by the nerve terminal or the release of ACh from the terminal; there are those that block at ganglia and those that block, via a competitive or depolarizing form of blockade, at neuromuscular junctions (Chapter 5). The drugs that form the subject for this chapter are those that block responses in muscarinic receptors and are essentially without effect, except at inordinately high doses, at the nicotinic receptors found in autonomic ganglia, skeletal muscle, and parts of the central nervous system.[22] Hence, these drugs are known as antimuscarinic or muscarinic blocking agents; the term *anticholinergic,* although often used for this class of drugs, incorrectly implies that they act at all cholinergic sites. They are also termed *belladonna alkaloids* or *atropine-like* because of their derivation from, or relation to, the oldest and best known member of the group.

The antimuscarinic drugs have a colorful, even sinister, history. They are derived from a number of plants, including *Atropa belladonna* (deadly nightshade), *Datura stramonium* also known as Jimsonweed or Jamestown weed, *Hyoscyamus niger* (henbane), and mandragora among others. Datura was used in India in antiquity; in fact, its name comes from the Sanskrit. These drugs are mentioned in the Ebers papyrus (circa 1550 B.C.), in the Greek herbal of Dioscorides, and by Galen.[2] In western civilization, the drugs came to be used by professional poisoners in the Middle Ages for slow poisoning because of the obscure symptoms and the slow course of illness. The Swedish botanist Linné named the shrub *Atropa belladonna* after Atropos, one of the three Fates, who cuts the thread of life. The term *belladonna* comes from the Italian "beautiful woman" and is so named because instillation of one of these drugs into the eyes was said to make women more attractive.[11]

CHEMISTRY AND CLASSIFICATION

The antimuscarinic drugs fall into four categories:

1. Naturally occurring belladonna alkaloids, atropine and scopolamine, which are organic esters. Atropine and scopolamine are composed of an aromatic acid, tropic acid, and a complex organic base (tropine or scopine, respectively). Atropine is a racemic mixture of *d* and *l* hyoscyamine; the *l* isomer is often used separately.

2. Semisynthetic derivatives, such as homatropine, which is produced by combining tropine with mandelic acid, or the quaternary ammonium derivatives of atropine, scopolamine, or homatropine (atropine methylnitrate, methscopolamine bromide, or homatropine methylbromide, respectively).

3. Synthetic quaternary ammonium compounds, such as methantheline and propantheline.

4. Synthetic antimuscarinic drugs that are not quaternary ammonium compounds, such as benztropine, trihexyphenidyl, and cyclopentolate.

An example of each of these is shown in Table 9-1.

MECHANISM OF ACTION

The antimuscarinic drugs, whether the naturally occurring alkaloid or the semisynthetic or synthetic derivatives, are competitive antagonists of ACh. They have an affinity for cholinergic muscarinic receptor sites but lack intrinsic activity.[3] Thus, they occupy the receptor sites and prevent access of ACh, creating a blockade that is difficult to reverse either in time or by increasing the amount of ACh

Table 9-1. Chemical structures of representatives of the four classes of antimuscarinic drugs

Type of compound	Example	Chemical structure
Naturally occurring alkaloid	Atropine	
Semisynthetic derivative of alkaloid	Methscopolamine	
Synthetic quaternary ammonium compound	Propantheline	
Synthetic but not quaternary ammonium compound	Benztropine	

in the area of the receptor by means of an anticholinesterase. In fact, atropine is an antagonist for the anticholinesterases and vice versa, so that each drug can be used as an antidote for the other in case of poisoning. In effect, the antimuscarinic drugs are capable of blocking responses of muscarinic receptors to nerve stimulation, to exogenous cholinergic drugs, and to the cholinomimetic alkaloids, although their capability for the latter two is greater than for the first.

PHARMACOLOGIC EFFECTS

Therapeutic doses of the antimuscarinic drugs produce effects attributable to the blockade of peripheral muscarinic receptors and similar receptors in the central nervous system, chiefly the medulla and higher cerebral centers. In the discussion that follows, the principal concern will be with atropine and scopolamine, but it must be emphasized that atropine and scopolamine differ in the relative intensity of their antimuscarinic effects on specific organs (Table 9-2) and that there is a difference in the susceptibility of various effectors to antimuscarinic agents in general. Thus, as is shown in Table 9-3, salivary glands respond to low doses of these drugs, whereas gastric secretion is inhibited only by very high doses. Finally, there are some major differences between antimuscarinic drugs in the onset and duration of their actions, as can be seen in Table 9-4.

Peripheral actions

The antimuscarinic drugs possess both peripheral and central actions, but the nature and intensity of these vary with the individual drug. The peripheral actions are caused by an interruption of cholinergic impulses to a given effector; where there is sympathetic innervation, this means that the effector is under the control of the sympathetic nervous system only.

Eye. Antimuscarinic drugs block parasympathetic receptors in the sphincter of the iris and in

Table 9-2. The relative effects of atropine and scopolamine on various effectors

	Iris	Ciliary body	Secretion: saliva, sweat, bronchial	Bronchial muscle	Gastrointestinal muscle	Heart	Central nervous system
Atropine	+	+	+	+ +	+ +	+ +	+
Scopolamine	+ +	+ +	+ +	+	+	+	+ +

Table 9-3. Order of susceptibility of effectors to increasing doses of antimuscarinic agents

Response	Dose
Secretion (saliva, sweat, bronchial)	Low
Mydriasis, cycloplegia, tachycardia	
Loss of parasympathetic control of urinary bladder and gastrointestinal smooth muscle	↓
Inhibition of gastric secretion	High

Table 9-4. Onset and duration of cycloplegia induced by some antimuscarinic drugs

Drug	Onset (min)	Duration
Atropine	30-40	6 days or longer
Scopolamine	20-30	3 days
Homatropine	40-60	36-48 hr
Cyclopentolate	25-75	6-24 hr
Tropicamide	20-35	2-6 hr

the ciliary muscle, thus leading to dilation of the pupil (mydriasis) and paralysis of accommodation (cycloplegia). There is photophobia and fixation of the lens for far vision, so vision for near objects is blurred. There is little effect on intraocular pressure, except in the case of narrow-angle glaucoma, where administration of these drugs may cause a dangerous rise in pressure. Onset and duration of action of the mydriatic and cycloplegic effects differ, as shown in Table 9-4, and to some extent the choice of an agent for an ophthalmologic procedure will be influenced by these differences.

Respiratory tract. After administration of antimuscarinic drugs, the bronchial smooth muscle is left under the sole control of the sympathetic nervous system and is therefore relaxed. This relaxation of the smooth muscle decreases the airway resistance. Sometimes there is an increase in respiratory minute volume resulting from medullary stimulation. The bronchoconstriction caused by ACh, serotonin, and pilocarpine is reversed, but that caused by histamine is not. Secretion of all glands in the nose, mouth, pharynx, and respiratory tract is inhibited. This suppression of secretory activity in the respiratory tract is the underlying reason for the effectiveness of atropine and scopolamine in preventing laryngospasm during general anesthesia[12]; these agents are not capable of blocking contraction of the laryngeal muscle.

Salivary glands. All parasympathetically mediated salivary secretion is completely abolished, while salivary gland vasodilation is unaffected. The mouth and throat become unpleasantly dry, to the point that speech and swallowing may become difficult.

Gastrointestinal tract. While the antimuscarinic drugs are quite effective in preventing the expected motor and secretory responses of the gastrointestinal tract to administered cholinergic drugs, their effects on vagal stimulation are more ambiguous. Antimuscarinic drugs have a marked inhibitory effect on motility throughout the gastrointestinal tract. Thus, interference with the normal parasympathetic impulses to the gastrointestinal tract, as would occur with the antimuscarinic drugs and the ganglionic blocking agents, will cause a profound decrease in the tone of gastrointestinal smooth muscle as well as in the frequency and amplitude of peristaltic contractions. With respect to secretion, gastric secretory activity in humans is inhibited only at very high doses of the belladonna alkaloids, when essentially all other parasympathetic function has been blocked and the patient has an extremely dry mouth, blurred vision, an increased heart rate, and marked inhibition of gastrointestinal motility. At these high doses, atropine reduces gastric acidity, pepsin secretion, and total gastric secretion. The fact that the gastrointestinal tract, particularly the secretory apparatus, is resistant to the belladonna alkaloids and the fact that the therapeutic use of these drugs as antiulcer and antispasmodic drugs has been so disappointing support the hypothesis that there are transmitters other than ACh involved in the regulation of secretion and motor activity in the gastrointestinal tract. Two of these transmitters are ATP[8] and histamine.[6] It should be noted that at high doses atropine has antihistaminic (H_1) activity, and the antihistamine diphenhydramine has marked antimuscarinic activity, one manifestation of which is xerostomia.

Cardiovascular system. The effects of these drugs differ according to the dose administered and whether the subject is in the erect or recumbent position. With oral doses employed to limit salivation (0.4 to 0.6 mg), a mild, centrally mediated bradycardia often results. In most cases, however, the heart rate increases significantly in humans given 1.0 mg or more. In the erect subject there is little or no change in cardiac output.[23] As is shown in Table 9-2, doses of scopolamine that cause mydriasis rarely cause tachycardia, whereas atropine at doses sufficient to have ocular effects will inevitably accelerate the heart.

Urinary tract. The pelvis of the kidney, the ureter, and the urinary bladder are relaxed by atropine, leading to urinary retention in humans. This retention is particularly likely in the presence of prostatic hypertrophy.

Body temperature. The belladonna alkaloids suppress sweating because the sweat glands are innervated by muscarinic cholinergic fibers of the sympathetic nervous system. The rise in body temperature that follows the administration of large doses of atropine or scopolamine has no central component and is caused only by the inhibition of sweating. It is also the most serious and life-threatening result of an overdose of one of these drugs.

Central effects

Central effects are produced only by those antimuscarinic drugs that can penetrate the blood-brain barrier. The quaternary amines, such as methscopolamine and propantheline, are thus without effect on the central nervous system.

Medulla and higher cerebral centers. Both scopolamine and atropine produce complex effects on the central nervous system. With small doses of atropine, there is direct stimulation of the central nervous system, which is generally manifested only as a mild stimulation of respiration via vagal nuclei in the medulla. In therapeutic doses, scopolamine can produce effects ranging from decreased psychologic efficiency, drowsiness, sedation, euphoria, and amnesia to excitement, restlessness, hallucinations, and coma. Atropine is much less active in this respect than is scopolamine.

Antitremor activity. The belladonna alkaloids were used in the treatment of Parkinson's disease in the mid 1800s, long before their mechanism of action was understood and before the biochemical nature of the defect in parkinsonism had been elucidated. Their efficacy in suppressing tremor was later suggested to be due to a "central atropine-acetylcholine antagonism,"[13] and more recently it has been proposed that the striatum is the site of cholinergic systems that in parkinsonism are released from an inhibitory control mediated by dopamine.[9]

Vestibular function. The belladonna alkaloids have been the basis of some very ancient anti–motion sickness drugs. Scopolamine is more effective than atropine, and it probably acts on vestibular end organs or the cortex, or both.[7]

ABSORPTION, FATE, AND EXCRETION

The belladonna alkaloids are readily absorbed from all parts of the gastrointestinal tract except the stomach, as would be expected with alkaloids that form acid salts. Absorption is more rapid from subcutaneous tissue or muscle than it is from the gastrointestinal tract. The drugs are rapidly distributed throughout the body, about 50% being bound to plasma protein. The metabolism of these drugs in humans is not well understood, but the kidney provides the main route for excretion of atropine in changed and unchanged form. Within 24 hours, 27% to 94% of a dose of labeled atropine will be excreted, and very little will be excreted after 24 hours. A third of the atropine will appear as unchanged atropine, the remainder as a metabolite of uncertain identity.[19] Data suggest that there may be genetic differences in the way different humans handle atropine,[20] and this evidence accords well with the finding some years ago that rabbits possess a genetically determined enzyme, atropinesterase, that explains their singular ability to tolerate large doses of atropine.[5] Various idiosyncratic responses or variations in sensitivity to one or another of the actions of these drugs are not uncommon. Young people show a high incidence of idiosyncratic responses; persons with Down's syndrome are more sensitive to the mydriatic effects, while blacks develop greater tachycardia.[11]

GENERAL THERAPEUTIC USES

The therapeutic uses, which will be briefly enumerated, are all based on the pharmacologic effects, peripheral and central, that were discussed above. However, as should be clear already, it is very difficult to obtain a high degree of selectivity in the organ or organs to be affected, since the antimuscarinic drugs tend to affect many muscarinic sites. Certain drugs, however, are more effective and therefore potentially more useful in a particular therapeutic role than others. It should also be noted that the quaternary ammonium compounds, two of which are shown in Table 9-1, differ from atropine and scopolamine in a number of important respects. Two important differences are (1) they do not readily pass the blood-brain barrier because they are ionized at all pH levels, and thus they have no effect on the central nervous system, and (2) they have greater ganglionic blocking properties than do the nonquaternary compounds. This latter point may explain why orthostatic hypotension and impotence are sometimes encountered in patients being treated with these agents. It has been claimed that these synthetic compounds possess a greater selectivity for the gastrointestinal tract than do the other antimuscarinic drugs and that therefore they are preferred agents for the treatment of gastrointestinal disorders because they cause fewer side effects. While it has been difficult to demonstrate that these synthetic compounds do in fact have fewer muscarinic side effects and are at the same time more selective for the gastrointestinal tract, it has been shown in patients with duodenal ulcer that low doses of propantheline are as effective as near-toxic doses of that drug in inhibiting food-stimulated gastric secretion. Furthermore, it was shown in the same experiment that when the low dose of propantheline was given with a conventional dose of the H_2 receptor antagonist cimetidine, the inhibitory effect on gastric secretion was significantly enhanced.[14]

Ophthalmology

By local administration of antimuscarinic drugs, it is possible to produce mydriasis and cycloplegia of very long duration (atropine), medium duration (scopolamine), and very short duration (tropicamide). Mydriasis is necessary for a thorough examination of the retina and optic disc; cycloplegia is necessary for measurement of the refractive powers of the lens. Mydriasis can be produced alternately with miosis for the purpose of breaking up adhesions that may have developed between the lens and the iris. The topical use of these drugs is strongly contraindicated in patients with a predisposition to narrow-angle glaucoma, and while systemic anticholinergic drugs are usually safe for patients with open-angle glaucoma, they may precipitate a first attack of acute angle-closure glaucoma.[10]

Respiratory tract

The belladonna alkaloids are of slight or no benefit in the relief of the bronchospasm of bronchial asthma. However, they do suppress secretion throughout the respiratory tract, an advantage during the administration of general anesthesia, because these drugs produce a dry field, lessen the danger of aspiration of fluid, and prevent laryngospasm.[11]

Salivary secretion

The antimuscarinic drugs are widely used to diminish salivary secretion before surgery, particularly oral surgical procedures. The use of atropine for this purpose not only provides a dry oral cavity but also diminishes the salivary response to irritating anesthetic gases. Occasionally atropine is used to reduce excessive salivary secretion in heavy metal poisoning and parkinsonism.

Gastrointestinal tract

The antimuscarinic drugs have been used extensively as antispasmodics, as antiulcer therapy, and for a variety of disorders characterized by the term *spasticity*. While their use is often attended by symptomatic relief, they have proved of questionable benefit in the treatment of peptic ulcer, severe dysenteries, and so-called spasticity syndromes. It has become popular to substitute the synthetic quaternary ammonium compounds for the naturally occurring alkaloids for these therapeutic goals on the questionable basis that side effects should be less severe with the synthetic compounds. Table 9-5 shows the dosages of atropine at which these effects appear, and it is clear that if reduction in intestinal peristalsis is a therapeutic aim, then tachycardia, blurring of vision, and dryness of

Table 9-5. Effects of atropine in relation to dosage

Dose	Effects
0.5 mg	Slight cardiac slowing; some dryness of mouth; inhibition of sweating
1.0 mg	Definite dryness of mouth; thirst; acceleration of heart, sometimes preceded by slowing; mild dilation of pupil
2.0 mg	Rapid heart rate; palpitation; marked dryness of mouth; dilated pupils; some blurring of near vision
5.0 mg	All of the above symptoms marked; disturbed speech; difficulty in swallowing; restlessness and fatigue; headache; dry, hot skin; difficulty in micturition; reduced intestinal peristalsis
10.0 mg and more	Above symptoms more marked; rapid, weak pulse; iris practically obliterated; very blurred vision; flushed, hot, dry, scarlet skin; ataxia, restlessness, and excitement; hallucinations and delirium; coma

From Gilman, A.G., Goodman, L.S., and Gilman, A., eds. Goodman and Gilman's The Pharmacological Basis of Therapeutics, ed. 6. New York, © 1980 Macmillan Publishing Co., Inc., 1980, p. 127.

mouth must be accepted as inevitable accompaniments.

Cardiovascular system

The application of the antimuscarinic drugs to treatment of cardiovascular disorders is limited. They can be used during anesthesia and surgery to prevent vagal reflexes, in cases of myocardial infarction in which there is excessive vagal tone causing sinus or nodal bradycardia, in cases of a hyperactive carotid sinus reflex producing bradycardia and syncope, or in cases of digitalis-induced heart block.

Genitourinary tract

The belladonna alkaloids have been used to treat a variety of urologic disorders, including renal colic (usually in combination with opioids), nocturnal enuresis, and other forms of urinary incontinence. Inasmuch as the bladder is not very susceptible to the action of muscarinic drugs (Table 9-3), these drugs have not proved very useful in the treatment of these disorders. Tricyclic antidepressants are currently the drugs of choice for nocturnal enuresis; belladonna tincture has some effect on daytime incontinence.

Preanesthetic medication

Preanesthetic medication constitutes a major use for the belladonna alkaloids. Scopolamine in particular provides the central effects of euphoria, amnesia, and sedation as well as the inhibition of salivary and other secretions and the protection that this inhibition provides against laryngospasm.[11] It should be pointed out that many of the newer inhalation anesthetics do not have the irritating properties that anesthetics like ether and chloroform have, so that the need for suppression of respiratory and salivary secretions is not as great as it was in the past.[16]

Central nervous system

Part of the rationale for the use of the belladonna alkaloids as preanesthetic medication is that they have outstanding CNS effects. Other uses for the antimuscarinic drugs based on their central action are to prevent motion sickness and to treat Ménière's disease and parkinsonism. Scopolamine is the drug most frequently chosen for the first two purposes, but it is not particularly effective in preventing nausea and vomiting due to most other causes, as for instance radiation sickness. Scopolamine has been prepared in a transdermal system for the prevention of motion sickness. The system is a flexible disk with an adhesive surface that, when placed on the skin behind the ear, will deliver 0.5 mg scopolamine over a period of 3 days. An effective concentration of the drug in the blood is achieved in 2 to 4 hours. Delivered this way, scopolamine has been shown, in various controlled trials, to be more effective than placebo but not significantly better than the antihistamine dimenhydrinate.[21] Also, the usual effects of cholinergic blockade are minimal, although there is occasional dryness of the mouth and drowsiness. In Parkinson's disease, as is discussed in Chapter 16, the anticholinergics not only are the oldest drugs to be used for this condition but also are still considered to be extremely useful in conjunction with levodopa, for the therapeutic goal in parkinsonism is to restore normal activity to the striatum by reducing cholinergic function or enhancing dopaminergic function, or both. The anticholinergic drugs favored for this purpose are the nonquaternary synthetic compounds that gain ready access to the brain and have greater central than peripheral effects. These include benztropine, biperiden, trihexyphenidyl, cycrimine, and such antihistamines as orphenadrine and diphenhydramine.[24]

Antidote to anticholinesterase poisoning

Toxicity from anticholinesterases may result from their use in the treatment of myasthenia gravis (particularly in the early phase of therapy when the patient is not yet tolerant to the muscarinic effects of these drugs) or from exposure to one of the organophosphate insecticides or anticholinesterase nerve gases. Typically, these anticholinesterases produce a spectrum of muscarinic, nicotinic, and CNS effects. Atropine is effective in antagonizing all the effects at muscarinic sites and thus will relieve hypersecretion of salivary and respiratory glands, bronchoconstriction, gastrointestinal symptoms, sweating, the various other manifestations of muscarinic stimulation, and some central actions. It will not interfere with the desired effects of anticholinesterases at neuromuscular junctions when these drugs are being used for myasthenia gravis, nor will it prevent the neuromuscular stimulation, followed by respiratory failure, that is characteristic of nicotinic stimulation. For treatment of acute toxicity with anticholinesterases, very large doses of atropine are used; for treatment of milder symptoms of muscarinic stimulation, as in myasthenia gravis, much lower doses suffice.[17]

Antidote to poisoning by mushrooms containing muscarine

As pointed out in Chapter 8, the mushroom *Inocybe lateraria* is poisonous because of its high content of the alkaloid muscarine. Atropine is a specific antagonist.

ATROPINE POISONING

Atropine and related drugs, despite wide availability in nature and in medicine cabinets (scopolamine is the principal ingredient in many OTC sleep preparations), have produced relatively few fatal cases of poisoning. In fact, atropine has an enormous margin of safety, as has been demonstrated in cases in which massive doses were used in so-called atropine toxicity therapy for schizophrenia.[15] Most of the reported cases have involved children who accidentally ingested eyedrops or other medicines that contained atropine or scopolamine. The colloquialism "hot as a hare, red as a beet, dry as a bone, blind as a bat, and mad as a wet hen" vividly conveys the symptoms of atropine intoxication, which are predictable extensions of the pharmacology of this group of drugs. There is dryness of the mouth, extreme thirst, a burning sensation in the throat, and difficulty in swallowing; dilation of the pupils and cycloplegia with severe impairment of vision and photophobia; flushing of the skin, vasodilation of skin vessels, and absence of sweating and a rise in body temperature to 105° F or more; urinary retention; and severe symptoms of CNS toxicity. A description of the toxic central effects of atropine and homatropine in children includes ataxia that becomes so severe that the patients are unable to sit or stand unassisted, a dysarthric quality of speech, restlessness with constant muttering, shouting, and singing, great confusion, visual hallucinations, and violent, aggressive, and maniacal behavior.[1,18] Mild toxic reactions may subside in a few hours; most cases require a day or more for complete recovery. Therapy for atropine poisoning is chiefly supportive, although the antianxiety drugs, such as chlordiazepoxide and diazepam, have been used to control CNS excitation. Physostigmine and neostigmine are also helpful in that they raise the amount of ACh in the vicinity of the receptors and act to terminate the atropine blockade more rapidly.

CONTRAINDICATIONS

Topical use of antimuscarinic drugs is absolutely contraindicated in cases of suspected or diagnosed glaucoma. Systemic doses of anticholinergic drugs can be used in patients with open-angle glaucoma but not in patients with narrow-angle glaucoma. As has already been pointed out, use of these drugs may precipitate the first attack of acute angle-closure glaucoma. In prostatic hypertrophy, anticholinergic drugs may cause urinary retention.

DRUG INTERACTIONS

The anticholinergic action of many of the atropine-like drugs is potentiated by antihistamines, which particularly accentuate the xerostomia, by the tuberculostatic drug isoniazid, by MAO inhibitors, and by tricyclic antidepressants. The phenothiazines tend to potentiate the CNS effects of the antimuscarinic drugs. When atropine is given in the presence of propranolol, it is likely to prevent the bradycardia for which propranolol may have been prescribed, and it may also block the vagal actions of the digitalis glycosides.

THERAPEUTIC USES IN DENTISTRY

The principal use of the anticholinergic drugs in dentistry is to decrease the flow of saliva during dental procedures and to decrease the secretion

Table 9-6. Preparations and dosages used in dentistry

Drug	Dose	Route of administration	Time of administration
Atropine sulfate	0.25-1.0 mg	Oral	1-2 hours before procedure
Belladonna tincture	0.6-1 ml	Oral	2½-3 hours
Glycopyrrolate	1-2 mg	Oral	30-45 minutes
Methantheline bromide	50-100 mg	Oral	30-45 minutes
Propantheline bromide	15-30 mg	Oral	30-45 minutes
Scopolamine hydrobromide	0.6 mg	Oral	30-60 minutes

from respiratory glands during general anesthesia. To reduce salivation, small doses given orally or parenterally about 30 minutes to 2 hours before the procedure will be effective, but the drug may also produce some unpleasant side effects that may be objectionable to patients. The same dose may be employed to diminish salivary flow in heavy-metal poisoning. With respect to use during general anesthesia, the anticholinergics will diminish secretion from the respiratory tract, thus lessening the likelihood of aspiration pneumonia and laryngospasm, but, as was pointed out earlier, the anesthetic gases in greatest use at the present time are not highly irritating to the respiratory tract. The antimuscarinic drugs also are used in conjunction with certain anesthetics to prevent reflex vagal slowing of the heart. Scopolamine can be used instead of atropine; it has the advantage over atropine in having a more rapid onset of action and more useful CNS effects. Table 9-6 lists some preparations and dosages used in dentistry.

IMPLICATIONS FOR DENTISTRY

Not only does the dentist occasionally have reason to use the anticholinergic drugs, but the dentist often encounters patients who are taking these drugs for any one of the reasons enumerated earlier. The most characteristic effects of these drugs that concern the dentist are xerostomia and the discomfort that this brings to the patient, as well as the deterioration in oral health. While a few dentists have reported using small doses of pilocarpine to stimulate salivary flow, most dentists advise their patients to drink water, suck on lemon drops, irrigate the mouth with glycerin solutions, and pay scrupulous attention to oral hygiene. Relief of xerostomia caused by radiation is considered in Chapter 45.

Antimuscarinic drugs

Nonproprietary name	Proprietary name
Naturally occurring alkaloids	
atropine	—
belladonna (tincture and extract)	—
l-hyoscyamine	Levsin
levorotatory alkaloids of belladonna	Bellafoline
scopolamine	—
scopolamine (transdermal therapeutic system)	Transderm-Scōp
Semisynthetic derivatives	
atropine methylnitrate	in Festalan
homatropine	Homatrocel Ophthalmic
methscopolamine	Pamine
Synthetic quaternary ammonium compounds	
anisotropine	Valpin 50
clidinium	Quarzan
glycopyrrolate	Robinul
hexocyclium	Tral Filmtabs
isopropamide	Darbid
mepenzolate	Cantil
methantheline	Banthine
oxyphenonium	Antrenyl
propantheline	Pro-Banthine
tridihexethyl	Pathilon
Synthetic nonquaternary ammonium compounds	
benztropine	Cogentin
cyclopentolate	Cyclogyl Ophthalmic
oxyphencyclimine	in Vistrax
procyclidine	Kemadrin
trihexyphenidyl	Artane
tropicamide	Mydriacyl Ophthalmic

CITED REFERENCES

1. Alexander, E., Jr., Morris, D.P., and Eslick, R.L. Atropine poisoning: report of a case, with recovery after the ingestion of one gram. New England Journal of Medicine **234:**258-259, 1946.
2. Ambache, N. The use and limitations of atropine for pharmacological studies on autonomic effectors. Pharmacological Reviews **7:**467-494, 1955.
3. Ariëns, E.J. Affinity and intrinsic activity in the theory of competitive inhibition. Part 1. Problems and theory. Archives Internationales de Pharmacodynamie et de Therapie **99:**32-49, 1954.
4. Berg, J.M., Brandon, M.W.G., and Kirman, B.H. Atropine in mongolism. Lancet **2:**441-442, 1959.
5. Bernheim, F., and Bernheim, M.L.C. The hydrolysis of homatropine and atropine by various tissues. Journal of Pharmacology and Experimental Therapeutics **64:**209-216, 1938.
6. Black, J.W., Duncan, W.A.M., Durant, C.J., Ganellin, C.R., and Persons, E.M. Definition and antagonism of histamine H_2-receptors. Nature **236:**385-390, 1972.
7. Brand, J.J., and Whittingham, P. Intramuscular hyoscine in control of motion sickness. Lancet **2:**232-234, 1970.
8. Burnstock, G. Cholinergic, adrenergic, and purinergic neuromuscular transmission. Federation Proceedings **36:**2434-2438, 1977.
9. Duvoisin, R.C. Cholinergic-anticholinergic antagonism in parkinsonism. Archives of Neurology **17:**124-136, 1967.
10. Effects of systemic drugs with anticholinergic properties on glaucoma. Medical Letter on Drugs and Therapeutics **16:**28, 1974.
11. Eger, E.I. II. Atropine, scopolamine, and related compounds, Anesthesiology **23:**365-383, 1962.
12. Eger, E.I. II., Kraft, I.D., and Keasling, H.H. A comparison of atropine, or scopolamine, plus pentobarbital, meperidine, or morphine as pediatric preanesthetic medications. Anesthesiology **22:**962-969, 1961.
13. Feldberg, W. Present views on the mode of action of acetylcholine in the central nervous system. Physiological Reviews **25:**596-642, 1945.
14. Feldman, M., Richardson, C.T., Peterson, W.L., Walsh, J.H., and Fordtran, J.S. Effect of low-dose propantheline on food stimulated gastric acid secretion. Comparison with an "optimal effective dose" and interaction with cimetidine. New England Journal of Medicine **297:**1427-1430, 1977.
15. Forrer, G.D. Symposium on atropine toxicity therapy: history and future research. Journal of Nervous and Mental Disorders **124:**256-259, 1956.
16. Greenblatt, D.J., and Shader, R.I. Anticholinergics. New England Journal of Medicine **288:**1215-1219, 1973.
17. Grob, D. Anticholinesterase intoxication in man and its treatment. In Koelle, G.B., ed. Cholinesterases and Anticholinesterases, Handbuch der Experimentellen Pharmakologie, vol. 15. Berlin, Springer-Verlag, 1963.
18. Hoefnagel, D. Toxic effects of atropine and homatropine eyedrops in children. New England Journal of Medicine **264:**168-171, 1961.
19. Kalser, S.C. The fate of atropine in man. In Vessell, E.S., ed. Drug Metabolism in Man. Annals of the New York Academy of Sciences **179:**667-683, 1971.
20. Paskind, H.A. Some differences in response to atropine in white and colored races. Journal of Laboratory and Clinical Medicine **7:**104-108, 1921.
21. Price, N.M., Schmitt, L.G., McGuire, J., Shaw, J.E., and Trobough, G. Transdermal scopolamine in the prevention of motion sickness at sea. Clinical Pharmacology and Therapeutics **29:**414-419, 1981.
22. Tvede, K.M., and Cahen, R.L. Action of atropine on sympathetic ganglia. Federation Proceedings **11:**398, 1952.
23. Weissler, A.M., Leonard, J.J., and Warren, J.V. Effects of posture and atropine on the cardiac output. Journal of Clinical Investigation **36:**1656-1662, 1957.
24. Yahr, M.D., and Duvoisin, R.C. Drug therapy of parkinsonism. New England Journal of Medicine **287:**20-24, 1972.

GENERAL REFERENCES

Clarke, R.S.J., Dundee, J.W., and Moore, J. Studies of drugs given before anaesthesia. IV. Atropine and hyoscine. British Journal of Anaesthesia **36:**648-654, 1964.

Krnjević, K. Central cholinergic pathways. Federation Proceedings **28:**113-120, 1969.

Paton, W.D.M., and Rang, H.P. The uptake of atropine and related drugs by intestinal smooth muscle of the guinea-pig in relation to acetylcholine receptors. Proceedings of the Royal Society of London; B: Biological Sciences **163:**1-44, 1965.

10 Ganglionic blocking drugs

Enid A. Neidle

It has been known for a long time that transmission of impulses from the preganglionic to the postganglionic neurons of the autonomic nervous system involves the transmitter ACh, and it has also been known that the ganglia constitute one of the so-called nicotinic sites on which both ACh and nicotine are effective. In fact, in 1889 Langley used nicotine to paralyze transmission from autonomic ganglia. Recently, sophisticated anatomical and electrophysiologic techniques have revealed that the ganglia are not a simple relay mechanism as was formerly thought, nor is it even certain that transmission in sympathetic ganglia is identical with that in parasympathetic ganglia. Interneurons mediating inhibitory mechanisms from both central and peripheral loci and interneurons mediating ganglionic reflexes have been identified. It is significant too that the ganglia represent a small organization of neurons that are not protected by a barrier membrane, such as the blood-brain barrier, which means that these nerve centers are affected by many drugs and chemicals that ordinarily never gain access to central synapses.

A variety of pharmacologic and electrophysiologic studies in sympathetic ganglia have led to two conceptions of ganglionic transmission in which at least three kinds of receptors are postulated: cholinergic nicotinic, cholinergic muscarinic, and adrenergic (possibly dopaminergic).[4] In one scheme, summarized in Figure 10-1, preganglionic stimulation activates, at a muscarinic cholinergic synapse, small intensely fluorescent (SIF) cells or interneurons to release dopamine, which acts on ionic channels in the ganglion cell to generate a hyperpolarizing potential or P wave. A second view is that the release of dopamine caused by preganglionic stimulation activates adenylate cyclase to increase the formation of cAMP, which

promotes the phosphorylation of the membrane structures and thus ganglionic hyperpolarization.[9] Studies of neurotransmission in the cat submandibular ganglion (parasympathetic) have revealed the existence of nicotinic, muscarinic, and adrenergic receptors, but not the presence of an interneuron.[15] Finally, while ACh is certainly recognized as the primary transmitter in sympathetic ganglia, and the presence of an adrenergic transmitter also appears to be well substantiated, evidence is accumulating that additional substances may modulate ganglionic activity. Thus, a substance P–like peptide, present in inferior mesenteric ganglia of the guinea pig[5] and in superior cervical sympathetic ganglia of the neonatal rat,[7] has been proposed as a transmitter. Other peptides identified in sympathetic ganglia include somatostatin, vasoactive intestinal polypeptide, and one or more enkephalins.[14]

While the exact details of ganglionic transmission remain to be elucidated, it is clear that only one transmitter, ACh, is of primary importance. Thus, any drug that interferes with the synthesis or release of ACh or with its interaction with the receptor has the theoretical capacity for interfering with ganglionic transmission (compounds having these actions are listed in Chapter 5). Between 1895 and 1926 a number of compounds having the generic structure shown in Table 10-1 and termed methonium compounds were synthesized, and in 1915 Burn and Dale[2] described the ganglionic blocking action of tetraethylammonium (TEA). In the 1940s an entire series of diiodide and dibromide derivatives of these methonium compounds were synthesized, and in 1946 Acheson and Moe[1] published a systematic and extensive pharmacologic study of TEA. Interest in these drugs arose because they could be used as pharmacologic tools for ex-

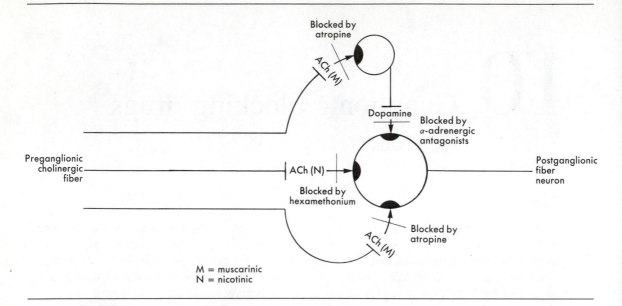

Figure 10-1. Schematic diagram of the principal synaptic connections in the mammalian superior cervical ganglion, which shows the relationship between the various neuronal elements, the neurotransmitters released at the different synapses, and the sensitivity of synaptic receptors to different antagonists. Activation of postjunctional adrenergic and muscarinic receptors respectively inhibits and facilitates transmission through the primary nicotinic pathway. (Adapted from Greengard, P., and Kebabian, J.W., Federation Proceedings **33:**1059-1067, 1974.)

Table 10-1. Some nondepolarizing ganglionic blocking agents

Agent	Chemical structure
Methonium compounds	
Methonium compounds	$(CH_3)_3 N^+ - (CH_2)_n - {}^+N (CH_3)_3$
Hexamethonium	$CH_3 - \underset{\underset{CH_3}{\mid}}{\overset{\overset{CH_3}{\mid}}{N^+}} - (CH_2)_6 - \underset{\underset{CH_3}{\mid}}{\overset{\overset{CH_3}{\mid}}{N^+}} - CH_3$
Pentolinium	
Mecamylamine	

ploring various aspects of autonomic pharmacology and because, at least at first, they offered the promise of being useful therapeutic agents in the treatment of hypertension, gastric ulcer, and other diseases that seemed to have an autonomic component and that had not yet yielded to therapeutic measures then available.

CHEMISTRY, CLASSIFICATION, AND MECHANISM OF ACTION

Classification of the ganglionic blocking agents can be based on their chemical structure or on their mechanism of action. Rossum's classification is based on mechanism and divides these drugs into three groups.[12]

1. Depolarizing agents, such as nicotine and dimethylphenylpiperazinium (DMPP), which produce initial stimulation and varying degrees of subsequent block, perhaps through a mechanism analogous to that of succinylcholine. At higher doses, these agents can stimulate other cholinergic receptors such as those at the neuromuscular junction and central nervous system.

2. Competitive agents, such as hexamethonium (C-6) and TEA.

Table 10-2. Usual predominance of sympathetic (adrenergic) or parasympathetic (cholinergic) tone at various effector sites, with consequent effects of autonomic ganglionic blockade

Site	Predominant tone	Effect of ganglionic blockade
Arterioles	Sympathetic (adrenergic)	Vasodilatation, increased peripheral flow, hypotension
Veins	Sympathetic (adrenergic)	Dilatation, pooling of blood, decreased venous return, decreased cardiac output
Heart	Parasympathetic (cholinergic)	Tachycardia
Iris	Parasympathetic (cholinergic)	Mydriasis
Ciliary muscle	Parasympathetic (cholinergic)	Cycloplegia
Gastrointestinal tract	Parasympathetic (cholinergic)	Reduced tone and motility, constipation
Urinary bladder	Parasympathetic (cholinergic)	Urinary retention
Salivary glands	Parasympathetic (cholinergic)	Xerostomia
Sweat glands	Sympathetic (cholinergic)	Anhidrosis

From Gilman, A.G., Goodman, L.S., and Gilman, A., eds. Goodman and Gilman's The Pharmacological Basis of Therapeutics, ed. 6. New York, © 1980 Macmillan Publishing Co., Inc., 1980, p. 216.

3. Noncompetitive agents such as chlorisondamine, a bisquaternary salt related to C-6, and mecamylamine, a secondary amine. Chlorisondamine is presumed to interfere with the normal sequence of events in ganglionic transmission, and mecamylamine appears to have some of the properties associated with the competitive blocking agents.[13]

The basic prototype for the methonium compounds is shown in Table 10-1. The length of the chain, or the number of hydrocarbon units between the quaternary nitrogen atoms, is a critical factor in the pharmacology of these compounds. As the chain is shortened, neuromuscular stimulating properties become less and less prominent, disappearing completely in hexamethonium. Peak ganglionic blocking potency appears at C-5 and C-6. Shortening the chain to less than four carbon atoms results in inactivity of the compound. Table 10-1 also shows the chemical structure of two nondepolarizing blocking agents that are not methonium compounds and whose mechanism of action is presumably not simply competitive blockade of the receptor.

PHARMACOLOGIC EFFECTS

This section will be restricted to a discussion of the pharmacology of the competitive and noncompetitive (nondepolarizing) blocking agents; the depolarizing agents such as nicotine will not be discussed. All of the ganglionic blocking agents, irrespective of their structure or their mechanism of action, have the same basic pharmacology, although a number of them have been demonstrated to have actions at sites other than ganglionic receptors. An ideal ganglionic blocking agent, according to Paton and Zaimis,[11] is a compound that interferes only with ganglionic transmission, blocks without previous excitation, and does not interfere with the release of transmitter. Hexamethonium is the prototype for these criteria. The pharmacology of this group of drugs is predictable because *all* ganglia, parasympathetic and sympathetic, are blocked by most of the commonly used agents. However, it is important to realize several facts about these drugs. First, ganglia are not equally sensitive to the blocking agents, so that it is easier, for instance, to eliminate the response of the salivary gland to chorda tympani stimulation than it is to eliminate the response of the nictitating membrane to stimulation of the cervical sympathetic nerve. Second, the effect of ganglionic agents is profoundly affected by the background tone or, expressed in another way, is proportional to the rate of nerve transmission through the ganglia at any given time. If vascular tone is high, as it would be in a standing individual, the ganglionic blocking agents will produce a profound fall in blood pressure, much greater than they would in a recumbent individual in whom vascular tone would be lower. Finally, as is shown in Table 10-2, the magnitude of the effect of these drugs is related to the question of which division of the autonomic nervous system, if any, provides the dominant control for a given organ.

Eye

The parasympathetic division plays a dominant role in the maintenance of pupillary diameter and activity in the ciliary muscle. Blockade of autonomic ganglia, therefore, leads to partial, but not maximal, dilation of the pupil and partial paralysis of accommodation.

Respiratory tract

There is inhibition of secretory activity in the respiratory tract and slight bronchial relaxation, but ganglionic blocking agents do not affect respiration directly.

Salivary glands

The salivary glands are predominantly under the control of the parasympathetic nervous system. Thus, ganglionic blockade results in very marked xerostomia.

Gastrointestinal tract

The volume and acidity of gastric secretions that occur spontaneously or in response to insulin are, respectively, strongly inhibited and modified by the ganglionic blocking agents, but there is little effect on secretion induced by histamine.[6] Marked inhibition of motility occurs throughout the gastrointestinal tract, leading to paralytic ileus, and propulsive movements may cease completely. Characteristically, most patients taking ganglionic blocking agents suffer from constipation, often alternating with diarrhea.

Cardiovascular system

There is a fall in blood pressure that is gradual in onset. Normotensive recumbent subjects show the least change; the most prominent alteration in blood pressure occurs in sitting or standing subjects for the obvious reason that vascular reflexes play such an important role in the maintenance of blood pressure in these circumstances. The fall in pressure may be as great as -35% of the control level. Changes in heart rate depend on the existing vagal tone, but generally cardiac rate rises slightly in humans. Cardiac output, on the other hand, tends to drop, mainly because of poor venous return and pooling of blood in the extremities. Blood flow alterations depend on the location of the vascular bed. In the skin there is an increase in blood flow that manifests itself as a rise in surface temperature and a pinkness of the skin. The effects on coronary, pulmonary, muscle, renal, cerebral, and splanchnic circulation are inconsistent because, although vascular resistance may drop in some of these organs, there is not necessarily a concomitant increase in blood flow.

Urinary tract

There is blockade of parasympathetic ganglia of the efferent arm of the spinal reflex normally responsible for micturition. As a result, distention of the bladder does not trigger the voiding response, and there is urinary retention because of incomplete bladder emptying.

Sweat glands

The sweat glands are inhibited so that the skin is dry as well as warm and flushed from the vasodilation of skin blood vessels.

Central nervous system

In therapeutic doses, hexamethonium and its congeners do not gain ready access to the central nervous system, and they usually have no central effects. At high doses, hexamethonium has been reported to depress respiration, particularly in the barbiturate-treated animal.[10] Mecamylamine and other secondary and tertiary amine blocking agents have been reported to produce prominent central effects, such as tremor, choreiform movements, mental aberrations, and convulsions.[3]

ABSORPTION, FATE, AND EXCRETION

The quaternary ammonium compounds are poorly absorbed when administered by the oral route. As pointed out in Chapter 1, the quaternary ammonium compounds have low membrane penetrability at any pH. Furthermore, gastrointestinal propulsive activity is so inhibited and gastric emptying so delayed that large amounts of an orally administered drug may be sequestered in the stomach. After absorption these drugs are restricted to the extracellular space and do not readily cross the blood-brain barrier. When hexamethonium is given parenterally, usually subcutaneously or intramuscularly, most of the drug—about 80% in the first 3 hours after intravenous injection and about 90% in the first 24 hours—is excreted unchanged by the kidney. Mecamylamine is well absorbed on oral administration and has therefore been the most widely used ganglionic blocking agent. Because it can exist in a nonionized state, it diffuses more readily across cell membranes and therefore is distributed in intracellular as well as extracellular spaces. Mecamylamine is excreted by the kidney in the unchanged form, and its excretion is affected by the pH of the urine.

GENERAL THERAPEUTIC USES

As was mentioned earlier in this chapter, it was anticipated when the ganglionic blocking agents were first developed that they would serve as valuable therapeutic agents in treating diseases possibly caused by hyperactivity of the autonomic nervous system (such as hypertension, peptic ulcer, and gastrointestinal spastic conditions) and in producing controlled hypotension for operative procedures in which it is extremely important to diminish the likelihood of bleeding. While the ganglionic blocking agents have been tried extensively in treating hypertension and ulcers, in the latter they have proved largely ineffective and in the former the side effects are so disturbing and the difficulty in adjusting the dose so great that their use has been supplanted by other agents (see Chapter 28). In cases in which controlled hypotension is the goal, trimethaphan and hexamethonium have been used with some success. In hypertensive emergencies, ganglionic blocking agents such as trimethaphan are sometimes used, although sodium nitroprusside and diazoxide are preferred agents.[8]

TOXIC REACTIONS AND SIDE EFFECTS

As is true of all the other autonomic drugs, toxicity from the ganglionic blocking agents can be extrapolated from their known pharmacologic effects. Some of these effects are annoying but bearable—xerostomia, blurring of vision, constipation. Other side effects present more severe problems—orthostatic hypotension, urinary hesitancy, sexual impotence.

Since considerable tolerance to these effects may develop, they may seem less of a problem as time goes on. However, the ganglionic blocking agents can produce peripheral circulatory collapse with cerebral and coronary insufficiency, as well as paralytic ileus and complete urinary retention. This extremely serious toxicity is a major reason for the gradual abandonment of these drugs in the treatment of hypertension.

DRUG INTERACTIONS

Mecamylamine, the only ganglionic blocking agent used to any extent for the ambulatory patient, is potentiated by a variety of drugs, including alcohol, general anesthetics, several diuretics (thiazides, chlorthalidone, and furosemide), antacids, and other antihypertensives. Sympathomimetic drugs administered to a patient taking mecamyl-

amine will produce exaggerated effects; the significance of these effects for the dental patient receiving a local anesthetic with epinephrine has not been described.

IMPLICATIONS FOR DENTISTRY

The ganglionic blocking agents are no longer in wide use with ambulatory patients; thus, patients with problems stemming from ganglionic blockade that might ordinarily prove troublesome to the dentist, namely xerostomia and orthostatic hypotension, are not likely to be encountered.

Ganglionic blocking agents

Nonproprietary name	Proprietary name
tetraethylammonium*	—
hexamethonium*	—
mecamylamine	Inversine
trimethaphan	Arfonad
pentolinium*	Ansolysen

*No longer available in the United States for clinical use.

CITED REFERENCES

1. Acheson, G.H., and Moe, G.K. The action of tetraethylammonium ion on the mammalian circulation. Journal of Pharmacology and Experimental Therapeutics 87:220-236, 1946.
2. Burn, J.H., and Dale, H.H. The action of certain quaternary ammonium bases. Journal of Pharmacology and Experimental Therapeutics 6:417-438, 1915.
3. Freis, E.D. Clinical uses of ganglionic blocking agents in the treatment of hypertension and a comparison of different blocking agents. In Moyer, J., ed. Hypertension. Philadelphia, W.B. Saunders Co., 1959.
4. Greengard, P., and Kebabian, J.W. Role of cyclic AMP in synaptic transmission in the mammalian peripheral nervous system. Federation Proceedings 33:1059-1067, 1974.
5. Jiang, Z.-G., Dun, N.J., and Karczmar, A.G. Substance P: a putative sensory transmitter in mammalian autonomic ganglia. Science 217:739-741, 1982.
6. Kay, A.W., and Smith, A.N. Effect of hexamethonium iodide on gastric secretion and motility. British Medical Journal 1:460-463, 1950.
7. Kessler, J.A., Adler, J.E., Bohn, M.C., and Black, I.B. Substance P in principal sympathetic neurons: regulation by impulse activity. Science 214:335-336, 1981.
8. Koch-Weser, J. Hypertensive emergencies. New England Journal of Medicine 290:211-214, 1974.
9. McAfee, D.A., Henon, B.K., Whiting, G.J., Horn, J.P., Yarowsky, P.J., and Turner, D.K. The action of cAMP and catecholamines in mammalian sympathetic ganglia. Federation Proceedings 39:2997-3002, 1980.
10. Paton, W.D.M., and Zaimis, E.J. Paralysis of autonomic ganglia by methonium salts. British Journal of Pharmacology 6:155-168, 1951.

11. Paton, W.D.M., and Zaimis, E.J. The methonium compounds. Pharmacological Reviews **4:**219-253, 1952.
12. Rossum, J.M. van. Classification and molecular pharmacology of ganglionic blocking agents. Part I. International Journal of Neuropharmacology **1:**97-110, 1962.
13. Rossum, J.M. van. Classification and molecular pharmacology of ganglionic blocking agents. Part II. International Journal of Neuropharmacology **1:**403-421, 1962.
14. Schultzberg, M., Hökfelt, T., Terenius, L., Elfvin, L.-G., Lundberg, J.M., Brandt, J., Elde, R.P., and Goldstein, M. Enkephalin immunoreactive nerve fibres and cell bodies in sympathetic ganglia of the guinea-pig and rat. Neuroscience **4:**249-270, 1970.
15. Suzuki, T., and Volle, R.L. Nicotinic, muscarinic, and adrenergic receptors in a parasympathetic ganglion. Journal of Pharmacology and Experimental Therapeutics. **211:**252-256, 1979.

GENERAL REFERENCES

Eccles, J.C. The Physiology of Synapses. New York, Academic Press, Inc., 1964.
Gyermek, L. Ganglionic stimulant and depressant agents. In Burger, A., ed. Drugs Affecting the Peripheral Nervous System. New York, Marcel Dekker, Inc., 1967.
Kharkevich, D.A. Ganglion-blocking and Ganglion-stimulating Agents. Oxford, England, Pergamon Press, 1967.
Riker, W.F., Jr., and Okamoto, M. Pharmacology of motor nerve terminals. Annual Review of Pharmacology and Toxicology **9:**173-208, 1969.
Volle, R.L. Ganglionic transmission. Annual Review of Pharmacology and Toxicology **9:**135-146, 1969.
Volle, R.L., and Hancock, J.C. Transmission in sympathetic ganglia. Federation Proceedings **29:**1913-1918, 1970.

11 Neuromuscular blocking drugs

Joel D. Schiff

Early in the sixteenth century, Spanish explorers of the New World encountered a plant extract used by South American natives to poison the tips of their hunting arrows. This extract, known as curare, was brought back to Europe, and its lethal mode of action was quickly found to depend on muscular paralysis. However, with the knowledge of their preparation shrouded in tribal lore, the samples available to Western civilization were crude. For many years the only classification of curares depended on their storage vessels, hence calabash curare, pot curare, and tube curare (tubocurarine). Further understanding of the actions of curare did not come for many years.

In 1856, Claude Bernard reported that the site of action of curare was the junction between nerve and muscle.[4] Bernard found that although neuromuscular transmission was blocked by curare, conduction of impulses along the motor nerve was unimpeded, and the muscle was still able to contract if stimulated directly. The substance used by Bernard in his studies, d-tubocurarine, was subsequently purified, and in 1942 it was administered for the first time to a patient undergoing surgery for appendicitis.[17] This drug, along with a number of other agents that similarly block neuromuscular transmission (Table 11-1), has since found widespread acceptance for its ability to produce muscular flaccidity and is frequently administered as an adjunct to general anesthesia during surgery.

NEUROMUSCULAR TRANSMISSION AND BLOCKADE

Nervous control of skeletal muscle contraction is mediated by the transmitter substance ACh. In response to a motor neuron action potential, ACh is released from the terminal region of the nerve fiber. The transmitter then diffuses across the junc-

Table 11-1. Effect of various agents on the depth of blockade produced by nondepolarizing and depolarizing blocking agents

Agent	Tubocurarine	Succinylcholine
Tubocurarine	+	−
Succinylcholine	−, then +	−, then +
Anticholinesterase	−	+
Hexafluorenium	0	+
Ether, halothane	+	0
Streptomycin, neomycin	+	0
Reduced temperature	−	+

Key: + = intensification of the blockade, − = reversal or lessening of the blockade, 0 = no major effect.

tional cleft and binds with specific receptor proteins on the postjunctional membrane (endplate) of the muscle fiber. The binding of ACh to the receptor brings about a nonspecific increase in the ionic permeability of the endplate membrane and a consequent depolarization (endplate potential) of the junctional region of the muscle fiber. Under normal conditions, the endplate potential is sufficient to trigger an action potential in the electrically excitable muscle fiber membrane, and muscular contraction follows.[21]

Neuromuscular blocking drugs interfere with the ability of ACh to evoke endplate depolarization. They are generally separated into two groups according to whether they themselves bring about endplate depolarization in the course of their action; as will be seen, the depolarizing and the nondepolarizing blocking agents differ in the mechanisms through which they produce neuromuscular blockade. Figure 11-1 shows the physiologic events that occur in a nerve, neuromuscular junction, and skeletal muscle that lead to contraction of muscle and the drugs that block these events.

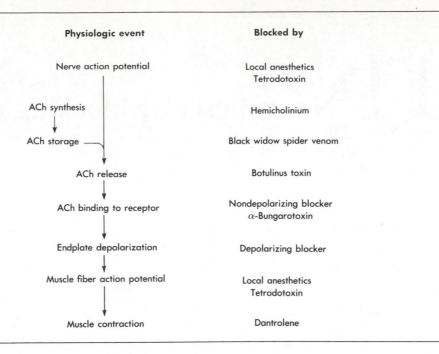

Physiologic event	Blocked by
Nerve action potential	Local anesthetics Tetrodotoxin
ACh synthesis	Hemicholinium
ACh storage	Black widow spider venom
ACh release	Botulinus toxin
ACh binding to receptor	Nondepolarizing blocker α-Bungarotoxin
Endplate depolarization	Depolarizing blocker
Muscle fiber action potential	Local anesthetics Tetrodotoxin
Muscle contraction	Dantrolene

Figure 11-1. Process of physiologic events that occur in a nerve, neuromuscular junction, and skeletal muscle leading to contraction of the muscle, and the drugs that block these events.

NONDEPOLARIZING BLOCKING AGENTS

The nondepolarizing, or competitive, neuromuscular agents, a group that includes tubocurarine (*d*-tubocurarine), metocurine (dimethyl-*d*-tubocurarine), pancuronium, atracurium, vecuronium, and gallamine, are molecules with multiple quaternary ammonium sites spaced 12 to 14 Å apart. All except gallamine, tubocurarine, and vecuronium are bisquaternary compounds with bridged, multiringed structures supplying structural rigidity; gallamine is triquaternary with a more flexible molecular structure, vecuronium is a monoquaternary derivative of pancuronium, and tubocurarine is a monoquaternary amine with a second nitrogen that is partially ionized at physiologic pH (Figure 11-2).

All of these agents act by occupying the endplate receptor sites of the muscle fiber and thus blocking access to these sites by ACh. The drugs themselves do not cause endplate depolarization.[6] Inhibition of neuromuscular transmission by these drugs is competitive, with the blocking agent and ACh competing for receptor sites on the muscle fiber. By interfering with nervous excitation of muscle without themselves producing any excitation, the nondepolarizing blocking agents cause flaccid paralysis.

DEPOLARIZING BLOCKING AGENTS

The major depolarizing blocking agents, succinylcholine and decamethonium (C-10), like the nondepolarizing blockers, are bisquaternary compounds with an interquaternary spacing of 12 to 14 Å. However, unlike the nondepolarizing agents, the depolarizing blockers have flexible chain linkages between their cationic moieties.

Depolarizing blocking agents act by binding to the cholinergic receptor at the muscle endplate. As the class name suggests, the initial effect of the binding of these agents is a depolarization of the muscle fiber. During the early phase of action, there is a period of excitation during which the sensitivity of the muscle to ACh is actually increased. Indeed, it is possible for the drug-induced depolarization to be great enough to trigger action potentials and spontaneous twitching—fasciculations—in the muscle fibers. The depolarization produced by the blocking agent gradually diminishes, but the endplate membrane potential does not completely return to its resting level. After the transient excitation and during the period in which endplate depolarization is still prominent, neuromuscular transmission is blocked in what is variously referred to as a depolarization, or phase 1, block. As the membrane repolarizes, there is a gradual transition to a desensitization, or phase 2, block.

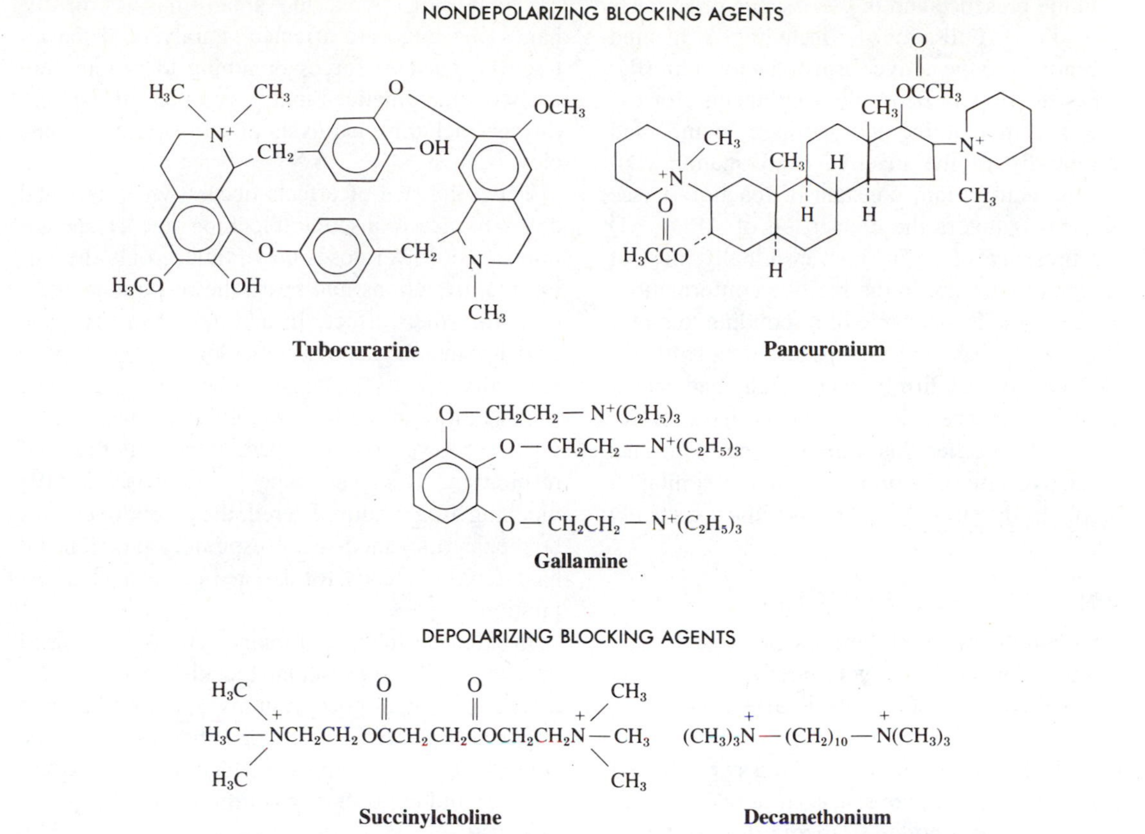

NONDEPOLARIZING BLOCKING AGENTS

Tubocurarine

Pancuronium

$$O-CH_2CH_2-N^+(C_2H_5)_3$$
$$O-CH_2CH_2-N^+(C_2H_5)_3$$
$$O-CH_2CH_2-N^+(C_2H_5)_3$$

Gallamine

DEPOLARIZING BLOCKING AGENTS

Succinylcholine

$$(CH_3)_3\overset{+}{N}-(CH_2)_{10}-\overset{+}{N}(CH_3)_3$$

Decamethonium

Figure 11-2. Structural formulas of neuromuscular blocking agents.

Whereas the former is a labile neuromuscular blockade readily reversed by removal of the depolarizing blocking drug, the latter is a longer lasting blockade that is only slowly reversed.[38]

A number of theories have been proposed to account for the endplate receptor desensitization of the phase 2 blockade produced by the depolarizing blocking agents. It should be noted that a similar receptor desensitization occurs under laboratory conditions when the presence of ACh is prolonged at the neuromuscular junction by exposure to anticholinesterase or by continuous perfusion with the transmitter.[2] Thus, the loss of the depolarizing ability of ACh may be considered a form of drug tachyphylaxis, and any model for the actions of the depolarizing blocking agents must also account for the more general phenomenon.

The currently accepted model for desensitization blockade of the endplate receptor is similar to that originally proposed by Katz and Thesleff[24] in 1957. Receptors can exist in either of two conformational states, active and inactive, and these interconvert

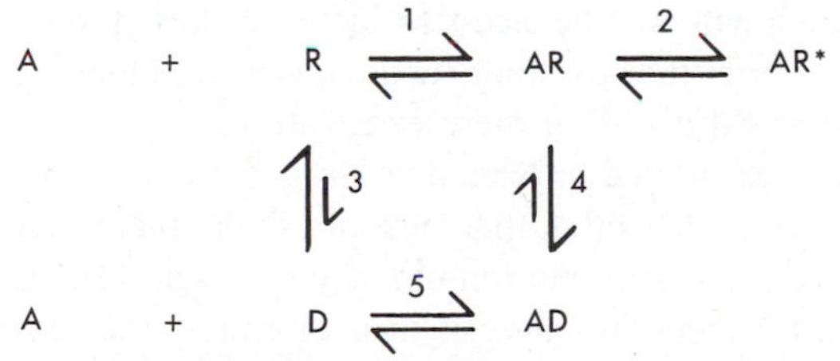

Figure 11-3. Scheme for desensitization blockade of endplate receptors. Reactions, 1, 2, and 5 are assumed to be in relatively rapid equilibrium, whereas reactions 3 and 4 are slower. A is the ligand, which may be ACh or a depolarizing blocking agent; R and D are, respectively, the active and inactive (desensitized) conformations of the receptor, and AR* is the high-permeability depolarizing state. The equilibrium constant of reaction 3 very likely favors the conversion of D to R; however, that of reaction 4 favors the formation of AD from AR. Thus, in the presence of the ligand, most receptors are inactivated to the AD state. Partial agonists such as the depolarizing blocking agents are characterized by a higher affinity for D than for R. (Modified from Katz, B., and Thesleff, S. Journal of Physiology (London) **138:**63-80, 1957.

both in the presence and in the absence of agonists (Figure 11-3). Full agonists, including ACh, bind preferentially to the active form of the receptor (R), whereas the depolarizing blocking agents, for example, succinylcholine and decamethonium, bind preferentially to the inactive conformation (D). Since the equilibrium constant of reaction 4 (see Figure 11-3) favors the conversion of AR to AD in the presence of an agonist, eventually most of the receptor sites are in the inactive conformation, and the muscle is incapable of responding to motor neuron ACh. Although the specific details of this model are not yet firmly established, and recent investigations have suggested on the basis of detailed kinetic studies that there may be more than one inactive conformation,[12] a scheme similar in principle to that in Figure 11-3 is almost certainly valid.

PHARMACOLOGIC EFFECTS

Although the major pharmacologic effects of the neuromuscular blocking agents are on the skeletal muscle endplate, these agents do affect other systems and effectors.

The ideal neuromuscular blocking agent would be rapid in onset and consistent in duration of action. It would be a nondepolarizing drug so that it would not cause muscle fasciculations, it would be free of autonomic and cardiovascular effects, and it would not liberate histamine from muscle or other tissues. In addition, it would not induce tachyphylaxis so that prolonged blockade could be maintained without the need to increase dose levels. None of the existing neuromuscular blocking agents fulfills all of these expectations. Pancuronium has proved an excellent drug for its relative lack of effects other than neuromuscular blockade. Atracurium and vecuronium may represent further improvements because of their more rapid action; however, at the time of this writing, clinical experience with these agents has been limited within the United States.

Neuromuscular junction effects

On administration, neuromuscular blocking agents of both classes first affect the facial muscles and then the other muscles of the head and neck. In the conscious subject, this action produces diplopia, dysarthria, and dysphagia; because of dysphagia, secretions accumulate in the throat, and breathing becomes difficult. In addition, there is an uncomfortable sensation of warmth. As the

blockade progresses, the small muscles of the hands and body are affected. Paralysis of the intercostal muscles forces breathing to become entirely diaphragmatic. Finally, complete flaccid paralysis, including paralysis of all respiratory muscles, occurs.

This sequence of effects occurs when maximal doses of neuromuscular blocking agents are administered; lower doses may produce only the earlier manifestations and spare the respiratory muscles from their effect. In addition, there is some evidence that the depolarizing blocking agents preferentially block transmission to white muscles, such as those of the limb musculature, while sparing the slower red muscles, including those of respiration. However, when any neuromuscular blocking drug is administered, the practitioner must be prepared for the loss of respiratory function and have facilities ready for assisted or controlled respiration.

In addition to their primary actions on striated muscle, the neuromuscular blocking agents affect a number of other body systems. Some of the more important of these actions on other sites must be considered in choosing the blocking agent to administer and in observing additional precautions in their use.

Central effects

None of the neuromuscular blocking drugs described here has any apparent influence on the central nervous system.[35] The reason for this is the inability of these compounds, all of which are cations with extremely low lipid solubility, to cross the blood-brain barrier.

Autonomic effects

Because of their relative specificity for the nicotinic cholinergic receptors of the muscle endplate, the neuromuscular blocking drugs as a group have no major influence on the autonomic nervous system. However, individual drugs of this category do exert certain specific autonomic influences.

Gallamine interferes with the vagal parasympathetic influence on the cardiac pacemaker and thus causes tachycardia[33]; it is not known whether this effect is a specific ganglionic blocking action or whether the drug possesses an atropine-like action confined to the muscarinic receptors of the sinoatrial node.

Pancuronium can also increase the heart rate, although less consistently than gallamine. The effect may result from inhibition of the vagus, disinhibition of sympathetic ganglia, prevention of norepinephrine reuptake, or some combination of these effects.

Succinylcholine causes a transient bradycardia as it is administered, probably through a vagomimetic action on the cholinergic receptors of the heart.[16] After administration of succinylcholine, there is a longer-lasting period of tachycardia that seems to be the result of stimulation of sympathetic ganglia.[36]

Tubocurarine (and, to some extent, metocurine) can block ganglionic transmission in the autonomic nervous system by interfering with the action of ACh at postganglionic nicotinic receptors, but this action requires doses several times higher than those used to induce muscle relaxation.[19] Nevertheless, autonomic tone and reflexes are probably depressed at clinical dosage levels.

Histaminic effects

All of the neuromuscular blocking agents, but most notably tubocurarine and, to a lesser extent, succinylcholine and metocurine, cause the release of histamine from mast cells into the circulation.[1] Thus, these drugs are capable of producing histamine-mediated symptoms such as hypotension, edema, bronchospasm, and increased salivary flow. The last two actions may introduce complications during performance of controlled respiration and can be prevented by prior administration of antihistamines. Pancuronium, gallamine, and especially vecuronium do not induce significant histamine release from muscle or other tissues.

Vascular effects

Although none of the neuromuscular blocking drugs has any direct effect on vascular tone, all can produce hypotension via a combination of indirect actions. The release of histamine, as described above, causes edema and vasodilation. The loss of skeletal muscle tone as a result of neuromuscular blockade eliminates the muscle pumping action in the veins of the lower extremities; hence, there is a pooling of blood in the veins of the legs and a concomitant reduction in venous return to the heart. In addition to these physiologic effects on the circulation, there is another factor that is a consequence of the use of assisted or controlled respiration during the period of muscular paralysis: the increased intrathoracic pressure produced by the respirator during its positive pressure phase ad-ditionally reduces venous return to the heart. In this respect, alternating positive and negative pressure respirators are less harmful than are intermittent positive pressure devices because of the increased venous return in the negative pressure phase of the former.

These causes of hypotension can be treated by positioning the patient with the lower extremities elevated slightly above the heart and by administering isotonic fluids intravenously, possibly in combination with sympathomimetic vasoconstrictors.

ABSORPTION, FATE, AND EXCRETION

All neuromuscular blocking agents are generally administered intravenously. Intramuscular administration is somewhat effective for most of the agents discussed and may be used in treating some pediatric patients in whom intravenous injection might present difficulties, but this route does not offer the precision of control or the rapidity of onset of action afforded by the intravenous route.

All of the agents discussed in this chapter are ineffective when given orally. This was known to be the case for tubocurarine by the South American hunters who readily ate prey felled by arrows laden with the drug.

All of the blocking agents discussed show their effects within a few minutes after administration and, with the exception of succinylcholine, persist for 20 to 60 minutes. Succinylcholine gives its maximal effect within 2 minutes of injection, and recovery is apparent after approximately 5 minutes. With any of the agents, blockade may be prolonged either by repeated injection of the agent or by the use of continuous intravenous infusion.

With the exception of succinylcholine, atracurium, and vecuronium, all of the agents mentioned are to a large extent excreted unchanged by the kidneys.[7] Succinylcholine is hydrolyzed by plasma pseudocholinesterase first to succinylmonocholine, a much weaker depolarizing blocking agent, and then to succinic acid and choline. It is possible to inhibit the plasma pseudocholinesterase by use of hexafluorenium.[29] Under these conditions, the action of succinylcholine is prolonged for 20 to 30 minutes, approximately the same duration as that of the other agents described.

It should be noted that in certain individuals who have an atypical plasma cholinesterase, succinylcholine will have a much lower effective dose and will persist in the body for at least 30 minutes. Such patients should be identified by assaying cholinesterase activity in isolated plasma before administering the blocking agent lest respiratory failure result from overdosage. If a neuromuscular blockade of short duration is desired in these individuals, purified cholinesterase can be injected intravenously before infusing succinylcholine.[15] Cholinesterase injection is ineffective after the succinylcholine blockade has set in.

Atracurium is unique in that it undergoes spontaneous, nonenzymatic degradation at physiologic temperature and pH. (A second major pathway of elimination is hydrolysis by nonspecific esterases.) Thus, atracurium is especially suited for patients with impaired hepatic and renal systems. Vecuronium may also be used in patients with kidney failure because it is largely eliminated by way of hepatic metabolism and biliary excretion.

GENERAL THERAPEUTIC USES

Since the first clinical use of tubocurarine in 1942,[17] a number of applications for the neuromuscular blocking agents have gained wide acceptance.[11,14] Some of these are described below.

Surgery

The most frequent use of neuromuscular blocking agents is as an adjunct to general anesthesia during surgical procedures. The most common indication under this heading is to relax the abdominal wall musculature during abdominal surgery. This application is especially useful in procedures such as appendectomy in which the underlying condition has produced reflex splinting of these muscles. During brain or cerebrovascular surgery in which the patient is sedated but conscious neuromuscular blockade is needed to suppress cough and sneeze reflexes so that the field of operation may remain immobilized.

Tetanus

In mild cases of tetanus, the patient is generally able to sustain respiration except during intermittent spasms. Here, neuromuscular blocking agents are administered to reduce the severity of these spasms. In severe cases of tetanus, in which the rigor of the patient extends to the respiratory musculature, blocking drugs are administered to induce flaccidity so that artificially assisted respiration may be used.

Electroconvulsive therapy

In the treatment of depressive psychoses with electroconvulsive therapy, the therapeutic result is a consequence of the electrical stimulation of the central nervous system; the massive muscle spasm that accompanies such treatment is of no therapeutic use and has the potential for producing bodily injury. Neuromuscular blockade is therefore induced by injection of succinylcholine before the electrical stimulation of the brain. Succinylcholine is used here because of its short duration of action and lack of residual side effects.

Other uses

Succinylcholine is used to produce a short-lived muscular relaxation to permit a number of brief nonsurgical manipulations such as the setting of fractures of the extremities or mandible or the insertion of an endotracheal tube; in the last case the drug prevents laryngospasm.

APPLICATIONS IN DENTISTRY

Dental practice holds few indications for the use of neuromuscular blocking agents. Among the situations in which use of these drugs might be appropriate are mandibular fractures, when muscle relaxation is needed to permit manipulation of bone fragments, and trismus, when no more conservative means exist to permit mouth opening for diagnosis and treatment. In addition, the short-acting neuromuscular blocker succinylcholine is used to facilitate the insertion of an endotracheal tube whenever the use of general anesthesia makes intubation appropriate. Indeed, in any office in which general anesthesia is used, succinylcholine should always be available to permit tracheal intubation should a patient suffer laryngospasm.

TOXICITY AND ANTIDOTES

The major threat of overdosage with neuromuscular blocking agents is death from respiratory failure. In cases of overdose, respiratory function must be maintained with external devices, either through an endotracheal tube or via tracheostomy. Overdosage of nondepolarizing blocking agents may be reversed to some extent through administration of anticholinesterases, generally accompanied by atropine to prevent excessive parasympathetic sequelae to these drugs. No treatment exists to reverse the phase 2 blockade of the depolarizing blockers.

DRUG INTERACTIONS

Many different classes of drugs are capable of interacting, either synergistically or antagonistically, with the neuromuscular blocking agents (Table 11-1). The following sections describe the actions of drugs likely to be administered in conjunction with neuromuscular blockers and their effects on the activities of the blocking agents.

Anticholinesterases

Inhibitors of acetylcholinesterase, by blocking the enzymatic hydrolysis of ACh at the motor endplate, increase the amount of transmitter available at the receptor sites. These drugs antagonize the blockade produced by the nondepolarizing blocking agents, which act by competing with ACh for occupancy of receptor binding sites. Their effect when administered during the action of a depolarizing neuromuscular blocker is more complex; after a brief period of antagonism, during which the blockade is reduced, they act to intensify the neuromuscular blockade by further desensitizing the receptors to transmitter.

Hexafluorenium, which specifically inhibits plasma pseudocholinesterase without affecting the endplate acetylcholinesterase, prolongs the presence of succinylcholine in the circulation. This action both extends the duration of the neuromuscular blockade by succinylcholine and decreases the dose necessary to obtain that blockade. In addition to its inhibitory effect on plasma cholinesterase, hexafluorenium is itself a nondepolarizing neuromuscular blocker and as such potentiates the blockade induced by other nondepolarizing blockers.[29]

General anesthetics

Anesthetics that stabilize excitable membranes, most prominently ether and the halogenated inhalation agents, tend to act synergistically with the nondepolarizing blocking agents.[22,23] When ether is used for general anesthesia, doses of tubocurarine must be reduced to one third to one half of the usual dose.[36]

Antibiotics

Some antibiotics, such as streptomycin and other aminoglycosides, reduce the amount of ACh released by the motor nerve terminal in response to an action potential and thus act synergistically with the nondepolarizing neuromuscular blocking drugs.[3,10,37] Other antibiotics that may lower dosage requirements for the neuromuscular blockers include the tetracyclines, clindamycin, lincomycin, and the polymyxins.

Sympathomimetics

Catecholamines and other sympathomimetic agents increase the amount of ACh released from the motor neuron and thereby antagonize the blockade produced by nondepolarizing blocking agents.[25]

Lithium

Lithium salts, used for the prophylaxis and treatment of manic-depressive illness, can, at therapeutic doses, slow the onset of neuromuscular blockade by the depolarizing agents but not that by the competitive blockers. Lithium also intensifies the blockade by gallamine and pancuronium but not that by tubocurarine or the depolarizing agents, and it prolongs the effect of depolarizing blockers and pancuronium but not that of gallamine or tubocurarine.[20]

Neuromuscular blocking agents

Administration of a nondepolarizing blocking agent to a patient under the influence of the same drug or a different nondepolarizing blocking drug simply augments the blockade: the agents act additively, with no evidence of either synergism or antagonism.

Administration of a depolarizing blocking agent to a patient already treated with another depolarizing blocker may lighten the blockade for a brief interval that would correspond to the period of early transient facilitation that follows administration of any of the depolarizing drugs. However, the ultimate effect of the second drug is augmentation of the neuromuscular blockade.

Combinations of depolarizing and nondepolarizing neuromuscular blocking agents are generally antagonistic and therefore have little clinical value. Use has been made of this antagonism, however, in the administration of low doses of succinylcholine to speed recovery from blockade by nondepolarizing blocking agents. It is a frequent practice to use succinylcholine to induce a rapid blockade for tracheal intubation prior to the production of a long-term blockade with tubocurarine. Here, the short lifetime of succinylcholine in the body effectively prevents any significant antagonism between the two drugs.[13] Interestingly, subsequent administration of the nondepolarizing drug generally gives evidence of enhanced neuromuscular blockade. Nondepolarizing blocking agents are occasionally used as pretreatment before infusion of succinylcholine to prevent the pain occasionally associated with fasciculations produced by the latter drug. In this case, the dose of succinylcholine must be increased for the drug to be effective.

OTHER AGENTS AFFECTING NEUROMUSCULAR TRANSMISSION

A number of substances, both synthetic and of biologic origin, have been found to act by affecting one or more of the processes involved in normal neuromuscular transmission. Although clinical applications have not yet been found for all of these drugs, it should be recalled that nearly a century elapsed between Bernard's discovery of the site of action of curare and the first use of that drug in surgery. As the mechanisms of action of each of the following drugs become more completely known, it is possible that useful applications for some or all of them will be found.

Hemicholinium

Most of the choline produced by the enzymatic hydrolysis of ACh is returned to the motor nerve terminal by a specific transport system and is then used in the synthesis of new transmitter.[32] Hemicholinium, by blocking the neuronal uptake of choline, interferes with the synthesis of ACh and thus acts to deplete the nerve terminal of this substance.[27] The resulting blockade of neuromuscular transmission is gradual in onset but is accelerated by increased motor neuron activity.

Botulinus toxin

The toxin produced by *Clostridium botulinum* acts on the motor nerve terminal to prevent the release of ACh in response to the arrival of an axonal action potential.[5] The toxin interferes with the influx of extracellular calcium ions into the nerve terminal[34]; calcium influx during the action potential is necessary for ACh release.[21]

Black widow spider venom

The venom of the black widow spider rapidly depletes the motor nerve terminal of its stores of ACh by causing complete exocytosis of transmitter independently of stimulation or calcium influx.[30]

α-Bungarotoxin

This peptide toxin isolated from the venom of the banded krait, as well as the similar if not identical neurotoxin from the venom of the cobra, is capable of binding irreversibly with the cholinergic receptor proteins of the muscle endplate.[8,26] The toxin does not cause endplate depolarization, and its effect is similar to that of the nondepolarizing blocking agents, although irreversible. The ability of radiolabeled α-bungarotoxin to bind stoichiometrically with cholinergic receptors makes it possible to locate and count receptor sites; this has provided a useful technique for research on a number of subjects ranging from denervation supersensitivity to myasthenia gravis.

Tetrodotoxin

Tetrodotoxin, found in a number of tissues of the puffer, or fugu, fish, prevents the propagation of both axon and muscle fiber action potentials by interfering with electrically activated sodium ion conductance. Saxitoxin, which is produced by certain strains of algae and has been implicated in the occasional contamination of shellfish that consume these algae, has a similar effect on sodium channels. The effect of these toxins is similar to that of local anesthetics, but their potencies are a millionfold greater, and they are only slightly reversible.

Dantrolene

Dantrolene (Figure 11-4) is an agent that acts within the skeletal muscle fiber rather than on the neuromuscualr junction. Its sites of action include the transverse tubular system and sarcoplasmic reticulum, where it inhibits the depolarization-induced release of Ca^{++} from the cisternae of the sarcoplasmic reticulum into the cytoplasm, thus interfering with excitation-contraction coupling.[28]

The principal therapeutic applications of dantrolene are for the relief of spasticities associated with upper motor neuron disorders (e.g., stroke, cerebral palsy, and multiple sclerosis[9,33]) and for prophylaxis and treatment of malignant hyperthermia.[18]

Spastic movements, clonus, and rigidities that result from stroke or cerebral palsy are often relieved by dantrolene; the spasticity of multiple sclerosis is relieved to a lesser extent, possibly because the lesions of this condition are more widespread.[31] On the other hand, dantrolene is actually contraindicated in amyotrophic lateral sclerosis because the muscular weakness associated with this condition, when exacerbated by the drug (see below), can lead to respiratory difficulty.[31]

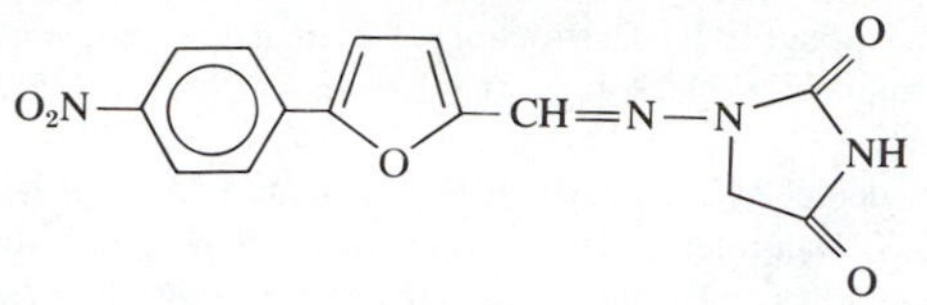

Figure 11-4. Structure of dantrolene.

Malignant hyperthermia (malignant hyperpyrexia) is a genetically transmitted condition in which there is an apparent reduction in the threshold for Ca^{++} release from the sarcoplasmic reticulum of skeletal muscle.[18] Drugs such as the depolarizing blocking agents succinylcholine and decamethonium and certain general anesthetics, most notably halothane and ether, can trigger an attack of malignant hyperthermia in which the increased release of Ca^{++} into muscle cytoplasm causes contracture and an enormous acceleration of the cellular metabolism of muscle; the latter generates heat (body temperature can rise by 1 C every 5 minutes and reach 43 C), carbon dioxide (arterial P_{CO_2} over 100 mm Hg), and lactic acid (arterial blood pH below 7.0) and the hyperthermia, hypoxemia, and acidosis, in turn, cause muscle edema and structural damage.[18] In addition, the hyperthermia and resultant sympathetic reflex response increase heart metabolism five- to eightfold and can lead to arrhythmias. Attacks of malignant hyperthermia are frequently fatal. Dantrolene, by blocking the precipitating event, the release of Ca^{++} from sarcoplasmic reticulum, can prevent or halt an attack of malignant hyperthermia.[18]

Side effects of dantrolene include muscle weakness and hepatotoxicity. The muscle weakness, which is simply an extension of its therapeutic action, generally does not appear at dosages used for treatment of spastic movements, although doses high enough to produce this effect are sometimes needed to achieve symptom remission. Doses of dantrolene that produce muscle weakness are routinely employed in prophylaxis of malignant hyperthermia before surgery on patients with a familial history of the condition.

Hepatotoxicity of varying degrees has been reported in about 1% of patients taking dantrolene for 60 days or longer. Accordingly, hepatic function should be monitored during long-term therapy with dantrolene.[31] Furthermore, the minimal effective dose should be used.

Dantrolene is effective when administered either orally, where about 20% is absorbed, largely via the small intestine, or intravenously.[31] Metabolism of dantrolene takes place in the liver, largely by 5-hydroxylation of the hydantoin moiety.[31]

Neuromuscular blocking agents

Nonproprietary name	Proprietary name
Nondepolarizing (competitive)	
atracurium	Tracrium
gallamine	Flaxedil
metocurine	Metubine
pancuronium	Pavulon
tubocurarine	—
vecuronium	Norcuron
Depolarizing (noncompetitive)	
decamethonium*	Syncurine
succinylcholine	Anectine, Quelicin, Sux-Cert, Incert
Other	
dantrolene	Dantrium
hexafluorenium	Mylaxen

*Not available for use in the United States.

CITED REFERENCES

1. Alam, M., Anrep, G.V., Barsoum, G.S. Talaat, M., and Wieninger, E. Liberation of histamine from the skeletal muscle by curare. Journal of Physiology (London) **95:**148-158, 1939.
2. Axelsson, J., and Thesleff, S. The ''desensitizing'' effect of acetylcholine on the mammalian motor endplate. Acta Physiologica Scandinavica **43:**15-26, 1958.
3. Barnett, A., and Ackermann, E. Neuromuscular blocking activity of gentamicin in cats and mice. Archives Internationales de Pharmacodynamie et de Therapie **181:**109-117, 1969.
4. Bernard, C. Analyse physiologique des propriétés de systèmes musculaire et nerveux au moyer du curare. Comptes Rendus Hebdomadaires des Seances de l'Academie des Sciences; D: Sciences Naturelles (Paris) **43:**825-829, 1856.
5. Burgen, A.S.V., Dickens, F., and Zatmen, L.J. The action of botulinum toxin on the neuro-muscular junction. Journal of Physiology (London) **109:**10-24, 1949.
6. Castillo, J. del, and Katz, B. A study of curare action with an electrical micromethod. Proceedings of the Royal Society of London; B: Biological Science **146:**339-356, 1957.
7. Chagas, C. The fate of curare during curarization. In de Reuck, A.V.S., ed. Curare and Curare-like Agents. Boston, Little, Brown & Co., 1962.
8. Chang, C.C., and Lee, C.Y. Isolation of neurotoxins from the venom of *Bungarus multicinctus* and their modes of neuromuscular blocking action. Archives Internationales de Pharmacodynamie et de Therapie **144:**241-257, 1963.
9. Dantrolene sodium for treatment of spasticity. Medical Letter on Drugs and Therapeutics **16:**61-62, 1974.

10. Enomoto, K.-I., and Maeno, T. Presynaptic effects of 4-aminopyridine and streptomycin on the neuromuscular junction. European Journal of Pharmacology **76:**1-8, 1981.

11. Feldman, S.A. Muscle Relaxants. Philadelphia, W.B. Saunders Co., 1973.

12. Feltz, A., and Trautmann, A. Desensitization at the frog neuromuscular junction: a biphasic process. Journal of Physiology (London) **322:**257-272, 1982.

13. Foldes, F.F. The choice and mode of administration of relaxants. In Foldes, F.F., ed. Muscle Relaxants. Philadelphia, F.A. Davis Co., 1966.

14. Foldes, F.F., ed. Muscle Relaxants. Philadelphia, F.A. Davis Co., 1966.

15. Goedde, H.W., and Altland, K. Suxamethonium sensitivity. Annals of the New York Academy of Sciences **179:**695-703, 1971.

16. Graf, K., Strom, G., and Wahlin, A. Circulatory effects of succinylcholine in man. Acta Anesthesiologica Scandinavica (Supplement) **114:**1-48, 1963.

17. Griffith, H.R., and Johnson, G.E. The use of curare in general anesthesia. Anesthesiology **3:**418-420, 1942.

18. Gronert, G.A. Malignant hyperthermia. Anesthesiology **53:**395-423, 1980.

19. Guyton, A.C., and Reeder, R.C. Quantitative studies on the autonomic actions of curare. Journal of Pharmacology and Experimental Therapeutics **98:**188-193, 1950.

20. Hill, G.E., Wong, K.C., and Hodges, M.R. Lithium carbonate and neuromuscular blocking agents. Anesthesiology **46:**122-126, 1977.

21. Hubbard, J.I. Microphysiology of vertebrate neuromuscular transmission. Physiological Reviews **53:**674-723, 1973.

22. Karis, J.H., Gissen, A.J., and Nastuk, W.L. Mode of action of diethyl ether in blocking neuromuscular transmission. Anesthesiology **27:**42-51, 1966.

23. Karis, J.H., Gissen, A.J., and Nastuk, W.L. The effect of volatile anesthetic agents on neuromuscular transmission. Anesthesiology **28:**128-133, 1967.

24. Katz, B., and Thesleff, S. A study of the "desensitization" produced by acetylcholine at the motor end-plate. Journal of Physiology (London) **138:**63-80, 1957.

25. Kuba, K. Effects of catecholamines on the neuromuscular junction in the rat diaphragm. Journal of Physiology (London) **211:**551-570, 1970.

26. Lester, H.A. Blockade of acetylcholine receptors by cobra toxin: electrophysiological studies. Molecular Pharmacology **6:**623-631, 1972.

27. MacIntosh, F.C. Effect of HC-3 on acetylcholine turnover. Federation Proceedings **20:**562-568, 1961.

28. Morgan, K.G., and Bryant, S.H. The mechanism of action of dantrolene sodium. Journal of Pharmacology and Experimental Therapeutics **201:**138-147, 1977.

29. Nastuk, W.L., and Karis, J.H. The blocking action of hexafluorenium on neuromuscular transmission and its interaction with succinylcholine. Journal of Pharmacology and Experimental Therapeutics **144:**236-252, 1964.

30. Okamoto, M., Longnecker, H.E., Jr., Riker, W.F., Jr., and Song, S.K. Destruction of mammalian motor nerve terminals by black widow spider venom. Science **172:**733-736, 1971.

31. Pinder, R.M., Brogden, R.N., Speight, T.M., and Avery, G.S. Dantrolene sodium: a review of its pharmacological properties and therapeutic efficacy in spasticity. Drugs **13:**3-23, 1977.

32. Potter, L.T. Synthesis, storage and release of (^{14}C) acetylcholine in isolated rat diaphragm muscles. Journal of Physiology (London) **206:**145-166, 1970.

33. Riker, W.F., Jr., and Wescoe, W.C. The pharmacology of Flaxedil, with observations of certain analogs. Annals of the New York Academy of Sciences **54:**373-392, 1951.

34. Simpson, L.L. Ionic requirements for the neuromuscular blocking action of botulinum toxin: implications with regard to synaptic transmission. Neuropharmacology **10:**673-684, 1971.

35. Smith, S.M., Brown, H.O., Toman, J.E.P., and Goodman, L.S. The lack of cerebral effects of *d*-tubocurarine. Anesthesiology **8:**1-14, 1947.

36. Taylor, P. Neuromuscular blocking agents. In Gilman, A.G., Goodman, L.S., and Gilman, A., eds. Goodman and Gilman's The Pharmacological Basis of Therapeutics, ed. 6. New York, Macmillan, Inc., 1980.

37. Wright, J.M., and Collier, B. The effects of neomycin upon transmitter release and action. Journal of Pharmacology and Experimental Therapeutics **200:**576-587, 1977.

38. Zaimis, E. Experimental hazards and artefacts in the study of neuromuscular blocking drugs. In de Reuck, A.V.S., ed. Curare and Curare-like Agents. Boston, Little, Brown & Co., 1962.

GENERAL REFERENCES

Bowman, W.C. Pharmacology of Neuromuscular Function. Baltimore, University Park Press, 1980.

de Reuck, A.V.S., ed. Curare and Curare-like Agents. Boston, Little, Brown & Co., 1962.

Katz, R.L., ed. Muscle Relaxants. New York, American Elsevier, 1975.

Kolb, M.E., Horne, M.L., and Martz, R. Dantrolene in human malignant hyperthermia. A multicenter study. Anesthesiology **56:**254-262, 1982.

Savarese, J.J., and Kitz, R.J. Does clinical anesthesia need new neuromuscular blocking agents? Anesthesiology **42:**236-239, 1975.

Tauc, L. The vesicular hypothesis of acetylcholine release from neurons: are there alternatives? In Kalsner, S., ed. Trends in Autonomic Pharmacology, Vol. 2. Baltimore, Urban & Schwarzenberg, 1982.

Zacks, S.I. The Motor Endplate. Huntington, N.Y., R.E. Krieger Publishing Co., Inc., 1974.

12 Psychopharmacology: antipsychotics and antidepressants

Leslie P. Felpel

As many as 8 million people in the United States suffer from psychiatric disorders, and approximately 2 million of these are receiving pharmacotherapy for their disorder at any given moment. Although drugs are not curative in themselves, their use has contributed much to our understanding of mental illness and has reduced hospital-bed occupancy by mental patients to a tenth of what it was in 1950. Effective drug therapy has permitted individuals who would otherwise have been chronically hospitalized to be useful members of society. Thus, in daily practice, the dentist can expect to treat individuals who are receiving a wide variety of psychotherapeutic agents, which, though not usually a complicating factor per se, may become a complication when other drugs are used concurrently. Understanding the pharmacology of these agents takes on new meaning when drug interactions are considered.

For the purposes of this discussion, psychiatric disorders will be classified as psychotic states (e.g., schizophrenia), which are treated therapeutically with the antipsychotic drugs, sometimes also referred to as neuroleptics, and affective disorders (e.g., depression), which are treated therapeutically with the antidepressant drugs and lithium. Neuroses (e.g., anxiety) are treated with antianxiety agents (Chapter 13). Often the term *major tranquilizer* is used for the antipsychotic drugs and *minor tranquilizer* for the antianxiety drugs. These terms should be discarded because they imply that the two groups of drugs have similar mechanisms of action, differing only in degree of activity or potency, which is not the case.

In schizophrenia, the patient's ability to function is markedly impaired because of disturbances in thought processes. Because of these disturbances, the patient is disorganized, may suffer from hallucinations and delusions, and may exhibit behavioral patterns suggestive of a loss of contact with reality. Neither the etiology nor the pathogenesis of schizophrenia is known. Many hypotheses have been offered to account for schizophrenia, and, not surprisingly, many of these emphasize the possible involvement of certain chemicals that are normally found within the brain. Most of these chemicals, at one time or another, have been proposed to be neurotransmitters in the central nervous system.

At the present time, perhaps the most popular (though not universally accepted) biochemical hypothesis for schizophrenia suggests that there is a hyperactivity of dopaminergic neurons and/or pathways in certain regions of the brain. There is no direct evidence to support this hypothesis, but it is known that drugs effective in the treatment of schizophrenia (the antipsychotics) decrease dopaminergic transmission,[27,42] increase the rate of dopamine synthesis and utilization,[8,26] antagonize the effect of iontophoretically applied dopamine on striatal neurons,[6,41,49] and inhibit dopamine-sensitive adenylate cyclase activity.[22] In addition, the parkinsonism-like motor disturbances, which are common side effects of the antipsychotics, are assumed to be due to decreased central dopaminergic activity resulting from blockade of dopamine receptors in the basal ganglia.

It is difficult to establish what area of the brain is involved in the pathologic process leading to schizophrenia, but it is known that numerous interconnections exist between neurons in the frontal cortex, the amygdaloid area, hippocampus, nucleus accumbens, and the limbic cortex, all of which contain dopamine. These same areas are considered to be involved in mood and thought processes. If dysfunction of these dopaminergic systems were to occur, it is not unreasonable to expect that alterations in mood, personality, and thought processes would follow. However, although dopaminergic systems appear to be involved in schizophrenia, it is still not clear whether such involvement is the cause or the result of schizophrenia.

The affective illnesses refer to those disorders that alter the mood of the individual. There are many classifications of the affective disorders, but for purposes of this discussion it is sufficient to consider only depression and mania. Most people have, at one time or another, suffered from feelings of sadness, loss, or grief. In normal circumstances, such feelings are related to specific causes, are not incapacitating, and are generally short-lived. In the mentally ill patient, however, depression is severe, disabling, and characterized by seclusiveness and nonverbalization. On the other hand, those individuals who suffer from mania exhibit a marked elevation of mood, typified by hyperactivity and an increase in verbalization. These same individuals may also suffer from alternating periods of depression, in which case the disorder may be referred to as a manic-depressive illness.

As with schizophrenia, various theories have been offered to explain the cause of affective disorders, again with attention focusing on putative neurotransmitters. At present, the most popular hypothesis for the biochemical basis of affective disorders suggests that a deficiency of norepinephrine or 5-hydroxytryptamine (serotonin) or both exists at central synaptic sites. There is little direct support for this biogenic amine theory, however, and, for the most part, evidence is based on the known mechanisms of action of drugs that are useful in treating the disorders. Although there are conflicting data, in general, those drugs that are effective against depression increase the activities of monoamines in the CNS, while drugs that are effective against mania do the opposite.

The first drugs to provide a basis for the biogenic amine hypothesis of affective disorders were reserpine and iproniazid. Reserpine can produce a depression-like state in normal individuals and is known to deplete central stores of catecholamines and serotonin. Iproniazid, an MAO inhibitor, improves the mood of depressed patients and increases the concentrations of monoamines in the brain by blocking the enzyme, MAO, which nor-

mally catabolizes them intraneuronally. The tricyclic antidepressants more recently introduced for the treatment of depression block the reuptake of monoamine neurotransmitters into presynaptic nerve terminals. Such an action would presumably increase the amount of neurotransmitter present at functionally deficient synapses. This mechanism of action also lends support to the biogenic amine hypothesis of affective disorders.

Currently, it is impossible to identify the areas of the central nervous system where monoamine concentrations are abnormal or where there is dysfunction. In fact, not all data support the biogenic amine hypothesis of affective disorders, and it is entirely possible that future studies will show that a variety of factors, other than or in addition to biochemical, are causative for manic-depressive illness.

Most of the psychotherapeutic properties of the psychoactive drugs were discovered by accident. In 1950, while attempting to develop antihistaminic agents, the Rhône-Pauline Laboratories in France synthesized chlorpromazine. The unusual "sedative" properties of chlorpromazine were soon noted, and the drug was first used to treat schizophrenic patients in 1952. The tricyclic antidepressants were synthesized in an attempt to produce more "specific" antipsychotic agents. (Note in Figures 12-1 and 12-3 the close resemblance in chemical structure with the phenothiazines.) However, it was soon recognized that imipramine, a prototypical antidepressant, was more beneficial in depression than in schizophrenia. The antidepressant properties of the MAO inhibitors were discovered when it was observed that isoniazid, a prototypical MAO inhibitor, produced a euphoric state in patients who were being treated for tuberculosis. Lastly, though the psychoactive properties of lithium were noted as early as 1949,[7] only since 1970 has this compound been widely recognized as an effective treatment for the manic phase of manic-depressive illness.

ANTIPSYCHOTICS

The principal drugs effective in the treatment of schizophrenia, the phenothiazines and butyrophenones, are dopamine antagonists (i.e., they block dopamine receptors) in the periphery and in the central nervous system. Direct evidence for this action being the mechanism by which these drugs exert their antipsychotic effect is lacking since a "schizophrenic" dopamine receptor has not been

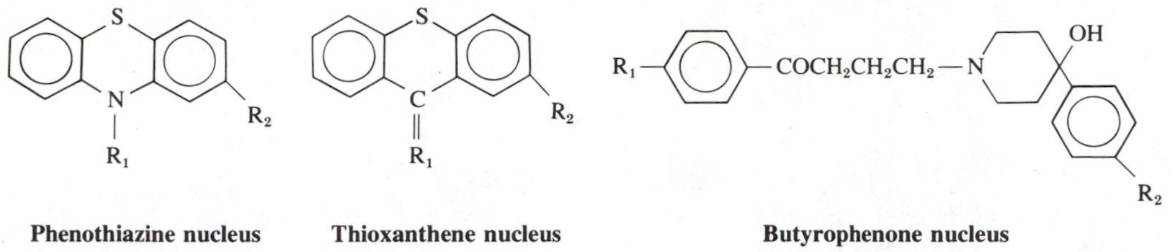

Figure 12-1. Structural formulas of representative antipsychotic drug groups.

identified. In addition to dopamine, neurochemicals such as norepinephrine,[46] the endogenous opioid peptides,[2] and the prostaglandins[19] have also been implicated in schizophrenia, suggesting that this is a very complex and multifaceted disease. Thus, although the dopamine theory of schizophrenia provides a good working hypothesis, it should be kept in mind that many other mechanisms may be involved in the disease process.[26]

Chemistry and structure-activity relationships

Of the several classes of antipsychotics, some are closely related structurally, others share a stereochemical resemblance, and still others appear to be chemically unrelated but nevertheless act similarly.

Phenothiazines and thioxanthenes. The basic ring structure of the phenothiazines is illustrated in Figure 12-1. Substitutions at R_1 divide the phenothiazine antipsychotics into three major groups. One group, represented by chlorpromazine, is derived when R_1 is an aliphatic chain. Compounds like chlorpromazine with three carbons in the chain (e.g., $-CH_2-CH_2-CH_2-N(CH_3)_2$) have antipsychotic properties, whereas those with only two carbons, such as promethazine, are usually antihistaminic and/or anticholinergic in nature. A second group, represented by thioridazine, is derived when the substituent group at R_1 is composed of a piperidine ring. These phenothiazines are usually less sedative than the aliphatic agents. A third group, represented by prochlorperazine, results when the substituent group contains a piperazine ring. Drugs in this group are the most active of the three as antipsychotic agents but are also most likely to produce extrapyramidal side effects.

Substitutions at the R_2 position can increase the potency of a given antipsychotic. Promazine, which lacks a substituent group at R_2, is made much more potent when a chlorine atom is placed at the R_2 position, resulting in chlorpromazine. Increasing the halogenation at R_2 (triflupromazine) increases the antipsychotic potency to an even greater extent. It should be noted that not all phenothiazines are antipsychotic. Minor structural changes, for example, the addition of a chlorine atom adjacent to R_2 on the phenothiazine ring, result in compounds devoid of antipsychotic activity. Obviously the therapeutic efficacy of these drugs depends on highly specific molecular properties.

The thioxanthene antipsychotics, represented by chlorprothixene, are closely related to the phenothiazines and are formed when the ring nitrogen adjoining R_1 is replaced by a carbon atom (Figure 12-1).

Butyrophenones. The butyrophenone antipsychotics are not chemically related to the phenothiazines but do contain a stereochemically related nucleus (Figure 12-1). These compounds share common pharmacologic properties and may therefore be used to treat the same clinical conditions. The only butyrophenone that will be discussed in this chapter is haloperidol. Droperidol, another butyrophenone, is used in the United States for its antinauseant properties and by anesthesiologists as a premedicant. It does have antipsychotic properties however.

Dihydroindolones. The only representative from the dihydroindolone class of antipsychotics currently available in the United States is molindone (Figure 12-2). This compound is not structurally related to the phenothiazines, thioxanthenes, or butyrophenones. Its structure resembles that of serotonin, but it is not clear whether this has any clinical significance. The pharmacologic and clinical profile of this compound very closely resembles that of the piperazine group of phenothiazines.

Dibenzoxazepines. Loxapine (Figure 12-2) is the only dibenzoxazepine available at present in

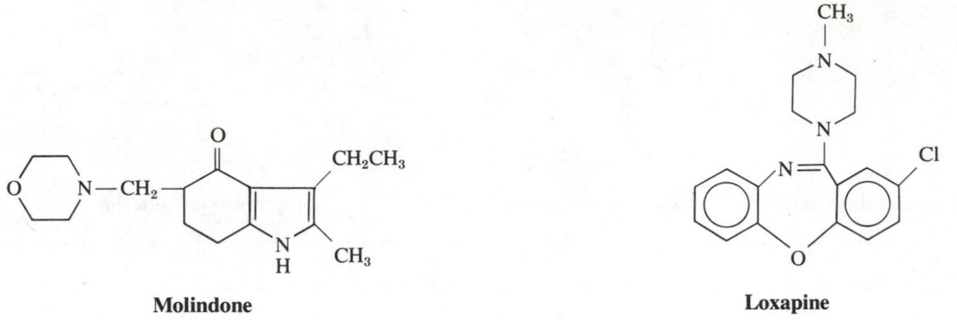

Figure 12-2. Structural formulas of molindone and loxapine.

the United States. The structure of this compound is interesting in that it contains seven members in its central ring and, as a result, resembles a tricyclic antidepressant (Figure 12-3). Loxapine, however, does not appear to have antidepressant activity. Like molindone, this drug has a clinical and pharmacologic profile similar to that of the piperazine phenothiazines.

Miscellaneous antipsychotics. There are a number of drugs that possess antipsychotic activity that are not yet approved for use in the United States, and, of course, many that are in the experimental stage. Some of these drugs have led to refinements in our concept of the underlying disorder of schizophrenia.

Clozapine is a dibenzodiazepine similar in chemistry and antipsychotic profile to loxapine. Although a tendency to elicit blood dyscrasias limits its clinical usefulness, clozapine is notable for the minimal nature of the extrapyramidal side effects it produces.[12] Pimozide, a diphenylbutylpiperidine derivative, resembles a butyrophenone in which the keto oxygen has been replaced by a 4-fluorophenyl moiety. Pimozide is a rather specific dopamine antagonist that has good antipsychotic properties but few or no parkinsonism-like side effects. Penfluridol, another diphenylbutylpiperidine, is undergoing clinical trials in the United States. Finally, the benzamide derivative sulpiride, which has been used clinically in Europe, appears to be a selective antagonist of mesolimbic dopaminergic transmission.

These drugs emphasize the possibility that multiple central dopamine receptors exist and that they may be differentially blocked by appropriate compounds. Presumably then, specific antipsychotic drugs could be developed that would avoid the ex-

trapyramidal side effects that plague all of the antipsychotic agents currently available in the United States.

Pharmacologic effects

The phenothiazines, thioxanthenes, butyrophenones, dihydroindolones, and dibenzoxazepines appear to have nearly identical neuropharmacologic properties. This is not to imply that there are no differences between these drugs, as differences do exist and will be mentioned wherever appropriate. Future studies will, no doubt, reveal a number of other, subtle differences. At the present time, however, it is appropriate to discuss these drugs as a single class.

Central nervous system. Although the precise mechanism of action of the antipsychotic drugs is not known, they all share the ability to block dopamine receptors at CNS sites.[44] If, as has been hypothesized, schizophrenia is associated with an excess of dopamine at certain CNS loci, then drugs capable of acting as dopamine antagonists should be effective in the treatment of schizophrenia. Furthermore, the characteristic extrapyramidal side effects of the antipsychotic drugs become explicable on the basis of blockade of dopamine receptors.

Experimental studies have focused on areas of the brain that are involved in behavior, emotion, and motor activity. Major areas associated with behavior and emotion are the limbic system, the reticular formation, and the hypothalamus. The basal ganglia are areas concerned with involuntary motor activity. The effect of the antipsychotic drugs on these various structures has been studied in detail, particularly for chlorpromazine, which will serve as the prototype for this class of compounds.

After high doses of chlorpromazine, seizure-like activity can be recorded from the amygdala,[31] a component of the limbic system. In animals, sham rage evoked by electrical stimulation of the amygdala is inhibited by chlorpromazine.[10] Chlorpromazine is also thought to increase dopamine turnover in the limbic system.[26] Although the clinical significance of these findings is unclear, it is interesting that dopamine is found within the limbic system where it presumably plays a role in emotion and behavior. The dopaminergic antagonistic activity of chlorpromazine in the limbic system could therefore partially account for its antipsychotic properties.

Unlike sedatives such as barbiturates, chlorpromazine does not depress the reticular formation. However, it does raise the threshold for incoming stimuli at the level of collateral input from sensory pathways to the reticular formation.[4] The output of the reticular formation in response to sensory stimuli is thus depressed by chlorpromazine. Because schizophrenia may in part be a result of continual "flooding" of the brain by afferent input, reduction of this input by chlorpromazine and related drugs may explain their usefulness in the treatment of the disorder.

In general, the phenothiazines produce sedation on initial administration, but tolerance develops to the sedative effects of these drugs in 1 to 4 weeks, and the patient becomes progressively more alert as treatment is continued.[29] Fortunately, tolerance does not seem to develop to the antipsychotic action of the phenothiazines.

Many of the autonomic manifestations of emotion and behavior are a function of the hypothalamus. Chlorpromazine exerts an inhibitory effect on adrenergic systems within the hypothalamus, which may contribute to a loss of thermoregulation, the development of postural hypotension, and alterations in the secretion of various pituitary hormones. With respect to the last point, antipsychotics decrease the secretion of corticotropin and growth hormone and increase that of prolactin.

The extrapyramidal side effects produced by the antipsychotic drugs include a parkinsonian-like syndrome, dyskinesias, akathisia, and tardive dyskinesia. The various types of phenothiazines produce varying degrees of extrapyramidal side effects; in descending order these are the piperazines, aliphatics, and piperidines. This order represents in reverse the anticholinergic potencies of these compounds.[43] Haloperidol, a weak anticholinergic, commonly produces extrapyramidal side effects, whereas clozapine, a potent anticholinergic, is virtually devoid of motor disturbances. The most recently approved antipsychotics, molindone and loxapine, are similar to chlorpromazine in causing extrapyramidal reactions. Antiparkinson drugs are sometimes administered to antagonize the antipsychotic-induced motor disturbances, though this practice is not universally accepted.

Tardive dyskinesia, as the name suggests, is an extrapyramidal disorder that appears after the patient has been treated with an antipsychotic for a long period of time. This condition is thought to reflect the development of supersensitivity resulting from chronic blockade of the dopamine receptors in the basal ganglia.[23] The signs of tardive dyskinesia consist of abnormal, rapid, and alternating movements of the tongue (thrusting) and perioral areas; facial grimacing, tics, nose twitching, and so on. Muscle activity can sometimes involve the extremities and torso and may become severe enough to disrupt eating and even breathing patterns. Unlike other extrapyramidal side effects, tardive dyskinesia does not necessarily regress on reduction of the dose or withdrawal of the drug. In fact, this side effect is frequently not seen until the antipsychotic is either withdrawn or reduced in dosage. The only consistently effective treatment for tardive dyskinesia seems to be an increase in the dose of the antipsychotic that caused it in the first place. Obviously, such a procedure leads to a vicious cycle and a serious dilemma therapeutically. All of the clinically available antipsychotics have this side effect, though results with some of the experimental compounds suggest that antipsychotic activity in the absence of extrapyramidal side effects may be a possibility.

Chlorpromazine is an effective antiemetic and was at one time commonly employed for this purpose. The antiemetic action is exerted on the chemoreceptive trigger zone rather than the vomiting center, since copper sulfate–induced emesis, which is caused by direct stimulation of the vomiting center, is not blocked by chlorpromazine. Nausea and vomiting caused by motion sickness are also not prevented by chlorpromazine.

Although medullary respiratory centers are slightly depressed by chlorpromazine, clinically effective doses have little effect on respiration. However, if a sedative-hypnotic, antianxiety, or opioid drug is given to a patient receiving antipsychotic medication, an additive depressant effect on respiration may result.

Vasomotor centers are depressed by the antipsychotics, which may contribute to the development of orthostatic hypotension. A second factor promoting orthostatic hypotension is the action of these drugs on the autonomic nervous system.

Autonomic nervous system. Chlorpromazine and other antipsychotics have potent α-adrenergic blocking properties that partially account for their hypotensive effects. Patients chronically treated with the antipsychotic drugs often exhibit slight tachycardia and increased coronary blood flow in response to the drug-induced hypotension. It should be stressed that because of the α-adrenergic blockade, the pressor effects of epinephrine may be diminished or even reversed in patients receiving chlorpromazine chronically.

The following side effects of the phenothiazines may be due to their weak anticholinergic properties: blurring of vision, constipation, and decreases in sweating, salivation, gastric secretion, and intestinal tone. Phenothiazines also have antihistaminic, antiserotonergic, and even adrenergic properties, which further complicate the interpretation and overall pattern of their central and peripheral activities. The autonomic effects of butyrophenones, molindone, and loxapine are similar, though weaker, than the phenothiazines. Although the autonomic effects of antipsychotics can be annoying, tolerance to these reactions does occur.

Cardiovascular system. Most of the cardiovascular effects of chlorpromazine have been mentioned. Orthostatic hypotension is a result of both central and peripheral actions of chlorpromazine, while tachycardia and increased coronary blood flow are due to central compensatory cardiovascular reflexes. The aliphatic and piperidine phenothiazines are the most likely, and the piperazines the least likely, to cause orthostatic hypotension. Chlorpromazine has a direct depressant effect on the heart, as well as an antiarrhythmic action, which may be due in part to its quite pronounced local anesthetic effect. Vascular reflexes mediated by vasomotor centers of the brainstem are depressed by chlorpromazine. The butyrophenones have slightly less pronounced hypotensive effects than the phenothiazines, but tachycardia is a common side effect.

Endocrine system. Most of the endocrine effects of chlorpromazine are related to disturbances in the secretion of pituitary hormones. Chlorpro-

mazine may cause lactation and amenorrhea or delay of ovulation and menstruation in women and gynecomastia and impotence or decreased libido in men.[33] The urinary excretion of estrogens, progestins, and 17-hydroxycorticoids is decreased by chlorpromazine. Both diuretic and antidiuretic effects have been demonstrated in animals and humans, though a weak diuresis seems to be the predominant effect in humans. A more complete discussion of the endocrine effects of phenothiazines may be found in a review by Domino.[13]

Absorption, fate, and excretion

Chlorpromazine is readily absorbed from the gastrointestinal tract, but most of the drug is inactivated in the gastrointestinal tract and liver before reaching the systemic circulation. More than 100 metabolites of chlorpromazine are thought to exist, many of which are still unidentified. These metabolites may remain in the body for up to months after chlorpromazine therapy has terminated. The metabolites of chlorpromazine are finally excreted in the urine and feces.

Haloperidol is rapidly absorbed from the gastrointestinal tract. The major metabolites are inactive and are excreted in the bile and urine.

Molindone and loxapine are rapidly absorbed after oral administration and metabolized in the liver. The resulting metabolites are excreted in the urine and feces. Approximately 3% of molindone is eliminated unchanged in the urine.

Toxic reactions and side effects

The most troublesome side effects of the antipsychotic agents, particularly the phenothiazines and butyrophenones, are tardive dyskinesia and the parkinsonian-like extrapyramidal disorders consisting of tremor, akathisia, dystonia, uncoordinated movements, torticollis, facial grimacing, and dysarthria. Therapy is often terminated in patients exhibiting motor disturbances. However, in cases of uncontrollable psychotic states, patients may have to remain on medication even if the extrapyramidal reactions are marked. Tardive dyskinesia has important implications in dentistry, as the facial musculature is particularly involved, and is discussed below in greater detail.

Allergic reactions, though less frequent than extrapyramidal symptoms, are serious enough to necessitate adjustment of the dosage or withdrawal of the medication. These reactions may be manifested as cholestatic jaundice, blood dyscrasias, or dermatologic responses. The latter may take the form of phototoxic or photoallergic eruptions, in which exposure to direct sunlight causes the skin to take on an unusual blue-gray pigmentation.

Other adverse effects of this group of drugs are extensions of their pharmacology. Thus, there may be endocrine effects, such as amenorrhea, gynecomastia, and impotence. Autonomic effects may result in orthostatic hypotension, faintness, xerostomia, nasal stuffiness, urinary retention, and constipation. Alterations in body temperature, particularly hypothermia, may also occur, and there have been reports of disturbances in cardiac function.

General therapeutic uses

At the present time, the antipsychotic drugs are primarily used for the treatment of psychotic states. However, the wide variety of pharmacologic effects of the phenothiazines has led to their use as antiemetics, preoperative medications to relax and calm the patient, antihistaminics, and antihelminthics (primarily in veterinary preparations). Other applications of the phenothiazines include the control of hallucinations associated with acute alcohol withdrawal and the treatment of intractable hiccough. The use of the butyrophenone droperidol in the production of neuroleptanalgesia is covered in Chapter 19.

There is perhaps no other class of drugs that has such a wide range of doses as the antipsychotics. Although dose requirements for most patients fall within a relatively narrow spectrum, treatment is highly individualized, and patients may be encountered who require doses differing by 20- to 30-fold. Adjustments in dose are frequently made, depending on the patient's plasma concentration of the drug, the clinical response, and the like. As a rule, treatment with the antipsychotic agents is uninterrupted and indefinite in duration.

Long-acting depot antipsychotic preparations, primarily in the form of fluphenazine enanthate and fluphenazine decanoate, are convenient in those individuals in whom compliance is a problem. These injectable forms are effective for a period of 2 to 3 weeks once therapeutic blood concentrations are obtained and stabilized. Frequently, a reduced total drug dose is possible because problems with absorption from the gastrointestinal tract are bypassed. In general, depot forms are safe for younger patients in good physical condition. A disadvantage to this mode of administration is that the

drug cannot be discontinued should side effects occur.

Currently, antipsychotics such as the phenothiazines, thioxanthenes, and butyrophenones are considered to be the more established agents. Molindone and loxapine are generally reserved for those patients who are refractory to the above compounds.

Implications for dentistry

Since it is estimated that 1 in every 20 individuals in the United States has received some pharmacotherapy for mental illness, it is inevitable that the dentist will encounter such individuals in his daily practice. Many of these patients will be receiving more than one drug for their condition, and, in addition, these patients may be taking a variety of other drugs (alcohol, cough remedies, aspirin, etc.) that may not be revealed in responses to a medical history questionnaire. Many of these drugs can add to the depressant effects of the antipsychotics and lead to complications if sedative-hypnotics, antianxiety agents, anesthetics, or narcotic analgesics are used in the course of dental treatment. Chlorpromazine is known to potentiate the effects of general anesthetics and to increase the analgesic and respiratory depressant responses to opioids (Table 12-1). The cardiac effects of thioridazine may be potentiated by hydroxyzine.[18]

Since the introduction of the antipsychotic drugs, it has been recognized that they cause a number of extrapyramidal syndromes. Most of these occur concomitantly with drug administration and disappear when the agent is withdrawn. However, as has already been mentioned, tardive dyskinesia develops only after prolonged use of the antipsychotic. Only recently has the prevalence of this condition been appreciated. Tardive dyskinesia has been estimated to occur in as many as 40% of patients receiving antipsychotic medication. Curiously, the abnormal movements of tardive dyskinesia often start in the orofacial musculature, particularly the tongue, which alternately protrudes, retracts, and undergoes a rolling movement. As time goes on, muscles of the extremities also become involved; however, because the orofacial muscles are primarily affected in the early development of tardive dyskinesia, the patient very often reasons that the dentist can correct the problem. At present, there is no cure for drug-induced tardive dyskinesia, and withdrawal of the causative drug does not always diminish the severity of the motor

Table 12-1. Interactions of antipsychotic drugs with other drugs

Antipsychotic drug	Drug used for dental or self-therapy*	Therapeutic intent	Possible response or effect†
Phenothiazines, thioxanthenes, butyrophenones, molindone, loxapine	Phenothiazines	Antinauseant, antiemetic	CNS depression
	Barbiturates	Sedation, hypnosis	CNS depression
	General anesthetics (inhalation and intravenous)	General anesthesia, conscious sedation	CNS depression (especially respiratory depression)
	Benzodiazepines	Antianxiety, intravenous sedation	CNS depression
	Antihistamines	Sedation, relief from colds, antiallergic, antianxiety	CNS depression
	Narcotic analgesics	Analgesia	CNS depression, respiratory depression (especially with meperidine), miosis
	Ethanol	Sedation	CNS depression

*Self-therapy refers to use of OTC drugs that contain ingredients that may interact with antipsychotic drugs.
†These drug interactions do not invariably occur, and they are not necessarily severe when they do occur.

disturbance. In fact, the persistence of tardive dyskinesia despite drug withdrawal suggests permanent drug-induced pathologic changes within the central nervous system. Although tardive dyskinesia was first observed after phenothiazine treatment, the butyrophenones appear to be even more active in causing this condition. The newer antipsychotics molindone and loxapine also produce extrapyramidal side effects, including tardive dyskinesia.

Unfortunately, individuals who require treatment with the phenothiazine antipsychotics usually must take these drugs for a long period of time, if not for life. Prolonged phenothiazine use can sometimes cause a reduction in leukocyte count, which predisposes the patient to infection, and oral candidiasis may be frequently observed in these patients. In addition, the reduced salivary flow due to the anticholinergic properties of the phenothiazines can result in xerostomia and an increased incidence of cervical caries.

Orthostatic hypotension may occur, particularly with the aliphatic phenothiazines and the thioxanthenes. In the emergency treatment of phenothiazine-induced vasomotor collapse, epinephrine is contraindicated because the α-receptor blocking action of the phenothiazines may cause "epinephrine reversal" and an even greater reduction in blood pressure. Norepinephrine or phenylephrine, which lack significant β_2-adrenergic activity, are preferred in these circumstances.

ANTIDEPRESSANTS

The development of antidepressant drugs, such as the tricyclics and the MAO inhibitors, and the elucidation of their pharmacologic actions, has led to the development of the amine hypothesis of affective disorders.[35] This hypothesis holds that depression is caused by a relative unavailability of biogenic amines, particularly norepinephrine and serotonin, at functionally significant sites in the central nervous system. The tricyclic antidepressants block the reuptake of central biogenic amines (especially norepinephrine and/or serotonin) into presynaptic nerve terminals,[15] whereas the MAO inhibitors prevent the degradation of these neurotransmitters by the enzyme MAO.[11] Both of these actions would presumably restore the relative availability of CNS amines to normal or near normal levels.

In the United States, depression is pharmacologically treated most commonly with tricyclic antidepressants and rarely with MAO inhibitors. Although this pattern generally holds true in other countries, the reluctance to use MAO inhibitors is not as great outside the United States. Several new antidepressants, including maprotiline and trazodone, were recently approved for clinical use. These drugs are structurally unrelated to the tricyclics and MAO inhibitors; however, they are as efficacious in the treatment of affective disorders and offer the benefit of having fewer side effects. While pharmacologically similar to the tricyclics

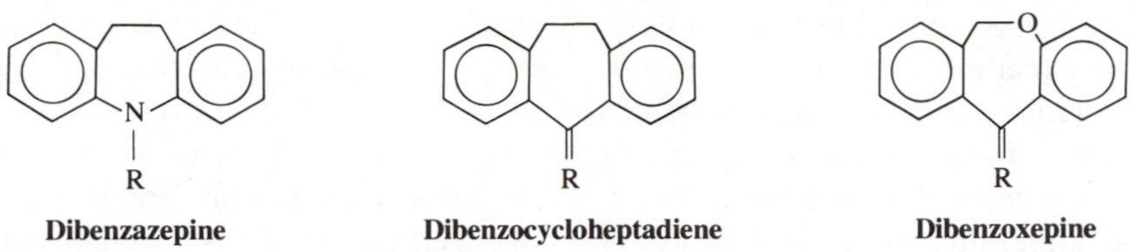

Dibenzazepine   Dibenzocycloheptadiene   Dibenzoxepine

Figure 12-3. Structural formulas of the tricyclic rings of dibenzazepine, dibenzocycloheptadiene, and dibenzoxepine antidepressants.

in terms of blocking biogenic amine uptake, maprotiline and trazodone are, respectively, more specific for norepinephrine and serotonin. There are, in addition, a large number of investigational antidepressants that exhibit a variety of mechanisms of action. The experimental drug iprindole, for instance, does not inhibit the uptake of either norepinephrine or serotonin.[32] Such findings suggest that depression may result from a variety of central neurochemical disorders and that the amine hypothesis should not be accepted as valid for all forms of depression. Alternatively, the amelioration of depressive illnesses could have a single cause, such as the reduction in the number or sensitivity of a particular monoaminergic receptor, which could be induced by several different methods. These might include direct effects of drugs or homeostatic reactions to prolonged increases in neurotransmitter concentration. This last possibility would explain the well-known several weeks delay between drug administration and therapeutic effect.

Tricyclic antidepressants

Chemistry and structure-activity relationships. A relatively small modification of the phenothiazine ring structure results in an entirely new group of drugs, the tricyclic antidepressants. The name of these compounds is derived from the triple-ring structure consisting of two benzene moieties connected through a seven-membered ring (Figure 12-3).

The first agent and prototype of the tricyclics is imipramine, a dibenzazepine derivative. Structural analogues of imipramine include the dibenzocycloheptadienes, in which a carbon atom is substituted for the nitrogen of the central ring, and the dibenzoxepines, in which one of the methylene groups of the center ring of the dibenzocycloheptadiene

molecule is replaced by an oxygen atom. A prototype drug for the dibenzocycloheptadienes is amitriptyline and for the dibenzoxepines, doxepin.

Substitutions at R (Figure 12-3) usually consist of aminopropyl groups that may be either dimethyl or monomethyl amino derivatives. Compounds such as imipramine, amitriptyline, and doxepin have two methyl substituents on the nitrogen atom of the side chain and are tertiary amines. Desipramine, nortriptyline, and protriptyline have one methyl group and are secondary amines.

Pharmacologic effects. As is true of the antipsychotic drugs, the tricyclic antidepressants have therapeutically useful effects on the central nervous system and a range of complex effects on other systems.

Central nervous system. When administered to a normal individual, the tricyclic antidepressants initially produce quietness, lethargy, and often an increased feeling of anxiety. With continued administration, the individual may experience thought disorders and become increasingly confused. After the tricyclic antidepressants have been administered for approximately 2 to 3 weeks, depressed patients, instead of showing evidence of mental confusion, are more able to consider their problems, usually feel better, and in general experience an elevation of mood. Untoward central side effects can include dizziness, lightheadedness, and even delirium and hallucinations.

All of the tricyclic antidepressants seem to have in common the ability to inhibit the reuptake of norepinephrine and/or serotonin into central presynaptic fibers.[15] Normally, after a nerve impulse releases a biogenic amine from synaptic vesicles in the nerve terminal, most of the transmitter is taken back into the terminal, stored, and made available for reuse. Tricyclic antidepressants, by blocking this reuptake, increase the concentrations of norepinephrine or serotonin at "critical" central synapses. Most data are compatible with this series of events, but in experimental studies in humans, brain titers of norepinephrine cannot be measured directly; thus, most investigations have primarily focused on measurements of amines and their metabolites in the urine after the administration of tricyclic antidepressants. Such measurements may not accurately reflect neurotransmitter concentrations in the central nervous system.

It should be noted that the secondary amino tricyclics are more effective inhibitors of norepinephrine uptake than are the tertiary amines. Conversely, tertiary amines inhibit serotonin uptake to a greater extent. These differences should theoretically be reflected in the cardiovascular responses to the two groups; however, the fact that tertiary amino antidepressants are demethylated to active secondary amino products (e.g., imipramine to desipramine) may obscure such differences clinically.

Autonomic nervous system. The tricyclic antidepressants are much more potent anticholinergics than their phenothiazine analogues. Thus, dry mouth, constipation, urinary retention, and ophthalmologic changes (blurred vision and mydriasis) are commonly observed. Paradoxically, excessive sweating is also reported.

Cardiovascular system. The tricyclic antidepressants can cause hypotension and compensatory tachycardia. Prolongation of the QT interval, flattening of the T wave, and various arrhythmias have been reported with these drugs. Postural hypotension, particularly in the elderly, is not uncommon.

Absorption, fate, and excretion. The tricyclic antidepressants are readily absorbed from the gastrointestinal tract. The drugs are distributed throughout the body and are tightly bound to plasma and tissue proteins. As previously mentioned, many pharmacologically active metabolites are formed in the liver by N-demethylation; microsomal oxidation and subsequent glucuronidation inactivate the agents and promote their excretion. Approximately two thirds of a single dose is eliminated in the urine and one third in the feces over the course of several days.

Toxic reactions and side effects. Initially, the tricyclics may cause insomnia and restlessness or feelings of fatigue and weakness, but tolerance develops to these effects. Although these agents do not elicit the extrapyramidal side effects of the antipsychotics, mild tremor may sometimes occur. In some individuals, tics, ataxia, and incoordination

have been reported. The anticholinergic effects result in dryness of the mouth, mydriasis, and urinary retention and may also contribute to cardiovascular disturbances.

Acute overdosage, which may be self-inflicted by the suicidal patient, presents a potentially life-threatening mix of CNS excitation and depression, anticholinergic effects, and cardiovascular derangements. Even in conventional doses, the incidence of sudden death from myocardial infarction or ventricular arrhythmias is increased fourfold in patients with cardiac disease. Blood dyscrasias, skin rashes, photosensitization, and cholestatic jaundice—all manifestations of allergic reactions—have been reported but are less frequent than with the phenothiazines.

A final danger to the patient is the possibility of adverse drug interactions. Coadministration with MAO inhibitors, for example, may cause anxiety, vomiting, tremor, convulsions, coma, and death. The tricyclics may also obtund the antihypertensive action of guanethidine and other adrenergic neuron blocking agents by preventing their uptake into nerve terminals. Drug interactions that the dentist must consider are discussed below.

Monoamine oxidase inhibitors

The MAO inhibitors include many chemically unrelated compounds that share the ability to antagonize the action of MAO, the enzyme responsible for the metabolic degradation of the naturally occurring monoamines: epinephrine, norepinephrine, dopamine, and serotonin. Some of these inhibitors, such as tranylcypromine, are structurally related to amphetamine (Figure 12-4).

Pharmacologic effects. Like the tricyclic antidepressants, the MAO inhibitors increase the concentration of norepinephrine and serotonin in the central nervous system. By preventing the catabolic action of MAO, the MAO inhibitors allow the buildup of monoamines in presynaptic nerve terminals. More transmitter is then available for subsequent release. Although these effects are compatible with the amine hypothesis of depression, it should be noted that the MAO inhibitors are not specific for MAO, that they affect other enzymes, and that they have nonenzymatic actions as well. In addition, there is a delay of up to several weeks between the time that enzyme inhibition occurs and mood elevation begins. Obviously, we do not have a clear understanding of the antidepressant action of this group of drugs. However, the existence of

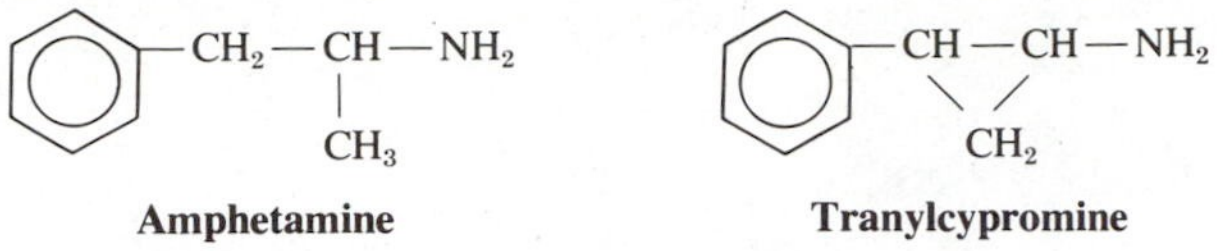

Figure 12-4. Structural formulas of amphetamine and the MAO inhibitor tranylcypromine.

at least two forms of MAO (MAO-A and MAO-B) in the brain and specific inhibitors of MAO-A, such as clorgyline, whch has been reported to be effective in some cases of depression,[30] and specific inhibitors of MAO-B, such as deprenyl, which is useful in Parkinson's disease (see Chapter 16), suggests that selective inhibition of specific forms of MAO may be of potential use in the future. At the present time, though, MAO inhibitors are, in general, less effective in the treatment of depression than are the tricyclic antidepressants and have the potential for more dangerous side effects. The use of MAO inhibitors is, therefore, mostly limited to patients refractory to other drugs.

The most prominent autonomic effects of the MAO inhibitors are exerted on the cardiovascular system, and hypotension is the main result. Tachycardia, dry mouth, sweating, hot flashes, diarrhea, constipation, difficulty in micturition, and impotence are less severe side effects. Transmission of nerve impulses through the autonomic ganglia is antagonized by the MAO inhibitors, and evidence suggests that the sympathetic ganglia are the more severely affected.

Absorption, fate, and excretion. The MAO inhibitors are rapidly absorbed from the gastrointestinal tract. The metabolic fate of the MAO inhibitors is relatively unknown, but the drugs are apparently rapidly metabolized and excreted. The long duration of effect is believed to be due to an irreversible inactivation of MAO.

Toxic reactions and side effects. Most of the MAO inhibitors intended for use as antidepressants have been withdrawn from the market because of their serious side effects. One important adverse reaction to the MAO inhibitors is hepatotoxicity. The MAO inhibitors may also cause orthostatic hypotension and, in overdosage, central excitatory manifestations of insomnia, agitation, hyperreflexia, and frank convulsions.

Drug interactions are of particular concern with the MAO inhibitors. Such interactions may result from enzyme inhibition, an increase in intraneuronal biogenic amines, or both and are likely to be serious and potentially fatal. Among the drugs with which the MAO inhibitors interact are the tricyclic antidepressants, opioid analgesics (especially meperidine), alcohol and other CNS depressants, direct-acting sympathomimetics like phenylephrine that are commonly used as nasal decongestants, amphetamine and similar indirect-acting adrenergics, and levodopa and other precursors of the biogenic amines. Acute hypertensive crises have been precipitated by the ingestion of foods containing pressor amines, such as tyramine, that release norepinephrine from nerve endings. In patients treated with the MAO inhibitors, increased stores of norepinephrine are available for release, and ingested tyramine, which is normally metabolized by enteric and hepatic MAO, reaches the systemic circulation in increased amounts. Foods that contain sympathomimetic amines and therefore should be avoided include aged cheeses (especially Cheddar and Swiss), alcoholic beverages (particularly Chianti wine), canned fish products, snails, liver, nuts, broad beans, citrus fruits, coffee, and almost any product made with yeast. Hypertensive crises precipitated by such foods are characterized by severe headaches, often localized in the occipital region, and frequently by fever.

Amoxapine, maprotiline, and trazodone

Amoxapine, maprotiline, and trazodone are recent additions to the antidepressant armamentarium (Figure 12-5). Amoxapine, a dibenzoxazepine resembling the tricyclics in chemical structure, is the N-demethylated derivative of the antipsychotic loxapine. Although related to the tricyclics, maprotiline is novel in that it is a tetracyclic antidepressant. Trazodone is a triazolopyridine derivative structurally dissimilar from other antidepressants.

Pharmacologic effects. These three compounds differ significantly in their selectivity of action on biogenic amine uptake. Maprotiline inhibits the up-

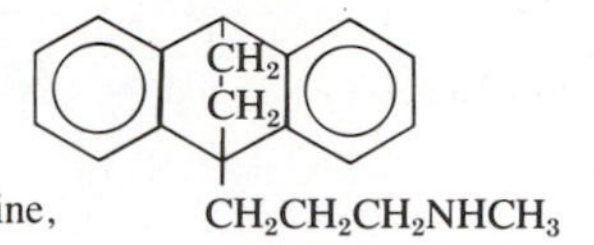

Figure 12-5. Structural formulas of amoxapine, maprotiline, and trazodone.

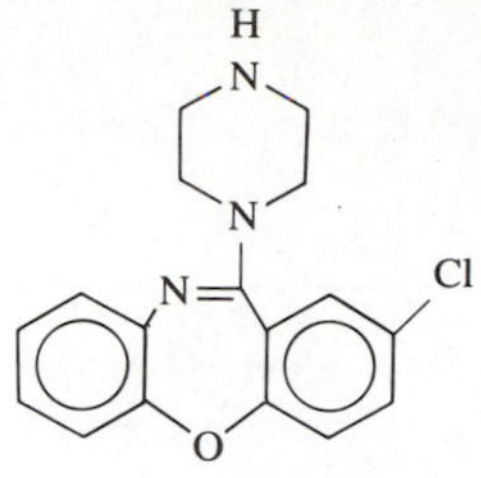

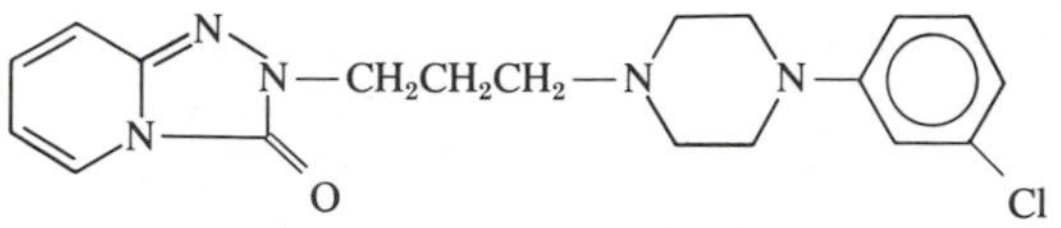

take of catecholamines but has little or no effect on serotonin. Trazodone, on the other hand, is a relatively selective serotonin uptake inhibitor. Both of these compounds have mild anxiolytic properties. Amoxapine resembles the tricyclics in pharmacologic activity, but it also blocks dopamine receptors. This latter action probably accounts for its antipsychotic effect, which is similar to that of loxapine.

Maprotiline, trazodone, and amoxapine all have anticholinergic properties; however, they are much less strong in this regard than the tricyclic antidepressants. Trazodone may actually lower intraocular pressure and thus may be the agent of choice in depressed patients with glaucoma. This fact might be particularly important in the treatment of the elderly.

Maprotiline has no effect on ventricular contractility and, unlike the tricyclic antidepressants, causes a slight bradycardia and a fall in blood pressure.[5] No effects are noted on respiration. Trazodone, like maprotiline, causes bradycardia, decreased blood pressure, and minimal electrocardiographic changes.[16] Although cardiac disturbances have yet to be reported, amoxapine should probably be used cautiously in patients with preexisting cardiovascular disorders.

Absorption, fate, and excretion. Maprotiline is readily absorbed after oral administration. High concentrations may be found within 30 minutes in the cortex, cerebellum, and medulla, whereas after 2 hours the hippocampus has the highest concen-

tration. The principal metabolite is the demethylated derivative, which is further metabolized and excreted in the urine and bile.

Trazodone and amoxapine are also well absorbed from the oral route. Peak concentrations are reached in 1 to 2 hours. Several metabolites of trazodone are formed, and 70% to 75% is excreted in the urine within 72 hours after administration. Amoxapine is almost completely metabolized and excreted in the urine.

Toxic reactions and side effects. While all three of these agents are supposed to have less severe side effects than the tricyclics, it should be noted that they do have mild to moderate anticholinergic properties. Sedation is a common side effect with all three compounds. Cardiovascular effects of maprotiline and trazodone are minimal, and they do not produce orthostatic hypotension. Skin rash, however, is not infrequent with maprotiline, trazodone, and amoxapine. Amoxapine, presumably because of its antidopaminergic activity, produces extrapyramidal side effects and, as a result of increased prolactin secretion, amenorrhea, gynecomastia, and galactorrhea.

New antidepressants

There are a large number of antidepressant drugs that are still being tested clinically or have been approved for use outside the United States. These compounds vary in mechanism of action, side effects, and potency. Many will no doubt become available for clinical use in the United States. A short list of these agents includes mianserin, a tetracyclic unrelated to maprotiline; ciclazindol, an analogue of maprotiline; fluvoxamine and a host of other selective inhibitors of serotonin uptake; bupropion and aletamine, structural analogues of amphetamine; nisoxetine, a specific inhibitor of norepinephrine reuptake; nomifensine, a reuptake inhibitor of norepinephrine, serotonin, and dopamine which also causes dopamine release; and iprindole, which blocks the uptake of neither norepinephrine nor serotonin.

The diversity of this group of drugs indicates either that structural requirements necessary for antidepressant activity are quite liberal or that there are several causes of depression. Although it might be frustrating to discover that depression may result from a variety of biochemical alterations, it is encouraging that such an impressive array of new and effective antidepressants, with potentially fewer side effects than available drugs, is being investigated and readied for clinical use.

General therapeutic uses

The tricyclic antidepressants are used primarily for the treatment of depression and are usually considered the agents of choice by most clinicians. The MAO inhibitors, as previously indicated, are more toxic than the tricyclic antidepressants and find use primarily in those patients who are refractory to the tricyclics. The MAO inhibitors were at one time used for the treatment of hypertension but have now been replaced by antihypertensives that have fewer drug interactions, are less toxic, and are equal or superior in therapeutic efficacy (see Chapter 28).

The tricyclic antidepressants are used with caution in the elderly, not because of age per se, but because of the possible exacerbation of cardiovascular disease. In patients over 50, initial doses may be approximately one third of the recommended dose and are then increased gradually over the next 7 to 14 days. Maprotiline and trazodone may be of benefit for the treatment of the elderly, since cardiovascular and anticholinergic side effects with both of these drugs are minimal.

Like the antipsychotics, the antidepressants may have to be administered over a long period of time and are often continued for several weeks after clinical remission to guard against relapse. Several weeks of continuous drug administration are usually necessary before therapeutic effects are noted. This slow onset in effect may be related to the alterations in brain neurochemicals or receptors, as discussed previously. While it is claimed that maprotiline, trazodone, and amoxapine have a more rapid onset of action than the tricyclics, this has yet to be confirmed in clinical studies.

Implications for dentistry

Tricyclic agents. The anticholinergic side effects of tricyclic drugs (e.g., xerostomia) and their tendency to be additive with CNS depressants are of concern for the dentist (Table 12-2). Frequently, candy is employed to stimulate salivation; overuse of this technique can, however, result in an increased incidence of caries. Anticholinergic agents should not be administered in conjunction with the tricyclics because additive effects can result in toxic reactions (confusion, agitation, and hyperthermia). The use of antianxiety agents, barbiturates, and other CNS depressants should be restricted in patients receiving tricyclics, because additive CNS depressive effects occur. The action of barbiturates may also be prolonged as a result of competition for hepatic microsomal enzymes.

Local anesthetics containing vasoconstrictors should be used with care in patients receiving tricyclic antidepressant therapy. Because of the cardiotoxic effects of the tricyclics, and their potentiation of adrenergic drugs, accidental intravascular injection could precipitate arrhythmias, hypotension, hypertension, or congestive heart failure.[3]

Monoamine oxidase inhibitors. A variety of drug interactions involve MAO inhibitors. One of the most troublesome drug interactions for the practicing dentist may be the prolongation and enhancement of the central effects of the narcotic analgesics, barbiturates, and other CNS depressants. MAO inhibitors given in conjunction with meperidine sometimes cause severe hyperthermia, seizures, and excitement, in addition to reactions that resemble a narcotic overdose. These interactions generally require a reduction in the dose of concomitantly administered CNS depressants; meperidine, however, should be avoided entirely. Phenylephrine is the only vasoconstrictor used in dentistry that is strongly potentiated by inhibition of monoamine oxidase.

Amoxapine, maprotiline, and trazodone. While the most recently approved antidepressants may have fewer side effects than the traditional antidepressants, their anticholinergic and sedative properties should be kept in mind. Conversely, while antidepressants in general produce few motor

Table 12-2. Interactions of antidepressants with other drugs

Antidepressant drug	Drug used for dental or self-therapy*	Therapeutic intent	Possible response or effect†
Tricyclic antidepressants or MAO inhibitors	Phenothiazines	Antinauseant, antiemetic, sedation	Increased antipsychotic effect, increased antidepressant effect, anticholinergic toxicity‡
	Barbiturates	Sedation, hypnosis	CNS depression, decreased antidepressant effect
	General anesthetics	General anesthesia, inhalation sedation	CNS depression
	Benzodiazepines	Antianxiety, intravenous sedation	CNS depression
	Antihistamines	Sedation, relief from colds, antiallergic, antianxiety	CNS depression, anticholinergic toxicity‡
	Ethanol	Sedation	CNS depression
	Direct-acting sympathomimetics§	Gingival retraction, vasoconstriction	Arrhythmia, hypertension
	Narcotic analgesics‖	Analgesia	Increased analgesic effect, respiratory depression

*Self-therapy refers to use of OTC drugs that contain ingredients that may interact with antidepressant compounds.
†These drug interactions do not invariably occur, and they are not necessarily severe when they do occur.
‡Anticholinergic reactions are limited to the tricyclic compounds.
§MAO inhibitor interactions restricted to phenylephrine.
‖Meperidine plus an MAO inhibitor may result in hyperthermia, CNS stimulation, and seizures.

disorders, the close structural relationship of amoxapine to the antipsychotics and the resultant increased risk of extrapyramidal disorders could be a factor to consider, especially in the patient requiring prosthodontic care. Until more is learned about these agents, it seems prudent to assume that drug interactions similar to those involving the tricyclics may occur.

LITHIUM

As mentioned earlier, the psychoactive properties of lithium have been known for decades. However, there has been a renewed interest in lithium because the cation's effectiveness in the treatment of mania suggests that the cause of mania may be a simple ionic imbalance. Elucidating the mechanism of action of lithium may help to clarify our understanding of the etiology of various mental disorders. Although lithium is most effective in the treatment of the manic phase of manic-depressive illness, it is also sometimes effective in the treatment of the depressive phase, as well as in selected forms of unipolar depression.

Pharmacologic effects

Even though the mechanism of action of lithium is not established, it is known that the lithium ion can compete with monovalent cations, such as Na^+, for ionic channels in nerve membrane.[17]

Since the molecular basis of mental disorders is unknown, it is difficult to predict the significance of these competitive actions of lithium; nevertheless, effects on ionic channel transport might be expected to alter the physiologic properties of nervous tissue.

Several putative neurotransmitters of the central nervous system, particularly the biogenic amines, are affected by lithium. Experimental studies have established that lithium increases the turnover of norepinephrine in the brain,[45] decreases the amount of norepinephrine, serotonin, γ-aminobutyric acid, and glutamic acid released from brain slices,[20,21] enhances uptake of serotonin and norepinephrine into neurons,[9] and accelerates the rate of synthesis of serotonin.[40] The net result of these alterations is presumably a reduction of monoamine activity at central synapses.

In human studies, indirect measurements must be utilized to assess the effects of drugs on biogenic amines within the central nervous system. Thus, cerebrospinal fluid titers of 5-hydroxyindoleacetic acid, the principal metabolite of serotonin, and homovanillic acid, the major metabolite of dopamine, were increased in manic patients treated with lithium.[14] Urinary concentrations of 3-methoxy-4-hydroxyphenylglycol, the principal CNS metabolite of norepinephrine, also rise in manic patients treated with lithium.[1,34] Because it is unclear what role these neurotransmitters play in mental disorders, it is difficult to assess the importance of their drug-induced alterations.

Clinically, lithium alleviates the manifestations of mania over the course of 1 to 2 weeks. Sleep and appetite disturbances abate, and swings in mood are prevented. Lithium is unique among the psychotherapeutic agents in that mental changes (e.g., euphoria, depression) are not observed in normal individuals.

Lithium may produce transient electrocardiographic changes[36]; however, in cases in which the lithium concentration remains in the therapeutic range, such changes are not significant. Cardiotoxicity, when it does occur, is usually the result of a lithium overdose.

Absorption, fate, and excretion

Lithium is readily absorbed from the gastrointestinal tract. The cation eventually equilibrates throughout the total body water; no particular affinity for the brain or a specific organ has been detected. Excretion of lithium is primarily via the kidney.

Toxic reactions and side effects

The most common side effects of lithium, including gastrointestinal irritation, fine hand tremor, muscular weakness, polyuria, thirst, sleepiness, and a sluggish feeling, are often associated with initial therapy and usually fade within 1 to 2 weeks. Occasionally, thirst, polyuria, and hand tremor may continue for several months or even years.[37] With continued lithium therapy, approximately 4% of patients develop diffuse, nontoxic goiters. The role lithium plays in this condition is still not clear, but the condition is successfully treated by the administration of thyroid hormone.

Lithium has been shown to inhibit the renal response to antidiuretic hormone[47] and to cause histologic changes in the kidney.[24] In general, these effects appear to be moderate and reversible.[37] Although the toxic action of lithium was at one time considered to be primarily renal in origin, this concept has been revised, and the principal site of untoward effects is now believed to be the central nervous system. Severe intoxication results in vomiting, diarrhea, unconsciousness, and convulsions.

Most adverse effects of lithium have been found to correlate very closely with serum lithium concentrations. As a result, simple and convenient methods for measuring lithium have been sought

that do not involve taking blood samples. One such method has been the utilization of salivary lithium titers to predict serum concentrations. To date, there is disagreement about whether this approach is accurate in humans.

General therapeutic uses

The primary therapeutic use of lithium is for the treatment of manic-depressive illness.[37] Initial high therapeutic doses are often adjusted downward to lower maintenance levels (which may partially account for the alleviation of initial feelings of tiredness). Even so, the dose response is such that 7 to 10 days are required before the antimanic effects are noted, and a short course of antipsychotic medication is normally required in cases of fully developed mania.

Lithium has been employed for a variety of other disorders, including depression, epilepsy, aggressive behavior, and alcoholism. The therapeutic effectiveness of lithium in these conditions ranges from little or no benefit to considerable improvement, but more carefully controlled therapeutic trials are necessary before any definitive conclusions can be drawn. Frequent measurements of lithium are required to maintain proper serum concentrations and are particularly important as a guard against lithium toxicity, which can occur during prolonged therapy.

Implications for dentistry

In experimental animals, the analgesic effect of codeine and dextropropoxyphene is decreased, while that of morphine is increased, by lithium. Whether these findings are applicable to humans is not known. Teratogenic effects, such as cleft palate and deformities of the ear and eye, occur in animals and in humans if lithium is administered during the first trimester of pregnancy.[38]

Patients taking lithium frequently complain of a metallic taste in their mouths, which can alter the taste of food. Probably because of drug-induced xerostomia, polydypsia is common. In early phases of lithium therapy, facial spasms and transient facial paralyses, especially of the lower jaw, have occurred.

Although there have been reports of reduced dental caries in experimental animals when lithium was administered in the drinking water[25] or in the diet,[39] others have not been able to confirm these observations.[48] Lithium has been found to have no significant effect on plaque or gingivitis in dogs.[28]

Antipsychotics

Nonproprietary name	Proprietary name
Phenothiazines	
acetophenazine	Tindal
carphenazine	Proketazine
chlorpromazine	Thorazine
fluphenazine	Permitil, Prolixin
mesoridazine	Serentil
perchlorperazine	Compazine
perphenazine	Trilafon
piperacetazine	Quide
promazine	Sparine
thioridazine	Mellaril
trifluoperazine	Stelazine
triflupromazine	Vesprin
Thioxanthenes	
chlorprothixene	Taractan
thiothixene	Navane
Butyrophenones	
haloperidol	Haldol
Dihydroindolones	
molindone	Moban
Dibenzoxazepines	
loxapine	Loxitane

Drugs for affective disorders

Nonproprietary name	Proprietary name
Tricyclics	
amitriptyline	Elavil, Endep
desipramine	Norpramin, Pertofrane
doxepin	Sinequan, Adapin
imipramine	Tofranil, Presamine, Janimine, SK-Pramine
nortriptyline	Aventyl, Pamelor
protriptyline	Vivactil
trimipramine	Surmontil
MAO inhibitors	
isocarboxazid	Marplan
phenelzine	Nardil
tranylcypromine	Parnate
Dibenzoxazepines	
amoxapine	Asendin
Tetracyclic	
maprotiline	Ludiomil
Triazolopyridines	
trazodone	Desyrel
Antimanics	
lithium carbonate	Eskalith
lithium citrate	Cibalith-S

CITED REFERENCES

1. Beckmann, H., St. Laurent, J., and Goodwin, F.K. The effect of lithium on urinary MHPG in unipolar and bipolar depressed patients. Psychopharmacologia **42**:277-282, 1975.
2. Bloom, F., Segal, D., Ling, N., and Guillemin, R. Endorphins: profound behavioral effects in rats suggest new etiological factors in mental illness. Science **194**:630-632, 1976.
3. Boakes, A.J., Laurence, D.R., Teoh, P.C., Barar, F.S.K., Benedikter, L.T., and Prichard, B.N.C. Interactions between sympathomimetic amines and antidepressant agents in man. British Medical Journal **1**:311-315, 1973.
4. Bradley, P.B. Tranquilizers. In Root, W.S., and Hoffmann, F.G., eds. Physiological Pharmacology, vol. 1. New York, Academic Press, Inc., 1963.
5. Brunner, H., Hedwall, P.R., Meier, M., and Bein, H.J. Cardiovascular effects of preparation CIBA 34,276-Ba and imipramine. Agents and Actions **2**:69-82, 1971.
6. Bunney, B.S., Walters, J.R., Roth, R.H., and Aghajanian, G.K. Dopaminergic neurons: effect of antipsychotic drugs and amphetamine on single cell activity. Journal of Pharmacology and Experimental Therapeutics **185**:560-571, 1973.
7. Cade, J.F.J. Lithium salts in the treatment of psychotic excitement. Medical Journal of Australia **2**:349-352, 1949.
8. Carlsson, A., and Lindqvist, M. Effect of chlorpromazine and haloperidol on formation of 3-methoxytyramine and normetanephrine in mouse brain. Acta Pharmacologica et Toxicologica **20**:140-144, 1963.
9. Colburn, R.W., Goodwin, F.K., Murphy, D.L., Bunney, W.E., Jr., and Davis, J.M. Quantitative studies of norepinephrine uptake by synaptosomes. Biochemical Pharmacology **17**:957-964, 1968.
10. Dasgupta, S.R., Mukherje, K.L., and Werner, G. The activity of some central depressant drugs in acute decorticate and diencephalic preparations. Archives Internationales de Pharmacodynamie et de Therapie **97**:149-156, 1954.
11. Davison, A.N. Physiological role of monoamine oxidase. Physiological Reviews **38**:729-747, 1958.
12. De Maio, D. Preliminary clinical evaluation of a new neuroleptic agent: HF-1854. In Cerletti, A., and Bové, F.J., eds. The Present Status of Psychotropic Drugs: Pharmacological and Clinical Aspects. Amsterdam, Excerpta Medica Foundation, 1969.
13. Domino, E.F. Human pharmacology of tranquilizing drugs. Clinical Pharmacology and Therapeutics **3**:599-664, 1962.
14. Fyrö, B., Petterson, U., and Sedvall, G. The effect of lithium treatment on manic symptoms and levels of monoamine metabolites in cerebrospinal fluid of manic depressive patients. Psychopharmacologia **44**:99-103, 1975.

15. Glowinski, J., and Axelrod, J. Inhibition of uptake of tritiated noradrenaline in the intact rat brain by imipramine and structurally related compounds. Nature **204:**1318-1319, 1964.

16. Gomoll, A.W., and Byrne, S.E. Trazodone and imipramine: comparative effects on canine cardiac conduction. European Journal of Pharmacology **57:**335-342, 1979.

17. Hodgkin, A.L., and Katz, B. The effect of sodium ions on the electrical activity of the giant axon of the squid. Journal of Physiology (London) **108:**37-77, 1949.

18. Hollister, L.E. Hydroxyzine hydrochloride: possible adverse cardiac interactions. Psychopharmacology Communications **1:**61-65, 1975.

19. Horrobin, D.F. Schizophrenia as a prostaglandin deficiency disease. Lancet **1:**936-937, 1977.

20. Katz, R.I., Chase, T.N., and Kopin, I.J. Evoked release of norepinephrine and serotonin from brain slices: inhibition by lithium. Science **162:**466-467, 1968.

21. Katz, R.I., Chase, T.N., and Kopin, I.J. Effect of ions on stimulus-induced release of amino acids from mammalian brain slices. Journal of Neurochemistry **16:**961-967, 1969.

22. Kebabian, J.W., Petgold, G.L., and Greengard, P. Dopamine-sensitive adenylate cyclase in caudate nucleus of rat brain and its similarity to the ''dopamine receptor.'' Proceedings of the National Academy of Sciences of the United States of America **69:**2145-2149, 1972.

23. Klawans, H.L., Jr. The pharmacology of tardive dyskinesias. American Journal of Psychiatry **130:**82-86, 1973.

24. Lindop, G.B.M., and Padfield, P.L. The renal pathology in a case of lithium-induced diabetes insipidus. Journal of Clinical Pathology **28:**472-475, 1975.

25. Malthus, R.S., Ludwig, T.G., and Healy, W.B. Effect of trace elements on dental caries in rats. New Zealand Dental Journal **60:**291-297, 1964.

26. Matthysse, S. Antipsychotic drug actions: a clue to the neuropathology of schizophrenia? Federation Proceedings **32:**200-205, 1973.

27. Matthysse, S., and Lipinski, J. Biochemical aspects of schizophrenia. Annual Review of Medicine **26:**551-565, 1975.

28. McDonald, J.L., Schemehorn, B.R., and Stookey, G.K. Effect of lithium upon plaque and gingivitis in the beagle dog. Journal of Dental Research **57:**474, 1978.

29. Mirsky, A.F., Primac, D.W., and Bates, R. The effects of chlorpromazine and secobarbital on the c.p.t. Journal of Nervous and Mental Disease **128:**12-17, 1959.

30. Murphy, D.L., Lipper, S., Campbell, I.C., Major, L.F., Slater, S., Buchsbaum, M.S., and Gordon, E. Comparative studies of MAO-A and MAO-B inhibitors in man. In Singer, T.P., von Korff, R.W., and Murphy, D.L., eds. Monoamine Oxidase: Structure, Function, and Altered Functions. New York, Academic Press, 1979.

31. Preston, J.B. Effects of chlorpromazine on the central nervous system of the cat: a possible neural basis for action. Journal of Pharmacology and Experimental Therapeutics **118:**100-115, 1956.

32. Ross, S.B., Renyi, A.L., and Ogren, S.O. A comparison of the inhibitory activities of iprindole and impramine on the uptake of 5-hydroxytryptamine and noradrenaline in brain slices. Life Sciences **10:**1267-1277, 1971.

33. Sachar, E.J. Neuroendocrine responses to psychotropic drugs. In Lipton, M.A., DiMascio, A., and Killam, K.F., eds. Psychopharmacology: A Generation of Progress. New York, Raven Press, 1978.

34. Schildkraut, J.J. The effects of lithium on norepinephrine turnover and metabolism: basic and clinical studies. Journal of Nervous and Mental Disease **158:**348-360, 1974.

35. Schildkraut, J.J., and Kety, S.S. Biogenic amines and emotion. Science **156:**21-30, 1967.

36. Schou, M. Electrocardiographic changes during treatment with lithium and with drugs of the imipramine type. Acta Psychiatrica Scandinavica **38:**331-336, 1962.

37. Schou, M. Lithium in psychiatric therapy and prophylaxis. Journal of Psychiatric Research **6:**67-95, 1968.

38. Schou, M., Goldfield, M.D., Weinstein, M.R., and Villeneuve, A. Lithium and pregnancy. I. Report from the register of lithium babies. British Medical Journal **2:**135-136, 1973.

39. Shaw, J.H., and Griffiths, D. Developmental and post-developmental influences on incidence of experimental dental caries resulting from dietary supplementation by various elements. Archives of Oral Biology **5:**301-322, 1961.

40. Sheard, M.H., and Aghajanian, G.K. Neuronally activated metabolism of brain serotonin: effect of lithium. Life Sciences **9:**285-290, 1970.

41. Siggins, G.R., Hoffer, B.J., and Ungerstedt, U. Electrophysiological evidence for involvement of cyclic adenosine monophosphate in dopamine responses of caudate neurons. Life Sciences **15:**779-792, 1974.

42. Snyder, S.H., Banerjee, S.P., Yamamura, H.I., and Greenberg, D. Drugs, neurotransmitters, and schizophrenia. Science **184:**1243-1253, 1974.

43. Snyder, S., Greenberg, D., and Yamamura, H.I. Antischizophrenic drugs and brain cholinergic receptors. Affinity for muscarinic sites predicts extrapyramidal effects. Archives of General Psychiatry **31:**58-61, 1974.

44. Snyder, S.H., Taylor, K.M., Coyle, J.T., and Meyerhoff, J.L. The role of brain dopamine in behavioral regulation and the actions of psychotropic drugs. American Journal of Psychiatry **127:**199-207, 1970.

45. Stern, D.N., Fieve, R.R., Neff, N.H., and Costa, E. The effect of lithium chloride administration on brain and heart norepinephrine turnover rates. Psychopharmacologia **14:**315-322, 1969.

46. Sternberg, D.E., Charney, D.S., Heninger, G.R., Leckman, J.F., Hafstad, K.M., and Landis, D.H. Impaired presynaptic regulation of norepinephrine in schizophrenia. Archives of General Psychiatry **39:**285-289, 1982.

47. Thomsen, K. Lithium-induced polyuria in rats. International Pharmacopsychiatry **5:**233-241, 1970.

48. Wisotzky, J., and Hein, J.W. Effects of drinking solutions containing metallic ions above and below hydrogen in the electromotive series on dental caries in the Syrian hamster. The Journal of the American Dental Association **5:**796-800, 1958.

49. York, D.H. Dopamine receptor blockade—a central action of chlorpromazine on striatal neurones. Brain Research **37:**91-99, 1972.

GENERAL REFERENCES

Aldenhoff, J.B., and Lux, H.D., eds. Basic Mechanisms in the Action of Lithium: Proceedings of a Symposium at Schloss Ringberg, Bavaria, Germany, October 4-6, 1981. Amsterdam, Excerpta Medica Foundation, 1982.

Born, G.V.R., Farah, A., Herken, H., and Welch, A.D., eds. Handbook of Experimental Pharmacology. New York, Springer-Verlag, 1980.

Grahame-Smith, D.G., Hippius, H., and Winokur, G., eds. Psychopharmacology 1, Part 1: Basic Preclinical Psychopharmacology. Amsterdam, Excerpta Medica Foundation, 1982.

Grahame-Smith, D.G., Hippius, H., and Winokur, G., eds. Psychopharmacology 1, Part 2: Clinical Psychopharmacology. Amsterdam, Excerpta Medica Foundation, 1983.

Palmer, G.C., ed. Neuropharmacology of Central Nervous System and Behavioral Disorders. (Physiologic & Pharmacologic Bases of Drug Therapy Series). New York, Academic Press, 1981.

Paykel, E.S., ed. Handbook of Affective Disorders. New York, Guilford Press, 1982.

Schwab, J., ed. Schizophrenia 1980: implications for psychopharmacology. In Psychiatry, Psychopharmacology and Alternatives: Trends for the 80's. New York, Marcel Dekker, 1981.

13 Antianxiety drugs and centrally acting muscle relaxants

Leslie P. Felpel

ANTIANXIETY AGENTS

The search for drugs that effectively treat anxiety without producing sedation has been characterized by enthusiastic reports of "miracle" drugs, followed either by denials of clinical efficacy or reports of sedation, addiction, or other dangerous side effects. Ethanol was perhaps the first substance used as an antianxiety agent, but its depressant effect on the central nervous system accounts for its antianxiety properties. Other general CNS depressants, such as chloral hydrate, paraldehyde, and the barbiturates, have also been employed (and sometimes still are); however, none of these agents act selectively to relieve fear and apprehension.

The first glimmer of hope that specific antianxiety actions might be obtainable was the discovery in 1955 of the behavioral effects of meprobamate. Meprobamate was originally developed as a centrally acting skeletal muscle relaxant, but its antianxiety properties were soon noted and used clinically. The fact that the central effects of meprobamate appeared to be similar to but less spectacular than those of chlorpromazine generated the terms *minor* and *major* tranquilizers as a distinction between the two classes of compounds these drugs represented. As emphasized in the previous chapter, this terminology should be abandoned because these two groups of drugs have entirely different mechanisms of action, and their behavioral effects, when closely examined, are dissimilar.

Antianxiety agents may be referred to by many other terms, including ataractics, anxiolytics, anxiolytic sedatives, and psychosedatives. Implicit in these terms is the basic underlying pharmacologic effect of all of these agents—sedation. Even the most popular antianxiety agents, the benzodiazepines, produce some degree of CNS depression, though there is evidence that the benzodiazepines have somewhat more specific antianxiety properties than do drugs like the barbiturates. The term *antianxiety* is therefore used with the understanding that drugs in this class do not have specific antianxiety effects but are the most selective of those currently available.

The dentist uses antianxiety drugs primarily for premedication of the nervous and apprehensive patient. Intravenously administered diazepam has also gained wide acceptance as an agent for so-called conscious sedation, as discussed in Chapters 19 and 44. The usefulness and effectiveness of any given antianxiety agent will vary, depending on the patient, the clinical surroundings, the "chair-side" manner of the dentist, and, of course, the properties of the chosen drug. A knowledge of the pharmacology of the various antianxiety agents is critical for the dentist in selecting the proper drug, avoiding drug interactions, and obtaining the desired therapeutic response with minimal deleterious side effects.

Benzodiazepines

The benzodiazepines are without doubt one of the most popular of all drug classes in the history of medicine. Diazepam was the most frequently prescribed drug in the United States for several years during the 1970s and remains so today. Over 68 million prescriptions were written for benzodiazepines in 1978; more than one half of these were for diazepam alone. Surveys indicate that approximately 15% of adults in the United States take one of the benzodiazepines at least once a year. In fact, both the lay press and members of the medical community have suggested that these and other antianxiety agents are overused, that they frequently serve either as a substitute for the practitioner's time or as a placebo for a population increasingly

Table 13-1. Chemical structures of benzodiazepines currently available in the United States

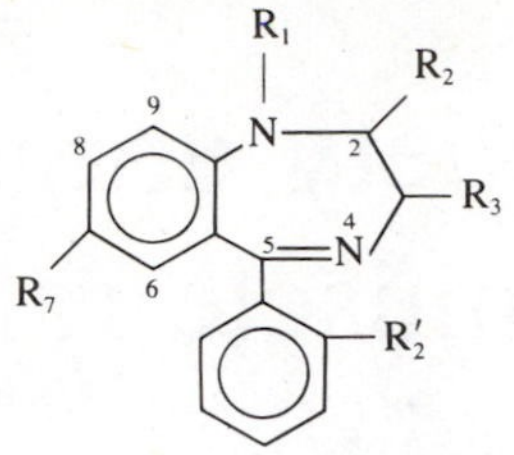

Drug	Substituent groups				
	R_1	R_2	R_3	R_7	R_2'
Chlordiazepoxide	See Figure 13-1				
Diazepam	— CH_3	= O	— H	— Cl	— H
Oxazepam	— H	= O	— OH	— Cl	— H
Flurazepam	— $CH_2CH_2N(C_2H_5)_2$	= O	— H	— Cl	— F
Clorazepate	— H	= O	— COOH	— Cl	— H
Clonazepam	— CH_3	= O	— H	— NO_2	— Cl
Lorazepam	— H	= O	— OH	— Cl	— Cl
Prazepam	— CH_2—◁	= O	— H	— Cl	— H
Temazepam	— CH_3	= O	— OH	— Cl	— H
Halazepam	— CH_2CF_3	= O	— H	— Cl	— H
Alprazolam	See Figure 13-1				
Triazolam	See Figure 13-1				

unwilling to accept a mild state of unhappiness without medication. In response to this problem, prescribing information in the package inserts for the benzodiazepines has been revised to warn the practitioner that these drugs should not be prescribed for longer than 4 months without a careful reassessment of the patient's status and that they should not be prescribed for the stress of everyday life. However, medical opinion is not unanimous regarding overuse of these antianxiety agents. There are those who believe that a number of patients who truly need them are so denied because of the bad publicity associated with their use and that the benzodiazepines may, in certain instances, be underprescribed.

Chemistry and structure-activity relationships. The basic structure of the pharmacologically active benzodiazepines is illustrated in Table 13-1. All of the benzodiazepines currently available in the United States are derived from this molecule by the addition of various substituent groups. A slight modification of the basic structure has produced a new class of compounds, the triazolobenzodiazepines, represented by alprazolam in Figure 13-1 (shown with chlordiazepoxide, the original benzodiazepine).

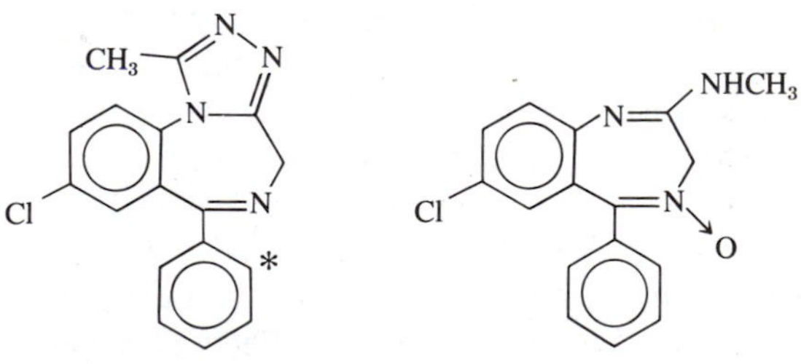

Alprazolam　　　　**Chlordiazepoxide**

Figure 13-1. Structural formulas of alprazolam and chlordiazepoxide. A third benzodiazepine, triazolam, is derived from alprazolam by the addition of a chloride atom on the ortho position of the phenyl group, as indicated by the asterisk(*).

All benzodiazepines with psychopharmacologic activity have an electronegative group at R_7. A chlorine atom appears to confer optimal activity, whereas bromo and nitro substitutions are only weakly anxiolytic. However, a nitro moiety at R_7 enhances anticonvulsant properties, as illustrated by clonazepam, which is used exclusively as an anticonvulsant. Hydrogen or methyl groups at R_7 or substitutions at positions 6, 8, or 9 reduce pharmacologic activity significantly. Substitution at position 5 with any group other than a phenyl ring also reduces efficacy. Halogenation at R_2 increases potency; larger alkyl substitutions decrease it. Substitution on the nitrogen at R_1 with a methyl group (but no other) enhances activity, as do methyl or hydrogen substitutions at R_3.

Pharmacologic effects. The most important pharmacologic effects of the benzodiazepines are on the central nervous system, but these drugs can have some effects, though often not clinically significant, on other systems as well.

Central nervous system. The benzodiazepines have clinically useful antianxiety, sedative-hypnotic, anticonvulsant, and skeletal muscle relaxant properties. Several neural mechanisms and neurotransmitters have been implicated to explain these properties. However, although benzodiazepine-induced changes in CNS neurotransmitters can be demonstrated experimentally, the full significance of these changes remains obscure.

The gross central effects of the benzodiazepines differ little from those of the older sedative-hypnotics, such as the barbiturates. All of the benzodiazepines depress the central nervous system to varying degrees, depending on the dose. Drowsiness and sedation are common manifestations of this central depressant action and may be considered a side effect in some instances and therapeutically useful in others. Some of the newer benzodiazepines, such as flurazepam and temazepam, are being promoted specifically as hypnotic agents. Whether their ability to promote sleep is significantly greater than that of other benzodiazepines is not clear. As will be discussed later, differences in the pharmacokinetics of the various benzodiazepines, rather than in supposed pharmacologic specificity, may be the most important consideration in the selection of one of these drugs over another.

Although it is difficult to differentiate clinically the central effects of the benzodiazepines from those of other sedative-hypnotics, there are certain experimental animal models that indicate that the benzodiazepines do in fact have "specific" antianxiety properties. For example, vicious macaque monkeys, when given chlordiazepoxide, become calm and tame.[35] Septal rats, which become highly irritable after lesions are placed in the septal area of the brain, are also rendered tranquil by the benzodiazepines.[35] The doses required to produce these effects are one-tenth those that cause ataxia and somnolence. The sedative-hypnotics, such as the barbiturates or meprobamate, will also tame these animals, but the doses required invariably produce incoordination and drowsiness.

In addition to behavioral investigations there are numerous studies that have examined the effects of benzodiazepines on the electrical activity of areas of the brain that are associated with emotion and behavior. In these studies too, the evidence suggests a somewhat more specific antianxiety action of the benzodiazepines as compared to the barbiturates or other sedative-hypnotics. The benzodiazepines, for example, depress the limbic system (an area of the brain associated with emotion and behavior) at doses lower than those that depress the reticular formation and cerebral cortex. The opposite is true for sedative-hypnotics like the barbiturates. The "specific" effects of benzodiazepines on the limbic system correlate with taming in experimental animals and anxiety relief in humans. Experimentally, spontaneous discharge, as well as aurally, visually, or tactually evoked activity of neurons in the hippocampus (a major structure of the limbic system), is depressed by the benzodiazepines.[1,7,32,50] Neurons of the amygdaloid nucleus, another major component of the limbic system, are also depressed by the benzodiazepines, as are the amygdaloid-evoked hippocampal responses.[30,39] Unfortunately, although these studies are interesting, the behavioral significance of these findings is not clear. The causes, mechanisms, and neural structures involved in anxiety are unknown, and a reliable, generally accepted animal model for anxiety is not yet available. Thus, results obtained in behavioral studies with animals are very difficult to interpret and even more difficult to extrapolate to humans.

The benzodiazepines interact with several putative neurotransmitter systems. Diazepam, for example, has a high affinity for glycine receptors,[57] and those benzodiazepines with the highest affinity are the most potent antianxiety agents in humans.[44] The biogenic amines have also been implicated in the mechanism of action of the benzodiazepines. Serotonin has been shown to decrease, and norepinephrine to increase, the antianxiety effects of the benzodiazepines.[49] In these same studies, norepinephrine antagonized the depressant effects of the benzodiazepines, thus implicating norepinephrine in benzodiazepine-mediated CNS depression.

Perhaps the most important and exciting advancement in our understanding of anxiety and the mechanism of action of the benzodiazepines came with the discovery of specific binding sites in the brain of several species including humans.[29,46,47] The high-affinity binding sites to benzodiazepines appear to be a part of the γ-aminobutyric acid (GABA) receptor, since benzodiazepines do not directly interfere with GABA binding. In fact, a reciprocal effect is noted, the binding of one agent to its site increasing the affinity of the other site to its ligand.[17] In autoradiographic studies, benzodiazepine receptors have been shown to be coupled to GABA receptors[53]; thus a functional link between the benzodiazepines and the GABA-ergic system seems to be established. These findings have led investigators to propose that the benzodiazepines are binding to a receptor normally available for binding by an endogenous ligand, in a manner analogous to the endogenous opioids, the enkephalins.

An ionic mechanism underlying the antianxiety action of the benzodiazepines has not been identified. However, it is known that benzodiazepines alter the kinetics of GABA-activated chloride ion channels in nerve membrane such that the frequency and duration of their opening are increased.[51] The mechanism by which this action occurs is unknown. Previous studies have shown that GABA-mediated presynaptic inhibition in the spinal cord could be potentiated by diazepam.[40] GABA-mediated postsynaptic inhibition in the cerebellum and substantia nigra is also potentiated by the benzodiazepines.[23] The benzodiazepines do not appear to have direct GABA-mimetic effects, however.[16]

To complicate the issue further, it is now evident that at least two types of benzodiazepine receptor sites exist in the central nervous system.[28,56] While the significance of this finding is not clear, it does raise the possibility that multiple receptor types, each with a different physiologic function, could subserve the antianxiety, sedative, anticonvulsant, and muscle relaxant properties of the benzodiazepines. It also suggests that drugs with more specific antianxiety effects and fewer side effects might be found in the future.

The anticonvulsant and skeletal muscle relaxant properties of the benzodiazepines will be discussed in Chapter 15 and at the end of this chapter, respectively. Suffice it to say here that the anticonvulsant effect may stem from actions on the amygdala, cerebellum, and cerebral cortex, and muscle relaxation from an attenuation of spinal and supraspinal reflexes (e.g., the linguomandibular reflex).[43]

Cardiovascular system. In normal therapeutic doses, the benzodiazepines cause few alterations in cardiac output or blood pressure when administered intravenously to healthy individuals.[36,48] Slightly greater than normal doses cause slight decreases in blood pressure, cardiac output, and stroke volume in normal subjects as well as patients with pulmonary disease, but these effects are usually not clinically significant. The benzodiazepines are often prescribed for cardiac patients in whom anxiety is a contributing factor to their symptoms.

Respiratory system. As is true of any sedative drug, the benzodiazepines are respiratory depressants. In normal doses, the benzodiazepines given alone have little effect on respiration in the healthy individual. However, there have been a few reports of respiratory failure caused by the benzodiazepines in patients with pulmonary disease. The benzodiazepines may also potentiate the respiratory depressant effects of other CNS depressant drugs if used concomitantly, though such potentiation is weak when the benzodiazepines are administered orally. Poor suckling, hypothermia, and a need for ventilatory assistance have been reported in the neonate after the intravenous injection of lorazepam to the mother shortly before delivery.[55]

Absorption, fate, and excretion. The pharmacokinetics of individual benzodiazepines differ such that there is a wide range in speed of onset and duration of action among these compounds. Frequently, the benzodiazepines are classified according to their elimination half-life, as illustrated in Table 13-2. This table should only serve as a general guideline, since the elimination half-life of a given drug may not correlate well with its clinical profile. The rates of drug absorption and tissue distribution are much more important factors in determining onset and duration of clinical effects after short-term administration.[22] Additionally, there is a wide variation in half-life among patients.

Following oral administration, most of the benzodiazepines are rapidly absorbed and highly bound to plasma protein. Peak blood concentrations are generally obtained in 1 to 3 hours. However, the lipid solubility of these compounds differs significantly, such that a highly lipid-soluble drug like diazepam exerts its effect quickly, whereas oxazepam, which is poorly lipid soluble, has a slow onset of action. Diazepam also accumulates in body fat because of its lipophilic properties, and it

Table 13-2. Classification of benzodiazepines based on elimination half-life after oral administration

Drug	Time to peak plasma concentration (hr)	Elimination half-life (hr)	Major active metabolites
Short- to intermediate-acting			
Alprazolam	1-2	12-15	None
Lorazepam	1-6	10-18	None
Oxazepam	1-4	5-15	None
Temazepam	2-3	10-20	None
Triazolam	1-2	1.5-5	α-hydroxytriazolam
Long-acting			
Chlordiazepoxide	0.5-4	5-30	Desmethylchlordiazepoxide Demoxepam Desmethyldiazepam
Clorazepate*	1-2	30-100	Desmethyldiazepam
Diazepam	0.5-2	20-50	Desmethyldiazepam
Flurazepam*	0.5-1	47-100	Desalkylflurazepam
Halazepam	1-3	14	Desmethyldiazepam
Prazepam*	2.5-6	30-100	Desmethyldiazepam

*Does not reach circulation as parent drug in clinically significant amounts. Values reflect the primary metabolite.

is slowly eliminated from these stores. This characteristic partially accounts for the prolonged half-life of diazepam, which can range in patients from 1 day to as much as 8 days.

Many of the benzodiazepines are converted to pharmacologically active metabolites that have long half-lives. Clorazepate and prazepam are inactive as the parent compound after oral administration because of an essentially complete conversion (in the stomach and liver, respectively) to the long-acting metabolite desmethyldiazepam. Note that many other benzodiazepines, including chlordiazepoxide, diazepam, and halazepam, are also converted, at least in part, to desmethyldiazepam. In general, the metabolites are conjugated with glucuronic acid and excreted in the urine and feces. Oxazepam and lorazepam are not converted to active metabolites but are simply conjugated and excreted. These drugs are therefore eliminated fairly rapidly and may be preferable in the elderly who may suffer a deficiency in hepatic metabolic enzymes.[41]

Toxic reactions and side effects. The most common side effect of the benzodiazepines is drowsiness. This may not be necessarily an unwanted reaction, but rather a desirable therapeutic result in the case of anxiety states that cause insomnia. Other side effects that are a result of CNS depression and are dose dependent include ataxia, incoordination, dysarthria, confusion, apathy, muscle weakness, dizziness, and somnolence. The elderly (over 65) appear to be particularly susceptible, and individuals with a history of alcohol or barbiturate abuse particularly resistant, to the CNS depressant properties of the benzodiazepines.

The elderly and the young, especially teenage girls, occasionally exhibit excitement rather than the expected depression of the central nervous system after administration of the benzodiazepines. Excitatory central effects of the benzodiazepines may include an increased incidence of nightmares, rage, and hostility. A paradoxical decrease in seizure threshold, particularly in patients with grand mal epilepsy, has also been observed. In addition to behavioral patterns indicative of stimulation, there have been several reports that the benzodiazepines can cause an increase in motor activity, such as hyperkinesis and agitation. These unusual occurrences of what appears to be a CNS excitatory action may be a disinhibitory effect not unlike that observed with alcohol.

The benzodiazepines, unlike the older sedative-hypnotics, cause only mild disturbances in normal sleep patterns. These alterations will be discussed further in Chapter 14. Patients seem to adapt fairly quickly to the nonspecific CNS depression of the benzodiazepines but somewhat less rapidly to the antianxiety effects. Nonetheless, daytime sedation following a nighttime dose, referred to as "hangover," is a common side reaction, especially of the long-acting benzodiazepines. This residual effect may be beneficial in some cases but undesirable in others.

Side effects of the benzodiazpines other than those referable to their CNS depressant actions are usually more irritating than life-threatening. Allergic reactions to the benzodiazepines are usually manifest as relatively minor skin rashes. Intramuscularly and intravenously administered diazepam can cause local pain, phlebitis, thrombosis, or all three.[26] Phlebitis is more likely to occur if a vein in the hand or wrist is used and may be more common following repeated injections, especially in heavy smokers, the elderly, and women taking oral contraceptives. A more severe complication arises if the injection has been inadvertently made into an artery. In such a case, the patient usually reports pain that radiates distally, and ischemic changes are noted in the digits. This reaction can occur up to 3 days after injection and may lead to gangrene, necessitating amputation. If an intraarterial injection is made, it has been suggested that the needle be left in place and the artery flushed with a vasodilator, such as papaverine or procaine.[37]

Tolerance and habituation occur rather frequently with the benzodiazepines, but physical dependence is somewhat less common. High doses, on the order of 10 to 20 times the therapeutic dose, must be taken for several months before dependence occurs.[38] Nevertheless, the abuse potential for some of the benzodiazepines is high; the rapid onset of action and euphoric properties of diazepam make it particularly popular as a drug of abuse. Because of the strong binding of diazepam to cellular membranes and plasma proteins, it is very difficult to remove the drug rapidly by dialysis or diuresis in patients with acute overdose.

Despite these problems, one of the major advantages of the benzodiazepines, as compared to other sedatives, is their margin of safety. Death is rare in cases of overdose and is usually the result of a combination of drugs, especially alcohol, along with the benzodiazepines. The few deaths associated with the use of a benzodiazepine alone have primarily involved either geriatric patients or very young children, which may reflect a deficiency of hepatic metabolic enzymes in these two populations.

The unborn child may be the most susceptible to benzodiazepine toxicity. Diazepam is teratogenic in animals and has been implicated as a cause of cleft lip and palate in humans. It is probable that other benzodiazepines have similar effects. In addition, frequent use of benzodiazepines during pregnancy may lead to a withdrawal syndrome in the neonate, and large doses given to the mother during labor and delivery may result in respiratory depression, hypotonia, and a tendency in the infant toward hypothermia.

New benzodiazepines. There are scores of benzodiazepines chemically related to those currently available in this country that are in various stages of clinical investigation. Many have already been approved for use in other countries. While these benzodiazepines share common pharmacologic properties, several of them seem to be more specific than others with regard to their sedative, muscle relaxant, anticonvulsant, or antianxiety actions. Such benzodiazepines include midazolam, used as an intravenous preanesthetic; estazolam, quazepam, flunitrazepam, nitrazepam, brotizolam, and lormetrazepam, promoted as hypnotics; tetrazepam and xilobam, for muscle relaxation; ketazolam, uldazepam, bentazepam, clobazam, oxazolam, and bromazepam, as antianxiety agents; and tofisopam, an anxiolytic with little or no sedative, muscle relaxant, or anticonvulsant properties. The spectrum of activity of this last benzodiazepine is interesting in that it suggests that compounds with specific antianxiety action (i.e., with little or no accompanying CNS depressant effects) might be obtainable. Continued drug development also indicates that the end to this large array of benzodiazepines is nowhere in sight.

Propanediol carbamates

Meprobamate was considered the agent of choice for the treatment of anxiety in the mid-1950s. However, with the discovery of the addictive properties of this compound, its popularity declined rapidly. The pharmacology of meprobamate differs little from the barbiturates, though, unlike the barbiturates, its antianxiety effects are demonstrable at doses that do not markedly diminish motor or intellectual performance.

The parent drug of the propanediol carbamates, meprobamate, is illustrated in Figure 13-2. Clinically useful derivatives of meprobamate are made by substitutions on the carbamyl nitrogen atoms.

Pharmacologic effects. The site and mechanism of action of meprobamate on the central nervous system are not established. Meprobamate is known to more readily depress polysynaptic than mono-

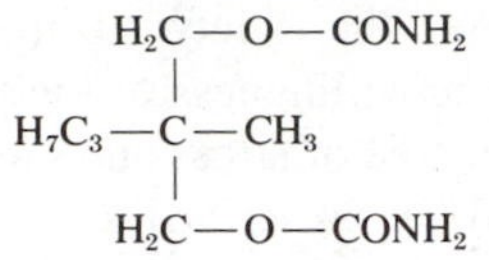

$$H_2C-O-CONH_2$$
$$H_7C_3-C-CH_3$$
$$H_2C-O-CONH_2$$

Meprobamate

Figure 13-2. Structural formula of meprobamate.

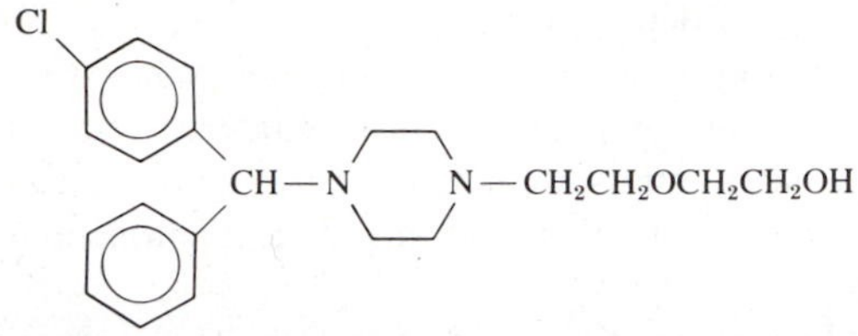

Figure 13-3. Structural formula of hydroxyzine.

synaptic pathways,[6,9,12] thus forming the basis for the classification of meprobamate as an interneuronal blocking agent and a centrally acting skeletal muscle relaxant. Whether the interneuronal depressant property of meprobamate plays a role in the antianxiety effect of this compound remains purely speculative.

Therapeutic doses of meprobamate have little effect on the cardiovascular or respiratory system, though slight hypotension may occur occasionally. As with other CNS depressants, marked cardiovascular and respiratory depression may occur with overdosage.

Tybamate, an analogue of meprobamate, has antianxiety and skeletal muscle relaxant properties at doses that cause little or no sedation. Tybamate has been shown to depress spinal polysynaptic reflexes preferentially over monosynaptic reflexes,[52] which may account for muscle relaxation but, as with meprobamate, leaves the question of mechanism of action for relief of anxiety open to speculation.

Absorption, fate, and excretion. Meprobamate is rapidly absorbed from the gastrointestinal tract and reaches a peak plasma concentration in 2 to 3 hours. The half-life of meprobamate is approximately 10 to 12 hours. Most of the drug is converted metabolically to hydroxymeprobamate, which is excreted along with a glucuronide and a small amount of free meprobamate in the urine. Like the barbiturates, meprobamate increases hepatic microsomal enzyme activity and thus accelerates its own metabolism, which may partially explain the development of tolerance to this drug after prolonged use. The metabolism of meprobamate may also be accelerated by the presence of aminopyrine, phenylbutazone, chlorpromazine, and the barbiturates. Other propanediol derivatives are metabolized much like meprobamate; however, they do not induce hepatic microsomal enzyme activity. Tolerance and physical addiction, which develop to meprobamate, do not occur with tybamate,

perhaps because of the relatively short half-life (3 to 6 hours) of the latter agent.

Toxic reactions and side effects. The CNS depressant properties of meprobamate account for most of its troublesome side effects, such as somnolence, dizziness, and, at high doses, ataxia and confusion. Allergic reactions consisting of skin eruptions, bronchospasm, hypotension, anuria, and fever have been observed. There have also been reports of blood dyscrasias (i.e., aplastic anemia, leukopenia, and agranulocytosis). Toxic doses result in marked respiratory and cardiovascular depression, while therapeutic doses produce mild hypotension and little effect on the respiratory system.

Perhaps the most serious side effect of meprobamate is the development of physical and psychologic dependence. Withdrawal symptoms, including insomnia, restlessness, tremor, and anxiety, may be precipitated when the drug is suddenly withdrawn from patients who have received 2 gm or more per day for prolonged periods.

Diphenylmethane antihistamines

The chemical structure of hydroxyzine, the most popular of this drug class, is shown in Figure 13-3. Hydroxyzine is similar in structure to the piperazine antihistamines (Chapter 23). Analogues of hydroxyzine are used primarily for their antihistaminic properties rather than for their ability to alleviate fear and apprehension.

Pharmacologic effects. The antihistamines all produce CNS depression with resultant sedation that in part accounts for their antianxiety effect. These drugs also have prominent and sometimes beneficial anticholinergic, antihistaminic, antiemetic, antiarrhythmic, and hypotensive properties. The mechanism of action responsible for the relief of anxiety is unknown. The only side reactions that may be of concern with these compounds are drowsiness and dry mouth. Additive effects occur if these drugs are used in conjunction with other CNS depressants.

Hydroxyzine has very slight depressant effects on the cardiovascular and respiratory systems. Like other antihistamines, hydroxyzine has antiarrhythmic properties and may cause bronchodilation.

Absorption, fate, and excretion. Hydroxyzine is rapidly absorbed from the gastrointestinal tract, and pharmacologic effects may begin within 15 to 30 minutes. The metabolic fate of hydroxyzine includes hepatic conversion to the lipid-soluble derivative *p*-chlorobenzhydrylpiperazine (also known as norchlorcyclizine), which may be toxic to the human fetus, and the water-soluble hydroxyzine N-oxide. The hydroxyzine N-oxide derivative is excreted rapidly, whereas norchlorcyclizine is excreted slowly and tends to accumulate in the body. Other metabolites include a lipophilic *p*-chlorobenzhydrol derivative and a hydrophilic *p*-chlorobenzhydrol glucuronide conjugate.

Toxic reactions and side effects. Hydroxyzine is generally considered to be relatively free of toxic side effects. The CNS depressant effect of hydroxyzine is additive with that of other CNS depressants. As described above, there are indications that a lipid-soluble metabolite of hydroxyzine may be dangerous to the fetus, but such an effect has been demonstrated experimentally only at doses 50 to 100 times therapeutic.

General therapeutic uses

Most people have experienced some anxiety in the course of daily life. Obviously, not everyone requires pharmacotherapy for fear and apprehension; anxious states are often brought on by a series of events that eventually pass, allowing the anxiety to subside. This is a natural sequence, and it is only when the anxious state remains after an adequate lapse of time, or when it interferes with the patient's functioning, that pharmacotherapy is indicated. It should be remembered that antianxiety agents are not curative but merely treat the symptoms of anxiety, permitting the patient to cope more effectively with the situation or respond more favorably to psychotherapy. The antianxiety agents are useful in the treatment of acute anxiety resulting from transient stress, whether environmental, physical, or psychologic in origin. Ideally, for the treatment of long-standing anxiety these agents should be employed only with the proper psycho-

therapy, but because of the demands placed on the physician's time, the safety of the antianxiety agents, and the unwillingness of the patient to endure a certain degree of stress and unpleasantness, these drugs may be prescribed too frequently and with too little supervision (though as discussed previously, this last point is somewhat controversial).

Because anxiety fluctuates from day to day and is usually episodic, the dose of these drugs must be individualized and adjusted more frequently than perhaps with any other type of pharmacotherapy. Unfortunately, this rule is not generally adhered to in practice. The elimination half-life of most of these compounds and their active metabolites is sufficiently long to cause an accumulation of the drug in the body if it is administered on the basis of the traditional regimen of two to three doses a day. It must also be remembered that the longer a patient is treated with antianxiety agents, the greater is the chance of developing dependence and withdrawal symptoms if the drug is discontinued.

In addition to anxiety, there are a number of other disease states for which these agents are extremely useful. Chlordiazepoxide has been found to be helpful in the treatment of alcohol and sedative-hypnotic withdrawal syndromes and, like most of the benzodiazepines, has been shown to have anticonvulsant properties. Clonazepam has been approved for use strictly as an anticonvulsant for several types of epilepsy (see Chapter 15), and diazepam appears to be the agent of choice for the control of status epilepticus. It may also be used in control of seizures caused by local anesthetics. The skeletal muscle relaxant properties of diazepam have led to the successful use of this agent in the treatment of tetanus and for the relief of the spasticity associated with cerebral palsy. Diazepam has also found widespread use as a premedicant in general anesthesia and obstetrics; however, midazolam (not yet approved for use in the United States) may supercede diazepam in this regard. Alprazolam may have antidepressant properties and has been useful in the treatment of panic attacks. Although temazepam and flurazepam have antianxiety properties, they are promoted primarily for the treatment of sleep disorders. Finally, hydroxyzine may be used as a premedicant for anesthesia and has been approved as adjunctive therapy for pruritus.

Therapeutic uses in dentistry

The antianxiety agents are important in dentistry for the premedication of the apprehensive patient, the patient exhibiting mild neurosis associated with the mouth, and the uncooperative child. Antianxiety agents, particularly intravenous diazepam, are also used with success as adjuncts to local anesthesia. The sedation achieved with diazepam lasts 30 to 60 minutes. Additionally, diazepam causes anterograde amnesia in approximately 50% of patients, so that the patient often cannot recall the procedures performed.

Perhaps one of the more perplexing questions the practicing dentist has regarding the use of the benzodiazepines is which agent to choose from the ever-expanding list of drugs. There is little doubt of the clinical efficacy of the benzodiazepines in a variety of dental procedures.[3,11,14,18,25] However, there are no unusual characteristics associated with any benzodiazepine that would make it the drug of choice in dentistry. Essentially, any benzodiazepine is suitable as an antianxiety agent *if* the pharmacokinetics of that drug are kept in mind. The major decision with regard to the use of benzodiazepines for the treatment of the anxious patient is therefore not so much which drug to use but rather when to administer it. While there is no simple solution for this problem, the pharmacokinetic characteristics of individual compounds will, to a large extent, dictate the optimal dose schedule. Clorazepate (which has desmethyldiazepam as its active metabolite) and diazepam both have very fast absorption rates after oral administration, so that antianxiety effects may be expected within ½ hour. These would be useful drugs to administer if an antianxiety agent were required just prior to initiating a dental procedure.

Although a single dose of diazepam may appear to have a short duration of action, it should be kept in mind that this result is in large part due to rapid and extensive distribution to fat tissue. The elimination half-life of diazepam is really quite long, and the patient should be cautioned as to the possibility of residual drug effect. A similar warning might be appropriate for any of the benzodiazepines that are converted to long-acting metabolites. For these benzodiazepines, a rational regimen might be to administer the compound prior to bedtime on the night before the dental procedure. This would offer at least two advantages: (1) a good night's sleep and (2) a "therapeutic" hangover of antianxiety effect in the morning. The use of benzodiazepines specifically promoted as hypnotics (i.e., flurazepam and temazepam) might be considered for those patients who complain of sleep irregularities prior to their dental appointment.

Benzodiazepines that are classified as short to intermediate acting in Table 13-2, such as oxazepam and lorazepam, might be the agents of choice in elderly patients or in patients with liver disease, because they do not require hepatic biotransformation before elimination. However, the onset of antianxiety effect is slower than with diazepam, and, therefore, these drugs would need to be administered 2 to 3 hours before dental surgery. Prazepam also requires several hours for antianxiety activity to begin. This is due to its slow absorption, and conversion to desmethyldiazepam. Peak plasma concentrations of the active metabolites are achieved after about 6 hours.[19]

Chlordiazepoxide, the oldest benzodiazepine used clinically, enjoys a pharmacologic profile similar to that of diazepam but has a slightly longer onset time. When allowances are made for this delay, it proves to be an excellent antianxiety agent. Chlordiazepoxide should still be considered for dental procedures because the availability of this compound in "generic" form offers the choice of an inexpensive benzodiazepine, which may indeed be a factor in some cases.

Table 13-3 lists preparations and dosages appropriate for mild to moderate anxiety. The doses indicated should be viewed only as guidelines, each patient will require individualized treatment, and the minimum effective dose should be administered.

Implications in dentistry

The primary concern of the dentist in using an antianxiety agent should be the CNS depression caused by the drug, either alone or when combined with other CNS depressants that the dentist may plan to give or that the patient may already have taken. The antianxiety agents have additive effects with other CNS depressants, such as the anesthetics, antipsychotics, antidepressants, opioid analgesics, sedatives, and particularly alcohol. (Alcohol appears to enhance the absorption of diazepam by a factor of nearly 2.[24]) Respiratory depression is the most serious consequence of the addition of a CNS depressant. The patient should be reminded that antihistamines, even the small amounts con-

Table 13-3. Preparations for the treatment of anxiety

Drug	Usual dose* (mg)	Route of administration
Alprazolam	0.75-1.5 (adult)	Oral
	0.5-0.75 (elderly)	Oral
Clordiazepoxide	15-100 (adult)	Oral
	50-100 (adult)	IM, IV
	10-20 (elderly)	Oral
	10-20 (children 6-10 years old)†	Oral
Clorazepate	15-60 (adult)	Oral
	7.5-15 (elderly)	Oral
	15 (children 9-12 years old)†	Oral
Diazepam	4-40 (adult)	Oral
	2-10 (adult)	IM, IV
	2-5 (elderly)	Oral
	3-10 (children 6 months and over)	Oral
Halazepam	60-160 (adult)	Oral
	20-40 (elderly)	Oral
Lorazepam	2-6 (adult)	Oral
	1-2 (elderly)	Oral
	2-4 (adult)	IM, IV
Oxazepam	30-120 (adult)	Oral
	30 (elderly)	Oral
Prazepam	20-40 (adult)	Oral
	10-15 (elderly)	Oral
Hydroxyzine hydrochloride	75-400 (adult)	Oral
	25-100 (adult)	IM
	50-100 (children over 6 years old)	Oral
	0.6-1.1 mg/kg (children)	IM
Hydroxyzine-pamoate‡	75-400 (adult)	Oral
	50-100 (children over 6 years old)	Oral
Meprobamate	1200-1600 (adult)	Oral
	200-600 (children 6-12 years old)	Oral

*Oral doses represent daily amounts given in divided doses. Parenteral doses reflect single administrations.

†Dosage not established in children under the age group shown.

‡The pamoate salt is reported to be converted to the hydrochloride salt in the stomach, with a resultant prolonged effect, but there is no experimental evidence to support this claim.

tained in OTC preparations promoted as cold remedies or for the treatment of insomnia, may add to the CNS depressant action of the antianxiety agents. The dentist should also caution the patient about the hazards of driving an automobile or operating potentially dangerous machinery up to 24 hours after drug administration.

Other drug interactions with which the dentist should be familiar include the simultaneous use of benzodiazepines and nicotine. Heavy smokers seem somewhat resistant to the CNS depressant properties of the benzodiazepines, and greater than normal doses may be required to obtain the desired degree of sedation or reduction in anxiety. The benzodiazepines have weak anticholinergic properties; thus, diazepam is contraindicated in patients with narrow-angle glaucoma. The anticholinergic action of the benzodiazepines may be additive with other drugs that have anticholinergic activity, such as the antipsychotics, antidepressants, and, obviously, the classic anticholinergic agents. Although xerostomia may be a common complaint with the chronic use of benzodiazepines, considering the short-term clinical use of these drugs by the dentist, it should rarely be a limiting factor and, in fact, may be beneficial for a number of operative procedures. The short-term clinical use of benzodiazepines in dentistry should also eliminate the problem of drug accumulation, since long-term therapy would rarely, if ever, be needed.

Diazepam is perhaps the most popular benzodiazepine used in dentistry. In light of the similarities in pharmacologic profile of the benzodiazepines, the reason for this is difficult to explain. It should be noted, however, that diazepam may be the agent of choice for the control of seizures caused by an overdose of local anesthetics,[10,31] and it depresses the gag reflex.[14] The more recently introduced benzodiazepines are said to be as effective as diazepam in the treatment of anxiety but have fewer side effects.[8] Undoubtedly, the trend over the next several years will be the development of benzodiazepines with greater selectivity with respect to their antianxiety, anticonvulsant, sedative, and muscle relaxant properties.

Although the benzodiazepines are the most popular of the currently available antianxiety agents, by no means does this imply that they are always the agents of choice. Patients who are sensitive to the benzodiazepines may be effectively relaxed and calmed by ethanol or hydroxyzine. Many clinicians consider ethanol or the antihistamine diphenhydramine as agents of choice for the treatment of anxiety in the elderly. The anticholinergic properties of hydroxyzine cause marked reduction in salivary flow, which makes this a particularly useful drug for dentistry. Higher doses of hydroxyzine also produce some degree of muscle relaxation, which is also often beneficial in dental procedures. The possibility of teratogenic effects of hydroxyzine, benzodiazepines, and meprobamate, though slight, precludes the use of all of these drugs in the pregnant patient, particularly during the first trimester. The antihistamines are an excellent choice for those patients who have tendencies to abuse psychoactive drugs. Hydroxyzine might also be considered in cases of severe pain in which morphine is being used. This combination may produce greater analgesia than either drug alone,[4] and the dose of each may therefore be reduced accordingly.

The sedative-hypnotics should not be totally overlooked as antianxiety agents because, as mentioned earlier, any sedative-hypnotic may relieve fear and apprehension in a high enough dose. Meprobamate might be used in those rare instances of hypersensitivity to the benzodiazepines, but its abuse potential, tendency to interact with other drugs, and limited efficacy as an antianxiety agent weigh against it in most cases. Pentobarbital and phenobarbital are inexpensive and often well-tolerated choices for relief of anxiety. Because of their respiratory depressant effects, however, the barbiturates are contraindicated in patients who suffer from asthma or other respiratory difficulties. The troublesome interactions of the barbiturates with other drugs, due to barbiturate stimulation of hepatic microsomal enzyme activity, also restricts their use. Administration of barbiturates as antianxiety agents may be indicated if the patient need not remain alert. Chloral hydrate is an excellent choice for the treatment of unmanageable children. This drug will be discussed in greater detail in Chapter 14.

The variety of factors that govern the choice of an antianxiety agent is endless. This section has attempted to illustrate some of the more important determinants of which the dentist should be cognizant when making his selection. In practice, the dentist should become familiar and comfortable with a limited number of antianxiety drugs and select from these according to the pharmacology of the drugs, the particular treatment to be rendered, and the needs of the patient. The obvious potential for the development of more specific antianxiety benzodiazepines should serve as a stimulus for the practicing dentist to stay current in the field of antianxiety medication. A knowledge of the pharmacologic profile of the benzodiazepines may also prevent the dentist from being misled by dubious claims of specificity for newly introduced benzodiazepines.

CENTRALLY ACTING MUSCLE RELAXANTS*

Certain conditions of skeletal muscle, such as muscle spasms or trismus, are believed to be the result of disturbed influences of the motor areas of the central nervous system on skeletal muscle. Drugs that could prevent or lessen these neurotropic influences on voluntary muscle would be extremely helpful in physical medicine and dentistry. The centrally acting muscle relaxants supposedly represent such a group of drugs, acting to diminish the tonic flow of nerve impulses to voluntary muscle. Although mephenesin and similar drugs have been shown to reduce polysynaptic spinal reflexes in experimental animals, in humans these drugs act primarily as mild sedatives and are never employed at doses that could cause flaccid paralysis of voluntary muscles.

Centrally acting muscle relaxants should be clearly distinguished from several other classes of agents that can reduce muscular activity. The neuromuscular blocking agents, such as tubocurarine and succinylcholine, act by blocking synaptic transmission at the neuromuscular junction. Dantrolene has been introduced as a peripherally acting muscle relaxant and is thought to block normal excitation-contraction coupling steps within the muscle[34] (Chapter 11). Baclofen, an analogue of the central inhibitory transmitter GABA, inhibits motor tone by an unknown mechanism.[2] These last two drugs are being investigated for treatment of spastic paralysis. None of these agents, however, is indicated in the treatment of skeletal muscle spasms.

Chemistry

The chemical structures of agents having centrally acting muscle relaxing properties vary, but groups of structurally similar compounds can be distinguished, as shown in Figure 13-4. In 1945, the muscle relaxant effects of aryl-glycerol esters in experimental animals were observed, and after evaluation of several analogues mephenesin was introduced for clinical use in 1948.[54] Mephenesin proved to be of limited usefulness because of its short duration of action. Carbamate esters of glycerol, exemplified by methocarbamol and chlorphenesin carbamate, had a more prolonged duration of action because of slow metabolic transformation and excretion. Meprobamate, tybamate, and ca-

---

*This section was written by Vahn A. Lewis.

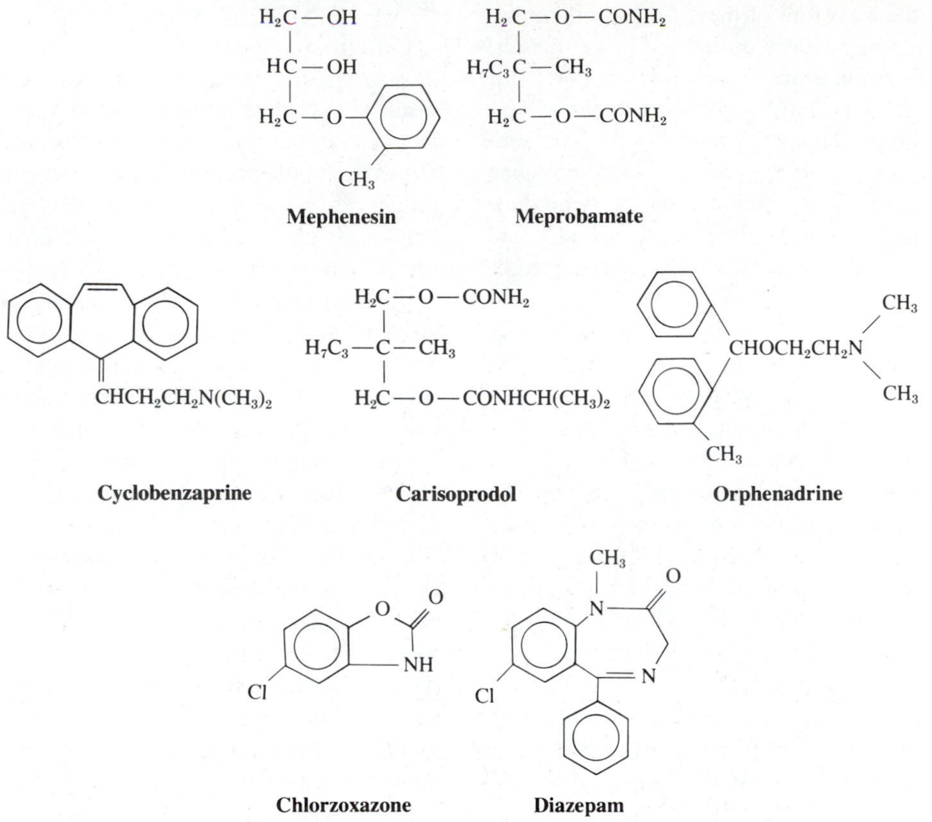

Figure 13-4. Structural formulas of some centrally acting muscle relaxants.

risoprodol are dicarbamate esters of glycerol; with the last two having additional substituents to increase their potency and absorption. Metaxalone and chlorzoxazone are heterocyclic carbamates that demonstrate muscle relaxing properties. Significantly different from the above glycerol derivatives, orphenadrine is an analogue of the antihistamine diphenhydramine. Cyclobenzaprine is a recent addition to the centrally acting muscle relaxant drugs and is a close structural analogue of the antidepressant amitriptyline. The benzodiazepines, while structurally different from muscle relaxants of the mephenesin type, have clinical actions that are in many ways parallel. Baclofen is the *p*-chlorophenyl analogue of GABA.

Pharmacologic effects

The pharmacologic effects of the mephenesin-like centrally acting muscle relaxants will be considered separately from those of the nonmephenesin group.

Mephenesin-like. The centrally acting muscle relaxants, of which mephenesin will be taken as the prototype, cause relaxation of voluntary muscle through a depressant action on the central nervous system. These depressant effects have not been associated with an action on any specific transmitter system or neurologic circuit. Rather, alteration of the excitability of neural membranes in general may be involved. Although early investigations emphasized depression of spinal interneurons as the site of action, these agents generally reduce neural activity in a variety of brain structures including the brain stem, thalamus, and basal ganglia. Furthermore, certain agents that do not produce muscle relaxation also show some preferential depression of polysynaptic reflexes; thus, depression of interneurons is not an identifying characteristic of this class.[15] At progressively larger doses sedation, hypnosis, unconsciousness, and death occur. Elevation of the convulsant threshold can be demonstrated. Table 13-4 compares some

Table 13-4. Pharmacologic comparison of centrally acting muscle relaxants, sedative-hypnotics, antianxiety drugs, and antihistamines

Pharmacologic properties	*Centrally acting muscle relaxants (prototype mepehenesin)*	*Sedative-hypnotics (prototype phenobarbital)*	*Antianxiety drugs (prototype diazepam)*	*Antihistamines (prototype diphenhydramine)*
Anticholinergic properties	No	No	Mild	Yes
Antihistaminic properties	No	No	No	Yes
Paradoxical low-dose excitement	Yes	Yes	Yes	No
Ataxia	Yes	Yes	Yes	No
Anesthesia	Yes	Yes	Variable	No
Arousal at high doses	Difficult	Difficult	Difficult	Easy
Lethal effect	Respiratory depression	Respiratory depression	Respiratory depression	Convulsions
Convulsant threshold	Raised	Raised	Raised	Lowered
Dependence-liability	Yes, but usually mild	Yes	Yes, but usually mild	No

pharmacologic characteristics of classes of drugs used for skeletal muscle relaxation. Qualitatively, sedative-hypnotics, centrally acting muscle relaxants, and antianxiety drugs are similar pharmacologically, while the antihistamines (and orphenadrine) produce sedation that is qualitatively different.

The cardiovascular effects of sedative doses of the centrally acting muscle relaxants of the mephenesin type are minimal. Adequate cardiovascular performance is usually maintained at doses higher than those that produce respiratory depression. The problems of shock and renal failure can complicate recovery from toxic doses of these agents, however.

Nonmephenesin-like. The pharmacology of orphenadrine citrate, an antihistamine analogue, differs from that of compounds similar to mephenesin. Conventional antihistamines, in addition to blocking histamine$_1$ receptors, are frequently anticholinergic and produce drowsiness and sedation. This sedation is of a different character than that produced by mephenesin-like drugs; increasing the dose leads to hallucinations, delusions, and convulsions. Nevertheless, because the dose-response curve for antihistamines is rather flat, these drugs have been considered relatively safe and have been widely used in OTC sleep aids for this reason. Physical dependence liability is also minimal. Orphenadrine has been employed primarily as an adjunct in the treatment of parkinsonism. Compared with the mephenesin group of drugs, no special advantage has been demonstrated for orphenadrine as a muscle relaxant.

Cyclobenzaprine, a structural and pharmacolog-

ic analogue of the tricyclic antidepressants, is used for the short-term (2 to 3 weeks) treatment of muscle spasm associated with acute painful musculoskeletal conditions. One hypothesis for its mechanism of action is that it increases brainstem norepinephrine-mediated inhibition of ventral motor neurons of the spinal cord. Its efficacy is similar to that of diazepam, but it produces more xerostomia, drowsiness, tachycardia, and dizziness. Many tricyclic antidepressants have significant antihistaminic effects, and the general pharmacologic properties of cyclobenzaprine are similar to those shown in Table 13-4 for the antihistamines.[13]

Although a considerable number of agents are available as centrally acting muscle relaxants, the agent of choice for many muscular problems is diazepam or another long-acting benzodiazepine.[45] Benzodiazepines, while tending to have more sedative properties than some of the agents classified as centrally acting muscle relaxants, are equal or better in their muscle-relaxing properties,[20] are low in toxicity,[42] have few side effects, and have a low physical dependence liability.

Toxic reactions and side effects

Muscle relaxants are used at sedative doses, and only when administered at concentrations several times greater will they produce ataxia and flaccid paralysis. Data obtained from experimental animals compare the relative safety of some commonly prescribed muscle relaxants (Table 13-5).[5,20] Doubling the dose of phenobarbital needed to produce ataxia results in death. With diazepam, lethality occurs at 20 times the ataxic dose, thus making diazepam a much safer drug for these pur-

Table 13-5. Comparison of the paralyzing and lethal doses of central depressant drugs in mice

Agent	LD50 (mg/kg)	Ataxia ED50 (mg/kg)	Therapeutic index
Phenobarbital	242	120	2.0
Mephenesin	610	178	3.4
Meprobamate	800	235	3.4
Carisoprodol	980	165	5.9
Chlordiazepoxide	720	100	7.2
Diazepam	620	30	20.7

poses. The clinically useful muscle relaxants have therapeutic indexes in between these extremes.

Tolerance and physical dependence develop with the chronic administration of muscle relaxants, but in general withdrawal is mild although qualitatively similar to that seen with other CNS depressant drugs.

Side effects associated with centrally acting muscle relaxants are primarily related to effects on the central nervous system: drowsiness, dizziness, headache, blurred vision, ataxia, lethargy, paradoxical excitement, and nystagmus. Gastrointestinal symptoms such as vomiting, heartburn, nausea, anorexia, and abdominal distress have been reported. Allergic reactions may also occur and include skin rash, pruritus, fever, and hair loss or color change.[15,54] Several animal studies have implicated diazepam, chlordiazepoxide, and meprobamate as being teratogenic or mutagenic, so the benefit-to-risk ratio should be carefully weighed for use of these agents in women of childbearing age. In addition, meprobamate has been shown to cross the placental barrier and to be excreted in the milk of lactating mothers at 2 to 4 times the maternal plasma concentration. Cyclobenzaprine, because of its actions on the autonomic nervous system, has some additional side effects. Since it has anticholinergic properties, its use should be avoided in conditions such as narrow-angle glaucoma and prostate hypertrophy. Because of its effect on norepinephrine reuptake, cyclobenzaprine may also be contraindicated in patients for whom increased sympathetic activity is to be avoided, as for instance those with hyperthyroidism or recovering from a myocardial infarction.

Drug interactions with the centrally acting muscle relaxants are of several kinds. First, these drugs potentiate the depressant actions of opioids, sedative-hypnotics, antianxiety drugs, antihistamines, and antidepressants. Second, drug interactions can occur when these agents induce drug- and hormone-metabolizing enzymes of the liver. For this reason, centrally acting muscle relaxants should be used with caution in patients taking anticoagulants and in those with the metabolic disorder porphyria. Third, increased skeletal muscle relaxation should be expected when the centrally acting muscle relaxants are given together with drugs whose primary pharmacologic activity is neuromuscular blockade (e.g., succinylcholine) or with drugs that have such an activity as a side effect (e.g., the aminoglycosides or certain general anesthetics). Fourth, cyclobenzaprine should not be given to patients taking MAO inhibitors or guanethidine and related drugs.

General therapeutic uses

Centrally acting muscle relaxants are used medically as adjuncts to rest, physical therapy, and other measures for the relief of discomfort associated with acute, painful musculoskeletal conditions. They have been promoted for use in skeletal muscle spasms of local origin, multiple sclerosis, cerebral palsy, sprains, strains, fibrositis, rheumatoid spondylitis, bursitis, and arthritis. Drugs such as salicylates and adrenal corticosteroids may be used concomitantly.

Uses in dentistry

Centrally acting muscle relaxants may be valuable agents for some dental procedures. Diazepam is generally preferred because of its good muscle-relaxing properties and its safety. It has been found to reduce postprocedural trismus and may be used as an adjunct for treating muscle spasms of the head and neck, as in the temporomandibular joint (TMJ) syndrome.[27,45] However, the etiology of TMJ pain is complex, involving interactions between patient anxiety, muscle spasms, occlusal problems, and joint dysfunction.[33] The efficacy of therapy with centrally acting muscle relaxants will be greater if the dysfunction is primarily due to anxiety or muscle spasm. Since the relationship between CNS activity and peripheral muscle tone is poorly understood, it is unlikely that the centrally acting muscle relaxants will produce either consistent or predictable results. There still exists a paucity of double-blind studies that demonstrate the efficacy of such treatment; the one thing that is clear from such studies is that the placebo cure rate is high.[21]

While combinations of centrally acting muscle relaxants and analgesic drugs may be valuable, fixed-dose combinations may provide suboptimal doses of analgesic. Prescribing full therapeutic doses of each agent is superior therapy, if the use of a combination is indicated. It should be noted that these agents are not primary treatment for every type of facial pain. Trigeminal neuralgia (tic douloureux) and pain of Bell's palsy require specific therapies.

Antianxiety agents

Nonproprietary name	Proprietary name
Benzodiazepines	
alprazolam	Xanax
chlordiazepoxide	Librium
clorazepate	Tranxene
diazepam	Valium
halazepam	Paxipam
lorazepam	Ativan
oxazepam	Serax
prazepam	Centrax
triazolam	Halcion
Diphenylmethane antihistamines	
hydroxyzine hydrochloride	Atarax
hydroxyzine pamoate	Vistaril
Propanediol carbamates	
meprobamate	Equanil, Miltown
tybamate*	Tybatran

Muscle relaxants

Nonproprietary name	Proprietary name
Mephenesin-like	
carisoprodol	Soma, Rela
chlorphenesin carbamate	Maolate
chlorzoxazone	Paraflex
mephenesin*	—
meprobamate	Miltown, Equanil
metaxalone	Skelaxin
methocarbamol	Robaxin
tybamate*	Tybatran
Benzodiazepines	
diazepam	Valium
Miscellaneous	
baclofen	Lioresal
cyclobenzaprine	Flexeril
dantrolene	Dantrium
orphenadrine	Norflex

*Not available in the United States

CITED REFERENCES

1. Arrigo, A., Jann, G., and Tonali, P. Some aspects of the action of Valium and of Librium on the electrical activity of the rabbit brain. Archives Internationales de Pharmacodynamie et de Therapie **154**:364-373, 1965.
2. Baclofen in spasticity. Lancet **2**:594-595, 1977.
3. Baird, E.S., and Curson, I. Orally administered diazepam in conservative dentistry: a double-blind trial. British Dental Journal **128**:25-27, 1970.
4. Bellville, J.W., Dorey, F., Capparell, D., Knox, V., and Bauer, R.O. Analgesic effect of hydroxyzine compared to morphine in man. Journal of Clinical Pharmacology **19**:290-296, 1979.
5. Berger, F.M. The muscle relaxant and analgesic properties of carisoprodol. In Miller, J.G., ed. The Pharmacology and Clinical Usefulness of Carisoprodol. Detroit, Wayne State University Press, 1959.
6. Berger, F.M. The pharmacological properties of 2-methyl-2-n-propyl-1,3-propanediol dicarbamate (Miltown), a new interneuronal blocking agent. Journal of Pharmacology and Experimental Therapeutics **112**:413-423, 1954.
7. Campbell, J.L., Sherman, A.D., and Petty, F. Diazepam anxiolytic activity in hippocampus. Communications in Psychopharmacology **4**:387-392, 1980.
8. Cooper, A.J., Magnus, R.V., Rose, M., Phanjoo, A., Lancaster, N.P., Pollard, P., and Knowlson, P. Controlled trial of dipotassium clorazepate (Tranxene) in anxiety. British Journal of Psychiatry **123**:475-476, 1973.
9. Crankshaw, D.P., and Raper, C. Mephenesin, methocarbamol, chlordiazepoxide, and diazepam: actions on spinal reflexes and ventral root potentials. British Journal of Pharmacology **38**:148-156, 1970.
10. de Jong, R.H., and Heavner, J.E. Local anesthetic seizure prevention; diazepam versus pentobarbital. Anesthesiology **36**:449-457, 1972.
11. Dental Practitioner Research Unit. Oxazepam before dental treatment. British Journal of Clinical Practice **24**:323-326, 1970.
12. DeSalva, S.J., and Ercoli, N. Differential action of styramate and meprobamate on spinal reflexes. Proceedings of the Society for Experimental Biology and Medicine **101**:250-252, 1959.
13. Flexeril—a new muscle relaxant. Medical Letter on Drugs and Therapeutics **20**:12, 1978.
14. Foreman, P.A. Control of anxiety/pain complex in dentistry: intravenous psychosedation with techniques using diazepam. Oral Surgery, Oral Medicine, and Oral Pathology **37**:337-349, 1974.
15. Franz, D.N. Centrally acting muscle relaxants. In Goodman, L.S., and Gilman, A., eds. The Pharmacological Basis of Therapeutics, ed. 5. New York, Macmillan, Inc., 1975.
16. Gallagher, D.W. Benzodiazepines: potentiation of a GABA inhibitory response in the dorsal raphe nucleus. European Journal of Pharmacology **49**:133-143, 1978.
17. Gavish, M., and Snyder, S.H. Soluble benzodiazepine receptors: GABA-ergic regulation. Life Sciences **26**:579-582, 1980.
18. Grant, G.H. Chlordiazepoxide used for apprehensive dental patients: preliminary observations. Journal of the American Dental Association **66**:182-185, 1963.

19. Greenblatt, D.J. Benzodiazepines 1980: current update: pharmacokinetic comparisons. Psychosomatics 21(Suppl): 9-16, 1980.

20. Greenblatt, D.J., and Shader, R.I., eds. Benzodiazepines in Clinical Practice. New York, Raven Press, 1974.

21. Greenblatt, D.J., and Shader, R.I. Meprobamate: a study of irrational drug use. American Journal of Psychiatry 127:1297-1303, 1971.

22. Greenblatt, D.J., Shader, R.I., Divoll, M., and Harmatz, J.S. Benzodiazepines: a summary of pharmacokinetic properties. British Journal of Clinical Pharmacology 11:11S-16S, 1981.

23. Haefely, W., Kulcsar, A., Mohler, H., Pieri, L., Polc, P., and Schaffner, R. Possible involvement of GABA in the central actions of benzodiazepines. Advances in Biochemical Psychopharmacology 14:131-151, 1965.

24. Hayes, S.L., Pablo, G., Radomski, T., and Palmer, R.F. Ethanol and oral diazepam absorption. New England Journal of Medicine 296:186-189, 1977.

25. Healy, T.E.J., Robinson, J.S., and Vickers, M.D. Physiological responses to intravenous diazepam as a sedative for conservative dentistry. British Medical Journal 3:10-13, 1970.

26. Hegarty, J.E., and Dundee, J.W. Sequelae after the intravenous injection of three benzodiazepines—diazepam, lorazepam, and flunitrazepam. British Medical Journal 2:1384-1385, 1977.

27. Libman, R.H. Pharmacology of sedatives for outpatient dentistry. Anesthesia Progress 23:144-149, 1976.

28. Lippa, A.S., Critchett, D., Sano, M.C., Klepner, C.A., Greenblatt, E.N., Coupet, J., and Beer, B. Benzodiazepine receptors, cellular and behavioral characteristics. Pharmacology, Biochemistry and Behavior 10:831-843, 1979.

29. Möhler, H., and Okada, T. Benzodiazepine receptor: demonstration in the central nervous system. Science 198:849-851, 1977.

30. Morillo, A. Effects of benzodiazepines upon amygdala and hippocampus of the cat. International Journal of Neuropharmacology 1:353-359, 1962.

31. Munson, E.S., and Wagman, I.H. Diazepam treatment of local anesthetic-induced seizures. Anesthesiology 37:523-528, 1972.

32. Olds, M.E., and Olds, J. Effects of anxiety-relieving drugs on unit discharges in hippocampus, reticular midbrain, and pre-optic area in the freely moving rat. International Journal of Neuropharmacology 8:87-103, 1969.

33. Pagonis, E. Current knowledge associated with temporomandibular joint syndrome. Ohio State Medical Journal 73:220-221, 1977.

34. Pinder, R.M., Brogden, R.N., Speight, T.M., and Avery, G.S. Dantrolene sodium: a review of its pharmacological properties and therapeutic efficacy in spasticity. Drugs 13:3-23, 1977.

35. Randall, L.O., Heise, G.A., Schallek, W., Bagdon, R.E., Banziger, R., Boris, A., Moe, R.A., and Abrams, W.B. Pharmacological and clinical studies on Valium, a new psychotherapeutic agent of the benzodiazepine class. Current Therapeutic Research 3:405-425, 1961.

36. Rao, S., Sherbaniuk, R.W., Prasad, K., Lee, S.J.K., and Sproule, B.J. Cardiopulmonary effects of diazepam. Clinical Pharmacology and Therapeutics 14:182-189, 1973.

37. Rees, M., and Dormandy, J. Accidental intra-arterial injection of diazepam. British Medical Journal 281:289-290, 1980.

38. Reggiani, G., Hurlimann, A., and Theiss, E. Some aspects of the experimental and clinical toxicity of chlordiazepoxide. In Baker, S.B.C., Bossier, J.R., and Koll, W., eds. Toxicity and Side Effects of Psychotropic Drugs, vol. 9, Proceedings of the European Society for the Study of Drug Toxicity. Amsterdam, Excerpta Medica Foundation, 1967.

39. Schallek, W., Kuehn, A., and Jew, N. Effects of chlordiazepoxide (Librium) and other psychotropic agents on the limbic system of the brain. Annals of the New York Academy of Sciences 96:303-314, 1962.

40. Schmidt, R.F., Vogel, E., and Zimmerman, M. Die Wirkung von Diazepam auf de präsynaptische Hemmung und andere Rückenmarksreflexe. Naunyn Schmiedebergs Archiv für Pharmakologie und Experimentelle Pathologie 258:69-82, 1967.

41. Shader, R.I., and Greenblatt, D.J. Clinical implications of benzodiazepine pharmacokinetics. American Journal of Psychiatry 134:652-656, 1977.

42. Shader, R.I., Greenblatt, D.J., Salzman, L., Kochansky, G.E., and Hartzman, A.B. Benzodiazepines: safety and toxicity. Diseases of the Nervous System 36:23-26, 1975.

43. Sinha, J.N., Dixit, K.S., Srimal, R.C., and Bhargava, K.P. Central muscle relaxant activity of a dozen CNS active agents and a correlation with their psychotropic activity. Japanese Journal of Pharmacology 18:48-53, 1968.

44. Snyder, S.H., and Enna, S.J. The role of central glycine receptors in the pharmacologic actions of benzodiazepines. Advances in Biochemical Psychopharmacology 14:81-91, 1975.

45. Somers, N. An approach to the management of temporomandibular joint dysfunction. Australian Dental Journal 23:37-41, 1978.

46. Speth, R.C., Wastek, G.J., Johnson, P.C., and Yamamura, H.I. Benzodiazepine binding in human brain: characterization using 3H-flunitrazepam. Life Science 22:859-866, 1978.

47. Squires, R., and Braestrup, C. Benzodiazepine receptors in rat brain. Nature 266:732, 1977.

48. Steen, S.N., and Martinez, L.R. Some pharmacologic effects of intravenous chlordiazepoxide. Clinical Pharmacology and Therapeutics 5:44-48, 1964.

49. Stein, L., Wise, C.D., and Berger, B.D. Antianxiety action of benzodiazepines: decrease in activity of serotonin neurons in the punishment system. In Garattini, S., Mussini, E., and Randall, L.O., eds. The Benzodiazepines. New York, Raven Press, 1973.

50. Steiner, F.A., and Hummell, P. Modification of spontaneous and evoked activity of hippocampal and lateral geniculate neurons by nitrazepam and phenobarbital. Electroencephalography and Clinical Neurophysiology 27:105, 1969.

51. Study, R.E., and Barker, J.L. Cellular mechanisms of benzodiazepine action. Journal of the American Medical Association 247:2147-2151, 1982.

52. Tseng, T., Przybyla, A.C., Chen, S.T., and Wang, S.C. Locus of central depressant action of tybamate. Neuropharmacology 9:211-218, 1970.

53. Unnerstall, J.R., Kuhar, M.J., Niehoff, D.L., and Palacios, J.M. Benzodiazepine receptors are coupled to a sub-

population of gamma-aminobutyric acid (GABA) receptors: evidence from a quantitative autoradiographic study. Journal of Pharmacology and Experimental Therapeutics **218:**797-804, 1981.

54. van Dijl, W. Muscle relaxant drugs. In Meyler, L., and Herxheimer, A., eds. Side Effects of Drugs, vol. 6. Baltimore, The Williams & Wilkins Co., 1968.

55. Whitelaw, A.G.L., Cummings, A.J., and McFayden, I.R. Effect of maternal lorazepam on the neonate. British Medical Journal **282:**1106-1108, 1981.

56. Williams, E.F., Rice, K.C., Paul, S.M., and Skolnick, P. Heterogeneity of benzodiazepine receptors in the central nervous system demonstrated with kenazepine, an alkylating benzodiazepine. Journal of Neurochemistry **35:**591-597, 1980.

57. Young, A.B., Zukin, S.R., and Snyder, S.H. Interaction of benzodiazepines with central nervous glycine receptors: possible mechanism of action. Proceedings of the National Academy of Sciences of the United States of America **71:**2246-2250, 1974.

GENERAL REFERENCES

Accepted Dental Therapeutics, ed. 39. Chicago, American Dental Association, 1982.

Baldessarini, R.J. Chemotherapy in Psychiatry. Cambridge, Harvard University Press, 1977.

Bloom, F.E. Neural mechanisms of benzodiazepine actions. American Journal of Psychiatry **134:**669-672, 1977.

Garattini, S., Mussini, E., and Randall, L.O., eds. The Benzodiazepines. New York, Raven Press, 1973.

Gilman, A.G., Goodman, L.S., and Gilman, A., eds. Goodman and Gilman's The Pharmacological Basis of Therapeutics, ed. 6. New York, MacMillan Publishing Co., 1980.

Greenblatt, D.J., and Shader, R.I. Benzodiazepines in Clinical Practice. New York, Raven Press, 1974.

Valzelli, L. Psychopharmacology. Flushing, New York, Spectrum Publications, 1973.

14 Sedative-hypnotics and central nervous system stimulants

Leslie P. Felpel

SEDATIVE-HYPNOTICS

The sedative-hypnotics compose a class of drugs that are used to produce varying degrees of CNS depression. As sedatives, these drugs produce drowsiness, relaxation, calmness, and decreased motor activity with no loss of consciousness. As hypnotics, they produce a state of unconsciousness that is similar, but not identical, to natural sleep. They also produce decreased motor activity and impaired, but not abolished, sensory responsiveness. The degree of CNS depression produced by the sedative-hypnotics is strongly dose dependent, and theoretically any CNS depressant could act either as a sedative or a hypnotic, depending on the dose administered. Practically speaking, however, not all CNS depressants can be used as sedative-hypnotics. For example, CNS depressants such as the general anesthetics would obviously not be useful sedative-hypnotics on an outpatient basis. The barbiturates are the classic sedative-hypnotics, but they have been replaced to a large extent by the benzodiazepines. Some of the advantages of the benzodiazepines over the barbiturates are (1) greater relative safety; (2) less additive effect when combined with other CNS depressants, especially ethanol; (3) slower development of tolerance and physical dependence; (4) minimal induction of hepatic enzyme activity; (5) fewer drug interactions; and (6) minimal effect on rapid-eye-movement (REM) sleep. The pharmacology of the benzodiazepines does not differ whether they are used as antianxiety agents or as sedative-hypnotics and is discussed in detail in Chapter 13. For this reason, the pharmacology of the barbiturates will be emphasized in this chapter, whereas the pharmacology of the benzodiazepines will be discussed as it relates to their use as hypnotics.

In practice, the major indication for the use of hypnotics is in the treatment of insomnia. The sedative-hypnotics are administered preoperatively in dentistry to relax and calm the anxious patient and to sedate and facilitate sleep in the pre- and postoperative patient. Such uses would suggest that the sedative-hypnotics are antianxiety agents, as indeed they are. The barbiturates were at one time the only drugs available for the treatment of anxiety, but their use for this purpose has declined with the introduction of the benzodiazepines. In fact, the greater margin of safety afforded by the benzodiazepines has led many clinicians to suggest that the older sedative-hypnotics are obsolete and should be restricted solely to the treatment of insomnia. There was a 40% decrease in the number of prescriptions written for hypnotic drugs during the 1970s, with the benzodiazepines accounting for approximately 50% of the total written. During this same period of time, there has been a 50% decline in barbiturate-related suicides. While this overall pattern certainly indicates a declining use of the barbiturates, it should be noted that the philosophy for the treatment of insomnia has changed from the casual prescribing of hypnotics to a more thoughtful and careful exploration and elimination, if possible, of the cause of the individual's insomnia. Evidence from sleep laboratories has shed new light on the physiologic role and mechanisms of sleep and, further, has dismissed some of the faulty, preconceived ideas about sleep. For example, every individual does not require 8 hours of sleep; many patients who complain of insomnia do not, in fact, suffer from it; sleep patterns, even in the normal individual, sometimes fluctuate; and frequently psychologic rather than pharmacologic intervention is the more rational and beneficial therapy.

Despite the overall declining use of barbiturate

drugs, there are several reasons why the dentist may still wish to prescribe them. They are, for instance, relatively inexpensive when compared to the nonbarbiturate sedative-hypnotics, particularly the benzodiazepines. They are also convenient to administer, and a wide range in duration of effect can readily be attained depending on the drug prescribed. Finally, the clinician may feel more comfortable using drugs for which a wealth of scientific and clinical literature exists. Such information allows the practitioner to make a more rational decision as to the type and quantity of drug to prescribe for a given clinical condition, what side effects might be expected, and what precautions to take in the use of a given drug.

For purposes of classification, the sedative-hypnotic drugs may be categorized as either barbiturates or nonbarbiturates. With the exception of the benzodiazepines, the nonbarbiturate sedative-hypnotics offer no advantages over the barbiturates. As will be discussed, all the nonbarbiturate sedative-hypnotics have abuse potential, can be addictive, depress the central nervous system, and may be more troublesome than the barbiturates when overdose occurs. Due to the widespread use of the sedative-hypnotics, the clinician would be wise to become experienced in the clinical use of the benzodiazepines and not more than two or three of the barbiturates, to prescribe sedative-hypnotics in rare instances in which acute insomnia is detrimental to the patient, and to prescribe or administer the sedative-hypnotic with which he feels most comfortable and that has the best therapeutic index for a given clinical condition.

Barbiturates

Chemistry and structure-activity relationships. Barbituric acid, which lacks CNS depressant properties, is formed by the condensation of urea and malonic acid, as illustrated in Figure 14-1. In order to obtain barbiturates that have CNS depressant properties, both hydrogens at C_5 must be replaced by organic groups. Depending on the substituents added, three types of barbiturates are formed (Table 14-1). In the first group, substitutions are made only at C_5, and, in general, increasing the chain length (up to a point) of these substituent groups (1) increases hypnotic activity, (2) decreases the latency of onset, and (3) decreases the duration of effect. If the chain length reaches eight carbon atoms, the drugs become more toxic and assume convulsant properties.

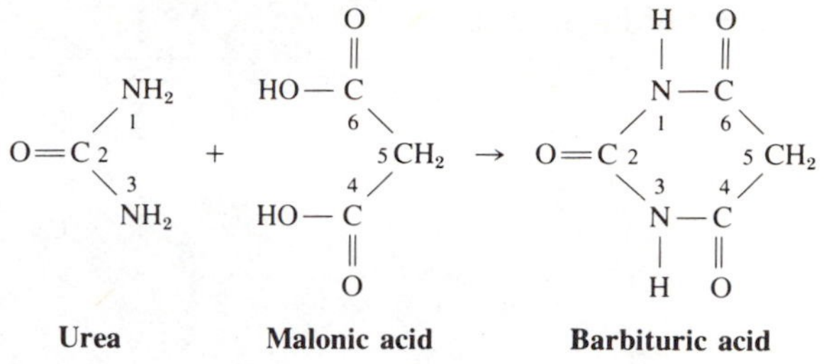

Figure 14-1. Chemical formation of barbituric acid.

A second group of barbiturates results when alkyl groups are substituted at N_3. These agents are commonly referred to as the N-alkyl barbiturates and, with the exception of meprobarbital, are not commonly used.

A third class of barbiturates is produced when the oxygen at C_2 of the barbiturate nucleus is replaced with a sulfur atom. These agents have an extremely short duration of action, are commonly employed as intravenous anesthetics, and are more appropriately discussed in Chapters 19 and 44. Technically, the sulfur-substituted drugs are not truly barbiturates because barbiturates by definition require oxygen at C_2. The sulfur-substituted barbiturates are commonly referred to as the thiobarbiturates, while the true barbiturates are sometimes called oxybarbiturates.

Pharmacologic effects

Central nervous system. As with all sedative hypnotics, the barbiturates produce varying degrees of CNS depression, ranging from mild sedation to death. Many factors contribute to the level of depression attained, for example, the drug used, its dose and route of administration, and the behavioral state as well as the environmental surroundings of the patient at the time of administration. With regard to the last point, it has long been known that the physical environment and the psychologic set of the patient influence the effectiveness of hypnotics and sedatives. Thus, a barbiturate taken prior to retiring in the evening at home is more likely to produce the desired sedative or hypnotic effect than the same drug taken at a rock concert.

The behavioral effects of the barbiturates indicative of general CNS depression include diminished responsiveness to external stimuli and diminished psychologic performance. Subjectively, the patient experiences relaxation, a feeling

Table 14-1. General barbiturate ring structure with examples of the chemical formulas of the three types of barbiturates

$$
\begin{array}{c}
\text{H} \quad\quad \text{O} \\
| \quad\quad\quad \| \\
\text{N} \!\!-\!\! \text{C} \quad\quad \text{R}_1 \\
/\,1 \quad\; 6\,\backslash \quad / \\
\text{R}_x \!\!=\!\! \text{C}\,2 \quad\quad\quad 5\,\text{C} \\
\backslash\,3 \quad\; 4\,/ \quad \backslash \\
\text{N} \!\!-\!\! \text{C} \quad\quad \text{R}_2 \\
| \quad\quad\quad \| \\
\text{R}_3 \quad\quad \text{O}
\end{array}
$$

Generic name	Type	R_1	R_2	R_3	R_x
Pentobarbital	Oxybarbiturate	Ethyl	*l*-Methylbutyl	H	O
Mephobarbital	N-alkylbarbiturate	Ethyl	Phenyl	CH_3	O
Thiopental	Thiobarbiturate	Ethyl	*l*-Methylbutyl	H	S

of well-being, and drowsiness. Coincident with these subjective feelings, the electroencephalogram (EEG) displays an increase in fast activity (25 to 35 Hz), which is commonly referred to as barbiturate activation. As the dose of the barbiturate increases and the patient goes to sleep, the EEG displays an increase in high-amplitude slow waves (2 to 8 Hz) that are similar to those observed during natural sleep. Frequently, these high-amplitude slow waves occur in bursts called spindles. At even higher doses, the EEG record displays occasional periods of electrical silence, which become longer as toxic doses are approached. If toxic doses are achieved, complete electrical silence occurs in the EEG.

Notwithstanding the fact that EEG patterns recorded after the administration of barbiturates are similar to those observed during natural sleep, important differences do occur. For example, during natural sleep, humans as well as lower animals cycle through several stages of sleep, ranging from the deepest stage (stage IV) to the most active stage in which dreaming and rapid eye movements occur (REM sleep). Numerous studies have established that the amount of time that an individual spends in REM sleep is critical, and if the individual is deprived of REM sleep or if the time spent in REM sleep is reduced, the individual will "make-up" or increase the time spent in REM sleep at a subsequent time (REM rebound). Barbiturates have been shown to decrease the amount of time spent in REM sleep, and, as a result, serious questions have been raised as to the true value of the barbiturates in the treatment of insomnia. With the exception of very low doses of both the benzodi-

azepines and chloral hydrate, all sedative-hypnotics reduce REM sleep. Therapeutic doses and continued use of the benzodiazepines reduce stage III, stage IV, and REM sleep, the significance of which is unknown.

Although the barbiturates appear to depress all levels of the central nervous system, a considerable body of scientific evidence suggests that the reticular formation—a complex network of neurons, nuclei, and neural pathways that extends throughout the brainstem from the medulla to the thalamus—is particularly sensitive to the depressant action of the barbiturates.[3,18] The reticular formation and its rostral and thalamocortical projections compose a "system" that is referred to as the ascending reticular activating system (ARAS). The term *ARAS* connotes the effect of this system on the cerebral cortex and the resultant behavioral response to this activity. The importance of the ARAS in the modulation of sleep and wakefulness has long been known. Stimulation of appropriate areas of the reticular formation in a sleeping animal causes behavioral arousal and converts the EEG from the characteristic sleep pattern to that of an awake animal. If the appropriate areas of the reticular formation are experimentally destroyed, the EEG pattern is that characteristic of a drowsy or sleeping animal, and the animal behaviorally appears to be asleep.[20] Though the classical concepts of the ARAS have been challenged in recent years, it is still thought that a major action of the barbiturates is exerted on the reticular formation.

Experimental studies indicate that the barbiturates exert their pharmacologic effects by actions on pre- and postsynaptic elements of the neuronal synapse. Pentobarbital, for example, has been shown to reduce the amount of neurotransmitter released from the presynaptic nerve terminals of the spinal cord[31] and cortex.[24] More recent investigations implicate a selective depressant effect of pentobarbital on excitatory postsynaptic activity.[1] In addition to actions on excitatory transmission, experiments in a variety of animals suggest that the barbiturates affect inhibitory mechanisms. A number of CNS depressants, including the barbiturates and chloral hydrate, prolong spinal presynaptic inhibition[19,28] as well as postsynaptic inhibition.[21,33] Although the significance of these findings is unclear, interaction of barbiturates with the inhibitory neurotransmitter GABA is likely because this amino acid appears to be the transmitter involved with spinal presynaptic inhibition. In vitro studies have demonstrated that phenobarbital increases the time that GABA-activated ionic channels of the membrane are open.[2] However, not all inhibitory synapses may be affected similarly by the barbiturates, since phenobarbital and pentobarbital depress GABA-mediated inhibitory responses in invertebrates.[6] As discussed in Chapter 13, the benzodiazepines are also known to interact with GABA systems, which suggests a common mechanism of action for many sedative-hypnotic drugs.

Cardiovascular system. At sedative doses, the barbiturates do not affect the cardiovascular system. At hypnotic doses, a mild hypotension and decrease in heart rate occur. Progressive depression of the cardiovascular system develops as the dose of barbiturates is increased beyond the hypnotic range.

Respiratory system. Sedative doses of barbiturates have little effect on respiration. At hypnotic concentrations and higher, the barbiturates are progressive respiratory depressants. Medullary respiratory centers are depressed as toxic levels of barbiturates are approached, and eventually even the carotid and aortic body receptors are depressed. A complication, and often a serious limitation, in the use of barbiturates in anesthesia is an increased incidence of respiratory reflex activity, such as cough, hiccough, sneezing, and laryngospasm.

Hepatic system. Chronic use of the barbiturates causes an increase in liver microsomal enzyme activity[5] that appears to be a result of increased synthesis of enzyme. The result is that the rate of metabolism of a number of drugs, including the barbiturates, is elevated. This action gives rise to a number of drug interactions which will be discussed later.

Absorption, fate, and excretion. The barbiturates are generally available as sodium salts and as such are completely absorbed from the gastrointestinal tract and distributed to nearly all tissues of the body.

One of the most important factors determining barbiturate distribution to the brain is the lipid solubility of the drug. Thiopental, for example, which is highly lipid soluble, readily crosses the blood-brain barrier, and high concentrations are reached in seconds. The high rate of blood flow to the brain also contributes significantly to the entry of thiopental into the brain. Other barriers, such as the placenta, are equally permeable to the barbiturates, and severe respiratory depression can occur in the fetus if a barbiturate is used during delivery.

Barbiturates with less lipid solubility, such as phenobarbital, slowly penetrate the blood-brain barrier. Thus, phenobarbital administered intravenously may require up to 15 minutes to produce maximal CNS depression. After oral administration of phenobarbital, sedative effects may be noted within 30 minutes.

The central actions of the long-acting barbiturates are terminated primarily by renal excretion. Barbital, for example, is excreted nearly totally unchanged in the urine. Approximately 50% of the total dose of phenobarbital is also eliminated in this fashion. The remaining phenobarbital, as is the case for most of the intermediate-acting and short-acting barbiturates, is transformed by the liver to inactive metabolites, which in turn are excreted by the kidney. The ultra-short-acting barbiturates, such as thiopental, are handled somewhat differently by the body. Physical redistribution from brain tissue to other tissues is the primary mechanism by which the central effects of the ultra-short-acting barbiturates are terminated. Storage of the ultra-short-acting barbiturates occurs primarily in muscle and body fat. From these depots, the ultra-short-acting barbiturates are slowly released, metabolized, and excreted. Such mechanisms account for a prolonged depressant aftereffect with the ultra-short-acting barbiturates, leading to the well-known barbiturate "hangover" following surgical anesthesia.

Currently, the Food and Drug Administration (FDA) is processing changes in the labeling of barbiturates. Such changes will emphasize the duration of action for which research has demonstrated the effectiveness of the various barbiturates and will include a comparison of the half-lives of the various barbiturates. New labeling information unrelated to the pharmacokinetics will include instructions to patients as to the indications and proper use of the barbiturates.

Benzodiazepines

The pharmacology of the benzodiazepines is discussed in detail in Chapter 13. Consideration here will be limited to the use of these drugs in sleep disorders.

Pharmacologic effects. Although the benzodiazepines are most commonly used as antianxiety agents, these drugs are CNS depressants and produce sedation and hypnosis. Some of the benzodiazepines, namely flurazepam, temazepam, and triazolam, are promoted specifically as hypnotics rather than as antianxiety agents. Nitrazepam and flunitrazepam are other benzodiazepines primarily prescribed for their hypnotic effects, but they are not yet available in the United States. As discussed earlier, the benzodiazepines do not suppress REM sleep as severely as do the barbiturates, but deep sleep (stages III and IV) is significantly suppressed. EEG alterations by the benzodiazepines are not the same as those caused by the barbiturates, indicating perhaps a different site or mechanism of action, though the significance of these EEG changes is unknown.

Absorption, fate, and excretion. The pharmacokinetic characteristics of the benzodiazepines employed as hypnotics are not significantly different from those used as antianxiety agents (and covered in Chapter 13). In fact, the pharmacokinetics of many of the benzodiazepines promoted for anxiety relief make them excellent hypnotic agents. Because hypnotics are most commonly used for the treatment of patients who have difficulty falling asleep, rapid absorption is essential. Most of the hypnotic benzodiazepines are rapidly absorbed after oral administration, and various dosage forms have been formulated to hasten absorption.

One of the major disadvantages of many benzodiazepines is their metabolic conversion to long-acting derivatives. This pattern leads to a "hangover" effect the day following the night of initial drug use and accumulation of metabolites on repeated administration. The major active metabolite of flurazepam, desalkylflurazepam, has an elimination half-life of 47 to 100 hours. In sleep laboratory studies, it has been shown that flurazepam

does not reach full effectiveness until the second or third consecutive night of intake.[16] Temazepam, on the other hand, has a half-life on the order of 10 hours because no active metabolites are formed, except very small amounts of oxazepam. Because of the lack of active metabolites and the short duration of action, temazepam appears to be useful and effective for repeated nightly use. Clorazepate, by virtue of its long-acting metabolite desmethyldiazepam, would be suitable when a prolonged effect is desired, but "hangover" and accumulation can be a therapeutic problem. Diazepam is a useful hypnotic, but daily ingestion also leads to the buildup of desmethyldiazepam. Because of its pharmacokinetic profile, diazepam should probably not be administered as a hypnotic more frequently than every 48 hours or more than twice in a 7-day period. Nitrazepam and flunitrazepam also accumulate in the body in the form of long-acting metabolites. One of the more promising hypnotic benzodiazepines, triazolam, has an elimination half-life of approximately 5 hours, and its active metabolites are rapidly eliminated. As a result of these pharmacokinetic characteristics, triazolam might prove to be a very effective hypnotic that can be used over prolonged periods of time.

Chloral hydrate and other nonbarbiturates

A variety of drugs of diverse chemical structures have sedative-hypnotic properties. Such drugs include chloral hydrate, triclofos sodium, paraldehyde, ethchlorvynol, methaqualone, glutethimide, methyprylon, antihistamines, anticholinergics, and the propanediol carbamates. Except for chloral hydrate and triclofos sodium these sedative-hypnotics have few clinical indications in dentistry and are not widely prescribed. These agents are, however, occasionally prescribed by physicians, and the dentist should recognize that all of them depress the central nervous system.

Pharmacologic effects. As was mentioned previously, the nonbarbiturate sedative-hypnotics differ little from the barbiturates in terms of their behavioral effects, subjective effects, and, in many cases, mechanisms of action. As a group, they offer no major advantages over the barbiturates, have been less well studied, and are associated with some additional toxicities. One of the oldest nonbarbiturate sedative-hypnotics that does have dental applications is chloral hydrate. Chloral hydrate is available in convenient liquid preparations and offers the advantage of minimal effects on REM sleep. It is sometimes asserted that chloral hydrate is a "safe" sedative-hypnotic. While its overall safety record is impressive, the therapeutic index of the drug is actually no better than that of the barbiturates. In addition, severe laryngospasm with cardiorespiratory arrest following aspiration of orally administered chloral hydrate in liquid form has been reported.[10]

In general, the nonbarbiturate sedative-hypnotics have minor cardiovascular effects when administered in therapeutic doses. As medication is increased beyond therapeutic levels, cardiovascular depression can occur with all the sedative-hypnotics.

The respiratory effects of therapeutic doses of the nonbarbiturates are minimal. These effects, however, become more severe as the dose is increased.

Absorption, fate, and excretion. Chloral hydrate is rapidly converted by the liver to trichloroethanol, which evidently is responsible for the central depressant properties of the parent compound. Triclofos sodium yields the same derivative during hydrolysis in the gastrointestinal tract; trichloroethanol is in turn conjugated with glucuronic acid and excreted in the urine. Like the barbiturates, chloral hydrate and other nonbarbiturates can induce liver enzymes, giving rise to several drug interactions.

Toxic reactions and side effects

The principal toxic reactions associated with the use of the sedative-hypnotics arise out of their effects on respiration and mentation (particularly when combined with other CNS depressants), their abuse potential (discussed in Chapter 46), and their ability to induce hepatic microsomal enzymes.

Sedative-hypnotics can depress respiration and should not be administered to patients whose respiration is compromised in any way. Additionally, the barbiturates increase the incidence of respiratory complications, such as laryngospasm, coughing, sneezing, and hiccough, when they are used as intravenous anesthetics. Confusion, somnolence, and impaired performance are other possible undesired consequences of CNS depression.

A number of unusual reactions have been attributed to the sedative-hypnotics, particularly to the benzodiazepines. Such reactions include depression, agitated toxic psychosis, manic behavior, increased anxiety, hostility, and rage.[7] Because these responses are unlike what would be expected of a sedative-hypnotic drug, they have been termed paradoxical reactions. After careful evaluation, however, it appears that the incidence of paradoxical responses to the benzodiazepines is very small and that, in many cases, the response may not be paradoxical, but rather predictable if the patient has a history of poor impulse control or aggressive and destructive behavior.[8] There is a greater tendency for paradoxical reactions to occur in young children and in the elderly (over 65 years old). The mechanisms responsible for such reactions are unknown, but several factors may play a role: (1) specific areas of the reticular formation are known to be differentially sensitive to the depressant effects of the barbiturates[18] and presumably other CNS depressants, (2) clearance of the benzodiazepines differs dramatically in the young and the old,[11] (3) receptor sensitivity may vary in the elderly,[23,29] and (4) hepatic enzyme function may not yet be fully developed in the young and may be impaired as a natural phenomenon of the aging process.

It has already been pointed out that the sedative-hypnotics potentiate the effects of other CNS depressants, including alcohol, phenothiazines, antihistamines, anesthetics, opioid analgesics, and antianxiety agents. In addition, a number of drug interactions with the barbiturate and nonbarbiturate sedative-hypnotics arise from the ability of these agents to induce hepatic microsomal activity. Because these drugs are administered to patients for short intervals by the dentist, this reaction should not be a problem in most clinical situations, unless the patient is already taking them on a long-term basis. If hepatic microsomal activity has been elevated, the effectiveness of anticoagulants, tricyclic antidepressants, quinidine, digitoxin, corticosteroids, antibiotics such as doxycycline, and other drugs will be decreased. Patients may, on the other hand, have reduced titers of drug-metabolizing enzymes because of hepatic disease, age (both very young and very old), or genetic factors, and thus an exaggerated depressant response to a given dose of sedative-hypnotic might be anticipated. Moreover, concurrent medication with a sedative-hypnotic can inhibit the metabolism of certain drugs (e.g., tricyclic antidepressants), leading to enhanced responses. Many of these potentially dangerous drug interactions may be prevented simply by obtaining an accurate medical history, keeping a continuous record of drugs (both prescribed and self-administered) taken by the patient, and consulting with the patient's physician when the patient's clinical status or drug history is uncertain.

Sedative-hypnotics that stimulate hepatic microsomal enzyme activity also have the potential for augmenting porphyrin synthesis. Their use is therefore strictly contraindicated in patients suffering from acute intermittent porphyria or porphyria variegata. Chloral hydrate and the benzodiazepines are probably the least likely to exacerbate these conditions.

Therapeutic uses in dentistry

There is little difference between the dental and medical uses of the sedative-hypnotics. Whether employed by the dentist or physician, the common desired therapeutic response is sedation or hypnosis. Therapeutic applications for the sedative-hypnotics have also been discussed in detail in Chapters 13 (antianxiety agents), 15 (anticonvulsant drugs), 19 (general anesthetics), and 44 (management of pain and anxiety).

The sedative-hypnotics are among the most useful drugs at the clinician's disposal to calm and relax the anxious patient. Not to be discounted in attaining the desired therapeutic effect with the sedative-hypnotics is the chairside manner of the clinician. The degree of confidence in the therapeutic efficacy of the sedative-hypnotics (or any drug) that the dentist conveys to the patient, the manner in which the drug is presented to the patient (including explicit instructions in the proper use of the agent), and the operatory environment are all important factors in determining the patient's response.

No other class of drugs is more useful than the sedative-hypnotics for the treatment of insomnia. If the insomnia is due to anxiety, it may be treated by a sedative-hypnotic alone. If pain is a contributing factor to insomnia, an analgesic should be prescribed with the sedative-hypnotic. The selection of the "best" sedative-hypnotic for a given clinical condition will be dependent on many factors, and at the present time there probably is no single best choice. It bears reiteration that the clinician should become familiar with the pharmacology and clinical use of a very limited number of drugs from each class of sedative-hypnotics rather than continually switching from one sedative-hypnotic to another. This procedure will result in nothing but frustration and a continuous search for an ideal sedative-hypnotic that does not, and probably will never, exist.

Table 14-2. Classification of barbiturates according to duration of action

	Onset of effect	Duration of effect
Long-acting Phenobarbital	2-3 hours*	>6 hours
Short-acting to intermediate-acting Amobarbital Pentobarbital Secobarbital	30-60 minutes*	3-6 hours
Ultra-short-acting Thiopental	Immediate†	15-30 minutes‡

*Oral administration.
†Intravenous administration.
‡After single intravenous dose.

The barbiturates offer the clinician the advantage of predictable therapeutic response and side effects and a history of therapeutic efficacy and safety, particularly in the case of short-term use. The barbiturates of choice for the dentist usually are the short-acting variety because the onset of sedation is short (approximately 30 minutes to 1 hour) and the duration of effect (3 to 4 hours) is more than sufficient for most dental applications. The traditional classification of the barbiturates on the basis of their duration of action is illustrated in Table 14-2.

Because barbiturates are used in limited quantities and for short periods of time in dental practice, the dentist need not be particularly concerned about the development of tolerance or addiction, which can be a problem with long-term use. The barbiturates, like the benzodiazepines, are contraindicated in pregnant women.

The use of nonbarbiturate sedatives other than the benzodiazepines or the chloral derivatives is not warranted for dental practice. None of the other sedative-hypnotics offers major advantages, and nearly all of them share the disadvantages of the barbiturates, benzodiazepines, and chloral hydrate. The clinician is best advised to recognize the names of the nonbarbiturate sedative-hypnotics and to be aware of the potential for drug interactions with other CNS depressants.

In terms of overall safety, the benzodiazepines are probably the safest sedative-hypnotics available. However, our knowledge of the pharmacologic and toxic effects of the benzodiazepines, especially those drugs like flurazepam and temazepam that are promoted as hypnotics, is still somewhat limited. A report of the Institute of Medicine has in fact challenged the impression that the benzodiazepine hypnotics are safer and more effective than the barbiturates.[14] The report indicates that the barbiturates and benzodiazepines are probably equally effective for short-term use. The potential risks of the benzodiazepines mainly devolve from their long-acting characteristics and include unwanted daytime carryover effects (''hangover'') and an increased likelihood of adverse reactions in elderly patients or those with diminished kidney function. The potentiation of the effects of ethanol, even when alcohol is consumed the day following the night of benzodiazepine intake, emphasizes the risks of drug interactions involving the long-acting metabolites of the benzodiazepines. The safety of the benzodiazepines has also not been established in the case of pregnant women. Indeed, there is some evidence of birth defects if the benzodiazepines are taken during the first trimester of pregnancy.[15] Some of the newer benzodiazepines are not recommended for long-term use in children because of the possibility of adverse effects during this stage of rapid development. Such effects might not be apparent for several years. Future clinical trials may provide evidence for the safety of benzodiazepines in pediatric dentistry, however, because diazepam has been approved for use in children as young as 6 months of age. Extensive clinical trials have not been carried out for flurazepam, temazepam, or triazolam, and thus it is recommended that they not be used in patients under the age of 18. The Institute of Medicine report also suggests that benzodiazepine suppression of stage III and stage IV sleep may be more significant than previously thought and may offset any advantage gained by the minimal suppression of REM sleep.

Chloral hydrate (or the closely related triclofos sodium) is an excellent choice as a sedative-hypnotic for patients allergic to or intolerant of the barbiturates or benzodiazepines. The onset and duration of action of chloral hydrate is approximately the same as that of the short- to intermediate-acting barbiturates. Chloral hydrate is frequently used to sedate children, though the impression that it is a safe agent must be questioned in light of reports of nearly fatal laryngospasm during aspiration of the irritant drug.[10] Chloral hydrate has an unpleasant taste, which is masked in commercially available syrups and elixirs or if it is mixed in orange juice.

The use of any of the hypnotic drugs for insomnia should be limited to short-term treatment. Research in sleep laboratories shows that most hyp-

Table 14-3. Preparations and doses of sedative-hypnotics

	Route of administration*	Adult dose (mg)	
		Sedation	*Hypnosis*
Barbiturates†			
Amobarbital	O, R, IM, IV	30-100	100-200
Pentobarbital	O, R, IM, IV	30-100	100-200
Secobarbital	O, R, IM, IV	30-100	100-200
Benzodiazepines			
Clorazepate	O	7.5-15	15
Diazepam‡	O, IM, IV	2-10	10
Flurazepam	O	15	15-30
Temazepam	O	15	30
Triazolam	O	0.25	0.25-0.5
Chloral derivatives			
Chloral hydrate§	O, R	250-500	500-2000
Triclofos sodium	O	—	1500

*O = oral, R = rectal, IM = intramuscular, IV = intravenous.
†Dose for children for preoperative sedation = 2 mg/kg body weight.
‡Dose for children for preoperative sedation = 0.04 to 0.2 mg/kg body weight.
§Dose for children for preoperative sedation = 50 mg/kg body weight.

notics lose their effectiveness in the treatment of insomnia within 3 to 14 days of continuous use. The benzodiazepines are the only drugs that have been proved to be effective in promoting sleep beyond 14 days of consecutive use. As discussed previously, new FDA-approved labeling will emphasize this point. An active ongoing FDA program will also continue to encourage physicians and dentists to restrict the prescribing of hypnotics and will advise that the underlying cause of insomnia be sought and treated by nonpharmacologic means.

Preparations and doses for clinically useful sedative-hypnotics are listed in Table 14-3. These doses should be used only as guidelines, as each patient will have different requirements, and dosages should be individualized.

Implications for dentistry

Many of the problems associated with the sedative-hypnotics, such as tolerance, addiction, abuse, and the induction of hepatic microsomal enzyme activity, are a result of chronic use. Fortunately, the sedative-hypnotics are indicated for only short-term use in dentistry; thus, many of the usual factors limiting their use are not pertinent. This is not to imply that problems do not arise with the administration of sedative-hypnotics in dental practice, but only that they are minimized. For example, although overdose with the sedative-hypnotics would be unlikely with the amount of drug required for most dental situations, a potential problem exists if the patient combines the prescribed sedative-hypnotic with large amounts of other CNS depressants, such as alcohol. The clinician and patient must also be constantly alert to the possibility of other drug interactions described previously.

It is the responsibility of the clinician to ensure that the patient who is receiving or about to receive a sedative-hypnotic be cognizant of the danger of combining other CNS depressants, particularly alcohol, with these agents. If the use of a sedative-hypnotic for any given patient is anticipated, the clinician should insist that the patient be accompanied to the dental appointment by a qualified driver or someone to assist the patient after the dental procedures are completed, and he should refuse to provide dental care until this instruction is met. Obviously the patient to whom a sedative-hypnotic is administered should be instructed not to operate dangerous machinery or perform otherwise potentially dangerous activities and to abstain from alcohol. The patient should also be made aware of the potential risks of self-administration of OTC preparations that contain CNS depressants, such as cold remedies containing antihistamines or preparations for insomnia formulated to include antihistamines or bromides. As a matter of fact, the antihistamines have sufficient CNS depressant properties that they are often used for sedation in dentistry. Diphenhydramine is particularly useful for those patients who are intolerant to other CNS depressants, and the elderly respond particularly well to this compound.

While the barbiturates produce significant depression of the CNS, even to the point of unconsciousness, it should be noted that they are not analgesics. In fact, there are indications that they may be antianalgesic in that the patient may exhibit increased responsiveness to painful stimuli. When pain is present or evoked, the patient may become aroused and agitated and experience delirium.[13] Obviously, if pain is a contributing factor to either anxiety or insomnia, an analgesic will be required in order to obtain sedation or hypnosis.

Throughout this chapter, the advantages of the short-term use and limited quantities of sedative-hypnotics prescribed in dentistry have been emphasized. There is, however, a serious disadvantage in using such limited quantities of drugs in

that the dentist, rather than writing a prescription for two or three capsules of a barbiturate, will instead dispense this quantity to the patient from office stock. If the drug is to be used outside the office, it must be placed in a suitable container and fully labeled according to state laws. Further restrictions and regulations regarding controlled substances are covered in Chapter 49.

CENTRAL NERVOUS SYSTEM STIMULANTS

There are a variety of drugs that stimulate the central nervous system, but few of these have ever been successfully used therapeutically for their stimulant effects per se. The CNS stimulants, also called analeptics, should theoretically have great therapeutic value in the treatment of respiratory depression that occurs after an overdose of CNS depressants. However, years of study and experience indicate that, in practice, patients overdosed with CNS depressants recover more readily and with fewer complications when they are treated with supportive measures rather than when CNS stimulants are used as antidotes. The pharmacologic response to CNS stimulants is so unpredictable, the margin of safety so small, and the danger of producing convulsions so great that, at the present time, there are no safe centrally acting respiratory stimulants.

There are few, if any, clinical indications for CNS stimulants in dentistry. Nonetheless, the probability of treating patients who have received a CNS stimulant is great. The CNS stimulants most widely used, but least likely to give rise to drug interactions or clinical problems, belong to the xanthine derivatives. The xanthine drugs include caffeine, present in coffee, tea, cola beverages, and cocoa; theophylline, present in coffee and tea; and theobromine, present in cocoa. Of these, caffeine is by far the most widely used and is in fact the most commonly used CNS stimulant in the world.

Another group of CNS stimulants commonly encountered in dental practice is the centrally acting sympathomimetic group, which includes such drugs as amphetamine, methylphenidate, and the diverse array of drugs used for diet suppression. As shown in Figure 14-2, these drugs are chemical derivatives of phenylethylamine and are thus closely related to the adrenergic neurotransmitters. Amphetamines and methylphenidate are used in the treatment of narcolepsy and, particularly the latter drug, in the treatment of MBD syndrome or hy-

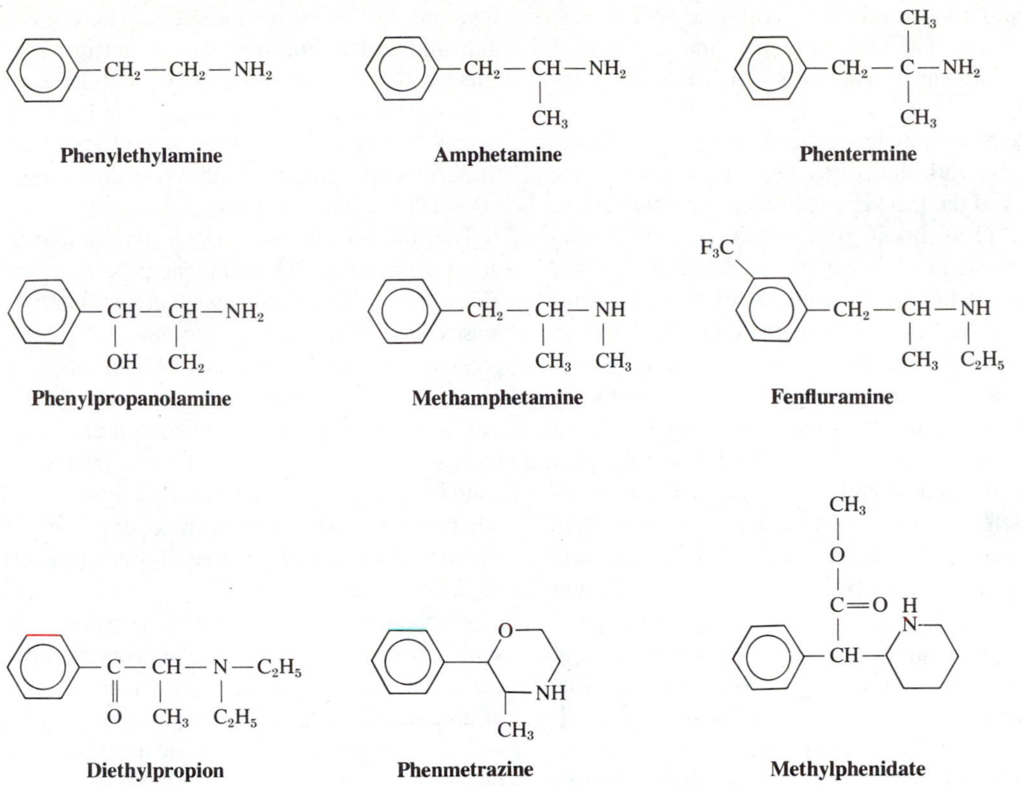

Figure 14-2. Structural formulas of phenylethylamine and related sympathomimetic CNS stimulants.

perkinetic child syndrome. Amphetamines have been employed as anorexiants or appetite suppressants, but the FDA has moved against this practice, citing the many risks and marginal benefits of these drugs in weight control. The sympathomimetic or adrenergic CNS stimulants, particularly amphetamine, continue to be popular drugs of abuse, and the present upsurge in their use and in the use of cocaine (see Chapter 45), another CNS stimulant with powerful effects on the sympathetic nervous system, is alarming. Hence an increasing number of patients under the influence of these drugs may be encountered in dental practice.

Compounds that have been used as "specific" respiratory stimulants compose yet another class of CNS stimulants. Drugs from this group are unlikely to be encountered in dental practice. These drugs include nikethamide, ethamivan, and doxapram. Of these drugs, doxapram is the most recent addition and appears to have a more favorable therapeutic index than the others. Doxapram is still somewhat controversial and not widely used, but

it does illustrate the point that specific respiratory stimulants have therapeutic potential, and the search for such agents continues.

Stimulants of the central nervous system that the dentist should almost never be faced with are those traditionally classified as the convulsant drugs. In this category are strychnine, picrotoxin, and pentylenetetrazol. All of these drugs find greatest value in the experimental study of neurophysiology and neuropharmacology and as laboratory tools for the study of epilepsy. Although all of these drugs were used therapeutically at one time, none remains available for use. Strychnine is, however, a major component of rat poison, and accidental poisoning, particularly of children, still occurs.

Xanthine derivatives

Caffeine, theophylline, and theobromine are methylated derivates of xanthine. Theobromine has no (or only slight) CNS stimulant properties, while theophylline and caffeine are potent stimulators. Because it is the only methylxanthine used primarily for its central effect, caffeine will be discussed here. (The use of theophylline and its salts in the treatment of asthma is considered in Chapter 32).

Caffeine stimulates the central nervous system unequally, with the cortex being the most and the spinal cord the least excited. A therapeutic dose of caffeine (100 to 250 mg), which is contained in one or two cups of strong coffee, acts at the cortical level to produce a clearer train of thought, a reduction in reaction time and drowsiness, and an increase in motor activity. Hyperesthesia, or increased reaction to sensory stimuli, is commonly experienced with caffeine and obviously has dental implications. The EEG is shifted toward higher frequencies and slightly increased voltage levels after caffeine. These EEG changes are indicative of an increase in "alertness," but they reveal little as to the mechanism of action of caffeine. Recent studies indicate that the xanthines alter cyclic nucleotide concentrations, interfere with the central actions of adenosine, and disturb intracellular calcium homeostasis.

Respiratory centers of the medulla are stimulated by caffeine in doses slightly greater than therapeutic, and it is this action, though nonspecific, that may offer some slight therapeutic value in the treatment of CNS depressant poisoning. At high doses caffeine stimulates the spinal cord to cause increased reflex activity; stimulation of motor centers leads to convulsions. Fatal poisoning by caffeine is extremely rare, as the oral lethal dose has been estimated to be 10 gm.

Caffeine has a variety of seemingly antagonistic effects on the cardiovascular system. It directly stimulates the myocardium, thus increasing its rate and force, and vascular smooth muscle, which leads to peripheral vasodilation. At the same time it probably stimulates both the vagal and vasomotor centers in the medulla. The net result of these cardiovascular effects on blood pressure is obviously not consistent, though in many cases a slight increase is usually noted. Arrhythmias have been known to occur if excessive coffee is consumed.

Amphetamine and related sympathomimetic agents

The central excitatory effects of amphetamine and amphetamine-like drugs may be noted at the level of the cerebral cortex, subcortical areas, and spinal cord. Therapeutic doses can improve physical performance, increase motor activity, induce

tremors, and cause restlessness. There are some indications that improvement in performance occurs particularly in those individuals whose performance is impaired as a result of fatigue or boredom.[17,32] Amphetamine also causes hyperreactivity to peripheral stimuli, alertness, wakefulness, and often elation and euphoria.

The mechanism by which the amphetamine drugs exert their CNS stimulant effect is unknown. However, evidence indicates that amphetamine releases and blocks the uptake of norepinephrine into presynaptic nerve terminals.[4] Additionally, amphetamine and related drugs may act as direct central adrenergic agonists. The central excitatory effects of amphetamine appear to be primarily mediated via a central noradrenergic system, though other neurotransmitters, such as dopamine, have also been implicated in some of the central effects of amphetamine.[30]

Amphetamine and related compounds, being sympathomimetic amines, have prominent peripheral cardiovascular actions. By causing the release of norepinephrine, amphetamine stimulates both α and β receptors and causes an increase in blood pressure, reflex slowing of the heart, and sometimes cardiac arrhythmias. A more detailed discussion of the sympathomimetic actions of amphetamine and other adrenergic drugs may be found in Chapter 6.

The excitatory effect of amphetamine on respiration, which results in an increase in both the depth and rate of respiration, is due to stimulation of the medullary respiratory centers. This action is much more prominent when the respiratory centers have been previously depressed by CNS depressant drugs.

Nikethamide, ethamivan, and doxapram

Nikethamide, ethamivan, and doxapram stimulate the entire central nervous system, although at one time each of these drugs was considered to be a "specific" respiratory stimulant and thus useful as an antidote in cases of CNS depressant overdose. Clinical use, however, has proved the nonselective nature of their stimulant properties, the narrow margin of safety between the respiratory stimulant dose and the dose that produces convulsions, and the more favorable prognosis in cases of CNS depressant overdose when these stimulants are not used. Respiratory stimulant effects appear to be exerted via a direct excitatory action on medullary respiratory centers, though all levels of the central nervous system are stimulated to some degree. Large doses of any of these drugs can produce tonic-clonic convulsions, and the dose at which convulsions occur is very near that which stimulates respiration. Of the three drugs, doxapram has the greatest margin of safety, but it is still not safe enough when used in cases of severe CNS depression. Other than the temporary use of doxapram in chronic obstructive pulmonary disease or to assist respiration during emergence from general anesthesia, there is little clinical use for any of these three drugs at present.

Strychnine, picrotoxin, and pentylenetetrazol

Strychnine, picrotoxin, and pentylenetetrazol are best classified as convulsants and are generally not used therapeutically. Because these drugs produce seizures, they have been used in screening procedures for the discovery of effective antiepileptic agents. They find greatest use as pharmacologic tools for the experimental study of the central nervous system.

Strychnine is thought to produce CNS stimulation by reducing the activity in certain inhibitory pathways. By this mechanism, unopposed excitatory input could then enhance neural activity to the point of convulsions. Picrotoxin interferes with inhibitory pathways that are different from those affected by strychnine. Interest has focused on the pharmacology of strychnine and picrotoxin because of their dissimilar effects on inhibitory pathways and the implication that different and identifiable neurotransmitters may account for the different types of inhibition. Obviously the actions of these drugs have greater experimental than clinical value.

Pentylenetetrazol is an experimental tool that may find occasional clinical application. Pentylenetetrazol can be administered in small doses to uncover latent epilepsy by causing epileptic-like discharges as recorded on the electroencephalogram. Before the introduction of the antipsychotic agents, pentylenetetrazol was used as a convulsant drug to treat certain mental disorders. Fortunately, the antipsychotic drugs have made this form of treatment obsolete.

Pentylenetetrazol reduces inhibitory transmitter-induced chloride conductance.[22] Picrotoxin and strychnine have similar effects, which suggests a common ionic mode of action for all three compounds.

Toxic reactions and side effects

The side effects of most of the CNS stimulants can readily be predicted as merely extensions of their CNS-stimulating properties. Insomnia, excitement, talkativeness, hyperreactivity, restlessness, irritability, tremor, muscle rigidity, and convulsions are toxic effects that might be observed with any of the CNS stimulants. Hypertension, tachycardia, arrhythmias, sweating, hyperthermia, and a number of visual, auditory, and tactile disturbances may also occur.

A correlation between coffee consumption and coronary disease has been reported, but this finding has been disputed by other studies. Pregnant women who drink more than six cups of coffee a day have a greater chance of miscarriage. An association between coffee intake and cancer of the lower urinary tract has also been suggested. While these effects cannot be attributed directly to caffeine, there is evidence that caffeine is teratogenic.[9] Although the toxic effects of caffeine appear to be controversial and somewhat difficult to document experimentally, the prolonged and excessive consumption of coffee and other products containing caffeine should be questioned.

The psychic effects of amphetamine and related drugs make these agents popular as drugs of abuse and thus have given rise to chronic toxicity. Oral amphetamine produces a prolonged euphoria, whereas intravenous administration produces the well-known "rush." The individual who abuses amphetamine on a long-term basis may display any or all of the signs of acute toxicity and, in addition, may suffer from drug-induced mental illness. Psychotic states closely resembling schizophrenia, as well as hallucinations and paranoia, are common side effects of chronic toxicity.[30]

Therapeutic uses

Few of the CNS stimulants find any clinical application that utilizes their central stimulatory effects. The use of the currently available CNS stimulants in the clinical situation in which they might be most beneficial (i.e., respiratory depression due to overdose of CNS depressants) is generally not safe, is not recommended, and only further complicates the clinical status of the patient. Doxapram finds clinical application as a respiratory stimulant after general anesthesia and for acute hypercapnia in patients with chronic pulmonary disease; however, it can only be considered as an adjunctive aid for temporary use. The major uses of the CNS stimulants at present are for the treatment of the MBD syndrome in children and as appetite suppressants for the treatment of obesity. It appears to be paradoxical that amphetamine and other CNS stimulants, such as methylphenidate and pemoline, are effective in the treatment of the hyperactive child. In these children, administration of these drugs results in an increase in the attention span, reduction in hyperactivity, and an improvement in behavior. Body growth appears to be normal[12] or perhaps retarded in children under therapy with the amphetamines,[25] which may be due simply to their anorexic side effect. Methylphenidate is the agent of choice for MBD syndrome because it does not suppress the appetite to the same degree as does amphetamine. Though not well documented, it appears that growth patterns revert to normal when children are taken off either drug.[26] The mechanism of action for the calming effect exerted by these stimulants in the hyperactive child is not clear. Caffeine is not particularly effective in MBD, indicating that a CNS stimulant action per se is not sufficient for this therapeutic effect.

Pemoline has stimulant properties and side effects (including insomnia and anorexia) similar to those of amphetamine. In the treatment of MBD, pemoline may be an alternative for patients who are refractory or cannot tolerate amphetamine or methylphenidate. The final clinical response to pemoline is the same as that to amphetamine or methylphenidate but takes longer to attain. There are several other centrally acting drugs used in the treatment of MBD that are not CNS stimulants, including chlorpromazine, thioridazine, imipramine, and desipramine.

Amphetamine-like drugs are used therapeutically to reduce weight. Weight loss appears to be due principally to a centrally mediated suppression of appetite. The mechanism by which the anorexiants suppress appetite is unknown, but, because of their structural similarity to the monoamines, interference with central monoamine neurotransmitters is probable.[27] Because tolerance develops to the appetite-suppressant action of CNS stimulants and because of their abuse potential, particularly for the amphetamines and phenmetrazine, their use in the control of obesity is extremely questionable. The risk of abuse is much less with drugs such as diethylpropion, phentermine, fenfluramine, and mazindol. However, their use is not without risk of abuse, and they should be prescribed only intermittently and with caution. In fact, it is generally agreed that the use of the anorexiants should be restricted to those patients whose obesity places them at serious medical or psychologic risk.

Implications for dentistry

Although the dentist may have to deal with patients who have received a CNS stimulant (in the form of caffeine in coffee) more often than any other centrally acting drug, it will be rare that this poses any significant problem. Side effects of the CNS stimulants that could be of concern to the dentist are primarily manifestations of the increased level of activity of the central nervous system, both sensory and motor. Patients exhibiting side effects of the CNS stimulants may be nervous, hyperexcitable, hyperreactive to peripheral stimuli, irritable, restless, and hyperactive; they also may display motor abnormalities, such as tremor and minor twitching of muscles. The clinician should keep in mind that CNS stimulation is followed by CNS depression. Such a phenomenon is minimal or questionable in the case of caffeine ingested in coffee. However, in cases of patients taking amphetamine, such depression can be significant, and a greater than expected CNS depression could occur if CNS depressants were to be used in this poststimulatory period.

Sedative-hypnotics

Nonproprietary name	*Proprietary name*
Barbiturates	
amobarbital	Amytal
aprobarbital	Alurate
butabarbital	Butisol
hexobarbital	Pre-Sed
mephobarbital	Mebaral
pentobarbital	Nembutal
phenobarbital	Luminal
secobarbital	Seconal
talbutal	Lotusate
thiopental	Pentothal
Benzodiazepines	
flunitrazepam*	Rohypnol
flurazepam	Dalmane
nitrazepam*	Mogadon
temazepam	Restoril
triazolam	Halcion

*Not available in the United States.

Nonproprietary name	Proprietary name
Others	
acetylcarbromol	Paxarel
chloral hydrate	Noctec
ethchlorvynol	Placidyl
ethinamate	Valmid
glutethimide	Doriden
methaqualone	Quaalude, Mequin
methyprylon	Noludar
paraldehyde	Paral
triclofos sodium	Triclos

Central nervous system stimulants

Nonproprietary name	Proprietary name
Methylxanthines	
caffeine*	NoDoz
Sympathomimetics	
amphetamine (racemic)	Benzedrine
benzphetamine	Didrex
dextroamphetamine	Dexedrine
diethylpropion	Tenuate
fenfluramine	Pondimin
mazindol	Sanorex
methamphetamine	Desoxyn
pemoline	Cylert
phendimetrazine	Anorex
phenmetrazine	Preludin
phentermine	Wilpowr
phenylpropanolamine*	Dietac
Respiratory stimulants	
doxapram	Dopram
ethamivan†	Emivan
nikethamide	Coramine
Convulsants	
pentylenetetrazol†	Metrazol
picrotoxin†	—
strychnine†	—

*Ingredients in many OTC preparations.
†No longer available clinically.

CITED REFERENCES

1. Barker, J.L., and Gainer, H. Pentobarbital: selective depression of excitatory postsynaptic potentials. Science **182:**720-722, 1973.
2. Barker, J.L., and McBurney, R.N. Phenobarbitone modulation of postsynaptic GABA receptor function on cultured mammalian neurons. Proceedings of the Royal Society of London. Series B. Biological Sciences **206:**319-327, 1979.
3. Bradley, P.B. The central action of certain drugs in relation to the reticular formation of the brain. In Jasper, H.H., Proctor, L.D., Knighton, R.S., Noshay, W.C., and Costello, R.T., eds. Reticular Formation of the Brain. Boston, Little, Brown & Co., 1958.
4. Carr, L.A., and Moore, K.E. Norepinephrine: release from brain by *d*-amphetamine in vivo. Science **164:**322-323, 1969.
5. Conney, A.H., Davidson, C., Gastel, R., and Burns, J.J. Adaptive increases in drug-metabolizing enzymes induced by phenobarbital and other drugs. Journal of Pharmacology and Experimental Therapeutics **130:**1-8, 1960.
6. Cote, I.L., and Wilson, W.A. Effect of barbiturates on inhibitory and excitatory responses to applied neurotransmitters in Aplysia. Journal of Pharmacology and Experimental Therapeutics **214:**161-165, 1980.
7. DiMascio, A., Shader, R.I., and Giller, D.R. Behavioral toxicity. Part IV: emotional (mood) states. In Shader, R.I., and DiMascio, A., eds. Psychotropic Drug Side Effects. Baltimore, The Williams & Wilkins Co., 1970.
8. DiMascio, A., Shader, R.I., and Harmatz, J. Psychotropic drugs and induced hostility. Psychosomatics **10**(section 2):46-47, 1969.
9. Fujii, T., Sasaki, H., and Nishimura, H. Teratogenicity of caffeine in mice related to its mode of administration. Japanese Journal of Pharmacology **19:**134-138, 1969.
10. Granoff, D.M., McDaniel, D.B., and Barkowf, S.P. Cardiorespiratory arrest following aspiration of chloral hydrate. American Journal of Diseases of Children **122:**170-171, 1971.
11. Greenblatt, D.J., Allen, M.D., Harmatz, J.S., and Shader, R.I. Diazepam disposition determinants. Clinical Pharmacology and Therapeutics **27:**301-312, 1980.
12. Gross, M.D. Growth of hyperkinetic children taking methylphenidate, dextroamphetamine, or imipramine/desipramine. Pediatrics **58:**423-431, 1976.
13. Harvey, S.C. Hypnotics and sedatives. In Gilman, A.G., Goodman, L.S., and Gilman, A., eds. Goodman and Gilman's The Pharmacological Basis of Therapeutics, ed. 6. New York, Macmillan, Inc., 1980.
14. Institute of Medicine. Report of a Study: Sleeping Pills, Insomnia, and Medical Practice. Washington, D.C., National Academy of Sciences, 1979.
15. Istvan, E.J. Drug-associated congenital abnormalities? Canadian Medical Association Journal **103:**1394, 1970.
16. Kales, A., Bixler, E.O., Scharf, M., and Kales, J.D. Sleep laboratory studies of flurazepam: a model evaluating hypnotic drugs. Clinical Pharmacology and Therapeutics **19:**576-583, 1976.
17. Laties, V.G., and Weiss, B. Performance enhancement by the amphetamines: a new approach. In Brill, H., and Cole, J.O., eds. Proceedings of the Fifth International Congress of Neuropsychopharmacology. Amsterdam, Excerpta Medica Foundation, 1967.

18. Magni, F., Moruzzi, G., Rossi, G.F., and Zanchetti, A. EEG arousal following inactivation of the lower brainstem by selective injection of barbiturate into the vertebral circulation. Archives Italiennes de Biologie 99:33-71, 1961.

19. Miyahara, J.T., Esplin, D.W., and Zablocka, B. Differential effects of depressant drugs on presynaptic inhibition. Journal of Pharmacology and Experimental Therapeutics 154:119-127, 1966.

20. Moruzzi, G., and Magoun, H.W. Brain stem reticular formation and activation of the EEG. Electroencephalography and Clinical Neurophysiology 1:455-473, 1949.

21. Nicoll, R.A. The effects of anaesthetics on synaptic excitation and inhibition in the olfactory bulb. Journal of Physiology (London) 223:803-814, 1972.

22. Pellmar, T.C., and Wilson, W.A. Synaptic mechanism of pentylenetetrazole: selectivity for chloride conductance. Science 197:912-914, 1977.

23. Reidenberg, M.M., Levy, M., Warner, H., Coutinho, C.B., Schwartz, M.S., Yu, G., and Cheripko, J. Relationship between diazepam dose, plasma level, age, and central nervous system depression. Clinical Pharmacology and Therapeutics 23:371-374, 1978.

24. Richards, C.D. On the mechanism of barbiturate anaesthesia. Journal of Physiology (London) 227:749-767, 1972.

25. Safer, D.J., and Allen, R.P. Factors influencing the suppressant effect of two stimulant drugs on the growth of hyperactive children. Pediatrics 51:660-667, 1973.

26. Safer, D.J., Allen, R.P., and Barr, E. Growth rebound after termination of stimulant drugs. Journal of Pediatrics 86:113-116, 1975.

27. Samanin, R., and Garrattini, S. Central Mechanisms of Anorectic Drugs, New York, Raven Press, 1979.

28. Schmidt, R.F. Pharmacologic studies on the primary afferent depolarization of the toad spinal cord. Pfluegers Archive European Journal of Physiology 277:325-346, 1963.

29. Sellers, E.M. Clinical pharmacology and therapeutics of benzodiazepines. Canadian Medical Association Journal 118:1533-1538, 1978.

30. Snyder, S.H., Banerjee, S.P., Yamamura, H.I., and Greenberg, D. Drugs, neurotransmitters, and schizophrenia. Science 184:1243-1253, 1974.

31. Weakly, J.N. Effect of barbiturates on "quantal" synaptic transmission in spinal motoneurones. Journal of Physiology (London) 204:63-77, 1969.

32. Weiss, B., and Laties, V.G. Enhancement of human performance by caffeine and the amphetamines. Pharmacological Reviews 14:1-36, 1962.

33. Westecker, M.E. Reciprocal activation of two evoked potential components in the olfactory bulb. Pfluegers Archive European Journal of Physiology 324:297-310, 1971.

GENERAL REFERENCES

Clark, D.L., and Rosner. Neurophysiologic effects of general anesthetics. I. The electroencephalogram and sensory evoked responses in man. Anesthesiology 38:564-582, 1973.

Finn, S.B. Cinical Pedodontics. ed. 4. Philadelphia, W.B. Saunders Co., 1973.

Franz, D.N. Central nervous system stimulants. Strychnine, picrotoxin, pentylenetetrazol, and miscellaneous agents. In Gilman, A.G., Goodman, L.S., and Gilman, A., eds. Goodman and Gilman's The Pharmacological Basis of Therapeutics. ed. 6. New York, Macmillan, Inc., 1980.

Harvey, S.C. Hypnotics and sedatives. In Gilman, A.G., Goodman, L.S., and Gilman, A., eds. Goodman and Gilman's The Pharmacological Basis of Therapeutics, ed. 6. New York, Macmillan, Inc., 1980.

Ho, I.K., and Harris, R.A. Mechanism of action of barbiturates. Annual Review of Pharmacology and Toxicology 21:83-111, 1981.

Jaffe, J.H. Hypnotic and sedative agents. In Jarvik, M.E., ed. Psychopharmacology in the Practice of Medicine. New York, Appleton-Century-Crofts, 1977.

Killam, E.K. Drug action on the brain-stem reticular formation. Pharmacological Reviews 14:175-223, 1962.

Levenson, H.S., and Bick, E.C. Psychopharmacology of caffeine. In Jarvik, M.E., ed. Psychopharmacology in the Practice of Medicine. New York, Appleton-Century-Crofts, 1977.

Rall, T.W. Central nervous system stimulants. The xanthines. In Gilman, A.G., Goodman, L.S., and Gilman, A., eds. Goodman and Gilman's The Pharmacological Basis of Therapeutics, ed. 6. New York, Macmillan, Inc., 1980

Rosner, B.S., and Clark, D.L. Neurophysiologic effects of general anesthetics. II. Sequential regional actions in the brain. Anesthesiology 39:59-81, 1973.

15 Anticonvulsants

Leslie P. Felpel

Epilepsy is a convulsive disorder characterized by periodic and irregular discharges of nervous tissue. There are many variations on this theme, but in general the irregular discharges are sufficient to cause cerebral disturbances, such as alterations in consciousness, as well as other clinical symptoms. A variety of seizure types exists, and the basic pathology of epilepsy is still not well understood; thus, classification of epilepsies has not been uniform.

CLASSIFICATION OF EPILEPSIES

In 1970 the International League Against Epilepsy adopted a classification for epileptic seizures based on clinical and electroencephalographic patterns. A modified version of this scheme is illustrated in Table 15-1, which also lists the more traditional but less specific terminology used in categorizing the epilepsies and the primary or most commonly used anticonvulsant drugs. The seizure patterns are broadly divided into three major groups: (1) generalized epilepsies, in which consciousness is lost, convulsions involve the entire body, and the EEG displays characteristic rhythms; (2) partial (focal) epilepsies, in which consciousness may be impaired but not lost (at least initially), convulsions involve restricted areas of the body and are initially unilateral, and the EEG displays rhythmic activity that initially is restricted to one hemisphere; and (3) unclassifiable epilepsies.

Generalized epilepsies

The most common type of generalized epilepsy is grand mal, which usually has a sudden onset (sometimes preceded by an aura), beginning with the so-called epileptic cry due to the forcing of air through the tonically contracted muscles of the larynx. This cry is followed by a loss of consciousness, loss of postural tone, and tonic-clonic con-

tractions of skeletal muscles. Autonomic responses commonly include sweating, loss of sphincter control (often resulting in urination and defecation), pupillary dilation, and loss of light reflexes. The EEG pattern displays bilateral synchronous high-voltage polyspike activity. The greatest danger to the patient during the seizure is injury as a result of the loss of postural tone. Tongue biting and even the fracturing of teeth may result from the powerful tonic contractions of facial musculature. After the tonic-clonic contractions of skeletal muscle, the patient usually awakens, is confused and lethargic, and then goes back to sleep for approximately 30 minutes. On reawakening, the patient is again lethargic, confused, and disoriented and often complains of headache and other muscular aches. Fortunately, grand mal epilepsy is usually responsive to pharmacotherapy.

A second common type of generalized epilepsy is petit mal, which characteristically occurs in childhood. There are several varieties of petit mal, but the most common form is characterized by an abrupt but very short (5 to 10 seconds) loss of consciousness with minor muscular twitching (often restricted to the eyelids and face), a three-per-second spike-and-wave EEG pattern, and no loss of postural control. Because of the brief loss of consciousness and a "vacant" look in the eyes of the patient, Calmeil, in 1824, introduced the term *absence* to identify this common variety of petit mal. Like grand mal, absence seizures are responsive to pharmacotherapy.

Other uncommon types of petit mal epilepsy that are classified as generalized are (1) myoclonic, characterized by a sudden, brief, and violent contraction of one or many muscles, and (2) akinetic, characterized by a sudden and brief loss of muscle tone. Usually these varieties of generalized epilepsy are associated with diffuse and severe progres-

Table 15-1. Classification of epilepsies

New classification	Traditional terminology	Characteristics	Primary anticonvulsants
Generalized epilepsies	Grand mal	Clinical—bilateral and symmetrical tonic-clonic seizures, generalized from the onset; EEG—bilateral synchronous spikes at approximately 10 Hz	Phenytoin, phenobarbital, primidone
	Petit mal	Clinical—temporary (but complete) loss of consciousness, minor motor seizures; EEG—bilateral, synchronous spike-and-wave complexes at approximately 3 Hz	Ethosuximide, valproic acid, clonazepam
Partial epilepsies	Focal (local, Jacksonian)	Clinical—no loss of consciousness, restricted area of onset (motor or sensory); EEG—local spikes and spike-and-wave complexes	Phenytoin, phenobarbital, primidone
	Temporal lobe (psychomotor)	Clinical—complex and variable behavioral alterations, impaired consciousness; EEG—abnormality localized over temporal region; neurologic status—evidence of brain damage	Phenytoin, primidone, phenobarbital, carbamazepine
Unclassifiable epilepsies		Atypical, irregular	

sive diseases of the brain and, in general, are refractory to drug treatment.

Generalized epilepsies may occur in the form of continuous seizures. This state is referred to as status epilepticus and, fortunately, is rare. If the seizure pattern is of the grand mal variety, the patient's life is in danger; death ensues if the seizures are not terminated. Petit mal status is less common than grand mal status and does not have the same acute morbidity and mortality. Status epilepticus may develop in patients with convulsive disorders, in patients who have had acute diseases that affect the brain (such as meningitis, encephalitis, toxemia of pregnancy, uremia, or acute electrolyte imbalances), and in patients for whom convulsant medication has been withdrawn too rapidly. Fortunately, status epilepticus is responsive to pharmacotherapy. The initial agent of choice for this condition is diazepam, although intravenous phenytoin and phenobarbital are also used. Because large doses of the depressant drug are usually required, there is the danger of severe respiratory depression and the possibility of respiratory arrest. In case of refractory status epilepticus, the patient may have to undergo general anesthesia. Obviously, grand mal status epilepticus is best treated in a hospital setting.

Partial epilepsies

The partial epilepsies are named according to the early clinical manifestations of the disorders. Thus,

what is now called jacksonian motor epilepsy, after Hughlings Jackson who first described the condition, begins with muscular contractions of isolated muscle, with involvement of other muscles as the abnormal discharge "marches" (spreads) over the motor cortex. Similarly, jacksonian sensory epilepsy, which "marches" over the sensory cortex, gives rise to sensations from various areas of the body. Psychomotor epilepsy characteristically is associated wtih lesions of the temporal lobe and a variety of bizarre behavioral patterns of which the patient is totally amnesic. Other areas of the central nervous system such as the hypothalamus, fornix, and cingulate cortex are also thought to play a role in psychomotor epilepsy.

An important facet of the partial epilepsies is that, although they normally begin with localized symptoms, any of them may progress to generalized seizures. The mechanisms responsible for such a pattern are unknown; however, much evidence supports the concept that an abnormal discharge from a locus of neurons spreads to other, "normal" populations of neurons, which in turn eventually broadcast the abnormal discharge to all areas of the brain. Unfortunately, partial seizures are generally more refractory to drugs than are generalized seizures.

For practical purposes, all patients with epilepsy will have to take medication for life in order to achieve some measure of control over the seizures. The only exception to this rule is that children often "outgrow" petit mal, but there are also indications that such individuals have a tendency to develop other forms of epilepsy in later years. It is important to realize that the anticonvulsants do not cure epilepsy but simply control the seizure. The primary objective of anticonvulsant therapy at the present time is to suppress completely all seizures without causing any impairment of CNS function or other deleterious side effects. With the currently available anticonvulsants, significant seizure control can be obtained in 70% to 80% of all cases.

CHEMISTRY AND STRUCTURE-ACTIVITY RELATIONSHIPS

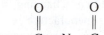

The chemical linkage $-\overset{\overset{\text{O}}{\|}}{\text{C}}-\text{N}-\overset{\overset{\text{O}}{\|}}{\text{C}}-$ is present in most of the effective anticonvulsants and is shown within the dotted lines in Figure 15-1, which represents the basic five-atom ring structure common to most clinically used anticonvulsants. Substitution at position 1 of the ring results in the various classes of anticonvulsants as indicated in Table 15-2.

A phenyl ring at R_1 or R_2, such as appears in phenytoin, is a highly desirable though not critical substituent for protection against grand mal epilepsy. An alkyl substituent at R_1 or R_2, such as appears in ethosuximide, is desirable (but again not critical) for control of petit mal epilepsy. Alkyl chains attached to either a nitrogen or a carbon of the basic ring structure tend to increase the sedative properties of anticonvulsants. These structure-activity relationships should be recognized as generalizations to which exceptions occur. Valproic acid, for instance, is a simple branched-chain carboxylic acid. However, it should also be noted that compounds (such as diazepam) that do not seem to share the basic anticonvulsant structure may have steric conformations that are very similar to the classic anticonvulsants.

HYDANTOINS

Phenytoin (or diphenylhydantoin) was one of the first drugs discovered as a result of an organized scientific search for a compound effective for a given disease. Introduced by Merritt and Putnam[20] in 1938, phenytoin was immediately recognized as a breakthrough in anticonvulsant therapy because prominent protection against seizures was obtained without accompanying sedation. Phenytoin has served not only as an effective anticonvulsant but

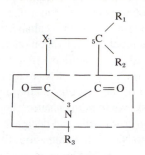

Figure 15-1. Basic ring structure common to anticonvulsants.

Table 15-2. Classes of anticonvulsants according to substitution at position 1 of the chemical structure shown in Figure 15-1

Anticonvulsant	Substitution
Barbiturates	— CO — NH —
Hydantoins	— NH —
Succinimides	— CH_2 —
Oxazolidinediones	— O —

also as an important pharmacologic tool that has increased our understanding of the underlying mechanisms responsible for the epilepsies.

Mephenytoin and ethotoin are chemically and pharmacologically related to phenytoin. In general, they offer the same spectrum of anticonvulsant properties as phenytoin but are either more toxic or less potent. Because of their limitations, these hydantoins are normally used in combination with other anticonvulsants.

Pharmacologic effects

Although the exact mechanism of action responsible for the anticonvulsant effect of phenytoin is not established, many of its pharmacologic properties are known, any or all of which may contribute to its anticonvulsant action. In neurophysiologic studies, phenytoin has been shown to prevent the spread of abnormal neuronal depolarizations from the epileptic focus to surrounding normal neuronal populations, yet the spontaneous discharges at the focus itself are not depressed.[21] Additionally, phenytoin suppresses the duration of afterdischarge of neurons. Reduction in the spread of neuronal activity and afterdischarge by phenytoin is, at least in part, due to a block of posttetanic potentiation.[9] Posttetanic potentiation refers to a phenomenon in which synaptic transmission is enhanced as a result of presynaptic repetitive activation (as would occur at an abnormally firing epileptic focus).

The major site of action of phenytoin appears to be at the level of the neuronal membrane. Phenytoin has been shown to both enhance[28] and suppress[3] Na^+ extrusion from cells and decrease membrane permeability to Na^+.[23] In summation, these actions favor an increase in the ratio of extracellular to intracellular Na^+, stabilizing the neuronal membrane, which in turn diminishes seizure propagation. At therapeutic concentrations, however, phenytoin does not alter either the stimulus threshold or the normal propagation of nervous impulses. The stabilizing effect on excitable membranes may account for the effectiveness of phenytoin in trigeminal neuralgia.[16] Phenytoin inhibits Ca^{++} influx across cellular and subcellular membranes.[26] It is unclear if this is a direct effect of phenytoin on Ca^{++} transport mechanisms or a secondary result of the inhibition of Na^+ influx. Phenytoin has also been shown to interfere with the interaction of Ca^{++} and calmodulin, which in turn disrupts Ca^{++}-dependent phosphorylation of proteins necessary for neurotransmitter release from presynaptic nerve terminals.[7]

Another action of phenytoin that may be important in terms of its anticonvulsant effect is its influence on the concentrations of cyclic nucleotides in brain cells. These nucleotides, specifically cAMP and cGMP, are vital regulators of neural transmission. Phenytoin, as well as carbamazepine, phenobarbital, and primidone, inhibits experimentally induced accumulations of cAMP and cGMP in brain tissue.[18]

Absorption, fate, and excretion

Phenytoin is slowly absorbed from the gastrointestinal tract and eventually metabolized in the liver to its primary metabolite, the parahydroxyphenyl derivative. After conjugation with glucuronic acid and excretion in the bile, the compound is then reabsorbed and eliminated in the urine. This metabolite is devoid of anticonvulsant activity. Several other metabolites of phenytoin and a small amount of the parent drug are found in the urine. Phenytoin is also excreted by the salivary glands, which may be a contributing factor in producing gingival hyperplasia as a side effect. The FDA now requires that phenytoin capsules be labeled as "extended"

or "prompt" depending on their absorption rate. Extended indicates slow absorption with peak blood concentrations obtained in 4 to 12 hours. Prompt indicates rapid absorption with peak concentrations in 1.5 to 3 hours. The half-life of phenytoin generally varies from 15 to 20 hours. Because noncompliance is such a major problem in anticonvulsant therapy, it is sometimes advisable to administer the total dose of phenytoin once a day. This dosing regimen is appropriate only if divided doses have been shown to control seizures. Once-a-day administration is not appropriate for tablets or suspensions of phenytoin because toxic plasma concentrations may be achieved, particularly in children. Changing from one dosage form or brand of manufacture to another may lead to suboptimal drug concentrations because of differences in bioavailability.

Toxic reactions and side effects

Symptoms associated with overdose of phenytoin include ataxia, nystagmus, incoordination, and unsteadiness. These symptoms may be the result of damage to Purkinje cells of the cerebellum, which has been reported with long-term use of phenytoin. Drowsiness, lethargy, diplopia, confusion, and (rarely) hallucinations are also manifestations of phenytoin toxicity. Phenytoin has little detrimental effect on the cardiovascular system unless administered intravenously in a massive dose. Under such conditions, cardiovascular collapse, irreversible coma, and death have occurred. (As discussed in Chapter 24, phenytoin is useful in the treatment of cardiac arrhythmias associated with digitalis intoxication.) Less serious side effects of phenytoin include gingival hyperplasia, which occurs in approximately 10% to 30% of patients, hirsutism, gastrointestinal disturbances, and drug allergy. Various blood dyscrasias, such as leukopenia, agranulocytosis, aplastic anemia, and megaloblastic anemia may occur. The latter condition is apparently due to altered folic acid metabolism and can be corrected by administration of folic acid. Phenytoin also disturbs the metabolism of vitamin D. Although the resultant effect on bone metabolism is usually subclinical, overt cases of rickets and osteomalacia have been observed.[13] The condition is treated and prevented by providing vitamin D supplements sufficient to restore the calcification of bone to normal. Other drugs implicated in anticonvulsant-induced osteomalacia include phenobarbital and, presumably, derivatives of phenobarbital and phenytoin.

Children born to mothers who have received phenytoin throughout their pregnancy are at a greater risk for congenital malformations.[2] The most common anomalies are cleft lip and cleft palate and congenital heart disease.[1] These developmental defects, as well as psychomotor delay, prenatal and postnatal growth deficiencies, impaired intellectual performance, and genitourinary and skeletal deformations, are collectively referred to as the fetal hydantoin syndrome. While none of the currently available anticonvulsants is completely devoid of teratogenic potential, some data suggest that carbamazepine and phenobarbital may be the safer anticonvulsants to use in pregnancy.[27]

BARBITURATES

Phenobarbital is one of the oldest, least expensive, least toxic, and most effective anticonvulsants available. Phenobarbital also offers one of the widest spectrums of anticonvulsant activity, being effective against grand mal epilepsy, focal seizures, and psychomotor epilepsy. It is the agent of choice for the initial treatment of children who have had their first grand mal attack, since it has low toxicity and, unlike phenytoin, does not promote hair growth (hirsutism) or gingival hyperplasia.

Barbiturates other than phenobarbital are occasionally employed for the treatment of epilepsy. Mephobarbital is said to be less sedating than phenobarbital, though the anticonvulsant properties of this compound are probably due to its metabolite, phenobarbital, to which it is converted by the liver.

Primidone is a deoxybarbiturate relative of phenobarbital and is effective in combination with phenytoin for generalized and psychomotor seizures, particularly those refractory to other drugs. Some hepatic conversion to phenobarbital occurs with primidone. The use of primidone is somewhat limited due to its sedative properties.

Pharmacologic effects

The barbiturates are CNS depressants and exert a marked inhibitory effect on repetitive activity in central pathways. Like phenytoin, phenobarbital limits the spread of seizure discharges, but it also raises the threshold for activation of epileptic foci. As discussed in Chapter 14, the synapse is the principal site of action of the barbiturates. Excitatory signals can be depressed by the barbiturates whereas inhibitory transmissions are prolonged.

These synaptic effects occur at low doses of barbiturates; higher doses depress all forms of neuronal activity. Barbiturates block the transcellular transport of sodium and potassium ions, which could explain the membrane-stabilizing properties of these compounds. The inhibition by phenobarbital of the accumulation of cAMP has already been mentioned. Another membrane effect that could account for the anticonvulsant properties of the barbiturates is the inhibition of Ca^{++} flux, similar to that described for phenytoin.

Absorption, fate, and excretion

Phenobarbital is completely, if slowly, absorbed from the gastrointestinal tract. About one half of the drug is bound to plasma protein. Approximately 30% of phenobarbital is excreted unchanged in the urine, and the rest is inactivated by the liver. Entry of phenobarbital into the brain is slow; therefore, the drug is not useful for the initial, emergency treatment of status epilepticus, even when administered intravenously. The plasma half-life of phenobarbital ranges between 50 and 160 hours. Because of its long half-life, very small fluctuations in plasma concentrations occur over a 24-hour period.

As mentioned earlier, primidone and mephobarbital are converted to phenobarbital in the liver. Phenobarbital can be detected in the plasma approximately 24 to 48 hours after initiation of primidone therapy. Another metabolite of primidone, which is formed more readily than phenobarbital, is phenylethylmalonamide. This compound is measurable within 1 to 2 hours after administration of primidone. Animal studies indicate that this metabolite possesses some anticonvulsant properties, which may contribute to the beneficial effect of primidone.

Toxic reactions and side effects

The major side effects of phenobarbital are covered in Chapter 14. When used as an anticonvulsant, the most common side effect of phenobarbital is, of course, sedation, although a paradoxical excitatory reaction may sometimes occur in children and the elderly. Tolerance usually develops to the sedative effects of phenobarbital. Like phenytoin, phenobarbital has been reported to cause megaloblastic anemia and osteomalacia, which have been successfully treated wtih folic acid and vitamin D, respectively. As previously discussed, phenobarbital appears to be relatively free of teratogenic effects. However, it should also be noted that, when it is combined with phenytoin (a commonly used combination), teratogenicity appears to increase.[10]

The most common side effects of primidone are primarily a result of its CNS depressant properties. Complications include sedation, dizziness, ataxia, and nystagmus. Various blood dyscrasias and rashes similar to those described for phenytoin and phenobarbital also occur with primidone.

SUCCINIMIDES

Fewer side effects and greater anticonvulsant properties have allowed ethosuximide to replace trimethadione (see below) as the agent of choice for petit mal epilepsy. Methsuximide and phensuximide preceded ethosuximide for the treatment of absence seizures, but because ethosuximide has proved to be more effective and less toxic, the use of the former compounds is restricted to patients refractory to first-line drugs.

Pharmacologic effects

Ethosuximide prevents petit mal (absence) seizures in approximately 50% of patients and reduces their frequency in another 40% to 45%. The pharmacologic properties of ethosuximide appear to be very similar to those of trimethadione. Ethosuximide elevates the threshold for electroshock seizures, depresses the firing of experimentally produced epileptic foci, antagonizes cortically evoked inhibition in the spinal nucleus of the trigeminal tract,[11] and depresses the release of excitatory neurotransmitters is significantly affected by trimeidence that ethosuximide has a significant action on the neuronal membrane. Thus, no effect has been reported on Na^+, K^+, Cl^-, or Ca^{++} fluxes.

Absorption, fate, and excretion

The succinimides are absorbed from the gastrointestinal tract, metabolized by the liver, and excreted either unchanged or as metabolites in the urine. The plasma half-life of ethosuximide is approximately 30 hours in children and 60 hours in adults. Ethosuximide passes membrane barriers rapidly and thus appears quickly in cerebrospinal fluid, milk, saliva, and the fetus. Because salivary titers accurately reflect plasma concentrations, samples are readily obtained for monitoring.

Toxic reactions and side effects

Common side effects of the succinimides include gastrointestinal distress, headache, dizziness, and skin rash. More serious reactions, blood dyscrasias in particular, have been reported but are rare. Nonetheless, blood counts are recommended at no greater than monthly intervals, since fatal cases of bone marrow depression have been reported. Patients suffering from such toxic effects may exhibit fever, sore throat, and cutaneous petechiae as well as other hemorrhages. These serious responses appear to be dose related.

There is little information available regarding the teratogenicity of ethosuximide. While apparently not without teratogenic potential, ethosuximide is less teratogenic than trimethadione, phenytoin, or primidone[27] and is probably the drug of choice for petit mal in pregnancy.

OXAZOLIDINEDIONES

Trimethadione was the first anticonvulsant agent specific for petit mal epilepsy. It and the closely related agent paramethadione are now reserved for treatment of absence seizures in patients refractory to other drugs.

Pharmacologic effects

Studies have shown that trimethadione is more effective in elevating seizure threshold and depressing the firing of experimentally produced foci than it is in preventing the local propagation of seizure activity.[21] Unlike phenytoin, trimethadione does not antagonize posttetanic potentiation. The prominent depressant effect of trimethadione on repetitive neuronal firing may result from the ability of this compound to reduce the permeability of neuronal membranes to potassium.[12] Trimethadione enhances both presynaptic and postsynaptic inhibition but does not alter GABA synthesis, concentrations, or metabolism. None of the other neurotransmitters is significantly affected by trimethadione either. Indeed, more is known about what trimethadione does not do than what it does; thus, its mechanism of anticonvulsant action remains obscure.

Absorption, fate, and excretion

The oxazolidinediones are absorbed from the gastrointestinal tract, metabolized by the liver, and excreted either unchanged or as metabolites in the urine. The metabolites accumulate in the body and are thought to be responsible for most of the anticonvulsant properties of these drugs. For example, trimethadione is almost completely converted to dimethadione, which is more potent than the parent drug. Dimethadione is not metabolized but is slowly excreted by the kidney. After several weeks of trimethadione administration, dimethadione attains concentrations over 20 times that of the administered drug.

Toxic reactions and side effects

A characteristic side effect of trimethadione is hemeralopia, also referred to as light blindness. This condition is characterized by visual disturbances in bright light or sunlight. Skin rashes and blood dyscrasias have also been reported. Periodic blood counts are recommended with the oxazolidinediones.

Trimethadione use should be held to an absolute minimum in pregnancy, as spontaneous abortions occur with increased frequency and the potential for teratogenesis is also greater than normal. Characteristic fetal anomalies include malformed or low-set ears, cleft lip and palate, delayed mental development, speech impairment, urogenital and skeletal malformation, and cardiac defects. The term *fetal trimethadione syndrome* has been used to describe these malformations. Most of the serious toxic effects of trimethadione do not seem to be dose related.

VALPROIC ACID

Valproic acid (dipropylacetic acid) was introduced in Europe (as sodium valproate) in 1963 and has been widely used since. It was approved for use in the United States in 1978. Valproic acid appears to be particularly effective for absence (petit mal) seizures, but it also antagonizes grand mal and psychomotor seizures. Interest has focused on valproic acid because of the simplicity of its structure (Figure 15-2) and the fact that it is chemically unrelated to all other anticonvulsant drugs currently available.

Pharmacologic effects

There are three major hypotheses for the mechanism of valproic acid's anticonvulsant activity. First, it has been suggested that valproate ions increase GABA concentrations in the brain. The drug then presumably acts by enhancing GABA-mediated neuronal inhibition. Unfortunately, a good correlation between increased brain levels of GABA and anticonvulsant activity has never been convincingly demonstrated, especially at therapeutic doses of valproic acid. Second, valproate may have a direct effect on the neuronal

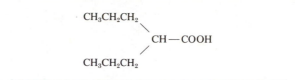

Figure 15-2. Structural formula of valproic acid.

membrane to diminish its excitability.[25] Last, valproate may potentiate GABA so that a given amount of GABA produces a greater inhibitory effect.[19] At present, it is probably safe to say that valproic acid exerts its anticonvulsant effect through the GABA system, even if the exact mechanism is unclear.

Absorption, fate, and excretion

Valproic acid is completely absorbed from the gastrointestinal tract, but absorption rates depend on the formulation (capsules, syrup, etc.) and whether the dose has been taken in the presence of food. Absorption is delayed if valproic acid is taken 2 to 3 hours after a meal. The drug exists in blood in the ionized form and is largely bound to plasma proteins. Valproic acid crosses membrane barriers freely and is thus found in the fetus, milk, blood, liver, kidney, and brain. It also accumulates in growing bone. Valproic acid undergoes extensive metabolic degradation before excretion in the urine. The half-life of valproate is approximately 10 hours, which may partially account for the fluctuations in plasma concentrations when it is administered on a long-term basis.

Toxic reactions and side effects

The most common manifestations of valproic acid toxicity are appetite disturbances, indigestion, heartburn, nausea, and weight change. Fortunately, the gastrointestinal reactions are temporary. Serious side effects, including hepatic, neurologic, or hematologic toxicity, are rare. High doses of valproic acid may give rise to platelet disorders, leading to bruising of the skin and, occasionally, gingival bleeding. Usually, however, the platelet disorders are not severe, and the patient is asymptomatic. Teratogenic effects have been demonstrated in animal studies, and reports from human use suggest that valproic acid is potentially teratogenic.[4]

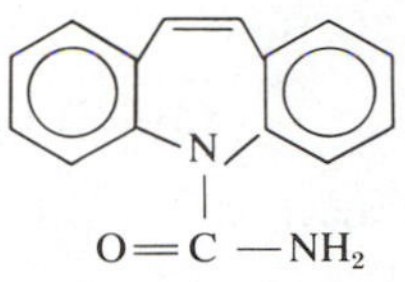

Figure 15-3. Structural formula of carbamazepine.

CARBAMAZEPINE

Carbamazepine is an iminostilbene derivative (Figure 15-3) closely related chemically to the tricyclic antidepressants. It differs from the tricyclic imipramine only by the presence of a double bond in the central ring and a shorter side chain. Carbamazepine is a major anticonvulsant drug, being most effective against generalized tonic-clonic seizures and partial seizures with complex symptoms. Like phenytoin, carbamazepine is indicated for the treatment of trigeminal neuralgia, but it is not an analgesic and is not effective for other types of pain.

Pharmacologic effects

The mechanism of action of carbamazepine is unknown. Certain thalamic nuclei implicated in the generalization and spread of seizure discharges are depressed by doses of carbamazepine that have no effect on other thalamic nuclei nor on the reticular formation, amygdala, hippocampus, and striatum.[15] Carbamazepine blocks posttetanic potentiation, but at doses higher than therapeutic. As would be expected by its structural resemblance to the tricyclic antidepressants, carbamazepine inhibits the uptake of norepinephrine into neuronal tissue. The potency of carbamazepine in inhibiting norepinephrine uptake is approximately one fourth that of imipramine, yet imipramine has only weak anticonvulsant properties. It is therefore unlikely that this mechanism contributes significantly to the anticonvulsant action of carbamazepine. Like phenytoin, carbamazepine reduces experimentally induced cAMP accumulation,[18] but again at higher than therapeutic doses.

Absorption, fate, and excretion

Carbamazepine is absorbed relatively slowly, with peak plasma concentrations obtained in 3 to 8 hours. It is distributed throughout the body, with highest concentrations occurring in liver, kidney, and brain. Several metabolites of carbamazepine are formed, some of which have anticonvulsant properties. The metabolites are excreted in the urine. Like phenobarbital, carbamazepine induces hepatic drug-metabolizing enzymes.

Toxic reactions and side effects

The most common signs and symptoms of overdose with carbamazepine are neurologic. These include dizziness, double vision, drowsiness, headache, ataxia, and slurred speech. Convulsions may be precipitated in the case of acute intoxication with carbamazepine. Various types of involuntary motor activity have been reported, but these are most common in the elderly. Psychologic effects might be predictable, due to the close structural relationship of carbamazepine to the tricyclic antidepressants, but this has been difficult to demonstrate clinically. Some improvement in mood and alertness, especially in patients previously sedated with depressant drugs, has been reported; on the other hand, so also have mental disorders, including psychoses. Hematologic reactions to carbamazepine are rare but serious. Bone marrow depression, aplastic anemia, leukopenia, and agranulocytosis have been associated with carbamazepine; however, a causal relationship needs to be critically documented.

BENZODIAZEPINES

Most of the benzodiazepines have some anticonvulsant properties. The pharmacology of these drugs is discussed in detail in Chapter 13. Of the benzodiazepines that are available in the United States, only diazepam, clonazepam, and clorazepate are used clinically as anticonvulsants. Diazepam is very effective in terminating the life-threatening continual convulsion of status epilepticus and for the treatment of local anesthetic–induced seizures,[22] whereas clonazepam is generally most effective for petit mal (absence) seizures and in the treatment of myoclonic epilepsy. Clorazepate is indicated as adjunctive therapy in the management of partial seizures. Complex partial seizures and reflex epilepsies, such as photosensitive epilepsy, may also respond to clonazepam. Though the site of action responsible for the anticonvulsant properties of the benzodiazepines is unknown, the cerebellum has been proposed as a possible site of action, because diazepam simultaneously increases the firing frequency of cerebellar Purkinje cells and decreases epileptiform discharge of the cerebral cortex.[17] Like phenytoin, the benzodiazepines prevent the spread of the seizure discharge but have little effect on the seizure focus. The anticonvulsant action of the benzodiazepines is thought to be exerted through modification of GABA-mediated systems, as is the case for their antianxiety action. The possibility that different receptors might be involved in these two pharmacologic effects is likely, however, and is of significant interest both pharmacologically and clinically. The absorption, fate, and excretion of the benzodiazepines are discussed in Chapter 13. There are no differences in these properties when these drugs are used as anticonvulsants, as opposed to when they are used as antianxiety agents, except that it should be noted that the major metabolite both of clorazepate and diazepam (desmethyldiazepam) has anticonvulsant properties, whereas that of clonazepam (the 7-amino derivative) is pharmacologically inactive.

The side effects predictable for CNS depressants, including drowsiness, dizziness, ataxia, nystagmus, dysarthria, and hypotonia, occur most commonly with the benzodiazepines. Serious side effects are very rare. Occasionally the administration of clonazepam precipitates a different variety of seizure than the one being treated. The potential teratogenicity of the benzodiazepines is discussed in Chapter 13. There is little evidence to date that clonazepam is teratogenic, but it is recommended that use of the compound during pregnancy be limited to those cases in which the clinical situation warrants the risk.

Nitrazepam is primarily used as a hypnotic. However, it is used in some countries as an anticonvulsant, particularly for the treatment of infantile spasms with hypsarrhythmia. This is, fortunately, a rare type of epilepsy; it is refractory to most anticonvulsants and, in general, the prognosis for these patients is poor.

OTHER ANTICONVULSANTS
Carbonic anhydrase inhibitors

The carbonic anhydrase inhibitors are primarily effective against petit mal epilepsy but are useful also for the control of seizures that have a tendency to recur at a specific time of the menstrual cycle. The mechanism by which the latter seizures are controlled is unclear; however, acetazolamide is known to reduce intracellular sodium and water retention, both of which increase during the premenstrual period. By inhibiting carbonic anhydrase (located in glial cells), carbon dioxide is allowed to accumulate in the brain. Carbon dioxide eleva-

tion causes a decrease in intracellular sodium and an increase in intracellular potassium. Neuronal hyperpolarization and decreased excitability are the net result that in turn is thought to block the spread of seizure discharges. Further research is needed to explain how this mechanism occurs.

The carbonic anhydrase inhibitors are primarily used as adjuncts to other anticonvulsants, such as ethosuximide or phenytoin. Tolerance to the anticonvulsant effect develops rapidly. There are few side effects with the carbonic anhydrase inhibitors, but skin rashes, gastrointestinal disturbances, and tingling of the hands and feet are the most common. Most symptoms disappear in 8 to 24 hours. Teratogenic effects have been demonstrated in experimental animals.

Phenacemide

The toxicity of phenacemide is such that it may be considered a "drug of the last resort." The use of phenacemide is restricted to those cases of psychomotor seizures that are refractory to all other drugs. Phenacemide is a very toxic agent; it can cause disorders of the blood-forming system, kidney, and liver. Behavioral and personality changes that have resulted in suicide have also been reported with phenacemide.

Experimental drugs

Because the currently available anticonvulsants effectively control seizures for a large percentage of patients, the impetus to develop new drugs is not as great as for many other classes of drugs. Nonetheless, there is still a need for agents with specific and potent anticonvulsant properties but free from complicating side effects. In this regard, derivatives of known anticonvulsants, as well as compounds chemically unrelated to currently available drugs, have been examined as potential anticonvulsants.

Eterobarb is a barbiturate derivative that appears to be as effective as phenobarbital for the control of tonic-clonic and partial seizures. The compound is metabolically converted to phenobarbital and other metabolites in the body. Eterobarb reportedly produces less sedation than phenobarbital, but few clinical trials have been conducted.

Cinromide is a cinnamamide derivative under investigation clinically as a broad-spectrum anticonvulsant. In limited clinical trials it appears to be a useful adjunct for therapy of patients with refractory partial seizures.

Table 15-3. Adverse effects of anticonvulsants

	Phenobar-bital	Phenyt-oin	Ethosux-imide	Trimetha-dione	Primi-done	Carbamaz-epine	Clonaz-epam	Valproic acid
Sedation	X	X*	X	X	X	X	X	X
Ataxia	X*	X*	X	X	X	X	X	X
Nystagmus	X*	X*			X	X	X	X
Dizziness	X*		X	X	X	X	X	X
Headache		X				X		X
Paradoxical excitation	X*				X	X		
Motor disorders		X	X			X	X	X*
Psychotic reactions				X	X	X	X	
Other behavioral changes	X	X	X	X	X	X	X	
Hepatoxicity		X				X		X
Megaloblastic anemia	X	X			X	X		
Other blood dyscrasias	X	X	X	X	X	X	X	X
Osteomalacia	X	X			?		X	
Lupus erythematosus syndrome		X	X	X	X	X		
Gastrointestinal disturbances	X	X	X		X	X	X	X
Skin rashes	X	X	X	X	X	X	X	
Alopecia	X			X		X	X	X
Hirsutism		X						
Gingival hyperplasia		X						
Hemeralopia				X				
Teratogenicity	?	X	?	X	?	?	?	?

*Only at high doses.

The anticonvulsant properties of the benzodiazepines and the elucidation of their pharmacologic actions have stimulated new interest in compounds that might be GABA agonists. A number of GABA agonists, such as progabide and muscimol, are currently being examined. Although toxicity, limited penetration of the brain, and a number of other deficiencies may limit the usefulness of these particular compounds, GABA agonists as a group represent a new approach to the treatment of epilepsy.

GENERAL THERAPEUTIC USE

The goal of anticonvulsant therapy is to obtain 100% control of epileptic seizures at the least toxic and lowest possible dose. Obviously these conditions cannot be met in all cases, but it is thought that with the currently available anticonvulsant drugs 80% of all patients can be seizure free if drug plasma concentrations are properly monitored and the appropriate dose adjustments are made. Initial anticonvulsant therapy sometimes necessitates not only frequent alterations in dose but also a seemingly trial-by-error approach until the seizure responds to a specific anticonvulsant.

Even after the epilepsy is initially controlled, the continued administration of the drug may lead to the development of tolerance. At this stage, an adjunctive agent or even another primary anticonvulsant may be added to the drug regimen. The addition of other anticonvulsants obviously necessitates dosage adjustments once again. Chronic administration of a given anticonvulsant, even if tolerance does not develop, may produce side effects that necessitate dosage changes or a substitution of another anticonvulsant. While these adjustments may not always be necessary, it is well to note that anticonvulsant therapy is not static, routine, and completely predictable but, rather, subject to a variety of factors that are ever changing.

IMPLICATIONS IN DENTISTRY

The most common adverse effects and some of the unusual side reactions of the primary anticonvulsant drugs are summarized in Table 15-3. This list is not intended to be comprehensive, and the clinician may find in practice or in the literature a variety of additional adverse effects. Included, however, are the common untoward effects that are pertinent for the day-to-day practice of dentistry. For example, most of the primary anticonvulsant drugs produce some degree of CNS depression, so the dentist must be aware of the additive effect of

CNS depressants likely to be used, such as anesthetics, antianxiety agents, and the opioid analgesics. Another common side effect of most of the anticonvulsant agents is the production of blood dyscrasias. Such disorders may increase the patient's susceptibility to infection. The fact that various anticonvulsants alter mineral metabolism should be considered when one is confronted with anomalies in tooth development.

A number of side effects specific to individual anticonvulsant agents are clinically relevant to dentistry. Phenytoin-induced gingival hyperplasia is a well-known example. Hyperplasia most commonly occurs in the anterior mandibular region, especially in the case of "mouth breathers," and develops to the greatest extent in the interdental papillae between the incisors. Edentulous areas of the alveolar mucosa do not undergo hypertrophy, or do so to a lesser extent than other areas. Histologically, hyperplasia is characterized by proliferation of connective tissue, but there is controversy as to the specific tissue component affected. Some studies suggest that the number[24] or activity[8] of fibroblasts increases. Whatever the mechanism, the phenytoin-induced hyperplasia may totally or partially obscure the crowns of teeth, which obviously hampers proper cleaning, is esthetically unpleasing, and necessitates periodic resection. The rate of development of the condition can be diminished by proper oral hygiene.

Phenobarbital increases hepatic microsomal enzyme activity, and, as a result, blood concentrations of drugs metabolized by these enzymes may be altered. For example, phenobarbital can increase the rate of metabolism of phenytoin, an effect that could theoretically result in a decreased anticonvulsant activity of phenytoin. Experimentally, however, the anticonvulsant properties of phenytoin and phenobarbital are additive when used in combination, and therapeutically these two drugs are often used in combination with beneficial results. The increased hepatic microsomal enzyme activity may diminish the antimicrobial effectiveness of antibiotics (e.g., tetracyclines) inactivated by the liver.

Carbamazepine induces liver microsomal enzymes, and it too can decrease the antimicrobial action of some antibiotics. Carbamazepine toxicity may be precipitated by the concomitant administration of propoxyphene (Darvon).[6] Temporary carbamazepine-induced taste disorders have been reported, but these apparently subside with time.[14]

An unusual side effect of primidone is localized gingival pain. Such a reaction could cause the patient, and the dentist, to assume falsely that the pain was of dental origin. A complete medical history is therefore essential for proper dental treatment.

It is often recommended that the patient who has epilepsy should be treated somewhat cautiously so as to reduce emotional upset and help prevent the precipitation of a seizure. However, except in cases of patients whose seizures are not well controlled, the patient with epilepsy need not be handled any differently from other patients. Indeed, due to the lingering stigma associated with epilepsy, these patients may be reluctant to reveal their disease, and a seizure disorder may only be ascertained by the clinician being alert to subtle clues offered by anticonvulsant-induced side effects or by designing a properly phrased and complete medical history.

Anticonvulsants used clinically

Nonproprietary name	Proprietary name
Hydantoins	
ethotoin	Peganone
mephenytoin	Mesantoin
phenytoin	Dilantin
Barbiturates	
mephobarbital	Mebaral
metharbital	Gemonil
phenobarbital	Luminal
primidone*	Mysoline
Succinimides	
ethosuximide	Zarontin
methsuximide	Celontin
phensuximide	Milontin
Oxazolidinediones	
paramethadione	Paradione
trimethadione	Tridione
Benzodiazepines	
clonazepam	Clonopin
clorazepate	Tranxene
diazepam	Valium
nitrazepam†	Mogadon
Miscellaneous	
acetazolamide	Diamox
carbamazepine	Tegretol
phenacemide	Phenurone
valproic acid	Depakene

*Not a true barbiturate.
†Not available in the United States.

CITED REFERENCES

1. Anderson, R.C. Cardiac effects in children of mothers receiving anti-convulsant therapy during pregnancy. Journal of Pediatrics **89**:318-319, 1976.
2. Biale, Y., Lewenthal, H., and Aderet, N.B. Congenital malformations due to anticonvulsive drugs. Obstetrics and Gynecology **45**:439-442, 1975.
3. Bittar, E.E., Chen, S.S., Danielson, B.G., and Tong, E.Y. An investigation of the action of diphenylhydantoin on sodium efflux in barnacle muscle fibres. Acta Physiologica Scandinavica **89**:30-38, 1973.
4. Brown, N.A., Kao, J., and Fabro, S. Teratogenic potential of valproic acid. Lancet **1**:660-661, 1980.
5. Capek, R., and Esplin, B. Effects of ethosuximide on transmission of repetitive impulses and apparent rates of transmitter turnover in the spinal monosynaptic pathway. Journal of Pharmacology and Experimental Therapeutics **201**:320-325, 1977.
6. Dam, M., and Christiansen, J. Interaction of propoxyphene with carbamazepine. Lancet **2**: 509, 1977.
7. De Lorenzo, R.J. Phenytoin: calcium- and calmodulin-dependent protein phosphorylation and neurotransmitter release. Advances in Neurology **27**:399-414, 1980.
8. Ebodi, M.S., and Scott, P.M. Increase in collagen level by diphenylhydantoin as possible mechanism of drug-induced gingival hyperplasia. Clinical Toxicology **4**:39-46, 1971.
9. Esplin, D.W. Effects of diphenylhydantoin on synaptic transmission in cat spinal cord and stellate ganglion. Journal of Pharmacology and Experimental Therapeutics **120**:301-323, 1957.
10. Fedrick, J. Epilepsy and pregnancy: a report from the Oxford Record Linkage Study. British Medical Journal **1**:442-448, 1973.
11. Fromm, G.H., and Kohli, C.M. The role of inhibitory pathways in petit mal epilepsy. Neurology **22**:1012-1020, 1972.
12. Gross, G.J., and Woodbury, D.M. Effects of pentylenetetrazol on ion transport in the isolated toad bladder. Journal of Pharmacology and Experimental Therapeutics **181**:257-272, 1972.
13. Hahn, T.J., Hendin, B.A., Scharp, C.R., Boisseau, V.C., and Haddad, J.G., Jr. Serum 25-hydroxycalciferol levels and bone mass in children on chronic anticonvulsant therapy. New England Journal of Medicine **292**:550-554, 1975.
14. Halbreich, U. Tegretol dependency and diversion of the sense of taste. Israeli Annals of Psychiatry **12**:328-332, 1974.
15. Holm, E., Kelleter, R., Heinemann, H., and Hamann, K.F. Elektrophysiologische Analyse der Wirkungen von Carbamazepine auf das Behirn der Katze. Pharmakopsychiatrie Neuro-psychopharmakologie **3**:187-200, 1970.
16. Iannone, A., Baker, A.B., and Morrell, F. Dilantin in the treatment of neuralgia. Neurology **9**:126-128, 1958.
17. Julien, R.M. Cerebellar involvement in the antiepileptic action of diazepam. Neuropharmacology **11**:683-691, 1972.
18. Lewin, E., and Bleck, V. Cyclic AMP accumulation in cerebral cortical slices: Effect of carbamazepine, phenobarbital, and phenytoin. Epilepsia **18**:237-242, 1977.
19. Macdonald, R.L., and Bergey, G.K. Valproic acid augments GABA-mediated postsynaptic inhibition in cultured mammalian neurons. Brain Research **170**:558-562, 1979.
20. Merritt, H.H., and Putnam, T.J. Sodium diphenyl hydantoinate in the treatment of convulsive disorders. Journal of the American Medical Association **111**:1068-1073, 1938.
21. Morrell, F., Bradley, W., and Ptashne, M. Effect of drugs on discharge characteristics of chronic epileptogenic lesions. Neurology **9**:492-498, 1959.
22. Munson, E.S., and Wagman, I.H. Diazepam treatment of local anesthetic-induced seizures. Anesthesiology **37**:523-528, 1972.
23. Pincus, J.H., and Rawson, M.D. Diphenylhydantoin and intracellular sodium concentration. Neurology **19**:419-422, 1969.
24. Shafer, W.G. Effect of Dilantin sodium on growth of human fibroblast-like cell cultures. Proceedings of the Society for Experimental Biology and Medicine **104**:198-201, 1960.
25. Slater, G.E., and Johnston, D. Sodium valproate increases potassium conductance in Aplysia neurons. Epilepsia **19**:379-384, 1978.
26. Sohn, R.S., and Ferrendelli, J.A. Inhibition of Ca^{++} transport into rat brain synaptosomes by diphenylhydantoin. Journal of Pharmacology and Experimental Therapeutics **185**:272-275, 1973.
27. Sullivan, F.M., and McElhatton, P.R. A comparison of the teratogenic activity of the antiepileptic drugs carbamazepine, clonazepam, ethosuximide, phenobarbital, phenytoin, and primidone in mice. Toxicology and Applied Pharmacology **40**:365-378, 1977.
28. Woodbury, D.M. Effect of diphenylhydantoin on electrolytes and radiosodium turnover in brain and other tissues of normal, hyponatremic and postictal rats. Journal of Pharmacology and Experimental Therapeutics **115**:74-95, 1955.

GENERAL REFERENCES

Glazko, A.J. Antiepileptic drugs: biotransformation, metabolism, and serum half-life. Epilepsia **16**:367-391, 1975.

Hassell, T.M. Epilepsy and the Oral Manifestations of Phenytoin Therapy. Basel, S. Karger AG, 1981.

Jasper, H.H., Ward, A.A., and Pope, A., eds. Basic Mechanisms of the Epilepsies. Boston, Little, Brown & Co., 1969.

Kutt, H. Interactions of antiepileptic drugs. Epilepsia **16**:393-402, 1975.

Pippenger, C.E., Penry, J.K., and Kutt, H. Antiepileptic Drugs: Quantitative Analysis and Interpretation. New York, Raven Press, 1978.

Schmidt, R.P., and Wilder, B.J. Epilepsy. Philadelphia, F.A. Davis Co., 1968.

Simon, D., and Penry, J.K. Sodium di-N-propylacetate (DPA) in the treatment of epilepsy; a review. Epilepsia **16**:549-573 1975.

van Duijn, H., and Beckmann, M.K.F. Dipropylacetic acid (Depakine) in experimental epilepsy in the alert cat. Epilepsia **16**:83-90, 1975.

Woodbury, D.M., Penry, J.K., and Pippenger, C.E., eds. Antiepileptic Drugs, ed. 2. New York, Raven Press, 1982.

16 Antiparkinson agents

Leslie P. Felpel

Parkinson's disease, first clearly described in 1817 by James Parkinson, is a chronic progressive degenerative disease of the central nervous system. The disease rarely occurs before the age of 40 but affects approximately 1% of the population over the age of 50. As a rule, Parkinson's disease has an insidious onset, beginning with a slight unilateral weakness of the hand and mild tremor. The most obvious clinical manifestations of parkinsonism are tremor, rigidity, and hypokinesia. Abnormalities of posture and balance, which impair righting reflexes, equilibrium adjustments, and locomotion, contribute to the disability of the patient. Control of the larynx and respiratory muscles is impaired, so that the voice loses volume and develops a monotonous quality, and maximum breathing capacity is reduced. Disorders of the autonomic nervous system, such as orthostatic hypotension, urinary retention or incontinence, and excessive sweating, are common. Drooling of saliva is also common but is mainly due to difficulty in swallowing (dysphagia) rather than to excessive secretion of saliva. Dysphagia may be severe and can result in death by asphyxia, aspiration, or pneumonia. The degenerative progression of the disease proceeds at irregular rates in different patients but, in general, continues over a period of 10 to 20 years before ultimately terminating in severe invalidism. Life expectancy is reduced in parkinsonian patients because of the usual complications associated with chronic invalidism, such as dehydration, pneumonia, and susceptibility to infections.

A causal relationship between Parkinson's disease and the great influenza pandemic of 1918 to 1926 (von Economo's encephalitis lethargica) has long been suspected but never completely proved. A parkinson-like syndrome may also be caused by syphilis, carbon monoxide poisoning, chronic manganese poisoning, cerebral hypoxia caused by arteriosclerosis, and most of the antipsychotic and some of the antidepressant drugs. The prototype of Parkinson's disease, however, is primary or idiopathic parkinsonism, a condition for which no inciting factor has been identified.

Though we are far from pinpointing the cause of Parkinson's disease, tremendous advances have been made in our understanding of the neuropathology of parkinsonism, the central control of movement, and the role of neurotransmitters in motor control and extrapyramidal function. One of the first findings that suggested a role for neurotransmitters in extrapyramidal function was the discovery of large amounts of dopamine in the corpus striatum,[2,20] an area that is an important part of the extrapyramidal system. At about the same time, the drug reserpine was reported to have characteristic extrapyramidal side effects that were similar to the bradykinesia of Parkinson's disease. When it was demonstrated that reserpine-induced bradykinesia was reversed by 3,4-dihydroxyphenylalanine (levodopa, L-dopa), the precursor of dopamine, a link between dopamine and extrapyramidal motor function was established.[7,8] Soon after these experimental findings in animals were reported, abnormally low levels of dopamine were measured in the brains of patients who suffered from Parkinson's disease.[12] Reports of the clinical effectiveness of intravenously administered levodopa on the bradykinesia of Parkinson's disease soon followed.[1,4] Finally, the oral dose regimen of levodopa was established after clinical trials indicated that massive oral doses were required in order to permit a small amount of drug to cross the blood-brain barrier and enter the central nervous system.[9,10] Levodopa, either alone or in combination with other agents, remains the most effective drug for the treatment of parkinsonism today.

Before the discovery of levodopa, the standard

drugs used in the treatment of Parkinson's disease were the anticholinergic agents. There is substantial evidence that a balance between cholinergic and dopaminergic mechanisms exists in the basal ganglia. For example, the substantia nigra inhibits the activity of many neurons of the neostriatum by means of a dopaminergic nigrostriatal pathway,[16] and cholinergic striatal pathways modulate the activity of an inhibitory GABA-containing striatonigral pathway. These reciprocating circuits form the basis for the concept of a feedback interaction between the substantia nigra and the striatum. In parkinsonism, degeneration of melanin-containing neurons of the substantia nigra is a characteristic finding.[24] Loss of these neurons forming the nigrostriatal pathway would release the neostriatum from the inhibitory effect of the substantia nigra, and thus the cholinergic striatonigral input would be unopposed, resulting in an imbalance of activity in both the striatum and the substantia nigra.

Although Parkinson's disease is no doubt more complicated than an imbalance between two neurotransmitters, the effectiveness of levodopa and the anticholinergic drugs in the treatment of this disease and the fact that cholinergic agents like physostigmine exacerbate the clinical symptoms of parkinsonism support this concept. Evidence for this theory is also provided by the fact that the antipsychotic agents (see Chapter 12), which are potent antagonists of dopamine, commonly produce a parkinson-like syndrome as a side effect. Moreover, all of the antihistamines that are effective in treating Parkinson's disease have some anticholinergic activity, and this property may be responsible for their antiparkinson effects.

The classic dopaminergic-cholinergic imbalance concept of Parkinson's disease explains a variety of clinical and pharmacologic responses. However, the identification of several dopamine receptor subtypes in the brain[17] has suggested that this concept may need to be revised and that dopamine may play an even greater role in brain function than previously thought. For example, the differential therapeutic efficacies of various dopamine agonists suggest that Parkinson's disease may not be a single entity but, rather, may consist of several varieties, depending on the receptor subtype involved. The fact that the three cardinal symptoms of parkinsonism (tremor, bradykinesia, and rigidity) do not respond uniformly to the antiparkinson drugs raises the possibility that these symptoms may be caused by different receptors. Further, the characteristic dementia of Parkinson's disease and the characteristic psychotic side effects of levodopa support the concept of a role for dopamine, and possibly for dopamine receptor subtypes, in emotion and behavior. The possible involvement of dopamine in schizophrenia, in the mechanism of action of the antipsychotic drugs, and in antipsychotic drug–induced extrapyramidal disorders (tardive dyskinesia, parkinsonism), has been discussed in Chapter 12. Because the functional development of dopamine receptors in experimental animals correlates fairly well with increasing motor activity, it has been suggested that dopamine may have a crucial function in the development of locomotion. The obvious relationship of dopamine to motor activity has also led to the suggestion of a possible role for dopamine in the hyperactivity syndrome (MBD) in children. Symptoms of motor hyperactivity in the elderly (oral-facial dyskinesias, "mouthing," and tremors) may also be, at least in part, a result of altered dopamine metabolism. Finally, dopamine is known to have an important physiologic role in the central regulation of endocrine function.

At present, most experimental studies have concentrated on the role of dopamine in Parkinson's disease. However, it should be noted that there are several other putative neurotransmitters and neuromodulators in the basal ganglia, including norepinephrine, serotonin, and GABA, and the peptides leu-enkephalin, met-enkephalin, and substance P. The possible interactions of these chemicals, and their role in parkinsonism, have yet to be explored. As our understanding of the pharmacology, anatomy, and physiology of the basal ganglia is improved, a variety of new therapeutic avenues for the treatment of Parkinson's disease will be opened.

LEVODOPA

Levodopa is a neutral amino acid formed from L-tyrosine, and it is a precursor of several endogenous catecholamines, including dopamine and norepinephrine, as shown in Figure 16-1. The major metabolic pathway for levodopa in the body is decarboxylation to dopamine by the enzyme dopa decarboxylase. This enzyme is distributed throughout the body, and its significance in levodopa therapy will be described.

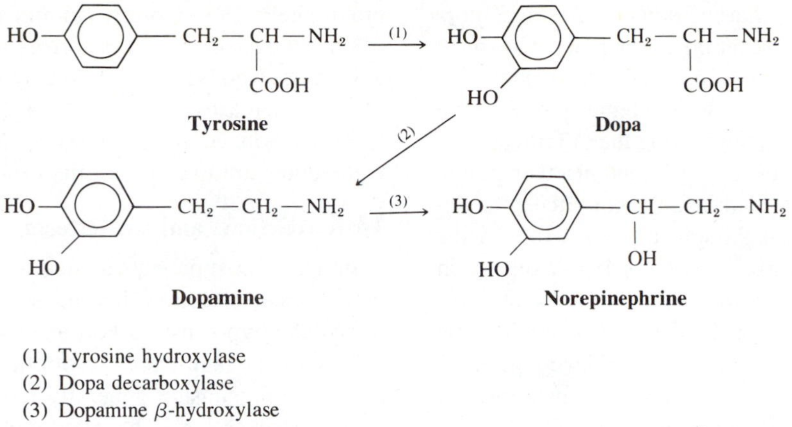

(1) Tyrosine hydroxylase
(2) Dopa decarboxylase
(3) Dopamine β-hydroxylase

Figure 16-1. Synthesis and metabolism of dopa.

Pharmacologic effects

Central nervous system. One of the most characteristic and constant findings in Parkinson's disease is degeneration of melanin-containing cells in the substantia nigra.[24] The major neuronal pathway from the substantia nigra to the neostriatum (caudate nucleus and putamen) contains dopamine,[16] and it is this pathway that appears to degenerate in Parkinson's disease, with a resultant loss of dopamine. The obvious therapy for such a condition would be to restore dopamine concentrations in the basal ganglia to normal. Dopamine, however, does not cross the blood-brain barrier and thus is not effective when administered systemically. The immediate amino-acid precursor of dopamine, levodopa, readily enters the brain, where it is presumably converted metabolically to dopamine. It must be emphasized that levodopa is not curative and does not markedly alter the course of the disease. Postmortem examinations of the brains of parkinsonian patients indicate that morphologic changes in the central nervous system are similar whether patients are treated with levodopa or not.

A beneficial response to levodopa is usually obtained in approximately 75% of parkinsonian patients. However, a decreasing therapeutic response and increasing extrapyramidal motor side effects develop over the course of several years of treatment. Rather bizarre episodes of akinesia occur with increasing frequency with long-term levodopa therapy. In such cases, the patient remains in a given position for various periods of time, as if he were "frozen" and unable to move. The most common form of akinesia is called the "end-of-dose akinesia," and this variety has been shown to correspond to decreasing blood concentrations of levodopa. Patients receiving long-term levodopa therapy also display a response that has been termed the "on-off" effect. This name is derived from the fact that the parkinsonian patient displays fluctuating responses that alternate between complete abolition of symptoms and the full-blown parkinsonian syndrome. This phenomenon occurs at a time corresponding to peak concentrations of levodopa. A third form of oscillation is hypotonia, in which the patient does not respond to levodopa, and no relationship has been found as yet between its occurrence and blood titers of levodopa. The mechanisms responsible for these unusual responses, for the gradual loss of therapeutic efficacy, and for the extrapyramidal side effects during long-term levodopa therapy are unknown. However, the identification of at least three types of dopamine receptors (D_1, D_2, and D_3) in the brain[17] has given new impetus to studies attempting to account for both levodopa-induced side effects and therapeutic responses. The three dopamine receptors types have been characterized with respect to their affinity (or ability to bind) for either dopamine or dopamine antagonists, whether they are adenyl cyclase dependent or independent, and their location (presynaptic, postsynaptic, striatum, cerebral cortex, etc.). The postsynaptic D_2 receptor appears to be particularly important in mediating dopaminergic behavior and responses.[17,22] Several studies have demonstrated that the density of D_2 receptors is reduced in the striatum of patients who have been treated on a long-term basis with levodopa[18,19] and who have become disabled and unresponsive to levodopa therapy, suggesting that a critical density of receptors is necessary to obtain a therapeutic response to the antiparkinson agent. Receptor desensitization is also thought to play a role in the diminishing response to levodopa, as well as in levodopa-induced dyskinesias and the "on-off" effect. Some support for this concept is provided by the observation that withdrawal of levodopa for 2 to 3 weeks (drug holiday) permits reinstitution of the drug at a greatly reduced dose and with less therapeutic fluctuation.[11] Because dopamine receptors that mediate dyskinesia may not be the same, or in the same brain area, as those subserving normal movement, there is currently an active search for drugs selective in stimulating or inhibiting the various dopamine receptors. These drugs offer great promise, but they are in the experimental stage at present.

All of the clinical manifestations of parkinsonism (i.e., tremor, rigidity, and hypokinesia) respond to some degree to levodopa therapy. There are some indications that tremor is less sensitive to levodopa than is rigidity or hypokinesia, but abnormalities of posture, equilibrium, and locomotion improve with treatment. Whereas levodopa initially improves the mental status of the parkinsonian patient, it appears that prolonged usage can induce dementia.

Cardiovascular system. A moderate degree of tachycardia, hypertension, and hypotension occurs with levodopa therapy. These effects are presumably caused by dopamine formed by the metabolism of levodopa. Dopamine may also be responsible for the increased incidence of arrhythmias reported after levodopa therapy. Because of the relatively high incidence of coronary heart disease in the age range of the typical parkinsonian patient, not all arrhythmias may necessarily be caused by levodopa. The levodopa-induced incidence of sinus tachycardia and atrial and ventricular extrasystoles is low and can be reduced further with the addition of a decarboxylase inhibitor, as will be discussed later.

Absorption, fate, and excretion

Levodopa is absorbed from the gastrointestinal tract, but over 90% of the drug is converted to dopamine by dopa decarboxylase in the liver. Approximately 1% of orally administered levodopa reaches the brain. When the drug is combined with a dopa decarboxylase inhibitor, however, this percentage increases significantly. Dopamine is further metabolized by the enzyme MAO, and the metabolites are excreted in the urine.

Toxic reactions and side effects

Initially, most patients treated with levodopa experience side effects such as nausea, vomiting, and orthostatic hypotension. Fortunately, tolerance develops to the nausea and vomiting, and the orthostatic hypotension generally requires no therapeutic intervention. The perplexing and perhaps most serious toxic effect of levodopa is the appearance of involuntary movements. These movements are initially restricted to the orofacial musculature and include abnormal mouth movements, such as chewing motions and protrusion and retraction of the tongue; facial grimacing; and abnormal movements of the head. Later in treatment, the limb and trunk musculature may also be involved. Unfortunately, these movements often occur at dosages of levodopa that are just threshold for control of the parkinsonian symptoms. To date, these dyskinesias cannot be controlled with pharmacologic agents. Although they are relieved somewhat by a reduction in levodopa administration, usually this approach also results in increased parkinsonian symptoms.

On initial therapy levodopa often produces various mental disturbances, such as anxiety, insomnia, nightmares, and nervousness. More serious psychiatric side effects occur in a small proportion of patients and can result in delirium, depression, and even full-blown psychotic states.

LEVODOPA COMBINED WITH DECARBOXYLASE INHIBITORS

Dopa decarboxylase is responsible for the enzymatic decarboxylation of levodopa to dopamine. Because dopa decarboxylase is widely distributed throughout the body, levodopa administered systemically is largely converted to dopamine in the periphery. Under these conditions, very small amounts of levodopa are available for penetration into the central nervous system. In order to increase circulating levels of levodopa, dopa decarboxylase inhibitors have been administered with levodopa. One of the commonly used dopa decarboxylase inhibitors is carbidopa. This drug allows a 60% to

80% decrease in the dose of levodopa necessary to control parkinsonian symptoms. The administration of carbidopa with levodopa also reduces the prominent gastrointestinal side effects of levodopa. Unfortunately, the abnormal involuntary muscle movements, particularly those of the orofacial muscles, are not significantly diminished by the administration of carbidopa with levodopa, and, in fact, there are indications that they become more frequent and start earlier. There also appears to be little difference between the mental disturbances produced by levodopa alone as opposed to those produced by this drug combination. Carbidopa is nontoxic and pharmacologically inactive in the absence of levodopa; nevertheless, carbidopa is not currently recommended in pregnancy or in patients under 25 years of age. Carbidopa is available as a single agent or in combination with levodopa in a fixed 1:10 (carbidopa:levodopa) ratio. Packaged alone (but used in combination with levodopa), carbidopa is useful for patients who require either greater or lesser amounts of the drug than is provided in the standard 1:10 ratio. Levodopa, combined with a peripheral decarboxylase inhibitor, remains the drug formulation of choice for the treatment of Parkinson's disease.

DRUGS WITH ANTICHOLINERGIC ACTIVITY

The pharmacology of the anticholinergic agents is discussed in Chapter 9. As was mentioned earlier, their mechanism of action as antiparkinson agents related to the blockade of cholinergic pathways in the basal ganglia, thus restoring the cholinergic-dopaminergic balance. The anticholinergics are not highly efficacious antiparkinson agents but decrease tremor, rigidity, and akinesia somewhat in some patients. All the anticholinergics produce sedation and, in high doses, can elicit euphoria, visual hallucinations, and changes in mood. Trihexyphenidyl has been reported to have abuse potential, and parkinsonian patients may "fake" parkinsonian signs in order to obtain the drug. Toxic doses of the anticholinergics can cause severe mental disturbances, including excitement, confusion, hallucinations, delirium, depression, coma, and medullary paralysis. Due to cholinergic blockade, the anticholinergics can produce xerostomia, increased intraocular pressure, tachycardia, palpitations, arrhythmias, urinary retention, constipation, and tachypnea.

The pharmacology of the antihistamines is cov-

ered in Chapter 23. These agents possess some degree of anticholinergic activity, and it is this property that is thought to be responsible for their antiparkinson properties.

MISCELLANEOUS ANTIPARKINSON AGENTS
Amantadine

The antiparkinson effects of amantadine, an antiviral agent, were discovered when the drug was used to treat a viral infection in a patient who had Parkinson's disease.[21] Amantadine appears to block dopamine reuptake or to release or facilitate release of dopamine from dopaminergic nerve terminals.[15,25] As with levodopa, these actions would result in increased dopamine activity in the basal ganglia, so long as there was dopamine available to be released. Amantadine is usually used in combination with levodopa, because an additive effect has been demonstrated when these two drugs are used together. When given alone, the efficacy of amantadine diminishes after several weeks of treatment. This fade lends support to the hypothesis that amantadine's mechanism of action is via the release or the inhibition of reuptake of dopamine. In the presence of levodopa, presumably dopamine would be replaced in the nerve terminals of the striatum and thus available for amantadine. Amantadine is probably best used (1) alone at the early stages of Parkinson's disease when symptoms are troublesome but not so severe as to interfere with the individual's employment or social activities; (2) alone for the management of patients who do not respond well to levodopa; or (3) in combination with levodopa when a more beneficial response is required.

Approximately 80% to 90% of amantadine is excreted unchanged in the urine, and thus build-up may occur in patients with impaired renal function. Such accumulation may lead to toxic manifestations: confusion, hallucinations, toxic psychosis, convulsions, and coma. An unusual side effect of amantadine is livedo reticularis. In this condition the skin becomes edematous and shiny. The small superficial blood vessels become more prominent, and the skin takes on a livid red color with a marbled, netlike appearance. The dorsum of the feet and hands are particularly susceptible, but the condition appears to have no pathologic significance. Common side effects include anorexia, insomnia, nausea, vomiting, dizziness, abnormal involuntary movements, lightheadedness, edema, and sweating. These side effects are not severe and are further limited by the development of tolerance.

Deprenyl

Deprenyl is a selective inhibitor of MAO-B, the predominant MAO in the brain and the enzyme that rather selectively oxidizes dopamine. The obvious rationale for the use of a selective MAO-B inhibitor would be to elevate dopamine concentrations at postsynaptic receptor sites in the brain, while at the same time causing little or no effect on norepinephrine or serotonin. Deprenyl finds greatest therapeutic value as an adjunct to conventional therapy of parkinsonism.[5] By prolonging the availability of dopamine, dosages of levodopa can be reduced by approximately 10%.[3]

Deprenyl is metabolized to amphetamine in the brain and liver. While the objective signs of parkinsonism may not be improved as assessed clinically, very often patients report that they feel better after deprenyl. It has been suggested that this effect might be due to an elevation of mood from a central amphetamine-like action.[13]

In the early stages of Parkinson's disease, deprenyl is effective in diminishing or preventing the occurrence of the "on-off" effect. After the disease has progressed, deprenyl becomes ineffective. If the patient is treated early enough, however, there is no doubt that deprenyl used as an adjunct to levodopa prolongs the improvement of the parkinsonian patient's condition,[6] but it is not known if the drug prolongs the patient's life.

Side effects attributable to deprenyl include nausea, dry mouth, confusion, occasional visual hallucinations, dizziness, headache, and insomnia, especially if doses exceed 10 mg daily. An increased incidence of hyperkinesia (dyskinesia) and levodopa-induced psychoses occurs following deprenyl, especially at higher doses. This may be due to the formation of the metabolite, amphetamine. Deprenyl is unique among the MAO inhibitors in that it does not potentiate the pressor response to tyramine and thus is devoid of interaction with various foods that contain tyramine. Deprenyl is not yet available in the United States but is being clinically evaluated.

Dopamine agonists

The finding of several subtypes of dopamine receptors in the brain, advances in our knowledge of the neurochemistry of the normal and the parkinsonian brain, and clinical findings have all given impetus to the search for selective dopamine agonists for the treatment of Parkinson's disease. Most of the compounds currently being tested are ergot, or semisynthetic ergoline, derivatives that share a common dopamine-like substructure, as shown in Figure 16-2. Of these agents, only bromocriptine is currently available for clinical use.

Apomorphine, another dopamine agonist, also contains the dopamine moiety. Apomorphine is an effective drug for some cases of Parkinson's disease, but its duration of effect is so short that the drug must be given repeatedly. This, plus a number of side effects—nausea, vomiting, sweating, weakness, and (particularly) azotemia—led to discontinuation of its use in parkinsonism.

Although all of the compounds listed in Figure 16-2 are dopamine agonists, they are not similarly effective in all cases of Parkinson's disease.[23] That is, in clinical trials comparing several of the dopamine agonists, one of the drugs may be effective in a given patient whereas another dopamine agonist may not. This nonuniformity supports the theory of multiple dopamine receptor sites and the possibility that one or several of these sites may be abnormal in Parkinson's disease. To date, none of the drugs is absolutely selective for a given subtype of dopamine receptor, but there is no doubt that the trend will be to develop just such agents. It is likely that selective dopamine agonists will be the next major breakthrough in the therapy of parkinsonism.

One of the first effective ergoline alkaloid derivatives, lergotrile causes clinically unacceptable hepatotoxicity. Bromocriptine, a more promising derivative, is an effective antiparkinson agent and probably the best studied of this group of drugs. Bromocriptine is currently available in the United States but has FDA approval only for the treatment of conditions resulting from hyperprolactinemia (e.g., galactorrhea and amenorrhea). It is useful in certain patients who are unresponsive to levodopa, but in advanced stages of parkinsonism, when mental deterioration is evident, bromocriptine is not particularly effective. It decreases the severity and frequency of levodopa-induced "on-off" effects in some patients. Adverse effects include abnormal involuntary movements, mental changes (confusion, schizophreniform psychosis), nausea, vomiting, hiccoughs, and orthostatic hypotension. All of the adverse effects are reversible on withdrawal of the drug. Bromocriptine is perhaps best used in combination with levodopa/carbidopa, in which

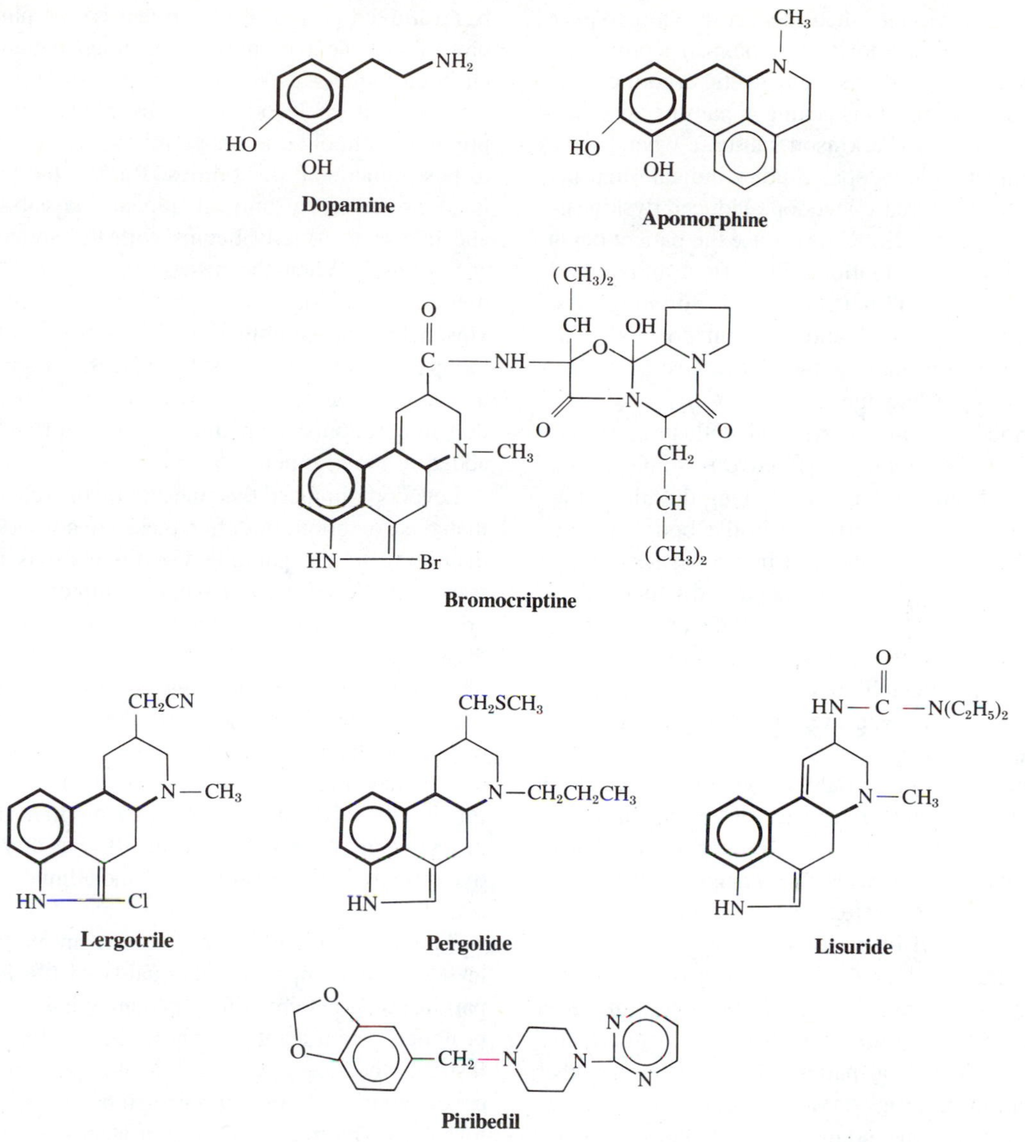

Figure 16-2. Structural formulas of dopamine agonists, with the dopamine moiety emphasized.

case the levodopa dose can be reduced 10% to 40%. It may also be used in patients who no longer are responsive to levodopa/carbidopa but who do not yet show signs of mental deterioration. The additive effect of bromocriptine with levodopa may result from the increased release and prevention of reuptake of dopamine or from the stimulation of different subtypes of dopamine receptors.

A third ergot derivative, lisuride, resembles bromocriptine structurally and shares the dopamine moiety but lacks the peptide moiety and the hal-

ogen. Lisuride is thought to function as a dopamine agonist, but it has potent actions on serotonin systems as well. Whether its serotonergic properties have any significance is unknown; however, serotonin is known to be deficient in the brains of patients with Parkinson's disease.[14] Lisuride resembles bromocriptine in its clinical and pharmacologic actions, but it is more potent. As with bromocriptine, lergotrile, and levodopa, the clinical effectiveness of lisuride wanes in time. Side effects, including nausea and mental changes, are similar to those described for bromocriptine. Unlike bromocriptine, lisuride causes somnolence, which may relate to its serotonin-like properties.

Pergolide, another semisynthetic ergoline derivative, is a potent, long-acting dopamine agonist. It is most useful in Parkinson's disease when used as an adjunct to levodopa. Studies indicate that pergolide may decrease levodopa-induced dyskinesias and increase the ''on'' time once the patient begins the ''on-off'' fluctuations. Side effects of pergolide are not severe and include nausea, vomiting, nasal stuffiness, sweating, and transient postural hypotension. Unfortunately, there have also been a few reports of cardiac and hepatic toxicity.

Piribedil, a nonergot derivative illustrated in Figure 16-2, appears to be effective in some cases of parkinsonism and has a fairly long duration of action. Piribedil is converted in the body to a metabolite that has antiparkinson properties. Tremor seems to respond better to piribedil than do the other signs of parkinsonism. Side effects of this drug include nausea, dyskinesia, drowsiness, and confusion, especially in the elderly. Unfortunately, it is the elderly who are most likely to have Parkinson's disease.

It might be appropriate to point out that although currently the clinical efficacy of the dopamine agonists does not appear to be as good as that of levodopa, this situation may change over the next few years. The development of selective dopamine agonists is still in its infancy, and many more of these drugs will undoubtedly be produced in the future. Additionally, it should be noted that most of the clinical trials with these compounds have been conducted on patients who are taking other antiparkinson drugs or who are either refractory or have reached the point of losing their initial responsiveness to conventional treatments. The fact that any of these patients responds to the dopamine agonists at all is encouraging and has given new hope for the treatment of Parkinson's disease. Furthermore, these compounds have served as pharmacologic tools in expanding our knowledge of the pathophysiology and pharmacology of Parkinson's disease.

GENERAL THERAPEUTIC USES

There can be little doubt that the combination of levodopa and carbidopa is the most effective antiparkinson treatment available to date. However, because of the serious side effects associated with levodopa therapy and the fact that levodopa has a limited period of effectiveness, the philosophy of treatment of the parkinsonian patient has changed somewhat. While in the past most patients were started on levodopa, many physicians now prefer to withhold that drug until the disease begins to pose functional disabilities. Rather, the patient is counseled as to future therapeutic possibilities, and treatment usually begins with the anticholinergic drugs. When the disease is adjudged to be moderate, levodopa may be added; for serious parkinsonism, the combination of levodopa and carbidopa is substituted. As the disease progresses, the adjunct agents, such as the anticholinergics, dopamine agonists, amantadine, or deprenyl, are added to the regimen.

Levodopa-induced dyskinesias are the rule rather than the exception, but often these are not seriously disturbing to the patient. The fluctuations in responsiveness of parkinsonian symptoms to levodopa and the progressively greater severity of these oscillations are a much greater hindrance to the patient, as is the progressive deterioration of mental function. The histopathology of the brain of the levodopa-treated parkinsonian patient is not unlike that of patients with Alzheimer's disease. Finally, the continual use of levodopa often results in unresponsiveness to the drug. It is at this stage that drug holidays are attempted and adjunct agents added.

Although antiparkinson therapy, in particular levodopa, has improved the quality of life for the parkinsonian patient, life expectancy has not been prolonged significantly. This limitation further illustrates the slow, persistent degenerative process occurring in the brain, a progression not responsive to current treatment. New approaches to therapy of parkinsonism will focus on the development of more specific dopamine receptor agonists and on the role of peptides in regulating dopamine function. The ultimate approach to therapy will be to elucidate the cause of Parkinson's disease.

IMPLICATIONS IN DENTISTRY
Levodopa

Facial movements induced by levodopa may cause a number of dental problems, including inflammation, damage to oral structures due to constant movement, damage to anterior teeth because of tongue thrusting, difficulty in wearing and retaining dentures, and an interesting but benign side effect called dysgeusia, or alterations in the sensation of taste. This last reaction is not seen when levodopa is combined with decarboxylase inhibitors.

A common side effect of levodopa, orthostatic hypotension may be treated simply by alterations in the dosage of levodopa. There is also some development of tolerance to this effect. However, despite therapeutic and physiologic adjustments, the patient sometimes still suffers from periodic episodes of hypotension. Orthostatic hypotension can be a particular problem to the dentist because of the reclining position of the patient during dental care. Patients known to be receiving levodopa therapy should therefore be allowed to sit up and leave the dental chair rather slowly, and precautionary measures should be taken to guard against the patient's falling.

There are a number of drug interactions involving levodopa with which the dentist should be acquainted. It is believed by some investigators that levodopa sensitizes the heart to epinephrine-induced arrhythmias. The mechanism responsible for the generation of these arrhythmias by epinephrine is unknown, but the excitatory action of levodopa on the heart is thought to be due to an action of dopamine on cardiac β-adrenergic receptors. Although some practitioners believe that this interaction provides a valid contraindication for the use of local anesthetics with vasoconstrictors in patients taking levodopa, as is pointed out in Chapter 17, the clinical significance of these interactions is not well established. The use of phenothiazines as antinauseants should be discouraged for patients on levodopa therapy. Such combinations can exacerbate the motor irregularities of Parkinson's disease, probably as a result of the dopamine antagonistic properties of the phenothiazines. Analgesics may be used with levodopa, but if general anesthesia is required, levodopa should be discontinued or the dosage reduced. Consultation with the patient's physician would probably be the wisest course of action in the event that general anesthesia is required. Though it is not usually a complication in dental practice, the dentist should be aware of other drug interactions with levodopa. Pyridoxine (vitamin B_6), which is present in OTC multivitamin preparations, can antagonize the antiparkinson effect of levodopa by enhancing its conversion to dopamine. Fortunately, this antagonism does not occur when the peripheral decarboxylase inhibitors are administered with levodopa. Because of the hypotensive effects of levodopa, patients with hypertension often require alterations in the dose of their antihypertensive medications.

Anticholinergic agents

Although the newer anticholinergic agents have fewer side effects than older drugs such as the belladonna alkaloids, the patient may still complain of typical anticholinergic side effects, including xerostomia. This condition may increase the incidence of caries and, if extreme, result in almost complete loss of teeth.[26] Other typical anticholinergic side effects are discussed in Chapter 9. Drugs with which the anticholinergics might interact include antihistamines, the butyrophenone and phenothiazine antipsychotics, tricyclic antidepressants, and other anticholinergics.

Amantadine, deprenyl, and ergot derivatives

To date, side effects of all of these drugs are generally not severe and have little clinical significance for the practicing dentist. If the patient has recently been started on any of these medications, transient nausea and vomiting may occur; thus, a patient scheduled for dental work at this time would be more susceptible to gagging, nausea, and vomiting. Because of hypotension on initial therapy, the same precautions indicated for levodopa regarding the patient's leaving the dental chair would apply to these agents, particularly with bromocriptine. Because all of these drugs are commonly used as adjuncts along with levodopa, the careful recording of the patient's medical history should reveal whether the patient is receiving combined therapy, and the appropriate precautions should then be observed.

Antiparkinson drugs

Nonproprietary name	*Proprietary name*
Anticholinergics	
benztropine	Cogentin
biperiden	Akineton
procyclidine	Kemadrin
trihexyphenidyl	Artane, Tremin

Antiparkinson drugs—cont'd

Nonproprietary name	Proprietary name
Other drugs with anticholinergic activity	
diphenhydramine	Benadryl
ethopropazine	Parsidol
orphenadrine	Disipal
Dopamine precursor and decarboxylase inhibitors	
carbidopa	Lodosyn
levodopa	Dopar, Larodopa
levodopa + benserazide*	Madopar
levodopa + carbidopa	Sinemet
Other drugs with dopaminergic effects	
amantadine	Symmetrel
bromocriptine	Parlodel
deprenyl*	—

*Not yet available clinically in the United States.

CITED REFERENCES

1. Barbeau, A., Sourkes, T.L., and Murphy, G.F. Les catecholamines dans la maladie de Parkinson. In de Ajuriaguerra, J., ed. Monoamines et Systeme Nerveaux Central. Paris, George, Geneve and Masson, 1970.
2. Bertler, Å., and Rosengren, E. Occurrence and distribution of dopamine in brain and other tissues. Experientia **15:**10-11, 1959.
3. Birkmayer, W. Long term treatment with L-deprenyl. Journal of Neural Transmission **43:**239-244, 1978.
4. Birkmayer, W., and Hornykiewicz, O. Der L-3,4-Dioxyphenylalanin(=DOPA)-Effekt bei der Parkinson-Akinese. Wiener Klinische Wochenschrift **73:**787-788, 1961.
5. Birkmayer, W., Riederer, P., Ambrozi, L., and Youdim, M.B.H. Implications of combined treatment with ''Madopar'' and L-deprenyl in Parkinson's disease. A long-term study. Lancet **1:**439-443, 1977.
6. Birkmayer, W., Riederer, P., and Youdim, M.B.H. (−) Deprenyl in the treatment of Parkinson's disease. Clinical Neuropharmacology **5:**195-230, 1982.
7. Carlsson, A. The occurrence, distribution, and physiological role of catecholamines in the nervous system. Pharmacological Reviews **11:**490-493, 1959.
8. Carlsson, A., Lindqvist, M., Magnusson, T., and Waldeck, B. On the presence of 3-hydroxytyramine in brain. Science **127:**471, 1958.
9. Cotzias, G.C., and Papavasiliov, P.S. Therapeutic studies of parkinsonian patients: long-term effects of D-L and L-dopa. In Barbeau, A., and Brunette, J.R., eds. Proceedings of the Second International Congress of Neuro-genetics and Neuro-ophthalmology of the World Federation of Neurology. Progress in Neurogenetics, vol. 1. Amsterdam, Excerpta Medica Foundation, 1969.
10. Cotzias, G.C., van Woert, M.H., and Schiffer, L.M. Aromatic amino acids and modification of parkinsonism. New England Journal of Medicine **276:**374-379, 1967.
11. Direnfeld, L., Spero, L., Marotta, J., and Seeman, P. The L-dopa on-off effect in Parkinson disease: treatment by transient drug withdrawal and dopamine receptor resensitization. Annals of Neurology **4:**573-575, 1978.
12. Ehringer, H., and Hornykiewicz, O. Verteilung von Noradrenalin und Dopamin (3-Hydroxytyramin) im Gehirn des Menschen und ihr Verhalten bei Erkrankungen des extrapyramidalen Systems. Klinische Wochenschrift **38:**1236-1239, 1960.
13. Eisler, T., Teräväinen, H., Nelson, R., Krebs, H., Weise, V., Lake, C.R., Ebert, M.H., Whetzel, N., Murphy, D.L., Kopin, I.J., and Calne, D.B. Deprenyl in Parkinson disease. Neurology **31:**19-23, 1981.
14. Fahn, S., Libsch, L.R., and Cutler, R.W. Monoamines in the human neostriatum: topographic distribution in normals and in Parkinson's disease and the role in akinesia, rigidity, chorea, and tremor. Journal of Neurological Sciences **14:**427-455, 1971.
15. Farnebo, L.-O., Fuxe, K., Goldstein, M., Hamberger, B., and Ungerstedt, U. Dopamine and noradrenaline releasing action of amantadine in the central and peripheral nervous system: a possible mode of action in Parkinson's disease. European Journal of Pharmacology **16:**27-38, 1971.
16. Hökfelt, T. *In vitro* studies on central and peripheral monoamine neurons at the ultrastructural level. Zeitschrift für Zellforschung und Mikroskopische Anatomie **91:**1-74, 1968.
17. Kebabian, J.W., and Calne, D.B. Multiple receptors for dopamine. Nature **277:**93-96, 1979.
18. Reisine, T.D., Fields, J.Z., Yamamura, H.I., Bird, E.D., Spokes, E., Schreiner, P.S., and Enna, S.J. Neurotransmitter receptor alterations in Parkinson's disease. Life Sciences **21:**335-343, 1977.
19. Rinne, U.K., Sonninen, V., and Laaksonen, H. Responses of brain neurochemistry to levodopa treatment in Parkinson's disease. Advances in Neurology **24:**259-274, 1979.
20. Sano, I., Gamo, T., Kakimoto, Y., Taniguchi, K., Takesada, M., and Nishinuma, K. Distribution of catechol compounds in human brain. Biochimica et Biophysica Acta **32:**586-587, 1959.
21. Schwab, R.S., England, A.C., Jr., Poskanzer, D.C., and Young, R.R. Amantadine in the treatment of Parkinson's disease. Journal of the American Medical Association **208:**1168-1170, 1969.
22. Seeman, P. Brain dopamine receptors. Pharmacological Reviews **32:**229-313, 1980.
23. Silbergeld, E.K., and Pfeiffer, R.F. Differential effects of three dopamine agonists: apomorphine, bromocriptine, and lergotrile. Journal of Neurochemistry **28:**1323-1326, 1977.
24. Turner, B. Pathology of paralysis agitans. In Vinken, P.J., and Bruyn, G.W., eds. Diseases of the Basal Ganglia. Amsterdam, American Elsevier, 1968.
25. Von Voigtlander, P.F., and Moore, K.E. Dopamine: release from the brain in vivo by amantadine. Science **174:**408-410, 1971.
26. Winer, J.A., and Bahn, S. Loss of teeth with antidepressant drug therapy. Archives of General Psychiatry **16:**239-240, 1967.

GENERAL REFERENCES

Calne, D.B., ed. Progress in the Treatment of Parkinsonism. Advances in Neurology, vol. 3. New York, Raven Press, 1973.

Fahn S., ed., Management of Parkinson's disease at different stages of the illness. Clinical Neuropharmacology 5(Suppl.):S1-S43, 1982.

Hornykiewicz, O. The mechanisms of action of L-DOPA in Parkinson's disease. Life Sciences **15:**1249-1259, 1974.

Lloyd, K.G., Davidson, L., and Hornykiewicz, O. The neurochemistry of Parkinson's disease: effect of L-DOPA therapy. Journal of Pharmacology and Experimental Therapeutics **195:**453-464, 1975.

Messiha, F.S., and Kenny, A.D., eds. Parkinson's Disease—Neurophysiological, Clinical, and Related Aspects. Advances in Experimental Medicine and Biology, vol. 90. New York, Plenum Press, 1976.

Pinder, R.M., Brogden, R.N., Sawyer, P.R., Speight, T.M., and Avery, G.S. Levodopa and decarboxylase inhibitors: a review of their clinical pharmacology and use in the treatment of parkinsonism. Drugs **11:**329-377, 1976.

Yahr, M.D. Levodopa. Annals of Internal Medicine **83:**677-682, 1975.

17 Local anesthetics

John A. Yagiela

Local anesthetics are agents that reversibly block nerve conduction when applied to a circumscribed area of the body. Although numerous substances of diverse chemical structure are capable of producing local anesthesia, most drugs of proven clinical usefulness (identified by the suffix ''caine'') share a fundamental configuration with the first true local anesthetic, cocaine.

For centuries, natives of the Peruvian highlands have relied on the leaves of the coca bush to prevent hunger, relieve fatigue, and uplift the spirit. Interest in the psychotropic properties of *Erythroxylon coca* led to the isolation of cocaine by Niemann in 1860 and to a study of its pharmacology by von Anrep in 1880. Although both men reported on the local anesthetic action of cocaine, credit for its introduction into medicine belongs to Carl Koller, a Viennese physician. In 1884, Koller was familiarized with the physiologic effects of cocaine by Sigmund Freud. Koller recognized the drug's great clinical significance and quickly demonstrated its pain-relieving action in several ophthalmologic procedures. The benefits of cocaine were widely appreciated; within a year local anesthesia had been successfully administered for a variety of medical and dental operations.

Knowledge of cocaine's potential for adverse reactions soon followed its general acceptance as a local anesthetic. Several deaths attributed to acute cocainization testified to the drug's low therapeutic index. The abuse liability of cocaine was dramatically illustrated by the self-addiction of Halsted, a pioneer in regional nerve blockade. A chemical search for safer, nonaddicting local anesthetics was instituted in 1892, culminating 13 years later in the synthesis of procaine by Einhorn and his associates. Since then, numerous improvements in the manufacture of local anesthetic solutions have been

made, and many useful agents have been introduced into clinical practice. However, as no drug is currently devoid of potentially serious toxicity, the search for new and better local anesthetics continues.

CHEMISTRY AND CLASSIFICATION

Certain physicochemical characteristics are required of a drug intended for clinical use as a local anesthetic. One obvious prerequisite is that the agent must depress nerve conduction. Since an axon whose cytoplasmic contents have been completely removed can still transmit action potentials, a drug must be able to interact directly with the axolemma in order to exert local anesthetic activity. A second important consideration is that the agent must have both lipophilic and hydrophilic properties in order to be effective by parenteral injection. Lipid solubility is essential for penetration of the various anatomic barriers existing between an administered drug and its site of action, including the nerve sheath. Water solubility ensures that, once injected in an effective concentration, a drug will not precipitate on exposure to interstitial fluid. These requirements have placed important structural limitations on the clinically useful local anesthetics.

Structure-activity relationships

The typical local anesthetic molecule can be divided into three parts: an aromatic group, an intermediate chain, and a secondary or tertiary amino terminus (Table 17-1). All three components are important determinants of a drug's local anesthetic activity. The aromatic residue confers lipophilic properties on the molecule, whereas the amino group furnishes water solubility. The intermediate portion is significant in two respects. First, it pro-

Table 17-1. Structural formulas of some commonly used local anesthetics

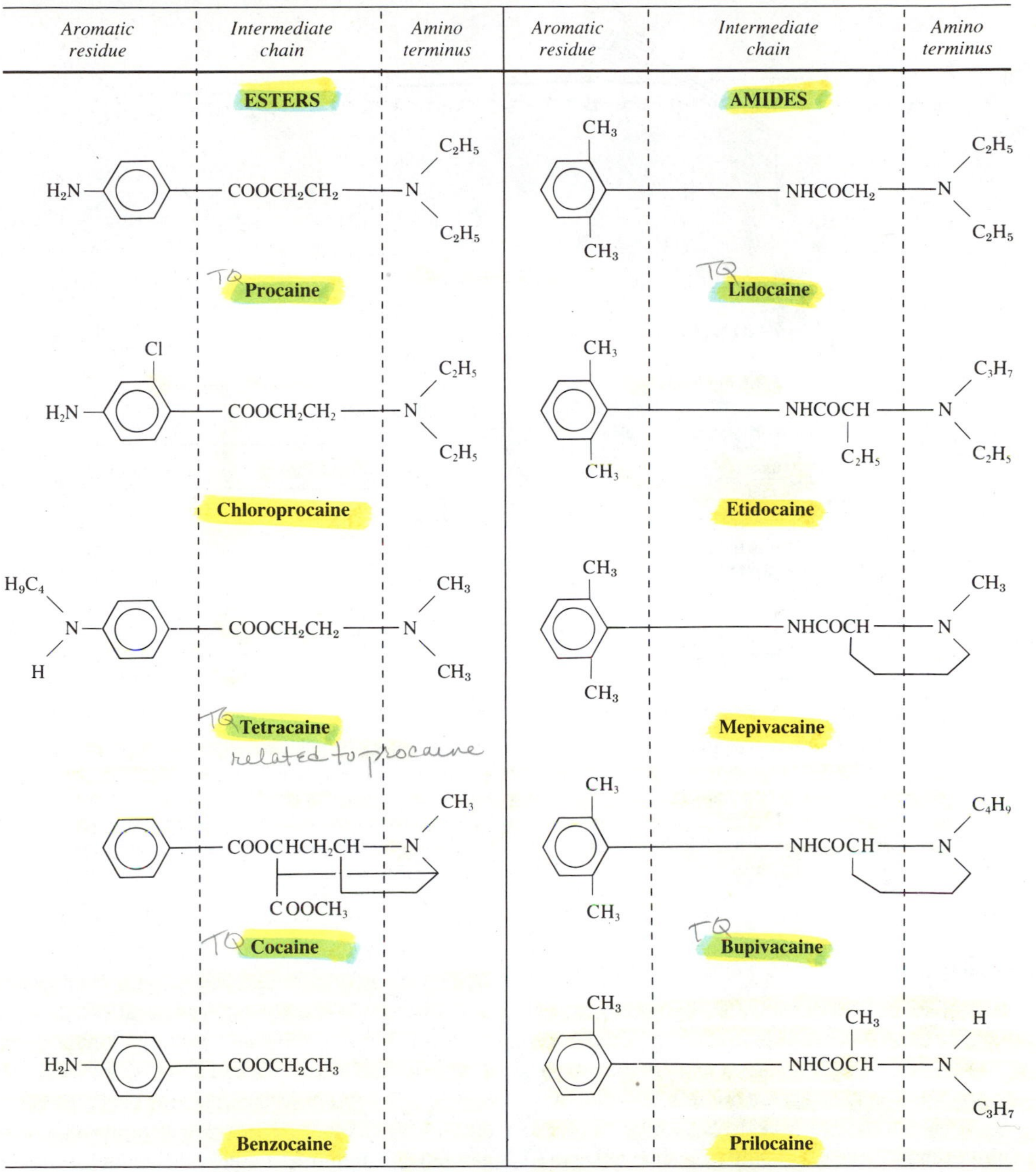

Aromatic residue	Intermediate chain	Amino terminus	Aromatic residue	Intermediate chain	Amino terminus
	ESTERS			**AMIDES**	
H_2N—⟨ring⟩—	$COOCH_2CH_2$—N	C_2H_5 / C_2H_5	CH_3 ⟨ring⟩ CH_3	$NHCOCH_2$—N	C_2H_5 / C_2H_5
	Procaine			**Lidocaine**	
H_2N—⟨ring, Cl⟩—	$COOCH_2CH_2$—N	C_2H_5 / C_2H_5	CH_3 ⟨ring⟩ CH_3	$NHCOCH$ / C_2H_5 —N	C_3H_7 / C_2H_5
	Chloroprocaine			**Etidocaine**	
H_9C_4 / H N—⟨ring⟩—	$COOCH_2CH_2$—N	CH_3 / CH_3	CH_3 ⟨ring⟩ CH_3	$NHCOCH$—N	CH_3
	Tetracaine			**Mepivacaine**	
⟨ring⟩—	$COOCHCH_2CH$ / $COOCH_3$ —N	CH_3	CH_3 ⟨ring⟩ CH_3	$NHCOCH$—N	C_4H_9
	Cocaine			**Bupivacaine**	
H_2N—⟨ring⟩—	$COOCH_2CH_3$		CH_3 ⟨ring⟩	$NHCOCH$ / CH_3 —N	H / C_3H_7
	Benzocaine			**Prilocaine**	

(handwritten annotations: "TQ" beside Procaine, Lidocaine, Tetracaine, Cocaine, Bupivacaine; "related to procaine" written below Tetracaine)

vides the necessary spatial separation between the lipophilic and hydrophilic ends of the local anesthetic. Second, the chemical link between the central hydrocarbon chain and the aromatic moiety serves as a suitable basis for classification of the local anesthetics into two groups, the esters (—COO—) and the amides (—NHCO—). This distinction is useful since there are marked differences in allergenicity and metabolism between the two drug categories. Minor modifications of any portion of the local anesthetic molecule can significantly influence drug action. For example, the addition of a chlorine atom to the ortho position on the benzene ring of procaine yields chloroprocaine, a local anesthetic 4 times as potent as the parent compound yet half as toxic when injected subcutaneously.

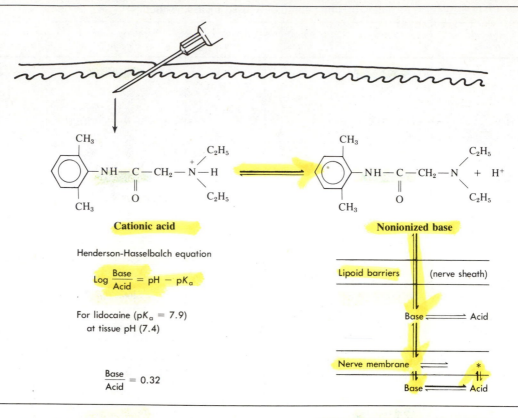

Figure 17-1. Distribution of a local anesthetic during nerve block. On injection of a local anesthetic solution, a portion of the cationic acid is converted to the free base. Calculated for lidocaine is the base/acid ratio in the extracellular fluid at equilibrium. Dark arrows depict the major pathway followed by a local anesthetic in reaching its site of action (*) within the nerve membrane. Although the acid form is presumed responsible for most of the blocking activity, the contribution of the nonionized base (represented by light arrows within the axolemma) must not be overlooked.

Influence of pH

By virtue of the substituted amino group, most local anesthetics are weak bases with pK_as ranging from 7.5 to 9.0. A local anesthetic intended for injection is usually prepared in salt form by the addition of hydrochloric acid. Not only is water solubility improved, but stability in aqueous media is also increased. Once injected, the acidic local anesthetic solution is quickly neutralized by tissue fluid buffers, and a fraction of the cationic form is converted to the nonionized base. As shown by the Henderson-Hasselbalch equation (Figure 17-1), the percentage of drug converted depends primarily on the local anesthetic pK_a and the tissue pH. Since only the base form can diffuse rapidly into the nerve, drugs with high pK_as tend to be slower in onset than similar agents with more favorable dissociation constants. Tissue acidity may also impede

the development of local anesthesia. Products of inflammation lower the pH of the affected tissue and limit formation of the free base. Ionic entrapment of the local anesthetic in the extracellular space not only delays the onset of local anesthesia but also may render effective nerve blockade impossible. In inflamed tissues, the failure to obtain satisfactory clinical pain relief is well known. (For the sake of completeness, it should also be mentioned that inflammatory exudates may inhibit local anesthesia directly by enhancing nerve conduction.[11])

Numerous attempts have been made to augment local anesthesia by capitalizing on the influence of pH. Alkalinization theoretically should increase local anesthetic activity by promoting tissue penetration and nerve uptake. Indeed, many topical agents are marketed in the base form to improve diffusion across epithelial barriers. Although it has been shown experimentally that alkalinization of local anesthetic solutions before use enhances nerve blockade, clinically results have been disappointing. Apparently, extracellular fluid has sufficient buffering capacity to negate differences in local anesthetic pH soon after injection. An alternative approach to modifying drug distribution is through the addition of carbon dioxide. Carbonation of a local anesthetic solution can substantially increase the rate of onset and sometimes the profundity of anesthesia. It has been suggested that the hydrocarbonate salt of the local anesthetic penetrates membranes more rapidly than does the conventional formulation and that the injected carbon dioxide diffusing into the nerve trunk lowers the internal pH and concentrates local anesthetic molecules by ion trapping.[37] Catchlove[12] has provided evidence that carbon dioxide may also potentiate local anesthetic activity by a direct effect on the nerve membrane. Though promising, carbonated local anesthetic solutions are not yet available in the United States.

MECHANISM OF ACTION

Local anesthetics block the sensation of pain by interfering with the propagation of peripheral nerve impulses. Both the generation and the conduction of action potentials are inhibited. Electrophysiologic data indicate that local anesthetics do not significantly alter the normal resting potential of the nerve membrane—instead they impair certain dynamic responses to nerve stimulation.

Effects on ionic permeability

The inactive nerve membrane is relatively impermeable to sodium ions. Excitation of the axolemma by an appropriate stimulus, however, will temporarily increase sodium conductance and cause the nerve cell to become less electronegative with respect to the outside. If the transmembrane potential is sufficiently depressed, a critical threshold is reached at which the depolarization becomes self-generating. A marked increase in sodium permeability induces a rapid influx of sodium through sodium-selective channels traversing the nerve membrane. The inward sodium current creates an action potential of approximately $+40$ mV that is then propagated down the nerve. The action potential is quite transient at any given segment of membrane; inactivation of sodium permeability (closure of the sodium channels) and an outward flow of potassium quickly repolarize the membrane.

Local anesthetics interfere with nerve transmission by blocking the influence of stimulation on sodium conductance.[50] A developing local anesthetic block is characterized by a progressive reduction in the rate of the depolarization phase of the action potential and a slowing of conduction. Since the onset and the rate of repolarization are not as greatly affected by local anesthetics, the safety factor for transmission decreases. When depolarization is retarded such that repolarization processes develop before the threshold potential can be reached, nerve conduction fails.[1]

Site of action

Several sites exist within the nerve membrane where local anesthetics could interfere with sodium permeability. Drugs capable of blocking conduction may be characterized according to their respective sites of action. The following classification of local anesthetics was proposed by Takman[52] and has been modified to reflect the findings of Hille[28] concerning drug-receptor reactions.

Class A—agents acting at a receptor site on the external opening of the sodium channel. Two marine biotoxins, tetrodotoxin and saxitoxin, are extremely potent local anesthetics. Both are positively charge guanidine-based compounds that bind specifically to an exterior protein constituent of the sodium channel, effectively ''plugging the pore.'' Although these drugs are quite selective in action, their limited penetrability of lipoid barriers has severely restricted clinical use.

Class B—agents acting at a receptor site accessible from the axoplasmic side of the sodium channel. Conversion of the amino terminus of certain local anesthetics to the quaternary form yields permanently charged cations largely incapable of crossing the nerve membrane. Although ineffective when applied externally to the axolemma, these experimental compounds demonstrate full blocking activity on internal administration. Studies involving stereoisomers and other local anesthetic derivatives indicate that a specific receptor is involved in the action of these drugs.[50]

Class C—agents affecting the sodium channel through a hydrophobic pathway. Numerous unrelated agents are capable of blocking nerve conduction. Examination of these drugs (alcohol, barbiturates, etc.) reveals that the only feature common to all is the lack of a positive charge at physiologic pH. Dissimilarity of molecular structures and direct correlation between local anesthetic potencies and membrane/buffer coefficients suggest that class C drugs may act in a manner analogous to the general anesthetics; that is, they may interact nonspecifically with hydrophobic regions of the axolemma, thereby causing an alteration of membrane structure and closure of the sodium channels. Benzocaine and several other class C drugs, however, closely resemble conventional local anesthetics in molecular configuration (Table 17-1). Experimental studies imply that at least part of the local anesthetic activity of these drugs results from binding to receptor sites identical with or similar to those responsive to class B compounds.[28,30] Although benzocaine and class B agents may both react with receptors in or adjacent to the sodium channel, marked differences exist in the way the drugs reach their locus of action. Whereas class B anesthetics are limited to diffusion up the sodium channel, benzocaine is able to penetrate the membrane directly to arrive at its receptor site.

Class D—agents acting by a combination of class B and class C mechanisms. Most of the clinically useful local anesthetics are in this category. Since these drugs exist as a mixture of cationic and neutral species at tissue pH, they are able to interfere with sodium conductance by combining with internal membrane receptors and perhaps by inducing membrane alterations through nonspecific hydrophobic binding. Both sodium channel and hydrophobic pathways are available to class D agents for gaining access to receptor sites. Although the preponderance of evidence indicates that most of the blocking action of these drugs is due to the attachment of local anesthetic cations to specific receptors, the neutral free base is also active (and of course largely responsible for efficient diffusion through the nerve sheath and membrane). A schematic representation of the interaction of a local anesthetic with its receptor in the sodium channel is presented in Figure 17-2. For purposes of illustration, it is assumed that the free base and cationic forms bind to the same receptor.

Influence on calcium

Much attention has focused on the interactions between local anesthetics and calcium ions. Conventional agents such as procaine and tetracaine inhibit the binding of calcium to phospholipids and displace calcium from artificial and natural membranes in direct relation to their respective anesthetic potencies. Moreover, local anesthetic inhibition of sodium conductance can be accentuated by removing calcium from the extraneuronal fluid or reversed by increasing the external calcium concentration. These findings serve as a basis for the theory that anesthetics and calcium ions compete for the same phospholipid receptor and that displacement of calcium is a prerequisite for local anesthesia. Several lines of evidence suggest, however, that the interaction with calcium is indirect and not related to the mechanism of local anesthetic action. First, calcium has been ruled out as a specific regulator of the sodium channel.[50] The influence of calcium on sodium conductance arises from a "surface charge" phenomenon in which external calcium ions partially neutralize fixed membrane anions, permitting increased sodium entry during depolarization. Second, calcium can reverse not only the nerve-blocking action of conventional local anesthetics but also that of neutral class C agents.[45] With these drugs, no obvious relationship exists between blockade reversal by calcium and drug displacement from membrane binding sites. Third, local anesthetic activity has been shown in certain nerve preparations to be unaffected by variations of the external calcium concentration.[40] Even when an antagonism does occur, it is probably only the result of calcium ions hindering the passage of the local anesthetic across glial membranes covering the axon.[36]

These determinations in toto support the argument that the inhibition of calcium binding, however important to other aspects of local anesthetic pharmacology, is not involved in the mechanism of nerve block.[50] Observed antagonisms occur simply because calcium and local anesthetics have opposite and unrelated effects on sodium conductance. It is not surprising, therefore, that other substances that promote nerve conduction (such as prostaglandins and adenine nucleotides) can also interfere with local anesthesia.[29,33]

Differential nerve block

Peripheral neurons vary according to fiber size and type in their susceptibility to local anesthetics. Autonomic functions subserved by preganglionic B and postganglionic C fibers are readily disrupted by local anesthetics, whereas motor control, dependent on larger Aα and Aγ fibers, is not. Sensory neurons are quite heterogeneous in size and therefore exhibit a wide range of sensitivity. Modalities listed in increasing order of resistance to conduc-

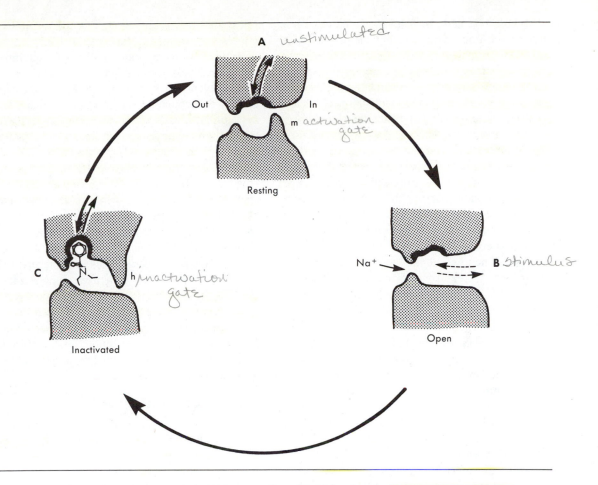

Figure 17-2. Effect of local anesthetic binding on sodium channel function. **A,** In the unstimulated nerve, most of the sodium channels are in a resting state. Sodium ions are prevented from passing through the channel by a barrier termed the activation gate (m). Only uncharged local anesthetic molecules can diffuse across the lipoid membrane to combine with the receptor (solid arrows). **B,** An appropriate stimulus (e.g., membrane depolarization) causes the sodium channel to open. In this configuration, local anesthetic cations are able to migrate up the sodium channel to bind with the receptor (broken arrows). Sodium channels free of the local anesthetic support nerve conduction by permitting sodium ions to flow into the axon. **C,** Soon after opening, the sodium channel becomes inactivated by the erection of a second barrier, the inactivation gate (h). This channel configuration is synonymous with the refractory period; sodium channels once inactivated cannot be induced to open by a depolarizing current until repolarization of the nerve membrane has permitted conversion from the inactive to the resting configuration. The normal conversion to the resting state is retarded by the presence of a local anesthetic (shown schematically), which also binds more avidly to the receptor when the channel is inactivated.

tion block include the sensations of pain, cold, warmth, touch, pressure, and proprioception. In general, the more susceptible a fiber is to a local anesthetic agent, the faster it is blocked and the longer it takes to recover.

Critical length. The clinical observations described above should not be construed as proof that large myelinated axons are inherently more resistant to local anesthetics than are smaller fibers. A careful study of individual axons by Franz and Perry[23] revealed that the minimal blocking concen-

tration of procaine is independent of fiber diameter. A differential block in which small C and Aδ fibers were affected but larger fibers were not could be obtained, but only when the length of compound nerve exposed to procaine was restricted to several millimeters. Based on these findings, the authors concluded that differential sensitivities of fibers of unequal diameter result from variations in the "critical length" that must be exposed to a local anesthetic for conduction to fail. In myelinated nerves, for instance, action potentials are propagated from one node of Ranvier to the next in a saltatory fashion, with a safety factor such that three consecutive nodes must be blocked in order for impulse transmission to be interrupted. Since internodal distance is directly related to fiber diameter, it is understandable that small neurons appear to be more sensitive clinically than large fibers to conduction block. As a local anesthetic diffuses into the nerve trunk, it reaches an effective concentration over a length required to inhibit small axons before it spreads sufficiently to block large fibers. Anatomic barriers to diffusion, nonuniform distribution of drug, or the use of a minimal amount of local anesthetic may even preclude some large axons from ever being affected. As local anesthesia fades, small neurons are the last to recover because circumscribed areas of drug concentrations adequate for their inhibition remain along the nerve after the more substantial areas required for large axons have broken up. The "critical length" hypothesis may also be applied to unmyelinated axons as a group. Differences in modes of impulse transmission, however, preclude direct comparisons based on fiber size between myelinated and unmyelinated axons. Smaller in diameter, C fibers nevertheless had about the same local anesthetic sensitivity, or critical length, as did small myelinated axons in the study by Franz and Perry.[23]

Margin of safety for nerve transmission. In apparent opposition to the clinical pattern of fiber susceptibility, Gissen and colleagues[25] have argued that sensitivity to local anesthetics is directly (not inversely) related to fiber diameter. These investigators examined the influence of various agents on the amplitude of the compound action potential of the rabbit sciatic and vagus nerves and concluded that the margin of safety for nerve transmission was less in large axons than in small fibers.[26] In other words, sodium permeability had to be depressed more in C fibers than in A fibers in order to prevent nerve conduction. The clinical pattern of differential block is attributed to the dynamics of local anesthetic distribution and the greater diffusion barrier surrounding large fibers. Although the design of their experiments has been questioned,[24] the findings of Gissen and colleagues are at least interesting and may be viewed as complementary to those of Franz and Perry.[23]

Frequency-dependent block. In addition to other variables, the pattern of impulse traffic normally carried in situ by the different nerve fibers contributes greatly to differential nerve block.[44] Local anesthetics inhibit high-frequency trains of impulses more readily than they do single action potentials. Variously called Wedensky inhibition, transition block, use-dependent block, or frequency-dependent block, this aspect of local anesthetic activity is accounted for by postulating that attachment of the drug to its receptor is favored when the sodium channel is in the inactivated configuration and that such binding retards conversion of the channel from the inactivated to the resting state (Figure 17-2).[28] Rapid firing increases sodium channel inactivation and therefore local anesthetic blockade. Although all conventional local anesthetics display some frequency dependence, the phenomenon is, of course, more pronounced with cationic agents, the very access to the receptor site of which depends on repetitive depolarization. Noxious stimuli and sympathetic nervous system transmissions, both of which are encoded in rapid bursts of impulses, are particularly susceptible to local anesthetics. Motor function, however, usually involves low-frequency discharges and is relatively resistant to drug interference.

PHARMACOLOGIC EFFECTS

Although primarily used to depress peripheral nerve conduction, local anesthetics are not selective and may interfere with impulse transmission in any excitable tissue. Most prominent of the systemic effects of local anesthetics are those related to the cardiovascular and central nervous systems, but virtually any organ dependent on nervous or muscular activity may be affected. Local anesthetics may also influence a variety of tissues through actions unrelated to specific disturbances in sodium conductance.

Central nervous system

Local anesthetics readily pass from the peripheral circulation into the brain. Because central neurons are particularly sensitive to local anesthetics, blood concentrations incapable of altering peripheral nervous activity may profoundly influence CNS function. Initial signs and symptoms of a CNS effect are usually excitatory in nature and consist of a feeling of light headedness and dizziness followed by visual and auditory disturbances, apprehension, disorientation, and localized involuntary muscular activity. Depressant responses such as slurred speech, drowsiness, and unconsciousness may also occur and are especially prominent with certain drugs (e.g., lidocaine). As higher blood concentrations of drug are attained, muscular fasciculations and tremors intensify and develop into generalized tonic-clonic convulsions. On termination, seizure activity is often succeeded by a state of CNS depression identical to general anesthesia. With excessively large doses, respiratory impairment becomes manifest; if untreated, death by asphyxiation may ensue.

The CNS excitation sometimes observed after local anesthesia is intriguing since the sole action ascribed to these agents is one of depression. Indeed, studies involving topical application of local anesthetics to exposed cortical or spinal cord neurons document that the only direct effect of procaine and related drugs is to inhibit electrical activity.[15] The apparent stimulation observed clinically is best explained on the basis that inhibitory cortical neurons or synapses are highly susceptible to transmission block. Initial disruption of these pathways results in a disinhibition of excitatory neurons, manifested clinically as stimulation. Considering these facts, it is not surprising that under appropriate conditions local anesthetics display considerable *anticonvulsant* activities. Hyperexcitable central neurons, for example, may be depressed at dosages much below those associated with seizure production.

Cardiovascular system

Local anesthetics can exert a variety of effects on the cardiovascular system. Some influences are beneficial and serve as a basis for the use of selected agents in the treatment of cardiac arrhythmias; others are not and merely serve to accentuate systemic toxicity.

Myocardium. At nontoxic concentrations, local anesthetics differ somewhat in their electrophysiologic influences on the heart. Whereas lidocaine shortens the action potential duration and the effective refractory period in Purkinje fibers, procaine acts in the opposite direction. Both drugs, however, increase the effective refractory period relative to the action potential duration and decrease cardiac automaticity, especially in ectopic pacemakers. Through a centrally mediated disinhibition of sympathetic nervous activity, heart rate and cardiac output may be elevated.

Local anesthetics in toxic doses are qualitatively similar in action. Membrane excitability and conduction velocity are depressed throughout the heart. Sinus bradycardia and impairment of myocardial contractility contribute to a reduction in cardiac output. These effects are magnified by hypoxia; but, even if respiration is supported artificially, circulatory collapse may occur after excessively large doses.

Peripheral vasculature. The effects of local anesthetics on blood vessels are complex and dose dependent.[4,8] Dilute solutions enhance spontaneous myogenic contractions and peripheral resistance in certain vascular beds, presumably by increasing the cytoplasmic concentration of ionic calcium within smooth muscle fibers. Coincidentally, local anesthetics reduce vascular tone related to autonomic function by diminishing neurotransmitter release and smooth muscle responsiveness. Concentrations employed clinically inhibit myogenic activity as well as autonomic tone and cause vasodilation in the area of injection. Subconvulsive doses of local anesthetics exert minor influences on the peripheral vasculature as a whole, but toxic blood concentrations may cause arteriolar dilation and profound hypotension.

Miscellaneous effects

Aside from their influences on cardiovascular and central nervous function, local anesthetics in concentrations compatible with life exert few systemic effects. Transmission at the neuromuscular junction and at autonomic ganglia may be affected, but intraarterial administration is usually required for these effects to be observed clinically. A variety of smooth muscle actions and antibacterial, antihistaminic, and antimuscarinic effects have also been reported.[16]

In tissue culture, local anesthetics are capable of disrupting numerous cellular functions: locomotion, endocytosis, exocytosis, axonal transport, cell fusion, and maintenance of normal morphology. These effects have been ascribed to disturbances of the cytoskeleton (microtubules and microfilaments). Various calcium- and calmodulin-dependent enzymic activities and membrane transport systems are also susceptible to local anesthetic influences.[53] The toxicologic and therapeutic implications of all these actions remain to be determined.

Vasoconstrictor effects

Vasoconstrictors are often added to local anesthetic solutions to impede systemic absorption of the anesthetic agent (see Chapter 6). Epinephrine in concentrations of 4 to 20 μg/ml (1:250,000 to 1:50,000) is most commonly used for this purpose, but other sympathomimetic amines including levonordefrin, norepinephrine, and phenylephrine are also employed. Localization of the anesthetic solution in the area of injection by epinephrine is often highly beneficial. The duration of local anesthesia may be prolonged severalfold, and even the success rate and intensity of nerve block may be improved. Systemic toxicity may be reduced because drug metabolism is more likely to keep pace with drug absorption. During surgery, hemostasis afforded by the infiltration of a local anesthetic solution containing epinephrine may also be advantageous.

Normally, sympathomimetic drugs included in anesthetic formulations produce no pharmacologic effects of consequence other than localized arteriolar constriction. Epinephrine may decrease total peripheral resistance by 20% to 30% and increase stroke volume commensurately, but there is no change in heart rate or mean blood pressure. Injudicious dosage, accidental intravascular injection, or adverse drug interactions, however, may promote clinically noticeable effects on the central and sympathetic nervous systems. Heart rate and systolic blood pressure may be elevated by epinephrine, causing uncomfortable palpitations and pain in the chest. Restlessness and apprehension similar to that produced by local anesthetics may also occur. Phenylephrine, a relatively pure α-adrenergic agonist, avoids the direct cardiac and CNS stimulation associated with epinephrine, but it may significantly elevate systolic and diastolic pressures and reflexly slow the heart for an extended period of time. Other sympathomimetics, such as norepinephrine and levonordefrin, are somewhat intermediate in their systemic effects.

Concern is often expressed about the use of epinephrine and other catecholamine vasoconstrictors in dental patients with cardiovascular disease. Although it is important to minimize myocardial stimulation in such patients, the minute amount of epinephrine used in local anesthesia does not usually increase the risk of dental treatment. In fact, the quantity of epinephrine released endogenously during stress is much greater than that present in any dental cartridge. As a guideline for cardiac patients, the New York Heart Association recommended in 1955 that the amount of epinephrine administered during any one session not exceed 0.2 mg.[49] This is equivalent to 20 ml of a 1:100,000 epinephrine solution. Current evidence suggests that this amount is excessive for patients with seriously compromised cardiovascular systems; the reader is referred elsewhere for a thorough review of vasoconstrictor use in the cardiac patient.[31]

ABSORPTION, FATE, AND EXCRETION

Pharmacokinetic considerations regarding local anesthetics are vital, since the balance between a local anesthetic's uptake into the systemic circulation and its removal through redistribution, metabolism, and excretion determines in large measure the drug's toxic potential. The rate of absorption is dependent on several factors, including the dosage and pharmacologic profile of the drug employed, the presence of a vasoconstrictor agent, and the nature of the administration site. Obviously, the more drug that is injected, the higher its resultant blood concentration will be. Less obvious are the qualitative influences of the anesthetic solution and how these interact with the site of administration. Drugs with potent vasodilating properties, such as procaine and lidocaine, may significantly enhance their own uptake, particularly when injected into a highly vascular space. Inclusion of epinephrine or another vasoconstrictor is especially important in these instances. Drugs that are not strong vasodilators, such as mepivacaine and prilocaine, do not markedly accentuate their own absorption and do not require as much epinephrine to limit uptake. Absorption after topical application varies widely. Although intact skin and oral mucosa are relatively impermeable, local anesthetics are readily absorbed from most mucosal surfaces. Instillation of tetracaine into the pyriform fossa, for instance, results in a peak plasma concentration one third to one half that obtained after rapid intravenous infusion. By comparison, absorption of lidocaine from the tracheobronchial tree is much slower. Regardless of the site of administration, sympathomimetic agents are topically ineffective in delaying absorption. Uptake may be minimized, however, by using local anesthetics prepared in the form of an ointment or gel instead of an aqueous spray.

On entering the circulation, a local anesthetic is partially bound by plasma proteins (α_1-acid glycoprotein in particular) and red blood cells. After distribution throughout the intravascular space, the unbound drug is free to diffuse into the various organs of the body. Since redistribution is a major mechanism for the removal of slowly metabolized drugs from the bloodstream, an anesthetic agent (e.g., prilocaine) that leaves the circulation quickly to enter muscle and other tissues will enjoy a reduced toxicity. So-called barriers to diffusion are relatively ineffective with the local anesthetics. In addition to entering the central nervous system, these drugs readily cross the placenta and may occasionally induce severe cardiac depression in the fetus.

The metabolic fate of a particular agent largely depends on the chemical linkage between the aromatic residue and the rest of the molecule. Ester drugs are inactivated by hydrolysis. Derivatives of p-aminobenzoic acid (e.g., procaine, tetracaine) are preferentially metabolized in the plasma by pseudocholinesterase; the ratio between plasma and liver hydrolysis with other esters is somewhat variable. Products of hydrolytic cleavage may undergo further biotransformation in the liver before being eliminated in the urine. Less than 2% of an administered dose of procaine is excreted unchanged by the kidneys. Metabolism of amide drugs occurs primarily in the liver. The initial reaction is usually N-dealkylation of the tertiary amino terminus. The resultant secondary amine is susceptible to hydrolysis by hepatic amidase activity, but conjugation, hydroxylation, or further dealkylation may also occur. Inactivation of prilocaine, a secondary amine, is relatively rapid because dealkylation is not required before hydrolysis can take place. Some metabolites retain significant pharmacologic activity and may contribute to drug toxicity. Much of the sedative effect of lidocaine, for example, has been attributed to its de-ethylated metabolites monoethylglycinexylidide and glycinexylidide.[51] As with ester compounds, minimal amounts (1% to 20%) of administered amides appear in the urine as unmetabolized compounds.

Differences in biotransformation of the various local anesthetics are at times clinically relevant. Individuals with certain genetically based defects in pseudocholinesterase activity are unusually sensitive to procaine and other esters; conventional doses of these drugs may occasionally lead to toxic reactions. Alternatively, severe hepatic disease or reduced hepatic blood flow may produce systemic intolerance to lidocaine and presumably to other local anesthetics dependent on adequate liver function for their metabolism.

TOXIC REACTIONS AND SIDE EFFECTS

Modern local anesthetic solutions are quite safe when employed by competent personnel. Nevertheless, a substantial literature describing various adverse reactions attests to the potential toxicity of these agents, particularly when they are used in a cavalier manner.

Systemic toxicity

Most toxic effects of a serious nature are related to excessive blood concentrations achieved through inadvertent intravascular injection or through the administration of large quantities of drug. Convulsions, respiratory depression, and cardiovascular collapse represent the greatest hazards to health. Such reactions can usually be prevented by observing three precautions: (1) *administer the smallest dose that will provide effective anesthesia*, (2) *employ proper injection techniques, including aspiration*, and (3) *use a vasoconstrictor-containing solution when indicated to retard drug absorption*. If an adverse response occurs in spite of these procedures, immediate therapy must be rendered. The patient should be placed in the supine position with the legs elevated, and oxygen should be administered. This procedure is often all that is needed for mild toxic reactions, epinephrine responses, or syncopal attacks.

Convulsions are usually self-limiting and require no treatment other than supporting ventilation and protecting the patient from bodily harm. Pharmacologic intervention is necessary, however, when seizures are so intense or prolonged that hypoxic injury threatens to ensue. Small intravenous doses of a rapidly acting barbiturate (e.g., 50 to 100 mg of thiopental) are often successful in terminating local anesthetic seizures. Barbiturates unfortunately tend to potentiate the postconvulsive depressant phase of local anesthetic toxicity. For this reason, succinylcholine, a neuromuscular blocker without CNS depressant action, is sometimes employed in lieu of a barbiturate. Seizure control with succinylcholine, though, is open to some criticism. Thorough training in artificial ventilation is a mandatory prerequisite for its use because the drug paralyzes the muscles of respiration. Furthermore, neuromuscular blockade treats only the outward manifestations of a convulsion; electrical disturbances within the central nervous system progress unimpeded. Perhaps the most satisfactory method of seizure control for the dentist is the intravenous administration of diazepam. Experimental evidence and clinical experience indicate that diazepam (0.1 to 0.2 mg/kg) can eliminate local anesthetic convulsions without producing significant effects on ventilation or circulation.[39] Various agents have also been used in attempts to *prevent* seizures. Most anticonvulsants examined have been disappointing in this regard, but diazepam has been shown in cats to double the convulsant ED50 of lidocaine without causing undesirable CNS disturbances.[18] Diazepam is consequently a premedication of choice when the administration of a large quantity of local anesthetic is anticipated. Surprisingly, some drugs commonly used for preoperative sedation, including meperidine and promethazine, may actually facilitate local anesthetic convulsions.[48]

Treatment of most severe toxic reactions is symptomatic and consists of reversing respiratory and circulatory disruptions as they occur. Since most deaths attributed to local anesthetics are related to tissue anoxia, support of ventilation is of paramount importance. Arterial hypotension is controlled by the coadministration of intravenous fluids and vasoconstrictor agents. Cardiopulmonary resuscitative techniques are necessary in situations where cardiac function is interrupted.

Local tissue responses

Commercially available local anesthetics are relatively nonirritating to tissues. Many reactions described in the past were caused not by local anesthetics but by metallic or alcoholic contaminants that gained access to the solutions during or after manufacture. Local anesthetic concentrations required to damage peripheral nerves usually far exceed those required for transmission blockade. Conventional preparations may, however, induce focal necrosis in skeletal muscle tissue approximating the injection site.[56] The damage occurs rapidly after a single administration and is completely reversed in a matter of several weeks. Local anesthetics may also impede cell motility, depress collagen synthesis, and perhaps delay wound healing.

Tissue responses to injected local anesthetic preparations are usually caused or augmented by vasoconstrictor additives. Epinephrine creates tissue hypoxia by reducing local blood flow while simultaneously increasing oxygen consumption. Although tissue injury may be induced by any of the sympathomimetics used currently, norepinephrine is particularly apt to cause ischemic necrosis. The injection of local anesthetic with vasoconstrictor is also especially hazardous in areas supplied by terminal arteries (e.g., nose, digits, and penis). In dentistry, tissue irritation is reflected by an increased incidence of postanesthetic pain at the injection site in patients receiving local anesthetic formulations that contain vasoconstrictors.

Idiosyncratic reactions

In rare instances, patients have experienced toxic reactions to very small amounts of local anesthetic. Some such reactions may represent an abnormal susceptibility to the drug.[27] Most often, however, these responses are anxiety related or the result of inadvertent intravascular injection. With respect to the latter possibility, it has been determined accidentally that the convulsant dose of lidocaine in humans is only 10 mg when the drug is injected into the vertebral artery.[32]

Amide local anesthetics are sometimes listed with other drugs as causative agents in malignant hyperthermia (MH). This inclusion is based on a few supposed cases of MH and on the ability of these drugs to potentiate contracture of skeletal muscle in various experimental situations. The preponderance of evidence indicates, however, that lidocaine is not a triggering agent. For example, lidocaine has no effect on porcine MH nor has it caused problems when used for local anesthesia in patients with a history of MH.[54] Although it may be prudent to avoid lidocaine during a fulminant attack, the drug appears quite safe for routine dental use in MH-susceptible patients.

Allergic phenomena

Local anesthetics rarely cause allergic reactions; however, when one does occur, an ester derivative of *p*-aminobenzoic acid is usually involved. Methylparaben, a preservative used in certain local anesthetic preparations, may also serve on occasion as an antigenic stimulant. Historically, most documented cases of allergy (in the form of contact dermatitis) occurred in dentists and other health professionals exposed to ester agents on a regular basis. Urticarial eruptions, erythematous rashes, and other dermatologic responses represent common manifestations of local anesthetic allergy in patients and are regularly treated with antihistamines. Anaphylactic responses of a serious nature require epinephrine.

In spite of the low incidence of verifiable allergy to local anesthetic solutions in patients, a relatively high percentage of individuals provide medical histories of presumptive local anesthetic hypersensitivity. Many of these cases undoubtedly represent anxiety or toxic reactions misdiagnosed as immunologic in origin. Such mistakes are particularly apparent where amides are concerned since most investigations have shown these compounds to be essentially nonallergenic.[5] When a single agent is involved, substitution with another local anesthetic is the simplest method of resolving the problem, if consideration is given to the fact that esters may exhibit cross-allergenicity with each other and with methylparaben. Drug selection becomes more difficult when a patient claims allergy to all conventional agents. Diphenhydramine (1% with or without 1 : 100,000 epinephrine) has been used with some success in such instances, but its suitability as a local anesthetic is limited. An alternative approach is to screen for drug allergy. Although sensitivity testing methods are generally somewhat unreliable and may be potentially dangerous, a regimen of intracutaneous injections graduating to full-challenge tests in a supervised medical setting has proved useful in identifying local anesthetic formulations that can be safely employed.[19]

DRUG INTERACTIONS

By virtue of their influences on excitable membranes, local anesthetics are potentially capable of interacting with a wide spectrum of therapeutic agents. Lidocaine combined with another antiarrhythmic drug may generate profound disturbances in cardiac automaticity and conduction, far in excess of what either compound would have caused if given alone. Though feeble by itself, the neuromuscular blocking activity of local anesthetics has been used to advantage in preventing succinylcholine-induced fasciculations and in reducing the dose of succinylcholine required during surgery for adequate muscle relaxation.

In coronary care units, where large doses of lidocaine are infused intravenously to prevent and to treat ventricular arrhythmias, the coadministration of an H_2-histamine receptor blocker (e.g., cimetidine)[22] or a β-adrenoceptor antagonist (e.g., propranolol)[13] may be a common cause of lidocaine toxicity and, perhaps, the reason for a number of unexplained deaths. These drugs reduce hepatic blood flow, the rate-limiting factor in lidocaine clearance. Moreover, they may also inhibit directly the uptake and metabolism of lidocaine by the liver.

A unique interaction may occur between certain esters and the sulfonamides. Procaine and several other local anesthetics (benzocaine, butacaine, and tetracaine) are metabolized to yield *p*-aminobenzoic acid. The antibacterial action of sulfonamides is competitively antagonized by this metabolite.

Although the potential for interactions involving local anesthetics is great, clinical manifestations appear infrequently outside the hospital and then only when very large doses are employed or when unusual patient factors are present. Much more likely to occur are interactions between various drugs and the vasoconstrictors employed during local anesthesia. Epinephrine, for example, may generate dangerous cardiac arrhythmias during halothane anesthesia or in patients with excessive concentrations of thyroid hormone in the blood. Similarly, catecholamines can induce undesirable changes in cardiac action and blood pressure in patients receiving tricyclic antidepressants, β-adrenergic blockers, or adrenergic neuron blocking drugs (e.g., guanethidine). Levodopa and the phenothiazines may also alter the effects of catecholamine vasoconstrictors, but the clinical significance of these interactions is not well established. Despite statements to the contrary,[14] local anesthetics containing epinephrine *may* be used without special reservation in patients taking MAO inhibitors.[41] Exogenous catecholamines are mostly degraded by the enzyme catechol-O-methyltransferase; inhibition of MAO has little impact on their respective metabolic fates[6] or cardiovascular actions.[9] Of the vasoconstrictors currently added to local anesthetic solutions, only phenylephrine is contraindicated with concomitant MAO therapy.

Certainly the most important interaction featuring vasoconstrictors is the intended one—inhibition of local anesthetic uptake from the injection site. Animal data suggest, however, that this is not the only interaction that can occur involving the anesthetic agent and its vasoconstrictor partner. Acute lethality studies document that epinephrine potentiates the toxicity of local anesthetics administered intravenously as a bolus.[2,55] By protecting against local anesthetic depression of the cardiovascular system, the vasoconstrictor allows a greater than normal fraction of anesthetic to reach the brain and spinal cord.[57] As a result, local anesthetic toxicity may be enhanced as much as twofold. This finding has important implications inasmuch as accidental intravascular injections are thought to be the most common cause of systemic toxicity, at least in adult patients.

Largely because of the drug interactions associated with the sympathomimetic amines, attention has been focused on noncatecholamine alternatives for vasoconstriction. Of these, several analogues of the antidiuretic hormone vasopressin have proved suitable, and one, felypressin (phenylalanine^2-lysine^8 vasopressin), is now in widespread use in Europe and elsewhere as a vasoconstrictor for local anesthesia. Although felypressin is not quite as effective as epinephrine and cannot be relied on for surgical hemostasis, it avoids the drug interaction problems of the catecholamines and is comparatively less toxic in the concentrations employed. Because felypressin does not stimulate tissue oxygen consumption, local toxicity is also reduced. Local anesthetics with felypressin are not currently available in the United States.

GENERAL THERAPEUTIC USES

Local anesthetics are widely employed for the relief of pain. By obviating the necessity of general anesthesia, these drugs have been instrumental in reducing the mortality and morbidity associated with a variety of operative procedures. They also render valuable though less conspicuous service by obtunding the pain of sunburn, toothache, and other mundane afflictions. In addition, local anesthetics are increasingly being used for purposes unrelated to pain control.

Techniques of anesthesia

The onset, quality, extent, and duration of local anesthesia vary markedly with the technique of administration employed. As might be expected, no single agent is capable of performing all of the clinical duties local anesthetics are expected to fulfill.

Surface application. Local anesthetics are prepared for topical use in several different forms. Aqueous solutions are especially suited for coverage of large surfaces; anesthesia of small areas is often best accomplished with an ointment or viscous gel. Although penetration of the intact epidermis is insignificant, uptake by injured skin or by mucous membranes can be rapid. It is suggested that no more than one fourth of the maximum recommended dosage for infiltration be employed when substantial absorption can be expected.[1] Topical activities are often not related to efficacies determined for other administration sites: tetracaine and lidocaine are useful topical agents, whereas mepivacaine, prilocaine, and procaine are not. Benzocaine, ineffective parenterally, is well adapted for surface anesthesia because of its slow absorption and lack of systemic toxicity.

Infiltration and nerve block. Inhibition of transmission in circumscribed portions of the peripheral nervous system is accomplished by the techniques of infiltration and nerve block. Infiltration anesthesia is performed by injecting a local anesthetic into the area to be anesthetized. In this manner, the nerve endings exposed to the anesthetic solution are quickly rendered unresponsive. Nerve block is produced by depositing a local anesthetic solution close to the appropriate nerve trunk but proximal to the intended area of anesthesia. After a certain latency period required for diffusion of the local anesthetic into the nerve interior, sensations will be lost in all tissues innervated by the distal portion of the affected nerve. Although infiltrations and single nerve blocks usually anesthetize discrete areas, compound injections (e.g., brachial plexus or sciatic-femoral blocks) may affect large segments of the body, including whole limbs. All of the many local anesthetics suitable for infiltration are also useful for nerve blockade.

Spinal anesthesia. Deposition of a local anesthetic solution in the subarachnoid space can be used to produce surgical anesthesia in all structures of the body below the diaphragm. Injection is ordinarily made inferior to the first lumbar vertebra to avoid possible injury to the spinal cord. Once introduced, the drug mixes with the cerebrospinal fluid and begins to spread throughout the subarachnoid space. The extent of cephalad diffusion of the local anesthetic, and therefore the level of anesthesia obtained, is governed by several factors: the dose, specific gravity, and volume of local anesthetic solution administered; the size and position of the spinal canal; and the degree of cerebrospinal fluid mixing imposed by the rate of injection and by movements of the patient. Tetracaine is most commonly used for spinal anesthesia, but numerous other agents are also employed.

Epidural block. Local anesthetic infusion into the potential space between the dura mater and the connective tissue lining of the vertebral canal provides an effective alternative to subarachnoid anesthesia. Patient resistance to epidural injection is less of a problem, and the neurologic difficulties sometimes encountered after spinal block are avoided. Epidural anesthesia is comparatively slow in onset, however, and requires considerably more total drug than does its subarachnoid counterpart. The level of anesthesia is also less predictable and more difficult to control. The clinical use of lidocaine, prilocaine, and other local anesthetics for epidural blockade has been reviewed by Lund and colleagues.[35]

Intravascular injection. Local anesthetics are sometimes introduced directly into a blood vessel to effect short-term regional analgesia. One popular technique consists of injecting an anesthetic solution (ordinarily 0.5% procaine or 0.5% lidocaine) intravenously into a limb previously exsanguinated by elevation or with an Esmarch bandage. Isolation of the local anesthetic solution from the systemic circulation is accomplished by placing a pneumatic tourniquet proximal to the injection site. Egress of the local anesthetic from the vascular compartment to peripheral tissues is so rapid that relasing the tourniquet as soon as 5 minutes after injection does not result in toxic blood concentrations. Other techniques using intravascular local anesthetics have also been practiced on occasion. For example, lidocaine may be mixed with irritating drugs in an attempt to alleviate the pain associated with intravascular injection.

Treatment of cardiac arrhythmias

Two local anesthetics, procainamide and lidocaine, have established roles in the therapeutic management of cardiac arrhythmias, especially of ventricular origin. The antiarrhythmic properties of these agents are discussed in Chapter 24.

Other uses

Local anesthetics are sometimes administered intravenously to produce or to supplement general anesthesia. As an adjunctive agent, lidocaine has been used to prevent postoperative muscle pain caused by succinylcholine and to depress airway reflexes and sympathetic nervous system responses during endotracheal intubation and extubation and other procedures affecting the bronchial tree. Local anesthetics have also been employed, with mixed success, as intravenous analgesic and anticonvulsant medications.

USES IN DENTISTRY

It would be difficult to overstate the profound influence of local anesthesia on the practice of dentistry. Many of the complex restorative procedures routinely performed on conscious patients would be inconceivable without effective pain control. By eliminating most nociceptive sensations associated with dental care, local anesthetics improve patient acceptance of dental treatment and, as a result, contribute significantly to oral health. Because local anesthetics are so frequently employed and, for many practitioners, represent the only drugs administered parenterally, the toxicity as well as efficacy of these agents is of particular interest and concern.

Safety in dentistry

Without question, local anesthesia is often considerably safer in dentistry than in medicine. Dosages employed for infiltration and nerve block in the oral cavity are often less than one tenth those used for compound nerve block or for epidural injection. Recipients of dental anesthesia are in better systemic health than some medical patients and usually undergo only minor operative stress. Reports, nevertheless, occasionally appear describing instances of death from local anesthesia in dental practice.

Statistics related to local anesthetic toxicity in dentistry are meager and subject to error. Mortality figures range from 1 death in 1.4 million local anesthetic administrations[46] to 1 in 45 million.[47] These values are open to question. It is possible that some deaths from local anesthetics go unreported and that others are mistakenly identified as myocardial infarctions, cerebrovascular accidents, or the like. It is also possible, however, that some deaths imputed to local anesthetics are caused by procedural stress or are merely accidents of time and place and are not causally related to drug administration at all. Tabulations of nonfatal adverse reactions directly attributable to local anesthetics are limited, but in one of the largest and best controlled investigations, Persson[42] recorded adverse effects in 2.5% of 2,960 patients given 1 to 2 cartridges of various anesthetic agents. Because most of the complications observed—pallor, unrest, sweating, fatigue, palpitations, nausea, and fainting—are common manifestations of acute anxiety, it is evident that many adverse effects ascribed to local anesthesia are actually generated by the process of injection and not by the drugs themselves.

Most severe systemic reactions in dentistry probably arise from accidental intravascular injections. In view of the small amounts of drug (<100 mg) routinely administered for most procedures, toxic

Table 17-2. Comparison of local anesthetics used in dentistry

Proprietary name	Preparation contents	Maximum dose		Duration of anesthesia (soft tissue)	
		In children (mg/kg)	In adults (ml)	Maxillary infiltration (min)	Inferior alveolar block (min)
Xylocaine with Epinephrine	2% lidocaine HCl; 1:100,000 epinephrine	7	15	170	200
Carbocaine with Neo-Cobefrin	2% mepivacaine HCl; 1:20,000 levonordefrin	6	15	140	210
Carbocaine	3% mepivacaine HCl	6	10	85	180
Citanest Forte	4% prilocaine HCl; 1:200,000 epinephrine	8	10	130	190
Citanest	4% prilocaine HCl	8	10	85	175
Marcaine with Epinephrine	0.5% bupivacaine HCl; 1:200,000 epinephrine	3	15	395	440
Ravocaine	0.4% propoxycaine HCl; 2% procaine HCl; 1:20,000 levonordefrin	0.2*	8	145	175

*Dosage in ml/kg.

overdosage in an adult patient seems very unlikely. Allergic responses are also considered rare, particularly with the amide drugs in current use. Aspiration tests indicate that the needle is placed inside a blood vessel in about 3% of all injections and much more frequently during blockade of the inferior alveolar and the posterior superior alveolar nerves. Negative aspiration, unfortunately, does not guarantee that the needle lumen is outside the vessel; using improper aspiration force or placing the lumen against a vessel's intimal lining can prevent blood from entering the anesthetic cartridge.

In view of the fact that lidocaine is routinely given intravenously in quantities that exceed the amount in a dental cartridge without producing toxic manifestations in cardiac patients, it has been proposed that local anesthetics injected intraarterially within the oral cavity may gain direct access to the central nervous system by passing regressively down the branches and trunk of the external carotid artery and into the internal carotid.[3] This hypothesis would seemingly account for adverse reactions associated with relatively small amounts of drug; however, studies in rats have shown that internal carotid injections are actually less toxic than intravenous administrations.[55] The explanation for this finding is that the circle of Willis is not patent physiologically in the normal brain, thus precluding drug entry into the medulla where it can depress respiration. It is possible that toxic reactions in dentistry might only occur in patients with an abnormal cerebral circulation, but a more plausible explanation is that intravenous injection of even the small amounts of drug in a single dental cartridge can cause adverse responses in sensitive individuals, particularly if the drug is given rapidly and a vasoconstrictor is present in the solution.[27,57]

Drug selection

Selection of a local anesthetic for dental application must include considerations of efficiency, safety, and individual patient and operative needs. That such factors are difficult to evaluate is illustrated by the diversity of results obtained in various clinical trials.[10,17,21,38] One of the few areas of agreement is that the introduction of the amide lidocaine in 1948 marked a significant advance over the ester preparations then available. Indeed, 2% lidocaine hydrochloride with 1:100,000 epinephrine remains unsurpassed as a dental anesthetic for routine use. Besides lidocaine, three additional amides have been developed and widely marketed that possess similar advantages in stability, nonallergenicity, and efficacy over the ester agents (Table 17-2). Mepivacaine, introduced in 1957, is generally equivalent to lidocaine in its pharmacologic profile. Two distinctive features of mepivacaine are its topical ineffectiveness and its use as a 3% solution without a vasoconstrictor. Prilocaine, used clinically for the first time in 1960, is a less potent and less toxic alternative to lidocaine. Like mepivacaine, it is not used topically but is effective for dental application without epinephrine. The most recently introduced local anesthetic for dentistry is bupivacaine. This drug is slightly slower in onset than the previous amides, but it is equally efficacious and has a longer duration of action, making it well suited for providing postoperative pain relief in oral surgery.

One significant dissimilarity among the amide preparations concerns the presence or absence of a vasoconstrictor additive. Local anesthetic formulations without epinephrine-like drugs are particularly useful in those instances in which sympathomimetic amines are contraindicated. Plain solutions are additionally promoted on the basis of a shorter duration of action. While it is true that soft-tissue anesthesia is comparatively brief after maxillary infiltration with 3% mepivacaine or 4% prilocaine (both without vasoconstrictor), differences in duration of mandibular injections are trivial (Table 17-2). Because the period of pulpal anesthesia is often 20% to 25% that of soft-tissue anesthesia, the limited maxillary duration of these agents is sometimes disadvantageous. For instance, 4% prilocaine, which compares favorably with 2% lidocaine with epinephrine in both onset and profundity of anesthesia, fails about one fifth of the time to provide adequate pain relief toward the end of restorative procedures averaging 25 minutes in length.[10]

The utility of local anesthetics without vasoconstrictors in pediatric dentistry deserves special comment. It is sometimes claimed that the shorter duration of soft-tissue symptoms with plain local anesthetic solutions should reduce the incidence of self-inflicted cheek and lip trauma. Such claims are dubious since blockade of the inferior alveolar and long buccal nerves that supply most of the tissues at risk is not significantly shortened by these preparations (Table 17-2). Furthermore, no studies relating a reduction in traumatic cheilitis to the use of plain solutions have been reported. Consideration of systemic toxicity should actually limit the pedodontic use of local anesthetics without vasoconstrictors. Two cartridges of 3% mepivacaine, for instance, exceeds the maximum recommended dose for a 15 kg child; inattention to the dosage limits of this preparation has needlessly resulted in a number of fatalities.[7] Because the safety margin of local anesthetics is quite low in small children, it is advisable to employ a preparation containing a vasoconstrictor if not doing so would result in more total drug being administered.

Other than amide compounds being advocated over esters, it is difficult to suggest a particular local anesthetic for routine dental application. Certainly, if a proposed treatment requires a considerable volume of drug or necessitates a relatively prolonged operation, formulations such as lidocaine with epinephrine are indicated. Bupivacaine with epinephrine would be a good choice if a truly prolonged effect is desired. A plain local anesthetic solution might be more appropriate, however, for short procedures involving the maxillary arch. When special patient factors or operative needs are not present, drug selection is best founded on the respective anesthetic efficacies and potential toxicities of the agents available. Since no local anesthetic preparation has emerged that is superior to the rest in affording pain relief, use of any particular drug should be dictated largely by its relative unlikelihood of producing untoward responses. Estimates of toxicity of local anesthetics used in dentistry unfortunately have not been made. Accepting that serious adverse reactions in most patients are caused by intravascular injections, one could predict by considering just the local anesthetic moieties involved that a 3% mepivacaine solution would be 50% more toxic than an equal volume of 2% mepivacaine with levonordefrin. As described previously, however, some evidence suggests that sympathomimetic amines may potentiate the intravascular toxicity of concomitantly administered local anesthetics, making conclusions at this point impossible. Until definitive information about the intravascular toxic potentials of the various local anesthetic formulations becomes available, recommendation of any single preparation for general use over all the others cannot be made.

PREPARATIONS AND DOSAGE
Agents for parenteral administration

Local anesthetics intended for injection within the oral cavity are supplied in 1.8 ml single-dose cartridges. Pyrogen-free distilled water with sodium chloride added for osmotic balance serves as the local anesthetic vehicle. Local anesthetic solutions range in pH from under 3.0 to over 6.0; generally, preparations with vasoconstrictors are adjusted to a lower pH than are plain formulations to enhance stability of the sympathomimetic amine constituents. Sodium metabisulfite or an equivalent antioxidant is also included to help prevent vasoconstrictor breakdown. Some local anesthetics contain methylparaben. Useful for its antimicrobial action in multidose vials, methylparaben serves no purpose in dental local anesthetic preparations, and its incorporation should be discontinued. Currently available local anesthetics accepted by the Council on Dental Therapeutics of the American Dental Association are described below.[14]

Procaine hydrochloride and propoxycaine hydrochloride. Procaine is the ester derivative of *p*-aminobenzoic acid and diethylaminoethanol. A 2% procaine hydrochloride solution with 1 : 50,000 epinephrine and a 4% solution with 1 : 2500 phenylephrine were formerly available, but procaine is now marketed only as a 2% concentration in combination with 0.4% propoxycaine hydrochloride and either 1 : 20,000 levonordefrin or 1 : 30,000 norepinephrine as the vasoconstrictor. Propoxycaine is a derivative of procaine in which a propoxy group is added to the ortho position on the aromatic ring. The procaine-propoxycaine formulation is the only ester preparation currently available in dentistry. Cross-allergenicity may occur between procaine, propoxycaine, and other derivatives of *p*-aminobenzoic acid.

Tetracaine hydrochloride. Tetracaine is an ester derivative of *p*-aminobenzoic acid in which a butyl chain replaces one of the hydrogens on the *p*-amino group. The drug has approximately ten times the toxicity and potency of procaine. Development of nerve block is unusually slow with tetracaine, so it was often combined with procaine to provide anesthesia that is quick in onset yet prolonged in duration. (The preparation used for injection in dentistry is no longer available.) For surface application, 0.5% to 2% tetracaine is included in spray, liquid, cream, and ointment formulations. Tetracaine is one of the most effective topical anesthetics, but the drug's toxic potential should dictate caution in its use.

Lidocaine hydrochloride. Lidocaine is an aminoethylamide derivative of xylidine. It is several times more potent and toxic than procaine and provides local anesthesia that is by comparison more prompt, more extensive, and longer lasting. The administration of 2% lidocaine hydrochloride with 1 : 100,000 epinephrine is most suitable for routine dental use, but the drug is also available as a plain solution and with 1 : 50,000 epinephrine. Although 2% lidocaine with vasoconstrictor provides satisfactory dental anesthesia in normal circumstances, it has sometimes proved ineffective in rendering extremely sensitive teeth completely pain free. A concentrated solution of 5% lidocaine with 1 : 80,000 epinephrine has been shown to produce effective anesthesia in most instances where conventional local anesthetic preparations have failed.[20] Lidocaine is the only amide used for top-

ical anesthesia in dentistry. Formulations available include a 2% viscous gel, 3% cream, 2% and 4% liquids, 5% ointment, and 10% aerosol spray.

Mepivacaine hydrochloride. Mepivacaine is an amide product of xylidine and N-methylpipecolic acid. Similar in many respects to lidocaine, mepivacaine hydrochloride is marketed in a 2% concentration with 1 : 20,000 levonordefrin and as a 3% solution without vasoconstrictor. In contrast to some ester local anesthetics, cross-allergenicity is rare between mepivacaine and related agents.

Prilocaine hydrochloride. Unlike other amide anesthetics, prilocaine is a secondary amino derivative of toluidine. Instances of cyanosis observed after large doses of prilocaine (>400 mg) probably result from its metabolic breakdown to *o*-toluidine, a known inducer of methemoglobin. Somewhat less potent than lidocaine, prilocaine hydrochloride is marketed as a 4% solution with and without 1 : 200,000 epinephrine. Since the toxicity of prilocaine is approximately one half that of lidocaine, relative toxicities on a milliliter basis are essentially equal.

Bupivacaine hydrochloride. Bupivacaine is a homologue of mepivacaine rendered highly lipid soluble by replacement of the N-methyl group with a butyl chain. Bupivacaine is about 4 times as potent and as toxic as mepivacaine; it also has a slightly higher pK_a and a slower onset of action. For dentistry, 0.5% bupivacaine hydrochloride is available as a plain solution or with 1 : 200,000 epinephrine. Clinical trials indicate that bupivacaine with epinephrine produces operative anesthesia several times longer than that afforded by other drugs.[34,43] Additionally, the formulation provides postoperative analgesia averaging 8 hours in the mandible and 5 hours in the maxilla. The plain solution is also long acting, but it may be less effective alone than with vasoconstrictor.

Although not yet available for dental use, etidocaine, a homologue of lidocaine, is similar to bupivacaine in being very lipid soluble and in having an extended duration of action. A 1.5% solution of the hydrochloride salt with 1 : 200,000 epinephrine is being evaluated for intraoral anesthesia. If marketed, it will have the same applications as bupivacaine but will enjoy a faster onset time.

Agents limited to surface application

Topical anesthetics are used in the oral cavity for a variety of purposes. Formulations marketed as pressurized sprays produce widespread surface anesthesia appropriate for making impressions or intraoral radiographs. Such preparations are potentially hazardous, however, and only products with metered valve dispensers to help prevent inadvertent overdosage should be employed. Topical liquids, which avoid the possibility of aerosol inspiration, may also be used for anesthetic coverage of large surface areas. Nonaqueous topical preparations are suitable for most other procedures. Common local anesthetic vehicles include lanolin, petrolatum, sodium carboxymethylcellulose, and polyethylene glycol.

Benzocaine. Benzocaine is a *p*-aminobenzoic acid ester lacking an amino terminus. Poorly soluble in aqueous fluid, benzocaine tends to remain at the site of application and is not readily absorbed into the systemic circulation. Because of its low toxic potential, benzocaine is especially useful for anesthesia of large surface areas within the oral cavity. Benzocaine is available in a variety of preparations ranging in anesthetic concentrations from 6% to 20%.

Butacaine sulfate. Butacaine is a *p*-aminobenzoic acid ester limited to surface application because of a high systemic toxicity. Proposed as an alternative to cocaine for anesthesia of the eye, ear, nose, and throat, 4% butacaine is marketed for dental use in a petrolatum-based ointment with 1% benzyl alcohol.

Dyclonine hydrochloride. Dyclonine is unusual in that it has a ketone linkage between the aromatic moiety and the rest of the anesthetic molecule. Available as a 0.5% solution with 0.3% chlorobutanol (see below) for topical use, dyclonine hydrochloride is not administered by injection because of its propensity for producing tissue irritation. Dyclonine may be used in patients allergic to derivatives of *p*-aminobenzoic acid.

Chlorobutanol. Chlorobutanol is a weak local anesthetic usually employed in combination with other agents. The drug is used primarily in obtundent dressings to relieve symptoms of acute pulpitis and postextraction wound pain.

Cocaine hydrochloride. Cocaine, the first anesthetic used in dentistry and medicine, is a naturally occurring benzoic acid ester. The pharmacology of cocaine is unique among the local anesthetics in that the drug inhibits the uptake of catecholamines by adrenergic nerve terminals. Cocaine, therefore, potentiates the action of endogenously released and exogenously administered sympathomimetic amines. As a result, cocaine may cause pupillary mydriasis, vascular constriction, and other manifestations of sympathetic nervous activity. Cocaine is also a powerful CNS stimulant and has become a popular drug of abuse (see Chapter 46). Restricted to therapeutic applications where its vasoconstricting property is of special benefit (e.g., topical anesthesia of the nasal mucosa before nasoendotracheal intubation), cocaine has no place in the routine practice of dentistry.

Other preparations

A number of local anesthetics not described above have been used in dentistry: butethamine (Monocaine), chloroprocaine (Nesacaine), isobucaine (Kincaine), meprylcaine (Oracaine), metabutethamine (Unacaine), piperocaine (Metycaine), and pyrrocaine (Dynacaine). None of these agents offers any advantage over the drugs previously discussed and need to be considered further.

Local anesthetics

Nonproprietary name	Proprietary name
Agents for parenteral administration	
bupivacaine	Marcaine, Sensorcaine
chloroprocaine	Nesacaine
dibucaine	Nupercaine
etidocaine	Duranest
lidocaine	Xylocaine, Octocaine, Alphacaine
mepivacaine	Carbocaine, Isocaine, Arestocaine
prilocaine	Citanest
procaine	Novocain
propoxycaine	Ravocaine
tetracaine	Pontocaine
Agents limited to surface application	
benzocaine	Americaine, Hurricaine
butacaine	Butyn
butamben	Butesin Picrate
chlorobutanol	in Dyclone
cocaine	—
cyclomethycaine	Surfacaine
dyclonine	in Dyclone
hexylcaine	Cyclaine
pramoxine	Tronothane
proparacaine	Alcaine

CITED REFERENCES

1. Adriani, J., and Naraghi, M. The pharmacologic principles of regional pain relief. Annual Reviews of Pharmacology and Toxicology **17:**223-242, 1977.

2. Åkerman, B. Effects of felypressin (Octopressin®) on the acute toxicity of local anesthetics. Acta Pharmacologica et Toxicologica **27:**318-330, 1969.

3. Aldrete, J.A., Narang, R., Sada, T., Liem, S.T., and Mller, G.P. Reverse carotid blood flow—a possible explanation for some reactions to local anesthetics. Journal of the American Dental Association **94:**1142-1145, 1977.

4. Altura, B.M., and Altura, B.T. Effects of local anesthetics, antihistamines, and glucocorticoids on peripheral blood flow and vascular smooth muscle. Anesthesiology **41:**197-214, 1974.

5. Arora, S., and Aldrete, J.A. Investigation of possible allergy to local anesthetic drugs: correlation of intradermal with intramuscular injections. Anesthesiology Review **3:**13-16, 1976.

6. Axelrod, J. Metabolism of epinephrine and other sympathomimetic amines. Physiological Reviews **39:**751-776, 1959.

7. Berquist, H.C. The danger of mepivacaine 3% toxicity in children. Journal of the California Dental Association **3**(9):13, 1975.

8. Blair, M.R. Cardiovascular pharmacology of local anaesthetics. British Journal of Anaesthesia **47:**247-252, 1975.

9. Boakes, A.J., Laurence, D.R., Teoh, P.C., Barar, F.S.K., Benedikter, L.T., and Prichard, B.N.C. Interactions between sympathomimetic amines and antidepressant agents in man. British Medical Journal **1:**311-315, 1973.

10. Brown, G., and Ward, N.L. Prilocaine and lignocaine plus adrenaline. British Dental Journal **126:**557-562, 1969.

11. Brown, R.D. The failure of local anaesthesia in acute inflammation: some recent concepts. British Dental Journal **151:**47-51, 1981.

12. Catchlove, R.F.H. Potentiation of two different local anaesthetics by carbon dioxide. British Journal of Anaesthesia **45:**471-474, 1973.

13. Conrad, K.A., Byers, J.M., III, Finley, P.R., and Burnham, L. Lidocaine elimination: effects of metoprolol and of propranolol. Clinical Pharmacology and Therapeutics **33:**133-138, 1983.

14. Council on Dental Therapeutics of the American Dental Association. Accepted Dental Therapeutics, ed. 39. Chicago, American Dental Association, 1982.

15. Covino, B.G. Local anesthesia. New England Journal of Medicine **286:**975-983, 1972.

16. Covino, B.G., and Vassallo, H.G. Local Anesthetics—Mechanisms of Action and Clinical Use. New York, Grune & Stratton, Inc., 1976.

17. Cowan, A. Minimum dosage technique in the clinical comparison of representative modern local anesthetic agents. Journal of Dental Research **43:**1228-1249, 1964.

18. de Jong, R.H., and Heavner, J.E. Local anesthetic seizure prevention: diazepam versus pentobarbital. Anesthesiology **36:**449-457, 1972.

19. deShazo, R.D., and Nelson, H.S. An approach to the patient with a history of local anesthetic hypersensitivity: experience with 90 patients. Journal of Allergy and Clinical Immunology **63:**387-394, 1979.

20. Eldridge, D.J., and Rood, J.P. A double-blind trial of 5 per cent lignocaine solution. British Dental Journal **142:**129-130, 1977.

21. Epstein, S. Clinical study of prilocaine with varying concentrations of epinephrine. Journal of the American Dental Association **78:**85-90, 1969.

22. Feely, J., Wilkinson, G.R., McAllister, C.B., and Wood, A.J.J. Increased toxicity and reduced clearance of lidocaine by cimetidine. Annals of Internal Medicine **96:**592-594, 1982.

23. Franz, D.N., and Perry, R.S. Mechanisms for differential block among single myelinated and nonmyelinated axons by procaine. Journal of Physiology (London) **236:**193-210, 1974.

24. Galindo, A. Conclusions concerning "differential sensitivities of nerve fibers to local anesthetics" may not be justified. Anesthesiology **55:**482-483, 1981.

25. Gissen, A.J., Covino, B.G., and Gregus, J. Differential sensitivities of mammalian nerve fibers to local anesthetic agents. Anesthesiology **55:**467-474, 1980.

26. Gissen, A.J., Covino, B.G., and Gregus, J. Differential sensitivity of fast and slow fibers in mammalian nerve. II. Margin of safety for nerve transmission. Anesthesia and Analgesia **61:**561-569, 1982.

27. Grenadier, E., Alpan, G., Keidar, S., and Palant, A. Respiratory and cardiac arrest after the administration of lidocaine into the central nervous system. European Heart Journal **2:**235-237, 1981.

28. Hille, B. Local anesthetics: hydrophilic and hydrophobic pathways for the drug-receptor reaction. Journal of General Physiology **69:**497-515, 1977.

29. Horrobin, D.F., Durand, L.G., and Manku, M.S. Prostaglandin E1 modifies nerve conduction and interferes with local anesthetic action. Prostaglandins **14:**103-108, 1977.

30. Huang, L.-Y.M., and Ehrenstein, G. Local anesthetics QX 572 and benzocaine act at separate sites on the batrachotoxin-activated sodium channel. Journal of General Physiology **77:**137-153, 1981.

31. Jastak, J.T., and Yagiela, J.A. Vasoconstrictors and local anesthesia: a review and rationale for use. Journal of the American Dental Association **107:**623-630, 1983.

32. Kozody, R., Ready, L.B., Barsa, J.E., and Murphy, T.M. Dose requirement of local anaesthetic to produce grand mal seizure during stellate ganglion block. Canadian Anaesthetists' Society Journal **29:**489-491, 1982.

33. Kraynack, B.J., and Gintautas, J. Reversal of procaine conduction blockade by adenine nucleotides *in vivo* and *in vitro*. Acta Anaesthesiologica Scandinavica **26:**334-336, 1982.

34. Laskin, J.L., Wallace, W.R., and de Leo, B. Use of bupivacaine hydrochloride in oral surgery—a clinical study. Journal of Oral Surgery **35:**25-29, 1977.

35. Lund, P.C., Cwik, J.C., and Gannon, R.T. Extradural anaesthesia: choice of local anaesthetic agents. British Journal of Anaesthesia **47:**313-321, 1975.

36. Marquis, J.K., and Deschenes, R.J. A reevaluation of calcium-local anesthetic antagonism. Experimental Neurology **76:**547-552, 1982.

37. Martin, R., Lamarche, Y., and Tétreault, L. Effects of carbon dioxide and epinephrine on serum levels of lidocaine after epidural anaesthesia. Canadian Anaesthetists' Society Journal **28:**224-227, 1981.

38. Mumford, J.M. and Geddes, I.C. Trial of Carbocaine in conservative dentistry. British Dental Journal **110:**92-94, 1961.

39. Munson, E.S., and Wagman, I.H. Diazepam treatment of local anesthetic-induced seizures. Anesthesiology **37:**523-528, 1972.

40. Narahashi, T., Frazier, D.T., and Takeno, K. Effects of calcium on the local anesthetic suppression of ionic conductances in squid axon membranes. Journal of Pharmacology and Experimental Therapeutics **197:**426-438, 1976.

41. Newcomb, G.M. Contraindications to the use of catecholamine vasoconstrictors in dental local analgesics. New Zealand Dental Journal **69:**25-30, 1973.

42. Persson, G. General side effects of local dental anaesthesia. Acta Odontologica Scandinavica Supplement **53:**1-140, 1969.

43. Pricco, D.F. An evaluation of bupivacaine for regional nerve block in oral surgery. Journal of Oral Surgery **35:**126-129, 1977.

44. Scurlock, J.E., Meymaris, E., and Gregus, J. The clinical character of local anesthetics: a function of frequency-dependent conduction block. Acta Anaesthesiologica Scandinavica **22:**601-608, 1978.

45. Seeman, P., Chen, S.S., Chau-wong, M., and Staiman, A. Calcium reversal of nerve blockade by alcohols, anesthetics, tranquilizers, and barbiturates. Canadian Journal of Physiology and Pharmacology **52:**526-534, 1974.

46. Seldin, H.M. Survey of anesthetic fatalities in oral surgery and a review of the etiological factors in anesthetic deaths. Journal of the American Dental Society of Anesthesiology **5**(2):5-12, 1958.

47. Seldin, H.M., and Recant, B.S. The safety of anesthesia in the dental office. Journal of Oral Surgery **13:**199-208, 1955.

48. Smudski, J.W., Sprecher, R.L., and Elliott, H.W. Convulsive interactions of promethazine, meperidine, and lidocaine. Archives of Oral Biology **9:**595-600, 1964.

49. Special Committee of the New York Heart Association, Inc. Use of epinephrine in connection with procaine in dental procedures. Journal of the American Dental Association **50:**108, 1955.

50. Strichartz, G. Molecular mechanisms of nerve block by local anesthetics. Anesthesiology **45:**421-441, 1976.

51. Strong, J.M., Parker, M., and Atkinson, A.J. Identification of glycinexylidide in patients treated with intravenous lidocaine. Clinical Pharmacology and Therapeutics **14:**67-72, 1973.

52. Takman, B.H. The chemistry of local anaesthetic agents: classification of blocking agents. British Journal of Anaesthesia **47:**183-190, 1975.

53. Volpi, M., Sha'afi, R.I., Epstein, P.M., Adrenyak, D.M., and Feinstein, M.B. Local anesthetics, mepacrine, and propranolol are antagonists of calmodulin. Proceedings of the National Academy of Sciences **78:**795-799, 1981.

54. Wingard, D.W., and Bobko, S. Failure of lidocaine to trigger porcine malignant hyperthermia. Anesthesia and Analgesia **58:**99-103, 1979.

55. Yagiela, J.A., and Belle, K.D. Local anesthetic toxicity: comparison of intravenous and intra-arterial routes. Journal of Dental Research **58**(A):209, 1979.

56. Yagiela, J.A., Benoit, P.W., Buoncristiani, R.D., Peters, M.P., and Fort, N.F. Comparison of myotoxic effects of lidocaine with epinephrine in rats and humans. Anesthesia and Analgesia **60:**471-480, 1981.

57. Yagiela, J.A., and Madsen, W.C. Mechanism of enhancement of lidocaine toxicity by epinephrine. Journal of Dental Research **61:**275, 1982.

GENERAL REFERENCES

Covino, B.G., and Vassallo, H.G. Local Anesthetics—Mechanisms of Action and Clinical Use. New York, Grune & Stratton, Inc., 1976.

de Jong, R.H. Local Anesthetics, ed. 2. Springfield, Ill., Charles C Thomas, Publisher, 1977.

Cousins M.J., and Bridenbaugh, P.O., eds. Neural Blockade in Clinical Anesthesia and Management of Pain. Philadelphia, J.B. Lippincott Co., 1980.

18 Principles of general anesthesia

Enid A. Neidle
Donald C. Kroeger
John A. Yagiela

It is especially fitting that this chapter on general anesthesia open by recognizing that the pioneering use of anesthetics is credited to two dentists, Horace Wells and his pupil and partner, William T.G. Morton, who practiced dentistry in New England in the early 1800s. Their work was preceded by the contributions of many others and came at a time when others were carrying out experiments that would lead them to compete for recognition as the discoverers of anesthesia. In fact, the competition over who should be credited with the discovery became so intense that in the 1840s a Congressional committee was established to examine the evidence. Despite political intrigue, the committee decided that Morton deserved credit for the discovery of general anesthesia and voted to grant him a handsome monetary award. Politics intervened again, however, and he never received the money.[4]

The history of anesthesia is no doubt as old as humankind itself, for surely since the dawn of time people have sought ways to alleviate pain. Records spanning thousands of years make it clear that they have had recourse to prayer, magic, the intervention of witch doctors and medicine men, techniques such as compression of nerves and blood vessels, and various plant products such as opium, mandragora, and cocaine. It was not until the eighteenth and early nineteenth centuries, however, that modern anesthesiology had its beginnings. The development of physics and chemistry led to the discovery of elements and simple molecules, including a number of gases. Joseph Priestley, an English scientist, is credited with the discovery of carbon dioxide, oxygen, and, in 1772, nitrous oxide. Although he thought oxygen might have some med-

ical use, Priestley was unaware of the anesthetic properties of nitrous oxide. In 1795, Humphry Davy, a 17-year-old surgeon's assistant in England who later became a distinguished scientist himself, began experiments with nitrous oxide. He inhaled the gas and used it on one occasion to relieve the pain of his erupting third molar (although at this time nitrous oxide was still considered to be extremely poisonous). He noted in his published studies of nitrous oxide the giddiness, pleasurable sensations, relaxation of muscles, and diminution of pain that were produced by inhalation of the gas. In 1799, Davy constructed the first anesthesia machine for the storage and inhalation of nitrous oxide.

The development of anesthesia was carried further by Michael Faraday, Davy's student, who in 1818 noted the anesthetic properties of diethyl ether (then known as "sweet vitriol"), and by Henry Hills Hickman, an English surgeon who carried out painless surgery on laboratory animals using carbon dioxide gas as the anesthetic. In 1824, Hickman published a pamphlet, *A Letter on Suspended Animation,* in which he suggested that patients could be made unconscious before surgery.

In the United States in the early 1800s, there was both scientific and popular interest in ether and nitrous oxide. Itinerant entertainers who called themselves professors went about delivering lectures on these gases and demonstrating their effects. One of the earliest of these demonstrations was conducted in 1824 by Joseph Dorfeuille, a museum director from Cincinnati, who gave nitrous oxide to a dozen spectators. "Laughing gas" parties and "ether frolics" became common among medical students, and because of his experiences at such an ether party, one medical student undertook to remove the tooth of a young woman while he administered ether from a towel. This use of ether in 1842 is the first on record.

Crawford W. Long, a Georgia physician who had been trained at the University of Pennsylvania Medical School, had attended ether frolics while a student, and, in 1842, he used ether when he removed two small tumors from the neck of a friend. The credit for the first use of ether in a nondental procedure belongs to Dr. Long. Because he wanted to include observations of the effects of ether in major surgical procedures, he did not publish reports of his pioneering use of ether until 1849, 3 years after the accounts of Morton's use of ether had appeared. A letter from Long, written in 1844, suggests that he was visited by a dentist and a surgeon from Boston, that the dentist was Morton or Wells, and that it was from Long that they learned the technique of administering ether during surgery.

In 1844 Horace Wells attended a demonstration in Hartford, Connecticut, of the effects of "laughing gas," and the subject who volunteered to take the gas injured himself badly. Wells noticed that he was unaware of his injury and apparently suffered no pain until the effects of the gas wore off. The next day Wells persuaded a prominent Hartford dentist to remove one of his own teeth while under nitrous oxide anesthesia, and Wells claimed that he felt no more than a pinprick. Wells then obtained permission to demonstrate his technique before a class at the Harvard Medical School and administered nitrous oxide to a young boy, who proceeded to scream loudly while his tooth was being removed; the boy later said he had felt no pain. Discouraged by the apparent failure of his demonstration and by the hostile reception that followed, Wells retired to his own practice and continued to use nitrous oxide through 1845, at which time its use was abandoned until 1863. Wells eventually became insane and committed suicide.

A former student and partner of Wells, William T.G. Morton of Boston, had begun to use ether topically for its local numbing effect on his denture patients. With the help of his chemistry professor at Harvard, Charles T. Jackson, Morton refined his technique and successfully administered anesthesia to a patient for the extraction of a molar tooth. Convinced of the importance of his discovery, he obtained an invitation to demonstrate his technique

for Dr. John C. Warren, a surgeon at the Massachusetts General Hospital. There, on October 16, 1846, Morton prepared a young patient for the surgical removal of a large mandibular tumor. To Morton is credited the discovery of anesthesia and the custom of saying, "Doctor, your patient is now ready."

Morton was anxious to patent the substance he called "Letheon," but several physicians from the Massachusetts General Hospital thought it unsuitable to patent a medical discovery and indicated that they would not continue to use it if its chemical nature remained a secret. Morton then offered to make known the nature of the substance and to serve as an anesthetist at various hospitals. He abandoned his medical studies and his dental practice and became the first professional anesthetist. In 1846, Oliver Wendell Holmes addressed a letter to Morton suggesting that the term *anesthesia* be given to the state produced by ether and that the agent itself be called an *anesthetic*.

Following Morton's demonstration in Boston, the use of anesthesia spread rapidly in spite of opposition from various groups, many of which still believed that there was something spiritually ennobling about pain, particularly the pain of childbirth. In 1847, Sir James Young Simpson first used ether in his obstetrical practice and in the same year successfully delivered a child using chloroform. Later, when Queen Victoria was delivered of her seventh child while under chloroform anesthesia, most ecclesiastic opposition was stilled.

No new agents were added until the 1920s and 1930s when ethylene, cyclopropane, and divinyl ether were introduced. Since the early 1950s a new series of halogenated agents containing fluorine have been introduced clinically and have largely replaced other inhalation agents except nitrous oxide.

Intravenous agents, mainly the thiobarbiturates (e.g., thiopental), became popular in the late 1930s. Other ultra-short-acting barbiturates were added to the list and were supplemented in the late 1960s by ketamine and the neuroleptanalgesic droperidol-fentanyl.

It is interesting to note that the use of nitrous oxide by dentists has exhibited a cyclical pattern of popularity every 25 to 30 years since Wells first used it. Currently, it is in the peak of its fifth cycle. With the development of new technologies and practices perhaps its use will stabilize.

GOALS OF ANESTHESIA

The primary goals of general anesthesia are to preserve the life of the patient, to provide the operator with an adequate surgical field, and to obtund pain. Ideally, a general anesthetic should (1) provide a smooth and rapid induction, (2) produce a state of unconsciousness or unresponsiveness, (3) produce a state of amnesia, (4) block a number of reflexes that might lead to bronchospasm, salivation, arrhythmias, and the like, (5) produce skeletal muscle relaxation, but preferably not of the respiratory muscles, through the blockade of various efferent impulses, (6) block the conscious perception of sensory impulses so that there is adequate analgesia to perform the procedure, and (7) provide a smooth, rapid, and uneventful emergence and recovery with no long-lasting adverse effects.

A "complete" anesthetic is one that produces unconsciousness, analgesia, and muscle relaxation by itself without undue risk to the patient. An example of such a complete anesthetic is diethyl ether (or simply ether). Although there are other complete anesthetics, the tendency in modern anesthesiology is to use a combination of drugs in order to take advantage of the best properties of each and to minimize unwanted side effects. Among the agents that are frequently used preoperatively are the antimuscarinic drugs to minimize salivation, laryngospasm, and reflex bradycardia and various analgesics and CNS depressants to provide preoperative sedation and amnesia. Drugs that are employed during the administration of general anesthesia in addition to the "primary" anesthetic include nitrous oxide, which lessens the total required dose of anesthetic and increases analgesia, drugs that paralyze skeletal muscle, and adrenergic drugs, which help maintain cardiovascular function.

The goals of anesthesia for general surgery also apply to dental surgery, but there are some important differences. Most dental patients are outpatients; in many dental procedures, particularly those not involving oral surgery, it is neither necessary nor desirable to render the patient unconscious. Usually the procedures are not as traumatic as those of general surgery. As is mentioned in Chapter 44, although general anesthesia is occasionally used in the hospital setting for dental patients, techniques have been developed for producing a state of *conscious sedation,* in which there is analgesia and relief from anxiety but no loss of consciousness.

TERMS USED IN ANESTHESIOLOGY

Consciousness is the mental state in which the person is capable of a rational response to commands and has all protective reflexes intact, including the ability to maintain a patent airway.

Sedation describes a state of partial or complete awareness of the environment but with a significant reduction of anxiety and restlessness.

Analgesia refers to a reduced perception of and responsiveness to noxious stimuli (i.e., stimuli that are described as painful) but without amnesia or loss of consciousness. Other modes of sensory perception remain intact (e.g., vision and hearing).

Amnesia refers to a loss of memory of the surgical experience, although the patient may be aware of the environment during surgery.

Induction is that phase of anesthesia beginning with the administration of anesthetic and continuing until the desired level of patient unresponsiveness is reached.

Unconsciousness is the state in which the patient is no longer aware of the environment and does not respond to familiar stimuli such as calling the patient's name.

Unresponsiveness refers to a loss of reaction to sensory stimuli, both noxious and nonnoxious.

Muscle relaxation is a reduction or loss of CNS regulation of skeletal muscle tone and reflexes which produces a state of flaccid paralysis and unresponsiveness of muscle to stretching and surgical cutting.

Surgical anesthesia is the state of unresponsiveness, analgesia, and muscle relaxation that allows the goals of surgery to be accomplished.

Maintenance is the process of keeping a patient in surgical anesthesia.

Recovery is the phase of anesthesia commencing when surgery is complete and the delivery of the anesthetic is terminated and ending when the anesthetic has been eliminated from the body.

Emergence delimits the stage of recovery during which the patient is regaining consciousness.

Minimum alveolar concentration (MAC) is used for quantifying the potency of anesthetic agents. MAC, as defined by Eger and colleagues,[14] is the alveolar concentration of anesthetic at which 50% of patients fail to respond to a standard surgical stimulus.

THEORIES OF ANESTHETIC ACTION

Since the introduction of general anesthesia, efforts have been directed toward discovering the mechanism of action of these agents. Our fragmentary knowledge of the structure of membranes, of neurologic circuits and neurotransmitters, and of behavioral states of clinical anesthesia such as consciousness, sleep, and pain makes the elucidation of the mechanism extremely difficult. Theories have been advanced for each of the above mentioned functions, however, and are summarized in the following sections.

Membrane theories

Membrane theories attempt to describe the action of the extremely diverse chemicals known to be general anesthetics on the basis of altering the molecular structure of the membrane. It is generally agreed that there are no specific receptors for anesthetics (and thus no direct antagonists) as there are for neurotransmitters. Anesthetic agents are rather indiscriminate in affecting the biophysical properties of membranes. The earliest theory, independently proposed by Meyer (1899)[25] and Overton (1901),[33] emphasized the correspondence between the lipid solubility of an agent and its anesthetic potency. The Meyer-Overton theory in essence states that anesthesia commences when any chemical substance has attained a certain molar concentration in the hydrophobic phase of the cell membrane. It is generally believed that the Meyer-Overton theory, though not actually explaining anesthesia, does account for the affinity of these agents for neural structures with their high concentration of lipid.

Mullins (1954),[31] in his critical volume fraction hypothesis, modified the original theory to include consideration of the volume of the membrane occupied by the anesthetic agent. It was reasoned that large molecules would have greater effects on the membrane than would smaller molecules. Indeed, the correlation between anesthetic potency and a function of both lipid solubility and molecular size is somewhat better than the correlation between anesthetic potency and lipid solubility alone.[6] A number of investigators have elaborated on Mullins' work in regard to the consequences of anesthetic uptake by the nerve membrane. Evidence was obtained that the absorption of anesthetic molecules causes expansion and disorder (fluidization) of the functional components embedded in the membrane matrix. Variations of Mullins' hypothesis involve the nature of the constituents most directly affected by the anesthetic, that is, lipids,[27,42] proteins (including lipoproteins),[35,48] or water.[28,34] Theories proposing a direct effect on water have the least support.

Several current theories suggest that anesthetics fluidize lipids in critical regions of the nerve membrane, leading to a disruption of the normal relationship between the fluid and solid phases of the lipid bilayer. It is postulated that as a result of this alteration in membrane structure, the nerve membrane is unable to facilitate the changes in protein configuration that are required for such essential steps in the transmission of nerve impulses as ion gating, synaptic transmitter release, and binding of the transmitter to the receptor.[42] These critical volume theories are supported by the fact that hyperbaric pressures and certain drugs antagonize anesthesia, presumably by reestablishing order and reversing membrane expansion.[26,36] Excessive compression or drug-induced ordering of the membrane matrix can lead to convulsions. It is interesting to note that closely related compounds (e.g., fluorinated ether congeners or stereoisomers of barbiturates) may produce opposing effects on membrane order.[11]

Recent studies have cast some doubt on membrane expansion as a cause of anesthesia. Direct measurements of expansion of lipid bilayers and red cell membranes in response to anesthetic concentrations of ethanol and halothane yield values that are effectively insignificant.[16] Moreover, the fact that congeners and even isomers of certain anesthetics have similar lipophilic properties but are nonanesthetic or excitatory in effect suggests that nonspecific absorption by membrane constituents is not relevant to general anesthesia. These and other lines of evidence point to functional membrane proteins (e.g., receptors or ion channels) with hydrophobic sites for drug association as the effectors of anesthetic action.[24]

Although most investigations have focused on the plasma membrane, it is equally possible that the membranes of mitochondria and synaptic vesicles are targets of anesthetic drugs. General anesthetics impair the ability of synaptosomes to sequester and to retain catecholamine neurotransmitters and of mitochondria to produce ATP and to take up calcium.[3,6] The latter effect has been used to explain the finding that anesthetics hyperpolarize cells in direct relation to their anesthetic potency.[32]

Neurophysiologic theories

Although membrane theories may provide a fundamental explanation of the pharmacodynamic actions of general anesthetics, they are not useful in describing the selective changes in consciousness, pain perception, and muscle relaxation observed clinically. Therefore, much research has been directed toward determining the neurologic sites and pathways that are affected by the various anesthetics. Some fundamental observations have established that fine diverging neural networks with terminals of a single axon distributed to a large number of polysynaptic elements, particularly those involving presynaptic inhibition,[37] have a low safety factor and are most sensitive to the actions of anesthetics.[2] Areas in the central nervous system having these features include the dorsal lamina of the spinal cord (substantia gelatinosa), the reticular system (including the midbrain reticular formation), and midline sensory relay nuclei of the thalamus.

Beginning with the studies of French and colleagues,[17] much attention has been directed toward the role of the mesencephalic reticular activating formation. This system, which receives a variety of nonspecific sensory inputs, is a major center responsible for initiating and maintaining consciousness and alertness of higher brain centers. As the activity of the system is depressed, the ascending influences on the limbic system and cortical structures are reduced until unconsciousness occurs. It is not surprising then that the reticular formation is one of the important sites to be affected by anesthesia, although this complex of neurons may respond quite differently to the various anesthetics.[10,12,21] Whereas barbiturates, ether, and halothane cause depression of spontaneous electrical activity, enflurane and cyclopropane may briefly enhance activity, and ketamine alters the pattern of firing.[30] All agents appear to block neuronal responses to sensory input.

The ascending influences from the mesencephalic reticular formation have marked effects on the intralaminar nuclei of the thalamus,[22,29] the hippocampus, and various circuits in the cerebral cortex. One of the earliest effects of anesthesia is the appearance of excitatory manifestations in the electroencephalogram. This increased activity of cortical neurons appears to result from a release of tonic inhibition arising from lower brain centers.

Although the reticular formation first attracted attention as the site of action of anesthetics, increasing interest is being directed to the laminar structures of the dorsal horns of the spinal cord (substantia gelatinosa).[23,40] It has been shown that the *analgesic* action of nitrous oxide involves the substantia gelatinosa, often referred to as the gateway for nociceptive impulses into the central nervous system.[13] The similarity of analgesia produced by opioids, nitrous oxide, cyclopropane, and ketamine suggests that a common mode of action may

be responsible.[5,20] Cross-tolerance to the analgesic effect of morphine and nitrous oxide, as well as the ability to block nitrous oxide analgesia with the opioid antagonist naloxone, gives further support to the theory that nitrous oxide may release endogenous morphine-like substances.[49] That the endogenous opioid system cannot be invoked as a mechanism of action generally, however, is demonstrated by the failure of naloxone to block the analgesic action of several anesthetics and the anesthetic action of nitrous oxide (as well as other drugs).[38,39]

Behavioral theories

Depressant-anesthesia theory. In 1920, Guedel[18] divided the course of ether anesthesia into a sequence of four stages and further subdivided the third, or surgical, stage into four planes (Figure 18-1). Each of these stages and planes represented a progressive and deepening depression of the central nervous system. In modern anesthesiology these observations are no longer used in their entirety because the anesthetic signs are obscured by the presence of other drugs used before and during the anesthetic period and because ether is seldom employed. Nevertheless, Guedel's scheme is useful in describing the effects of many of the depressant anesthetics used today. The classic stages of anesthesia, as described by Guedel, are stage I/analgesia, stage II/delirium, stage III/surgical anesthesia (planes 1, 2, 3, and 4), and stage IV/medullary paralysis.

Stage I starts with the beginning of anesthetic administration and ends with the loss of consciousness. The patient is unresponsive to mild pain-provoking stimuli and is able to respond to verbal commands. This stage is followed by delirium in stage II, during which violent thrashing and vomiting can occur. It is desirable to traverse this stage rapidly; for this reason, thiopental is often given intravenously before the administration of the general anesthetic agent. Stage III has been subdivided, as indicated above, into four planes in order of increasing depth of anesthesia, using a variety of indexes, including the diameter of the pupil, loss of ocular, oropharyngeal, and other reflexes, muscle relaxation, depth and regularity of respiration, and separation of the thoracic and abdominal (diaphragmatic) phases of respiration. Stage IV begins with the disappearance of the purely diaphragmatic respiration of stage III, plane 4 and ends with complete respiratory and circulatory col-

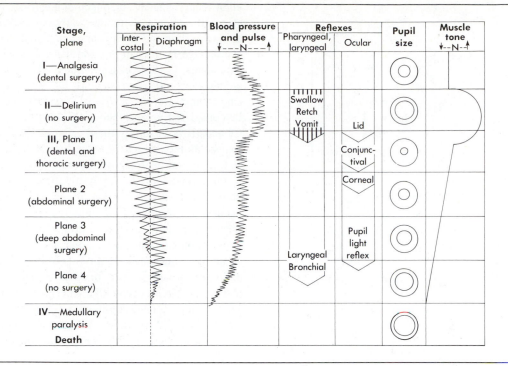

Figure 18-1. Guedel's scheme of progressive CNS depression produced by the anesthetic ether. Changes in physiologic functions are shown for the different stages and planes of Guedel's classification. Examples of surgery that can be performed at these anesthetic levels are given in parentheses.

lapse, culminating in death if the anesthetic is not discontinued and the patient given support for the cardiopulmonary systems.

The recovery from general anesthesia is the reverse of the process of induction. The patient progressively regains reflexes, and a short period of excitement similar to that previously encountered during stage II may occur, followed by emergence to consciousness with residual analgesia.

Whereas the stages of anesthesia can be useful in a descriptive sense, the further subdivision of the surgical stage into planes is not always as useful. This is primarily true because many of the more widely used anesthetics bring the patient to stage III very rapidly, making it difficult to judge the subtle differences between the planes of anesthesia, and because so many drugs are used as adjuncts to anesthesia and tend to obscure some of the signs described by Guedel. For instance, muscular relaxation can hardly be used to gauge the depth of anesthesia if a neuromuscular blocking agent has been administered, nor can the level of blood pressure be useful if an adrenergic amine has been given to prevent hypotension. Nevertheless, indexes of

autonomic function, such as progressive lowering of blood pressure and alterations in heart rate, can be valuable guides to the patient's status during anesthesia in the absence of medications that specifically obscure these functions.

In modern anesthesiology, the depth of anesthesia is to some extent determined by the needs of surgery. Since there is a diversity of purposes in surgery, along with a variety of types of anesthetic agents, an assessment of the desirable depth of anesthesia is made for each type of procedure. For example, if the procedure necessitates a bloodless field, as in plastic surgery, halothane may be used for its hypotensive properties. The endpoint of anesthesia becomes the production of hypotension, and other indexes of depth, such as respiratory movements, have little direct bearing on the choice of anesthetic depth for surgical procedures.

The effects of anesthetic agents are dependent on the degree of sensory input as well as on the dose of the anesthetic used. After surgical stimulation, the respiratory and cardiovascular systems tend to be less depressed, and the patient can appear

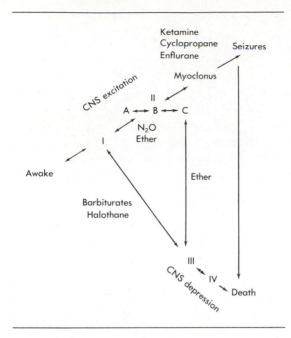

Figure 18-2. Scheme of reversible progression of states induced by various anesthetic agents. Stages I, II (A, B, C), myoclonus, and seizures indicate CNS excitation. Stages I, II, III, and IV refer to terminology used by Guedel. Some drugs that induce the various stages of CNS excitation and depression are indicated.

to be in a lighter level of anesthesia than the dose would indicate.

Cataleptic-anesthesia theory. In general, the older anesthetic agents follow Guedel's scheme of the stages of ether anesthesia. Certain discrepancies of these agents as well as experience with several newer drugs (e.g., ketamine and the neuroleptanalgesics) have led to the formulation of a multidimensional scheme that includes the concept of cataleptic anesthesia.[45] This scheme is based on the demonstration that anesthetics may produce surgical anesthesia by any of several different pathways (Figure 18-2). Some drugs (e.g., barbiturates, halothane) move the patient directly from the conscious state, or stage I, to stage III. Other anesthetics (e.g., ether) traverse stage II, moving directly to stage III. Stage II is characterized by hallucinatory (A, B) and then cataleptoid (C) behavior. At this time the subject is relatively unresponsive to stimuli.

The scheme of CNS excitation and depression suggests a progression of changes to different levels of excitability or depression, with some anesthetics sharing initial properties with drugs of opposite action. For example, both ether and ketamine can elicit stage II anesthesia, but ether goes on to induce stage III, whereas ketamine can proceed to generalized seizures.[46] It appears that a hallucinatory state (stage II, B) can precede the myoclonus-seizure states, CNS depression (stage III), or the cataleptic anesthetic state (stage II, C). Any agent that causes amnesia and a loss of responsiveness can be considered an anesthetic[47]; therefore, stages II, C, and III both satisfy these criteria. With agents like ketamine, which produce hyperexcited CNS states, central neurons become activated, and their responsiveness to stimuli is facilitated. The psychomotor unresponsiveness of surgical anesthesia occurs as a result of functional disorganization of the activated neurons' interaction with one another. While motor output may be enhanced, as demonstrated by muscular rigidity, coordinated motor activity is gone, resulting in an unresponsive surgical patient. With agents like ether, the diminished sensory input, integration, and motor output resulting from depression of neurons supply the conditions necessary for the production of anesthesia.

UPTAKE AND DISTRIBUTION OF ANESTHETIC GASES

The depth of anesthesia produced by the inhalation anesthetics depends on the partial pressure (or tension) of the anesthetic agents in the brain. The speed of induction and of recovery depends on the rate of change of partial pressure of the gas in the brain. This means that during induction the gas must move from the anesthetic apparatus to the pulmonary alveoli, from the alveoli to the blood, and from the blood to the brain. During the period of emergence, the anesthetic gas will move in the opposite direction but again will cross the same interfaces. The principal force governing this movement of anesthetic gas is the diffusion or concentration gradient, and the behavior of the gases as they move from one compartment to another across biologic interfaces is defined by two gas laws. Dalton's law deals with the partial pressure of gases and states that in a mixture the partial pressure of each component gas is directly related to its concentration in the mixture. Henry's law describes the solubility of gases in liquids and states that the quantity that will dissolve in a liquid is proportional to the partial pressure of that gas in contact with the liquid, or the partial pressure of the gas in the gas phase.

The Ostwald partition coefficient is an expression of the relative solubility of a substance in two

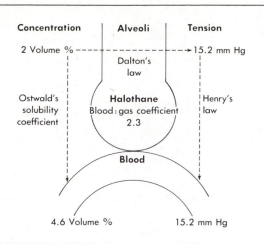

Figure 18-3. Effect of the blood/gas coefficient and the tension (partial pressure) exerted by halothane, 2 vol %, in the inspired air. Across the top of the diagram is the statement of Dalton's law that 2 vol % of halothane will exert 15.2 mm Hg pressure (0.02 × 760 mm Hg = 15.2 mm Hg) at 1 atmosphere pressure. Down the left-hand side, Ostwald's solubility coefficient states that 4.6 vol % of halothane will be dissolved in blood (2 vol % × 2.3 = 4.6). Down the right-hand side, Henry's law states that at equilibrium, the tension (partial pressure) of the gas in the gaseous phase (inspired air) will be equal to the tension of the gas in the liquid phase.

immiscible phases. When applied to anesthetic gases, it compares the amount of gas present in the first phase when one part is dissolved in the second phase. Thus, the blood/gas coefficient of 2.3 for halothane indicates that 2.3 parts of halothane are dissolved in blood for every part contained in an equal volume of alveolar air. These relationships are shown schematically in Figure 18-3.

As was mentioned earlier, during induction the various compartments of the body are brought into equilibrium with respect to the anesthetic gas. When equilibrium is reached, the tensions of the anesthetic gas in the inspired air, alveolar air, arterial blood, body tissues, and mixed venous blood are equal. The speed with which this equilibrium is achieved is affected by a number of factors, each of which will be considered in turn.

Concentration in inspired air

The greater the concentration of the anesthetic gas in inspired air, the more rapid will be the induction. This inspired tension normally is not held constant during induction. With irritating agents like ether, the tension is raised slowly. With halothane, which is nonirritating, or in situations in

which it is desired to accelerate the speed of induction, the concentration at the outset may be 2 to 3 times what it will be at the maintenance phase of anesthetic administration.

Alveolar concentration

The anesthetic tension in alveolar air is influenced by the tension in inspired air, the rate and depth of respiration (ventilation), the solubility of the anesthetic in the blood, cardiac output, pulmonary capillary flow, and the rate of tissue uptake. The alveolar tension is of particular importance because it is readily measured and, in most circumstances, is most representative of the brain concentration (which cannot be measured).

Ventilation rate and depth

The greater the ventilation of the lungs, the more anesthetic is delivered to the alveoli and thence to the brain, resulting in a more rapid induction. This factor is most significant during the initial phase of induction when uptake by the blood is very rapid. It is of less importance with insoluble agents like nitrous oxide and cyclopropane, which achieve high blood tensions rapidly, than it is with the more soluble drugs like ether and halothane, which equilibrate with the blood more slowly.

Concentration and second gas effects

The concentration effect occurs with relatively nonpotent anesthetics, such as nitrous oxide, that are administered in high concentrations (e.g., 75%) during induction of general anesthesia. Initially, nitrous oxide is taken up rapidly by the pulmonary circulation. This uptake would create a vacuum in the lungs were it not for the fact that fresh gas flows into the alveoli to replace the absorbed gas. The net result is that alveolar ventilation is effectively increased, the alveolar concentration rises more rapidly than would otherwise be the case, and general anesthesia is hastened.

With potent drugs given in lower concentrations (e.g., 2% to 5%) the concentration effect is negligible. However, if the anesthetic is administered along with nitrous oxide, then it too will be delivered to the alveoli in increased amounts as gas rushes inward to replace the nitrous oxide absorbed by pulmonary blood. This phenomenon is called the second gas effect.

Solubility in blood

Blood solubility is a major factor in the rate of induction of anesthesia. Solubility is generally ex-

Table 18-1. Some properties of inhalation anesthetics

Anesthetic	Blood/gas coefficient*	Brain/blood coefficient	Fat/blood coefficient	MAC vol %†
Nitrous oxide	0.47	1.1	3	110
Cyclopropane	0.46	1.5	21	9.2
Isoflurane	1.4	2.6	45	1.15
Enflurane	1.8	1.5	55	1.68
Halothane	2.3	2.6	60	0.77
Ether	12.1	1.0	5	1.92
Methoxyflurane	13.0	1.8	49	0.16

*All coefficients are taken at 37 C.

†MAC—minimum alveolar concentration is defined as that alveolar concentration of a gas necessary to prevent a skeletal muscle response to a standard surgical stimulus in 50% of patients.

pressed as the blood/gas partition coefficient, which is the ratio of the concentration of the anesthetic gas in arterial blood to that in the alveolar air at 37 C and at a time when the partial pressures in each compartment are the same. The anesthetic gases are generally divided into three groups: agents of low solubility in blood, those of intermediate solubility, and those of high solubility. This classification and the blood/gas coefficients for the respective anesthetics are shown in Table 18-1. If an agent is poorly soluble in blood, as is true of nitrous oxide and cyclopropane, only a small percentage of it will be removed from the alveolar air before an equilibrium between arterial blood and alveolar air will be reached. Thus, the attainment of anesthetic concentrations in the tissues will be rapid and the induction phase short. With agents of very high blood solubility, such as ether. The rate of change of alveolar tension for will be removed from the alveolar air, and relatively large amounts will have to be delivered from the inspired air. Therefore, the alveolar tension will rise slowly and induction will be similarly slow. Agents of intermediate solubility obviously will have an induction time somewhat slower than that of nitrous oxide and somewhat faster than that of ether. The rate of change of alveolar tension for an anesthetic gas from each of these groups, during both induction and emergence, is shown in Figure 18-4.

Inasmuch as recovery or emergence is a reversal of the process of induction, those anesthetics that are insoluble in blood will leave the blood very rapidly after the anesthetic gas is removed from the inspired air, and recovery will be very rapid. Conversely, recovery is slow with ether. High solubility is not completely disadvantageous, how-

ever, because small fluctuations in the concentration in the inspired air during maintenance will have little effect on the depth of anesthesia.

Cardiac output and blood flow

Cardiac output influences anesthetic uptake in opposite ways. On the one hand, if the cardiac output is very large, it will remove large quantities of gas from the alveoli and lower alveolar tension, thereby delaying the achievement of equilibrium between inspired air and arterial blood. On the other hand, a large cardiac output will deliver a greater amount of anesthetic to the tissue, thereby hastening the rate at which the tissues come to equilibrium with the arterial blood. Because the brain follows the arterial partial pressure of anesthetics closely, increasing total cardiac output generally slows the induction of general anesthesia.

The tissue uptake of an anesthetic agent is dependent on the blood flow, the arterial gas tension, and the blood/tissue coefficient, which varies according to the amount of lipid present. As shown in Table 18-1, halothane is 2.6 times as concentrated in the brain and 60 times as concentrated in fat as it is in blood. Muscle tissue has an affinity for anesthetic agents similar to that of blood, and the ratio is approximately 1:1. Lipids have a high affinity for anesthetic agents, and fatty tissues therefore act as a reservoir for anesthetic gases.

The uptake of anesthetic gases proceeds sequentially into three main compartments of the body, depending on the vascularity and lipid content of the tissue. Initially, the most active compartment is the vessel-rich group (VRG), consisting of the heart, liver, kidney, lungs, and brain. In fact, equil-

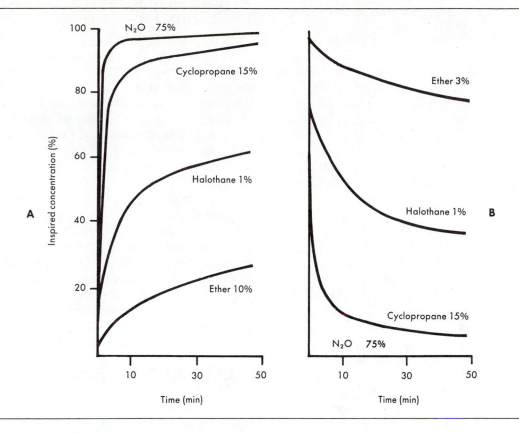

Figure 18-4. Rate of change of alveolar anesthetic tension during induction, **A,** and recovery, **B.** The *y* axis represents alveolar concentration as a percentage of inspired concentration. Note the rapid rise of alveolar tension during induction with agents of low blood solubility (nitrous oxide, cyclopropane), the slow rise of alveolar ether concentration, and the intermediate place of halothane. Recovery rates are a near mirror image of induction. (Adapted from Eger, E.I. Applications of a mathematical model of gas uptake. In Papper, E.M., and Kitz, R.J., eds. Uptake and Distribution of Anesthetic Agents. New York, McGraw-Hill Book Co., 1963.)

ibration between blood and brain is usually very rapid because the brain receives the largest share of the cardiac output and because the brain/blood coefficient is relatively low (Table 18-1). Nitrous oxide is initially absorbed into the VRG compartment at a rate of 1 to 2 L per minute for the first 10 to 15 minutes. At this time, the uptake drops to less than 0.5 L per minute over the next 1 to 1½ hours, during which time the anesthetic fills the muscle compartment. If anesthetic administration is continued beyond this time, the uptake rate drops still further (under 0.2 L/min) until the fat group of tissues is equilibrated. The time sequence of halothane uptake is very similar to that of nitrous oxide, except that nearly 2½ hours are needed to fill the muscle group.

ELIMINATION AND METABOLISM OF ANESTHETIC GASES

The same factors that determine the uptake of anesthetic gas and the rate of induction are also important during the elimination phase. This process is initiated by the removal of the gas from the inspired air mixture, so that the inspired air tension of anesthetic gas falls to zero. When this happens, the anesthetic begins to diffuse from the blood through the alveoli, and as the blood tension falls there is a fall in tissue tension. The less soluble the agent, the more completely and quickly the anesthetic will be removed from the blood and tissues and the more rapid will be the recovery. Although some anesthetics are metabolized, this process has little significance insofar as anesthetic recovery is concerned, although it does present problems of toxicity.

It was believed that inhalation anesthetics were eliminated via the lungs without any metabolic transformation. It has now been shown, however, that anesthetics (e.g., ether, halothane, and methoxyflurane) are chemically modified, some to an extensive degree.[7,41] Approximately 20% of administered halothane is metabolized in humans to trifluoroacetic acid and bromide.[41] About 50% of methoxyflurane is metabolized, resulting in plasma fluoride concentrations that can cause nephrotoxicity.[50]

CHEMICAL PROPERTIES OF INHALATION ANESTHETICS

The wide diversity of chemical substances capable of producing the anesthetic state precludes any uniform statements regarding their chemical properties. Although there are a number of drugs capable of producing general anesthesia, the volatile liquids or gases are usually preferred because the administration by inhalation permits rapid and precise control of the dose since termination of anesthesia depends on elimination of the vapor by expiration rather than by metabolism or excretion.

None of the current halogenated anesthetics nor the obsolete agents chloroform and trichloroethylene present a flammability or explosion hazard. Ether, however, is flammable and explosive. Cyclopropane, a three-carbon cyclic hydrocarbon, is a highly explosive gas. The only other gas commonly used is nitrous oxide, an inorganic compound that, although not explosive, will support combustion of other substances.

Other chemical reactions, besides fire and explosion, can occur with anesthetic agents. Chloroform in the presence of high temperature or flame will be converted to phosgene, an extremely toxic, irritating gas. Trichloroethylene is decomposed by soda lime used to absorb carbon dioxide in closed systems; the resultant product is both toxic and explosive. Ether when exposed to air (oxygen) and light forms peroxides that lower the ignition temperature for the anesthetic. Brass and aluminum are subject to corrosion when exposed to halothane and water. Finally, the volatile inhalation agents are absorbed in the rubber connections used in the administration system and are difficult to leach out of the anesthetic circuit.

PHARMACOLOGIC EFFECTS OF INHALATION ANESTHETICS
Cardiovascular system

All agents cause depression of myocardial contractility, the extent being related to the potency of the particular agent used, its concentration, and the duration of anesthesia. As a group, the halogenated anesthetics are the worst offenders in affecting contractility as well as in sensitizing the automaticity and conducting properties of the myocardium to the β-receptor stimulating properties of norepinephrine and epinephrine. Cyclopropane, which not only sensitizes the myocardium but also causes stimulation of the sympathetic nervous system, is very prone to produce arrhythmias. Cardiac rates are variably influenced, and the anesthetic effects are often masked by the preoperative administration of atropine or scopolamine, which block activity of the vagus nerve. Agents that directly excite the discharge of the sympathoadrenal axis are ether, isoflurane, nitrous oxide, and cyclopropane. Other agents may indirectly cause discharge by depressing respiration.

Respiration

The effect of most anesthetics on the respiratory centers in the brain is depression; the amount of respiratory depression is related to the amount of anesthetic used. Dissociative anesthetics may cause increased rigidity of the respiratory musculature, causing a condition called ''stone chest.'' In either case, ventilatory rates are diminished, and increased oxygen tensions or mechanical respiratory assistance may be required. Hypercarbia resulting from depressed ventilatory exchange excites the sympathoadrenal system, thereby causing a release of catecholamines.

Liver

Liver function tests indicate that almost all anesthetic agents cause some alterations. In most cases, the effects are reversible and not serious. Halothane, however, has produced a significant incidence of serious hepatic necrosis, especially if the patient has had prior anesthesia with halothane or is a carrier of hepatitis virus. There is evidence that hypoxia and reductive metabolic products play a role in hepatic toxicity.[19]

Kidney

The urine output during anesthesia is decreased by the release of antidiuretic hormone from the pituitary gland. Most general anesthetics also depress glomerular filtration by reducing renal blood flow. Fortunately, these alterations in renal function are transitory and readily reversible. The release of fluoride ion from certain halogenated anesthetics (e.g., methoxyflurane) has occasionally produced serious renal damage.

Skeletal muscle

Although most general anesthetics produce muscle relaxation by their actions on spinal cord and brainstem motor reflex centers, several agents have an additional effect on the neuromuscular junction. Ether is most prominent in this respect and can reduce the amount of a neuromuscular blocking agent required by as much as 50%. Agents with a lesser degree of action include enflurane, halothane, isoflurane, and cyclopropane. Cholinesterase inhibition by neostigmine does not antagonize this effect as it does for such nondepolarizing blocking agents as tubocurarine and pancuronium.

Smooth muscle

The smooth muscle of various organs is variably affected by anesthetic agents, but the effect is largely dependent on the depth of anesthesia. When it was in widespread use, cyclopropane was preferred for patients in shock states because of its minimal effect on vascular smooth muscle. Halothane, on the other hand, relaxes vascular smooth muscle, producing a hypotension that can be useful in producing bloodless surgical fields. Intestinal and bronchial smooth muscle are generally not adversely affected by light levels of surgical anesthesia.

ADMINISTRATION OF ANESTHETIC GASES

A variety of delivery systems have been used since the inception of anesthesia, and these range from simple techniques such as the open-drop method on a face mask or nose cone to anesthetic machines that incorporate a considerable number of technical devices. Figure 18-5 illustrates the major types of delivery systems, including the recently developed scavenger mask. It should be recognized that the requirements for dental anesthesia preclude a number of systems that are applicable to general surgery.

The systems fall into three general categories: open, semiopen or semiclosed, and closed. With the last system, in which the patient rebreathes the anesthetic mixture, the following mechanical devices are required: (1) gases, including oxygen, stored in either local tanks or a central delivery system, (2) flowmeters to measure the quantity of gases delivered, (3) vaporizers to volatilize anesthetic liquids, (4) mixing valves to regulate percentages of gases and oxygen, (5) carbon dioxide absorber system, (6) rebreathing bag or ventilators, or both, (7) assorted tubing and one-way valve systems, and (8) face mask or endotracheal tube.

Several features of the administration of anesthetic gases in modern anesthesiology should be mentioned. First, whereas several older agents (e.g., ether and cyclopropane) are highly effective agents, certain deficits have caused a marked decrease in their use and their replacement by newer agents, such as halothane, which do not share the same problems. In particular, the explosive character of cyclopropane has caused its use to be banned in most operating rooms. Second, some of the newer agents, such as enflurane and isoflurane, are extremely expensive, so closed or semiclosed systems for their administration are favored. Third, recent studies have provided evidence that operating room personnel (surgeons, anesthesiologists, nurses, etc.) and dentists who use nitrous oxide in their offices may be adversely affected by trace amounts of anesthetics in the operatory.[8,9,44] These findings have prompted the Occupational Safety and Health Administration (OSHA), in conjunction with several academic institutions, to attempt to determine the maximum allowable concentrations of anesthetic agents in the operating and recovery rooms. It should be mentioned that the potential risk of long-term, low-dose anesthetic exposure is subject to debate[15,43]; nevertheless, most authorities favor rebreathing systems in conjunction with scavenger masks and systems that remove anesthetic gases from the vicinity of the patient's mouth and nose.[1,44] Finally, because many dentists function as both anesthetist and surgeon, the nonrebreathing flow machine is most commonly used. Its simplicity in operation, however, has the major disadvantage of causing a high level of exposure of operatory personnel to anesthetic gases. The development of the scavenger mask and improved ventilation systems have helped to minimize such exposure.

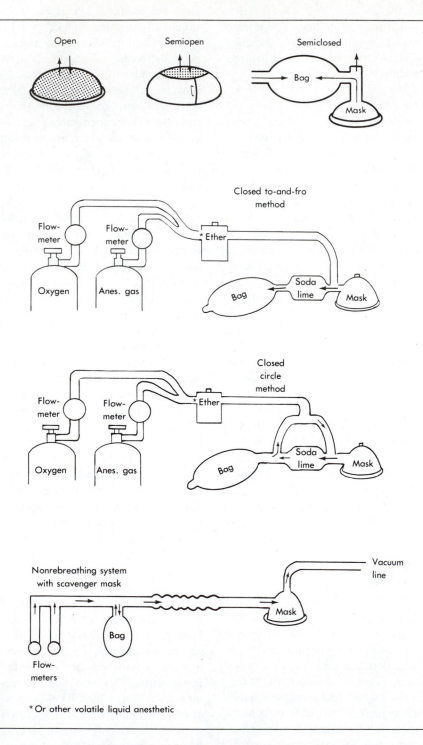

Figure 18-5. Major delivery systems for anesthesia.

CITED REFERENCES

1. Adams, D., Allen, G.D., and Scaramella, J. Modifying nitrous oxide analgesia circuits to reduce pollution in the dental operatory. Anesthesia Progress **23**:176-180, 1976.

2. Albe-Fessard, D., Beeson, J.M., and Abdelmoumene, M. Action of anesthetics on somatic evoked activities. In Yamamura, H., ed. Anesthesia and Neurophysiology. International Anesthesiology Clinics, Boston, Little, Brown & Co., 1970.

3. Bangham, A.D., and Mason, W.T. Anesthetics may act by collapsing pH gradients. Anesthesiology **53**:135-141, 1980.

4. Bankoff, G. The Conquest of Pain: The Story of Anesthesia. London, MacDonald and Co., Ltd., 1946.

5. Berkowitz, B.A., Finck, A.D., and Ngai, S.H. Nitrous oxide analgesia: reversal by naloxone and development of tolerance. Journal of Pharmacology and Experimental Therapeutics **203**:539-547, 1977.

6. Burnie, J.P. Molecular mechanisms of general anaesthesia. Anaesthesia **36**:1027-1039, 1981.

7. Cascorbi, H.F. Biotransformation of drugs used in anesthesia. Anesthesiology **39**:115-125, 1973.

8. Chenoweth, M.B. Inhalation anesthetics. Federation Proceedings **37**:2501-2503, 1978.

9. Cohen, E.N., Brown, B.W., Wu, M.L., Whitcher, C.E., Brodsky, J.B., Gift, H.C., Greenfield, W., Jones, T.W., and Driscoll, E.J. Occupational disease in dentistry and exposure to trace anesthetic gases. Journal of the American Dental Association **101**:21-31, 1980.

10. Cohen, P.J. The reticular activating system revisited. Anesthesiology **39**:1-2, 1973.

11. Cohen, S., Goldschmid, A., Shtacher, G., Srebrenik, S., and Gitter, S. The inhalation convulsants: a pharmacodynamic approach. Molecular Pharmacology **11**:379-385, 1975.

12. Darbinjan, T.M., Golovchinsky, V.B., and Plehotkina, S.I. The effects of anesthetics on reticular and cortical activity. Anesthesiology **34**:219-229, 1971.

13. de Jong, R.H., Robles, R., and Morikawa, K.-I. Actions of halothane and nitrous oxide on dorsal horn neurons ("the spinal gate"). Anesthesiology **31**:205-212, 1969.

14. Eger, E.I., II, Brandstater, B., Saidman, L.J., Regan, M.J., Severinghaus, J.W., and Munson, E.S. Equipotent alveolar concentrations of methoxyflurane, halothane, diethyl ether, fluroxene, cyclopropane, xenon, and nitrous oxide in the dog. Anesthesiology **26**:771-777, 1965.

15. Ferstandig, L.L. Trace concentrations of anesthetic gases: a critical review of their disease potential. Anesthesia and Analgesia **57**:328-345, 1978.

16. Franks, N.P., and Lieb, W.R. Is membrane expansion relevant to anaesthesia? Nature **292**:248-251, 1981.

17. French, J.D., Verzeano, M., and Magoun, H.W. A neural basis of the anesthetic state. Archives of Neurology and Psychiatry **69**:519-529, 1953.

18. Guedel, A.E. Inhalation Anesthesia: A Fundamental Guide. New York, Macmillan, Inc., 1937.

19. Harper, M.H., Collins, P., Johnson, B., Eger, E.I., II, and Biava, C. Hepatic injury following halothane, enflurane, and isoflurane anesthesia in rats. Anesthesiology **56**:14-17, 1982.

20. Hynes, M.D., and Berkowitz, B.A. Nitrous oxide and ketamine produce an opiate-like locomotor response in mice. Pharmacologist **20**:1543, 1978.

21. Julien, R.M., and Kavan, E.M. Electrographic studies of a new volatile anesthetic agent: enflurane (Ethrane). Journal of Pharmacology and Experimental Therapeutics **183**:393-403, 1972.

22. Kayama, Y., and Iwama, K. The EEG, evoked potentials, and single-unit activity during ketamine anesthesia in cats. Anesthesiology **36**:316-328, 1972.

23. Kitahata, L.M., Kosaka, Y., Taub, A., Bonikos, K., and Hoffert, M. Lamina-specific suppression of dorsal-horn unit activity by morphine sulfate. Anesthesiology **41**:39-48, 1974.

24. LaBella, F.S. Is there a general anesthesia receptor? Canadian Journal of Physiology and Pharmacology **59**:432-442, 1981.

25. Meyer, H. Zur Theorie der Alkoholnarkose. I. Welche Eigenschaft der Anästhetica bedingt ihre narkotische Wirkung? Archiv für Experimentelle Pathologie und Pharmakologie **42**:109-137, 1899.

26. Miller, K.W. Inert gas narcosis, the high pressure neurological syndrome, and the critical volume hypothesis. Science **185**:867-869, 1974.

27. Miller, K.W. Towards the molecular bases of anesthetic action. Anesthesiology **46**:2-4, 1977.

28. Miller, S.L. A theory of gaseous anesthetics. Proceedings of the National Academy of Sciences of the United States of America **47**:1515-1524, 1961.

29. Mori, K. Excitation and depression of CNS electrical activities induced by general anesthetics. In Miyazaki, M., Iwatsuki, K., and Fujita, M., eds. Proceedings of the Fifth World Congress of Anaesthesiologists. Amsterdam, Excerpta Medica Foundation, 1973.

30. Mori, K., Winters, W.D., and Spooner, C.E. Comparison of reticular and cochlear multiple unit activity with auditory evoked responses during various stages induced by anesthetic agents. II. Electroencephalography and Clinical Neurophysiology **24**:242-248, 1968.

31. Mullins, L.J. Some physical mechanisms in narcosis. Chemistry Review **54**:289-323, 1954.

32. Nicoll, R.A., and Madison, D.V. General anesthetics hyperpolarize neurons in the vertebrate central nervous system. Science **217**:1055-1057, 1982.

33. Overton, E. Studien über die Narkose zugleich ein Beitrag zur allgemeinen Pharmakologie. Jena, Germany, G. Fischer, 1901.

34. Pauling, L. A molecular theory of general anesthesia. Science **134**:15-21, 1961.

35. Seeman, P. The membrane actions of anesthetics and tranquilizers. Pharmacological Reviews **24**:583-655, 1972.

36. Seeman, P. Anesthetics and pressure reversal of anesthesia: expansion and recompression of membrane proteins, lipids and water. Anesthesiology **47**:1-3, 1977.

37. Shimoji, K., Ito, Y., Ohama, K., Sawa, T., and Ikezono, E. Presynaptic inhibition in man during anesthesia and sleep. Anesthesiology **43**:388-391, 1975.

38. Smith, E.H., and Rees, J.M.H. The effects of naloxone on the analgesic activities of general anesthetics. Experientia **37**:289-290, 1981.

39. Smith, R.A., Wilson, M., and Miller, K.W. Naloxone has no effect on nitrous oxide anesthesia. Anesthesiology **49**:6-8, 1978.

40. Taub, A., and Kitahata, L.M. Modulation of spinal-cord function by anesthesia. Anesthesiology **43**:383-385, 1975.

41. Tinker, J.H., Gandolfi, A.J., and Van Dyke, R.A. Elevation of plasma bromide levels in patients following halothane anesthesia: time correlation with total halothane dosage. Anesthesiology **44:**194-196, 1976.

42. Trudell, J.R. A unitary theory of anesthesia based on lateral phase separations in nerve membranes. Anesthesiology **46:**5-10, 1977.

43. Vessey, M.P. Epidemiological studies of the occupational hazards of anaesthesia—a review. Anaesthesia **33:**430-438, 1978.

44. Whitcher, C., Zimmerman, D.C., and Piziali, R.L. Control of occupational exposure to nitrous oxide in the oral surgery office. Journal of Oral Surgery **36:**431-440, 1978.

45. Winters, W.D. Effects of drugs on the electrical activity of the brain: anesthetics. In Elliott, H.W., ed. Annual Review of Pharmacology and Toxicology **16:**413-426, 1976.

46. Winters, W.D., Ferrar-Allado, T., Guzman-Flores, C., and Alcaraz, M. The cataleptic state induced by ketamine: a review of the neuropharmacology of anesthesia. Neuropharmacology **11:**303-315, 1972.

47. Winters, W.D., Mori, K., Spooner, C.E., and Bauer, R.O. The neurophysiology of anesthesia. Anesthesiology **28:**65-80, 1967.

48. Woodbury, J.W., D'Arrigo, J.S., and Eyring, H. Molecular mechanism of general anesthesia: lipoprotein conformation change theory. In Fink, B.R., ed. Molecular Mechanisms of Anesthesia. Progress in Anesthesiology, vol. 1. New York, Raven Press, 1975.

49. Yang, J.C., Clark, W.C., and Ngai, S.H. Antagonism of nitrous oxide analgesia by naloxone in man. Anesthesiolgy **52:**414-417, 1980.

50. Yoshimura, N., Holaday, D.A., and Fiserova-Bergerova, V. Metabolism of methoxyflurane in man. Anesthesiolgy **44:**372-379, 1976.

GENERAL REFERENCES

Clark, D.L., and Rosner, B.S. Neurophysiologic effects of general anesthetics. I. The electroencephalogram and sensory evoked responses in man. Anesthesiology **38:**564-582, 1973.

Davis, A.B. The development of anesthesia. American Scientist **70:**522-528, 1982.

Dripps, R.D., Eckenhoff, J.E., and Vandam, L.D. Introduction to Anesthesia: The Principles of Safe Practice, ed. 6. Philadelphia, W.B. Saunders Co., 1982.

Fink, B.R., ed. Molecular Mechanisms of Anesthesia. Progress in Anesthesiology, vol. 1. New York, Raven Press, 1975.

Greene, N.M. Symposium on metabolism. Anesthesiology **39:**111-255, 1973.

Greenfield, W. Anesthesiology in dentistry—past, present and future. Anesthesia Progress **23:**104-132, 1976.

Kaufman, R.D. Biophysical mechanism of anesthetic action: historical perspective and review of current concepts. Anesthesiology **46:**49-62, 1977.

Keys, T.E. The History of Surgical Anesthesia. New York, Dover Publications, Inc., 1963.

Roth, S.H. Mechanisms of anaesthesia: a review. Canadian Anaesthetists' Society Journal **27:**433-439, 1980.

Scaramella, J., Allen, G.D., Adams, D., and Randall, F. Nitrous oxide pollution levels in oral surgery offices. Journal of Oral Surgery **36:**441-443, 1978.

19 Agents used in general anesthesia and conscious sedation

Enid A. Neidle
John A. Yagiela
Donald C. Kroeger

Compounds of diverse chemical structure, ranging from elemental gases like xenon to more complex molecules like ketamine, can induce general anesthesia. General anesthetics are available as gases, volatile liquids, or solutions suitable for parenteral injection. In the discussion that follows, individual anesthetic agents will be considered from the point of view of their physical and chemical characteristics, anesthetic properties, pharmacology, toxicity, and therapeutic advantages and disadvantages. It should be emphasized at the outset that volatile liquids and gases are not only the oldest known anesthetic agents but also the most widely used, because administration by inhalation permits rapid induction, precise control over the dose, and rapid termination of anesthetic effects. Although inhalation anesthetics are often divided into gases and volatile liquids, there are few differences between these two classes of substances other than boiling point and solubility in various tissues (Table 19-1). With regard to boiling point, which determines the vapor pressure of the gaseous phase, liquids need special devices (vaporizers) to produce and maintain an adequate amount of anesthetic in the inspired air. Tissue solubility, however, is greater with the volatile liquids, and a smaller concentration of drug is therefore required to produce general anesthesia.

GASES

Of the gases that have been used as inhalation anesthetics, only nitrous oxide and cyclopropane will be discussed below. The structural formulas of these two anesthetics are shown in Figure 19-1.

Table 19-1. Physical and solubility properties of inhalation anesthetics

Agent	Boiling point (C)	Vapor pressure mm Hg 20 C (atm)	Brain/gas coefficient 37 C
Gases			
Nitrous oxide	−89	760	0.52
Cyclopropane	−33	760	0.69
Volatile liquids			
Ether	35	450	12.1
Halothane	50	243	6.0
Enflurane	57	175	2.5
Methoxyflurane	105	22.5	23.4
Isoflurane	49	250	3.7

Nitrous oxide

Physical and chemical properties. Nitrous oxide (N_2O) is a colorless, nonirritating gas with a pleasant, mild odor and taste. It has a blood/gas partition coefficient of 0.47 and is thus poorly soluble in blood. Nitrous oxide is excreted unchanged by the lungs. It is nonflammable but can support combustion in the absence of oxygen. It is available as a liquid in pressurized steel cylinders.

Anesthetic properties. Nitrous oxide is the oldest gaseous anesthetic in use today. It is also the only inorganic substance used as an anesthetic. Because of its very low solubility in blood, a state of equilibrium between alveolar and arterial tension is quickly reached; thus, induction and awakening occur very rapidly. Its primary disadvantage as a general anesthetic is its lack of potency. In order to ensure adequate oxygenation of the patient, nitrous oxide is normally not used at a concentration greater than 70%, the remainder being oxygen. At this concentration, it is incapable of inducing stage III, or surgical, anesthesia, and, in the absence of any premedication, stage I analgesia is produced. If, on the other hand, 85% nitrous oxide is administered, or if brief inhalations of 100% anesthetic gas are permitted, stage II anesthesia, marked by a dreamy or hallucinatory state, can be achieved. Administration of nitrous oxide under hyperbaric conditions (e.g., at 2 atmospheres) can produce a cataleptic-anesthetic state that may progress to convulsions.[34] When nitrous oxide is employed with other anesthetic agents, the maintenance concentration normally used is 60% to 70%. However, during the brief induction phase, it is safe to use a concentration of 85%. At subanesthetic concentrations (30% to 40%), nitrous oxide is an excellent analgesic. The maximum concentration that will provide good analgesia and at the same time allow most patients to remain in verbal communication with the clinician is about 60%.

Because of its lack of potency, nitrous oxide is unable to produce full surgical anesthesia by itself and is most commonly used as a supplement to other anesthetic agents, such as thiopental or halothane. When nitrous oxide is used with a more potent agent, it is possible to lower the concentration of the other drug and still achieve a more rapid induction and a shorter recovery period. This phenomenon is a reflection of the fact that nitrous oxide lowers the minimum alveolar concentration (MAC) of the other anesthetic. In the presence of adequate oxygenation, nitrous oxide does not usually produce any clinically significant respiratory or cardiovascular effects. (Nitrous oxide is a direct myocardial depressant; however, it also stimulates the sympathetic nervous system such that cardiac output remains unchanged.) Consequently, when it is combined with other inhalation agents, there is likely to be less cardiovascular and respiratory depression than would be caused by an equal depth of anesthesia induced by a single potent anesthetic drug.

Toxic reactions and side effects. Nitrous oxide is not acutely toxic to hepatic, renal, or other organ systems. Tissue damage has occurred, but it has usually been attributed to inadequate oxygenation resulting from the use of 100% nitrous oxide. Although nitrous oxide has little effect on respiration in normal individuals, whose ventilation is regulated by the arterial carbon dioxide tension, patients with chronic obstructive pulmonary disease, whose ventilatory drive is dependent on arterial oxygen, may become severely hypoxic on exposure to even sedative concentrations of anesthetic.[35] Thus, nitrous oxide should not be administered to such patients unless controlled respiration is planned.

Because high concentrations (50% to 70%) are used and because its solubility in blood greatly exceeds that of nitrogen, nitrous oxide will increase the volume of any air pockets in the body. This can occur, for instance, after injections of air into the ventricles during a pneumoencephalogram. The accumulation of nitrous oxide may also distend an obstructed bowel or increase the volume of air behind the tympanic membrane. In addition, the high concentration of nitrous oxide required during anesthesia results in the accumulation of a considerable quantity of dissolved gas within the body. When the administration of gas is stopped, large volumes of nitrous oxide diffuse from the blood into the alveoli, washing out oxygen. This temporary reduction in the amount of alveolar oxygen is termed diffusion hypoxia and can be prevented by administering pure oxygen for 3 to 5 minutes after the cessation of nitrous oxide inhalation.

In recent years, increasing attention has been given to the possible chronic toxicity of nitrous oxide. Cell division in tissue cultures exposed to nitrous oxide under hyperbaric pressure is interrupted in the presynthetic (G-1) phase.[3] Prolonged inhalation of analgesic concentrations of nitrous oxide leads to altered spermatogenesis and hematopoiesis in vivo.[17] Epidemiologic studies of operating room personnel indicate a significant increase of spontaneous abortion in women and in wives of men exposed to trace amounts of nitrous oxide and other anesthetics and a higher incidence of birth defects in their offspring. Although nitrous oxide is but one possible explanation for these findings, similar effects have been noted in rats exposed to nitrous oxide[19] and in dental practitioners,[5] who are more likely to be exposed to nitrous oxide alone, albeit in relatively high concentrations.[18] Further studies are needed to substantiate the occupational health hazard of nitrous oxide, but the evidence to date certainly calls for the development of methods to minimize nitrous oxide pollution within the operatory.[1]

The finding that nitrous oxide analgesia may involve the release of endogenous opioid-like substances (enkephalins) raises the possibility of a drug abuse problem.[2] The relationship between enkephalins and opioids suggests that tolerance and "addiction" to the opioids may also be caused by these and similar polypeptides. Further research is needed in this field, but it is well known that nitrous oxide is abused by some members of the dental profession, and evidence is mounting that this abuse is associated with deleterious effects.[20]

Therapeutic uses. Despite its lack of potency, nitrous oxide is one of the most widely used inhalation anesthetics. It is employed in surgery to provide rapid induction and is generally administered in conjunction with other, more potent anesthetic agents, as well as with a number of preanesthetic medications discussed later in this chapter. At a 40% concentration, there is good soft-tissue and periosteal analgesia. Awareness of sensory input is reduced, with the exception that sounds may seem louder and qualitatively different.[32] Historically, nitrous oxide was first used for dental surgery, but with the advent of local anesthetics it has been largely replaced as the drug of choice for providing analgesia sufficient for most dental procedures. More recently there has been an upsurge in the use of nitrous oxide, not to effect dental anesthesia but to provide relief from anxiety by the production of the euphoric, dreamy state of late stage I analgesia. In this use of nitrous oxide, which is described in greater detail in Chapter 44, local anesthesia is generally employed to complement the analgesia provided by nitrous oxide.[15]

Cyclopropane

Physical and chemical properties. Cyclopropane (trimethylene) is a three-carbon cyclic hydrocarbon that exists as a colorless gas with a slight odor. It has a low blood/gas partition coefficient (0.46), is flammable and explosive, and is available as a liquid in pressurized steel cylinders.

Anesthetic properties. Because of its insolubility in blood, cyclopropane is a very rapidly acting anesthetic, with induction occurring in 1 to 3 minutes and recovery in 5 to 10 minutes after administration is terminated. In contrast to nitrous oxide, cyclopropane is sufficiently potent that the deeper planes of anesthesia can easily be achieved. In concentrations as low as 1%, cyclopropane can produce analgesia without loss of consciousness or risk of explosion. The gas is nonirritating, so salivation and respiratory irregularities do not occur to any great extent. Laryngospasm and delirium may occur but can be avoided by first administering thiopental to produce unconsciousness, intubating the patient, and only then beginning the administration of gas. Cyclopropane produces good muscle relaxation during surgical anesthesia.

Blood pressure and cardiac output are well maintained during anesthesia because cyclopropane causes sympathoadrenal discharge. If an elevation of blood pressure occurs, it is the result of an increase in peripheral resistance. Since cyclopropane supports blood pressure even in the deeper planes of anesthesia, it has been particularly employed for patients in shock. Of all the anesthetic agents in current use, cyclopropane is most likely to sensitize the myocardium to circulating catecholamines. Like other anesthetics, it tends to depress respiration by reducing the ventilatory response to carbon dioxide.

Traditionally, the surgical anesthetic state induced by cyclopropane has been thought to be the result of CNS depression. However, evidence exists that CNS excitation occurs and that the surgical state is one of cataleptic anesthesia.[23] Its analgesic action on spinal neurons bears a striking resemblance to that produced by nitrous oxide.[31]

Toxic reactions and side effects. Nausea, vomiting, and headache during the recovery period are common. Emergence delirium, as well as postanesthetic hypotension, occasionally occurs. The normal or slightly elevated blood pressure during anesthesia, combined with an increased blood flow to skin and muscle, is said to lead to a greater than usual blood loss during surgery. Cyclopropane is neither hepatotoxic nor nephrotoxic.

The anesthetic's primary disadvantage is its explosive nature, and this has markedly limited its use. When cyclopropane is administered, great care must be exercised to reduce static electricity in the operating room, and the gas is not recommended for use in locales that have low humidity.

Therapeutic uses. Cyclopropane has virtually disappeared from the operating room in the past 10 years.[8] Reasons for its abandonment include the risks of fire and explosion, introduction of suitable nonflammable alternatives, and various economic and medicolegal considerations. Although cyclopropane in subanesthetic concentrations offers many of the advantages of nitrous oxide and has some potential for therapeutic application in conscious sedation without the danger of explosion, it is not currently used for dental procedures in any fashion.

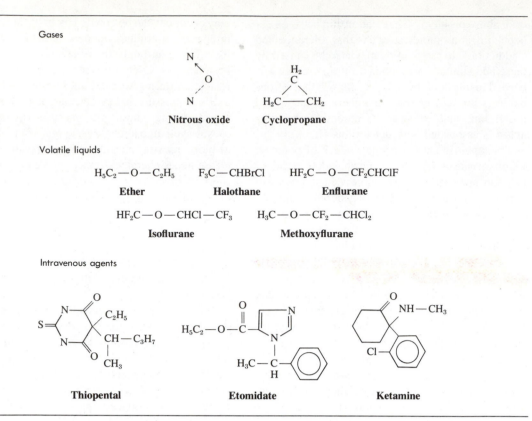

Figure 19-1. Structural formulas of anesthetic drugs.

VOLATILE LIQUIDS

The volatile liquids most commonly used as inhalation anesthetics, along with their clinical advantages and disadvantages, are discussed below. The structural formulas of these five anesthetics are illustrated in Figure 19-1.

Ether

Physical and chemical properties. Ether (diethyl ether) is an irritating liquid with a pungent odor. Its blood/gas partition coefficient is 12.1. It is flammable and explosive and is available in metal containers.

Anesthetic properties. Ether has traditionally been the anesthetic with which all others have been compared, since it has been the safest and most widely used anesthetic for over a hundred years. However, this agent is now rarely used alone, primarily because its induction is slow and unpleasant. This problem can be overcome by the use of other agents, such as thiopental or nitrous oxide, to produce rapid induction and atropine to inhibit excessive salivation and mucus secretion by the irritated respiratory tract epithelium. The recovery period is likewise slow and is accompanied by nausea and vomiting, even after relatively light levels of anesthesia. Because ether produces good analgesia and muscle relaxation and has no special toxicity for the respiratory or circulatory systems, some anesthesiologists believe that with proper management it is as good as or superior to other agents currently available.

Therapeutic uses. Ether is used infrequently as a general anesthetic in the United States and is not employed in dentistry at all.

Halothane

Physical and chemical properties. Halothane is a halogenated hydrocarbon with a blood/gas partition coefficient of 2.3. It is nonflammable, has a characteristic "sweet" odor, and is available in brown glass bottles.

Anesthetic properties. Halothane has become one of the most widely used anesthetics since its introduction in the early 1950s. It is a potent agent capable of inducing any depth of anesthesia required. With its moderate blood/gas partition coefficient, the induction time of halothane is intermediate: faster than ether but slower than nitrous oxide. It has poor analgesic properties, and even at surgical anesthetic levels the unconscious patient may respond to a noxious stimulus. For this reason, halothane is most often used with nitrous oxide or a narcotic analgesic. Since halothane produces incomplete muscle relaxation, it is also often combined with neuromuscular blocking agents.

Halothane has a direct depressant effect on myocardial contractility and, to a lesser degree, on vascular smooth muscle. Unlike ether and cyclopropane, halothane does not stimulate sympathoadrenal discharge; in fact, compensatory baroreceptor reflexes are blunted. Sympathetic nervous system activity is therefore unable to counteract the vascular and myocardial depression, which becomes more pronounced with increasing depth of anesthesia.

Halothane depresses respiration at all anesthetic concentrations. At light anesthetic levels, breathing becomes rapid and shallow, but arterial carbon dioxide is maintained at normal or slightly higher than normal concentrations. At deeper levels of anesthesia, the respiratory response to carbon dioxide is progressively lost, and controlled ventilation is frequently necessary.

It should be pointed out that unlike nitrous oxide and cyclopropane, which are excreted entirely unchanged by the lungs, as much as 20% of the administered halothane may be metabolized.[25]

Toxic reactions and side effects. Although halothane does not stimulate sympathoadrenal activity, cardiac arrhythmias can occur after the injection of pressor agents during surgery to augment blood pressure or as a result of catecholamines released endogenously in reponse to elevated carbon dioxide tension.

Halothane has been implicated in a delayed hepatic failure called *halothane hepatitis,* which may range from a very mild form of liver dysfunction to massive hepatic necrosis.[10] This adverse effect of halothane is extremely rare. There is evidence that it may occur after repeated administrations of halothane and that an allergic phenomenon, hypoxia, and/or volatile reductive metabolites may be involved. For these reasons, halothane is contraindicated in patients who have shown any signs of liver toxicity on previous exposure to halothane or related anesthetics, and it is considered undesirable to use halothane repeatedly in any patient.[29]

The condition known as malignant hyperthermia, in which the body temperature progressively increases to alarming and sometimes fatal levels, was once a very rare side effect of general anesthesia. With the advent and expanded use of halothane, however, its occurrence appears to have increased, although it is still rare. Elevated heat production associated with altered muscle metabolism appears to be responsible for the hyperthermia.[14] Discontinuing the anesthetic and packing the patient in ice, lavage, or even extracorporeal cooling may be required. The intravenous administration of the muscle relaxant dantrolene is also indicated to reduce the increases in myoplasmic Ca^{++} that support the metabolic derangements.[13] Malignant hyperthermia appears to have a genetically linked cause.

Therapeutic uses. Halothane is one of the most widely used anesthetics for general surgical anesthesia. Although it has the disadvantage of causing a decrease in blood pressure, it is a desirable anesthetic agent for operations in which a relatively bloodless field is necessary, as in plastic surgery. Halothane has at the present time limited application to the practice of dentistry in the outpatient setting.

Enflurane

Enflurane is a halogenated ether with properties similar to those of halothane. It has a blood/gas partition coefficient of 1.8, which makes it less soluble in blood than halothane; it is also less potent than halothane. Chemically, it is an ether and thus produces better muscle relaxation than does halothane. During stage II anesthesia, enflurane produces high-voltage discharges on the EEG, and the excitatory effect can progress to a state in which electrical seizures with convulsive activity occur.[16] Although clinical anesthesia with enflurane resembles that produced by halothane, the EEG and behavioral evidence suggest that a cataleptic-anesthetic state may occur. Enflurane is metabolized to a lesser extent than is halothane, and hepatotoxicity has not been associated with its use. It is employed for the same purposes as halothane, but it may have some advantages: better analgesia and muscle relaxation, lower liver toxicity, and less sensitization of the heart to the arrhythmogenic action of catecholamines. On the other hand, enflurane has a strong odor and is thus less suitable as an induction agent.

Isoflurane

Isoflurane, an isomer of enflurane, is a halogenated methyl ethyl ether. Released for use in 1979, it has become, with nitrous oxide, halothane, and enflurane, one of the most widely used inhalation anesthetics. Its blood/gas partition coefficient of 1.4 is the lowest of any of the potent inhalation anesthetics in widespread use today. Induction therefore should theoretically be very rapid, but in fact it is somewhat limited by the pungent odor of isoflurane, which, if induction is allowed to proceed too rapidly, leads to breath holding and coughing. This problem is usually overcome by the use of preanesthetic medications or by inducing with nitrous oxide and/or an intravenous agent. As with other general anesthetics, the MAC for isoflurane varies with age (e.g., 1.28% at ages 19 to 30 and 1.15% at ages 30 to 55) and is lowered in the presence of such drugs as morphine, lidocaine, and alcohol.[11] The chronic ingestion of alcohol raises the MAC for isoflurane, suggesting that alcoholics will be resistant to the effects of the anesthetic. Anesthesia with isoflurane is not associated with EEG and overt seizure activity.

Isoflurane is sufficiently potent to provide muscle relaxation adequate for any surgical procedure, but muscular blocking agents are normally used instead of the higher concentrations of anesthetic needed to secure muscle relaxation. Isoflurane, like other potent inhalation anesthetics, increases the action of the nondepolarizing neuromuscular blocking drugs.

Isoflurane produces a dose-related direct depression of myocardial contractility, which is exaggerated by preexisting congestive heart failure. The myocardial depression, however, is considerably less than that seen with halothane and enflurane. Cardiac output is well maintained even though stroke volume is decreased by virtue of an increase in heart rate. Arterial blood pressure and total peripheral resistance decline as dose is raised. Isoflurane does not sensitize the heart to arrhythmias; indeed, approximately 3 times the injected dose of epinephrine is tolerated during isoflurane as during halothane anesthesia. The anesthetic, however, does produce respiratory depression, which manifests itself as a decreased ventilatory response to hypercapnia and hypoxia.

In contrast to halothane, methoxyflurane, and enflurane, biotransformation of isoflurane is negligible (less than 0.2%). This finding suggests that it is neither nephrotoxic nor hepatotoxic, and this is confirmed by observations that repeated and prolonged exposures to isoflurane have not caused hepatorenal injury in animals. The fact that isoflurane is relatively insoluble in blood and that it undergoes virtually no biotransformation in the liver would suggest that halothane hepatitis will not likely be associated with isoflurane.[6]

Isoflurane has a number of advantages: it is chemically stable, nonflammable, and potent; induction is rapid and muscle relaxation adequate; and it is not arrhythmogenic and does not injure the kidneys or liver. On the other hand, isoflurane is continuously depressing to the cardiovascular and respiratory systems. It has also been associated wtih several cases of malignant hyperthermia, so it is absolutely contraindicated in any patient suspected of being susceptible to this condition.

Methoxyflurane

Methoxyflurane is a halogenated ether similar to enflurane. With a MAC of 0.16%, it is the most potent agent currently available. The blood/gas partition coefficient is high, so that induction is slow, taking up to 20 minutes if the drug is used by itself. As with other soluble anesthetics that require a prolonged induction period, methoxyflurane is generally used as a maintenance agent after induction is accomplished by a relatively insoluble compound, such as nitrous oxide, or by one of the intravenous agents (e.g., thiopental). The anesthetic action is similar to that of halothane, except that there is less respiratory depression and more muscle relaxation and analgesia. The major reason for methoxyflurane's relative disuse is that it is metabolized to a large extent (up to 50%), and plasma inorganic fluoride concentrations become elevated, sometimes high enough to produce renal failure (fluoride diabetes insipidus).[36] Although it is still available, methoxyflurane is rarely used other than as an inhalational analgesic in obstetrics and has little or no use in dentistry.

INTRAVENOUS AGENTS

Intravenous agents have become widely used in anesthesiology, but they lack the precise control of the anesthetic state provided by the inhalation anesthetics. Once an intravenous drug has been injected, practically nothing can be done to terminate its action. The time course of effect produced after injection is influenced by the distribution of the drug in the body and by its metabolic inactivation. On the other hand, interest in techniques of intra-

Table 19-2. Dosages of some parenteral drugs used to produce sedation, analgesia, or anesthesia

Drug	Route of administration	Dose* (mg)	Effect
Thiopental	Intravenous	150-500	Induction of anesthesia
Etomidate	Intravenous	15-30	Induction of anesthesia
Diazepam	Intravenous	5-10	Sedation
	Intravenous	10-20	Sedation with amnesia
Midazolam	Intravenous	15-20	Induction of anesthesia
Hydroxyzine	Intramuscular	50-100	Sedation
Scopolamine	Intramuscular	0.4-0.6	Sedation with amnesia
Morphine	Intravenous	10-15	Sedation analgesia
	Intravenous	35-200	Anesthesia
Fentanyl	Intravenous	0.05-0.1	Analgesia
Droperidol	Intravenous	2.5-5	Neurolepsis
Fentanyl + droperidol	Intravenous	†	Neuroleptanalgesia
Ketamine	Intravenous	70-150	Anesthesia
	Intramuscular	300-500	Anesthesia

*The dosages shown in this table are for a person weighing approximately 70 kg.
†The average volume of the commercial combination (Innovar) required is 4 to 8 ml, corresponding to 0.2 to 0.4 mg fentanyl and 10 to 20 mg droperidol.

venous anesthesia has been heightened by the rising cost of volatile anesthetics and concern about the effects of anesthetic trace gases on operating room personnel. The intravenous agents are of considerable use for induction of anesthesia and as the sole anesthetic in minor but painful procedures such as laceration and wound repair, changing of burn dressings, endoscopy, cardiac catheterization, and dental treatment. During therapy, they are also helpful in controlling otherwise unmanageable patients. In most cases, the intravenous agents are used to provide sedation and analgesia when other measures, for example oral sedative and opioid drug therapy, local anesthesia, or patient counseling, would be ineffective or unreliable in meeting the needs of the patient or practitioner. Although the short- and ultra-short-acting barbiturates were once widely used for these purposes, drugs from other classes are now employed more frequently. These agents include various combinations of antianxiety or antipsychotic tranquilizers, opioids, and drugs such as ketamine (Table 19-2). The relatively short action of most of these drugs, together with the light level of CNS depression used (i.e., in which the patient is awake and able to respond to verbal commands), makes their use especially suited for conscious sedation in dentistry. The basic pharmacology of most of the intravenous agents is presented elsewhere in this book, and a more complete discussion of the use of these agents in the control of anxiety and pain for the dental patient is provided in Chapter 44.

Barbiturates

The ultra-short-acting barbiturates include thiopental, methohexital, and thiamylal. Thiopental is the thiobarbiturate analogue of pentobarbital, and thiamylal is the thio-derivative of secobarbital. The actions of thiopental are typical of the barbiturates in this class. Despite claims to the contrary, the others offer no advantages over thiopental. Thiopental will therefore be discussed as a representative of the ultra-short-acting barbiturates. Its molecular structure is depicted in Figure 19-1.

Anesthetic effects. Thiopental is a potent anesthetic agent capable of producing stage III anesthesia. Its use is limited by its poor analgesic effect; even the unconscious patient may respond to a painful stimulus. For this reason, it is seldom relied on alone for anesthesia but is used primarily as an induction agent. For relatively short surgical procedures, thiopental has been used with nitrous oxide, which provides an analgesic effect. The induction period is smooth and very quick. The patient loses consciousness within several seconds after a rapid intravenous injection. Generally, however, induction is accomplished by administering the drug over a 15- to 30-second period. When consciousness is lost, inhalation anesthesia is begun.

Because of their high lipid solubility, the ultra-short-acting barbiturates have the ability to penetrate all tissues after injection. The amount of drug entering a given tissue is primarily dependent on the regional blood flow. Since the brain and viscera receive most of the cardiac output, they attain the highest concentration of the drug. Later, as the agent is redistributed to the more poorly perfused tissues, such as muscle and then fat, a progressive decline in the blood and brain concentrations occurs. The barbiturate concentration in the central nervous system diminishes to 50% of the initial peak level in 5 minutes and to less than 10% after 30 minutes. The gradual decline in plasma concentration after 30 minutes is caused by continued uptake into fat and by metabolism of the drug. The patient regains consciousness after a single dose in 10 to 20 minutes. Repeated doses required for extended anesthesia may cause cumulative effects and a prolonged recovery period.

Toxic reactions and side effects. Respiratory depression accounts for the major toxic effects of the barbiturates. After an injection, respiratory rate and volume are depressed, and apnea and coughing may occur. Laryngospasm may develop as a result of irritation from premature insertion of the tracheal cannula. Bronchospasms are occasionally observed, especially in the bronchial asthmatic patient.

At ordinary doses, moderate decreases in cardiac output occur but there is little change in systemic blood pressure because of a compensatory increase in total peripheral resistance. After high doses, the direct depressant effect of thiopental on the myocardium will lower blood pressure and may alter the redistribution pattern of the drug.

In a standard concentration of 2.5%, thiopental is irritating to tissue, so care must be taken to prevent intraarterial injection or extravasation, either of which may result in tissue necrosis. Both the high alkalinity of the solution (pH 11) and the chemical nature of the drug itself are responsible for this effect.

Therapeutic uses in dentistry. In dentistry the ultra-short-acting barbiturates are principally used in a slow intravenous infusion of a dilute solution to produce a sedative-hypnotic or sleeplike state in which the patient is able to maintain partial contact with the environment. Because these drugs have poor analgesic properties, painful procedures require that additional medication (i.e., local anesthetics, nitrous oxide, or narcotic analgesics) be given. Although consciousness is not lost in this technique, amnesia is produced; hence, the patient may have little or no recollection of the procedure. Care must be taken, however, to avoid stage I excitation or stage II delirium in sensitive patients.

Etomidate

Etomidate, a carboxylated imidazole derivative, represents a new class of intravenous anesthetics. Although unrelated chemically to thiopental (or to any other agent), etomidate exhibits a pharmacologic profile similar to that of the ultra-short-acting barbiturates.[9] As with thiopental, the onset of anesthesia after a bolus injection is nearly instantaneous, limited only by the circulation time of blood from the injection site to the brain. Likewise, anesthesia is brief after conventional doses, with recovery following redistribution of the agent from the central nervous system to muscle and fat. Unlike the barbiturates, however, the primary site of action of etomidate appears to be in the neocortex, where the drug mimics the inhibitory neurotransmitter GABA.

Etomidate enjoys several advantages over conventional induction agents. Although respiratory depression can occur, it is less frequent and intense than that associated with thiopental. Because etomidate is rapidly metabolized (half-life of about 1 hour), drug hangover is minimized. The most conspicuous advantage of etomidate is its freedom from cardiovascular toxicity. Induction doses cause a mild (15%) drop in total peripheral resistance, which is mirrored by similar decrements in cardiac output and myocardial oxygen consumption. Coronary blood flow is mildly increased. Unlike other intravenous anesthetics, etomidate does not appear to cause histamine release.

These beneficial features notwithstanding, it is unlikely that etomidate will replace the ultra-short-acting barbiturates in clinical practice. Etomidate has two significant liabilities: pain on injection and involuntary motor effects. Depending on variables such as the rate of injection, the size of the vein, and the premedication used, the incidence of phlebitis is 10% to 60%. Excitatory motor responses (myoclonus, hypertonus, hiccough) have been reported with similar frequency. Although the majority of such episodes are inconsequential or of only minor inconvenience, spontaneous motor activity has occasionally been prominent enough to complicate the intraoperative care of the patient.

Etomidate is currently recommended for the induction of general anesthesia in patients with cardiovascular derangements. Its role, if any, in dentistry has not been established.

Benzodiazepines

Diazepam, given intravenously in a dose of 5 to 10 mg, will normally sedate the mildly apprehensive patient. Increasing the dose to 10 to 20 mg produces, within 5 minutes, profound sedation with partial amnesia, which is present only during the early phase of sedation. There is no true analgesia, but the anxiety component of pain is diminished sufficiently to make the drug useful in procedures that are more anxiety-provoking than painful. If true analgesia is necessary, as for dental extractions and other surgery, local anesthetics, opioids, or nitrous oxide can be added. In susceptible individuals, excitation or delirium may occur at conventional doses. Recovery takes about 1 hour, but drowsiness and ataxia may persist for much longer. A euphoric state may develop, lasting up to 6 hours.

Slight respiratory and cardiovascular depression can occur. As compared with the barbiturates, a wide margin exists between the therapeutic dose and the dose producing serious respiratory depression. As a consequence, deaths due to respiratory arrest are rare. Nevertheless, hypoxia can occur, especially in patients with pulmonary disease or when the drug is administered together with other CNS depressants.

Antihistamines and antimuscarinic drugs

Hydroxyzine injection is suitable only for intramuscular administration. By this route, titrated dosing is not possible, and therefore the control afforded by intravenous injection is not achieved. Like most antihistamines, hydroxyzine is able to induce sedation, and with large doses some analgesia has been claimed. The sedation produced is essentially the same as that resulting from an equally effective dose of barbiturate or diazepam. A clinical impression exists, although unproved, that excitation or delirium is less likely to occur, especially in children. Like most antihistamines, hydroxyzine has some antimuscarinic actions, so antisialagogic and antiemetic effects are seen. Cardiovascular and respiratory effects are slight; however, toxic doses produce excitation that can lead to convulsions.

Scopolamine, like atropine, is generally used as a premedication for its antimuscarinic properties, usually in combination with an opioid or barbiturate. However, it can also be used to produce conscious sedation with marked amnesia. Scopolamine has no analgesic properties and may produce excitation and delirium in a painful situation.

Opioids

Morphine is the prototype of the group of opioid analgesics used to induce sedation-analgesia. Other commonly used drugs in this class that, aside from onset and duration differences, have essentially the same pharmacologic actions as morphine include meperidine, hydromorphone, alphaprodine, and fentanyl. Morphine is used most commonly for sedation-analgesia, but it has also gained acceptance for use in major surgery, especially open heart surgery. Extremely large doses are used in conjunction with oxygen and are usually supplemented with nitrous oxide or intravenous agents. Assisted ventilation is necessary during surgery and up to 48 hours afterward. Morphine is useful in heart surgery because the drug has very little depressant effect on the myocardium, although the blood pressure may be lowered. During the anesthetic period, cardiac patients have profound analgesia and a clouded consciousness with partial awareness of the surroundings. Amnesia may or may not occur. The use of increasingly large doses of morphine has been shown to cause a progressive central excitatory effect,[26] including convulsive activity.[33] The central state seen in patients undergoing major surgery with high doses of morphine appears to be one of excitation and cataleptic anesthesia.

In minor painful procedures (including dental surgery), morphine and other opioids in combination with one or more sedative compounds are useful in producing a state of sedation-analgesia, which can lessen anxiety and tension. There are two notable side effects associated with this use of morphine. First, there may be itching of the upper lip as the drug is being injected. This pruritus appears to be caused by the release of histamine from mast cells; the vasculature of the lips is an especially sensitive indicator of this phenomenon. The second problem is dysphoria, nausea, and vomiting that occur in many patients 2 to 3 hours after surgery. At this time, the effects of the sedative have worn off, leaving a predominance of opioid action. Morphine nausea is aggravated by motion and activity, which increase the sensory input from the vestibular apparatus of the ear. Patients are advised to remain quiet and in bed during this time.

The respiratory depressant effect of the opioids has somewhat limited their use, but the opioid antagonist naloxone can immediately reverse this and other effects of the opioids. However, the duration of action of naloxone (1 to 4 hours) is relatively short when compared with morphine (up to 5 hours), so additional postoperative doses of naloxone may be necessary.

Fentanyl is a synthetic opioid that is estimated

to be 80 to 100 times more potent than morphine. An advantage of fentanyl over the other opioids is its short duration of action (30 to 60 minutes), but repeated administration can prolong the duration of action and the recovery time. High doses of fentanyl used alone produce muscular rigidity through an action on the central nervous system.[30] Recently oxygen–high dose fentanyl anesthesia has been adopted for use during valvular and coronary artery surgery because it provides stable hemodynamic conditions.[21] However, reports of tachycardia and hypertension during surgery, as well as of myocardial ischemia, have led to the recommendation that the oxygen–high dose fentanyl anesthesia be supplemented with nitrous oxide, diazepam, or a neuroleptic, as for instance, droperidol.

Neuroleptic-opioid combinations

Opioid analgesics are used in combination with potent antipsychotic or neuroleptic agents to produce a state described as neuroleptanalgesia. Under the influence of this combination, the patient is sedated and demonstrates psychic indifference to the environment yet remains conscious and can respond to questions and commands. A mixture containing droperidol and fentanyl in a 50:1 fixed-dose combination is marketed as Innovar. The antipsychotic agents themselves can produce a state of sedation and quiescence in which the patient is indifferent to his surroundings. The addition of an opioid agent provides analgesia through modification of psychic and sensory components of pain. The combination of fentanyl (100 μg/kg), 100% oxygen, and droperidol (0.15 mg/kg) has been reported to provide stable hemodynamics during coronary bypass surgery.[27] However, nitrous oxide can be added in lieu of these high doses to achieve a deeper state of anesthesia.

After intravenous injection, 2 to 5 minutes are required before the peak effect is reached. Cardiovascular and respiratory depression occurs, and vagal blockade with atropine and assisted ventilation may be required to counteract respiratory depression. Postoperative respiratory depression caused by fentanyl frequently occurs and may be countered with naloxone. One problem with Innovar is that the durations of action of the two drugs differ, that of fentanyl being much shorter than that of droperidol. Fentanyl is available separately, however, and can be used to prolong and supplement the analgesic action. Droperidol, like the phenothiazines, may produce delayed extrapyramidal movements that can be controlled by anticholinergic drugs used in the treatment of parkinsonism.

Another mixture used to produce a similar state of neuroleptanalgesia contains two phenothiazines and meperidine. It is known by the proprietary names of its ingredients—Demerol, Phenergan, and Thorazine (or DPT). This combination may produce prolonged respiratory depression and orthostatic hypotension.

Sedative-narcotic combinations

Diazepam-morphine, diazepam-meperidine, diazepam-fentanyl, pentobarbital-meperidine-scopolamine (used in the Jorgensen technique), and a variety of other sedative-opioid mixtures have been used to provide sedation-analgesia. The rationale for the use of these combinations is to provide an antianxiety effect along with analgesia. However, in the case of diazepam-morphine, the duration of action of morphine is much longer than that of diazepam, and the recovery period, with its accompanying respiratory depression, nausea, and some hypotension, may be unnecessarily prolonged. Of course, analgesia lasting well into the postsurgical period is often advantageous, but fentanyl can be used when short-term opioid coverage (less than an hour) is desired.

Ketamine

Ketamine became available as a result of a study of compounds derived from phencyclidine. The molecular structure of ketamine is shown in Figure 19-1. Phencyclidine (otherwise known as "angel dust") has never been approved for human use because it commonly produces hallucinations and acute psychotic reactions during emergence; it has subsequently become a serious drug of abuse (see Chapter 46). Although it is not devoid of these properties, ketamine is sufficiently free of undesirable effects to be useful clinically. The anesthetic state produced by ketamine (termed dissociative anesthesia) has been characterized as a state of catalepsy, an excitatory state completely dissimilar from that seen after administration of agents such as ether and halothane (see Figure 18-2).[24] The patient is awake but appears to be unaware of the environment. The eyes remain open with a slow nystagmus, and the corneal and pupillary reflexes remain intact.[22] The dissociative state produced by ketamine is the result of a functional and electrophysiologic dissociation between the thalamoneocortical and limbic systems.[7] Excitatory activity in both the thalamus and limbic system, without clinical evidence of seizure activity, has been demonstrated following ketamine injection. This seizure activity does not seem to spread to the cortex, and paradoxically ketamine has been demonstrated to have anticonvulsant properties.[28] Adequacy of anesthesia is determined by the absence of purposeful responses to painful stimuli.

The onset of action of ketamine is about 1 minute after intravenous and 5 minutes after intramuscular injection; duration of anesthesia is about 5 to 10 minutes and 10 to 20 minutes, respectively; recovery takes much longer. Anesthesia can be maintained by repeated injections or by using a continuous infusion. Ketamine produces profound analgesia, but most protective reflexes are maintained. It causes no muscle relaxation; indeed, frequently there is an increase in muscle tone and sometimes muscle spasms. Rapid infusion of ketamine may lead to a transient respiratory depression; high doses may also depress respiration and obtund laryngeal reflexes. Blood pressure and cardiac output are elevated, which may increase cerebrospinal fluid pressure. Premedication with antimuscarinic drugs will prevent the reflex bradycardia and the copious secretory activity in the upper respiratory tract. The benzodiazepines (diazepam, flunitrazepam, and midazolam) have been shown to block the cardiovascular stimulation induced by ketamine.

On recovery, the patient experiences mild amnesia, forgetting the events of surgery that occurred during the deeper levels of anesthesia. However, the vivid dreams, hallucinations, and delirium that can arise during either induction or emergence are often recalled, sometimes causing unacceptable mental distress. The frequency of emergence delirium is reported to be less in children than in adults, possibly because children are less able to relate their experiences, especially those with a psychic component. Recurrence of hallucinations, similar to the flashbacks associated with the use of LSD may occur for up to 1 year in both adults and children. A number of drugs have been evaluated for their ability to alter the unpleasant emergence effects. Atropine and droperidol increase the frequency of vivid dreams, whereas thiopental and the benzodiazepines, especially lorazepam, diazepam, and midazolam, decrease the incidence of dreams and illusions. A recovery period with a minimum of sensory stimulation and other disturbances is also helpful. The lack of muscle relaxation and the ineffective block of visceral pain

make ketamine unsuitable for abdominal surgery, unless it is supplemented with agents such as nitrous oxide and tubocurarine. Although the cataleptic-anesthetic state induced by ketamine is one of central excitation, there is evidence that natural sleep is a more potent stimulator of convulsions than is ketamine in the epileptic patient.[4] Ketamine is contraindicated in patients with cardiovascular disease and cerebral trauma (i.e., increased intracranial pressure) and probably should not be used in patients with increased intraocular pressure, thyrotoxicosis, schizophrenia, or a history of adverse reactions to ketamine.

ANESTHETIC ADJUVANTS AND PREMEDICATION

The pharmacology of the neuromuscular blocking agents, which are frequently used during anesthesia to provide greater muscle relaxation, is discussed in Chapter 11. Many of the sedatives, analgesics, antihistamines, and antimuscarinics previously mentioned in this chapter and covered elsewhere in the book are administered to the patient minutes to several hours before anesthesia and surgery. Premedication is thought to help prepare the patient for the induction and maintenance of anesthesia, although certain of the supposed benefits have been challenged.[12]

Agents used in general anesthesia and conscious sedation

Nonproprietary name	Proprietary name
Inhalation agents	
Gases	
cyclopropane	—
nitrous oxide	—
ethylene	—
Volatile liquids	
enflurane	Ethrane
ether	—
halothane	Fluothane
isoflurane	Forane
methoxyflurane	Penthrane
Parenteral agents	
Barbiturates	
methohexital	Brevital
thiamylal	Surital
thiopental	Pentothal

*Not available in the United States.

Agents used in general anesthesia
and conscious sedation—cont'd

Nonproprietary name	Proprietary name
Parenteral agents—cont'd	
Carboxyimidazole	
etomidate	Amidate
Benzodiazepines	
diazepam	Valium
lorazepam	Ativan
midazolam*	—
Antihistamines	
hydroxyzine	Vistaril
Antimuscarinics	
scopolamine	—
Opioids	
alphaprodine	Nisentil
fentanyl	Sublimaze
hydromorphone	Dilaudid
meperidine	Demerol
morphine	—
Arylcycloalkylamines	
ketamine	Ketalar
Combinations	
droperidol + fentanyl	Innovar

CITED REFERENCES

1. Allen, G.D., Adams, D., and Scaramella, J. An inhalation analgesia circuit to minimize nitrous oxide pollution. Anesthesia Progress **23**:7-12, 1976.
2. Berkowitz, B.A., Finck, A.D., and Ngai, S.H. Nitrous oxide analgesia: reversal by naloxone and development of tolerance. Journal of Pharmacology and Experimental Therapeutics **203**:539-547, 1977.
3. Brinkley, B.R., and Rao, P.N. Nitrous oxide: effects on the mitotic apparatus and chromosome movement in HeLa cells. Journal of Cell Biology **58**:96-106, 1973.
4. Celesia, G.G., Chen, R.C., Bamforth, B.J. Effects of ketamine in epilepsy. Neurology **25**:169-172, 1975.
5. Cohen, E.N., Brown, B.W., Jr., Bruce, D.L., Cascorbi, H.F., Corbett, T.H., Jones, T.W., and Whitcher, C.E. A survey of anesthetic health hazards among dentists. Journal of the American Dental Association **90**:1291-1296, 1975.
6. Cohen, E.N., and Van Dyke, R.A. Metabolism of Volatile Anesthetics: Implications of Toxicity. Reading, Mass., Addison-Wesley Publishing Co., Inc., 1977.
7. Corssen, G., Miyasaka, M., and Domino, E.F. Changing concepts in pain control during surgery: dissociative anesthesia with CI-581. Anesthesia and Analgesia **47**:746-759, 1968.
8. Duncalf, D. Flammable anesthetics are nearing extinction. Anesthesiology **56**:217-218, 1982.
9. Dundee, J.W. Intravenous Anesthetic Agents. London, Edward Arnold (Publishers) Ltd., 1979.
10. Dykes, M.H.M. Is halothane hepatitis chronic active hepatitis? Anesthesiology **46**:233-235, 1977.
11. Eger, E.I., II. Isoflurane: a review. Anesthesiology **55**:559-576, 1981.
12. Forrest, W.H., Jr., Brown, C.R., and Brown, B.W. Subjective responses to six common preoperative medications. Anesthesiology **47**:241-247, 1977.
13. Gronert, G.A., Milde, J.H., and Theye, R.A. Dantrolene in porcine malignant hyperthermia. Anesthesiology **44**:488-495, 1976.
14. Gronert, G.A., Milde, J.H., and Theye, R.A. Role of sympathetic activity in porcine malignant hyperthermia. Anesthesiology **47**:411-415, 1977.
15. Himes, R.S., Jr., DiFazio, C.A., and Burney, R.G. Effects of lidocaine on the anesthetic requirements for nitrous oxide and halothane. Anesthesiology **47**:437-440, 1977.
16. Julien, R.M., and Kavan, E.M. Electrographic studies of a new volatile anesthetic agent: enflurane (Ethrane). Journal of Pharmacology and Experimental Therapeutics **183**:393-403, 1972.
17. Kripke, B.J., Kelman, A.D., Shah, N.K., Balogh, K., and Handler, A.H. Testicular reaction to prolonged exposure to nitrous oxide. Anesthesiology **44**:104-113, 1976.
18. Lane, G.A. Measurement of anesthetic pollution in oral surgery offices. Journal of Oral Surgery **36**:444-446, 1978.
19. Lane, G.A., Nahrwold, M.L., Tait, A.R., Taylor-Busch, M., Cohen, P.J., and Beaudoin, A.R. Anesthetics as teratogens: nitrous oxide is fetotoxic, xenon is not. Science **210**:899-901, 1980.
20. Layzer, R.B., Fishman, R.A., and Schafer, J.A. Neuropathy following abuse of nitrous oxide. Neurology **28**:504-506, 1978.
21. Lunn, J.K., Stanley, T.H., Eisele, J., Webster, L., and Woodward, A. High dose fentanyl anesthesia for coronary artery surgery: plasma fentanyl concentrations and influence of nitrous oxide on cardiovascular responses. Anesthesia and Analgesia **58**:390-395, 1979.
22. Miyasaka, M., and Domino, E.F. Neural mechanisms of ketamine-induced anesthesia. International Journal of Neuropharmacology **7**:557-573, 1968.
23. Mori, K., Iwabuchi, K., Kawamata, M., Ohta, K., and Fujita, M. The neural mechanism of cyclopropane anesthesia in the rabbit. Anesthesiology **36**:228-237, 1972.
24. Mori, K., Kawamata, M., Miyajima, S., and Fujita, M. The effects of several anesthetic agents on the neuronal reactive properties of thalamic relay nuclei in the cat. Anesthesiology **36**:550-557, 1972.
25. Mukai, S., Morio, M., Fujii, K., and Hanaki, C. Volatile metabolites of halothane in the rabbit. Anesthesiology **47**:248-251, 1977.
26. Nakamura, J., and Winters, W.D. Attenuation of the morphine EEG continuum following a repeat dose within 16 days: delayed tolerance in the rat. Neuropharmacology **12**:607-617, 1973.
27. Quintin, L., Whalley, D.G., Wynands, J.E., Morin, J.E., and Mayer, R. Oxygen-high dose fentanyl-droperidol anesthesia for aortocoronary bypass surgery. Anesthesia and Analgesia **60**:412-416, 1981.
28. Reder, B.S., Trapp, L.D., and Troutman, K.C. Ketamine suppression of chemically induced convulsions in the two-day white leghorn cockerel. Anesthesia and Analgesia **59**:406-409, 1980.

29. Reynolds, E.S., and Moslen, M.T. Halothane hepatotoxicity: enhancement by polychlorinated biphenyl pretreatment. Anesthesiology **47:**19-27, 1977.

30. Sokoll, M.D., Hoyt, J.L., and Gergis, S.D. Studies in muscle rigidity, nitrous oxide, and narcotic analgesic agents. Anesthesia and Analgesia; Current Researches **51:**16-20, 1972.

31. Taub, A., and Kitahata, L.M. Modulation of spinal cord function by anesthesia. Anesthesiology **43:**383-385, 1975.

32. Tekavec, M.M. Nitrous oxide sedation with auditory modification. Anesthesia Progress **23:**181-186, 1976.

33. Wikler, A., and Altschul, S. Effects of methadone and morphine on the electroencephalogram of the dog. Journal of Pharmacology and Experimental Therapeutics **98:**437-446, 1950.

34. Winters, W.D. Neuropharmacological studies and postulates on excitation and depression in the central nervous system. Recent Advances in Biological Psychiatry **9:**313-345, 1966.

35. Yacoub, O., Doell, D., Kryger, M.H., and Anthonisen, N.R. Depression of hypoxic ventilatory response by nitrous oxide. Anesthesiology **45:**385-389, 1976.

36. Yoshimura, N., Holaday, D.A., and Fiserova-Bergerova, V. Metabolism of methoxyflurane in man. Anesthesiology **44:**372-379, 1976.

GENERAL REFERENCES

Attia, R.R., and Grogono, A.W., eds. Practical Anesthetic Pharmacology. New York, Appleton-Century-Crofts, 1978.

Lichtiger, M., and Moya, F., eds. Introduction to the Practice of Anesthesia, ed. 2. New York, Harper & Row, Publishers, 1978.

Marshall, B.E., and Wollman, H. General anesthetics. In Gilman, A.G., Goodman, L.S., and Gilman, A., eds. Goodman and Gilman's The Pharmacological Basis of Therapeutics. ed. 6. New York, Macmillan, Inc., 1980.

Miller, R.D., ed. Anesthesia. New York, Churchill Livingstone, Inc., 1981.

Wade, J.G., and Stevens, W.C. Isoflurane: An anesthetic for the Eighties? Anesthesia and Analgesia **60:**666-682, 1981.

20 Opioid analgesics and antagonists

Gerald F. Gebhart

Opioid (narcotic) analgesics are primarily employed for relief from pain and consequently find widespread application in dentistry. Opioids, however, are not restricted to use as analgesics; they also have therapeutically useful antitussive and constipative effects in addition to undesirable effects, including respiratory depression, pupillary constriction, and at times unwanted constipation. Moreover, repeated use of opioids for relief from pain will produce a tolerance to their analgesic effect as well as physical and sometimes psychologic dependence. These shortcomings notwithstanding, no other drugs are more efficacious as analgesics than the opioids. In addition to the pharmacology of the opioid analgesics, or opioid *agonists,* agents classed as opioid *antagonists* are also considered in this chapter.

OPIOID ANALGESICS

Morphine, the prototypical opioid, and codeine are both natural products contained in opium, which is derived from the poppy plant, *Papaver somniferum.* The unripe seed capsules of the plant are incised, and the milky exudate is collected, dried, and powdered. This opium powder contains approximately 10% to 12% morphine and 0.5% to 1.0% codeine as well as many other alkaloids. None of the other alkaloids is therapeutically useful except papaverine, which is employed as a smooth muscle relaxant. Other currently available opioid analgesics are either semisynthetic modifications of the morphine molecule (e.g., hydromorphone, oxymorphone, hydrocodone, and oxycodone) or entirely synthetic (e.g., meperidine, fentanyl, methadone, and propoxyphene).

Generally, the first knowledge of opium is erroneously credited to Sumeria, one of the first civilizations. There is no acceptable evidence, however, that the Sumerians were familiar with opium or its properties; the first documented descriptions of *Papaver somniferum* do not appear until about 1550 B.C. in the Ebers papyrus of ancient Egypt.[17] Later, in the third century B.C., the writings of the Greek philosopher Theophrastus contained unequivocal references to poppy juice. The active analgesic and constipative principle of the poppy plant, though, was not isolated nor was the drug named (after Morpheus, the Greek god of sleep) until 1803, when Sertürner first isolated and described this active alkaloid from opium. Since then, many semisynthetic and wholly synthetic opioids have been introduced into medicine.

The opioids all share with morphine the ability to produce analgesia, respiratory depression, constipation and gastrointestinal spasm, and physical dependence; none has yet been demonstrated to be significantly different from or superior to morphine with respect to its important pharmacology. The incidence of untoward effects (e.g., respiratory depression) and the intensity of action of the opioids as a group are qualitatively similar and differ but little when compared at equipotent analgesic doses. Consequently, morphine will be discussed in greater detail than any of the other analgesics, and what is stated for morphine will apply in general to these opioids. Significant differences that do exist between morphine and other opioids will be introduced as each individual agent is discussed.

Basis of opioid action

The mechanisms by which opioids act at specific central and peripheral sites to produce their effects are not yet completely understood. Recent discoveries, however, have led to a much clearer understanding of the pharmacology of the opium alkaloids. In the early 1970s, sites in the central nervous system were discovered that stereospecifically

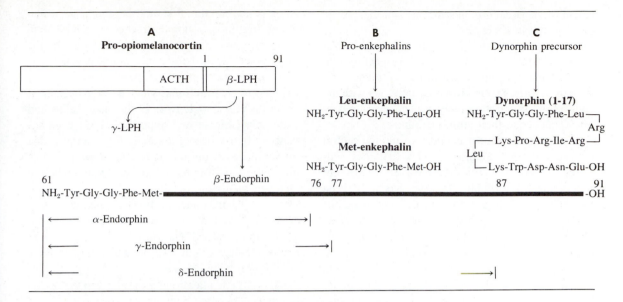

Figure 20-1. Derivation and structure of endogenous opioids. **A,** Endorphins, proteolysis products of the pituitary hormone β-lipotropin (β-LPH), are ultimately derived from the precursor molecule pro-opiomelanocortin. Other peptides of biologic importance obtained from pro-opiomelanocortin include adrenocorticotropin (ACTH), γ-lipotropin (γ-LPH), and several melanotropins (not shown). The initial amino acid sequence of β-endorphin is listed to illustrate its structural relationship to the enkephalins; the numbers refer to amino acid residues of β-LPH. **B,** Enkephalins. In addition to met- and leu-enkephalin, pro-enkephalins may give rise to at least two other biologically active molecules, a heptapeptide and an octapeptide, both of which contain met-enkephalin as part of their structure. **C,** Dynorphins. A common precursor is believed to yield the primary natural dynorphin (1-17, depicted above), a smaller dynorphin (1-8), and at least two other peptides: α-neo-endorphin and β-neo-endorphin.

and reversibly combine with opioids. These opiate receptors, as they were called, were later demonstrated to be the natural effectors of opioid action; that is, specific pharmacologic responses resulted from the binding of opioids to these receptors. The discovery of opioid receptors naturally raised questions as to their biologic significance and spurred research that led to the discovery of the endogenous opioid peptides in the brain. Subsequently, several families of endogenous peptides as well as a number of opioid receptor subtypes have been characterized.

Endogenous opioids. The three families of endogenous opioid peptides are the endorphins, the enkephalins, and the more recently identified dynorphins. Figure 20-1 illustrates the biologic derivations and structural relationships of the currently known opioid peptides. The pentapeptide enkephalins were the first opioid peptides to be discovered: methionine-enkephalin (met-enkephalin) and leucine-enkephalin (leu-enkephalin).[10] These endogenous peptides were subsequent-

ly demonstrated to be potent opioid agonists in the same biologic system in which morphine is active. At first, the enkephalins were thought to be derived from a larger 91–amino acid peptide, β-lipotropin, but it is now clear that β-lipotropin gives rise to a separate group of opioid peptides, the endorphins. The precursors for enkephalins are pro-enkephalin A and pro-enkephalin B, polypeptides containing repeated sequences of met- and leu-enkephalins plus several other active peptides.

The endorphins are a group of endogenous peptides that are larger in molecular size and are distributed differently in the central nervous system than the enkephalins. The parent protein molecule for the endorphins, pro-opiomelanocortin, gives rise to several important hormones, including ACTH and β-lipotropin, which in turn are further processed to form biologically active products. The most important opioid derived from β-lipotropin is β-endorphin, which constitutes the carboxy terminal 30–amino acid sequence of the peptide precursor. Other endorphins, α, γ, and δ, are contained in the β-endorphin structure, but their function is unclear at present.

The precursor for the dynorphins has not yet been characterized. However, with respect to both structure and distribution within the central nervous system, it differs from pro-enkephalin. As with the endorphins, dynorphins contain an enkephalin peptide sequence at their amino terminus.

The location of these peptides within the central nervous system supports the idea that these endogenous opioid peptides are involved in different functions. β-Endorphin, to date, has only been identified in neurons in the medial hypothalamus whose axons terminate in the amygdala, the periaqueductal gray, and the brainstem reticular formation. This peptide is also found in the anterior and intermediate lobes of the pituitary gland, from which it may be released into the general circulation. Its limited distribution in the brain and relatively long duration of action (½ hour for analgesia), suggest that β-endorphin acts more as a neurohormone than as a neurotransmitter.

Neurons containing enkephalins are widely distributed throughout the brain (e.g., periaqueductal gray and limbic system) and the spinal cord where they are considered to be neurotransmitters.[13] In contrast to the endorphins, enkephalins are stored in nerve terminals and are rapidly destroyed when released, as are most neurotransmitters.

Opioid receptors. In addition to discoveries regarding the sources of endogenous opioids, it is now established that there are several subtypes of opioid receptors. Whether these are different receptors or different binding sites on the same receptor is unclear at the present time. Each of the receptor types is distributed differently in the central and peripheral nervous systems and in the smooth muscle of the gastrointestinal tract. The subclasses of receptors are designated mu (μ), kappa (κ), and delta (δ); receptors designated sigma (σ), and epsilon (ε) have also been proposed.[22] The prototypical opioid agonist for the μ receptor is morphine, and its analgesic activity is considered to depend on its binding to the μ receptor. The enkephalins, on the other hand, are considered the typical agonist for the δ receptor, although they also interact with μ receptors. Dynorphin (1-17), representing the third class of opioid peptides, is thought to be the natural ligand for the κ receptor, an opioid receptor present in smooth muscle.[2] Selective ligands for the other receptors have been described, but the existence of these receptor sub-

types is not certain. It should be emphasized that neither the ligands nor the receptors exhibit total selectivity, and morphine, although it may be the prototypical agonist for μ receptors, produces effects at the other opioid receptors as well.

Physiologic functions. Much is yet to be learned about the physiologic roles of the enkephalins and endorphins, but several hypotheses have been advanced. It has been proposed, for example, that the endogenous opioids regulate the secretion of gonadotropins from the pituitary. When the opioid antagonist naloxone is administered to normal subjects, the plasma concentrations of luteinizing hormone (LH) and follicle-stimulating hormone (FSH) are increased. Naloxone apparently releases the hypothalamic neurons from a tonic endogenous opioid inhibition.

Considerable attention has been given to the theory that endogenous peptides influence nociception and that morphine and other centrally acting analgesics interact with the endogenous opioid system at specific receptors to modulate responses to pain. Although it is clear that morphine exerts its analgesic effect by binding to specific receptors in the brain and spinal cord, it has not been conclusively demonstrated that endogenous opioids normally play a significant role in pain reactions. The endogenous opioids and their receptors are present in the anatomic loci considered important to the perception of pain (spinal cord, brainstem reticular formation, periaqueductal gray, etc.); nevertheless, administration of naloxone does not affect resting pain thresholds or responses in human volunteers. One would expect that occupation of the opioid receptors by naloxone, thus preventing any action by the endogenous opioid peptides, would lower the response threshold for pain if endogenous opioids play a tonic role in pain perception. However, naloxone has been shown to negate the analgesic effects of acupuncture and of placebo administration after minor oral surgery and to be hyperalgesic in humans after major surgery. It would appear, therefore, that the endogenous opioid system affecting nociception is normally quiescent but becomes physiologically active in certain situations.

Sites and mechanisms of action. Among the many effects of the exogenous opioids, analgesia has been most thoroughly studied. Early investigators attempted to determine the locus of morphine's analgesic action by administering morphine to selected brain sites. These studies succeeded in

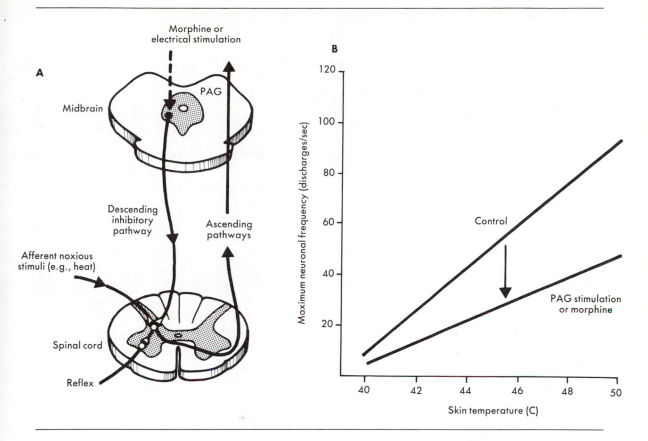

Figure 20-2. Effect of periaqueductal gray (PAG) activation by electrical stimulation or by morphine on the responses of dorsal horn spinal cord neurons to noxious peripheral stimuli. **A,** Activation of a descending pathway by morphine or by electrical stimulation in the periaqueductal gray inhibits neurons in the dorsal horn, attenuating the transmission of noxious signals to the brain and minimizing spinal reflexes. **B,** In the example of noxious heat, periaqueductal gray activation provides analgesia by reducing the slope of the linear relationship between the intensity of thermal stimulation and the rate of dorsal horn neuronal discharge.

identifying the area of brainstem surrounding the cerebral aqueduct as a site involved with morphine analgesia. Evidence from several other avenues of research has also implicated the periaqueductal gray as important to opioid-induced analgesia as well as to the perception of pain.[5] Electrical stimulation of this area in animals and humans produces a strong and long-lasting analgesia.[8] Corollary studies showing that the sites where analgesia can be produced by morphine injection or electrical stimulation are similar to sites containing endogenous opioids[19] and receptors[20] seem to explain the analgesic effect produced by these two forms of stimulation. Indeed, it has been shown that tolerance develops to repeated electrical stimulation just as it does to repeated injections of opioids.[8]

Naloxone antagonizes both the analgesia elicited by electrical stimulation and that produced by opioids.[8] Moreover, both morphine and stimulation in the periaqueductal gray similarly affect transmission of noxious stimuli in the spinal cord.[6] As shown in Figure 20-2, information about pain from peripheral receptors can be influenced at the level of the spinal cord by a descending system of inhibition activated by either morphine or electrical stimulation. Noxious afferent inputs excite and increase the discharge rate of certain spinal neurons, their frequency of discharge varying proportionally with the intensity of the noxious stimulus. Morphine or electrical stimulation in the periaqueductal gray diminishes this response.[3] Morphine administered intravenously has the same effect as the intracerebrally injected morphine.[6] It is well established that, in addition to a direct effect in the brainstem, opioids are capable of producing analgesia when injected directly into the spinal cord;

they may also have a direct action on peripheral nerve transmission.[23]

In summary, the sites of analgesic action of the opioids appear to be widely distributed throughout the nervous system. Knowledge about these sites and about opioid analgesia has been significantly advanced by elucidation of the endogenous opioid system. That is not to say, however, that opioid interactions with other putative neurotransmitters (e.g., norepinephrine, serotonin, ACh, and GABA) are not of equal importance. Opioid effects are complex, and a full understanding of the mechanisms of opioid action awaits further research.

Morphine

The structure of morphine is shown in Figure 20-3. Morphine can be synthesized only with great difficulty. Thus, morphine is extracted from opium, and semisynthetic congeners of morphine are produced by modification of either morphine or thebaine, a structurally related alkaloid present in opium.

Pharmacologic effects

Central nervous system. The CNS effects of morphine are a combination of stimulation and depression and include analgesia, drowsiness, euphoria-dysphoria, respiratory depression, suppression of the cough reflex, pupillary constriction, suppression of the secretion of some (luteinizing hormone) and enhancement of other (prolactin) pituitary hormones, and initial stimulation of the medullary chemoreceptor trigger zone for emesis followed by depression of the vomiting reaction.

Analgesia. The analgesia produced by morphine and its congeners occurs without loss of consciousness. When opioids are administered for relief of pain (or for a cough or diarrhea, for that matter), it must be appreciated that they provide only symtomatic relief without alleviation of the cause of the pain (or cough or diarrhea). The analgesia produced by opioid analgesics is selective in that other sensory modalities (e.g., vision, audition) are unaffected at therapeutic doses. As previously indicated, the central sites and mechanisms of opioid-produced analgesia are incompletely understood. It is believed, however, that brain and spinal sites as well as perhaps a peripheral action on nerve transmission are important to the analgesia produced by morphine and its congeners. It is generally accepted that, in addition to raising the threshold for pain perception, the opioids also alter the reaction to pain. Thus, opioid-induced anal-

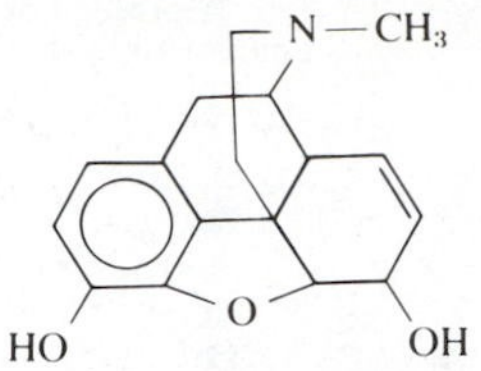

Figure 20-3. Structural formula of morphine.

gesia involves both the sensory-discriminative component (i.e., pain identification and localization) and the motivational-affective component (i.e., reaction to pain) of the pain experience. In fact, the perception of a noxious stimulus may not be as much affected by the opioid analgesics as is the reaction to it, since a common report from patients after receiving an opioid for relief of pain is that the pain is still present but that it is not discomforting. Thus, clinical impressions and patients' reports suggest a prominent action by narcotic analgesics within the motivational-affective component of the pain experience, presumably resulting from opioid action within the limbic system of the brain.

An additional significant feature of the opioid analgesics is that they are generally considered to be more effective against continuous, dull, aching pain than against sharp, intermittent pain. Regardless, morphine and its congeners are the most efficacious analgesics known; they are without peer in relieving pain. The standard parenteral analgesic dose of morphine, 10 mg per 70 kg body weight, is considered near optimal and will relieve moderate to severe pain. Higher doses will provide greater efficacy. It is also known that sensitivity to pain decreases with age and thus the pain relief provided by morphine or other opioids increases with age.

Respiratory depression. Morphine and its congeners depress respiration in a dose-related fashion. This respiratory depression is discernible even with therapeutic doses of morphine and represents the principal undesirable effect, and a potentially life-threatening aspect, of the opioids as a group. The opioids are capable of depressing all three measures of respiration: rate, minute volume, and tidal exchange. In humans, it is believed that the most significant effect of morphine is exerted on the pontine and medullary centers regulating respiratory frequency.[1] The opioid analgesics also act to decrease the response of brainstem respiratory centers to the carbon dioxide tension of the blood. Thus, irregular rhythms and periodic breathing are not uncommon even at therapeutic doses; after toxic doses of morphine or its congeners, the normal respiratory rate of 18 to 20 breaths per minute may be reduced to as low as 3 to 4 per minute. It is important to emphasize that all opioid analgesics are capable of depressing respiration to the same extent when administered in equianalgesic doses.

Cough suppression. Morphine and its congeners are effective antitussives; codeine, for example, is widely employed in cough preparations for this purpose. Morphine itself, however, is not commonly used as a cough suppressant. The opioids exert their antitussive effect by depression of an area within the brainstem. Although the brainstem sites for the respiratory depressant and antitussive effects of the opioids are anatomically close, there is no apparent relationship between opioid depression of one or the other, since nonanalgesic, nonrespiratory-depressant opioid analogues (e.g., dextromethorphan) are effective antitussives. In addition, suppression of the cough reflex occurs at opioid doses lower than that required to produce an analgesic effect or to depress respiration.

Pupillary reaction. At therapeutic doses, morphine and most of its congeners produce pupillary constriction (miosis) in humans. The emphasis on humans is significant, because in some other species, such as cats, in which opioids exert primarily an excitatory effect, the pupils are dilated by morphine and its congeners. The miosis produced by the opioids results from a central effect on the oculomotor nerve and not from an action on the circular or radial muscles of the iris of the eye. Although tolerance to the opioids has not yet been discussed, it is appropriate to indicate at this point that tolerance to the pupillary-constricting effect of morphine and some other opioids does not develop to any appreciable extent. Consequently, chronic users of morphine and heroin, for example, will continue to have constricted pupils although they will have developed a tolerance to many of the other opioid effects.

Nausea and vomiting. The opioids directly stimulate the chemoreceptor trigger zone in the medulla and can produce nausea and vomiting. However, after the initial period of stimulation, the opioids will depress the brainstem medullary center for vomiting. This subsequent depression occurs at therapeutic concentrations and is virtually total; other opioid analgesics or emesis-inducing agents administered during this time are generally ineffective. There is also apparently a vestibular component of the nausea produced by morphine and its congeners, since nausea occurs more frequently in ambulatory than in recumbent patients.

Gastrointestinal tract. The use of opium for relief of diarrhea and dysentery antedated by centuries the use of opium for relief of pain. Indeed, the opioids exert significant effects on smooth muscle all along the gastrointestinal tract. The overall action of morphine and its congeners is constipating, an effect long appreciated and used therapeutically. Opioid analgesics increase smooth muscle tone and decrease propulsive motility throughout the gastrointestinal tract. The opioids produce the most marked delay in gastrointestinal transit at the union of the stomach and the duodenum; opioid effects on the smooth muscle of the small intestine distal to the duodenum do not contribute as much to the delayed gastrointestinal emptying. In the large intestine, muscle spasms can result from the marked increase in muscle tone and nonpropulsive muscle contractions. Spasm of the smooth muscle of the biliary tract, which is often very painful, can also occur after the administration of therapeutic doses of morphine and some of its congeners.

Other smooth muscle. Morphine and other opioids also increase muscle tone in smooth muscle of organs other than those of the gastrointestinal tract, such as the ureters, urinary bladder, uterus, and bronchioles. At therapeutic doses, the effect of opioids on these muscles is generally unremarkable. Therapeutic doses of morphine may contribute to a reduced urine flow, but in addition to effects on tone and contractility of smooth muscle there is an antidiuretic effect of opioids. Opioids also will increase the tone of the uterus, but therapeutic doses of morphine do not generally influence the duration of labor. Likewise in the bronchial musculature, opioids administered at usual therapeutic doses do not produce significant bronchoconstriction, but they may aggravate an asthmatic condition or precipitate an asthmatic attack. In large doses, opioid effects on all of these smooth muscles may be significant: contraction of the ureter will contribute to cessation of urine flow, increased uterine tone will significantly prolong labor and may increase neonatal mortality, and bronchoconstriction will occur.

Cardiovascular system. The effects of morphine and its congeners on blood pressure, heart rate, and cardiac work are generally minor at therapeutic doses. The vasomotor center of the medulla is relatively unaffected by the opioid analgesics, and blood pressure is maintained near normal even after intoxicating doses of opioids. The fall in blood pressure that is observed during acute opioid intoxication is primarily caused by the hypoxia resulting from the opioid-induced respiratory depression.

Morphine and most other opioid analgesics release histamine and produce some vasodilation of the peripheral vasculature, often resulting in an overall sensation of warmth accompanied occasionally by itching of the face and nose. There also appears to be a poorly understood contribution by the central nervous system to the peripheral vasodilation. The resultant fall in peripheral resistance is the primary cause of the orthostatic hypotension and fainting that occur occasionally in some recumbent patients when the head-up position is suddenly assumed. The opioids have no direct effect on the vasculature and circulation of the brain, but cerebral vasodilation is not an uncommon consequence of opioid administration. The cerebral vasodilation is considered to be secondary to the depression of respiration produced by morphine and its congeners and to the consequent retention of carbon dioxide in the blood. The result is an increase in cerebrospinal fluid pressure, which prohibits the use of opioids in cases of cranial trauma and head injury in which cerebrospinal fluid pressure may already be elevated. Morphine also is occasionally employed in the treatment of pulmonary edema, where it is quite effective. The mechanism by which morphine exerts this beneficial action is unclear, but morphine appears to inhibit adrenergic tone centrally, promoting redistribution of blood to the periphery and reducing pressure in the pulmonary veins and capillaries without causing concomitant reduction of the systemic arterial pressure.[21]

Acute opioid intoxication. Death from acute intoxication by an opioid analgesic is most frequently the result of profound, direct respiratory depression. The signs of opioid overdose represent an extension of the pharmacology of these agents. The intoxicated individual is stuporous or asleep and has constricted pupils and depressed respiration. As the severity of intoxication increases, coma ensues and the blood pressure, initially maintained near normal levels, steadily falls if the hypoxia associated with the respiratory depression is unaltered. Measures must be instituted to support

respiration in cases of toxicity; pupillary dilation and shock, both caused by persistent hypoxia, precede death in the absence of an alteration in the respiratory status of the intoxicated individual.

The essential principle of treatment of acute opioid toxicity is restoration of adequate ventilation. This is most rapidly and dramatically achieved by administration of an opioid antagonist (e.g., naloxone), but in the absence of immediately effective opioid antagonism, a patent airway must be established and efficient pulmonary gas exchange must be restored by artificial respiration if necessary. Restoration of adequate pulmonary ventilation will prevent the hypoxic cardiovascular sequelae of opioid intoxication. Although opioid antagonists have not yet been discussed, it is important to interject two notes of caution regarding their use in cases of opioid overdose. First, the duration of most opioid antagonists is shorter than that of most opioid analgesics (which, moreover, have been given or taken in excess). Consequently, the opioid-intoxicated individual requires continued monitoring and readministration of additional opioid antagonist as necessary. Second, administration of an opioid antagonist to an acutely intoxicated, opioid-dependent individual must be initiated with great care. When administered to opioid-dependent individuals, opioid antagonists can precipitate a withdrawal syndrome of great severity that cannot be readily attenuated during the period of action of the antagonist.

Tolerance and physical dependence. Tolerance is defined as the decreased responsiveness to any pharmacologic effect of a drug as a consequence of prior administration of that drug. Consequently, increasingly larger doses must be administered over time to produce an effect equivalent to that produced on initial administration of the drug. Tolerance does not develop uniformly to all opioid effects. In general, tolerance develops to the depressant effects of the opioids but not to the stimulant effects. Thus, tolerance occurs to opioid-induced analgesia, euphoria, drowsiness, and respiratory depression but not, to any appreciable extent, to opioid effects on the gastrointestinal tract or the pupil.

In the therapeutic setting, the initial indication that tolerance has developed will generally be reflected in a shortened duration or reduced efficacy of analgesic effect. The rate at which tolerance emerges to the effects of opioids is a function of the dose and the frequency of administration as well as perhaps other, nonpharmacologic factors.

In general, the greater the opioid dose and the shorter the interval between doses, the more rapid is the development of tolerance. Tolerance, in fact, can occur to such an extent that the lethal dose of the opioid is increased significantly. It should be emphasized, however, that there always exists an opioid dose capable of producing death by respiratory depression regardless of the extent to which tolerance has developed.

Physical dependence refers to an abnormal physiologic state produced by repeated administration of a drug, which then makes its continued use necessary to prevent the appearance of a withdrawal or abstinence syndrome. Just as the rate of development of tolerance to the opioids is dose related, so too is the development of physical dependence. The greater the opioid dose and the longer the duration of administration, the greater is the degree of physical dependence and the more intense is the withdrawal syndrome. The mechanisms underlying the development of tolerance to and physical dependence on the opioids are not understood at present, although various "homeostatic" mechanisms, such as that of Goldstein and Goldstein,[7] have been proposed. Employing a cell culture possessing a large number of opioid receptors, Sharma and colleagues[18] demonstrated that opioid receptors are coupled with adenylate cyclase and that opioids exert a dual regulation: an initial, immediate inhibition of adenylate cyclase followed by a slowly developing increase in total activity. This dual regulation has been suggested to account for all of the known effects of opioids, but it does not rule out other contributing mechanisms.

Opioid analgesics are often rated in terms of "dependence liability" to indicate those agents that are considered to be more likely to produce significant physical dependence than others (see Table 20-1). It is not clear, however, how significant the differences are among opioid analgesics when they are compared at equianalgesic doses via the same route of administration. However, when opioid analgesics are compared in terms of how they are generally used therapeutically, important differences among them arise regarding the development of physical dependence. Thus, morphine has a greater dependence liability than codeine when both are employed in traditional therapeutic modes (i.e., morphine given parenterally for moderate to severe pain and codeine given orally for mild to moderate pain).

Absorption, fate, and excretion. Morphine in particular and most opioids in general are not nearly as effective when given orally as when given parenterally in the same dose. For morphine, oral administration for relief of pain is approximately one tenth as potent as parenteral injection. Since enteral absorption of morphine is good, most of the difference in efficacy between oral and parenteral administration is caused by metabolic inactivation during the first pass through the gastrointestinal tract and liver. The primary pathway for the metabolism of morphine is conjugation with glucuronic acid. Most of the conjugated morphine is eliminated from the body by glomerular filtration; only small amounts of free morphine are found in the urine. Some morphine glucuronide also appears in the bile, and a small percentage is eventually excreted in the feces. Morphine does not generally accumulate in tissues; the total excretion of an administered dose is usually about 90% complete in the first 24 hours.

General therapeutic uses. The opioid analgesics are employed primarily for the relief of pain. As indicated earlier, morphine and its congeners provide only symptomatic relief of pain without influencing its underlying cause. The opioids, when administered at therapeutic doses for the production of analgesia, also produce a drowsiness from which the patient is generally easily aroused as well as a "tranquilization." There is without doubt a significant antianxiety or "tranquilizing" contribution made by the opioids to what is considered to be their analgesic effect. This point was indirectly addressed previously when opioid effects on the motivational-affective component of the pain experience were discussed. Thus, although tolerance, physical dependence, and other undesirable effects (e.g., nausea and vomiting, respiratory depression, and constipation) are drawbacks to opioid use, the opioids undeniably produce a useful combination of desirable effects (e.g., analgesia and sedation).

Aside from their application for pain relief, the opioids are useful in inducing sleep, provided the sleeplessness is due to pain or coughing. Opioid analgesics should not be used for nighttime sedation in the absence of coughing or pain. As mentioned, morphine is also effective in the treatment of pulmonary edema.

Codeine

Codeine, like morphine, is a naturally occurring alkaloid present in opium powder. It differs from morphine in that a methoxy ($-OCH_3$) substitution replaces the hydroxyl ($-OH$) group on the aro-

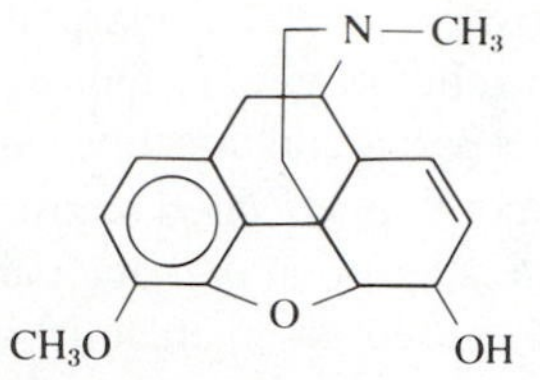

Figure 20-4. Structural formula of codeine.

matic ring of the molecule (Figure 20-4). This relatively minor structural change provides codeine with significant oral effectiveness. In fact, codeine is primarily employed as an orally administered analgesic and antitussive. Like morphine, codeine is metabolized primarily by the liver and is excreted chiefly in the urine, largely in inactive forms. Additionally, a small percentage (approximately 10%) of codeine is demethylated to form morphine in vivo, and both free and conjugated morphine are found in small quantities in the urine after therapeutic doses of codeine.

As with all opioid analgesics, the analgesic and antitussive actions of codeine (as well as respiratory depression, sedation, etc.) are central in origin. Codeine is frequently classified as a "mild analgesic," having an analgesic efficacy significantly less than that of morphine, primarily because codeine is used orally and is recommended for relief of mild to moderate pain. That codeine is a mild analgesic incapable of providing an analgesic effect equivalent to morphine is an erroneous, but widely held, impression. Morphine has an analgesic effect 12 to 13 times more potent than codeine when both drugs are administered intramuscularly. This simply means that approximately 120 mg of codeine is required to produce an analgesic effect equivalent to 10 mg of morphine. Both morphine and codeine are capable of producing significant analgesia. At the present time, however, doses of codeine in excess of 60 mg (orally) are not commonly used and, moreover, are not officially recognized as safe and effective by the Food and Drug Administration. Consequently, the impression remains that codeine has limited analgesic efficacy and that a dose of 60 mg of codeine represents an "analgesic ceiling" above which increased doses of codeine will not provide greater analgesic effect. This generally held impression, while supported by legal regulations, is not consistent with clinical evaluations regarding codeine's analgesic efficacy.[9]

The recommended analgesic dose of codeine is 30 to 60 mg orally; the recommended antitussive dose is 15 to 20 mg orally. At these doses, the side effects of codeine are relatively few and generally insignificant; nausea, constipation, dizziness, and sedation are the effects most frequently observed. At high doses, the frequency of nausea and vomiting is increased, a particularly undesirable effect in individuals who have undergone dental surgery. Among the opioids, codeine is particularly suitable for relief of pain in the ambulatory individual because it is orally effective, can provide significant analgesia and relief of dull, continuous pain, and can be taken for relatively long periods of time with little or no risk of physical dependence. For example, a dose of 60 mg of codeine taken three to four times daily over a period of 6 to 8 weeks is not associated with the development of significant physical dependence. Tolerance will, however, develop to the analgesic effect of codeine over time, and the doses must therefore be gradually increased. The prolonged use of codeine, with gradually increasing doses for the continuous production of analgesia, is associated with some risk of physical dependence. Codeine's demonstrated analgesic usefulness in some situations that show little or limited response to nonopioid analgesics makes codeine a drug of choice for certain pain states. It should be emphasized, however, that cases of dental pain associated with inflammation are best treated by aspirin or other nonopioid analgesics, since neither codeine nor any of the other opioids is antiinflammatory. Thus, aspirin alone or an aspirin-codeine combination is most appropriate for cases of dental pain involving or arising from inflammation; the use of codeine as the sole analgesic in such cases is not recommended.

Oxycodone and hydrocodone

Oxycodone (contained in Percodan) and hydrocodone (contained in Hycodan) are opioids similar in structure to morphine and codeine. Like codeine, both oxycodone and hydrocodone have a methoxy substitution for the phenolic hydroxy group of the morphine molecule. There are also other minor differences from codeine and morphine in the structures of these two agents. The methoxy substitution apparently protects these agents from rapid biotransformation by the liver. Thus, these compounds have good oral efficacy, and they are primarily employed as oral analgesics and antitussives. They do not differ significantly from morphine in terms of their important pharmacology. Oxycodone is approximately equipotent with morphine when given parenterally; it is employed, however, only in oral analgesic preparations. Hydrocodone is generally used as an antitussive and, as such, is approximately 2½ times as potent as codeine.

Meperidine

Meperidine is a synthetic analgesic agent that is structurally dissimilar to morphine. Meperidine was initially evaluated as an atropine-like agent but was subsequently discovered to possess significant analgesic efficacy. In 1939 it was introduced as an analgesic, sedative, and antispasmodic agent effective against most types of pain and supposedly free of many of morphine's undesirable properties. Over time, however, it has been demonstrated that meperidine does not significantly differ from morphine in its pharmacology, and in therapeutic doses (80 to 100 mg parenterally) meperidine produces analgesia, sedation, and respiratory depression, as well as the other CNS actions common to the opioids as a class. Furthermore, meperidine is not the antispasmodic agent it was once believed to be. Like other opioid analgesics, it is spasmogenic to the smooth muscle of the gastrointestinal tract but differs from other opioids in that it is generally not considered to be of value in the treatment of diarrhea. Also, meperidine generally is not associated with the same incidence of spasm of the biliary tract as is morphine, the opioid with which meperidine is most frequently compared. Although meperidine is not used in the treatment of diarrhea, a meperidine congener, diphenoxylate (contained in Lomotil), is widely employed for that purpose.

Morphine is approximately 8 to 10 times more potent than meperidine; when given parenterally at equianalgesic doses, the degree of sedation and respiratory depression is the same for both agents. Meperidine is often mistakenly considered to be a very useful oral analgesic agent at approximately the same dose recommended for parenteral administration (50 to 100 mg). Its oral efficacy, however, is about one fourth its parenteral efficacy; thus, approximately 4 times the dose of meperidine must be administered orally to produce analgesia equivalent to that achieved with parenteral meperidine. The duration of action of meperidine is slightly shorter than that of morphine, necessitating more frequent administration of the drug for relief of continuing pain. Acute intoxication associated with meperidine also differs from that with morphine in

that meperidine sometimes causes CNS excitation, manifested as tremors and convulsions, instead of the profound narcosis and coma usually associated with opioid overdosage.

Regarding the supposed lack of undesirable properties (e.g., physical dependence) associated with meperidine, it is important to note that meperidine is the opioid most commonly abused by health professionals, who still mistakenly believe that meperidine has a lower dependence liability and is easier to stop using than morphine. In fact, meperidine dependence has been widely documented since the drug was first introduced, and it is now recognized that meperidine has a significant abuse potential.

Alphaprodine

Alphaprodine is a phenylpiperidine opioid similar in structure and pharmacology to meperidine. The drug was first used clinically in 1949 and subsequently became a popular premedicant in pediatric dentistry. Alphaprodine is generally administered subcutaneously or intravenously, but many pedodontists favor injecting the drug into the buccal submucosa.

An advantage of alphaprodine over meperidine for preoperative sedation is its greater lipid solubility and hence faster rate of onset. The drug also has a shorter duration of action, which makes it well suited for outpatient surgical procedures. There is surprising disagreement concerning the relative potency of alphaprodine as an analgesic. Published potency values range from 1.5 to 3 times that of meperidine. In a well-controlled study, alphaprodine was found to be 3.7 times more potent than meperidine in causing respiratory depression.[12] Since the drug was often administered in doses more than one-half those normally used for meperidine, it is understandable that some clinicians considered alphaprodine to be more effective than other opioids, whereas other clinicians found it to be more dangerous. In 1980, alphaprodine was voluntarily withdrawn from the market; it was reintroduced in 1982 with a dosage recommendation for pediatric dentistry (0.3 to 0.6 mg/kg) significantly less than that previously used (approximately 1 mg/kg).

Methadone

Methadone is a synthetic opioid analgesic qualitatively similar to other opioids in its pharmacology. The structure of methadone is shown in Figure

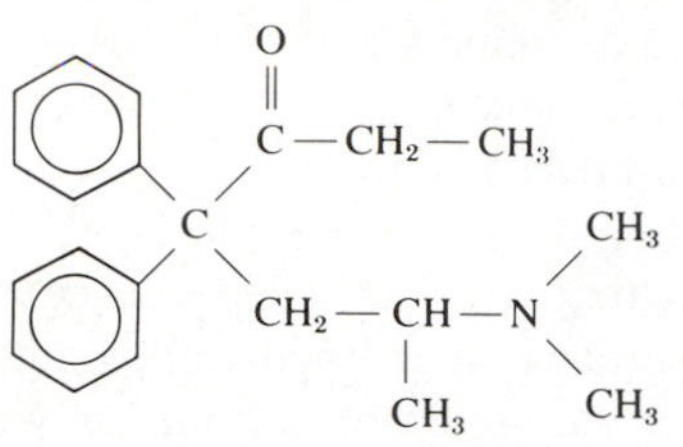

Figure 20-5. Structural formula of methadone.

20-5, and although it does not resemble that of morphine, methadone is induced by steric factors to assume the piperidine-like ring configuration that apparently is required for opioid-like activity. Methadone is approximately equipotent to morphine and, aside from methadone's greater oral efficacy, differs very little from morphine. Methadone, like morphine, produces analgesia, sedation, respiratory depression, miosis, and antitussive effects, as well as subjective effects similar to those of morphine. It also is constipating and causes biliary tract spasm. It is well absorbed from the gastrointestinal tract and eventually becomes localized in the lung, kidney, and liver, where it undergoes extensive biotransformation. The major metabolites of methadone are excreted in the urine and in the bile, along with small quantities of unchanged drug.

While methadone is a potent, orally effective analgesic agent, its primary use at present is replacement for heroin in the treatment of opioid addiction. Methadone possesses a combination of properties that make its application in the treatment of heroin addiction superior to other opioids. As already indicated, methadone has significant oral efficacy and, although its duration of action is similar to that of morphine after a single administration, exhibits a persistent effect when given repeatedly. Thus, methadone's duration of action is effectively increased, permitting a single daily dose in suppressing withdrawal symptoms in opioid-dependent individuals.

The term "blockade" unfortunately was employed when the utility of methadone in maintenance programs for heroin addicts was initially reported. Dole and colleagues[3,4] reported a "blockade" of the effects of heroin and a disappearance of "drug hunger" in heroin addicts after administration of relatively high doses of methadone. The term "blockade" is misleading because it promotes the interpretation that methadone's action is equivalent to antagonism, thus endowing methadone with a pharmacologic property it does not in fact possess. Methadone is *not* an opioid antagonist; it is an opioid *agonist* as are the other opioids discussed in this section. The utility of methadone (or any other opioid, for that matter) in maintenance programs relates to cross-tolerance and cross-dependence and not to some unique ability of methadone to "block" heroin's effects. Cross-tolerance among the opioids means that if an individual has become tolerant to the effects of one opioid (heroin, for example), the individual will also exhibit tolerance to the effects of other opioids. When cross-dependence exists, an individual physically dependent on one opioid will also exhibit physical dependence on other opioids. Thus, the withdrawal syndrome of the heroin-dependent individual can be prevented or reversed by administration of another opioid. These are general statements of principles that apply to the opioids as a class. In practice, the cross-tolerance and cross-dependence among the opioids are incomplete. As used in maintenance programs, methadone simply represents the substitution of one opioid for another, and methadone is employed rather than other opioids primarily because of its oral efficacy and the extended duration of action associated wth repeated administration.

Propoxyphene

Propoxyphene is a synthetic opioid analgesic structurally related to methadone. Propoxyphene was initially introduced and legally classified as a "nonnarcotic" analgesic. At present, it is listed within Schedule IV of the Controlled Substances Act of 1970, whereas codeine, the opioid with which propoxyphene is usually compared, is classed within Schedule II. It has now been amply demonstrated that propoxyphene is subject to abuse and that physical dependence does develop during high-dose, long-term use. Propoxyphene's dependence liability is considered to be slightly less than codeine's.

There is considerable disagreement regarding the analgesic efficacy of propoxyphene. Undeniably, propoxyphene produces CNS effects that appear qualitatively similar to those of codeine and other opioids. However, it is not generally agreed that analgesia is one of those central actions produced by propoxyphene (at the doses commonly employed). Critical reviews of the published literature

Table 20-1. Comparison of opioid analgesics

Nonproprietary name	Proprietary name	Usual therapeutic dose (mg)	Route of administration*	Duration (hours)	Dependence liability
Alphaprodine	Nisentil	40-60	SC	1-2	High
Buprenorphine†	Temgesic	0.3-0.6	IM	6-8	Moderate
Butorphanol†	Stadol	1-4	IM	3-4	Low
		0.5-2	IV		
Codeine	—	30-60	Oral	4-6	Low to moderate
Fentanyl	Sublimaze	0.05-0.1	IM	1.0-1.5	High
		0.05-0.1‡	IV	0.5-1.0	
Heroin§	—	3-5	IM	3-4.5	High
Hydrocodone	Dicodid	5-10	Oral	4-6	Moderate
Hydromorphone	Dilaudid	2	IM	4-5	High
		2-4	Oral	4-5	
Levorphanol	Levo-Dromoran	2-3	SC	4-7	High
		2-3	Oral	4-7	
Meperidine	Demerol	50-100	IM	2-4	High
		50-100	Oral‖	2-4	
Methadone	Dolophine	2.5-10	IM	4-5	Moderate
		5-15	Oral	4-6	
Morphine	—	10-15	IM	4-5	High
Nalbuphine†	Nubain	10	IM	3-6	Low
Oxycodone	In Percodan	5-10	Oral	4-5	High
Oxymorphone	Numorphan	1.0-1.5	IM	4-6	High
Pentazocine†	Talwin	30	IM	2-4	Low
		25-50	Oral	3-5	
Propoxyphene	Darvon	32-65	Oral‖	4-6	Low to moderate

NOTE: Estimates of duration and dependence liability are based on information in the literature and do not pretend to be definitive.
*IM = intramuscular; SC = subcutaneous; IV = intravenous.
†Mixed agonist-antagonist.
‡Much larger doses (e.g., 5 mg) may be used for general anesthesia.
§Heroin is a Schedule I drug and therefore not available for routine clinical use.
‖The efficacy of oral meperidine and propoxyphene is a matter of controversy.

on propoxyphene lead to the conclusion that the drug is no more efficacious an analgesic than aspirin and perhaps is even inferior to aspirin for relief of pain.[14] Nevertheless, propoxyphene is still widely employed, and it is claimed that approximately 65 mg of propoxyphene hydrochloride or 100 mg of propoxyphene napsylate is equivalent in analgesic efficacy to 65 mg of codeine. The currently recognized use of propoxyphene is for the treatment of mild to moderate pain; because of initial claims of an absence of dependence liability, propoxyphene is often prescribed in place of codeine as a centrally acting oral analgesic. As previously indicated, there appears to be no significant difference between the dependence liability of codeine and of propoxyphene, and the continued use of propoxyphene appears to derive from unjustified overconcern regarding codeine's addiction potential. Acute intoxication with propoxyphene can produce respiratory and CNS depression, confusion, hallucinations, and occasionally convulsions.

Fentanyl

Fentanyl is a relatively new synthetic opioid employed primarily as an anesthetic supplement. It is approximately 80 times more potent than morphine, but its duration of analgesic action is approximately one-third that of morphine. In combination with droperidol, fentanyl is available as Innovar and is employed for neuroleptanalgesia. Fentanyl is described in further detail in Chapter 19.

Other agents

A number of opioid analgesics, some listed in Table 20-1, have been omitted from discussion in this chapter on the basis that they offer no therapeutic advantage over morphine or codeine and for the most part are not widely used. New opioid analgesics continue to be developed, however, and it is likely that some of these will find clinical application. One promising group of drugs includes various analogues of fentanyl.[11] Sufentanil, one such drug, is approximately 10 times more potent than fentanyl and may be more effective in preventing sympathetic nervous system responses to surgical stimuli during general anesthesia. Of special interest to dentistry is alfentanil. This analgesic is remarkable in its brief duration of action and short metabolic half-life, both of which are less than one-half that of fentanyl. Alfentanil may be particularly well suited for outpatient intravenous sedation.

A second source of new analgesics is in analogues of the endogenous opioids. Although the naturally occurring enkephalins are quickly destroyed by various enzymes after injection, replacement of one or more amino acid residues with synthetic derivatives results in compounds that are effective parenterally and even retain some activity after oral administration.[16] Similar peptides may find use, not as analgesics per se, but rather as inhibitors of enzymes normally responsible for inactivation of endogenous opioids.

OPIOID ANTAGONISTS

Agents classed as opioid antagonists can be divided into two groups: "pure" antagonists and mixed antagonists (or agonist-antagonists). Naloxone is the only pure opioid antagonist currently available; however, a second drug, naltrexone, is being evaluated for clinical use. The group of agents possessing both agonist and antagonist efficacy can be further subdivided into drugs used as opioid antagonists and those administered for their agonist (i.e., analgesic) efficacy. Nalorphine and levallorphan are drugs that have been used to block opioid effects; pentazocine and the newer agonist-antagonists are marketed as analgesics.

The number of agonist-antagonists has grown considerably since the early 1950s, when it became widely appreciated that appropriate chemical manipulation of the opioid structure produced compounds that possessed most actions of the opioids but were also capable of reversing or antagonizing the effects of opioids given concomitantly. It was quickly learned, however, that agents having both agonist and antagonist properties were often unsuitable for clinical use as analgesics because of an undesirably high incidence of dysphoric side effects. New compounds continue to be synthesized and tested for use as analgesics, since it is believed that agents with an appropriate balance of agonist-antagonist properties should have a low dependence liability as well as utility in the treatment of heroin addiction. Several such drugs are now available for clinical use.

Although it was hoped that agonist-antagonists would not be abused and would have little or no dependence liability, the opioid-blocking aspect of their pharmacology does not prevent their abuse nor does it free these compounds of tolerance and dependence. Tolerance will develop to the agonist but not antagonist effects of these drugs. Subjects who repeatedly use these agents may become physically dependent, just as can occur with repeated use of morphine. Naloxone is an exception among the opioid antagonists; having no agonist effects, naloxone can be repeatedly given without either loss of efficacy or development of physical dependence. Among those agents classed as mixed antagonists, physical dependence has not been a problem with the use of nalorphine, primarily because it does not produce subjective effects that would encourage an individual to abuse the drug. All agonist-antagonists used for analgesia, however, can cause physical dependence, although the withdrawal symptoms differ somewhat from those produced by opioid agonists such as morphine.

As previously indicated, morphine is the prototypical opioid analgesic. All of its actions (analgesia, respiratory depression, gastrointestinal effects, etc.) are agonistic. When administered in the absence of an opioid, the agonist-antagonists also produce analgesia, respiratory depression, etc. When administered in the presence of an opioid, however, these agents may (1) prevent opioid effects if given just before or at the same time as the opioid analgesic, (2) reverse the effects if given after the administration of the opioid, as in acute opioid intoxication, or (3) precipitate a withdrawal syndrome in the opioid-dependent individual.

In addition to their potential utility as analgesic agents with a low dependence liability, antagonists have other uses. A primary therapeutic application of some agents in this class is in the treatment of opioid-induced respiratory depression. In acute opioid intoxication, the opioid antagonists are specific and will rapidly improve ventilation. It must be emphasized, however, that opioid antagonists are not general respiratory stimulants, as is sometimes assumed. Opioid antagonists will not alter respiratory depression produced by other drugs (e.g., barbiturates and alcohol) and in fact may worsen the respiratory depression associated with these other centrally acting drugs because of their own opioid agonist effect on respiration. Naloxone is exceptional in that it will not further embarrass respiration if administered to individuals suffering from respiratory depression produced by agents other than opioid analgesics. Opioid antagonists have also been employed in the diagnosis of opioid physical dependence. A final, potential application of opioid antagonists is in the possible prevention of relapse to opioid dependency. In general, they have been unsuccessful when evaluated for prevention of relapse to heroin addiction primarily because of their undesirable psychotomimetic and dysphoric effects. However, naltrexone, which combines oral efficacy, a long duration of action, and a lack of agonist characteristics, may prove to be a useful adjunct in the maintenance program of detoxified opioid addicts.

Nalorphine and levallorphan

Nalorphine was the first opioid antagonist. It differs in structure from morphine only in that an allyl group ($-CH_2CH = CH_2$) replaces the methyl group ($-CH_3$) at the nitrogen atom of the morphine molecule (Figure 20-6). This single alteration in structure endows nalorphine with both agonist and antagonist efficacy. Although no longer available in the United States, the drug will be discussed because of its historical importance.

Nalorphine is equipotent to morphine as an analgesic and also has agonist effects on the gastrointestinal tract as well as on respiration. When administered immediately before or shortly after an opioid, nalorphine will antagonize most of the gastrointestinal and CNS effects of that opioid. It will effectively reverse profound opioid-induced respiratory depression within minutes after intravenous administration of a 5 to 10 mg dose. Depending on the severity of the acute opioid intoxication, nalorphine may have to be readministered to maintain satisfactory pulmonary ventilation because nalorphine's duration of action is shorter than that of most opioids. Levallorphan remains the only mixed antagonist on the market that is used for its morphine-blocking action. It is approximately 7 to 10 times more potent an antagonist than nalorphine but is less active as an analgesic. Otherwise, levallorphan is similar to nalorphine in its pharmacologic profile.

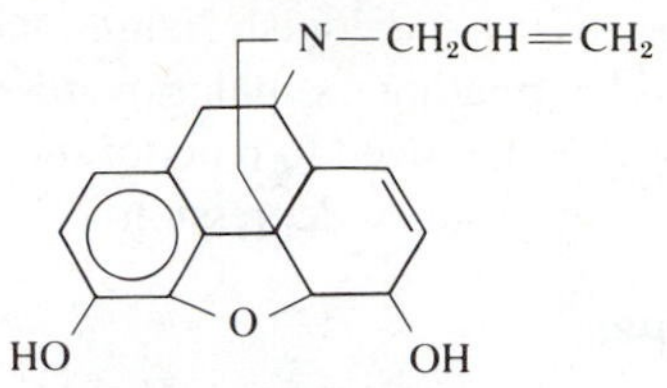

Figure 20-6. Structural formula of nalorphine.

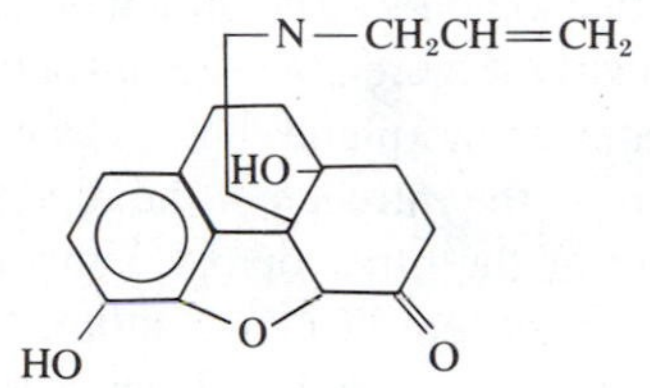

Figure 20-7. Structural formula of naloxone.

Naloxone and naltrexone

Naloxone is the only opioid antagonist currently available that is essentially devoid of opioid agonist effects (Figure 20-7). Naloxone is approximately 8 times more potent an opioid antagonist than nalorphine. In addition to antagonizing the effects of opioids, naloxone can block the agonist actions of most agonist-antagonists. This is an important point, since the respiratory depression produced by pentazocine, an agonist-antagonist, is reversible by naloxone but not by nalorphine. As mentioned previously, because naloxone lacks opioid agonist effects, its administration will not further compromise the respiratory status of an individual who has taken a nonopioid intoxicant. Like nalorphine and levallorphan, the duration of action of naloxone is relatively short (between 1 to 4 hours), and the drug is ineffective orally.

Naltrexone is a pure antagonist currently in the investigational stage of drug development. Although similar in most respects to naloxone, naltrexone is orally active and has a remarkably long duration of action for an opioid antagonist. As previously stated, these attributes suggest that naltrexone may be of use in the rehabilitation of some opioid addicts. Indeed, single daily administration of the drug can effectively block the action of 25 mg of heroin injected intravenously 24 hours after the last dose of the antagonist. Naltrexone may also prove useful in treating morphine overdose because it might obviate the need to monitor the patient for a relapse of respiratory depression.

Pentazocine

Pentazocine is an opioid agonist with very weak opioid antagonist activity. It is approximately one fiftieth as potent an opioid antagonist as nalorphine; however, because of its low antagonist activity pentazocine cannot be appropriately classed with the morphine-like opioids. The structure of pentazocine is shown in Figure 20-8. Pentazocine is structurally related to morphine, but it has an allyl-like substitution on the nitrogen of the piperidine ring, as do many of the other opioid antagonists. This compound is the product of continued efforts to develop efficacious opioid analgesics with little or no abuse potential or dependence liability. Pentazocine is promoted as such, but like other opioids it produces its major effects on the central nervous system and gastrointestinal tract and induces morphine-like subjective effects and euphoria. Thus, physical dependence can develop to pentazocine, and the drug is subject to abuse. Unlike codeine or propoxyphene (or other opioids), however, pentazocine will not suppress withdrawal symptoms in individuals dependent on other opioids, but neither can it antagonize morphine-induced respiratory depression. Pentazocine, however, can precipitate an abstinence syndrome in an opioid-dependent individual because of its residual antagonist activity, thus reemphasizing pentazocine's status among the mixed antagonists.

Pentazocine is well absorbed from the gastrointestinal tract; it is metabolized primarily in the liver, and glucuronide conjugates and small quantities of free pentazocine are excreted in the urine. It is approximately one third as potent an analgesic as morphine when given intramuscularly and approximately equipotent to codeine as an analgesic when given orally. Pentazocine is extensively used orally, generally in place of codeine; approximately 50 mg of pentazocine is considered equivalent to 60 mg of codeine for relief of pain. Like codeine, pentazocine's ability to obtund pain at higher doses is comparable to that of morphine (i.e., they have approximately equivalent analgesic efficacy). At therapeutic doses, pentazocine exhibits effects on the central nervous system and gastrointestinal tract that are qualitatively similar to those of other opioids (e.g., dizziness, nausea, and sedation as

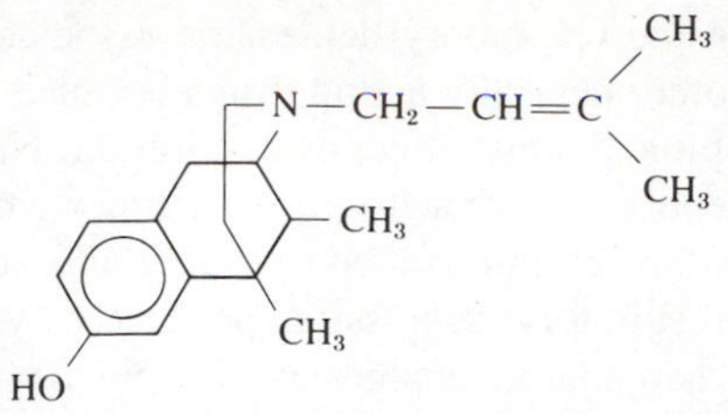

Figure 20-8. Structural formula of pentazocine.

well as analgesia). Unlike most other opioids, however, pentazocine can increase both heart rate and blood pressure. In toxic doses, it produces both nalorphine-like dysphoric effects and characteristic opioid-like respiratory depression, though the respiratory depression does not increase proportionately with increasing doses as it does for the opioid agonists. It should be reiterated that pentazocine is somewhat unusual in that only naloxone can counteract the agonist effects of pentazocine.[15]

Nalbuphine, buprenophine, and butorphanol

Nalbuphine, buprenorphine, and butorphanol are further examples of drugs with a mixture of agonist and antagonist properties. Nalbuphine is approximately as potent as morphine and has one fourth the antagonist activity of nalorphine; butorphanol is equipotent to morphine and has an antagonist potency one fortieth that of naloxone. It is claimed that these two drugs have the advantage over morphine of having low abuse potential. In addition, although at therapeutic doses they cause respiratory depression equivalent to that produced by 10 mg of morphine, the depression does not increase proportionately with increasing doses. In at least one third of patients there is significant sedation with both these drugs; other effects commonly associated with pentazocine and the opioid analgesics, such as nausea and vomiting, dizziness, hallucinations, and confusion, are less frequent. Butorphanol shares with pentazocine a tendency in analgesic doses to increase cardiac work. Nalbuphine and butorphanol have rapid onsets of action after intravenous administration (2 to 3 minutes) and only modest delays in onset (less than 30 minutes) after intramuscular or subcutaneous injection. The duration of action for butorphanol is 3 to 4 hours; for nalbuphine it is approximately 3 to 6 hours. The effects of both drugs are antagonized by naloxone.

Buprenorphine, the newest analgesic with opioid antagonist properties, is 25 to 50 times more potent an agonist than morphine and has approximately 10 times the antagonist activity of nalorphine. Its agonist effects are qualitatively similar to those of morphine, and buprenorphine produces a physical dependence described by addicts as morphine-like. Like butorphanol, nalbuphine, and pentazocine, however, buprenorphine may precipitate an abstinence syndrome in an opioid-dependent individual because of its residual antagonistic efficiency. In contrast to butorphanol and nalbuphine, buprenorphine has a long duration of action, with its nonanalgesic effects (e.g., miosis and respiratory depression) exhibiting maximal intensities long after administration. Even large doses of naloxone may fail to block the respiratory depression caused by an overdose of this drug.

USES IN DENTISTRY

Opioids used in dentistry are primarily those available for oral administration: codeine, meperidine, oxycodone, propoxyphene, and pentazocine. (In addition, alphaprodine, morphine, and fentanyl are used parenterally, as described in Chapter 44.) While these agents all possess therapeutically useful actions in addition to analgesia, they are employed in dentistry exclusively for pain relief. It should be recognized, however, that pain of dental origin frequently arises from or is accompanied by inflammation. Since opioids are not antiinflammatory, nonopioid analgesic agents with antiinflammatory efficacy (e.g., aspirin) are often the first avenue for relief of pain. Opioids are particularly useful when additional relief of pain is required; the opioids are capable of providing significantly greater analgesic relief than are the nonopioid analgesics (i.e., the opioids possess significantly greater analgesic efficacy). Combinations of opioids with aspirin, for example, are commonly employed and are rational, since both central and peripheral mechanisms of analgesia, respectively, are invoked.

Among the opioids available for use in dentistry, codeine is commonly the drug of choice. As previously indicated, the analgesic efficacy of propoxyphene is somewhat controversial, as is that of meperidine given orally in conventional doses.

IMPLICATIONS FOR DENTISTRY

The opioid analgesics are, of course, subject to abuse, and both significant physical dependence and addiction can develop. These aspects of the pharmacology and sociology of opioids are discussed in Chapter 46. Additional implications for dentistry relate to the possible interactions of opioids with other drugs that dentists may prescribe or that their patients may be taking for medical reasons. Drug interactions with orally administered opioids are not common nor usually of great clinical importance when they do occur. There are, however, recognized interactions between opioids and phenothiazine neuroleptics, tricyclic antidepressants, MAO inhibitors, and oral anticoagulants that can be clinically significant, particularly if the opioids are given parenterally. In general, the coadministration of CNS depressants often produces at least an additive depression and occasionally a greater than anticipated depression (i.e., potentiation). Opioids and phenothiazines (e.g., chlorpromazine) are known to produce an additive CNS depression as well as occasional enhancement of the actions of opioids (e.g., respiratory depression). Moreover, this combination may also produce a greater incidence of orthostatic hypotension than either agent administered alone. Increased hypotension has also been reported with combinations of opioids and tricyclic antidepressants. While combinations of opioids and either phenothiazines or tricyclic antidepressants have been reported to result in interactions, there are contradictions in the literature and the evidence is not conclusive. Thus, the clinical significance of these interactions, particularly at the doses of opioids employed orally in dentistry, is uncertain.

Interaction of opioids with oral anticoagulants has been reported to result in an enhanced response to the latter, but the clinical significance has not been established, and it is not likely that short-term opioid administration has an appreciable effect on the patient's response to oral anticoagulants.

A well-documented interaction of meperidine and MAO inhibitors results in severe and immediate reactions that include excitation, rigidity, and hypertension. Chemically unrelated opioids are not likely to cause a similar reaction.

Opioid analgesics and antagonists	
Nonproprietary name	*Proprietary name*
Agonist analgesics	
alphaprodine	Nisentil
codeine*	—
fentanyl	Sublimaze

*Also used as antitussives or cough suppressants.
†Not currently available in the United States.

Opioid analgesics and antagonists—cont'd

Nonproprietary name	Proprietary name
Agonist analgesics—cont'd	
hydrocodone*	Dicodid
hydromorphone	Dilaudid
levorphanol	Levo-Dromoran
meperidine	Demerol
methadone	Dolophine
morphine	—
opium	Pantopon
oxycodone	in Percodan
oxymorphone	Numorphan
propoxyphene	Darvon
Mixed agonist/antagonist analgesics	
buprenorphine†	Temgesic
butorphanol	Stadol
nalbuphine	Nubain
pentazocine	Talwin
Antagonists	
levallorphan	Lorfan
nalorphine†	Nalline
naloxone	Narcan
naltrexone†	—

CITED REFERENCES

1. Borison, H.L. Central nervous respiratory depressants—narcotic analgesics. Pharmacology and Therapeutics **3**:227-237, 1977.
2. Chavkin, C., James, I.F., and Goldstein, A. Dynorphin is a specific endogenous ligand of the kappa opioid receptor. Science **215**:413-415, 1982.
3. Dole, V.P., and Nyswander, M.E. Heroin addiction: a metabolic disease. Archives of Internal Medicine **120**:19-24, 1967.
4. Dole, V.P., Nyswander, M.E., and Kreek, M.J. Narcotic blockade. Archives of Internal Medicine **118**:304-309, 1966.
5. Gebhart, G.F. Opiate and opioid peptide effects on brain stem neurons: relevance to nociception and antinociceptive mechanisms. Pain **12**:93-140, 1982.
6. Gebhart, G.F., Sandkuhler, J., Thalhammer, J.G., and Zimmermann, M. Inhibition in the spinal cord of nociceptive information by electrical stimulation and morphine microinjection at identical sites in the midbrain in the cat. Journal of Neurophysiology **51**:75-89, 1984.
7. Goldstein, D.B., and Goldstein, A. Possible role of enzyme inhibition and repression in drug tolerance and addiction. Biochemical Pharmacology **8**:48, 1961.
8. Hosobuchi, Y., Adams, J.E., and Linchitz, R. Pain relief by electrical stimulation of the central gray matter in humans and its reversal by naloxone. Science **197**:183-186, 1977.
9. Houde, R.W., Wallenstein, S.L., and Beaver, W.T. Clinical measurement of pain. In deStevens, G., ed. Analgesics. New York, Academic Press, Inc., 1965.
10. Hughes, J. Isolation of an endogenous compound from the brain with pharmacological properties similar to morphine. Brain Research **88**:295-308, 1975.
11. Janssen, P.A.J. Potent, new analgesics, tailor-made for different purposes. Acta Anaesthesiologica Scandinavica **26**:262-268, 1982.
12. Kaufman, R.D., Aqleh, K.A., and Bellville, J.W. Relative potencies and durations of action with respect to respiratory depression of intravenous meperidine, fentanyl and alphaprodine in man. Journal of Pharmacology and Experimental Therapeutics **208**:73-79, 1979.
13. Miller, R.J. Peptides as neurotransmitters: focus on the enkephalins and endorphins. Pharmacology and Therapeutics **12**:73-108, 1981.
14. Miller, R.M., Feingold, A., and Paxinos, J. Propoxyphene hydrochloride—a critical review. Journal of the American Medical Association **213**:996-1006, 1970.
15. Payne, J.P. The clinical pharmacology of pentazocine. Drugs **5**:1-5, 1973.
16. Roemer, D., Buescher, H.H., Hill, R.C., Pless, J., Bauer, W., Cardinaux, F., Closse, A., Hauser, D., and Huguenin, R. A synthetic enkephalin analogue with prolonged parenteral and oral analgesic activity. Nature **268**:547-549, 1977.
17. Sapira, J.D. Speculations concerning opium abuse and world history. Perspectives in Biology and Medicine **18**:379-398, 1975.
18. Sharma, S.K., Klee, W.A., and Nirenberg, M. Dual regulation of adenylate cyclase accounts for narcotic dependence and tolerance. Proceedings of the National Academy of Sciences of the United States of America **72**:3092-3096, 1975.
19. Simantov, R., Kuhar, M.J., Pasternak, G.W., and Snyder, S.H. The regional distribution of a morphine-like factor enkephalin in monkey brain. Brain Research **106**:189-197, 1976.
20. Simon, E.J. The opiate receptors. Neurochemical Research **1**:3-28, 1976.
21. Ward, J.M., McGrath, R.L., and Weil, J.V. Effects of morphine on peripheral vascular response to sympathetic stimulation. American Journal of Cardiology **29**:659-666, 1972.
22. Wood, P.L. Multiple opiate receptors: support for unique mu, delta and kappa sites. Neuropharmacology **21**:487-497, 1982.
23. Yaksh, T.L. Spinal opiate analgesia: characteristics and principles of action. Pain **11**:293-346, 1981.

GENERAL REFERENCES

Adler, M.W., Manara, L., and Samanin, R. Factors Affecting the Action of Narcotics. New York, Raven Press, 1978.
Beers, R.F., Jr., and Bassett, E.G., eds. Mechanisms of Pain and Analgesic Compounds. New York, Raven Press, 1979.
Bonica, J.J., ed. Pain. New York, Raven Press, 1980.
Bonica, J.J., Albe-Fessard, D.G., and Liebeskind, J.C., eds. Advances in Pain Research and Therapy, vol. 4. New York, Raven Press, 1983.
Martin, J.B., Reichlin, S., and Bick, K.L., eds. Neurosecretion and Brain Peptides: Implications for Brain Functions and Neurological Disease. New York, Raven Press, 1981.

21 Peripherally acting (nonopioid) analgesics

Stephen A. Cooper
Paul J. Desjardins

Aspirin and acetaminophen have been recognized for many years as prototypes for the peripherally acting, nonopioid analgesics. Today there are several other drugs challenging the clinical status of these prototypes. Some of the claims made for these agents are a greater peak analgesia, a longer duration of action, and a lower incidence of side effects. Because the dentist must treat acute pain on a daily basis, the peripherally acting analgesics are of particular importance, and the primary objective of this chapter will be to present the most current information on the drugs, with the goal of providing a rational basis for their use in clinical practice.

ETIOLOGY OF PAIN

The initial event for most painful conditions is a noxious stimulus that results in the destruction or injury of tissue. The trauma may be initiated by a disease process, such as an apical abscess, or by surgical intervention, such as the extraction of a tooth. In either case, the resultant cellular destruction causes the release or synthesis of several biochemical mediators involved in the pain process (e.g., histamine, bradykinin, and other short-acting substances). Lysosomal proteins from the ruptured cells release histamine from storage sites in mast cells. Histamine causes increased capillary permeability that results in edema, redness, sensitization of nerve endings, and migration of cells such as polymorphonuclear (PMN) leukocytes and lymphocytes into the area. Histamine plays a major role in the early stages of tissue injury, but because it is quickly metabolized, it is not thought to play a key role in the later and more prolonged stages of the pain response.[16,47] Bradykinin also is found wherever there is tissue injury. Bradykinin is a nonapeptide that normally exists in a precursor form (kininogen) in the plasma α-globulin fraction. After tissue injury, an inactive enzyme, prekallikrein, is activated to kallikrein, which then transforms the kininogen to free bradykinin. Bradykinin diffuses throughout the area of injury and is involved in edema formation and sensitization of free nerve endings. Like histamine, it also has a short half-life and plays its major role in the early phases after injury.[16]

The more prolonged periods of pain and inflammation appear to be integrally involved with the reactions leading to the formation of prostaglandins. These reactions are complex and not completely understood, but an attempt will be made to present their role, as it is currently envisaged, in the overall picture of the pain response. When cells are ruptured, arachidonic acid, as well as other long-chain fatty acids, is released from cellular membranes as they become exposed to plasma phospholipases. Free arachidonic acid is highly reactive and is rapidly biotransformed by cyclooxygenase (prostaglandin synthetase) enzymes to cyclic fatty acids known as endoperoxides. The endoperoxides are unstable and through a cascade of reactions eventually form the prostaglandins. Many of the intermediates, as well as the prostaglandin products PGE_1 and PGE_2, are potent mediators of pain and inflammation.[16,47,48] There is an abundance of experimental evidence showing that when arachidonic acid or prostaglandins are injected into various tissues, prolonged pain and inflammation occur. However, if the animals are pretreated with inhibitors of prostaglandin synthesis, then the injection of arachidonic acid will not cause pain or inflammation. It is equally important that in vivo the prostaglandins are present at physiologically active concentrations as long as tissue debris, PMN cells, macrophages, and lymphocytes are present at the site of injury.[47]

The prostaglandins cause hyperalgesia by sensitizing nociceptive (pain) receptors in the periphery to other algesic mediators, such as bradykinin, and to physical forces. Once these receptors are stimulated, impulses are sent to the central nervous system where the brain interprets them and signals the appropriate response.

PHARMACOLOGIC APPROACHES TO CONTROLLING PAIN

There are three groups of drugs widely used in dentistry to control pain. The local anesthetics are administered parenterally or topically to block the propagation of nerve impulses so that the impulses arising from nociceptive stimuli at the peripheral site do not reach the brain, where they would normally be interpreted as pain. The centrally acting (opioid) analgesics affect the interpretation of and reaction to the impulses that reach the brain but have no proven analgesic effect at the site of injury or on nerve conduction. The local anesthetics and the centrally acting analgesics are discussed in Chapters 17 and 20, respectively. A few of the opioid analgesics will be mentioned in this chapter, because they are frequently used in combination with the peripherally acting analgesics.

Peripherally acting analgesics reduce or control pain by directly inhibiting the biochemical mediators of pain at the site of injury. In addition to their analgesic property, the majority of drugs in this class have antiinflammatory and antipyretic activity. In fact, they are often referred to as the nonsteroidal antiinflammatory drugs (NSAIDs). Occasionally, these drugs are referred to as ''mild analgesics,'' but this is a misnomer, and the use of this term should be discontinued.

Lim and colleagues,[28] in a cross-perfusion experiment using dogs, clearly demonstrated that certain drugs do indeed work in the brain, whereas other analgesics are active at the site of injury. Since these early experiments, there has been an accumulation of evidence supporting the classification of analgesics as either centrally acting or peripherally acting.

The primary mechanism of action of the peripherally acting analgesics is inhibition of the cyclooxygenase enzyme system that metabolizes arachidonic acid to its endoperoxide intermediates. Once formed, the endoperoxides are converted to thromboxanes, prostacyclin, and prostaglandins. Various intermediates and end products of this arachidonate cascade interact with other local mediators, such as bradykinin, histamine, and 5-hydroxytryptamine, to promote erythema, edema, and pain. Some evidence suggests that several recently introduced analgesics may owe their exceptional efficacy not only to a more effective inhibition of important isoenzymes of the cyclooxygenase system at the site of injury but also to secondary effects of cyclooxygenase inhibition within the central nervous system. Of course, unknown peripheral and central mechanisms also may contribute to their efficacy.

Differences in the clinical efficacy and side effects between aspirin and acetaminophen and the more recent analgesics may additionally be the result of variations in lipid solubility, protein binding, penetration of the blood-brain barrier, and liver metabolism. These differences will be mentioned as the particular drugs are discussed.

The peripherally acting analgesics are extremely important to pain control in dentistry because they can be taken orally, they do not cause CNS or respiratory depression at therapeutic doses (as do the centrally acting drugs), and, most important, they are very effective pain relievers.

ASPIRIN AND RELATED SALICYLATES

Aspirin has been commercially available since 1899, and until the late 1970s no peripherally acting analgesic could claim greater efficacy. The fact that the American public consumes in excess of 20 tons of aspirin each day and that aspirin or a closely related salicylate is found in over 400 different proprietary compounds justifies a thorough review of this drug.[45]

Chemistry and classification

Aspirin belongs to the salicylates, a class of compounds that were originally obtained from botanical sources. The first active substance of this group, salicin, was isolated from the bark of the willow tree. From salicin were synthesized salicylic acid, sodium salicylate, and finally acetylsalicylic acid (aspirin).[41,45] The structures of aspirin and related drugs are shown in Figure 21-1. The acetylsalicylic acid form was found to be preferable to its predecessors, and since the turn of the century its value as an antipyretic and antirheumatic agent has been firmly established.

Salicylamide is an amide derivative of salicylic acid. This drug has never been shown to have any clinically useful activity nor does it release salic-

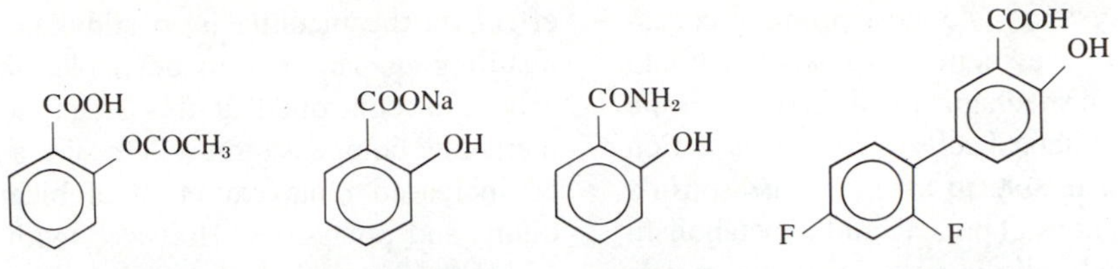

Figure 21-1. Salicylates and related structures.

ylate during metabolism. The rationale for including it as part of an analgesic or antipyretic combination is that salicylamide is rapidly transformed in the liver by conjugation and therefore saturates this biotransformation system, prolonging the half-lives of the other analgesic constituents. However, there is no experimental evidence to support this mechanism, and in all likelihood salicylamide makes little, if any, pharmacologic contribution to an analgesic mixture.

Pharmacologic effects

As has already been pointed out, aspirin has clinically useful analgesic, antipyretic, antiinflammatory, and antirheumatic effects. In the section that follows, its action on specific organs and systems will be considered.

Antipyretic effects. The antipyretic properties of aspirin are well documented. However, antipyresis is best demonstrated in febrile patients, since normal subjects show no marked change in body temperature when aspirin is administered. The primary mechanism for antipyresis appears to be related to the inhibition of synthesis of prostaglandin-like substances in the brain. Prostaglandins are potent pyrogens, and a prostaglandin-like substance has been isolated from febrile animals.[16,47] Other experimental evidence suggests that the reduction of temperature may be caused in part by a peripherally mediated superficial vasodilation or by a centrally mediated resetting of the temperature control center in the hypothalamus.[20,36]

Antiinflammatory effects. It is difficult to separate the analgesic and antiinflammatory effects of aspirin, since the vast majority of painful conditions have an inflammatory component. There is little doubt that the cascade of reactions leading to the formation of prostaglandins is integrally in-

volved with the inflammatory response and that aspirin's efficacy in treating inflammation is closely related to its inhibition of prostaglandin synthetase. This mechanism is attractive because aspirin is an effective antiinflammatory agent, regardless of the etiology of the inflammation. The fact that aspirin appears to inhibit the formation of common mediators of inflammation rather than the specific causes of various inflammatory reactions may explain why aspirin reduces inflammation in such diverse conditions as rheumatoid arthritis, postsurgical inflammation, and the inflammation that occurs in response to foreign bodies or musculoskeletal injuries. Other mechanisms that may be involved in aspirin's antiinflammatory effect include inhibition of leukocyte phagocytosis, suppression of immunologic processes, stabilization of lysosomal membranes, and a suppressive effect on the synthesis of mucopolysaccharides in connective tissue.

Cardiovascular system. Aspirin, in therapeutic doses, has no important direct or indirect effects on the heart or vascular system. In overdose, secondary effects on the cardiovascular system can result from severe alteration of electrolyte balance or dehydration. Although sodium salicylate is used infrequently, large doses can increase plasma volume as a result of the sodium load.[45]

Respiratory system. In therapeutic doses, aspirin has no appreciable effect on respiration. In overdose, aspirin initially stimulates respiration by a direct effect on the respiratory center in the medulla. This action can lead to respiratory alkalosis and an acid-base imbalance. In the later stages of aspirin poisoning or when exceedingly large doses are ingested, the respiratory center may be depressed, leading to fatal respiratory paralysis.[45,46]

Gastrointestinal tract. Aspirin has been reported to have three kinds of adverse effects on the gastrointestinal system. The most common is gastric distress. There is evidence suggesting that both local and systemic mechanisms interfere with the ability of gastric mucosal cells to resist penetration by acid. It is reasonable to assume that aspirin's interference with normal prostaglandin metabolism in gastric mucosal cells is a cause of the gastric distress. A second effect is occult gastric bleeding, resulting from cellular and capillary damage along the gastrointestinal tract. The third effect, which is very rare and idiosyncratic, is a sudden acute hemorrhage. These gastrointestinal effects are discussed in greater detail in the section on toxic reactions and side effects.

Blood. Aspirin significantly increases bleeding time by inhibiting the aggregation of platelets. As little as one 325 mg aspirin tablet can double the normal bleeding time for several days. This protracted inhibition of platelet adhesion appears to correlate with the ability of aspirin to irreversibly acetylate cyclooxygenase. Platelets lack the capability to regenerate this enzyme, and the synthesis of new platelets is required for recovery to occur. Sodium salicylate, which cannot acetylate other molecules, is much less active in prolonging bleeding time. When normal platelet prostaglandin metabolism is inhibited, the prostaglandin intermediates and thromboxane A_2 are decreased, and a substance known as prostacyclin, which is produced in the vascular wall and which prevents platelet aggregation and causes vasodilation, predominates. It is now thought that normal vascular hemostasis depends on a balance between thromboxane A_2 and prostacyclin.[33,49]

When used in high doses over long periods, aspirin can reduce plasma prothrombin. This effect can be reversed by administering vitamin K.[45] Also, when aspirin is used on a long-term basis, hematocrit and iron levels can be depressed, and the survival time of red blood cells may be shortened. In certain patients with a deficiency of glucose-6-phosphate dehydrogenase, a mild hemolytic anemia may appear.[45]

Kidney. Salicylates in therapeutic doses may cause the appearance of albumin, casts, and red and white blood cells in the urine and inhibit the tubular reabsorption of uric acid. However, with continued therapy the abnormal cells disappear, and there is no effect on renal function.

Acid-base equilibrium. As with respiration, aspirin significantly alters the acid-base balance only with greater than therapeutic doses. Aspirin's direct effect on the medulla is to stimulate respiration, resulting in carbon dioxide depletion. If the response is controlled at this stage, a physiologic metabolic compensation will ensue, and there will be increased renal excretion of bicarbonate, sodium, and potassium. However, with large doses of aspirin, a metabolic acidosis will eventually occur because of the uncoupling of oxidative phosphorylation and the inhibition of carbohydrate metabolism, leading to increasing blood concentrations of pyruvic, lactic, and acetoacetic acids.[50]

Absorption, fate, and excretion

When aspirin is taken orally, it is rapidly absorbed from the stomach and small intestine. Aspirin is a weak acid, with a pK_a of approximately 3.0, which favors absorption in the stomach. However, most absorption takes place in the small intestine because of its much larger surface area. The rate-limiting steps in the absorption of aspirin are the disintegration and dissolution of the tablet. These two steps can be greatly influenced by the manufacturing process, which determines such factors as particle size and compression of the tablet. Buffering the tablet increases the rate of dissolution, but the fastest absorption is obtained when aspirin is dissolved in hot water before ingestion. Other factors, such as gastric emptying time, gastric contents, and psychologic state of the patient, may also influence the rate of absorption.[25-27]

Acetylsalicylic acid has only a 20- to 30-minute half-life. It is quickly metabolized by gastric and plasma esterases to salicylic acid or the salicylate ion (Figure 21-2). Although very little of the acetylsalicylate becomes bound to plasma proteins, approximately 60% of the salicylate ion is bound to plasma proteins. Salicylate is distributed throughout most body fluids and tissues.[24] It can be isolated from spinal, peritoneal, and synovial fluids, saliva, breast milk, and sweat. The salicylate ion freely crosses the placenta from mother to fetus.[45]

The half-life of sodium salicylate is 3 to 4 hours; the main site of biotransformation is the liver by conjugation. The three metabolic products of salicylate are salicyluric acid (the glycine conjugate), the ether or phenolic glucuronide, and the acyl or ester glucuronide. A small portion, less than 10%, is oxidized to gentisic acid. Free salicylate and the salicylate metabolites are excreted both by glomerular filtration and by active proximal tubular

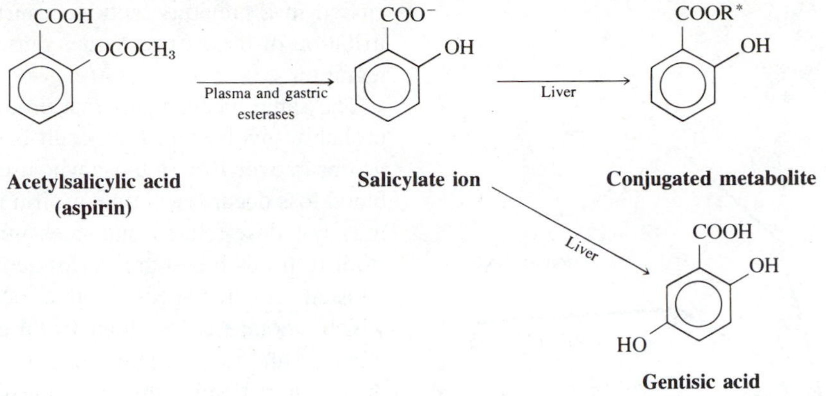

Figure 21-2. Metabolic fate of aspirin. *R = Glycine or glucuronate. (The phenolic glucuronide metabolite is not shown.)

secretion in the kidney. In normal humans, approximately 10% of ingested salicylate appears unchanged in the urine; however, this fraction may fall to 5% or rise to 85% during acidosis and alkalosis, respectively.

General therapeutic uses

The enormous use of aspirin by the general populations attests to its wide therapeutic applications. Its principal uses, both in medicine and dentistry, are to relieve pain, to reduce inflammation, and to reduce fever of almost any etiology.

There is some confusion between the analgesic and antiinflammatory effects of aspirin. In order to obtain antiinflammatory effects, large daily doses (up to 5 gm) must be taken on a long-term basis, whereas a single 650 mg dose of aspirin is sufficient to provide analgesia. The antiinflammatory property of aspirin may be of some benefit in short-term analgesic therapy, but it is incorrect to assume that aspirin's total analgesic effect is caused only by antiinflammatory activity. Certainly, patients with rheumatoid arthritis who are treated with aspirin will have pain relief long before there is any measurable reduction in joint swelling. Aspirin is used for almost all painful conditions, including orthopedic, postpartum, postoperative, cancer, and dental pain. However, aspirin is not recommended for pain from gout. At analgesic doses of 650 to 1000 mg, aspirin competes with uric acid for secretion by the proximal tubule. This could raise serum concentrations of uric acid, precipitating an acute attack of gout.

The antipyretic dose of aspirin is also 650 mg. At the present time there is no drug considered more efficacious than aspirin for reducing fever.[41,45]

There has been some interest in the possibility that aspirin, because it suppresses platelet aggregation, may interfere with abnormal coagulation of blood around the atheromatous plaques in arteries and arterioles and therefore might be useful in the prophylaxis against myocardial infarction and stroke. Existing data on this effect are inconclusive; large prospective studies are now in progress. Some of the results of these studies are discussed in Chapter 22.

Therapeutic uses in dentistry

Aspirin is an effective analgesic for almost any dental situation. Double-blind, controlled studies of the relief of pain following extraction of third molars demonstrated that 650 mg of aspirin was substantially more effective than 60 mg of codeine in relieving postoperative pain (Figure 21-3).[11] In fact, most controlled clinical studies have established that, regardless of the etiology of the pain, aspirin (650 mg) provides equal or greater pain relief than codeine (60 mg).[3] A problem with aspirin is that it has a rather flat dose-response curve, with near-maximal analgesia occurring at approximately 650 mg. Increasing the dose to 1000 mg may slightly increase analgesic efficacy and prolong the duration of effect. Clinically, this means that if 650 to 1000 mg of aspirin fails to relieve the discomfort, increasing the dose will be of little help. However, it cannot be overemphasized that

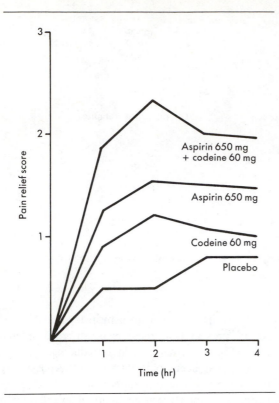

Figure 21-3. Time-effect curves for placebo, aspirin, codeine, and an aspirin-codeine combination. The mean pain relief scores are plotted against time in hours. (Adapted from Cooper, S.A., Engel, J., Ladov, M., Precheur, H., Rosenheck, A., and Rauch, D. Pharmacotherapy **2:**162-167, 1982.)

at this ceiling dosage, taken every 4 hours, aspirin is a very effective analgesic for most painful dental conditions.

Toxic reactions and side effects

Aspirin has numerous side effects at therapeutic doses, most of which are more annoying than serious. The most commonly reported side effect is nausea. It is difficult to estimate accurately the incidence, which may vary from 1% to 10% or more. It is important to realize that many procedures or illnesses may cause nausea by themselves and that the analgesic may be blamed unjustly. Certainly, many dental surgical procedures have the potential for causing nausea because of the swallowing of blood and debris, the use of sedative or anesthetic drugs, and the anxiety associated with dental surgery. However, it is also clear that aspirin can cause gastric irritation that leads to nausea and, occasionally, vomiting. In addition to the effects of aspirin on the gastric mucosa, which were discussed in a previous section, aspirin causes local irritation of the gastric tissues during tablet disintegration.

The same mechanisms that produce nausea are probably involved in the occult bleeding that develops in over 70% of those who use the drug. This blood loss occurs each time aspirin is ingested, but it is not dose-related and goes unnoticed unless stool tests for blood are performed. Only in very unusual circumstances is this occult bleeding, which amounts to less than 10 ml per day, of any clinical significance. However, aspirin is contraindicated in patients with gastrointestinal ulcers, especially those with peptic ulcers, because the normally innocuous bleeding may lead to severe internal hemorrhaging. A very few patients who have experienced severe gastric hemorrhaging for no apparent reason have been classified as having an aspirin idiosyncrasy.[45]

Aspirin significantly increases bleeding time by inhibiting the aggregation of platelets. In a clinical study, 20 minutes after ingestion of a single dose of aspirin, the bleeding time of the subjects was increased 2 to 3 times and did not return to baseline for several days. Although the prolongation of bleeding might seem alarming, it has apparently not caused any clinical problems.[49] Nevertheless, the possibility does exist that aspirin could promote postoperative hemorrhaging, especially if the clot has not fully formed. In view of these experimental findings, it may be prudent to recommend that aspirin therapy be discontinued before surgical procedures such as tooth extraction and that aspirin not be used prophylactically before any procedure that may involve postoperative bleeding. However, once the clot has formed, there should be no problems caused by the administration of aspirin or related salicylates.

Toxicity caused by aspirin overdose is common. Next to the barbiturates, aspirin holds the dubious distinction of being the most frequently used drug for attempted suicides. The drug is commonly involved in accidental poisoning, especially in children, because it is found in almost every household and proper precautions for storage are not taken. The cardinal signs of aspirin toxicity, called salicylism, include nausea, vomiting, tinnitus, hyperthermia, and hyperventilation. The hyperventilation eventually can lead to respiratory alkalosis, which may be followed by a metabolic acidosis accompanied by dehydration. The metabolic acidosis results from the uncoupling of oxidative phosphorylation and the disruption of both lipid and carbohydrate metabolism. By this stage, impaired vision, hallucinations, delirium, and other CNS effects may be evident, and the situation is considered life threatening.[45]

The treatment of aspirin overdose is primarily palliative and supportive. Gastric lavage, maintenance of electrolyte balance, and alkalinization of the urine are some common measures to be taken.

Allergy to aspirin has been reported but is rare considering the huge amount of this drug that is consumed. Many patients confuse side effects, such as nausea or tinnitus, with true allergic responses manifested by skin rashes, angioneurotic edema, or anaphylactic reactions. Patients with a history of skin eruptions caused by aspirin ingestion should be cautioned to avoid all proprietary compounds containing aspirin or any salicylate in order to avoid the more serious anaphylactic reaction.

Idiosyncratic reactions closely resembling the anaphylactic phenomenon have been noted in patients with asthma or histories of allergic reactions to other drugs.[30] The incidence of this kind of reaction in asthmatic patients has been reported to be as high as 20%, but this is probably an exaggerated estimate. Nevertheless, patients with histories of asthma or allergic disorders should be questioned to be sure that they can tolerate aspirin. The asthma-like attack is caused by a shift in the arachidonic acid cascade when the cyclooxygenase enzyme is blocked. This inhibition prevents arachidonate metabolism from producing bronchodilating prostaglandins, primarily PGE_2.[44] The lipoxygenase pathway then predominates and produces substances known as leukotrienes, previously known as slow-reacting substance of anaphylaxis (SRS-A). The leukotrienes constrict bronchioles in sensitive individuals, mimicking the asthmatic attack.[6,14]

Contraindications

Aspirin is contraindicated in a number of medical conditions (Table 21-1). Serious internal bleeding can result from the ingestion of aspirin by a patient with an ulcer condition. Patients with compromised liver function should use aspirin cautiously because, when used on a long-term basis, aspirin raises prothrombin time, which could lead to bleeding problems. Low doses of aspirin can exacerbate gouty arthritis as a result of competition between

Table 21-1. Contraindications to the use of aspirin and other salicylates

Disease state	Possible adverse effect of aspirin
Ulcer	Internal bleeding, possible hemorrhaging
Asthma	Asthmatic attack resembling an allergic reaction
Diabetes	Low doses may cause hyperglycemia, high doses may cause hypoglycemia
Gout	Low doses increase plasma urate, high doses lower plasma urate
Influenza	Reye's syndrome in children

salicylate and uric acid at the active secretion sites in the proximal tubule of the kidney. This competition causes an increase in the already high titers of plasma urate. In diabetes, high doses of aspirin may lower plasma glucose, whereas low doses may have the opposite effect. Asthma patients should use aspirin cautiously, since, as previously mentioned, 4% to 20% of asthmatic patients have reported intolerance to aspirin or other salicylate drugs.

Aspirin is not contraindicated in pregnancy, but it should be used with caution. In the third trimester, aspirin has been reported to delay parturition by inhibiting the synthesis of prostaglandins involved in initiating uterine contractions. There also is some evidence that in very high doses aspirin can have teratogenic effects.[45]

Aspirin should also be avoided in children with influenza or chickenpox (varicella). There are epidemiologic data suggesting that aspirin usage during these viral diseases increases the risk of developing Reye's syndrome.[21] This poorly understood disease produces a rapidly developing encephalopathy and fatty degeneration of the viscera that is lethal in 20% to 40% of cases.

A number of drug interactions may involve aspirin (Table 21-2). Because of its effects on blood glucose, aspirin can interact adversely with insulin or oral hypoglycemic agents, causing unpredictable changes in blood glucose concentrations. A dangerous drug interaction may occur if aspirin is used in conjunction with an anticoagulant such as dicumarol. Aspirin's acute effects of local irritation and inhibition of platelet aggregation could precipitate serious internal bleeding. Another potentially dangerous drug combination is aspirin and alcohol. Alcohol sensitizes the gastric mucosa to aspirin, and serious internal bleeding may result. As a gen-

Table 21-2. Some drug interactions involving aspirin

Drug	Possible interaction with aspirin
Dicumarol*	Internal bleeding, possible hemorrhaging
Heparin	Internal bleeding, possible hemorrhaging
Insulin	Enhancement of hypoglycemic effect
Sulfonylureas (oral hypoglycemic agents)	Enhancement of hypoglycemic effect
Phenytoin*	Increased free plasma concentration of phenytoin
Methotrexate*	Increased free plasma concentration of methotrexate
Alcohol	Internal bleeding, possible hemorrhaging
Probenecid	Decreased uricosuric effect, reappearance of gout

*Salicylates, which bind to protein, are capable of displacing other drugs that bind to protein, thus raising the free plasma concentration of these drugs.

eral rule, since about 60% of salicylate is bound to plasma protein, aspirin can interact with any drug that binds to protein by competing for binding sites on the protein molecules.

It should be obvious that aspirin is not an innocuous drug. It is fair to say that if aspirin were being introduced today as a new drug, it would not be sold over the counter and possibly would not even be approved by the FDA. However, this is more a reflection of the current rigorous standards of the FDA than an indictment of aspirin. Actually, aspirin's clinical record over the past 100 years far outweighs any experimental evidence that may cause aspirin to look like a dangerous drug. There are relatively few instances in which clinically significant side effects occur, and if reasonable precautions are taken to avoid aspirin when its use is contraindicated, the drug is indeed an extremely effective and safe analgesic.

ACETAMINOPHEN AND RELATED ANILINE DERIVATIVES

Acetaminophen and phenacetin are the only aniline derivatives currently in clinical use. Acetaminophen's claim to fame as an analgesic and antipyretic is as an aspirin substitute. Since 1949 it has been widely promoted as the drug of choice when aspirin cannot be used because of gastric problems or some other contraindication.

For many years phenacetin was a constituent of numerous analgesic preparations, including the well known APC (aspirin-phenacetin-caffeine) combination. Phenacetin has recently almost disappeared from use because of several studies linking long-term administration of such combinations with renal damage. Phenacetin is also capable of producing CNS disturbances (e.g., sedation) and hemolytic anemia and is more likely than acetaminophen to cause methemoglobinemia.

Chemistry and classification

The history of acetaminophen dates back to the late 1800s, when the antipyretic activity of aniline derivatives was discovered and several congeners, including acetaminophen, were synthesized. For some reason two other aniline derivatives, acetanilid and phenacetin, became popular and acetaminophen was put aside. Chemists eventually realized that acetaminophen was an active metabolite of both of these drugs (Figure 21-4), but it was not until the mid-1900s that acetaminophen became commercially successful.[43]

Mechanism of action

Acetaminophen has both analgesic and antipyretic activity that is essentially equivalent to that of aspirin. Phenacetin is also active in this regard, but the majority of its therapeutic effects are provided by acetaminophen, to which most of it is transformed by plasma and liver esterases. The mechanism of action also appears to be the same as that of aspirin, although there may be some differences in the spectrum of prostaglandin synthetases (cyclooxygenase enzymes) that are inhibited.[42] This reasoning is based largely on the differences in the therapeutic and toxic effects of aspirin and acetaminophen rather than on direct experimental evidence. Acetaminophen appears to be more active than aspirin as an inhibitor of CNS prostaglandin synthetases and less active in the periphery. A central component to the pain relief afforded by acetaminophen cannot therefore be discounted.

Pharmacologic effects

Compared to aspirin, acetaminophen has relatively few important effects on specific organs or systems. Therefore, the discussion of its pharmacologic effects will be noticeably shorter.

The potency and efficacy of acetaminophen as an antipyretic are similar to those of aspirin. It is probable that aspirin and acetaminophen have the

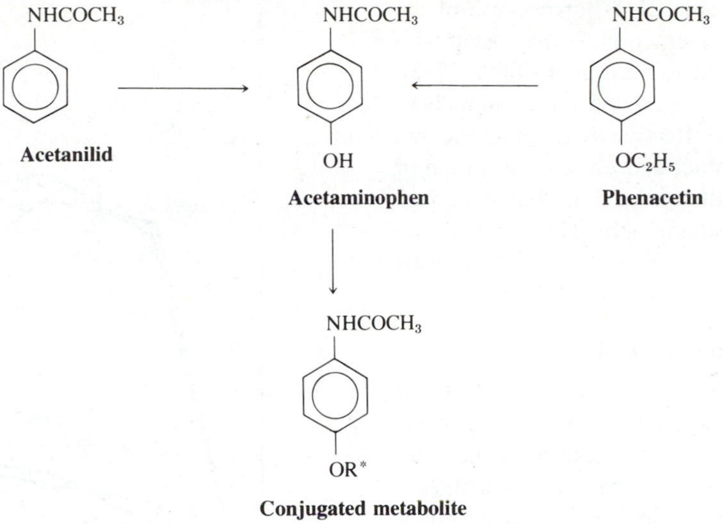

NHCOCH$_3$ NHCOCH$_3$ NHCOCH$_3$

Acetanilid   OH   OC$_2$H$_5$

Acetaminophen   **Phenacetin**

NHCOCH$_3$

OR*

Conjugated metabolite

Figure 21-4. Structure and major metabolic pathway of acetaminophen, phenacetin, and acetanilide. *R = Glucuronate (major), sulfate (minor).

same mechanism of action. For unknown reasons, acetaminophen is much less potent than aspirin as an antiinflammatory. However, it does have some activity in reducing postoperative edema.[40] In therapeutic concentrations, acetaminophen has no effect on the cardiovascular or respiratory systems. Acetaminophen does not inhibit platelet aggregation, cause occult bleeding or gastric irritation, nor does it have any renal effects. Even in overdose, most systems remain unaffected, with the primary target of toxicity being the liver.

Absorption, fate, and excretion

Acetaminophen is a weak base and is well absorbed in the small intestine after oral administration. The drug is evenly distributed throughout the body fluids and tissues, and it freely crosses the placenta. The half-life is approximately 3 to 4 hours, and the primary site of biotransformation (by glucuronide conjugation) is the liver (Figure 21-4). Other minor metabolites include a conjugate with sulfate and various hydroxylated metabolites. The binding of acetaminophen to plasma proteins is variable but rarely exceeds 40% of the total drug. Elimination is via the kidney by glomerular filtration and active proximal tubular secretion. The active secretion process is specific for organic bases, and there is no competition with organic acids like uric acid and aspirin.[43]

General therapeutic uses

Acetaminophen is approximately equipotent to aspirin as both an analgesic and an antipyretic. However, it is not classified as an antiinflammatory drug, and there is no question that aspirin is far superior in this regard. Nevertheless, there are some reports that acetaminophen does possess some antiinflammatory properties.[22] One study compared the effects of aspirin and acetaminophen on postoperative swelling after oral surgery.[39] When patients were treated with equal doses of either aspirin or acetaminophen, the acetaminophen treatment resulted in substantially less swelling. This finding may reflect an antiinflammatory effect of acetaminophen; it may also indicate a detrimental influence of aspirin on postoperative hemostasis.

It is not known why acetaminophen, as an analgesic and antipyretic, is as efficacious as aspirin and yet, as an antiinflammatory, is less effective. Perhaps when a basic compound like acetaminophen enters synovial fluid it is inactivated, masking its antiinflammatory effects. However, as noted above, postoperative swelling after dental surgery may not be analogous to the swelling of rheumatic disease.

Acetaminophen is the drug of choice when a peripherally acting analgesic or antipyretic is needed for a patient who should not take aspirin because of some disease state, such as a history of allergy or a peptic ulcer (Table 21-1), or because of the possibility of a drug interaction, as may occur with uricosuric agents used to treat gout (Table 21-2). In fact, it may even be argued that acetaminophen, because it is equally effective as an analgesic and antipyretic and does not cause gastric irritation or inhibition of platelet aggregation, should be preferred to aspirin. Acetaminophen, however, has no place in long-term therapy for rheumatoid arthritis or other inflammatory conditions.

Therapeutic uses in dentistry

The wide publicity given to the toxic effects of aspirin has caused increasing numbers of dentists to substitute acetaminophen for aspirin in the treatment of postoperative dental pain. Because the antiinflammatory effects of acetaminophen are minor and since much of dental pain is presumed to reflect inflammation, acetaminophen might not be expected to be as effective as aspirin in controlling such pain. Yet, in two independent studies, aspirin and acetaminophen were found equally effective in relieving pain after the extraction of third molars (Figure 21-5).[9,10]

Until recently, acetaminophen was thought to have a plateau for analgesia at about 650 mg, but it is now established that acetaminophen does have a linear dose-effect curve for analgesia up to 1000 mg.[23] Based on this finding, some clinicians are recommending the use of 1000 mg of acetaminophen rather than the customary 650 mg dose.

Toxic reactions and side effects

The potential for adverse effects from acetaminophen seems to be singularly confined to the situation in which there is an acute overdose, and herein lies its main therapeutic advantage over aspirin. In therapeutic doses, acetaminophen does not cause nausea, inhibit platelet aggregation, prolong prothrombin time, or produce any of the other side affects associated with the use of aspirin. Allergy to acetaminophen is rare and is generally manifested as skin eruptions. Unlike phenacetin, acetaminophen very rarely produces methemoglobinemia or blood dyscrasias.

Acute overdose from acetaminophen has become a problem, however, since mass advertising has made the drug so popular.[43] Pharmacologically, neither aspirin nor acetaminophen is a good choice for suicide, yet they are frequently so used because of their availability in sizable quantities in almost

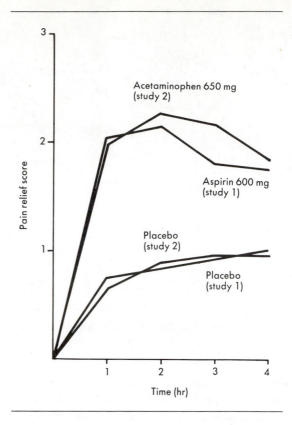

Figure 21-5. Time-effect curves for placebo, aspirin, and acetaminophen. The mean pain relief scores are plotted against time in hours. (Adapted from Cooper, S.A., Breen, J.F., and Guiliani, R.L. Journal of Clinical Pharmacology **19:**151-159, 1979; Journal of Oral Surgery **39:**21-25, 1981.)

every household. The therapeutic index for acetaminophen is high, so an amount well in excess of the therapeutic dose must be taken before clinical signs of toxicity appear. It is estimated that 6 gm or more must be taken within a relatively short time for toxicity to occur.

The most serious manifestation of acetaminophen overdose is hepatotoxicity. The degree of liver damage is directly related to the amount of drug ingested, and people with preexisting liver disease are most susceptible. Hepatotoxicity appears to result from a normally innocuous metabolite that is usually rapidly reduced by glutathione and eliminated. In overdose, this metabolite accumulates and alkylates intracellular organelles, crippling their ability to synthesize protein. When enough liver cells are damaged, clinical signs of toxicity, such as nausea and jaundice, appear.[37,43] In contrast to the rapid onset of toxic signs seen after an overdose with aspirin, clinical manifestations of acetaminophen poisoning may not appear until several days after ingestion of the drug, thus making diagnosis and treatment much more difficult than with aspirin overdose. Since the liver is a vital organ, severe hepatotoxicity must be regarded as a life-threatening situation.

Unfortunately, there is no satisfactory treatment for acetaminophen overdose. If it can be diagnosed within a few hours of ingestion, even though no clinical signs of toxicity have yet appeared, gastric lavage may be of some benefit. There is evidence that acetylcysteine or methionine will inactivate the destructive metabolite and ameliorate the condition. However, clinical reports have stated that administration of these agents must begin with 10 to 24 hours of the overdose to be of any benefit. At present, acetaminophen overdose presents a more dangerous and difficult management problem than does aspirin overdose. The clinician should not be lured into a false sense of security because of acetaminophen's freedom from toxic effects at therapeutic doses. To some extent, the dramatic rise in reported cases of acetaminophen overdose is due to a reluctance of the health professions to realize the potential hazards of this drug and to warn their patients of the consequences of misuse.

ANALGESIC ALTERNATIVES TO THE SALICYLATES AND ANILINE DERIVATIVES

Until the late 1970s, no single-entity oral analgesic had consistently demonstrated greater analgesic efficacy than 650 mg of aspirin or acetaminophen. Several new peripherally acting analgesics, most of which had earlier been approved for use as antiinflammatory drugs, have now been evaluated in postoperative dental pain and found to be superior to the standard drugs in peak analgesic effect, duration of effect, or both. The analgesic efficacy of these drugs will be discussed individually. However, because of their similarity, the general pharmacology and toxicology will be summarized as a group. A discussion of their antiinflammatory properties is provided in Chapter 22. Table 21-3 presents the structures and dosage regimens for these peripherally acting analgesics.

Phenylpropionic acid derivatives

The phenylpropionic acid derivatives constitute the largest group of aspirin alternatives. Three of these drugs—ibuprofen, naproxen, and fenoprofen—are currently available as analgesics.

Ibuprofen. Ibuprofen was the first single-entity oral analgesic to be approved by the FDA that showed a greater peak effect than 650 mg of aspirin.[12] It has also been approved for sale as a nonprescription drug. The recommended analgesic dose of ibuprofen is 400 mg every 4 to 6 hours. In one study, this dose was more effective than a combination of 650 mg aspirin with 60 mg codeine (Figure 21-6).[11] Doses larger than 400 mg have not been demonstrated to have any enhanced analgesic efficacy in nonrheumatic pain. Preoperative administration of ibuprofen can delay the onset and lessen the severity of postoperative pain.[15] Such pretreatment may be particularly useful when there is a high likelihood of moderate to severe discomfort postoperatively.

Ibuprofen is a weak organic acid and is strongly (>90%) bound to plasma albumin. It is extensively metabolized and then excreted in the urine, with a serum half-life of approximately 2 hours.

Naproxen. Naproxen is approved for a variety of inflammatory illnesses and for the relief of pain. It is available as both the free acid and as the sodium salt, the latter of which is more rapidly absorbed from the gastrointestinal tract and may be the preferred form for analgesic use. Its half-life is approximately 13 hours; the drug is partially metabolized, and its clearance is almost entirely renal. Like ibuprofen, naproxen is highly bound to plasma albumin but does not appear to interact with warfarin or oral hypoglycemics.[1,38]

The recommended analgesic regimen for naproxen is 500 mg initially, followed by 250 mg every 6 to 8 hours. (Respective doses for naproxen sodium are 550 mg and 275 mg.) The initial "loading" dose is presumably to achieve quickly a therapeutic blood concentration. However, a definitive relationship between analgesia and blood concentration has not been established.

The recommended dose of naproxen provides peak analgesia comparable to and longer in duration than that of aspirin (650 mg).[5] Definitive studies comparing naproxen to analgesic combinations with centrally acting drugs are not yet available.

Fenoprofen. Fenoprofen is marketed with both analgesic and antiinflammatory indications. Although not yet proved by clinical trials, the recommended dose of 200 mg every 4 to 6 hours is likely to be superior to 650 mg of aspirin. As with the other phenylpropionic acid derivatives, fenoprofen is extensively and reversibly protein bound

Table 21-3. Peripherally acting analgesics

Nonproprietary name	Chemical structure	Proprietary name	Recommended adult dose
Phenylpropionic acid derivatives			
Ibuprofen		Motrin	400 mg every 4-6 hr
Naproxen		Naprosyn	500 mg to start, then 250 mg every 6-8 hr
		Anaprox (Na⁺ salt)	550 mg to start, then 275 mg every 6-8 hr
Fenoprofen		Nalfon	200 mg every 4-6 hr
Pyrrole acetic acid derivatives			
Zomepirac		Zomax	50 to 100 mg every 4-6 hr
Salicylic acid derivatives			
Diflunisal		Dolobid	1000 mg to start, then 500 mg every 8-12 hr

(99%). It has a mean serum half-life of about 2.5 hours in healthy adults. Most of the drug is excreted renally as hydroxylated and conjugated metabolites.[19]

Pyrrole acetic acid derivatives

Zomepirac and tolmetin are structurally similar drugs that have analgesic, antipyretic, and antiinflammatory properties. Tolmetin is marketed as an antiinflammatory drug and is discussed in Chapter 22.

Zomepirac has been widely studied in postoperative dental pain. The recommended analgesic doses of 50 to 100 mg every 4 to 6 hours have consistently proved to be more effective than 650 mg of aspirin. Zomepirac 100 mg also was shown to be comparable to optimal doses of standard combinations of peripherally acting and centrally acting analgesics in a variety of clinical situations.[2,7,29,35]

Zomepirac clearance is primarily renal, with an elimination half-life of about 4 hours. Although it is extensively bound (>98%) to plasma proteins, studies in vitro and in normal volunteers have failed to find a significant drug interaction with concomitantly administered warfarin.[34]

Several deaths attributed to zomepirac "hypersensitivity" prompted its manufacturer to withdraw the drug in 1983. As of this writing it is not clear

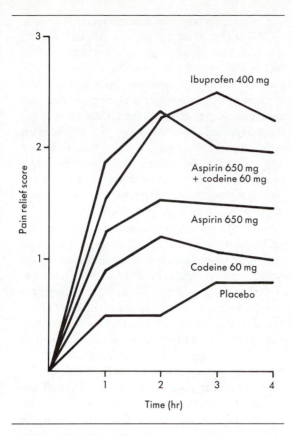

Figure 21-6. Time effect curves for placebo, codeine, aspirin, aspirin plus codeine, and ibuprofen. Mean pain relief scores are plotted against time in hours. (Adapted from Cooper, S.A., Engel, J., Ladov, M., Precheur, H., Rosenheck, A., and Rauch, D. Pharmacotherapy **2:**162-167, 1982.)

when zomepirac will be reintroduced and if the revised prescribing information will support its use in dentistry.

Diflunisal

Diflunisal is a difluorophenyl derivative of salicylic acid, but it is not metabolized to salicylate. It is slowly eliminated by the kidneys as both the unchanged drug and the glucuronide conjugate. In healthy adults, its plasma half-life is 10 to 11 hours.

Diflunisal has been studied in postoperative dental pain. In one series of investigations, 500 to 1000 mg of diflunisal produced greater analgesia than did aspirin or acetaminophen (both 650 mg), and peak effects were comparable to those obtained with fixed combinations containing optimal doses of opioids.[17,18] Diflunisal had an extended duration of action; the recommended dosage regimen of a 1000 mg "loading" dose followed by 500 mg

every 8 to 12 hours is the longest dosing interval of any marketed analgesic.

Pharmacologic effects

Like aspirin, each of these analgesics inhibits the cyclooxygenase enzyme system, thus preventing the formation of endoperoxides, prostaglandins, thromboxanes, and similar metabolites. This inhibition presumably contributes to their analgesic, antipyretic, and antiinflammatory properties. These drugs, again like aspirin, appear to have a "ceiling" effect or maximally effective dose, beyond which greater doses do not appreciably improve the analgesic response. All of these drugs are weak acids or salts of weak acids and are well absorbed after oral administration. They are highly bound to plasma albumin and the plasma half-lives range from 2 hours for ibuprofen to 10 to 13 hours for naproxen and diflunisal. These drugs are predominantly metabolized by the liver and eliminated by the kidney.

Toxic reactions and side effects

The side effects of these new peripherally acting analgesics are similar to those produced by aspirin; however, these drugs are said to have a more favorable therapeutic index. Gastric irritation (nausea and abdominal pain) is usually the most troublesome adverse effect. Dizziness, gastrointestinal bleeding, fluid retention, and nephrotoxicity have also been reported. Many adverse effects that limit the long-term use of these drugs in arthritis and other rheumatic diseases are of minimal consequence when the agents are used in the short-term treatment of acute pain. Inhibition of platelet aggregation is transient and reversible. In overdose, the clinical signs are similar to those produced by salicylates (tinnitus, nausea, vomiting, and electrolyte disturbances).

These peripherally acting analgesics should be avoided in patients whose medical conditions contraindicate the use of aspirin. Of particular concern are patients with gastrointestinal ulcers, coagulation disorders, asthma, or aspirin intolerance. The anaphylactoid responses to zomepirac underscore this warning; half of the patients who died were found retrospectively to be aspirin sensitive.

MISCELLANEOUS AGENTS WITH ANALGESIC ACTIVITY

Several inhibitors of cyclooxygenase have measurable analgesic activity but are limited in use because of their toxic potential. Examples include mefenamic acid, phenylbutazone, indomethacin, and sulindac.

Mefenamic acid, a derivative of anthranilic acid, is a mild analgesic that inhibits both prostaglandin synthesis and activity. In doses of 250 to 500 mg, its analgesic properties are comparable to those of aspirin. However, it has limited use because of reports of severe gastrointestinal side effects and blood dyscrasias. One indication for mefenamic acid is the treatment of severe dysmenorrhea, for which the drug is more effective than aspirin.

Phenylbutazone and indomethacin have been used exclusively as antiinflammatory agents for many years. These drugs must be administered cautiously because they can cause severe gastric irritation and occasionally blood dyscrasias. Although they have analgesic properties, they should never be used for this purpose because of their toxicity. Sulindac, a congener of indomethacin, is also not indicated for use as an analgesic.

COMBINATIONS OF PERIPHERALLY ACTING DRUGS

Aspirin and acetaminophen are often combined in proprietary compounds (Table 21-4). There is no evidence, however, that either analgesia or antipyresis is enhanced by such combinations. A ceiling effect still occurs when the total amount of aspirin and acetaminophen approaches 1 gm. The rationale for combining the various drugs in this class with each other does not appear to be based on sound clinical evidence of either improved efficacy or reduced toxicity, but rather on tradition.

Many of these combinations also contain caffeine. There is some evidence that stimulants such as amphetamines may potentiate the analgesic effects of aspirin-like drugs, but clear-cut evidence is lacking. The FDA has removed potent stimulants from all OTC and prescription analgesics but for the present has continued to permit the inclusion of caffeine.

COMBINATIONS OF PERIPHERALLY AND CENTRALLY ACTING ANALGESICS

There is a sound scientific basis for combining peripherally acting analgesics with centrally acting analgesics. The peripherally acting drugs combat pain by directly interfering with the biochemical mediators that cause sensitization of nerve endings at the site of injury, whereas the centrally acting drugs alter CNS perception of and reaction to pain. In addition to the fact that these combinations seem reasonable, an abundance of clinical data exists to support the validity of these combinations.[3,31,32] However, there is a common misconception that such combinations produce a synergistic phenomenon, that is, an effect greater than the sum of effects expected from both drugs. No evidence currently supports this belief, and, at best, there is a purely additive effect when drugs from these two classes of analgesics are combined. Indeed, if any synergism does exist, it is probably with the toxic effects rather than with analgesic efficacy.

Another misconception is that the centrally acting component in the combination is the major contributor to the overall efficacy of the drug preparation. Clinical studies indicate quite the opposite, showing that the peripherally acting component is an equal or, more often, greater contributor to the overall efficacy of the combination. When one limits the comparison to those studies evaluating pain of dental etiology, there is no question that the aspirin-like drugs provide the bulk of the pain relief, whereas the centrally acting drugs are of less benefit.[8] When side effects are compared, however, the centrally acting drugs are most often the cause.[3,13] The clinical significance of the centrally acting analgesics is that they provide additional analgesia beyond the ceiling effect of the peripherally acting component, and they also contribute a centrally mediated sedative effect. Therefore, the best combinations are those that use the optimal amount of an aspirin-like drug combined with the appropriate dose of a centrally acting drug.

ORAL ANALGESIC COMBINATIONS USED IN DENTISTRY

Although the centrally acting analgesics are discussed thoroughly in Chapter 20, it is appropriate to mention here some of the combinations of centrally and peripherally acting analgesics that are widely employed in dentistry.

In general, the opioid analgesics have poor oral/intramuscular (PO/IM) potency ratios, because after oral administration they are rapidly absorbed into the portal system and mostly transformed to inactive metabolites on their first pass through the liver. For example, to equal the effect of 10 mg of morphine administered intramuscularly, about 100 mg would have to be given by the oral route, resulting in a PO/IM ratio of approximately 0.1. A low PO/IM ratio also means that unpredictable and

Table 21-4. Some analgesic combinations commonly used in dentistry*

Nonproprietary name	Proprietary name	Contains (in mg)			Average adult dose
		ASA	APAP	Other ingredients	
ASA, caffeine	Anacin	400	—	Caffeine, 32	2 q4h
ASA, APAP	Gemnisyn	325	325		1-2 q4h
ASA, APAP, caffeine	Excedrin	250	250	Caffeine, 65	1-2 q4h
ASA, codeine	Empirin with codeine				
	#2	325	—	Codeine, 15	2 q4h
	#3	325	—	Codeine, 30	1-2 q4h
	#4	325	—	Codeine, 60	1 q4h
APAP, codeine	Tylenol with codeine				
	#2	—	300	Codeine, 15	2 q4h
	#3	—	300	Codeine, 30	1-2 q4h
	#4	—	300	Codeine, 60	1 q4h
ASA, oxycodone	Percodan-demi	325	—	Oxycodone, 2.44†	2 q6h
	Percodan	325	—	Oxycodone, 4.88†	1 q6h
APAP, oxycodone	Tylox	—	500	Oxycodone, 4.88†	1 q6h
	Percocet-5	—	325	Oxycodone, 5.0	1 q6h
APAP, hydrocodone	Vicodin	—	500	Hydrocodone, 4.88†	1-2 q6h
APAP, propoxyphene N	Darvocet N 100	—	650	Propoxyphene N, 100	1 q4h
ASA, propoxyphene HCl	Darvon with A.S.A	325	—	Propoxyphene HCl, 65	1 q4h
ASA, pentazocine	Talwin Compound	325	—	Pentazocine, 12.5	2 q4-6 h
ASA, caffeine, butalbital	Fiorinal	325	—	Caffeine, 40 Butalbital, 50	1-2 q4h
ASA, caffeine, butalbital, codeine	Fiorinal with codeine	Same as Fiorinal, plus			
	#1			Codeine, 7.5	1-2 q4h
	#2			Codeine, 15.0	1-2 q4h
	#3			Codeine, 30.0	1-2 q4h
ASA, caffeine, dihydro-codeine	Synalgos-DC	356	—	Caffeine, 30 Dihydrocodeine, 30	1-2 q4h
ASA, meprobamate	Equagesic	325	—	Meprobamate, 200	1-2 q4h

*ASA = aspirin; APAP = acetaminophen; N = napsylate; HCl = hydrochloride.
†Formulation contains a mixture of two different oxycodone salts.
Note: No attempt has been made to present a complete listing of drug combinations or proprietary preparations (which are available in a dazzling variety of dosage forms). Such listings can be found in a variety of sources, including *Facts and Comparisons* and *Physician's Desk Reference*. It should be noted that a number of the combinations provide less than optimal amounts of aspirin or acetaminophen. In such cases, taking two tablets instead of one would remedy this problem. However, with some drug preparations, such as Empirin or Tylenol with codeine #4, this would result in administration of an excessive amount of the narcotic analgesic, and unwanted side effects could occur.

sometimes dangerous effects may occur since individuals show great variability in their metabolic efficiencies. The best PO/IM ratio for any of the commonly used centrally acting analgesics is about 0.5.

Another general problem with the opioid analgesics is their relatively high incidence of undesirable side effects. They all cause nausea and CNS depression that becomes more intense as the dosage is increased. Mild CNS depression manifested as sedation may sometimes be useful, but ambulatory dental patients generally prefer being able to function normally once they leave the dental office.

Codeine is the most commonly used centrally acting agent in combination analgesics. Its effective oral dose range is 30 to 90 mg, 30 mg providing only minimal analgesia, 60 mg providing a little more analgesia with considerably more nausea and sedation, and 90 mg approaching the dose at which intolerable side effects appear. Codeine is available as a combination with aspirin or acetaminophen. For most patients, 600 to 650 mg of the peripherally acting component combined with either 30 to 60 mg of codeine should provide adequate pain relief for almost any dental condition.[3,4,13]

Propoxyphene (hydrochloride or napsylate) was also very popular in analgesic combinations. However, its therapeutic efficacy is open to considerable question. Some investigators have found that it is slightly less potent than codeine, whereas others claim that it has no greater effectiveness than a placebo.[3] Propoxyphene hydrochloride is available as 32 or 65 mg capsules and in combination with either aspirin or acetaminophen. The napsylate salt is available in 50 and 100 mg doses, which supply the equivalent, respectively, of 32 and 65 mg of propoxyphene hydrochloride. The napsylate salt is also available as an oral suspension.

Pentazocine, a centrally acting analgesic with opioid antagonist activity, is available in combination with aspirin and with acetaminophen. It offers no therapeutic advantages over codeine. At the recommended dose of 50 mg, pentazocine is about as effective as 60 mg of codeine. However, the combinations only provide for 25 mg of pentazocine.

Oxycodone and hydrocodone are close analogues of codeine but are approximately 10 to 12 times as potent.[4] In patients with very severe pain, 10 mg of oxycodone combined with either aspirin or acetaminophen is a most effective oral analgesic combination, although side effects such as nausea, dizziness, and sedation should be expected. Oxycodone is not marketed as a single entity; both hydrocodone and oxycodone are available in combination with other drugs (Table 21-4).

There are other centrally acting analgesics used in combination, but the vast majority of the market comprises codeine, oxycodone, propoxyphene, and pentazocine combined with either aspirin or acetaminophen (Table 21-4). Centrally acting analgesics such as morphine and oxymorphone have such low PO/IM ratios that they are of little use in oral analgesic therapy.

ANALGESIC COMBINATIONS THAT INCLUDE A SEDATIVE

Some proprietary compounds combine peripherally acting analgesics with either a sedative or both a sedative and a centrally acting analgesic. The rationale is that since patients with pain usually are suffering from anxiety, a sedative drug is indicated. Such fixed-dose combined drugs provide a convenient method to administer an analgesic and sedative with one prescription. On the other hand, the use of fixed-dose combinations makes it difficult to properly adjust the dosage of the various constituents to the individual needs of a patient. Another good argument against the fixed-dose combined drugs is that they increase the potential for adverse drug interactions. This problem is compounded further if the patient received psychoactive drugs during treatment that could have effects that carry over into the postoperative period.

Examples of sedatives found in the fixed-dose combined drugs are butalbital, meprobamate, and pyrilamine. There is little published evidence that sedative drugs either adversely affect the pain threshold or in any way contribute to the analgesic efficacy of the combination. However, like alcohol, they are capable of decreasing central inhibition, causing an increase in behavioral responses that sometimes may be mistaken for a decrease in the pain threshold.

IMPLICATIONS FOR DENTISTRY

There is abundant evidence that pain of dental etiology is most amenable to treatment by peripherally acting analgesics. Aspirin and acetaminophen continue to be the standards against which any oral analgesic should be compared. Clinical studies have shown these two drugs to be equally potent and equally effective analgesics. Either drug alone is usually adequate to relieve mild or moderate pain. It is critical, however, that the dosage be at least 650 mg.

If the pain is more severe and enhanced analgesia beyond the maximal effects of aspirin or acetaminophen are required, two options exist. First, the optimal amount of aspirin or acetaminophen can be combined with an effective dose of a centrally acting opioid analgesic. This is especially useful if mood alteration is also desired. Many fixed-combination products are available (Table 21-4). Unfortunately, not all combinations contain even the minimum amount of peripherally acting component.

The second option is to select a more efficacious peripherally acting analgesic. Several drugs have been demonstrated to have significant advantages over aspirin and acetaminophen in peak effect and duration of activity. In many situations, these peripherally acting drugs can be substituted for fixed-dose combinations containing an opioid such as codeine. The use of either a centrally acting drug alone or a fixed-dose combination that includes a sedative is not encouraged.

In clinical practice, many issues play a role in the clinician's choice of an analgesic. Psychology can be as important to the overall efficacy of an analgesic as its pharmacologic activity. If the clinician and patient are convinced a certain drug will work, that drug may be the most practical choice, regardless of what clinical trials have proved. Other nonpharmacologic factors such as the drug's name, appearance, and taste may also influence a drug's efficacy.

The pharmaceutical industry spends huge sums annually to convince the public and the profession that certain drugs are the most effective. The clinician should choose analgesic drugs and their proper dosages on the basis of sound scientific data and a critical review of past clinical experience. It is axiomatic that the patient deserves not only good psychology but also the most efficacious and safest analgesics available.

Peripherally acting analgesics and analgesic combinations

Nonproprietary name	Proprietary name
Single-entity analgesics	
acetaminophen	Anacin-3, Tylenol
aspirin	Empirin, Ecotrin, A.S.A.
diflunisal	Dolobid
fenoprofen	Nalfon
ibuprofen	Motrin, Rufen, Advil, Nuprin
mefenamic acid	Ponstel
naproxen	Naprosyn
naproxen sodium	Anaprox
salicylamide	Uromide
zomepirac*	Zomax
Analgesic combinations	
acetaminophen, codeine	Tylenol with Codeine, Empracet with Codeine
acetaminophen, hydrocodone	Vicodin
acetaminophen, meperidine	Demerol APAP
acetaminophen, oxycodone	Percocet-5, Tylox
acetaminophen, pentazocine	Talacen
acetaminophen, propoxyphene napsylate	Darvocet N 100
aspirin, caffeine	Synalgos
aspirin, caffeine, butalbital	Fiorinal
aspirin, caffeine, dihydrocodeine	Synalgos-DC
aspirin, caffeine, propoxyphene HCl	Darvon Compound
aspirin, codeine	Empirin with Codeine
aspirin, oxycodone	Percodan, Percodan-demi
aspirin, pentazocine	Talwin Compound
aspirin, phenacetin, caffeine	A.P.C.

*Not currently available in the United States.

CITED REFERENCES

1. Baele, G., DeWeerdt, G.A., and Barbier, F. Preliminary results of platelet aggregation before and after administration of ibuprofen. Rheumatology and Physical Medicine **10**(suppl):108-114, 1970.
2. Baird, W.M., and Turek, D. Comparison of zomepirac, APC with codeine, codeine and placebo in the treatment of moderate and severe postoperative pain. Journal of Clinical Pharmacology **20**:243-249, 1980.
3. Beaver, W.T. Mild analgesics: a review of their clinical pharmacology. American Journal of Medical Sciences **250**:577-604, 1965.
4. Beaver, W.T., Wallenstein, S.L., Rogers, A., and Houde, R.W. Analgesic studies of codeine and oxycodone in patients with cancer. I, II. Journal of Pharmacology and Experimental Therapeutics **207**:92-108, 1978.
5. Bloomfield, S.S., Barden, T.P., and Mitchell, J. Naproxen, aspirin, and codeine in postpartum uterine pain. Clinical Pharmacology and Therapeutics **21**:414-421, 1977.
6. Burka, J.F., and Paterson, N.A.M. Evidence for lipoxygenase pathway involvement in allergic tracheal contraction. Prostaglandins **19**:499-515, 1980.
7. Cooper, S.A. Efficacy of zomepirac in oral surgical pain. Journal of Clinical Pharmacology **20**:230-242, 1980.
8. Cooper, S.A., and Beaver, W.T. A model to evaluate mild analgesics in oral surgery outpatients. Clinical Pharmacology and Therapeutics **20**:241-250, 1976.
9. Cooper, S.A., Breen, J.F., and Giuliani, R.L. Replicate studies comparing the relative efficacies of aspirin and indoprofen in oral surgery outpatients. Journal of Clinical Pharmacology **19**:151-159, 1979.
10. Cooper, S.A., Breen, J.F., and Giuliani, R.L. The relative efficacy of indoprofen compared with opioid-analgesic combinations. Journal of Oral Surgery **39**:21-25, 1981.
11. Cooper, S.A., Engel, J., Ladov, M., Precheur, H., Rosenheck, A., and Rauch, D. Analgesic efficacy of an ibuprofen-codeine combination. Pharmacotherapy **2**:162-167, 1982.
12. Cooper, S.A., Needle, S.E., and Kruger, G.O. Comparative analgesic potency of aspirin and ibuprofen. Journal of Oral Surgery **35**:898-903, 1977.
13. Cooper, S.A., Precheur, H., Rauch, D., Rosenheck, A., Ladov, M., and Engel, J. Evaluation of oxycodone and acetaminophen in treatment of postoperative dental pain. Oral Surgery, Oral Medicine, Oral Pathology **50**:496-501, 1980.
14. Dahlen, S.-E., Hedqvist, P., Hammarström, S., and Samuelsson, B. Leukotrienes are potent vasoconstrictors of human bronchi. Nature **288**:484-486, 1980.
15. Dionne, R.A., and Cooper, S.A. Evaluation of preoperative ibuprofen for postoperative pain after removal of third molars. Journal of Oral Surgery **45**:851-856, 1978.
16. Ferreira, S.H., and Vane, J.R. New aspects of the mode of action of nonsteroid anti-inflammatory drugs. Annual Review of Pharmacology **14**:57-73, 1974.
17. Forbes, J.A., Beaver, W.T., White, E.H., White, R.W., Neilson, G.B., and Shackleford, R.W. Diflunisal: a new oral analgesic with an unusually long duration of action. Journal of the American Medical Association **248**:2139-2142, 1982.
18. Forbes, J.A., Foor, V.M., Bowser, M.W., Calderazzo, J.P., Shackleford, R.W., and Beaver, W.T. A 12-hour evaluation of the analgesic efficacy of diflunisal, propoxyphene, a propoxyphene-codeine combination, and placebo

in postoperative oral surgery pain. Pharmacotherapy **2**:43-49, 1982.

19. Gruber, C.M., Jr. Clinical pharmacology of fenoprofen: a review. Journal of Rheumatology **3**(suppl. 2):8-17, 1976.

20. Guerra (Perez-Carral), F., and Brobeck, J.R. The hypothalamic control of aspirin antipyresis in the monkey. Journal of Pharmacology and Experimental Therapeutics **80**:209-216, 1944.

21. Halpin, T.J., Holtzhauer, F.J., Campbell, R.J., Hall, L.T., Correa-Villanasenor, A., Lanese, R., Rice, J., and Hurwitz, E.S. Reye's syndrome and medication use. Journal of the American Medical Association **248**:687-691, 1982.

22. Hanjal, J., Sharp, J., and Popert, A.J. A method for testing analgesics in rheumatoid arthritis using a sequential procedure. Annals of the Rheumatic Diseases **18**:189-205, 1959.

23. Hopkinson, H.J. III, Smith, M.T., Bare, W.W., Levin, H.M., and Posatke, R.J. Acetaminophen (500 mg) versus acetaminophen (325 mg) for the relief of pain in episiotomy patients. Current Therapeutic Research **16**:194-200, 1974.

24. Lange, W.E., and Bell, S.A. Fluorometric determination of acetylsalicylic acid and salicylic acid in blood. Journal of Pharmaceutical Sciences **55**:386-389, 1966.

25. Leonards, J.R. The influence of solubility on the rate of gastrointestinal absorption of aspirin. Clinical Pharmacology and Therapeutics **4**:476-479, 1963.

26. Levy, G., and Hollister, L.E. Dissolution rate limited absorption in man: factors influencing drug absorption from prolonged-release dosage form. Journal of Pharmaceutical Sciences **54**:1121-1125, 1965.

27. Levy, G., and Leonards, J.R. Absorption, metabolism, and excretion of salicylates. In Smith, M.J.H., and Smith, P.K., eds. The Salicylates. New York, Interscience Publishers, 1966.

28. Lim, R.K.S., Guzman, F., Rodgers, D.W., Goto, K., Braun, C., Dickerson, G.D., and Engle, R.J. Site of action of narcotic and non-narcotic analgesics determined by blocking bradykinin-evoked visceral pain. Archives Internationales de Pharmacodynamie et de Therapie **152**:25-58, 1964.

29. Mehlisch, D.R., Joy, E.D., Moore, T.E., Porter, K., Stumpf, A.J., and Wolfe, S.H. Clinical comparison of zomepirac with APC/codeine combination in the treatment of pain following oral surgery. Journal of Clinical Pharmacology **20**:271-278, 1980.

30. Miller, F.F. Aspirin-induced bronchial asthma. Journal of the Oklahoma State Medical Association **60**:122-124, 1967.

31. Moertel, C.G., Ahmann, D.L., Taylor, W.F., and Schwartau, N. A comparative evaluation of marketed analgesic drugs. New England Journal of Medicine **286**:813-815, 1972.

32. Moertel, C.G., Ahmann, D.L., Taylor, W.F., and Schwartau, N. Relief of pain by oral medications: a controlled evaluation of analgesic combinations. Journal of the American Medical Association **229**:55-59, 1974.

33. Moncada, S., Higgs, E.A., and Vane, J.R. Human arterial and venous tissues generate prostacyclin (prostaglandin X), a potent inhibitor of platelet aggregation. Lancet **1**:18-20, 1977.

34. Muschek, L.D., and Grindel, J.M. Review of the pharmacokinetics and metabolism of zomepirac in man and animals. Journal of Clinical Pharmacology **20**:223-229, 1980.

35. Pruss, T.P., Gardocki, J.F., Taylor, R.J., and Muschek,

L.D. Evaluation of the analgesic properties of zomepirac. Journal of Clinical Pharmacology **20**:216-222, 1980.

36. Randall, L.O. Non-narcotic analgesics. In Root, W.S., and Hofmann, F.G., eds. Physiological Pharmacology. New York, Academic Press, Inc., 1963.

37. Rumack, B.H., and Matthew, H. Acetaminophen poisoning and toxicity. Pediatrics **55**:871-876, 1975.

38. Segre, E.J. Naproxen sodium (Anaprox) pharmacology, pharmacokinetics and drug interactions. Journal of Reproductive Medicine **25**:222-225, 1980.

39. Skjelbred, P., Album, B., and Løkken, P. Acetylsalicylic acid vs. paracetamol: effects on post-operative course. European Journal of Clinical Pharmacology **12**:257-264, 1977.

40. Skjelbred, P., and Løkken, P. Paracetamol versus placebo: effects on post-operative course. European Journal of Clinical Pharmacology **15**:27-33, 1979.

41. Smith, M.J.H. Anti-inflammatory activity of salicylates. In Smith, M.J.H., and Smith, P.K., eds. The Salicylates. New York, Interscience Publishers, 1966.

42. Symposium on analgesics. Archives of Internal Medicine **141**(special issue):271-406, 1981.

43. Symposium on paracetamol and the liver—overdosage and its management. Journal of International Medical Research **4**(suppl.):149-154, 1976.

44. Szczeklik, A., and Grylglewski, R.J. Prostaglandins and aspirin-sensitive asthma. American Review of Respiratory Disease **118**:799-800, 1978.

45. Tainter, M.L., and Ferris, A.J. Aspirin in modern therapy: a review. New York, Bayer Co., Division of Sterling Drug, Inc., 1969.

46. Tenney, S.M., and Miller, R.M. The respiratory and circulatory actions of salicylates. American Journal of Medicine **19**:498-508, 1955.

47. Vane, J.R. The mode of action of aspirin and similar compounds. Hospital Formulary **10**:618-629, 1976.

48. Vane, J.R., Weissman, G.W., and Zurier, R.B. Pain and prostaglandins: new clinical perspectives. Research Triangle Park, N.C., Medical Education Service, Burroughs Wellcome Co., 1977.

49. Weiss, H.J. Platelet physiology and abnormalities of platelet function. New England Journal of Medicine **293**:531-541, 580-588, 1975.

50. Winters, R.W., White, J.S., Hughes, M.C., and Ordway, N.K. Disturbances of acid-base equilibrium in salicylate intoxication. Pediatrics **23**:260-285, 1959.

GENERAL REFERENCES

Cooper, S.A. Peripherally-acting oral analgesics. Annual Review of Pharmacology and Toxicology **23**:617-647, 1983.

Flower, R.J., Moncada, S., and Vane, J.R. Analgesic-antipyretics and anti-inflammatory agents; drugs employed in the treatment of gout. In Gilman, A.G., Goodman, L.S., and Gilman, A., eds. Goodman and Gilman's The Pharmacological Basis of Therapeutics, ed. 6. New York, Macmillan, Inc., 1969.

Review of Biological Information on Acetaminophen and Aspirin. Fort Washington, Pa., McNeil Laboratories Science Information Division, 1972.

Robinson, H.J., and Vane, J.R., eds. Prostaglandin Synthetase Inhibitors. New York, Raven Press, 1974.

Smith, M.J.H., and Smith, P.K., eds. The Salicylates. New York, Interscience Publishers, 1966.

22 Antiinflammatory drugs

Clarence L. Trummel

An essential property of the tissues of animals is the ability to respond defensively to injurious stimuli. This property is discernible in some form in most species and is manifested in increasingly complex ways as the biologic specialization increases. It is seen perhaps in its simplest form in the phagocytosis and intracellular digestion of bacteria and other noxious materials by specialized cells in marine invertebrates lacking even a rudimentary vascular system. Response to injury reaches its ultimate expression in vertebrates as the complex series of humoral and cellular events known as inflammation.

Although inflammation has been recognized since antiquity, the notion that it is a normal, basically defensive, and thus usually desirable reaction to cellular injury is a rather recent development. The clinical features of inflammation—*tumor* (swelling), *rubor* (redness), *calor* (hotness), and *dolor* (pain)—led the early Greek physicians to regard it as a pathologic entity. This thinking persisted essentially unchanged until the work of Virchow, Cohnheim, Metchnikoff, and others in the late nineteenth century. Their investigations provided the first descriptive information of the cellular and vascular events occurring in inflammation and also gave impetus to a search for further knowledge on which our present concepts of the mechanisms and purpose of this vital phenomenon are based.

Formal definitions of inflammation are numerous and diverse, and none appears to have universal acceptance. Most emphasize one or another facet of inflammation, reflecting the particular interests or bias of the originator. A definition proposed recently by Ebert and Grant[18] seems as useful as any: *Inflammation is a process which begins following sublethal injury to tissue and ends with permanent destruction of tissue or with complete healing.*

This definition of inflammation points out several important features of the phenomenon. Inflammation is a unique biologic process, not a state, that is triggered by injury and proceeds toward some eventual conclusion. Normally, the tissue injury elicits a series of apparently well-regulated humoral and cellular events leading to localization of injury, removal of noxious agents, repair of physical damage, and restitution of function in the injured tissue. In this respect, inflammation is clearly essential for the well-being and even the survival of the host. Thus, in such injuries as those resulting from mechanical wounds, thermal or chemical burns, invasion by certain microorganisms, or a single, temporary exposure to an antigen, the resultant inflammatory process moves smoothly from initial reaction to complete healing. Except in the case of massive injuries, the form and function of the injured tissues are returned to a normal or near normal condition. It has been noted that "without inflammatory responses, we would go through life bearing all the open wounds of the past, a body unable to heal itself, quite like a machine that functions until a part wears out or breaks."[59] The importance of inflammation is well illustrated by the serious consequences of diseases, such as agranulocytosis, in which elements of the inflammatory process are absent or defective.

The inflammatory response to injury, however, is not always beneficial to the host. If inflammation becomes chronic, it may result in progressive destruction rather than repair of tissue. The basis for a persistent inflammatory response is not always apparent. In some conditions, such as tuberculosis, the injurious agent persists because it cannot be neutralized or eliminated by the host; inflammation

331

will then continue for as long as the agent is present. In other cases, particularly where an injurious stimulus has not been identified, the possibility exists that chronic inflammation results from a loss of homeostatic control of the inflammatory process. Regardless of their cause, unchecked inflammation and associated tissue destruction are the major pathologic features of numerous diseases, such as rheumatic fever, tuberculosis, glomerulonephritis, rheumatoid arthritis, psoriasis, ulcerative colitis, gout, and periodontitis. Diverse in many respects, these diseases have the common feature of persistent inflammatory lesions in one or more organ systems leading to progressive loss of the structural elements and functional capacity of the involved tissues. The association between chronic inflammation and tissue destruction is quite apparent in periodontitis. Here, oral bacteria continuously adjacent to the gingiva initiate and perpetuate an inflammatory reaction in this tissue. In one sense, the reaction is successful, because the bacteria are largely prevented from invading the host. The price paid for this protection, however, is progressive and irreversible destruction of the tooth-supporting tissues.

The potential sites in the multifactorial process of inflammation at which drugs could act to obtund the process are numerous; the actual sites at which drugs in current use do act are largely unidentified. Since the multiple events of the inflammatory process seem to be initiated and integrated by locally generated chemical mediators, it is often assumed that antiinflammatory drugs inhibit the production or activity of one or more of these mediators. For some agents at least, this assumption is supported by experimental evidence. To understand this evidence and appreciate its relevance to the rational use of these drugs, an understanding of the mediators and mechanisms at work in the inflammatory process is required. A synopsis of mediators follows, and the reader is referred to any of several recent monographs or reviews of inflammation (see General References).

MEDIATORS OF THE INFLAMMATORY PROCESS

Inflammation is a consistent and orderly progression of events initiated and presumably controlled by endogenous chemical mediators. These mediators, generated at the site of injury, normally exist as inactive precursors in plasma or are sequestered in cells. A stimulus that elicits inflam-

Table 22-1. Classification of endogenous mediators of inflammation

Origin	Major groups	Major mediators
Tissue	Vasoactive amines	Histamine
		5-Hydroxytryptamine
	Acidic lipids	Prostaglandins
		Leukotrienes (slow-reacting substances; SRSs)
	Lysosomal contents	Cationic proteins
		Enzymes (acidic and neutral proteases and others)
	Lymphocyte products	Migration inhibition factor
		Macrophage activating factor
		Chemotactic factors
		Histamine-releasing factor
		Lymphotoxin
		Skin reactive factor
		Mitogenic factors
	Others	Endogenous pyrogens from leukocytes
		Leukocytosis factors
Plasma	Kinin system	Bradykinin
	Complement system	C3 fragments
		C5 fragments
		C567 complex
	Clotting system	Fibrinopeptides
		Fibrin degradation products

mation does so by either activating extracellular mediators or causing the release of intracellular mediators. Release occurs by cytotoxic mechanisms, in which the cell is destroyed and its contents of mediators released, or by noncytotoxic mechanisms, in which the mediators are actively secreted, or by both. Other mediators are produced after the inflammatory response begins and contribute to subsequent events. The two most fundamental events in inflammation—the increased permeability of the microvasculature and the accumulation and activation of leukocytes—can both be largely attributed to the action of specific chemical agents. The endogenous mediators of inflammation, classified according to their place of origin (tissue or plasma), are shown in Table 22-1.

The appearance of these endogenous substances occurs in a time-related pattern. The first stage of inflammation can be defined as the amine stage, during which small, preformed biologic amines are released as a result of tissue damage. The second, or polypeptide, stage occurs when serum proteins are converted into vasoactive and neuroactive polypeptides by enzymes derived from blood. The third stage is associated with the release of intracellular enzymes that begin to attack the tissue debris. One such enzyme, phospholipase A_2, liberates from the cell membrane acidic lipids, which are then converted into prostaglandins and leukotrienes. The last stage of inflammation involves the lymphocytic phase of injury cleansing and repair.

Tissue mediators

Histamine. Histamine is the one mediator for which a role in the inflammatory process has been clearly established. This vasoactive amine is formed by decarboxylation of histidine and is widely distributed in the body. Although some free histamine exists in tissues, most is stored in mast-cell granules in a physiologically inactive form. (For a more complete discussion, see Chapter 23.) A variety of physical and chemical stimuli—antigens, complement fragments, a cationic protein from neutrophils, or simple mechanical trauma—can cause extrusion of the granules and release of active histamine into the extracellular fluid. One of the most characteristic actions of histamine is dilation of vessels of the microcirculation and a marked, but transient, increase in the permeability of capillaries and postcapillary venules. These vascular changes are similar to those that occur in tissue after injuries of all sorts. The evidence that histamine released from the ubiquitous mast cell is responsible for the initial permeability changes seen in an inflammatory response is extensive. For example, the histamine content of tissue fluid at the site of injury rises within minutes after the insult and then falls. Concurrent with these changes, mast cells in the area of damage are found to be degranulated. Furthermore, it has been shown that prior depletion of tissue histamine stores by various means or pretreatment with classic antihistamines will reduce the initial vascular response to injury.[37] However, it should be noted that inhibition of initial histamine-dependent events does not block the further development of the inflammatory response. Thus, the role played by histamine in inflammation is early, transient, and nonessential for subsequent events that may lead to lasting tissue alterations.

Antihistamines have little use as general antiinflammatory agents. In certain situations, such as immediate allergic reactions, large amounts of histamine are released locally or systemically from sensitized mast cells and basophils as a consequence of antigen-antibody reactions. In these instances, antihistamines may be useful in reducing symptoms attributable to histamine.

5-Hydroxytryptamine. 5-Hydroxytryptamine (5-HT, or serotonin) is a biogenic amine whose role in the inflammatory process in humans is not clear. The amine is synthesized by hydroxylation of tryptophan to give 5-hydroxytryptophan; this compound is then decarboxylated to yield 5-HT. After its release from storage sites, 5-HT is oxidized by MAO to 5-hydroxyindoleacetic acid, which is then excreted in the urine. In humans, most 5-HT (about 90%) is synthesized and stored in the enterochromaffin cells of the gastric mucosa. The remainder is found largely in the central nervous system and in platelets. The mast cells of rodents and a few other species contain large amounts of 5-HT, but those of humans normally contain none.

Like histamine, 5-HT has potent effects on smooth muscles and small blood vessels in some species. In rodents, subcutaneous injection of 5-HT causes arteriolar dilation, venular constriction, and separation of endothelial cells. However, in humans, the effects of 5-HT on vascular permeability are minimal. Although 5-HT is present in inflammatory exudates after injury, it appears to be of little importance, since the vascular changes of the inflammatory response are unaffected by 5-HT inhibitors. At present, the role of 5-HT in mediating inflammation appears to be minor.

Prostaglandins. The prostaglandins (PG) are a unique family of closely related acidic lipids found in all tissues. Like the leukotrienes, described below, prostaglandins are derived from arachidonic acid and similar 20-carbon polyunsaturated fatty acids that are liberated from the cell membrane by the action of phospholipase enzymes. There is currently much interest in the role of these substances in diverse physiologic and pathologic processes, including inflammation.

All of the prostaglandins can be considered as analogues of the hypothetical compound prostanoic acid, a 20-carbon unsaturated fatty acid with a cyclopentane ring at C_8-C_{12} (Figure 22-1). The different prostaglandins fall into several classes—A through F—according to the specific structure of the cyclopentane ring. They are further identified by a subscript (1, 2, or 3) indicating the number of double bonds in the side chains. PGE_2, therefore, represents a prostaglandin with an E-type ring structure and two double bonds in the side chains. Prostaglandins of the E and F series are considered to be the compounds of primary interest since they

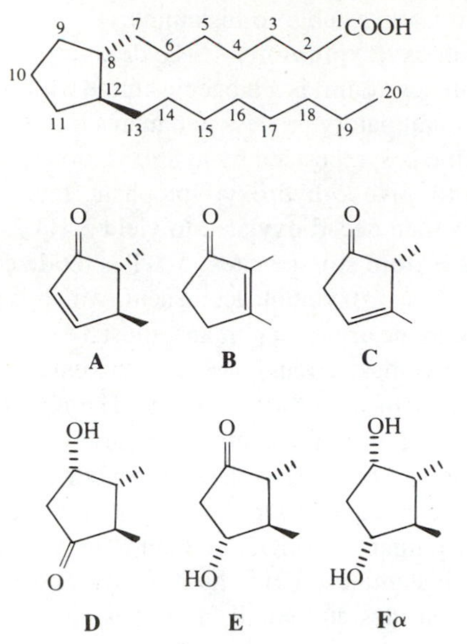

Figure 22-1. Molecular structure of prostaglandins. At top is the structure of prostanoic acid, a hypothetical compound of which the prostaglandins can be considered analogues. At bottom are the basic ring structures of prostaglandin groups A through F.

are the most abundant in mammalian systems. Consequently, they have been studied the most extensively. Prostaglandins A, B, and C can be derived chemically from PGE, but only PGA occurs naturally to any extent in humans.

Prostaglandins are synthesized from fatty acids by a microsomal enzyme complex (loosely termed "prostaglandin synthetase") found in all mammalian tissues. In humans, the most abundant precursor is arachidonic acid, which forms prostaglandins of the 2 series. Arachidonic acid is first oxidized by a cyclooxygenase to an intermediate endoperoxide, PGG_2, which is then converted to PGH_2. This latter compound is isomerized enzymatically or nonenzymatically to give PGE_2, $PGF_{2\alpha}$, or PGD (Figure 22-2). PGH_2 can also be metabolized to other biologically active compounds that differ structurally from the primary prostaglandins.[45] These include prostacyclin (PGI_2) and thromboxane A_2 (TXA_2). PGI_2 has a double ring formed by an oxygen bridge between C_6 and C_9, and TXA_2 contains an oxane rather than a pentane ring (Figure 22-2). Both compounds are unstable at physiologic temperatures and pH (half-life is 3

minutes for PGI_2 and 30 seconds for TXA_2) and change spontaneously to stable forms (6-keto-$PGF_{1\alpha}$ and TXB_2).

Although all tissues have the ability to convert arachidonic acid to the intermediate endoperoxides, the factors that control subsequent synthetic events and thus the types of compounds produced by a given tissue are largely unknown. Since the prostaglandins are not stored to any extent, their appearance in a tissue represents de novo synthesis. Following formation, they are rapidly metabolized, either locally at the site of origin or in the liver, lungs, and other tissues after uptake into the circulation. The initial inactivation step for prostaglandins of the E and F series is oxidation of the alcohol group at C_{15} by the enzyme prostaglandin dehydrogenase. Further reduction and eventual oxidation of the side chains occur, and the resultant metabolites are largely eliminated in the urine. Similar pathways of biotransformation and excretion appear to operate for PGI_2 and TXA_2.

Prostaglandins and the other active metabolites of the intermediate endoperoxides (PGI_2 and TXA_2) have a multitude of effects in almost every biologic process examined so far. These processes include smooth muscle contraction and relaxation, vascular permeability, renal electrolyte and water transport, gastrointestinal and pancreatic secretions, various central and autonomic nervous functions, release of hormones (e.g., ACTH, steroids, and insulin), luteolysis and parturition, lipolysis, bone resorption, and platelet aggregation. Not only are the affected processes diverse and the effects complex, but also the different prostaglandins sometimes appear to have antagonistic actions. For example, PGE_2, $PGF_{2\alpha}$, and PGI_2 in general cause vasodilation and inhibit platelet aggregation, whereas TXA_2 causes vasoconstriction and induces platelet aggregation. Qualitative and quantitative differences in responses to the prostaglandins exist among mammalian species, further complicating elucidation of the biologic role of these substances. It is thus axiomatic that generalizations about the actions of prostaglandins and related compounds are hazardous; the response to a given agent must be considered in the context of the particular tissue involved, the assay system used, and the species of experimental animal.

There is abundant evidence that prostaglandins and the intermediate endoperoxides are mediators of inflammation.[36,45] Arachidonic and other fatty acid precursors of prostaglandins present in the

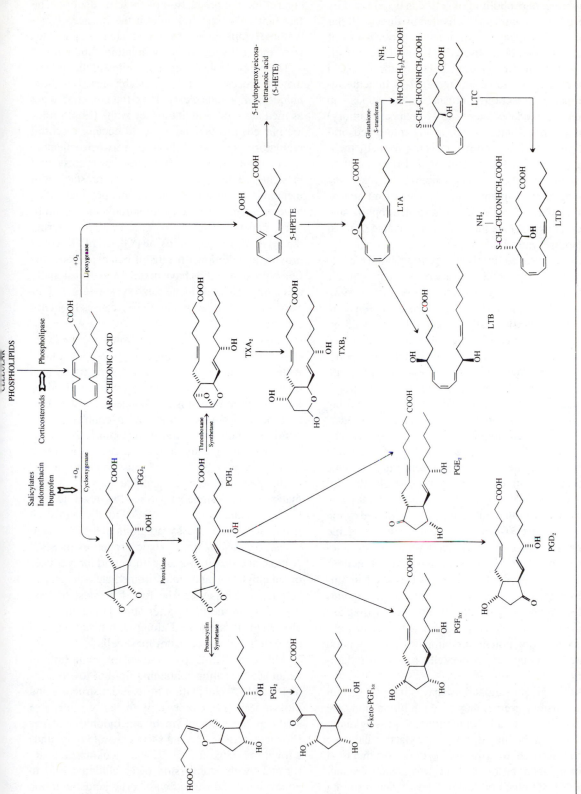

Figure 22-2. Pathways of arachidonic acid metabolism to prostaglandins (PG) and related compounds and to leukotrienes (LT). The cyclooxygenase pathway leads to formation of the cyclic endoperoxides PGG₂ and PGH₂ and subsequently to prostacyclin (PGI₂), thromboxane (TX), or the stable prostaglandins (E₂, F₂ₐ, and D₂). The lipoxygenas pathway results in formation of 5-hydroperoxyeicosatetraenoic acid (5-HPETE) and subsequently to leukotrienes A, B, C, and D. The open arrows indicate the metabolic steps that are inhibited by corticosteroids or nonsteroidal antiinflammatory agents, such as aspirin and indomethacin.

membrane phospholipid of cells can be released by phospholipase enzymes activated by direct cellular damage or by any nondestructive perturbation of the membrane, be it physical, chemical, hormonal, or neurohumoral. Prostaglandin synthesis could then ensue, as shown in Figure 22-2. In acute inflammatory reactions, prostaglandins appear in fluids and exudates later (6 to 12 hours after injury) than other mediators, such as histamine and bradykinin.[38] Prostaglandins are being formed, then, at a time when tissue damage and disintegration are more prominent. It is possible that some of the prostaglandin content found in sites of inflammation is derived from infiltrating neutrophils and macrophages, since these cells are capable of prostaglandin synthesis.[1,31]

Once released in tissue, prostaglandins could contribute to the inflammatory response in multiple ways. The evidence that they do so can be summarized as follows[9,22,36]: (1) prostaglandins are found in experimentally or naturally produced inflammatory fluids, (2) prostaglandins are involved in platelet aggregation, (3) platelets, neutrophils, and macrophages produce prostaglandins, with production in platelets occurring during aggregation and in neutrophils and macrophages during phagocytosis, (4) prostaglandins injected intradermally are potent inducers of vasodilation as well as of increased vascular permeability, an effect that is greatly augmented by the presence of histamine or 5-HT, (5) minute amounts of prostaglandins injected intradermally markedly increase the pain sensitivity to other mediators, such as bradykinin or histamine, (6) prostaglandins are pyrogenic when injected into the cerebral ventricles or anterior hypothalamus, suggesting a mediator function, (7) a severe disabling arthritis is produced in animals by injecting prostaglandins into the knee joint, and rheumatoid synovial cells produce prostaglandins in culture, and (8) certain antiinflammatory drugs that are potent inhibitors of prostaglandin synthesis reduce experimentally produced inflammation.

Although prostaglandins may stimulate certain inflammatory events, they may inhibit or modulate others. For example, inhibition of prostaglandin synthesis in the lung during anaphylactic challenge or in response to aspirin-like drugs or the food coloring agent tartrazine leads to a greater production of histamine and leukotrienes.[38] The resulting asthmatic reaction suggests that prostaglandins may be involved in a negative feedback mechanism controlling the production of these mediators. The fact that prostaglandins inhibit the release of mediators (lymphokines) from activated lymphocytes is further evidence of a modulating function.[11,46]

The precise role of prostaglandins in the inflammatory process is far from established, but these unique compounds clearly have the potential to act as mediators or modulators, or both. If both roles are played, prostaglandins could occupy a central regulatory position. A balance between enhancement and suppression of inflammatory events could be achieved by local regulation of prostaglandin metabolism, since in some systems prostaglandins have been shown to be either stimulatory or inhibitory, depending on their concentration. Altering the relative concentrations of PGE and PGF could provide an additional means of balance, since different prostaglandins have diverse and occasionally antagonistic actions in the same system (e.g., PGE_2 causes bronchodilation and $PGF_{2\alpha}$ causes bronchoconstriction).[3,33]

Leukotrienes. The term *slow-reacting substance* (SRS) was first applied to a lipid-soluble material produced by treatment of lung tissue with cobra venom. This material was characterized by its production of a slow, prolonged contraction of a smooth muscle preparation, in contrast to the rapid and transient action of histamine. A chemically and biologically similar material was subsequently found in the lungs of sensitized guinea pigs challenged with specific antigen in vitro.[55] This material was designated as the slow-reacting substance of anaphylaxis (SRS-A) to distinguish it from SRSs produced by nonimmunologic mechanisms. Studies of the biologic properties of SRS-A indicated that it might be an important mediator of anaphylactic and other immediate allergic reactions.[3,51] SRS-A can be found in most tissues, especially in the lung, after appropriate antigenic challenge. It is released along with histamine and other active products from mast cells.

Although SRS-A was known for some time to be an acidic, sulfur-containing lipid of low molecular weight,[49] elucidation of its exact structure and biosynthesis has come only recently. Intensive study of the metabolism of arachidonic acid has shown that SRS-A belongs to a class of compounds known as leukotrienes.[54] The leukotrienes are formed by the conversion of arachidonic acid to noncyclized, 20-carbon carboxylic acids with one or two oxygen substituents and three conjugated double bonds (Figure 22-2). The initial step in the biosynthetic pathway is generation of a 5,6-epoxide of arachidonic acid (leukotriene A) by the action of a lipoxygenase. Leukotriene A may be converted to the 5,12-dihydroxy acid (leukotriene B) or alternatively to leukotriene C by the addition of glutathione. Removal of glutamate from leukotriene C generates leukotriene D. These lipid-peptide structures appear to account for all of the biologic activity of SRSs found in immediate allergic reactions.[53] Although it has been proposed that leukotriene D is specifically responsible for the activity of SRS-A, the possibility that SRS-A is a mixture of leukotrienes has not yet been ruled out.[44,52] The ability of various cells to produce leukotrienes appears to be limited to the lung, leukocytes, blood vessels, and epicardium. In contrast, all cells except erythrocytes can convert arachidonic acid to prostaglandins and related compounds via the action of cyclooxygenase.

Leukotrienes C and D are potent in vivo and in vitro constrictors of bronchial smooth muscle in the guinea pig. Both compounds have similar effects in human bronchial muscle preparations, in which they are about 1000 times more potent than histamine.[53] Since these leukotrienes also increase vascular permeability, it seems likely that either one or both play a role in the bronchial constriction and mucosal edema of asthma. In addition to changes in vascular permeability, the leukotrienes can enhance chemotactic and chemokinetic responses in human polymorphonuclear leukocytes.[10,24] This finding suggests that these agents may be involved in localized inflammatory processes as well as in asthma.

Lysosomal products. The lysosomes of neutrophils contain a variety of enzymatic and nonenzymatic factors that play important roles in the manifestations and sequelae of inflammatory reactions (Table 22-2).[4,26] During phagocytosis of bacteria or foreign material by neutrophils, the contents of lysosomes are released into the extracellular environment. They are also released on lysis of the cell. Cationic proteins from lysosomes contribute to the inflammatory process by triggering mast cell degranulation, which in turn leads to increased vascular permeability. Lysosomal enzymes may contribute in several ways.[59] First, several of these enzymes have the potential to damage host tissues and probably do so. Thus, collagen, elastin, mucopolysaccharides, basement membrane, and other structural elements may be degraded. Second, lysosomal proteases cause the production of

Table 22-2. Factors in the neutrophil with inflammatory potential

Permeability factors	Leukokinin-forming enzyme
	Basic peptides
Leukotactic factors	C5-cleaving enzyme
	Basic peptides (chemotactic for monocytes)
Tissue-damaging enzymes; hydrolases for:	Elastin
	Basement membrane
	Collagen
	Other structural proteins

kinin-like substances from plasma kininogen and can generate chemotactic factors for neutrophils from complement, as is described in a succeeding section. Neutrophils thus may play a central role in perpetuating the inflammatory response by their dual ability to cause tissue damage and to elaborate specific mediators of inflammation. Another source of lysosomal factors, especially in chronic inflammatory lesions, may be the mononuclear phagocyte, or macrophage, the lysosomes of which contain substances similar to those of the neutrophil.[1]

Lymphocyte products. Delayed allergic reactions may be involved in some inflammatory processes, especially those of a chronic nature in which there is a persistent antigenic stimulus (e.g., in tuberculosis). These reactions are mediated by factors called lymphokines, which are produced by sensitized thymus-dependent lymphocytes after specific antigenic challenge.[7] Although a large number of putative lymphokines have been described in recent years, their role in inflammatory reactions with an immune component is unknown. Some of the better studied lymphokines that may function in inflammation-related events are (1) macrophage migration inhibition factor, which promotes the accumulation of macrophages in the area of injury, (2) macrophage activating factor, which stimulates various functional activities of these cells, including phagocytosis, (3) lymphotoxin, which is nonspecifically toxic to other cells, (4) chemotactic factors, which are specific attractants for neutrophils, macrophages, basophils, and eosinophils, (5) mitogenic factor, which causes proliferation of unsensitized lymphocytes, and (6) skin reactive factor, which mimics a delayed allergic reaction when injected into normal skin; that is, it causes increased vascular permeability and immigration of mononuclear cells.

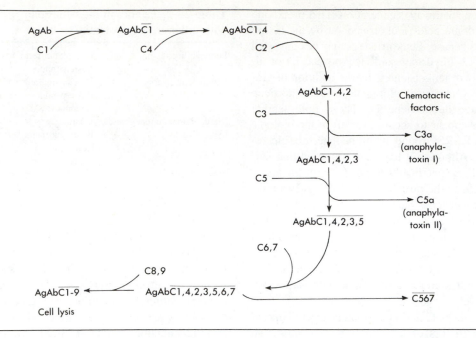

Figure 22-3. Complement fixation (classic pathway).

Plasma mediators

Kinins. The term *kinins* refers to various small peptides that are similar in structure and actions, including bradykinin, lysyl-bradykinin, and methionyllysyl-bradykinin. Bradykinin can be considered the prototype. It is a linear nonapeptide with a molecular weight of 1060. As with the release of histamine, almost any process causing tissue injury can trigger the series of events leading to the production of bradykinin. Bradykinin exists in plasma as an inactive precursor (kininogen) and is released in a cascade of reactions beginning with activation of Hageman factor (clotting factor XII). Hageman factor can be activated by a host of substances, including cartilage, collagen, basement membrane, sodium urate crystals, proteolytic enzymes, and bacterial lipopolysaccharides. Hageman factor in turn activates an enzyme called prekallikrein to yield kallikrein. Kallikrein then cleaves bradykinin from kininogen, an α_2-globulin precursor. (In addition, activated Hageman factor triggers both the clotting cascade by activating factor XI and the fibrinolytic system by activating plasminogen proactivator, ultimately yielding plasmin.) Kinins may also be produced extravascularly from tissue kininogen. After release, bradykinin is rapidly metabolized by enzymes present in both plasma and tissues.

Bradykinin has striking pharmacologic effects in humans and animals.[17] It is a potent but transient vasodilator of both arteries and veins by a direct action on smooth muscle. Intradermal injection of bradykinin causes marked increases in vascular permeability; in this respect it is more potent than histamine on a molar basis. Bradykinin applied to a blister base or injected intradermally or intraarterially in humans evokes sharp pain. Experimental pain can also be produced by a bradykinin-like substance isolated from human blister fluid and from synovial fluid obtained from acutely inflamed joints.[62] All of these phenomena implicate bradykinin in various aspects of acute inflammatory reactions. Proving this implication experimentally, however, has been frustrated by the short half-life of bradykinin and the complexity of the kinin generation mechanism and its interactions with other plasma systems.

Complement system. The complement system plays an important role in the inflammatory process. In humans, this system consists of 11 component proteins that react in a fixed sequence (Figure 22-3). An immune complex on a cell surface activates the first component, C1, and a cascade of events results in the formation of a complex that leads to membrane damage and cell lysis.

This so-called classic pathway of complement

activation can be initiated by most antigen-antibody complexes and such nonimmune factors as trypsin and plasmin. Other substances, such as complex polysaccharides, aggregated IgA, and bacterial endotoxin, may trigger an alternate pathway in which the first component to be activated is C3, followed then by the usual components in the activation scheme.[50]

In addition to the direct cellular damage cited above, certain fragments produced during the cascade of complement activation have biologic properties of importance.[5] Two of them (C3a and C5a) cause increased vascular permeability by inducing the release of histamine from mast cells. These substances are, therefore, referred to as anaphylatoxins and have been implicated in anaphylaxis and other allergic reactions. Three different chemotactic factors (C3a, C5a, and C$\overline{567}$ complex) have also been identified in complement. Neutrophils, monocytes, and eosinophils exhibit directed locomotion in response to these factors. Enhancement of phagocytosis and release of lysosomal enzymes have been attributed to other components of the activation scheme.

Complement fragments can be produced by mechanisms extrinsic to the complement system (e.g., by plasmin, trypsin, and bacterial proteases). This action suggests that complement fragments may participate in tissue injury and in the subsequent inflammatory response without classic or alternative complement activation.[58]

ANTIINFLAMMATORY AGENTS

Attempts to modify the inflammatory process with chemical agents date from antiquity. Although most measures historically have been aimed at reducing inflammation, it should be noted that a number of chemicals and treatments have been used to increase certain aspects of it. The use of liniments, counterirritants, and "antiphlogistics" may actually intensify some inflammatory reactions so as to bring about resolution of a lesion and subsequent healing. Although most of these practices were discarded along with bleeding and "drastic catharsis," a process formerly known as franking is still being used in which a chronic inflammation is made more acute in order to activate tissue repair. The incorporation of eugenol in periodontal packs involves this philosophy of therapy, as does the inhalation of irritant vapors for the treatment of bronchial congestion caused by viral infections.

The antiinflammatory properties of botanical preparations containing salicylates were known and utilized well before the Christian era. Although today considerably more and perhaps somewhat better drugs are available, an important feature of these agents remains unchanged: antiinflammatory drugs are palliative but not curative. Even though antiinflammatory agents may completely alleviate all of the discomforting signs and symptoms of inflammation, they are not likely to significantly affect either the cause or course of the disease. For example, the treatment of rheumatoid arthritis with corticosteroids may reduce or eliminate redness, swelling, and pain, but the destruction of the affected joints continues. Nonspecificity is such a constant characteristic of antiinflammatory drugs that agents that truly eliminate inflammation by acting on the causative factor (e.g., antibiotics) are not ordinarily considered to be antiinflammatory drugs.

In addition to their failure to eliminate specifically the inflammatory stimulus, antiinflammatory drugs pose other problems. By suppressing the inflammatory response, some of these agents can seriously compromise the body's defensive mechanisms. The price paid for symptomatic relief of inflammation at one site may be an acute infection at another. Most antiinflammatory drugs have a high incidence of adverse effects. In fact, in this group of agents, efficacy and toxicity are usually closely associated. The chronic use of these drugs further contributes to the possibility that toxic effects will occur.

The decision to treat an inflammatory process with drugs should not be made lightly. The causative agent must first be sought and eliminated, if possible. The desirability of suppressing inflammatory symptoms must be weighed against the possibility of unwanted effects. Such factors as the nature and anticipated course of the inflammatory disease and the degree of pain, disability, and deformity present are considered in making this decision. Finally, nondrug measures—orthopedic and physical therapy, surgery, and nutritional or psychologic counseling—may substitute for or reduce the need for antiinflammatory drugs.

Salicylates

The salicylates are among the oldest known drugs. Ancient physicians used preparations of willow and poplar bark, which contain salicin (a glycoside of salicylic alcohol), to treat sepsis, pain, gout, and fever. In 1838, the active principle in these preparations was identified as salicylic acid. This acid was synthesized in 1860, and the sodium

Table 22-3. Antiinflammatory and fatty acid cyclooxygenase inhibitory activity of nonsteroidal antiinflammatory drugs

Compound	Inhibition of prostaglandin synthesis (ED_{50}, μM)	Reduction of carrageenin-induced rat paw edema ($ED50$, moles/kg)	Peak plasma concentration (μM)	Plasma-protein binding (%)
Indomethacin	0.17	0.017	5.0	90
Phenylbutazone	7.25	0.325	230-500	98
Aspirin	37.0	0.833	280-300	50-80
Acetaminophen	660.0	Inactive	350	25

Adapted from Arrigoni-Martelli, E. Inflammation and Antiinflammatories. New York, Spectrum Publications, Inc., 1977.

salt was introduced into medicine in 1875. The antiinflammatory, antipyretic, and analgesic properties of salicylic acid were obvious, but so too was its toxicity. This shortcoming led to a search for safer but equally effective derivatives, which culminated in the preparation and introduction of aspirin (acetylsalicylic acid) in 1899 by Dreser of the Bayer Company of Germany. The popularity of aspirin was immediate, and today it remains one of the most widely used drugs in the world.[43] Aspirin may be considered a prototype of the nonsteroidal antiinflammatory drugs and is the standard of reference against which these agents are compared and evaluated. The pharmacology of aspirin and other salicylates is presented in Chapter 21; the following discussion will center on the antiinflammatory actions of these drugs.

The efficacy of salicylates as antiinflammatory agents has been solidly established by a century of experimental observation and many centuries of clinical experience. The mechanism by which this most useful clinical action is produced has so far eluded identification. A variety of mechanisms have been proposed, including interference with oxidative phosphorylation, inhibition of leukocyte migration or phagocytic activity, displacement of an endogenous antiinflammatory peptide from plasma proteins, and stabilization of lysosomal membranes.[19] Yet, the experimental evidence supporting these proposals is not impressive. Current attention is focused on the possibility that the antiinflammatory action of salicylates is due, at least in part, to inhibition of prostaglandin production, since not only salicylates but also certain other nonsteroidal antiinflammatory drugs have been shown to be potent inhibitors of prostaglandin synthetase prepared from many different tissues.[19] Furthermore, the potency of these agents as inhibitors of prostaglandin synthetase in vitro correlates well with their ability

to alleviate carrageenin-induced inflammation in animals (Table 22-3). In humans, antiinflammatory doses of aspirin (3 gm daily), salicylate (3 gm daily), or indomethacin (200 mg daily) reduce the output of prostaglandin metabolites in the urine by 77% to 98%.[27]

Inhibition of prostaglandin synthesis can explain other actions of aspirin. Although prostaglandins themselves do not appear to cause pain when injected locally, they do sensitize pain receptors to other mediators such as histamine or bradykinin.[9] The analgesic action of drugs like aspirin could thus be due to reduction of prostaglandin production. In this connection, it is of interest to note that such drugs can prevent the writhing response elicited by bradykinin but not that produced by prostaglandins.[19] Since a role for prostaglandins in temperature elevation has been suggested, it is also likely that the well-known antipyretic effect of aspirin and similar drugs is mediated by inhibition of prostaglandin synthetase.

It seems certain that prostaglandins and most likely their intermediates are involved in the inflammatory process. It is also clear that inhibition of prostaglandin biosynthesis is a general and unequivocal characteristic of aspirin and other nonsteroidal antiinflammatory drugs. Nevertheless, it is not possible at present to attribute all of the antiinflammatory effects of these drugs to inhibition of prostaglandin synthetase. Some antiinflammatory activity may be related to the ability of the salicylates to act as scavengers for tissue-destructive free radicals produced by the cyclooxygenase and lipoxygenase enzymes. These agents also affect numerous components of the inflammatory process (e.g., inhibition of lysosomal proteolytic enzymes) in which prostaglandins are not known to be involved.

General therapeutic uses. The antiinflammatory properties of the salicylates are clinically employed in a wide variety of inflammatory conditions, ranging from the simple, benign, and limited to the complex, serious, and chronic. Since it is effective, inexpensive, and readily obtained, aspirin is the standard remedy for pain of low to moderate intensity, regardless of cause, and for fever associated with minor infections, such as the common cold and influenza. The analgesic effect sought and attained with aspirin is probably caused in many cases by its antiinflammatory actions, a fact not usually appreciated by its users.

In addition to its widespread use for the symptomatic relief of aches, pains, and general malaise, salicylate is a drug of major importance in the treatment of several chronic inflammatory diseases.[2]

Rheumatic fever. The well-known "antirheumatic" effect of the salicylates is commonly utilized in the management of rheumatic fever. Aspirin markedly reduces the acute inflammatory components of the disease, such as fever and joint pain, swelling, and immobility. However, the salicylates do not affect other aspects of the disease, such as the proliferative reaction in the myocardium leading to scarring, nor do they alter the progression of the disease. Corticosteroids may be used instead of or in conjunction with salicylates and are especially valuable when serious myocarditis occurs. In the absence of acute cardiac complications, however, intensive salicylate therapy (5 to 8 gm/day for adults) is still the preferred treatment in most cases.[43]

Rheumatoid arthritis. Rheumatoid arthritis is a chronic systemic disease of unknown etiology. Several tissues and organs may be involved, but in most patients the chief clinical and pathologic features are a result of chronic inflammation of synovial membranes. Irreversible joint injury (subluxation, loss of motion, or ankylosis) results from formation of chronic granulation tissue that causes erosion of articular cartilage, subchondral bone, ligaments, and tendons. Extraarticular manifestations, such as subcutaneous or subperiosteal nodules of granulation tissue, peripheral neuropathy, and chronic skin ulcers, occur to a variable extent and appear to result from generalized focal vasculitis.

The etiology of the inflammatory response in rheumatoid arthritis is obscure, as are the factors that relate synovial inflammation to the eventual destruction of the joint. One proposal is that the synovitis is initiated by an autoimmune reaction.[13]

Antiimmunoglobulins, referred to as the rheumatoid factor and found in rheumatoid synovial fluid, can form complexes with IgG. These complexes may activate complement, which in turn triggers a number of inflammatory phenomena in the joint tissues, including histamine release, production of factors chemotactic for neutrophils and mononuclear cells, cell membrane damage, and prostaglandin synthesis. Both neutrophils and macrophages accumulate in the synovium and are found to contain aggregated IgG, rheumatoid factor, complement fragments, and fibrin; these substances are apparently acquired by phagocytosis. Lysosomal materials are released that amplify the inflammatory reaction and may directly damage tissues. Lymphokines produced by the lymphocytic cell infiltrate may also help propagate the reaction and participate in tissue destruction.

Salicylates (usually as aspirin) are still heavily used in the clinical management of rheumatoid arthritis. The majority of cases of rheumatoid arthritis can be controlled with salicylates alone.[43] Salicylates produce a measurable reduction of inflammation in the joints and associated tissues, a lessening of symptoms, and improved mobility. Clinical observation suggests that salicylate therapy can diminish or delay the development of crippling. This is probably not a direct effect of the drug on the progression of the disease but relates more to reduction of pain and subsequent facilitation of mobility. In addition to salicylates, the basic therapeutic regimen in rheumatoid arthritis includes rest, physical measures (primarily heat), and exercise.[13] In cases in which salicylate therapy is inadequate, other drugs may be used. These compounds include nonsteroidal agents such as indomethacin, phenylbutazone, gold salts, and newer compounds such as ibuprofen, as well as the corticosteroids and antimalarial drugs (i.e., chloroquine and hydroxychloroquine), penicillamine, and various immunosuppressants (e.g., azathioprine).

In rheumatoid arthritis, salicylates are given in doses sufficient to control the symptoms, usually 3 to 5 gm per day. The degree of suppression of inflammation increases with the plasma salicylate concentration even beyond the point of toxicity. Thus, patients with severe arthritis will tolerate tinnitus and other mild toxic manifestations in order to obtain the antiinflammatory effects gained by high plasma titers of salicylate. A regular dose interval to maintain constant effective blood concentrations is important. Evaluation of drug therapy in rheumatoid patients may be complicated by the spontaneous remissions and exacerbations characteristic of this disease.

Other rheumatic diseases. Aspirin is a preferred antiinflammatory agent in various other inflammatory diseases, including juvenile rheumatoid arthritis, ankylosing spondylitis, psoriatic arthritis, Reiter's syndrome, and degenerative joint disease (osteoarthritis). The arthralgia and fever of mild lupus erythematosus may be alleviated by aspirin. Acute episodes of inflammation in isolated joints, tendons, or bursae caused by trauma are also best treated with aspirin given in full doses immediately after the injury.

New uses for aspirin. The well-documented inhibition of platelet aggregation by aspirin provides the rationale for a potential new use of this drug. There is evidence that platelet aggregation and subsequent thrombogenesis are important processes in the production of stroke (cerebral vascular occlusion) and heart attack. It is theoretically possible that long-term treatment with a platelet antiaggregant, such as aspirin, could block this process and thereby reduce the incidence of infarction. Several studies have tested this possibility, and the results, taken together, indicate that it may be a valid approach. A Canadian trial of nearly 600 patients treated with aspirin for 26 months showed an overall reduction of 31% in stroke and death rates.[6] In five of six randomized trials of the effect of aspirin in patients with coronary artery disease, total mortality was reduced 15% to 30% in the patients given aspirin compared with the placebo group.[48] Several large trials now in progress in the United States and Europe should provide data that will further delineate the efficacy of aspirin in reducing both morbidity and mortality in thromboembolic disease.

Therapeutic uses in dentistry. The major use of aspirin in dentistry is to relieve pain associated with pathologic processes (pulpitis, dentoalveolar abscesses, etc.) or following surgical procedures. In both situations, the antiinflammatory actions of aspirin may contribute significantly to the therapeutic effect sought. There are few chronic inflammatory diseases per se solely limited to the oral structures and amenable to therapy with antiinflammatory agents. The temporomandibular joint may be involved in systemic rheumatic diseases, which would be treated with aspirin. The joint can also be singly affected by an acute or chronic inflammatory process, the etiology of which may be

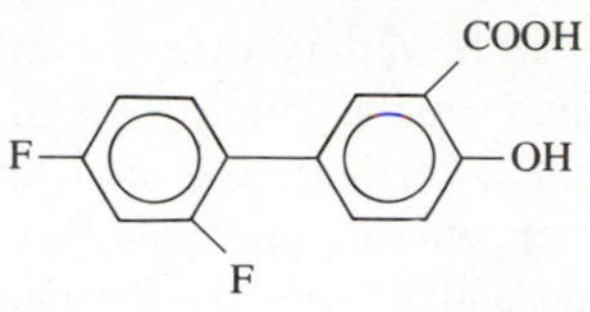

Figure 22-4. Structural formula of diflunisal.

known (trauma, immobilization, or malocclusion) or unknown (nonspecific osteoarthritis). In these cases, aspirin is used in conjunction with other therapies such as heat, exercise, correction of occlusal abnormalities, and joint surgery.

Diflunisal. Diflunisal is a recently marketed compound with antiinflammatory, analgesic, and antipyretic activity. It is a difluorophenyl derivative of salicylic acid (Figure 22-4). Like other salicylates, diflunisal inhibits the synthesis of prostaglandins. This is presumed to be the basis of its analgesic and antiinflammatory properties.

Diflunisal is indicated for the treatment of mild to moderate pain and for osteoarthritis. It appears to offer several advantages over aspirin. The drug is well absorbed after oral administration, with peak blood concentrations occurring in 2 to 3 hours. Although gastrointestinal symptoms can develop, diflunisal is less problematic in this respect than aspirin. It has a long plasma half-life (8 to 12 hours versus 2.5 hours for salicylate), which permits dose intervals of up to 12 hours. The drug is excreted in the urine as two soluble glucuronide conjugates accounting for about 90% of the administered dose. In plasma, it is highly protein bound.

The analgesic efficacy if diflunisal has been demonstrated in several published studies. These studies show that 500 mg diflunisal gives pain relief that is longer lasting and generally superior to that of 600 mg aspirin or acetaminophen in various pain states. In one study of postoperative tooth extraction pain, single doses of 500 or 1000 mg diflunisal were equivalent in peak analgesia to a combination of 600 mg acetaminophen with 60 mg codeine.[23] The effectiveness of diflunisal in osteoarthritis appears to be comparable to that of aspirin.

In terms of adverse effects, diflunisal qualitatively resembles aspirin. Effects on the gastrointestinal tract range from nausea and epigastric pain to peptic ulcer and gastrointestinal bleeding. Platelet function and bleeding time are affected in a

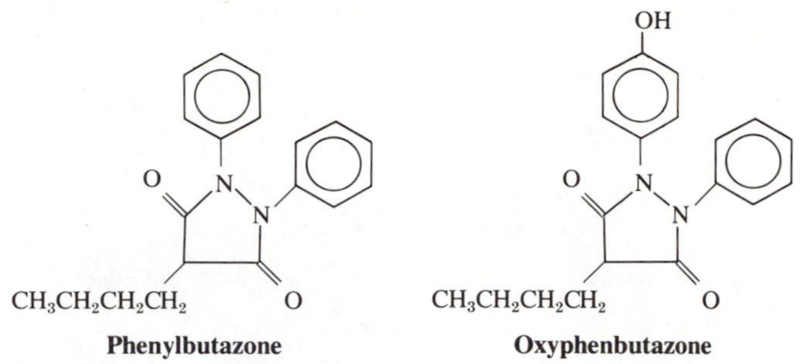

Figure 22-5. Structural formulas of phenylbutazone and oxyphenbutazone.

dose-related fashion. Like aspirin, diflunisal prolongs the prothrombin time in patients receiving oral anticoagulants, perhaps by competitive displacement of coumarins from protein binding sites. However, in all of these respects, diflunisal seems to be less troublesome than aspirin. This does not mean, of course, that this agent is without risk. As with any drug, the contraindications and precautions for its use must be carefully considered and the patient's response to treatment closely monitored. This is especially true if therapy of more than a few days' duration is undertaken.

As an antiinflammatory agent, diflunisal has limited use in dentistry. As a postoperative analgesic, however, it offers advantages when a nonopioid analgesic effective against moderate pain is required. It is more effective than aspirin and has a longer (8 to 12 hours) duration of action. It is unfortunately also much more expensive.

Other nonsteroidal antiinflammatory agents

During the last quarter century, the search for more specific, more potent, and less toxic antiinflammatory agents has produced a number of useful drugs. None of these, however, is an ideal agent; potency has been increased but so too has toxicity. As a group, these drugs offer limited advantages over aspirin in specific situations, and like aspirin they have no effect on the underlying cause or course of the disease.

Phenylbutazone. Phenylbutazone, a pyrazolone derivative (Figure 22-5), is a congener of antipyrine and aminopyrine. The latter agents were once used as analgesics, antipyretics, and antiinflammatory drugs, but their toxicity and the introduction of phenylbutazone in 1948 led to their abandonment.

Phenylbutazone resembles the salicylates in many respects. Its antiinflammatory effects can readily be demonstrated in laboratory animals and in patients with acute or chronic inflammatory conditions. Phenylbutazone has antipyretic effects and relieves pain, especially of rheumatic origin. It also has mild uricosuric properties. Furthermore, like the salicylates, phenylbutazone has inhibitory effects on prostaglandin synthesis, and this is presumed to be its mechanism of action.[21]

Phenylbutazone given by mouth is rapidly absorbed, with peak plasma concentrations attained in 2 hours. It is slowly transformed in the liver to oxyphenbutazone, an active metabolite (Figure 22-5). The parent compound and the metabolite have half-lives of about 72 hours, and both are extensively bound to plasma albumin.

Clinical use of phenylbutazone is associated with a high incidence of adverse effects. The most serious of these is bone marrow depression, leading to agranulocytosis, thrombocytopenia, leukopenia, or aplastic anemia. Leukemic changes have also been reported. Blood dyscrasias occur most frequently during high-dose therapy and may be manifested initially by fever, stomatitis, and sore throat. Gastrointestinal disturbances are common and range from mucosal irritation to frank ulceration and hemorrhage. Other adverse reactions include skin rashes, hepatitis, jaundice, purpura, and hematuria. Phenylbutazone causes sodium retention by the kidney; the resultant edema may be significant in persons with borderline or overt congestive heart failure. Oxyphenbutazone is said to cause less gastric irritation, but otherwise its pharmacologic, therapeutic, and toxic effects are the same.

There are few clinical situations in which either phenylbutazone or oxyphenbutazone would be the agent of choice. They may be useful in the treatment of acute gout or exacerbations of rheumatoid

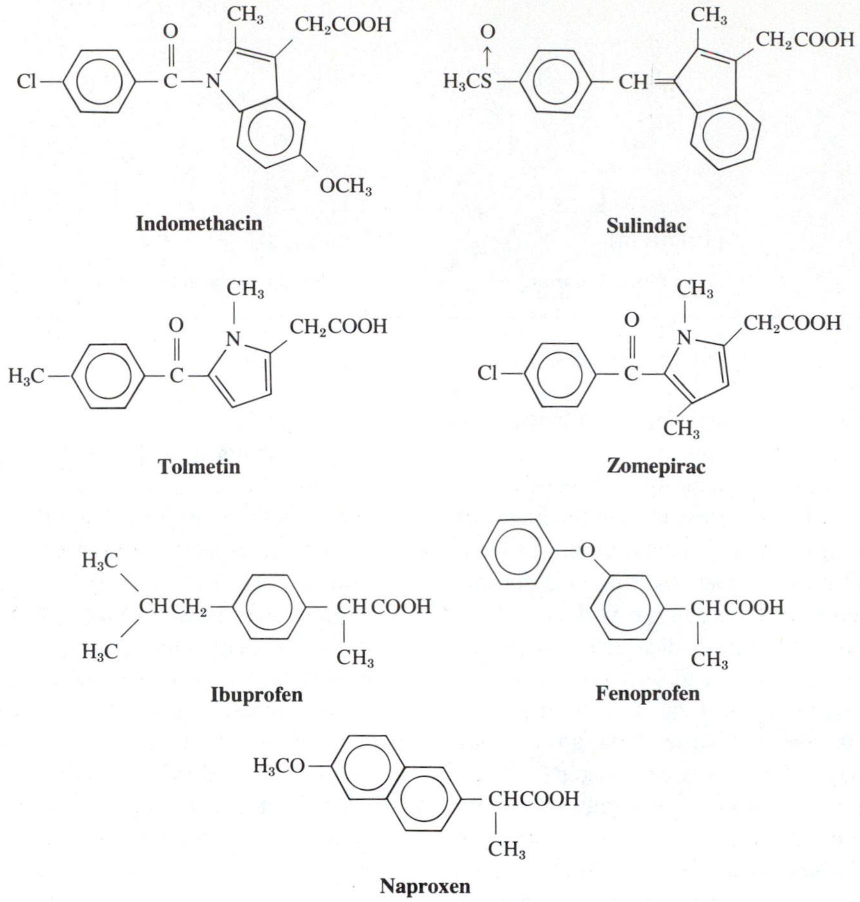

Figure 22-6. Arylalkanoic acid derivatives.

arthritis or other inflammatory diseases affecting the joints. They may also relieve the signs and symptoms of acute superficial thrombophlebitis. Whatever the reasons for their use, the duration of therapy with either drug should be limited to 1 week. Neither drug has any indications in dentistry.

Phenylbutazone and oxyphenbutazone are good candidates for drug interactions because of the high degree of plasma protein binding, their tendency to promote bleeding, and their gastrointestinal effects. Other antiinflammatory agents, oral anticoagulants, and sulfonamides compete with phenylbutazone for its protein binding sites. A beneficial antiinflammatory effect occurs when the nonsteroidal antiinflammatory drugs are given with the corticosteroids, because the nonsteroidal drugs displace the corticosteroids from secondary binding sites. Phenylbutazone is also known to induce hepatic microsomal enzymes.

Arylalkanoic acid derivatives. The arylalkanoic acid derivatives are nonsteroidal antiinflammatory, analgesic, and antipyretic agents. Indomethacin was the first of these drugs, and it will be considered separately from the newer agents.

Indomethacin. Indomethacin is a derivative of indoleacetic acid with potent antiinflammatory properties. Its chemical structure is shown in Figure 22-6. Like the salicylates, indomethacin has antipyretic and analgesic effects, the latter being most notable when the pain is associated with an inflammatory condition. Because of its serious toxicity, however, indomethacin should never be employed as an antipyretic or simple analgesic. Its use is reserved for those cases of rheumatoid arthritis, ankylosing spondylitis, and osteoarthritis in which less toxic drugs are ineffective or not tolerated. Indomethacin has also been used as a short-term antiinflammatory agent in the treatment of bursitis, tendonitis, and acute attacks of gouty arthritis. Although indomethacin is a more potent antiinflammatory agent both in vivo and in vitro than aspirin, its toxicity severely limits its clinical usefulness. There are no indications for the use of indomethacin in dentistry.

Indomethacin is a potent inhibitor of fatty acid cyclooxygenase in vitro. It markedly reduces the manifestations of inflammation in several animal models.[19] Like the salicylates, it has effects on numerous biochemical and cellular events that may be involved in the inflammatory process; some of these events may or may not be mediated by prostaglandins.

Indomethacin is well absorbed from the gastrointestinal tract, and peak plasma concentrations are reached in 2 to 4 hours. The drug is largely bound to plasma proteins. Following a single dose, most of the drug is eliminated in the urine as conjugated metabolites during the next 24 hours.

Adverse effects are common with indomethacin therapy. Gastrointestinal disturbances, such as epigastric pain, nausea, and diarrhea, occur frequently. The drug may also cause perforation of the esophagus, stomach, and duodenum, and the resultant hemorrhage can be fatal. The drug is thus contraindicated in patients with active gastrointestinal lesions or a history of such lesions. CNS effects such as severe headache and confusion also occur. In addition to dermatologic and allergic reactions, leukopenia, aplastic anemia, thrombocytopenia, and hepatitis have been reported; some of these reactions have proved fatal.[2]

As is the case for phenylbutazone and oxyphenbutazone, indomethacin has the potential for interacting with many drugs. Simultaneous administration of indomethacin and oral anticoagulants may be hazardous.

Newer derivatives. Beginning with ibuprofen in 1974, a number of arylalkanoic acid derivatives have been approved for marketing in the United States. Ibuprofen, fenoprofen, and naproxen are substituted phenylpropionic acids; tolmetin and sulindac are complex aromatic derivatives of acetic acid (Figure 22-6). Like other nonsteroidal drugs useful in the treatment of rheumatoid arthritis and degenerative joint disease, these drugs inhibit prostaglandin synthetase.[12,41]

In patients with rheumatoid arthritis, the arylalkanoic acid derivatives reduce joint swelling, pain, and morning stiffness, and they improve mobility as measured by an increase in walking time. When used in patients treated with corticosteroids, these agents may permit reduction of the steroid dose. With the exception of recommended doses of ibuprofen,[32] these agents are as effective as aspirin in treating rheumatoid arthritis and osteoarthritis. Because they are less likely to cause gastrointestinal or bleeding disturbances, their use in this regard will undoubtedly increase. Sulindac and naproxen are also indicated for symptomatic relief of tendonitis, bursitis, alkylosing spondylitis, and acute gouty arthritis. As described below, zomepirac was used for a short time as an analgesic, but it is not currently on the market.

These drugs are rapidly and almost completely absorbed from the gastrointestinal tract. Peak blood concentrations are reached in 30 to 60 minutes with tolmetin and between 1 and 2 hours with the other drugs. All of these agents are highly bound to plasma proteins; they are theoretically capable of interfering with the binding of other drugs, such as phenytoin or the sulfonamides. The drugs are variably metabolized and are then excreted in the urine as either the unchanged drug or as inactive metabolites. Ibuprofen, fenoprofen, and tolmetin all have short plasma half-lives (1 to 3 hours), while zomepirac and naproxen have plasma half-lives of about 4 and 12 hours respectively. Sulindac is unique among these agents in that the drug itself is inactive and must be metabolically reduced to the sulfide in order to exert biologic activity. The half-life of the sulfide is approximately 16 hours. More than half of the absorbed drug is excreted in the urine as unchanged sulindac or as a sulfone metabolite, and the remainder is eliminated through the feces.

Although the incidence is less than with aspirin, these agents produce a variety of gastrointestinal disturbances (epigastric pain, nausea, vomiting, bleeding, and constipation or diarrhea) and should be used with caution in patients with a history of peptic ulcer. CNS effects may include headache, dizziness, drowsiness, vertigo, and visual and auditory disturbances. Skin rashes are relatively common, and immediate allergic reactions have been reported. These agents decrease platelet aggregation and adhesiveness and increase bleeding time; they should be avoided in patients with bleeding disorders and used with caution in patients receiving anticoagulants. Because these drugs promote sodium retention, their use may lead to the formation of edema in susceptible individuals.

In 1978, zomepirac was approved by the FDA for oral use as an analgesic. A number of well-controlled trials in a variety of situations, including

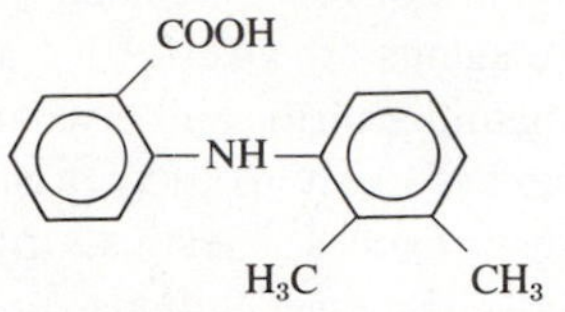

Figure 22-7. Structural formula of mefenamic acid.

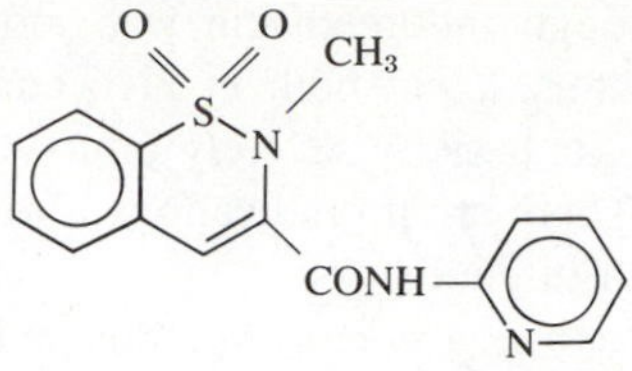

Figure 22-8. Structural formula of piroxicam.

acute postoperative pain and pain associated with cancer and chronic orthopedic conditions, clearly showed that zomepirac is an effective analgesic.[41] In most of these trials, 100 mg zomepirac consistently performed better than placebo, 650 mg aspirin, or 60 mg codeine. The maximal analgesic effect appeared to be equivalent to 650 mg aspirin or acetaminophen combined with 60 mg codeine. Since zomepirac was free of any opioid liabilities, its clinical use as an analgesic rapidly increased. In early 1983, several deaths caused by anaphylaxis were reported in patients receiving zomepirac. The drug was consequently withdrawn voluntarily from the market by the manufacturer. It may possibly be reintroduced with new warnings concerning this serious but unforeseen adverse effect; however, positive results concerning the analgesic efficacy of ibuprofen[14] and other phenylpropionic acid derivatives have lessened the need for zomepirac. (The analgesic use of these drugs in dentistry is covered in Chapter 21.)

Fenamates. The fenamates are a group of aspirin-like drugs derived from N-phenylanthranilic acid. Although at least a half-dozen fenamates are known, only mefenamic acid and meclofenamic acid are available in the United States. The structure of mefenamic acid is shown in Figure 22-7.

Both mefenamic and meclofenamic acids are potent antiinflammatory agents with analgesic and antipyretic properties. Clinical use, however, is limited by a high (approximately 25%) incidence of gastrointestinal symptoms ranging from gastric pain to diarrhea. In addition, the fenamates have all the liabilities of aspirin (tinnitus, gastric bleeding, and impairment of platelet function). More serious toxicity in the form of abnormal renal and hepatic function and hemolytic anemia have been documented.

Of these two agents, only meclofenamic acid is currently approved for treatment of inflammatory

disorders, specifically acute and chronic rheumatoid arthritis and osteoarthritis. Mefenamic acid is limited to use as an analgesic for moderate pain and for the treatment of primary dysmenorrhea. Neither agent has notable utility in dental medicine.

Oxicams. The oxicams are the newest group of nonsteroidal antiinflammatory drugs to be developed. Piroxicam, the first member of this class (Figure 22-8), was recently approved for the treatment of rheumatoid arthritis and osteoarthritis. A second drug, isoxicam, is expected to be marketed in the near future.

These drugs are similar to aspirin in many respects. They are analgesic, antipyretic, and antiinflammatory; they also inhibit platelet aggregation and promote gastrointestinal bleeding. All of these effects are attributed to inhibition of prostaglandin synthesis.

Piroxicam and isoxicam are at least as effective as aspirin for the treatment of rheumatoid arthritis, and they appear to be better tolerated. Their major advantage, however, is pharmacokinetic in nature. Both drugs are well absorbed, with peak plasma concentrations occuring several hours after administration (3 to 5 hours for piroxicam, 4 to 8 hours for isoxicam). The drugs are highly bound to plasma protein and are eventually eliminated in the urine after being extensively metabolized. The approximate plasma half-lives for piroxicam and isoxicam are, respectively, 50 and 30 hours. This slow elimination rate permits administration of a single daily dose, an advantage for drugs that must be taken on a long-term basis.

The side effects of these drugs are similar to those of other nonsteroidal antiinflammatory agents. In addition to gastrointestinal upset and the possibility of ulceration and hemorrhage, peripheral edema and, rarely, aplastic anemia may occur. Neither drug should be administered to a patient susceptible to aspirin-induced bronchospasm. There is currently no indication for these drugs in dentistry, and their proper role in medicine must await further experience with their use.

Miscellaneous agents for rheumatoid arthritis

Several groups of compounds unrelated to the aspirin-like drugs described above and to the adrenal corticosteroids considered below are useful in suppressing the signs and symptoms of rheumatoid arthritis. These drugs are relatively toxic, and they are for the most part restricted to refractory cases of arthritis and patients unable to tolerate standard medications.

Gold compounds. Gold salts have been employed clinically (chrysotherapy) for 50 years to treat certain inflammatory conditions. Because of their toxicity, their use is restricted to rheumatoid arthritis. They are generally indicated in active cases in which the arthritis steadily progresses despite an adequate regimen of salicylates, rest, and exercise therapy. In such cases, chrysotherapy (using either aurothioglucose or gold sodium thiomalate) usually induces a partial or complete remission of symptoms. The duration of these remissions is highly variable.

The mechanism by which gold salts suppress inflammation is unknown. Gold compounds inhibit prostaglandin synthesis, suppress cellular immune reactions, uncouple oxidative phosphorylation, stabilize lysosomal membranes, and inhibit lysosomal hydrolases. The relationship of these diverse actions to the observed clinical effects is not clear. Unlike other nonsteroidal antiinflammatory drugs, gold salts have no antipyretic or analgesic properties in nonrheumatic conditions.

Since the conventional gold salts are not well absorbed by the gastrointestinal tract, they are given by intramuscular injection. Their distribution and fate are complex and depend on the dose and dosage interval. The plasma half-life initially increases with each subsequent dose, and months may be required for mean blood concentrations to reach a plateau. After some period of constant weekly injections, gold accumulates in various tissues to such an extent that it may be continuously excreted for many months after administration has ceased. More than half of an administered dose is eventually eliminated in the urine and the remainder in the feces.

Chrysotherapy is complicated by a number of occasionally serious adverse reactions. Toxicity of gold salts may be initially manifested by mucocutaneous lesions. These include pruritus, dermatitis (ranging from mild to severe), stomatitis (including glossitis), colitis, and vaginitis. Blood dyscrasias, including leukopenia, agranulocytosis, and aplastic anemia, have been reported. Toxic effects involving the liver, kidney, and central nervous system can also occur. These adverse effects appear to be dose related and may develop at any time during chrysotherapy.

An orally effective form of gold, auranofin, is currently under investigation and will likely be approved for use in the near future. It appears to be less toxic than parenteral chrysotherapy, the major toxicity being diarrhea rather than skin rash and marrow depression. Since its antiarthritic effects appear to be equivalent to the conventional parenteral forms, auranofin may represent an important advance in those cases in which chrysotherapy is indicated.[42]

Antimalarial agents. Both chloroquine and more frequently hydroxychloroquine have been used in the treatment of rheumatoid arthritis and lupus erythematosus. They are generally administered in conjunction with other antiinflammatory drugs for relief of mild, early rheumatoid arthritis. Clinical improvement is usually very slow, requiring 3 to 6 months. After this time, if there is no evidence of benefit, the drug is discontinued.

Serious ocular toxicity has been caused by these drugs; the retinopathy is dose related and may progress even after therapy is discontinued. This effect has made the antimalarial drugs controversial as antirheumatic agents and mandates regular ophthalmologic testing during therapy. Other toxic effects include gastrointestinal, dermatologic, and neuropsychiatric disturbances.

Penicillamine. Penicillamine, a breakdown product of penicillin used in the treatment of heavy metal poisoning (Chapter 47), was first reported to be effective in rheumatoid arthritis in 1970. Its mode of action is unknown; penicillamine has both immunosuppressive and immunostimulant properties. As with chrysotherapy, penicillamine must be administered for several months before clinical improvement is noted. Side effects are frequent, usually occurring early in therapy. Skin rash similar to that caused by ampicillin is common, as are gastrointestinal disturbances and, to a lesser extent, nephropathy and thrombocytopenia. The drug must be withdrawn from about a third of patients because of adverse reactions.

Immunosuppressants. The immunosuppressant azathioprine (Chapter 39) and the antineoplastic cyclophosphamide (Chapter 40) are effective in relieving rheumatoid arthritis. Obviously, inhibition of the cellular elements of the inflammatory process can have multiple effects on inflammatory reactions, and it is not surprising that the exact mechanism by which such drugs ameliorate rheumatoid arthritis is unknown. It is also obvious that these drugs can cause severe adverse effects, such as promoting infections, blood dyscrasias, and neoplastic transformation, and that they should be used only in patients with the most debilitating disease and then only in its active stages.

Drugs used to treat gout

Gout is an inflammatory disease that stems from elevated concentrations of uric acid in blood and other body fluids. Such elevations may be the result of either an increased production (metabolic gout) or a decreased rate of excretion (renal gout). However, in most patients with gout, overproduction of uric acid rather than decreased elimination is the major contributing factor. Overproduction may be due to a primary defect in purine metabolism, such as a deficiency in the enzyme phosphoribosyl transferase, or secondary to certain hematologic disorders, cancer chemotherapy, or therapy with other drugs.

Essentially all of the clinical manifestations of gout derive from the precipitation of sodium urate from extracellular fluids when and where it exceeds the limits of solubility. These manifestations can be divided into four categories: acute gouty arthritis, tophaceous deposits (sodium urate deposits in and around joints in cartilage, bone, bursae, and subcutaneous tissue), uric acid nephrolithiasis, and gouty kidney with various degrees of impairment of renal function. Of all these, gouty arthritis is most frequently the first clinical manifestation of the disease. Intensive study of the mechanism of gouty arthritis has shown it to be an inflammatory reaction to sodium urate microcrystals deposited in synovial fluid.[63] Precisely how these crystals initiate inflammation is not known. The crystals can activate Hageman factor and in this way initiate the chain of events leading to bradykinin formation. In any case, large numbers of neutrophils accumulate in the synovium, possibly because of a chemotactic effect of uric acid. These neutrophils actively phagocytize urate crystals, leading to release of lysosomal enzymes and increased lactic acid production. Both of these events tend to propagate the inflammatory response, the former by damaging tissue and the latter by lowering the local pH and thus fostering further urate deposition.

Although the overall pathogenesis of gouty arthritis is understood, many specific events are still obscure. It is known that acute gouty arthritis often follows a precipitating event—surgery, injury, alcohol ingestion, dietary excess, emotional crisis, even the minor stress of walking—but it is not known how these events are related to urate crystal deposition. Another unknown is the sex distribution: less than 10% of gout occurs in women.[63]

Acute gouty arthritis is characterized clinically by severe inflammation of the joint and periarticular tissues. One or several joints may be involved simultaneously, as shown by marked swelling, redness, heat, and intense pain. Lymphangitis is occasionally present. There may also be systemic signs of inflammation, including fever, leukocytosis, and increased sedimentation rate. Without treatment, the arthritis gradually subsides over a period of 1 to 2 weeks. The rate of recurrence is variable after an initial attack, but in most patients recurrence is common, usually within a year. With increasing age, the incidence of attacks increases, as does the severity, duration of inflammation, and number of joints affected. The patient may in time rarely be free of gouty arthritis, and the pain, swelling, and stiffness can result in total and permanent disability.

The treatment of gout may involve multiple agents acting at different sites and having distinctly different objectives. Since the pathologic manifestations of the disease result from an elevated extracellular uric acid, a rational therapeutic maneuver is to lower urate concentrations. Two approaches toward this end are currently available: the use of uricosuric drugs to increase renal urate clearance, and the use of allopurinol to inhibit urate synthesis.

The uricosuric agents most often employed are probenecid and sulfinpyrazone (Figure 22-9). Both of these compounds can actually enhance urate retention by blocking its renal tubular secretion. At higher doses, however, these agents also block tubular reabsorption of urate, thus increasing urinary excretion of uric acid and lowering serum urate concentrations. Uricosuric drugs are used primarily in chronic gout to prevent formation of new tophi and to slowly mobilize urate deposits in old lesions.

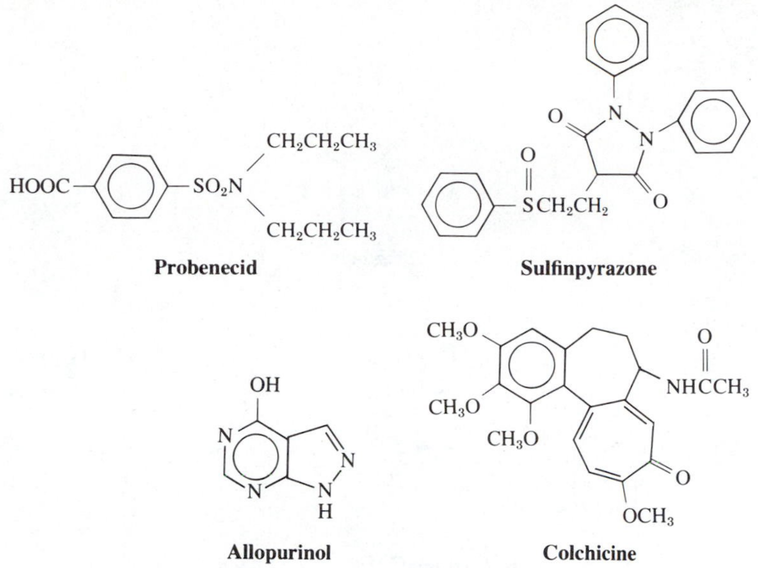

Figure 22-9. Agents used in the treatment and prevention of gout.

They are not useful in treating attacks of gouty arthritis, since mobilization of previously deposited urates may initially increase the severity of the attack. Maintenance of an alkaline diuresis during therapy with uricosuric agents is important. The pK_a of uric acid is 5.6, and the solubility of the nonionized form is low. Thus, an alkaline environment will minimize intrarenal deposition. Both probenecid and sulfinpyrazone are initially given in low doses, which are gradually increased until the desired serum urate concentration is obtained (usually 6 mg/100 ml); a maintenance dose is then established. Both drugs are generally well tolerated. The most common adverse effects are gastrointestinal disturbances and allergic reactions ranging from dermatitis to anaphylaxis. Although the salicylates are uricosuric at high doses, they are no longer used for this purpose. Since salicylates at ordinary doses may decrease urate excretion, they should be used cautiously in patients with gout.

Originally developed as an antineoplastic agent, allopurinol (Figure 22-9) is a relatively new drug in the treatment of gout. Allopurinol and its metabolite alloxanthine are competitive inhibitors of the enzyme xanthine oxidase. This enzyme catalyzes the oxidation of hypoxanthine to xanthine and then to uric acid. The action of allopurinol, therefore, is to reduce the biosynthesis of uric acid and

lower both blood and urine concentrations. The uric acid precursors do not accumulate in body fluids since they are sufficiently cleared by the kidney. Like the uricosuric agents, allopurinol is indicated for chronic rather than acute gout. It may be preferred in the more severe forms over the uricosuric agents. As with the uricosuric agents, allopurinol may initially increase the number of acute attacks of gouty arthritis unless colchicine prophylaxis, as described below, is used. The toxic effects of allopurinol include allergic reactions involving the skin (e.g., exfoliative, urticarial, and purpuric lesions) and blood (e.g., agranulocytosis, anemia, and thrombocytopenia). There is a modest incidence of gastric irritation.

In addition to efforts aimed at reducing the extracellular uric acid concentration, another aspect of therapy for gout is management of acute arthritis. This goal entails the short-term use of antiinflammatory agents, some of which (phenylbutazone, indomethacin, sulindac, and naproxen) have already been described. Although these drugs have no specific actions in gouty arthritis, they can effectively relieve the pain, tenderness, and swelling in affected joints.

The drug of choice in treating gouty arthritis is colchicine, a plant alkaloid with a long history of use in gout (Figure 22-9). When given at the first indication of an attack, colchicine effects a striking

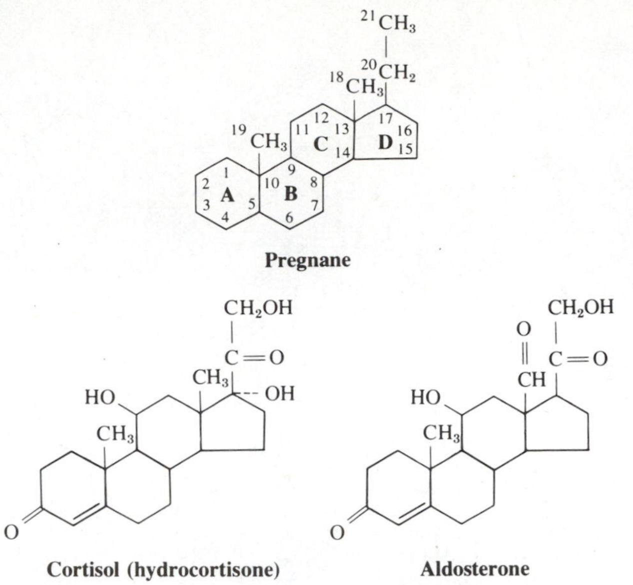

Figure 22-10. Structural formulas of pregnane, the basic corticosteroid nucleus, and cortisol and aldosterone, the prototypical glucocorticoid and mineralocorticoid, respectively.

reduction of the emerging signs and symptoms of arthritis. Pain usually disappears within 4 to 12 hours after intravenous doses and 24 to 48 hours after oral doses. It is relatively specific for this condition; the drug has little effect on other inflammatory conditions, nor does it have inherent analgesic properties. Colchicine may also be given prophylactically to prevent recurrent attacks.

The antiinflammatory effects of colchicine may be related to its well-known antimitotic activity.[21] It arrests mitosis in metaphase by binding to microtubular protein and preventing spindle formation. By a similar action, colchicine disrupts fibrillar microtubules in neutrophils and other motile cells. The involvement of the microtubular system in cell locomotion could explain colchicine inhibition of neutrophil migration and phagocytic activity in inflamed joints.

Colchicine is rapidly absorbed from the gastrointestinal tract and widely distributed in the body. The drug is partially metabolized in the liver, and the metabolites and unchanged drug are excreted in the feces. This action may explain why the gastrointestinal tract is a frequent site of adverse reactions.

The most common untoward effects of colchicine are nausea, vomiting, and diarrhea. Diarrhea is an important sign, since it may signal more serious toxic reactions, such as hemorrhagic gastroenteritis. The gastrointestinal effects of colchicine may be due to direct toxicity to intestinal mucosal cells. Long-term use of colchicine may lead to bone marrow depression, myopathy, and alopecia.

Adrenal corticosteroids

Certain adrenal corticosteroids and their synthetic analogues are widely used in medicine for their potent antiinflammatory properties. These agents are also referred to as glucocorticoids because of their profound effects on intermediary metabolism. Unfortunately, when the glucocorticoids are administered over long periods, as they often are, severe and even lethal toxic reactions can occur. To understand properly the therapeutic applications and limitations of this group of drugs, the physiologic role of the corticosteroids must be reviewed.

General physiologic and pharmacologic actions. Using cholesterol as a substrate, the adrenal cortex synthesizes and secretes two types of steroid hormones, the 19-carbon androgens and the 21-carbon corticosteroids. The latter group can be considered as derivatives of pregnane (Figure

22-10). The corticosteroids can be further classified on the basis of their major actions. Some compounds, such as cortisol, have relatively greater effects on carbohydrate metabolism, as measured by liver glycogen deposition, and are thus termed *glucocorticoids*. Others, represented by aldosterone, are most active in enhancing sodium retention and are referred to as *mineralocorticoids*. These designations are somewhat misleading, since all of the natural and most of the synthetic corticosteroids possess both actions to some degree, as can be seen in Table 22-4. Even so, this division is useful from a pharmacologic standpoint, since the antiinflammatory activity correlates well with glucocorticoid potency. The structures of cortisol and aldosterone are shown in Figure 22-10.

The corticosteroids are not stored to any extent in the adrenal gland but are continuously synthesized and secreted. There is a strong diurnal variation in this process; plasma concentrations of cortisol are severalfold higher at 8:00 A.M. than at 4:00 P.M.[29] Production of all corticosteroids except aldosterone is directly regulated by the blood concentration of ACTH secreted by the anterior pituitary (adenohypophysis). In turn, circulating corticosteroids act on the adenohypophysis to suppress the release of ACTH, completing the control loop linking the pituitary and the adrenal cortex. By this negative feedback mechanism, the administration of large doses of corticosteroids can deprive the adrenal cortex of the tropic influence of this hormone, thus completely suppressing adrenal production of corticosteroids. Control of aldosterone secretion is less clearly understood but appears to involve a direct effect of angiotensin on the adrenal cortex, leading to a rather selective stimulation of aldosterone synthesis and secretion with relatively little effect on the output of other corticosteroids.

The corticosteroids play diverse and complex roles in the body economy of mammalian organisms. They are involved in carbohydrate, protein, lipid, and purine metabolism; electrolyte and water balance; and the functions of the cardiovascular system, kidney, muscle, nervous system, and most other organs and tissues. It is not surprising, then, that the hormones of the adrenal cortex have a major impact on the ability of animals to withstand stressful events. Without the adrenal cortex, life is possible only when food and large amounts of sodium chloride and water are regularly ingested, a constant ambient temperature prevails, and infection and other perturbing events are absent.

Table 22-4. Potencies of some commonly used corticosteroids (relative to cortisol)

	Liver glycogen deposition*	Sodium retention
11-Desoxycorticosterone	0	100
Aldosterone	0.1	3000
Cortisone	0.8	0.8
Cortisol	1	1
Prednisolone	4	0.8
Triamcinolone	5	0
Fludrocortisone	10	3000
Dexamethasone	25	0
Betamethasone	30	0

*Generally paralleled by antiinflammatory activity.

All of the diverse actions of the corticosteroids are achieved by regulating the rate of certain cellular events, such as protein synthesis. Depending on the tissue involved, the corticosteroids can be either anabolic or antianabolic in regard to protein synthesis. This variability has led to a common assumption that the corticosteroids, like other steroid hormones, act by controlling RNA transcription and thereby the production of specific proteins. The evidence supporting this hypothesis is reviewed elsewhere.[28] How regulation of protein synthesis is related to the ultimate effects of the corticosteroids is largely unknown.

The pharmacologic effects of the glucocorticoids are largely exaggerations of the physiologic functions of the endogenous corticosteroids. These effects thus simulate the pathologic features of Cushing's syndrome, a metabolic disorder resulting from an excess of corticosteroids, primarily cortisol. A review of these features and their pathophysiologic basis is helpful in understanding the pharmacologic and toxic actions of the glucocorticoids.

Carbohydrate and protein metabolism. Through several actions, glucocorticoids exert prominent antiinsulin effects. There is a definite, but poorly understood, decrease in the peripheral utilization of glucose that may be due to the antagonism of the action of insulin at the cellular level. In the liver, glucocorticoids specifically stimulate glucose synthesis from amino acids; concurrently, they mobilize amino acids by inhibiting protein synthesis in muscle, connective tissues, and skin (the so-called antianabolic effect). These actions are reflected in the parallel increases in blood glucose, liver glycogen, and urinary nitrogen excretion seen after the administration of glucocorticoids. As a consequence of these actions, prolonged high titers of glucocorticoids cause clinical manifestations of protein wasting: retardation of linear growth in children, wasting of the skin and increased capillary fragility resulting in ecchymoses, loss of muscle tissue leading to weakness (which may be extreme), and osteoporosis associated with enhanced bone resorption.

Lipid metabolism. The action of glucocorticoids on lipid metabolism also antagonizes that of insulin. They inhibit fatty acid synthesis and exert a permissive action on fatty acid mobilization from adipose tissue by lipolytic hormones. Long-term administration of large doses of glucocorticoids causes redistribution of fat from peripheral stores to more central locations on the back, shoulders, abdomen, and face; the result is termed centripetal obesity. Cutaneous striae form on areas of the trunk where the skin is stretched by accumulation of fat.

Electrolyte and water balance. Excesses or deficiencies of corticosteroid hormones are associated with severe disturbances in electrolyte and fluid balance. These disturbances result from three actions of the corticosteroids on the kidney: enhanced reabsorption of sodium from the tubular fluid and increased urinary excretion of potassium and hydrogen ions. Thus, excessive levels of corticosteroids lead to sodium retention, hypokalemia, alkalosis, and expanded extracellular fluid volume. These changes are manifested clinically by edema and hypertension; they may lead to left ventricular hypertrophy and predispose the patient to congestive heart failure and stroke. In corticosteroid deficiency (Addison's disease), essentially the opposite occurs (loss of sodium, hyperkalemia, reduced extracellular fluid volume, and generalized cellular hydration) and, if severe, may quickly lead to death.

Antiinflammatory properties. In nonphysiologic doses, the glucocorticoids are potent nonspecific inhibitors of the inflammatory response. This antiinflammatory activity is independent of the initiating stimulus and occurs at multiple events throughout the course of the process. There are several prominent actions in this process. First, cortisol blocks the increased capillary permeability produced by such factors as histamine and kinins, thus reducing the formation of edema. Kinin generation is also inhibited. Second, cortisol interferes with the migration of neutrophils and mononuclear phagocytes into a site of inflammation; the phagocytic and digestive ability of macrophages is also reduced. Finally, cortisol inhibits formation of granulation tissue by retarding capillary and fibroblast proliferation and collagen synthesis. In general, the antiinflammatory potency of the glucocorticoids closely parallels their ability to inhibit protein synthesis. This relationship suggests that diminished protein synthetic capacity in tissues and inflammatory cells is basic to the action of glucocorticoids in inflammation. How this action relates to the various inflammatory events that are affected by glucocorticoids is not clear. Since glucocorticoids are known to stabilize the membranes of lysosomes, it has been proposed that these agents act by preventing the release of lysosomal enzymes and the subsequent development of inflammation[61]; however, the evidence supporting this view is weak. The possibility exists that some of the antiinflammatory effects of glucocorticoids are due to influences on the prostaglandin system.[39] Experiments have demonstrated that glucocorticoids can block the generation of prostaglandins and related compounds.[20,60] This effect is not caused by inhibition of cyclooxygenase but seems to be related to inhibition of the release of the fatty acid substrate. It is not known at present whether this effect is related to a direct or indirect inhibition of phospholipase A_2 or to stabilization of membrane phospholipids by glucocorticoids. As an example of indirect inhibition, steroids may stimulate in leukocytes the synthesis of macrocortin, a phospholipase A_2 inhibitor. Regardless of mechanisms, the finding that glucocorticoids can block arachidonic acid metabolism at this level may explain not only the inhibition of prostaglandin, thromboxane, and prostacyclin synthesis but also the inhibition of leukotriene synthesis seen with these drugs.

Immune responses. The glucocorticoids are widely used to suppress undesirable immune reactions, such as graft rejection. Despite intensive investigation, the basis of this effect is largely unknown. Glucocorticoid inhibition of immune phenomena may result from one or more actions on lymphoid cells: alteration in production or release of cells from the bone marrow, modification of their ability to migrate into sites of immunologic or inflammatory reactions, removal of cells from the circulation by destruction or sequestration in various tissue compartments, or direct suppression of their physiologic functions, such as lymphokine and antibody production. There is evidence to support all of these possibilities.[34] Another mechanism may be inhibition of phagocytosis and subsequent digestion (processing) of antigen by macrophages, an event necessary for development of some immune responses.[25] Finally, by virtue of their antiinflammatory actions, the glucocorticoids could also suppress immune reactions that lead to a nonspecific inflammatory response. This latter mechanism is generally presumed to be important in glucocorticoid suppression of cell-mediated immune reactions, such as graft rejection.

Absorption, fate, and excretion. All of the natural and synthetic corticosteroids except desoxycorticosterone are well absorbed from the gastrointestinal tract. Significant amounts of these drugs may also be absorbed from sites of local application, such as skin, mucous membranes, and the eye. In normal circumstances, more than 95% of circulating corticosteroids are bound to a plasma globulin with high affinity but low capacity for these compounds.[16]

Cortisol is rapidly degraded in the liver by reduction, conjugated with glucuronic acid, and excreted in the urine. Most other corticosteroids are similarly metabolized, although at different rates. The plasma half-life of cortisol is about 90 minutes. Synthetic analogues of cortisol generally have greater half-lives; for example, the potent long-acting compound dexamethasone has a plasma half-life of 200 minutes and a tissue half-life of approximately 72 hours. The persistence of such corticosteroid analogues in the body may explain their greater glucocorticoid potency relative to cortisol.[16]

The major metabolic products of corticosteroid metabolism found in the urine—the so-called 17-hydroxycorticosteroids and 17-ketosteroids—were formerly measured by clinical laboratories to assess adrenal-pituitary function. This method has been largely supplanted by direct measurement of plasma cortisol concentrations by radioimmunoassay.

General therapeutic uses. The glucocorticoids are used clinically in two ways. The first and most logical of these is replacement therapy. Insufficient production of corticosteroids can result from a defect in either the adrenal cortex or the anterior pituitary; these defects may be congenital or acquired. Depending on the degree of insufficiency, the outcome may be either acute or chronic. Acute adrenal insufficiency (adrenal crisis) is a life-threatening emergency characterized by extreme weakness, gastrointestinal symptoms, dehydration, and hypotension. It frequently follows abrupt cessation

of long-term high-dose therapy with glucocorticoids and stems from a drug-induced suppression of adrenal-pituitary function (which may require up to 2 years for full recovery).[29] The features of chronic adrenal insufficiency (Addison's disease) are similar to but milder than those of the acute state. The definitive treatment of adrenal insufficiency is administration of an appropriate agent to simulate the normal daily secretion of corticosteroids.

In addition to replacement therapy, the glucocorticoids are used on a purely empirical basis in a large number of conditions (Table 22-5). These disturbances have little in common except that most are characterized by chronic inflammatory and immune phenomena and are associated with tissue destruction and functional impairment. For this reason, it is generally assumed that the salutary effects of glucocorticoid therapy in these diseases are related to suppression of inflammation and immune reactions. In none of these conditions do the corticosteroids have specific actions on the basic disease process, in spite of their ability in some cases to produce dramatic improvement and even remission of signs and symptoms. The destructive aspects of the primary disease may continue unchecked; in rheumatoid arthritis, for example, cortisol can effectively relieve the distressing inflammation and pain, but deterioration of affected joints progresses. The use of corticosteroids in other than replacement therapy must therefore be considered as palliative in nature.

Because of their lack of specificity and their considerable potential for causing harm, the long-term use of corticosteroids to treat inflammatory disorders should be viewed with caution. Before corticosteroids are considered, less toxic agents and nondrug measures should be used to the maximum extent possible. This approach is well illustrated in rheumatoid arthritis. Corticosteroids should seldom be necessary in this disease and, in any case, should not be employed as the initial agent.[25] Most patients will improve considerably with large, regular doses of aspirin or a similar nonsteroidal antiinflammatory drug combined with splints, application of heat, and rest. This program may be supplemented by other drugs, such as gold salts. Patients in whom these drugs are ineffective or intolerable are candidates for corticosteroid therapy, but corticosteroids should be used in the smallest possible dosage for the shortest period of time as adjuncts to other measures.

Table 22-5. Some conditions treated
with corticosteroids

Adrenal insufficiency (acute or chronic, primary or secondary
    to anterior pituitary insufficiency)
Cerebral edema and increased intracranial pressure (brain tu-
    mors, meningitis, trauma, cerebrovascular accidents)
Collagen-vascular diseases
    Lupus erythematosus
    Polymyositis
    Polyarteritis nodosa
    Chronic granulomatous disorders (sarcoidosis and others)
    Temporal (giant cell) arteritis
    Mixed connective tissue disease syndrome*
Dermatologic disturbances
    Psoriasis
    Dermatitis (atopic, allergic, irritant)
    Pemphigus
    Lichen planus
Gastrointestinal diseases
    Ulcerative colitis
    Crohn's disease
    Celiac disease
Hematologic diseases
    Malignancies (acute and chronic lymphocytic leukemia, lym-
        phoma, multiple myeloma)
    Hemolytic anemia (autoimmune or drug-induced)
    Idiopathic thrombocytopenic purpura
Hepatic diseases
    Chronic active hepatitis
    Alcoholic hepatitis (severe forms with hepatic encephalop-
        athy)
Hypercalcemia (sarcoid, malignancies, vitamin D intoxication)
Multiple sclerosis (acute episodes)
Nephrotic syndrome
Ocular diseases with inflammatory or allergic components
Pulmonary disorders
    Asthma
    Chronic bronchitis (acute episodes)
    Aspiration pneumonia
Rheumatic diseases and joint ailments
    Rheumatic arthritis
    Rheumatic carditis
    Osteoarthritis (intraarticular administration)
    Bursitis (intracapsular administration)
Shock
Solid tumors (breast, prostate)
Tissue grafts and organ transplants

*Must be differentiated from scleroderma, which is usually not altered
by corticosteroids.

When corticosteroids are employed on a long-term basis, they are often administered on alternate days to minimize suppression of the pituitary-adrenal axis.[16] Giving a glucocorticoid every other day between 6 and 9 A.M. mimics the normal diurnal pattern of corticosteroid secretion. Such a regimen appears to lessen suppression of the adrenal cortex and permits increased endogenous corticosteroid production in response to stress. Unfortu-nately, alternate day therapy may not adequately control symptoms in some cases, especially in patients with rheumatoid arthritis and ulcerative colitis. Large doses of glucocorticoids for periods up to 1 week usually do not cause significant suppression of pituitary or adrenal function.

Therapeutic uses in dentistry. The glucocorticoids have rather limited applications in dentistry. Here, as in other branches of medicine, they are used largely to reduce the signs and symptoms of unwanted inflammatory reactions. This use falls into the following general categories: oral ulcerations, pulpal hypersensitivity, temporomandibular joint pain, postoperative sequelae, and anaphylaxis and other allergic reactions.

Oral ulcerations. A variety of ulcerative lesions of the oral mucosa may be treated by the application of glucocorticoids.[64] Relief of symptoms and abbreviation of the clinical course is usually obtained, regardless of the etiology of the ulceration. Applicable conditions are denture-induced and other traumatic ulcers, recurrent ulcerative (aphthous) stomatitis, erosive lichen planus, erythema multiforme, pemphigus, desquamative gingivitis and stomatitis, geographic tongue, and angular stomatitis (cheilitis). Although diseases such as pemphigus are usually treated with systemic glucocorticoids, further improvement of associated oral ulceration may be obtained by topical application of glucocorticoids. Despite the fact that herpetic ulcers may respond favorably, the use of glucocorticoids to treat this condition is contraindicated, since suppression of the host response may allow dissemination of the herpes virus. It is thus important for the therapist to make a careful diagnosis of oral ulcers before instituting glucocorticoid therapy.

The benefit of glucocorticoids applied topically is greatest when the period of contact with the tissue is maximal. This is difficult, of course, in the oral cavity. A partial solution is to apply the drug in a paste that adheres to the mucosa and resists dissolution and displacement. One such vehicle is carboxymethylcellulose in a base of polyethylene resin and mineral oil (Orabase); it is available with or without a glucocorticoid. Symptomatic relief of many oral ulcers, particularly those likely to be limited in duration, may be obtained with the adhesive paste alone.

Pulpal hypersensitivity. Hypersensitivity of the dental pulp can result from a variety of conditions that induce an inflammatory response in the pulp; these include operative trauma, invasion of the pulp by bacteria or their products, and exposure of dentin to the oral environment. Glucocorticoids have been variously applied directly or indirectly to the pulp to reduce pain.[47,56] Although success has been claimed, the efficacy of this therapy is not established and therefore cannot be recommended. Indeed, there is evidence that glucocorticoid suppression of inflammation in infected pulp may promote dissemination of bacteria into the blood.[35]

Temporomandibular joint pain. Inflammation in the temporomandibular joint causes variable degrees of pain and dysfunction. Initial treatment of temporomandibular joint arthralgia should be conservative in nature, with the objective of permitting natural resolution of the inflammatory process. Therapy would include any or all of such measures as reduction of functional stress by voluntary limitation of motion and a soft diet, application of heat, intensive treatment with a nonsteroidal antiinflammatory agent (such as aspirin) and antianxiety (muscle relaxant) drugs (such as diazepam), disarticulation of the teeth by a bite plane appliance, and adjustment of the occlusion. If this approach fails to relieve pain or if the pain is initially so severe as to preclude a course of conservative therapy, intraarticular injection of a glucocorticoid into the affected joint may be beneficial. Cortisol (hydrocortisone) and prednisolone are the agents most frequently used for this purpose. Complete or partial relief is obtained in most cases within 1 to 2 days. Relief of symptoms may be permanent or the condition may recur, especially if the underlying cause of the arthritis is not corrected. If the injection is properly done, there are few adverse effects of this form of treatment. Although deterioration of articular surfaces of the joint has been claimed to result from intraarticular injection of corticosteroid, the weight of available evidence does not support such an association.[57] Intraarticular injections into the temporomandibular joint require considerable skill and should not be attempted by those who lack experience in this technique, the details of which are found in standard texts of oral surgery.[30]

Postoperative sequelae. Glucocorticoids are occasionally used to lessen postoperative complications, mainly edema and trismus, following dental surgical procedures. Although the risk of adverse effects from a short intensive course of glucocorticoid is slight, the equivocal benefits obtained do not justify such "prophylactic" use. Emphasis should be placed instead on careful surgical technique and other nondrug measures to reduce uncomfortable postoperative sequelae.

Anaphylaxis and other allergic reactions. The immunosuppressant and antiinflammatory effects of the glucocorticoids may be used to treat the manifestations of various allergic reactions, such as urticaria, contact dermatitis, angioneurotic edema, allergic rhinitis and conjunctivitis, insect bites, drug reactions, and serum sickness. Since histamine is an important mediator in most of these conditions, H_1 antihistamines are the drugs of choice in their treatment. In anaphylaxis, large doses of glucocorticoids may be beneficial in reducing bronchospasm and laryngeal edema. In this situation, the glucocorticoids also act to increase cardiac contractility and enhance the vascular effects of catecholamines.[29] However, the maximal effects of glucocorticoids do not occur until several hours after administration. The glucocorticoids are thus not primary drugs in treating the life-threatening cardiovascular and respiratory failure of anaphylaxis; they should be given only after more important measures, such as administration of epinephrine and establishment of an airway, have been completed.

Toxic reactions and side effects. Although glucocorticoids are valuable agents in some situations, they have considerable potential to cause greater harm than good. Actualization of this potential depends on, among other factors, the intensity and duration of therapy. A single large dose or a short course of moderate doses of cortisol will cause few adverse effects. If, however, more than 20 to 30 mg of cortisol (or its equivalent) is given daily for more than a week, some manifestations of glucocorticoid toxicity will likely appear. In general, these manifestations are predictable from a knowledge of the pathologic features of endogenous Cushing's disease.[40]

The complications of glucocorticoid therapy are summarized below; the reader is referred elsewhere for a more comprehensive review.[15] The frequency and severity of adverse effects correlate with the dose and duration of therapy, the age and condition of the patient, and the disease being treated.

Hyperglycemia and glycosuria. A diabetic-like state stems from the antiinsulin action of the glucocorticoids. It is usually mild and controllable with diet or insulin or both. In diabetics, the requirement for insulin or oral hypoglycemic agents will be increased.

Myopathy. Large doses of glucocorticoids, especially the more potent fluorinated synthetic compounds, variably cause muscle wasting, manifested chiefly as weakness of the musculature of the limbs. Significant reduction of muscle mass in the extremities can occur. Recovery may be incomplete after cessation of therapy.

Osteoporosis. Osteoporosis is a common sequel of long-term glucocorticoid therapy and can lead to compression fractures of the vertebrae and to an increased susceptibility to traumatic fractures. In postmenopausal women and others prone to develop osteoporosis, this complication may be especially serious.

Suppression of growth. In growing individuals, glucocorticoids can inhibit skeletal growth and maturation.

Negative nitrogen balance. A net nitrogen loss results from the imbalance between protein synthesis and degradation. It reflects the antianabolic effects of the glucocorticoids in cutaneous and musculoskeletal tissues.

Peptic ulcer. There is an increased incidence of gastric ulcers in patients treated with glucocorticoids, especially in those with rheumatoid arthritis. Since such patients are almost always receiving aspirin or other nonsteroidal antiinflammatory drugs concurrently, it is difficult to directly implicate the glucocorticoids in the pathogenesis of these ulcers. Nonetheless, when they occur, ulcers associated with glucocorticoid therapy have a high incidence of complications, such as hemorrhage and perforation.

Ocular effects. Increased intraocular pressure, which may produce irreversible damage, and posterior subcapsular cataracts can result from either topical or systemic administration of glucocorticoids. Children and diabetic individuals are particularly susceptible to untoward ocular effects.

CNS effects. Psychologic disturbances can occur during glucocorticoid therapy. These reactions are reversible and range in severity from mild (euphoria, insomnia, or nervousness) to pronounced (manic-depressive or schizophrenic psychosis).

Edema and hypokalemia. Although water retention with hypokalemia is a potentially serious complication of glucocorticoid therapy, the incidence and severity can be greatly minimized by dietary sodium restriction and by the use of a synthetic glucocorticoid essentially devoid of mineralocorticoid activity.

Altered distribution of body fat. Chronic treatment with glucocorticoids often causes changes in distribution of body fat deposits, leading to the classic "cushingoid" appearance. The most characteristic of these changes are a round ("moon") face, supraclavicular fat pads ("buffalo hump"), and increased abdominal fat. The obese trunk may markedly contrast with the thin, wasted extremities.

Increased susceptibility to infection. The body's reaction to infectious agents is depressed by glucocorticoids. Fungal, bacterial, and viral pathogens that would otherwise cause localized or no infection may become widely disseminated with serious or fatal consequences. Latent tuberculosis may be reactivated after initiation of glucocorticoid therapy.

Suppression of pituitary-adrenal function. Prolonged administration of glucocorticoids (greater than physiologic amounts for more than 1 week) will result in suppression of ACTH and, consequently, adrenal corticosteroid production; the degree of suppression is dose related. Abrupt withdrawal or significant reduction of glucocorticoid dosage can thus precipitate acute adrenal insufficiency. Moreover, acute exacerbation of the disease being treated may occur during withdrawal. Cessation of glucocorticoid therapy or reduction must therefore be done slowly and with great caution to permit the recovery of normal pituitary and adrenal function.[15]

Miscellaneous effects. Acne, thinning of the skin, hirsutism, weight gain, intestinal perforation, pancreatitis, hyperlipidemia, hypertension, hepatomegaly, and poor wound healing may occur during long-term glucocorticoid therapy.

Implications for dentistry. Patients treated with large doses of glucocorticoids for long periods present special problems in dentistry. As noted above, such patients are likely to have a decreased resistance to infection and a poor wound healing response. Actual or potential sources of infection in the oral cavity, such as carious teeth and inflamed tissues, should be treated promptly. If surgical procedures are necessary, they should be as conservative, atraumatic, and aseptic as possible. Prophylactic antimicrobial coverage commencing before the surgical procedure is indicated in most cases.

A second consideration in patients treated with glucocorticoids is suppression of the pituitary-adrenal function. The degree of adrenal suppression depends on the length of treatment, the frequency and manner of administration, and the glucocorticoid preparation used (potency of individual agents may vary more than 25-fold; see Table 22-4). An individual with intact adrenal function will respond to a stressful situation such as anxiety, an acute infection, or a surgical procedure with an increased release of ACTH and production of cortisol. Subjects with suppressed adrenal function, however, are unable to increase cortisol production when required and may develop signs and symptoms of adrenal insufficiency.[40] In assessing the degree of suppression, a good guideline is to assume that any patient who has received 30 mg hydrocortisone or its equivalent for 4 or more weeks or 80 mg of hydrocortisone for more than 2 weeks should be assumed to be adrenally suppressed.[8] Therefore, during stressful dental situations (surgery or acute infections), the dose of glucocorticoids must be increased in such patients to compensate for the lack of endogenous hormone. The dose is usually at least double or triple the maintenance dose, depending on the degree of suppression of adrenal function and the severity of the stressful event. When the period of stress is over, the dose is gradually reduced over several days to the maintenance level.

A dental procedure done under general anesthesia constitutes a maximally stressful episode and requires essentially complete corticosteroid replacement in a patient with adrenal suppression. One commonly accepted approach is to give 100 mg cortisone acetate intramuscularly approximately 8 hours before the procedure. Sufficient hydrocortisone or its equivalent is then given intravenously during the procedure so that the total dose on the day of the operation is 300 mg cortisol or its equivalent. If the postoperative course is uneventful, corticosteroid dosage is tapered off over a 2- to 3-day period (e.g., 300 mg cortisol on the day of the procedure, 150 mg the following day, 75 mg on the next day, and the usual maintenance dose on the third postoperative day).[8] Since recovery of glucocorticoid-induced adrenal suppression may be very slow, dental patients formerly treated for prolonged periods with glucocorticoids and assumed to have adrenal suppression by the above criteria should receive glucocorticoids during stressful situations for 1 year after cessation of glucocorticoid therapy. It is obvious that consultation with the patient's physician is essential for the safe and effective management of an individual who is receiving or has received long-term glucocorticoid therapy.

Preparations. A large number of glucocorticoids are available in various forms for local, oral, and parenteral administration. These include the

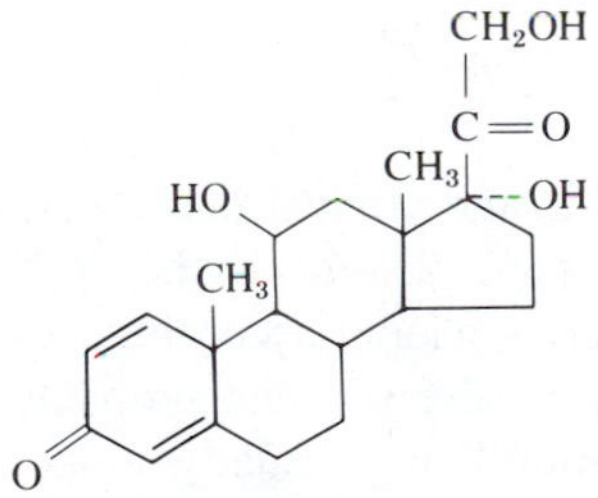

Prednisolone

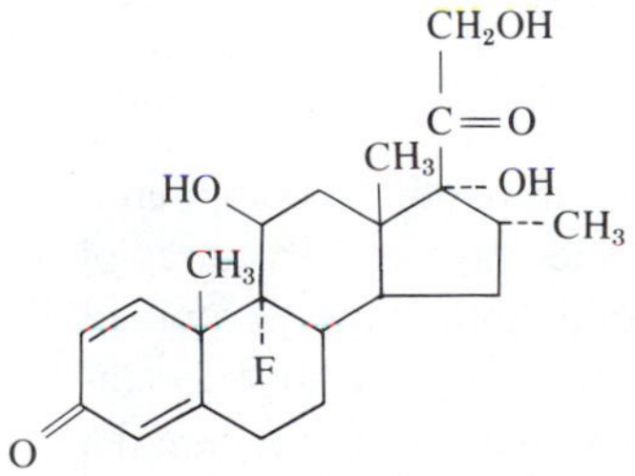

Dexamethasone

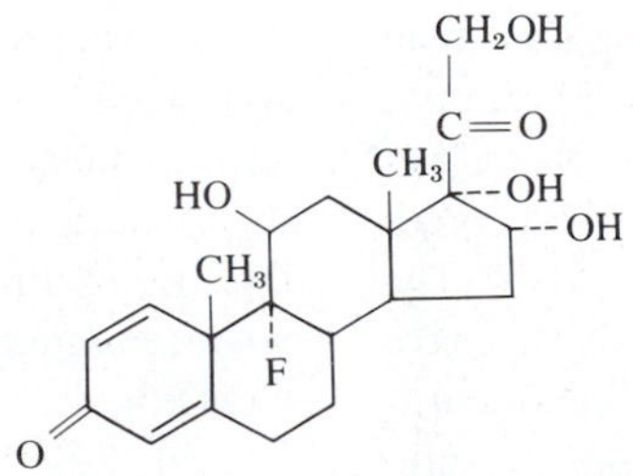

Triamcinolone

Figure 22-11. Structural formulas of the synthetic glucocorticoids: prednisolone, dexamethasone, and triamcinolone. Relative to the short-acting cortisol, prednisolone is classified as intermediate-acting and dexamethasone and triamcinolone are classified as long-acting.

Table 22-6. Some commonly used corticosteroid preparations

Nonproprietary name	Proprietary name	Relative potency	Usual adult dose	Route of administration	Preparations
Hydrocortisone	Hydrocortone	1	20-240 mg/day	Oral	Tablets: 5, 10, and 20 mg
Hydrocortisone acetate	Orabase HCA	1	2-3 times daily	Topical	Paste: 0.5%, containing gelatin, pectin, and sodium carboxymethylcellulose in a polyethylene and mineral oil base
	Hydrocortone Acetate	1	5-50 mg	Intraarticular	Suspension: 25 and 50 mg/ml
Hydrocortisone sodium succinate	Solu-Cortef	1	100-500 mg	Intravenous or intramuscular	Powder: 100, 250, 500, and 1000 mg
Prednisone	Deltasone	4	5-60 mg/day	Oral	Tablets: 1, 2.5, 5, 10, 20, and 50 mg
Prednisolone	Delta-Cortef	4	5-60 mg/day	Oral	Tablets: 1 and 5 mg
Prednisolone acetate	Meticortelone Acetate	4	5-10 mg*	Intraarticular	Suspension: 25 mg/ml
Triamcinolone acetonide	Kenalog in Orabase	5	2-3 times daily	Topical	Paste: 0.1%, with gelatin, pectin, and sodium carboxymethylcellulose in a polyethylene and mineral oil base
Triamcinolone diacetate	Aristocort Forte	5	5-40 mg every 1-8 weeks	Intraarticular	Suspension: 25 and 40 mg/ml
Dexamethasone	Decadron	25	0.5-9 mg/day	Oral	Tablets: 0.25, 0.5, 0.75, 1.5, 2, 4, and 6 mg
Dexamethasone acetate	Decadron-LA	25	1-5 mg*	Intraarticular	Suspension: 8 mg/ml
Betamethasone	Celestone	30	0.6-7.2 mg/day	Oral	Tablets: 0.6 mg

*Dose recommended for the temporomandibular joint.

natural hormone cortisol and synthetic compounds prepared by modifying the chemical structures of cortisol and other natural hormones. Several of these are shown in Figure 22-11. Relative to cortisol, the synthetic compounds are, in varying degree, longer acting and more potent on a weight basis. These differences are the basis for classifying the glucocorticoids as short acting (less than 12 hours), intermediate acting (12 to 36 hours), and long acting (more than 36 hours). Representatives of these three categories are cortisol, prednisolone, and dexamethasone, respectively.[15] The intermediate- and long-acting compounds also have a greater ratio of glucocorticoid to mineralocorticoid activity. Consequently, these agents are preferred for long-term use in the treatment of chronic inflammatory disorders, since they cause less disturbance of electrolyte and fluid balance than does cortisol.

In the clinical management of inflammatory or allergic disorders, the dosage of glucocorticoids varies widely according to such factors as the nature, severity, and probable duration of the condition being treated and the patient's response. In acute or life-threatening situations, a glucocorticoid should be given in sufficient doses to control the disorder quickly; treatment should then be discontinued as soon as possible. In the long-term management of chronic diseases, such as rheumatoid arthritis, alternate day therapy using the minimum dosage that achieves an acceptable reduction of symptoms is the regimen of choice.

Table 22-6 lists a few of the many different preparations currently available, some of the dosage forms, and a range of doses for a given route of administration.

Antiinflammatory drugs

Nonproprietary name	Proprietary name
Salicylates	
aspirin	—
choline salicylate	Arthropan
diflunisal	Dolobid
magnesium salicylate	Magan
salsalate	Disalcid
sodium salicylate	Uracel 5
sodium thiosalicylate	Arthrolate
Salicylate-like nonsteroidal agents	
fenoprofen	Nalfon
ibuprofen	Motrin, Nuprin, Advil
indomethacin	Indocin
isoxicam*	Maxicam
meclofenamate	Meclomen
mefenamic acid	Ponstel
naproxen	Naprosyn
oxyphenbutazone	Tandearil
phenylbutazone	Butazolidin
piroxicam	Feldene
sulindac	Clinoril
tolmetin	Tolectin
zomepirac*	Zomax
Other antirheumatic drugs	
auranofin*	Ridaura
aurothioglucose	Solganal
azathioprine	Imuran
chloroquine	—
cyclophosphamide	Cytoxan
gold sodium thiomalate	Myochrysine
hydroxychloroquine	Plaquenil
penicillamine	Cuprimine
Antigout drugs	
allopurinol	Zyloprim
colchicine	Colsalide
probenecid	Benemid
sulfinpyrazone	Anturane
Steroids	
betamethasone	Celestone
cortisone	Cortone Acetate
dexamethasone	Decadron
fludrocortisone	Florinef Acetate
fluprednisolone	Alphadrol
hydrocortisone (cortisol)	Cortef, Hydrocortone
methylprednisolone	Medrol
paramethasone	Haldrone
prednisolone	Delta-Cortef
prednisone	Deltasone
triamcinolone	Aristocort, Kenacort

*Not currently available in the United States.

CITED REFERENCES

1. Allison, A.C., Ferluga, J., Prydz, H., and Schorlemmer, H.U. The role of macrophage activation in chronic inflammation. Agents and Actions; Swiss Journal of Pharmacology **8:**27-35, 1978.
2. AMA Drug Evaluations, ed. 5. Chicago, American Medical Association, 1983.
3. Austen, K.F. Homeostasis of effector systems which can also be recruited for immunologic reactions. Journal of Immunology **121:**793-805, 1978.
4. Baggiolini, M., Bretz, U., Dewald, B., and Feigenson, M.E. The polymorphonuclear leukocyte. Agents and Actions; Swiss Journal of Pharmacology **8:**3-10, 1978.
5. Barkas, T. Biological activities of complement. Biochemical Society Transactions **6:**798-807, 1978.
6. Barnett, H.J.M. Platelet antiaggregants in stroke: a review of rationale and results. In Barnett, H.J.M., Hirsh, J., and Mustard, J.F., eds. Acetylsalicylic Acid: New Uses for an Old Drug. New York, Raven Press, 1982.
7. Bendtzen, K. Biological properties of lymphokines. Allergy **33:**105-119, 1978.
8. Blonde, L., Ré, R., Tullman, M.J., and Redding, S.W. Endocrinologic disease. In Tullman, M.J., and Redding, S.W., eds. Systemic Disease in Dental Treatment. New York, Appleton-Century-Crofts, 1982.
9. Bonta, I.L., and Parnham, M.J. Prostaglandins and chronic inflammation. Biochemical Pharmacology **27:**1611-1623, 1978.
10. Borgeat, P., and Samuelsson, B. Arachidonic acid metabolism in polymorphonuclear leukocytes: unstable intermediate in formation of dihydroxy acids. Proceedings of the National Academy of Sciences of the United States of America **76:**3213-3217, 1979.
11. Bourne, H.R., Lichtenstein, L.M., Melmon, K.L., Henney, C.S., Weinstein, Y., and Shearer, G.M. Modulation of inflammation and immunity by cyclic AMP. Science **184:**19-28, 1974.
12. Brogden, R.N., Heel, R.C., Speight, T.M., and Avery, G.S. Tolmetin: a review of its pharmacological properties and therapeutic efficacy in rheumatic diseases. Drugs **15:**429-450, 1978.
13. Christian, C.L. Joint diseases. In Wyngaarden, J.B., and Smith, L.H., Jr., eds. Cecil Textbook of Medicine, ed. 16. Philadelphia, W.B. Saunders Co., 1982.
14. Cooper, S.A., Needle, S.E., and Kruger, G.O. Comparative analgesic potency of aspirin and ibuprofen. Journal of Oral Surgery **35:**898-903, 1977.
15. David, D.S., Grieco, M.H., and Cushman, P., Jr. Adrenal glucocorticoids after 20 years; a review of their clinically relevant consequences. Journal of Chronic Diseases **22:** 637-711, 1970.
16. Dluhy, R.G., Newmark, S.R., and Lauler, D.P. Pharmacology and chemistry of adrenal glucocorticoids. In Azarnoff, D.L., ed. Steroid Therapy. Philadelphia, W.B. Saunders Co., 1975.
17. Douglas, W.W. Polypeptides—angiotensin, plasma kinins, and others. In Gilman, A.G., Goodman, L.S., and Gilman, A., eds. Goodman and Gilman's The Pharmacological Basis of Therapeutics, ed. 6. New York, Macmillan, Inc., 1980.
18. Ebert, R.H., and Grant, L. The experimental approach to the study of inflammation. In Zweifach, B.W., Grant, L.,

and McCluskey, R.T., eds. The Inflammatory Process, vol. 1, ed. 2. New York, Academic Press, Inc., 1974.

19. Ferreira, S.H., and Vane, J.R. New aspects of the mode of action of nonsteroid anti-inflammatory drugs. Annual Review of Pharmacology and Toxicology **14:**57-73, 1974.

20. Flower, R.J. Steroidal anti-inflammatory drugs as inhibitors of phospholipase A$_2$. Advances in Prostaglandin and Thromboxane Research **3:**105-112, 1978.

21. Flower, R.J., Moncada, S., and Vane, J.R. Analgesic-antipyretics and anti-inflammatory agents; drugs employed in the therapy of gout. In Gilman, A.G., Goodman, L.S., and Gilman, A., eds. Goodman and Gilman's The Pharmacological Basis of Therapeutics, ed. 6. New York, Macmillan, Inc., 1980.

22. Flower, R.J., and Vane, J.R. Inhibition of prostaglandin synthesis. Biochemical Pharmacology **23:**1439-1450, 1974.

23. Forbes, J.A., Calderazzo, J.P., Bowser, M.W., Foor, V.M., Shackleford, R.W., and Beaver, R.T. A 12-hour evaluation of the analgesic efficacy of diflunisal, aspirin and placebo in postoperative dental pain. Journal of Clinical Pharmacology **22:**89-96, 1982.

24. Ford-Hutchinson, A.W., Bray, M.A., Doig, M.V., Shipley, M.E., and Smith, M.J.H. Leukotriene B, a potent chemokinetic and aggregating substance released from polymorphonuclear leukocytes. Nature **286:**264-265, 1980.

25. Gifford, R.H. Corticosteroid therapy for rheumatoid arthritis. In Azarnoff, D.L., ed. Steroid Therapy. Philadelphia, W.B. Saunders Co., 1975.

26. Goldstein, J.M. Lysosomal hydrolases and inflammatory materials. In Weissman, G., ed. Mediators of Inflammation. New York, Plenum Press, 1974.

27. Hamberg, M. Inhibition of prostaglandin synthesis in man. Biochemical and Biophysical Research Communications **49:**720-726, 1972.

28. Haynes, R.C., Jr. Biochemical mechanisms of steroid effects. In Azarnoff, D.L., ed. Steroid Therapy. Philadelphia, W. B. Saunders Co., 1975.

29. Haynes, R.C., Jr., and Murad, F. Adrenocorticotropic hormone: adrenocortical steroids and their synthetic analogs; inhibitors of adrenal cortical steroid biosynthesis. In Gilman, A.G., Goodman, L.S., and Gilman, A., eds. Goodman and Gilman's The Pharmacological Basis of Therapeutics, ed. 6. New York, Macmillan, Inc., 1980.

30. Henny, F.A. The temporomandibular joint. In Kruger, G.O., ed. Textbook of Oral Surgery, ed. 5. St. Louis, The C.V. Mosby Co., 1979.

31. Higgs, G.A., McCall, E., and Youlten, L.J.F. A chemotactic role for prostaglandins released from polymorphonuclear leukocytes during phagocytosis. British Journal of Pharmacology **53:**539-546, 1975.

32. Huskisson, E.C., Hart, F.D., Shenfield, G.S., and Taylor, R.T. Ibuprofen: a review. Practitioner **207:**639-643, 1971.

33. Hyman, A.L., Spannhake, E.W., and Kadowitz, P.J. Prostaglandins and the lung. American Review of Respiratory Diseases **117:**111-136, 1978.

34. Kirkpatrick, C.H., and Rosenthal, A. Glucocorticoids and allergic reactions. In Azarnoff, D.L., ed. Steroid Therapy. Philadelphia, W. B. Saunders Co., 1975.

35. Klotz, M.D., Gerstein, H., and Bahn, A.N. Bacteremia after topical use of prednisolone in infected pulps. Journal of the American Dental Association **71:**871-875, 1965.

36. Kuehl, F.A., Jr., and Egan, R.W. Prostaglandins, arachidonic acid, and inflammation. Science **210:**978-984, 1980.

37. Levy, D.A. Histamine and serotonin. In Weissman, G., ed. Mediators of Inflammation. New York, Plenum Press, 1974.

38. Lewis, G.P. Prostaglandins in inflammation. Journal of the Reticuloendothelial Society **22:**389-402, 1977.

39. Lewis, G.P., and Piper, P.J. Two sites of action of steroids on the prostaglandin system. In Willoughby, D.A., Giroud, J.P., and Velo, G.P., eds. Perspectives in Inflammation. Baltimore, University Park Press, 1977.

40. Liddle, G.W. Adrenal cortex. In Wyngaarden, J.B., and Smith, L.H., Jr., eds. Cecil Textbook of Medicine, ed. 16. Philadelphia, W.B. Saunders Co., 1982.

41. McLeod, D.C. Zomepirac. Drug Intelligence and Clinical Pharmacy **15:**522-530, 1981.

42. Meyers, O.L., and Klemp, P. An oral formulation of gold for the treatment of rheumatoid arthritis. South African Medical Journal **59:**969-971, 1981.

43. Miller, R.L., Insel, P.A., and Melmon, K.L. Inflammatory disorders. In Melmon, K.L., and Morrelli, H.F., eds. Clinical Pharmacology: Basic Principles in Therapeutics, ed. 2. New York, Macmillan, Inc., 1978.

44. Moncada, S. Biological importance of prostacyclin. British Journal of Pharmacology **76:**3-31, 1982.

45. Moncada, S., Flower, R.J., and Vane, J.R. Prostaglandins, prostacyclin, and thromboxane A$_2$. In Gilman, A.G., Goodman, L.S., and Gilman, A., eds. Goodman and Gilman's The Pharmacological Basis of Therapeutics, ed. 6. New York, Macmillan, Inc., 1980.

46. Morley, J. Prostaglandins and lymphokines in inflammation. Rheumatology and Rehabilitation **17**(suppl.):18-24, 1978.

47. Mosteller, J.H. The ability of a prednisolone solution to eliminate pulpal inflammation. Journal of Prosthetic Dentistry **13:**754-760, 1963.

48. Mustard, J.F. The use of acetylsalicylic acid in the management of coronary artery disease. In Barnett, H.J.M., Hirsh, J., and Mustard, J.F., eds. Acetylsalicylic Acid: New Uses for an Old Drug. New York, Raven Press, 1982.

49. Orange, R.P., Murphy, R.C., Karnovsky, M.L., and Austen, K.F. The physicochemical characteristics and purification of slow-reacting substance of anaphylaxis. Journal of Immunology **110:**760-770, 1973.

50. Osler, A.G., and Sandberg, A.L. Alternate complement pathways. Progress in Allergy **17:**51-92, 1973.

51. Parker, C.W. Prostaglandins and slow-reacting substance. Journal of Allergy and Clinical Immunology **63:**1-14, 1979.

52. Piper, P.J., Samhoun, M.N., Tippins, J.R., Morris, H.R., Jones, C.M., and Taylor, G.W. SRS-A and SRS: their structure, biosynthesis and actions. International Archives of Allergy and Applied Immunology **66**(suppl. 1):107-112, 1981.

53. Samuelsson, B. Leukotrienes: mediators of allergic reactions and inflammation. International Archives of Allergy and Applied Immunology **66**(suppl. 1):98-106, 1981.

54. Samuelsson, B., and Hammarström, S. Leukotrienes: a novel group of biologically active compounds. Vitamins and Hormones **39:**1-30, 1982.

55. Stechschulte, D.J., Orange, R.P., and Austen, K.F. Detection of slow-reacting substance of anaphylaxis (SRS-A) in plasma of guinea pigs during anaphylaxis. Journal of Immunology **111**:1585-1589, 1973.

56. Swerdlow, H., Stanley, H.R., and Sayegh, F.S. Minimizing pulpal reactions with prednisolone therapy. Journal of Oral Therapeutics and Pharmacology **1**:593-601, 1965.

57. Toller, P.A. Use and misuse of intra-articular corticosteroids in treatment of temporomandibular joint pain. Proceedings of the Royal Society of Medicine **70**:461-463, 1977.

58. Ward, P.A. Complement-derived leukotactic factors in pathological fluids. Journal of Experimental Medicine **134**:109S-113S, 1971.

59. Ward, P.A. Inflammation. In LaVia, M.F., and Hill, R.B., Jr., eds. Principles of Pathobiology, ed. 2. New York, Oxford University Press, 1975.

60. Weissman, G. Prostaglandins as mediators of inflammation. In Barnett, H.J.M., Hirsh, J., and Mustard, J.F., eds. Acetylsalicylic Acid: New Uses for an Old Drug. New York, Raven Press, 1982.

61. Weissman, G., and Thomas, L. The effect of corticosteroids upon connective tissue and lysosomes. Recent Progress in Hormone Research **20**:215-245, 1964.

62. Wilhelm, D.L. Kinins in human disease. Annual Review of Medicine **22**:63-84, 1971.

63. Wyngaarden, J.B. Disorders of purine and pyrimidine metabolism: gout. In Wyngaarden, J.B., and Smith, L.H., Jr., eds. Cecil Textbook of Medicine, ed. 16. Philadelphia, W.B. Saunders Co., 1982.

64. Zegarelli, E.V., Kutscher, A.H., Silvers, H.F., Beube, F.E., Stern, I.B., Berman, C.L., and Herlands, R.E. Triamcinolone acetonide in the treatment of acute and chronic lesions of the oral mucous membranes. Oral Surgery, Oral Medicine, and Oral Pathology **13**:170-175, 1960.

GENERAL REFERENCES

Houck, J.C., ed. Chemical Messengers of the Inflammatory Process. Amsterdam, Elsevier/North Holland Biochemical Press, 1979.

Nickander, R., McMahon, F.G., and Ridolfo, A.S. Nonsteroidal anti-inflammatory agents. Annual Review of Pharmacology and Toxicology **19**:469-490, 1979.

Ryan, G.B., and Majno, G. Inflammation. Kalamazoo, Mich., The Upjohn Company, 1977.

Weissman, G., ed. The Cell Biology of Inflammation. Amsterdam, Elsevier/North Holland Biochemical Press, 1980.

23 Histamine and histamine antagonists

Clarence L. Trummel

HISTAMINE

Histamine, or β-aminoethylimidazole, is one of a heterogeneous group of biologically active, naturally occurring substances whose physiologic roles are largely undefined. In addition to histamine, this group includes another amine (5-HT, or serotonin), polypeptides (angiotensin, bradykinin, and kallidin), and lipid-derived substances (prostaglandins and SRS-A). These compounds have been collectively designated *autacoids*.[12] This term, derived from the Greek *autos* ("self") and *akos* ("cure"), is sufficiently nonspecific yet still acknowledges the endogenous origin and biologic activities of these substances as well as their certain, although uncharacterized, role in the body's economy.

Histamine was the first autacoid to be discovered. After its synthesis in 1907, a series of studies by Dale and Laidlaw[11] of the pharmacologic properties of histamine suggested that this substance might be involved in inflammatory and anaphylactic reactions. These workers observed that the local application of histamine caused redness, swelling, and edema, mimicking a mild inflammatory reaction. They also determined that large doses of histamine given systemically produced profound vascular changes very similar to those seen in shock of traumatic or anaphylactic origin. Although the presence of histamine in animal tissues had been suggested, it was not until 1927 that histamine was conclusively shown to be a natural constituent of mammalian tissues and not the result of bacterial action.[5] This finding provided important support for the work of Lewis and Grant,[20] who had demonstrated earlier that a histamine-like substance was released in the skin after various injuries, including antigen-antibody reactions.

These early studies and those that followed clearly established that histamine is involved in various pathophysiologic phenomena seen after injury to tissue. Since then, a large amount of detailed information regarding the synthesis, storage, release, and actions of histamine has been generated. In spite of this, our understanding of the role of histamine in the complex response of cells to injurious stimuli and the relation of this compound to other

Table 23-1. Distribution and content of histamine in various human tissues and cells

Tissue or cell	Histamine content*
Lung	33 ± 10
Mucosa (nasal)	15.6 (range 5.0-38.5)
Stomach	14 ± 4.0
Duodenum	14 ± 0.9
Skin (face)	30.4
Skin (abdomen)	6.6
Pancreas	4.8 ± 1.5
Spleen	3.4 ± 1.0
Bone marrow	3.3 ± 1.5
Kidney	2.5 ± 1.2
Liver	2.2 ± 0.8
Heart	1.6 ± 0.1
Thyroid	1.0 ± 0.1
Skeletal muscle	0.9 ± 0.1
Peripheral nerves	2-11
Central nervous system tissue	0-0.2
Whole blood	16-89 µg/L
Plasma	2.6 µg/L (range 0-15)
Basophils	1080 µg/10^9 cells
Eosinophils	160 µg/10^9 cells
Neutrophils	3.0 µg/10^9 cells
Lymphocytes	0.6 µg/10^9 cells
Platelets	0.009 µg/10^9 platelets

From Van Arsdel, P.P., Jr., and Beall, G.N. The metabolism and functions of histamine. Archives of Internal Medicine **106**(5):714-733, 1960. Copyright 1960, American Medical Association.

*Means or means ± standard error expressed as µg/gm unless otherwise indicated.

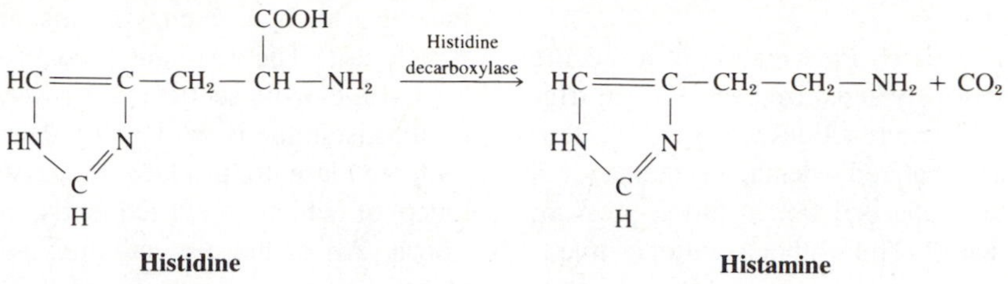

$$\text{Histidine} \xrightarrow{\text{Histidine decarboxylase}} \text{Histamine} + CO_2$$

Figure 23-1. Conversion of histidine to histamine.

autacoids is meager. Furthermore, it is increasingly evident that this ubiquitous amine is involved in physiologic processes other than reaction to injury. These processes may include gastric secretion,[10] neurotransmission in the central nervous system,[33] local control of the microcirculation,[37] and regulation of growth of rapidly proliferating cells, as in granulation tissue, bone marrow, and healing wounds.[17]

Formation, distribution, and release

Histamine is widely distributed in nature and is found in plants, bacteria, and animals. Nearly all mammalian tissues contain histamine or have the ability to form it. The histamine content of different tissues varies greatly. In humans and most other mammals, the highest concentrations are found in lung, skin, and intestinal mucosa; such organs as the pancreas, spleen, liver, and kidney have a low histamine content (Table 23-1). The physiologic significance of this pattern of distribution is not known. Although some tissue histamine may be derived from dietary sources or synthesized by bacteria in the gastrointestinal tract, most of it appears to be formed in situ.

Histamine is synthesized in mammalian tissues by the intracellular decarboxylation of the amino acid histidine (Figure 23-1). This conversion may be catalyzed either by aromatic L-amino acid decarboxylase or by histidine decarboxylase. Histidine decarboxylase is specific for L-histidine, requires pyridoxal phosphate, and appears to be primarily responsible for the synthesis of histamine in humans.

Histamine is associated in most tissues with the mast cell and in blood with a related cell, the basophil.[28] These cells synthesize histamine and store it as a proteinaceous complex with heparin in membrane-bound secretory granules. Histamine in this form is physiologically inactive but can be dis-

charged from the cell by a process commonly called degranulation. The first step in this process is activation of the cell by an appropriate stimulus. Once the cell is activated, a complex series of events leading to degranulation occurs.[3] These events require ionic Ca^{++} and metabolic energy and involve changes in intracellular cyclic nucleotide concentrations, assembly of microtubules, aggregation and coalescence of individual granules, and finally fusion of the perigranular membrane with the cell membrane. The granule contents are then released into the extracellular environment and dissociate to yield histamine and heparin.

A variety of conditions (or stimuli) can trigger the release of histamine from mast cells and basophils. These can be grouped into three categories.

1. *Tissue injury.* Any physical or chemical agent that injures tissue, particularly skin or mucosa, causes the immediate release of histamine from mast cells in the affected area. Depending on the severity of injury, histamine continues to be released for several minutes and appears to be largely responsible for the initial sharp increase in vascular permeability that is characteristic of acute inflammation. This histamine-dependent change in permeability is transient (up to 30 minutes) but is followed in 2 to 4 hours by a more prolonged increase in permeability lasting up to 4 hours. Although inhibitors of histamine release or inhibitors of the subsequent action of histamine can block the initial phase of vascular permeability after injury, they have little effect on the secondary or delayed phase, suggesting that autacoids or factors other than histamine mediate the secondary phase.[36] The mechanism by which a nonspecific injury triggers mast cell degranulation is not clear. It could depend on direct physical damage to mast cells or alternatively may involve the initial production of factors such as activated complement components or

vasoactive polypeptides that then stimulate histamine release.[22]

2. *Allergic reactions.* Presentation of a specific antigen to a previously sensitized subject can trigger immediate allergic reactions, ranging in intensity from mild (localized edema, erythema, and itching) to severe (marked fall in blood pressure and bronchospasm). The pathophysiologic manifestations of such reactions are caused in large measure by the release of histamine. This release occurs as a consequence of the binding of specific antigens to reaginic (IgE) antibodies attached to the plasma membranes of mast cells and basophils.[22] Binding of antigen and antibody may cause conformational changes in the membrane leading to an increase in Ca^{++} permeability. In any case, this antigen-antibody interaction is an appropriate stimulus for the series of events leading to degranulation of these cells.

3. *Drugs and other foreign compounds.* Although drugs that are antigenic (e.g., penicillin) can cause histamine release, there is also a large group of drugs and other chemicals that can trigger histamine release directly without a requirement for previous sensitization. For convenience, these agents can be classed as basic histamine releasers, macromolecular compounds, and enzymes.[15] The basic histamine releasers include aliphatic and arylalkyl amines, amides, amidines, diamidines, quaternary ammonium compounds, alkaloids, piperidine derivatives, pyridinium compounds, antimalarial drugs, dyes, and antibiotic bases. The prototypical histamine releaser, compound 48/80, and a number of therapeutic agents of interest, such as curare and morphine, fall into this category. Dextran is an example of a macromolecular compound that causes histamine release. Several enzymes, such as phospholipase A, have been shown to initiate mast cell degranulation, a fact that may explain the release of histamine caused by various insect and snake venoms. The mechanisms by which chemicals trigger histamine release vary. Some agents, typified by compound 48/80, act by stimulating an energy-dependent degranulation process with characteristics similar to anaphylactic histamine release. Other histamine releasers are effective in the absence of energy sources and seem to act with a detergent-like effect on cell membranes.

Metabolism

Histamine of either exogenous or endogenous origin is rapidly inactivated by two routes.[31] The more important of these is methylation of the imidazole ring by the enzyme histamine-N-methyltransferase. The resultant product is converted to methylimidazole acetic acid by MAO. In the other route, histamine is oxidatively deaminated by diamine oxidase to produce imidazole acetic acid, much of which is subsequently conjugated with ribose. All of these metabolites are inactive and, along with a small amount of free histamine, are excreted by the kidney.

Large oral doses of histamine have little effect, since histamine is largely degraded by intestinal bacteria. Any free histamine that is absorbed is largely inactivated in the intestinal wall and in the liver.

Pharmacologic effects

Most of the important effects of histamine can be attributed to its actions on smooth muscle and glands. In general, histamine causes relaxation of vascular smooth muscle, contraction of nonvascular smooth muscle, and stimulation of secretion of exocrine glands, especially those of the gastric mucosa. These actions are direct and independent of innervation. Different species show considerable variation in the sensitivity of target tissues to histamine. For example, the bronchial smooth muscle of the guinea pig is highly sensitive to histamine, and fatal bronchospasm occurs at doses that have minimal effects in other species, including humans. Within a single species, the actions of histamine are usually reproducible.

The existence of compounds that can specifically block the actions of histamine strongly supports the existence of specific histamine receptors. Furthermore, the differential effects of histamine antagonists suggest that there are two types of histamine receptors, termed H_1 and H_2. H_1 receptors primarily mediate effects on smooth muscle leading to vasodilation, increased vascular permeability, and contraction of nonvascular smooth muscle. These effects are blocked by the "classic" antihistamines, such as pyrilamine. H_2 receptors mediate histamine stimulation of gastric acid secretion and may be involved in other histamine effects such as direct cardiac stimulation. The more recently discovered H_2 blocking agents antagonize these effects.[6,7]

Cardiovascular system. The effects of histamine on the circulatory system are complex and vary markedly according to species. In most mammals, histamine causes some constriction of large vessels, both arterial and venous. Histamine also constricts arterioles and increases blood pressure in rats and rabbits. In contrast, the intravenous administration of histamine in humans and carnivores causes dilation of terminal arterioles, capillaries, and postcapillary venules and leads to a sharp decrease in peripheral resistance and a consequent fall in blood pressure. The dilation of these vessels is largely caused by the inhibitory action of histamine directly on the smooth muscle of the arterioles and precapillary sphincters. The subsequent increase in arteriolar and capillary blood flow causes, in turn, a passive dilation of postcapillary venules that is accompanied by an increase in their permeability. This increased permeability is caused by distension or stretching of the venules as well as by a contractile response of the endothelial cells caused directly by histamine; both phenomena contribute to "gaps" between the endothelial cells of the venules with exposure of the basement membrane. These gaps permit the movement of plasma protein and fluid through the basement membrane into the extravascular space, thus allowing the formation of edema.[36]

In addition to hypotension, arteriolar dilation induced by histamine leads to cutaneous flushing, especially over the face and upper trunk, and a rise in skin temperature. A short-lived but intense headache caused by dilation of cerebral vessels also occurs. This "histamine headache" is similar in quality and duration to the headache produced by other potent vasodilators, such as amyl nitrite.

The effect of histamine on the terminal vasculature can be graphically illustrated by injection of 10 to 20 μg of the amine into the skin. At the site of the injection, there is first immediate reddening, reflecting vasodilation. This reddening is followed shortly by a zone of erythema, or "flare," extending as an irregular halo for 1 cm or more beyond the original red spot. The flare is presumed to be caused by reflex vasodilation of adjacent small vessels, since it is abolished by disruption of the peripheral sensory nerves. Finally, the central spot is replaced by a disk of localized edema, or wheal, resulting from increased capillary permeability, and is accompanied by pain and itching. These events constitute the classic triple response, first described by Lewis and Grant.[20] It is worthwhile to note that a very similar response is elicited by the intradermal injection of antigen in a sensitized individual.

Hypotension resulting from moderate doses of histamine is quite transient, because reflex circulatory mechanisms come into play and the drug is rapidly inactivated. However, when histamine is given in large doses, there is a progressive fall in blood pressure that resembles that of traumatic or surgical shock. This fall is a consequence of both vasodilation and increased capillary permeability. The increased capillary permeability, in turn, leads to loss of plasma from the vascular compartment and a decrease in the effective blood volume. Venous return to the heart is diminished, and thus cardiac output declines in spite of a compensatory tachycardia. There may also be dyspnea caused by bronchoconstriction, but in normal humans circulatory depression is predominant. Without adequate treatment, death may ensue from histamine shock.

In the intact animal, histamine can cause cardiac stimulation. This response is largely the result of reflex mechanisms triggered by a histamine-induced fall in peripheral vascular resistance. However, there is evidence that histamine does have some direct positive chronotropic and inotropic effects on the heart. Although the cardiac stimulation may be caused in part by release of catecholamines, it is probable that histamine receptors in the myocardium are also involved.[19]

Nonvascular smooth muscle. Histamine generally stimulates contraction of nonvascular smooth muscle to a variable degree, depending on species and tissue. In humans, the smooth muscle of the bronchioles and gastrointestinal tract is most sensitive to this action; the smooth muscle of other organs, such as the uterus and bladder, is affected to a much lesser extent. Subjects with asthma are highly susceptible to histamine and may experience marked bronchial constriction from doses that would cause only minor increases in the airway resistance of a normal subject.

Exocrine glands. Histamine is a potent stimulator of gastric secretion in most species. Low doses of histamine that have minimal effects on blood pressure will elicit near maximal secretion of both hydrochloric acid and pepsin by the gastric glands. Based on this sensitivity of the gastric secretory cells to histamine and the presence of histamine in both gastric mucosa and gastric fluid, it has been suggested that histamine plays a physiologic role in gastric secretion.[10] The relationship between the polypeptide hormone gastrin, a potent gastric secretagogue, and histamine is unclear. The fact that H_2-receptor antagonists block stimulation of gastric secretion by both gastrin and histamine lends fresh support to the notion that gastrin acts by releasing histamine, which then acts directly on the parietal cell.[24]

Histamine also stimulates secretion of catecholamines by the chromaffin cells of the adrenal medulla. Although it can enhance salivary and lacrimal gland secretion, this effect is minimal unless large doses are used.

General therapeutic uses

There are currently no valid therapeutic applications for histamine. It is of some use, however, as a diagnostic tool in several diseases. The most important of these is the assessment of gastric acid production. In this test, histamine is given subcutaneously in a dose (usually 1 mg) that will stimulate gastric secretion without causing major effects on blood vessels or smooth muscle. The gastric fluid is subsequently sampled and its acid content determined. An isomer of histamine, betazole, can also be used in this test and offers the advantage of causing a lesser degree of unwanted side effects for a given degree of gastric stimulation.

Since histamine stimulates the chromaffin cells in the adrenal medulla to secrete catecholamines, it can be used in the diagnosis of chromaffin cell tumors (pheochromocytomas). If such a tumor is present, a rise rather than a fall in blood pressure will occur after a moderate intravenous dose of histamine. However, safer tests for pheochromocytoma, such as measurement of urinary catecholamine excretion, are available.

Toxic reactions and side effects

The toxic effects of histamine are largely predictable on the basis of its pharmacologic actions. In normal persons, these effects are dose dependent. The more prominent manifestations of histamine toxicity are cutaneous flushing, hypotension, headache, visual disturbances, dyspnea, and gastrointestinal disturbances such as nausea, vomiting, and diarrhea. Massive doses may lead to shock and circulatory failure. Histamine, even in low doses, may have serious adverse consequences in elderly persons or those with cardiovascular disease, asthma, or recent gastrointestinal bleeding.

HISTAMINE ANTAGONISTS

Histamine antagonists, or antihistamines, encompass a large group of compounds with the characteristic ability to block the actions of histamine. These compounds do not alter the formation, release, or degradation of histamine but competitively antagonize it at receptor sites. As described earlier, two classes of antihistamines are now defined on the basis of their ability to block different effects of histamine. Since the receptors mediating the vascular and smooth muscle effects and those mediating the gastric effects of histamine have been termed H_1 and H_2, respectively, these two groups of antihistamines are called H_1- and H_2-receptor antagonists or, more simply, H_1 and H_2 antihistamines.

The early interest in histamine as a mediator of certain pathologic processes of an allergic nature spurred interest in agents that could block histamine. The first such compound, a derivative of phenoxyethylamine, was reported by Bovet and Staub in 1937.[8] Although this substance could adequately protect guinea pigs against injected histamine or anaphylactic shock, it was too toxic for human use. Other less toxic compounds with antihistaminic activity were immediately sought. By 1946, numerous compounds with therapeutically useful properties had been found, including phenbenzamine, pyrilamine, diphenhydramine, and tripelennamine. During the following 20 years, hundreds of other compounds with antihistaminic properties were developed. Although many of these found their way into the drug market, few of them offer significant advantages over the original drugs.

As the pharmacologic properties of the antihistamines were studied, it became apparent that they had no effect on histamine-induced gastric acid secretion. In 1972, a potent antagonist of histamine-induced gastric secretion was reported.[6] This compound, burimamide, and its subsequently developed congeners offered great potential as therapeutic agents as well as tools for further investigation of the role of histamine in health and disease.

H_1-Receptor antagonists

Chemistry and classification. Most antihistamines with the ability to block H_1 receptors contain an ethylamine group and thus resemble histamine. These H_1-receptor antagonists, or H_1 antihistamines, can be represented by the general formula:

$$R_1 - X - \overset{|}{\underset{|}{C}} - \overset{|}{\underset{|}{C}} - N \overset{\displaystyle R_2}{\underset{\displaystyle R_3}{<}}$$

In this representation, R_1 is the nucleus of the compound and consists of one or more carbocyclic or

Table 23-2. Chemical classification of representative structures and dosages of major H_1 antihistamines

Class	Representative compound* (proprietary name)	Usual adult dose (oral)	Duration of action	Other compounds in same class
Alkylamines	**Chlorpheniramine maleate** (Chlor-Trimeton, others)	2-4 mg	4-8 hr	Brompheniramine maleate (Dimetane): 4 mg, 4-6 hr; Dexchlorpheniramine maleate (Polaramine): 2 mg, 4-6 hr; Dimethindene maleate (Triten): 2.5 mg, 12-24 hr; Tripolidine hydrochloride (Actidil): 2.5 mg, 6-8 hr
Ethanolamines	**Diphenhydramine hydrochloride** (Benadryl)	25-50 mg	6-8 hr	Carbinoxamine maleate (Clistin): 4-8 mg, 6-8 hr; Doxylamine succinate (Decapryn): 12.5-25 mg, 4-6 hr; Dimenhydrinate (Dramamine): 50-100 mg, 4-6 hr; Clemastine fumarate (Tavist): 1.34-2.68 mg, 8 hr
Ethylenediamines	**Tripelennamine citrate** (PBZ, others)	25-50 mg	4-6 hr	Pyrilamine maleate 25-50 mg, 6-8 hr
Piperazines	**Meclizine hydrochloride** (Bonine, others)	25-50 mg	24 hr	Cyclizine hydrochloride (Marezine): 50 mg, 4-6 hr; Buclizine hydrochloride (Bucladin-S): 50 mg, 4-12 hr
Phenothiazines	**Promethazine hydrochloride** (Phenergan)	12.5-25 mg	4-12 hr	Methdilazine hydrochloride (Tacaryl): 8 mg, 6-12 hr; Trimeprazine tartrate (Temaril): 2.5 mg, 6 hr

*Each structural formula is of the free base form.

heterocyclic aromatic systems; R_1 may or may not be separated from X by a methylene group. X is a carbon, oxygen, or nitrogen atom that connects the side chain to the nucleus. R_2 and R_3 are usually but not always methyl groups. The ethylene group in the side chain may also be part of a heterocyclic system containing nitrogen, as in cyclizine. A general conclusion from examination of structure-activity relationships is that a basic nitrogen atom is essential, whether it exists in the side chain alone, as in diphenhydramine, or in the ring structure alone, as in meclizine (Table 23-2).

By using the general formula above, the classic antihistamines can be grouped according to the substitution made at the X position. Five distinct classes are recognized: (1) alkylamines, in which X is carbon, (2) ethanolamines, in which X is oxygen, (3) ethylenediamines, in which X is nitrogen, (4) piperazines, in which X is carbon linked to a piperazine ring, and (5) phenothiazines, in which X is nitrogen as part of a phenothiazine nucleus.

There are other compounds with antihistamine activity that do not fit into this classification (e.g., phenindamine), but they are of little importance in therapeutics. The chemical structures of representative compounds of each of the major classes of H_1 antihistamines are shown in Table 23-2. Despite their structural heterogeneity, all of the classic antihistamines have only minor differences in pharmacologic properties. Such differences as do exist are mainly in potency, duration of action, and relative degree of effects on other systems.

Pharmacologic effects. The H_1 antihistamines exert a variety of effects. Although the basis of some of these effects is obscure, many clearly result from histamine antagonism. With the important exception of stimulation of gastric secretion, these agents can inhibit the contraction of gastrointestinal and bronchial smooth muscle, the increase in capillary permeability, the flare and itch components of the "triple response," and the vasodilation produced by histamine. Although H_1 antihistamines do not block histamine-induced gastric secretion, they do antagonize the increased secretions of the salivary and lacrimal glands and the increased release of epinephrine from the adrenal medulla stimulated by histamine. As with many other pharmacologic inhibitors, the mechanism of this action can be explained in terms of a competitive blockade of receptors; that is, the antihistamines appear to interact with a histamine receptor

on the target cell, resulting in a decreased availability of these receptors for histamine. This interaction is reversible, or competitive, since the inhibition produced by a given concentration of antihistamine can be overcome by increasing the concentration of histamine (Figure 23-2). There is no evidence that the antihistamines interfere with the synthesis, release, or biotransformation of histamine.

The action of the H_1 antihistamines in antagonizing histamine is specific; that is, the antihistamines "reverse" the effects of histamine by inhibiting its further action, but they have no directly opposing actions of their own. In contrast, epinephrine nonspecifically antagonizes histamine by exerting its own distinct effects, e.g., vasoconstriction, bronchodilation, cardiac stimulation, and decreased gastrointestinal motility. This type of antagonism is sometimes referred to as physiologic. This distinction is important in understanding why a physiologic antagonist such as epinephrine is a more effective agent than an antihistamine in treating systemic histamine toxicity.

As previously indicated, the bronchial smooth muscle of the guinea pig is quite sensitive to histamine, and low doses can trigger lethal bronchospasm. However, the prior administration of an H_1 antihistamine such as pyrilamine can protect the respiratory smooth muscle of these animals from a dose of histamine that is more than 100 times the lethal dose. These agents can similarly protect guinea pigs against histamine released during experimental anaphylaxis. A quite different situation prevails in humans. Although H_1 antihistamines can antagonize histamine-induced contraction of human respiratory muscle in vitro, these agents are relatively ineffective in relieving bronchospasm associated wtih asthma, anaphylaxis, and other allergic reactions. This ineffectiveness is caused in part by the involvement of autacoids other than histamine in mediating allergic bronchospasm in humans. These substances include SRS-A and kinins, against which the classic antihistamines show little antagonism.

In the human vascular system, H_1 antihistamines are quite effective in antagonizing the increased capillary permeability and consequent edema formation induced by histamine. However, these agents have less ability to inhibit the vasodilation caused by histamine. Since a combination of H_1 and H_2 antihistamines is more effective than either alone, it is possible that both H_1 and H_2 receptors

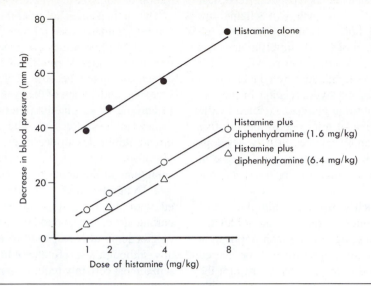

Figure 23-2. Log dose-response curves illustrating competitive antagonism of histamine by diphenhydramine. Decreases in blood pressure (ordinate) induced by graded intravenous doses of histamine (abscissa) were determined in anesthetized dogs. The animals then received diphenhydramine (1.6 or 6.4 mg/kg) followed by the same graded doses of histamine. (From Chen, G., and Russell, D. A quantitative study of blood pressure response to cardiovascular drugs and their antagonists. Journal of Pharmacology and Experimental Therapeutics **99:**401-408, 1950. © 1950, The Williams & Wilkins Co., Baltimore.)

may be involved in histamine-induced vasodilation.[26] The minor cardiac stimulation produced by histamine is little affected by antihistamines.

H₁ antihistamines have certain actions that are not obviously related to their ability to antagonize histamine. The most prominent and important of these is the depression of various CNS functions. Sedation is a common feature of therapeutic doses of all H₁ antihistamines and is usually manifested by drowsiness but may also be accompanied by lassitude, fatigue, dizziness, and incoordination. The ability to cause sedation varies widely among the available H₁ antihistamines; the most potent are the ethanolamines and phenothiazines, whereas the alkylamines have the lowest incidence of drowsiness. Another clinically useful central action of these agents is inhibition of nausea and vomiting, especially that associated with motion sickness. The H₁ antihistamines also exert some mild antiparkinson activity. Large doses of H₁ antihistamines can cause central stimulation that may result in convulsions. Some degree of stimulation—restlessness or insomnia—may occasionally be encountered even at therapeutic doses.

The mechanism of the CNS effects of the H₁ antihistamines is unknown. Although histamine is present in the brain and has been thought to play a role there as a neurotransmitter,[33] there is no firm evidence to suggest that the central effects of antihistamines are related to histamine antagonism. It has been suggested that both the anti-motion-sickness and the antiparkinson activities of the H₁ antihistamines could be caused by a central cholinergic blocking action.

Most H₁ antihistamines have some degree of local anesthetic activity. This property is most notable in diphenhydramine, promethazine, and pyrilamine and has been explored clinically in dentistry.[23,35] Consistent with this local anesthetic activity, these compounds also have a quinidine-like effect on conduction in the myocardium.

Mild antimuscarinic activity is another feature of most H₁ antihistamines. The decrease in salivary secretions that commonly occurs during antihistamine therapy is probably largely related to this action.

Absorption, fate, and excretion. As a class, the H₁ antihistamines are well absorbed after either oral or parenteral administration. Peak blood concentrations are achieved in 15 to 30 minutes after an oral dose. After absorption, the H₁ antihistamines are widely distributed in body fluids. For most of these agents the therapeutic effects last from 3 to 6 hours; a few, such as meclizine, are effective up to 24 hours (Table 23-2). Although the biotransformation of the H_1 antihistamines has not been intensively studied, the activity of this group appears to be terminated by conversion to inactive metabolites via hydroxylation in the liver.[25] These metabolites are largely excreted by the kidney. Some degree of tolerance to the sedative effects of the H_1 antihistamines usually develops with chronic use, but no concomitant decrease in their purely antihistaminic effects has been observed.

General therapeutic uses. The introduction of the antihistamines into clinical medicine stimulated great interest in these agents and their application in those pathologic states presumed to be caused by histamine release. The early enthusiasm for the antihistamines often led to their irrational use in various clinical situations. Although experience gained during the past 25 years has brought about a better appreciation of the therapeutic indications and limitations of the antihistamines, they are still often employed in instances in which their efficacy is doubtful or other agents might be more appropriate.

The most prominent use of the H_1 antihistamines is in countering the manifestations of various allergic conditions, that is, the reactions resulting from antigen-antibody combination in the body. The antihistamines have no effect on the interaction of antigens and antibodies or on the release of histamine that may be triggered by this interaction but act by competitively antagonizing the binding of liberated histamine to its receptor. This mechanism of action has several implications for the therapeutic use of the antihistamines. It means that these agents cannot alter the allergic basis of a given disease but can only provide relief from some of the symptoms. It also means the antihistamines are most effective when given before the release of histamine. Once histamine release has occurred, an antihistamine can only reduce further undesirable effects, unlike physiologic antagonists that can reverse them. Finally, the competitive nature of antihistamine action means that the effectiveness of these agents in a given situation depends on the relative concentrations of agonist versus antagonist. Thus, when substantial amounts of histamine are released either locally or systemically, the adverse effects of the antihistamine may preclude attainment of the sufficient concentration of antagonist to be clinically effective.

The clinical applications of the H_1 antihistamines can be summarized as follows.

1. H_1 antihistamines are generally useful in the treatment of allergic rhinitis of either a seasonal or an episodic nature because they relieve rhinorrhea, sneezing, and itching of the eyes and nasal mucosa. In chronic or vasomotor rhinitis, these drugs are somewhat less effective. The antihistamines are often combined with decongestants such as phenylpropanolamine for the management of allergic symptoms in the upper respiratory tract.

2. A number of allergic dermatoses can be treated with the H_1 antihistamines. Both acute and chronic urticaria respond favorably to these agents. Angioedema also responds to antihistamine therapy, although a severe attack involving the larynx will almost certainly require epinephrine for proper management of this serious complication. The H_1 antihistamines may be useful in controlling the itching associated wtih eczematous pruritus, atopic or contact dermatitis, and insect bites. However, in some situations (e.g., atopic dermatitis), topical corticosteroids are usually more effective. Although the antihistamines are topically effective in treating pruritus and urticaria, it should be noted that topical application can also cause an allergic dermatitis.

3. In systemic anaphylaxis, the H_1 antihistamines have no primary therapeutic role since they cannot control either the marked hypotension or the bronchospasm associated with a severe anaphylactic reaction. Here, the agent of choice is the physiologic antagonist, epinephrine. Antihistamines as well as corticosteroids may be given parenterally as an adjunct to the physiologic antagonist, but only after life-threatening problems are controlled. The antihistamines are of some value in treating the itching and urticarial lesions of serum sickness, although other manifestations such as arthralgia are little affected.

4. The H_1 antihistamines have little effect on the acute manifestations of bronchial asthma. The pathogenesis of bronchial asthma is complex, and, as indicated earlier and in Chapter 22, mediators of bronchial muscle constriction other than histamine are probably involved. Epinephrine, isoproterenol, and theophylline are the primary agents used to alleviate an acute asthmatic episode. Antihistamines have been used in an attempt to decrease preasthmatic cough in children, although the efficacy of this therapy is not established.

5. H$_1$ antihistamines, particularly chlorpheniramine, combined with nasal decongestants and analgesics are widely used for symptomatic relief of the common cold. There are currently more than 100 such preparations on the market, which indicates the popularity of these nostrums. Unless the cold is superimposed on an allergic rhinitis, any relief obtained from this combination stems largely from the drying of the mucosa caused by the anticholinergic action of the antihistamine and the actions of the vasoconstrictor and analgesic. Antihistamines alone are of no proven value in either preventing or shortening the duration of the common cold.

6. A central action of the H$_1$ antihistamines can be used to prevent or treat nausea and vomiting induced by motion. In general, these agents exert less anti-motion-sickness activity than do anticholinergics such as scopolamine. The effectiveness of individual antihistamines varies widely; promethazine, diphenhydramine, dimenhydrinate, and cyclizine are probably the most effective of all. However, the more potent agents tend to have greater sedative effects, a fact that must be considered in selecting an anti-motion-sickness drug. The H$_1$ antihistamines may also be useful in counteracting nausea and vomiting in vestibular disturbances such as Ménière's disease and other forms of vertigo. They are less effective than chlorpromazine or other phenothiazines for the control of nausea and vomiting following general anesthesia or associated wtih pregnancy, malignant diseases, radiation sickness, and various drugs.

7. Various OTC preparations sold as hypnotics include H$_1$ antihistamines because of their sedative effect. Since the dosages of antihistamine in such preparations are low, they are of limited value in inducing sleep. However, even in higher doses the antihistamines are less effective sedatives than barbiturates. Promethazine is widely used as an adjunct to general anesthesia to produce drowsiness as well as to prevent or control nausea and vomiting induced by anesthetic agents and narcotic analgesics.

8. Some miscellaneous uses of the H$_1$ antihistamines include reduction of tremors and muscle rigidity in Parkinson's disease, treatment of headaches of unknown etiology, such as migraine, and control of nonhemolytic, nonpyrogenic reactions to blood transfusion.

Uses in dentistry. The H$_1$ antihistamines are used in dentistry primarily for their central actions rather than for their specific antihistaminic effects. Promethazine and occasionally dimenhydrinate are used for preanesthetic sedation and for the prevention of nausea and vomiting induced by the anesthetic agent. The sedative effect is increased by the concomitant administration of a narcotic analgesic; meperidine is commonly used for this purpose.[4] The preoperative administration of promethazine may also achieve some inhibition of salivary and bronchial secretions, although more effective anticholinergic drugs should be used if control of secretions is essential.

Although H$_1$ antihistamines have some local anesthetic activity and their feasibility as local anesthetic agents for dental procedures has been demonstrated,[23,35] they have been little used for this purpose because far more effective agents (e.g., lidocaine) are available. Still, the local anesthetic activity of the antihistamines may be useful in cases where a patient is allergic to both amide- and ester-based local anesthetics.

The H$_1$ antihistamines can be used as secondary agents in the management of systemic anaphylactic reactions that may occur in the course of dental therapy. They can also be of value in the treatment of allergic lesions of the oral mucosa and angioneurotic edema of the orofacial region.

Toxic reactions and side effects. At therapeutic dose levels, the H$_1$ antihistamines are relatively free of serious adverse reactions. The most common side effects result from CNS depression, which is generally manifested as drowsiness, diminished alertness, lethargy, and decreased motor coordination. The incidence of sedation varies with individual agents, but in general the ethanolamines and the phenothazines are the most potent, the ethylenediamines are intermediate, and the alkylamines and piperazines tend to be relatively low in potency. Sedation caused by antihistamines may be a serious liability in a patient whose daily activities require mental alertness and coordination. In such cases, a reduction of dosage or substitution of agents may be necessary. Gastrointestinal disturbances such as nausea, vomiting, and epigastric distress also occur but are not common. The anticholinergic properties of the antihistamines occasionally cause insomnia, tremors, nervousness and irritability, palpitation, tachycardia, dry mouth, blurred vision, urinary retention, and constipation. The incidence of these effects increases with higher doses.

Large doses of antihistamines can cause marked

stimulation of the central nervous system manifested by hallucinations, excitement, and motor disturbances such as tremors and convulsions. Deaths have resulted from overdosage.

Allergic reactions to the H_1 antihistamines can occur; they are more frequent after topical application than after oral administration. Allergic lesions of the skin or oral mucosa should therefore not be treated by topical application of these agents. These reactions take the form of urticarial, eczematous, bullous, or petechial rashes, fixed drug eruptions, or, more rarely, anaphylaxis.

As with most drugs, various blood dyscrasis (hemolytic anemia, agranulocytosis, pancytopenia, and thrombocytopenia) have been reported after the use of antihistamines. Patients receiving long-term antihistamine therapy should thus be monitored periodically. Recently, meclizine and cyclizine have been shown to be teratogenic in laboratory animals. Until their potential for causing birth defects in humans is determined, their use is not advisable during the first trimester of pregnancy. Laboratory tests have also recently detected a carcinogenic potential for methapyrilene, an ethylenediamine-type antihistamine; this finding prompted its removal from the U.S. market in 1981.

Because of their sedative actions, the H_1 antihistamines can potentiate the CNS depressant effects of other agents, such as barbiturates, opioid analgesics, general anesthetics, and alcohol. Although such an interaction may be deliberately sought, as in the preanesthetic use of promethazine, these combinations should otherwise be avoided or monitored closely. Because the antihistamines have anticholinergic properties, they can produce manifestations of excessive cholinergic blockade if given during therapy with other anticholinergic drugs. Such manifestations (e.g., dry mouth, constipa-

tion, or blurred vision) are more likely to be troublesome than serious. The H_1 antihistamines can induce the hepatic microsomal enzymes responsible for their own degradation, and this has been shown in experimental animals to increase the metabolism of other agents, such as steroids and phenytoin.[18] Such an increase in the rate of metabolism could have clinical implications, but thus far none has been reported.

Antihistamines are variably excreted in breast milk. Because infants, especially newborn and premature, are at higher risk of adverse effects, the use of antihistamines in nursing women should be avoided. Furthermore, antihistamines, like other anticholinergic agents, may inhibit lactation.

Preparations and doses of drugs used in dentistry. The therapeutic value of the H_1 antihistamines can be encompassed by relatively few agents. Since a large number of preparations are available, the clinician has the task of selecting the most efficacious agent with minimal side effects. Because there is little quantitative data on which to base this choice, it is best for the clinician to select one or two well-known representatives of each class and become familiar with their therapeutic indications and limitations. These selections can be modified when convincing evidence of an advantage offered by another agent becomes available.

Oral doses of established examples of each of the major classes of H_1 antihistamines are given in Table 23-2. For more prescribing information the reader should consult a more detailed discussion of these agents.[1]

H_2-receptor antagonists

Chemistry and classification. The H_2-receptor antagonists, or H_2 antihistamines, are basically

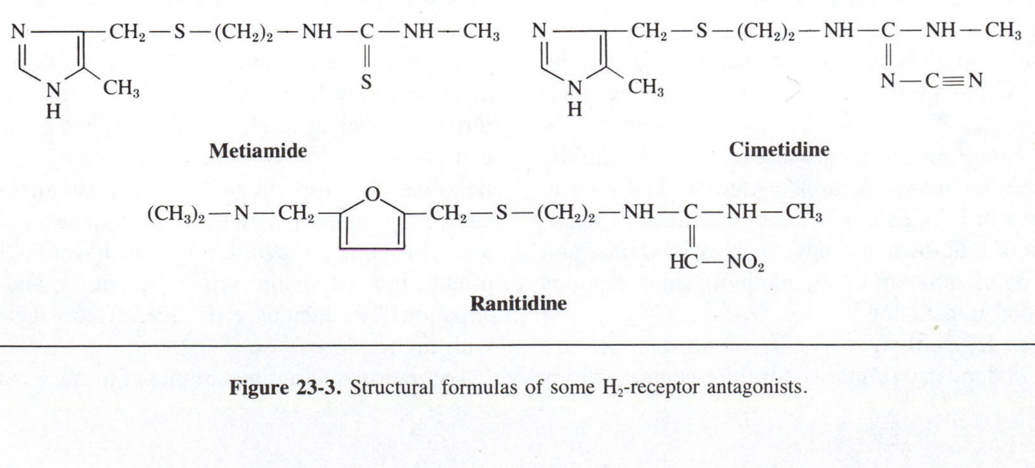

Figure 23-3. Structural formulas of some H_2-receptor antagonists.

structural analogues of histamine (Figure 23-3). Two changes in the histamine molecule are necessary to achieve H_2-receptor blocking activity.[14] One is modification of the imidazole ring, which results in a compound with greatly reduced histamine agonist properties but little antagonistic activity at H_2 receptors. The other is obtained by lengthening the side chain and reducing its basicity.

The first compound discovered to have the ability to block H_2 receptors was burimamide.[6] Its poor oral absorption and partial agonist properties led to a search for active congeners. The first of these to be tested was metiamide.[7] Although metiamide is orally effective, it caused a reversible neutropenia during clinical trials. Since the thiourea moiety in the side chain of metiamide was believed to be responsible for this adverse effect, the thiourea group was replaced by a cyanoguanidine group. The resultant compound, cimetidine, became available for clinical use in 1977.[16] More recently, ranitidine has been approved. It differs from cimetidine and earlier H_2 antagonists in that it is not an imidazole derivative but instead contains a furan ring.

Several differences between the H_1 and H_2 antihistamines are obvious. The H_1 antihistamines have aryl or heteroaryl rings that are highly lipophilic and bear little resemblance to the imidazole ring of histamine. Their side chains usually have an ammonium group and are positively charged at physiologic pH. In contrast, H_2 antihistamines have a modified imidazole or other heterocyclic ring and a polar but uncharged side chain. The H_2 antihistamines are hydrophilic; this property may account for their rather weak CNS and local anesthetic properties.[14]

Pharmacologic effects. The H_2 antihistamines are potent competitive antagonists of histamine. Since H_2 receptors are strongly implicated in the secretory function of the gastric mucosa, it is not surprising that these compounds cause a marked reduction in H^+ output, pepsin activity, and the total volume of gastric secretion. Inhibition of secretion can be attained in the fasting state or after stimulation with food, histamine, pentagastrin, and caffeine (Figure 23-4).[24] The ability of the H_2 antihistamines to block pentagastrin-induced gastric secretion supports the notion that the action of gastrin is mediated by the release of endogenous histamine.

There is some evidence that H_2 antihistamines

may enhance the metabolism of histamine. Increased amounts of methylated histamine were detected in the gastric mucosa of pigs and in the urine of humans after the administration of metiamide or cimetidine.[16] The contribution of this effect to the action of the H_2 antihistamines awaits further study.

The H_2 antihistamines have few effects other than those on gastric secretion. In certain situations, such as antagonism of a histamine-induced decrease in blood pressure, a combination of H_1 and H_2 antihistamines is more effective than either alone, which suggests that in such situations both H_1 and H_2 receptors are involved.[26]

Absorption, fate, and excretion. Cimetidine and ranitidine are both well absorbed after oral administration. Cimetidine can also be given intravenously. After absorption, the H_2 antihistamines are generally distributed in the total body water.[16] Therapeutic levels of cimetidine are reached in 1 to 1½ hours after an oral dose of 300 mg, and these levels persist for 6 to 8 hours. Cimetidine is largely eliminated unchanged (80% to 90%) in the urine.[16] The remainder of the drug is metabolized to sulfoxide and hydroxymethyl derivatives and excreted in the urine and feces. Ranitidine has a half-life of 2 to 3 hours; about 25% is excreted unchanged.

General therapeutic uses. Cimetidine and ranitidine are approved for the treatment of duodenal ulcers and pathologic hypersecretory states, such as the Zollinger-Ellison syndrome.[9,27] The usual dosage of cimetidine for treatment of an active ulcer is 1 gm per day, 200 mg taken after each meal and 400 mg at bedtime; for prophylaxis of recurrence, 400 mg is taken at bedtime. Although qualitatively similar to cimetidine in its effects on gastric secretion, ranitidine is 3 to 5 times more potent and thus can be given in a lower dosage. Cimetidine and ranitidine have been shown to decrease gastric acid secretion significantly (up to 90%) and to promote healing of duodenal and perhaps gastric ulcers.[9,27,32] They may also be effective in the management of gastric, or reflux, esophagitis. Although cimetidine has been used to treat upper gastrointestinal bleeding caused by ulcers or secondary liver disease and nonulcer dyspepsia and gastritis, there is little evidence to support its efficacy in these conditions. Finally, cimetidine is employed before surgery, particularly in patients with gastrointestinal obstruction, to elevate gastric pH and reduce the danger of aseptic pneumonia

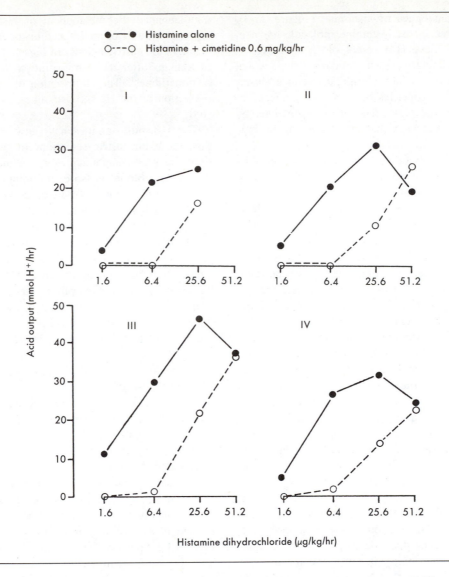

Figure 23-4. Inhibition of histamine-stimulated gastric acid production by cimetidine in humans. Histamine dihydrochloride in doses from 1.6 to 51.2 µg/kg/hour was infused intravenously with or without cimetidine at a dose of 0.6 mg/kg/hour for 105 minutes. When cimetidine was given, its administration was begun 15 minutes before the histamine infusion was started. Gastric juice was collected at 15-minute intervals and analyzed for acid concentration; the last four 15-minute intervals were used to establish the dose-response curves. Data shown are individual results from four normal adult subjects (I to IV). (From Aadland, E., and Berstad, A. Inhibition of histamine- and pentagastrin-stimulated gastric secretion by cimetidine in man. In Creutzfeldt, W., ed. Cimetidine, pp. 47-52, Amsterdam, Excerpta Medica Foundation, 1978.)

from aspiration of chyme during induction of general anesthesia.

Cimetidine is a widely prescribed drug; in 1980, total sales amounted to more than $500 million, making it one of the best selling drugs in the world. There are, however, sufficient data to indicate that much of the use of H_2 antihistamines might be inappropriate and unwarranted. In a recent study of 200 patients treated with cimetidine at a university hospital, only 7.5% had an approved indication (i.e., duodenal ulcer disease or pathologic gastric hypersecretion).[30] The drug was most frequently administered (52% of the time) to prevent upper gastrointestinal-tract bleeding in patients without a defined gastrointestinal lesion. Because cimetidine therapy is not free of adverse effects, there is a clear need to limit the drug to approved uses until its efficacy in ulcer prophylaxis, gastritis, acute gastrointestinal bleeding, and other conditions is proved.[13]

Toxic reactions and side effects. Early reports on cimetidine indicated that it was remarkably free of adverse effects. With the passage of time and extensive clinical use, it has become apparent that cimetidine can cause a variety of toxic reactions and side effects ranging from mild to severe. These problems have recently been reviewed.[21,29] Most untoward responses appear to have no obvious relation to blockade of H_2 receptors. This impression may simply be a result of an incomplete understanding of the presence and function of H_2 receptors in tissues other than the gastric mucosa.

The most common adverse effects of cimetidine are manifested in the central nervous system. These are highly variable and range from minor (headache, dizziness, lethargy, and fatigue) to more serious (mental confusion, delirium, focal twitching, hallucinations, and seizures). The CNS effects often appear to be dose related and are most commonly seen in elderly patients or those with impaired liver or kidney function. Cimetidine exerts a number of effects on endocrine function, most of which are both minor and reversible on cessation of therapy. The most notable of these is gynecomastia; others are elevation of serum prolactin, galactorrhea, loss of libido, impotence, and reduction in sperm counts. Small but definite increases in serum creatinine levels occur in most patients treated with cimetidine. This effect is not associated with other changes in renal function and ceases when the drug is withdrawn. The depression of granulocytes associated with metiamide does not appear to be a problem with cimetidine, but transient leukopenia, granulocytopenia, and thrombocytopenia have been reported. It is difficult to implicate cimetidine as a direct bone marrow suppressant, since the cases reported almost always involve the concomitant use of other drugs or the existence of other serious systemic diseases. Although cimetidine enhances cell-mediated immune reactions, there is no evidence that this phenomenon is related to any of the observed clinical responses. The occurrence of gastric cancer in patients treated with cimetidine has led to the suggestion that the agent may be carcinogenic. This has not been proved, and present information is insufficient to label cimetidine as a carcinogen.

Although cimetidine initially appeared to have no drug interactions of consequence, recent clinical reports and laboratory studies indicate that this is not the case. Cimetidine has been shown to increase blood concentrations of several drugs, including anticoagulants of the warfarin type, benzodiazepines, theophylline, propranolol and other β-blockers, lidocaine, and phenytoin, thus creating a risk of toxicity. The basis of these interactions appears to be competitive inhibition by cimetidine of the hepatic mixed-function oxidase system responsible for the metabolism of these drugs.[2,34] A cimetidine-induced decrease in hepatic blood flow may depress the entry of drugs into the liver and also slow metabolism. Patients receiving cimetidine together with any of the above drugs should be carefully monitored and, if appropriate, reduction of dosages or use of alternative agents should be considered.

Ranitidine appears to have fewer adverse effects than cimetidine. Unlike cimetidine, it has no antiandrogenic effects and thus far has not been reported to cause mental confusion or elevate serum creatinine activities.[9] Further investigation and clinical experience are necessary to establish these differences more conclusively.

Antihistamines

Nonproprietary name	Proprietary name
H_1-receptor antagonists	
Alkylamines	
brompheniramine	Dimetane
chlorpheniramine	Chlor-Trimeton
dexchlorpheniramine	Polaramine
dimethindene	Triten
triprolidine	Actidil
Ethanolamines	
bromodiphenhydramine	Ambodryl
carbinoxamine	Clistin
clemastine	Tavist
dimenhydrinate*	Dramamine
diphenhydramine	Benadryl
doxylamine	Decapryn
Ethylenediamines	
pyrilamine	—
tripelennamine	PBZ
Piperazines	
buclizine	Bucladin-S
cyclizine	Marezine
meclizine	Bonine

*The chlorotheophylline salt of diphenhydramine.

Antihistamines—cont'd

Nonproprietary name	Proprietary name
Phenothiazines	
methdilazine	Tacaryl
promethazine	Phenergan
trimeprazine	Temaril
Miscellaneous	
azatadine	Optimine
cyproheptadine	Periactin
diphenylpyraline	Hispril
phenindamine	Nolahist
H_2-receptor antagonists	
cimetidine	Tagamet
ranitidine	Zantac

CITED REFERENCES

1. AMA Department of Drugs. AMA Drug Evaluations, ed. 5. Chicago, American Medical Association, 1983.

2. Bauman, J.H., and Kimelblatt, B.J. Cimetidine as an inhibitor of drug metabolism: therapeutic implications and review of the literature. Drug Intelligence and Clinical Pharmacy **16**:380-386, 1982.

3. Beaven, M.A. Histamine. New England Journal of Medicine **294**:30-36, 320-325, 1976.

4. Bennett, C.R. Conscious Sedation in Dental Practice, ed. 2. St. Louis, The C.V. Mosby Co., 1978.

5. Best, C.H., Dale, H.H., Dudley, H.W., and Thorpe, W.V. The nature of the vaso-dilator constituents of certain tissue extracts. Journal of Physiology **62**:397-417, 1927.

6. Black, J.W., Duncan, W.A.M., Durant, C.J., Ganellin, C.R., and Parsons, E.M. Definition and antagonism of histamine H_2-receptors. Nature **236**:385-390, 1972.

7. Black, J.W., Duncan, W.A.M., Emmett, J.C., Ganellin, C.R., Hasselbo, T., Parsons, E.M., and Wyllie, J.H. Metiamide—an orally active histamine H_2-receptor antagonist. Agents and Actions; Swiss Journal of Pharmacology **3**:133-137, 1973.

8. Bovet, D., and Staub, A. Action protectrice des ethers phenoliques au cours de l'intoxication histaminique. Comptes Rendues des Seances de la Société de Biologie et de Ses Filiales (Paris) **124**:547-549, 1937.

9. Cimetidine and ranitidine (editorial). Lancet **1**:601-602, 1982.

10. Code, C.F. Reflections on histamine, gastric secretion, and the H_2 receptor. New England Journal of Medicine **296**:1459-1462, 1977.

11. Dale, H.H., and Laidlaw, P.P. Histamine shock. Journal of Physiology **52**:355-390, 1919.

12. Douglas, W.W. Histamine and 5-hydroxytryptamine (serotonin) and their antagonists. In Gilman, A.G., Goodman, L.S., and Gilman, A., eds. Goodman and Gilman's The Pharmacological Basis of Therapeutics, ed. 6. New York, Macmillan, Inc., 1980.

13. Fleshler, B. The impact of cimetidine on the treatment of acid-peptic disease. Primary Care **8**:195-203, 1981.

14. Ganellin, C.R., Durant, G.J., and Emmett, J.C. Some chemical aspects of histamine H_2-receptor antagonists. Federation Proceedings **35**:1924-1930, 1976.

15. Goth, A. Histamine release by drugs and chemicals. In Schachter, M., ed. Histamine and Antihistamines, vol. 1. International Encyclopedia of Pharmacology and Therapeutics, sect. 74. Oxford, England, Pergamon Press, Ltd., 1973.

16. Jacobs, R.S., and Catania, H. Cimetidine. Drug Intelligence and Clinical Pharmacy **11**:723-726, 1977.

17. Kahlson, G., and Rosengren, E. New approaches to the physiology of histamine. Physiological Reviews **48**:155-196, 1968.

18. Kuntzman, R. Drugs and enzyme induction. Annual Review of Pharmacology and Toxicology **9**:21-36, 1969.

19. Levi, R., Allan, G., and Zavecz, J.H. Cardiac histamine receptors. Federation Proceedings **35**:1942-1947, 1976.

20. Lewis, T., and Grant, R.T. Vascular reactions of the skin to injury. II. The liberation of a histamine-like substance in injured skin; the underlying causes of factitious urticaria and of wheals produced by burning; and observations upon the nervous control of certain skin reactions. Heart **11**:209-265, 1924.

21. McGuigan, J.E. A consideration of the adverse effects of cimetidine. Gastroenterology **80**:181-192, 1981.

22. McIntire, F.C. Histamine release by antigen-antibody reactions. In Schachter, M., ed. Histamines and Antihistamines, vol. 1. International Encyclopedia of Pharmacology and Therapeutics, sect. 74. Oxford, Pergamon Press, Ltd., 1973.

23. Meyer, R.A., and Jakubowski, W. Use of tripelennamine and diphenhydramine as local anesthetics. Journal of the American Dental Association **69**:112-117, 1964.

24. Parsons, M.E. The antagonism of histamine H_2-receptors *in vitro* and *in vivo* with particular reference to the actions of cimetidine. In Burland, W.L., and Simkins, M.A., eds. Cimetidine. Proceedings of the Second International Symposium on Histamine H_2-receptor Antagonists. Amsterdam, Excerpta Medica Foundation, 1977.

25. Peets, E.A., Jackson, M., and Symchowicz, S. Metabolism of chlorpheniramine maleate in man. Journal of Pharmacology and Experimental Therapeutics **180**:464-474, 1972.

26. Powell, J.R., and Brody, M.J. Identification and blockade of vascular H_2 receptors. Federation Proceedings **35**:1935-1941, 1976.

27. Ranitidine (Zantac). The Medical Letter on Drugs and Therapeutics **24**:111-113, 1982.

28. Riley, J.F., and West, G.B. The occurrence of histamine in mast cells. In Rocha e Silva, M., ed. Histamine and Antihistaminics, pt. 1. Handbook of Experimental Pharmacology, vol. 18, Berlin, Springer-Verlag, 1966.

29. Sawyer, D., Conner, C.S., and Scalley, R. Cimetidine: adverse reactions and acute toxicity. American Journal of Hospital Pharmacy **38**:188-197, 1981.

30. Schade, R.R., and Donaldson, R.M., Jr. How physicians use cimetidine: a survey of hospitalized patients and published cases. New England Journal of Medicine **304**:1281-1284, 1981.

31. Schayer, R.W. Catabolism of histamine in vivo. In Rocha e Silva, M., ed. Histamine and Antihistaminics, pt. 1. Handbook of Experimental Pharmacology, vol. 18. Berlin, Springer-Verlag, 1966.

32. Schlippert, W. Cimetidine: H_2-receptor blockade in

gastrointestinal disease. Archives of Internal Medicine **138:**1257-1260, 1978.

33. Schwartz, J.-C., Barbin, G., Duchemin, A.-M., Garbarg, M., Llorens, C., Pollard, H., Quach, T.T., and Rose, C. Histamine receptors in the brain and their possible functions. In Ganellin, C.R., and Parsons, M.E., eds. Pharmacology of Histamine Receptors. Bristol, John Wright & Sons, Ltd, 1982.

34. Somogyi, A., and Gugler, R. Drug interactions with cimetidine. Clinical Pharmacokinetics **7:**23-41, 1982.

35. Welborn, J.F., and Kane, J.P. Conduction anesthesia using diphenhydramine hydrochloride. Journal of the American Dental Association **69:**706-709, 1964.

36. Willoughby, D.A. Mediation of increased vascular permeability in inflammation. In Zweifach, B.W., Grant, L., and McClusky, R.T., eds. The Inflammatory Process, vol. 2, ed. 2. New York, Academic Press, Inc., 1973.

37. Zweifach, B.W. Microcirculation. Annual Review of Physiology **35:**117-150, 1973.

GENERAL REFERENCE

Douglas, W.W. Histamine and 5-hydroxytryptamine (serotonin) and their antagonists. In Gilman, A.G., Goodman, L.S., and Gilman, A., eds. Goodman and Gilman's The Pharmacological Basis of Therapeutics, ed. 6, New York, Macmillan, Inc., 1980.

24 Introduction to cardiovascular pharmacology: antiarrhythmic drugs

James L. Matheny

INTRODUCTION TO CARDIOVASCULAR PHARMACOLOGY

The following eight chapters describe the pharmacology of drugs that affect therapeutically the functioning of the cardiovascular system. Several classes of these drugs are used clinically to treat a variety of cardiovascular disorders. Generally speaking, drugs initially approved for use as antihypertensives, antianginals, or antiarrhythmics have been used for any of these disorders and sometimes for unrelated medical problems, as illustrated in Table 24-1. This situation exists because these drugs modify basic electrophysiologic and biochemical events that support the rhythm and force of cardiac contraction and the contractile tone of the peripheral vasculature. It follows that a basic understanding of cardiovascular physiology is a prerequisite for comprehending the pharmacologic effects of these drugs and their clinical uses.

Basic cardiac electrophysiology

Under normal conditions, the chambers of the heart contract as synchronized rhythmic units driven by electrical impulses generated in and conducted throughout the heart. The normal pacemaker impulse is generated in the sinoatrial (S-A) node and travels through the atria to each muscle cell, to the atrioventricular (A-V) node, and then through specialized conduction pathways in the common bundle of His, bundle branches, and the ventricular Purkinje network.

Three experimental measures are used to describe the normal electrophysiologic events in the heart as well as the dysrhythmias. These are automaticity, refractoriness, and responsiveness.

Automaticity. Automaticity is the unique property of cells of the S-A node and specialized conducting system to exhibit spontaneous phase 4 depolarization and thus impulse generation (Figure 24-1). Therefore, an increase in automaticity refers to an increase in the rate of impulse generation, and conversely a decrease in automaticity refers to a decrease in the rate of impulse generation. Under normal conditions, the pacemaker cells of the S-A node exhibit the most rapid phase 4 depolarization rate and thus control heart rate. The rate at which pacemaker cells generate impulses is a function of the rate of phase 4 depolarization, the maximum diastolic potential (MDP), and the magnitude of the threshold potential. For example, an increase in the rate of phase 4 depolarization results in an increased heart rate; an increase in the threshold potential results in a decreased heart rate; and an increase in MDP, or hyperpolarization, results in a decreased heart rate. These functions are under nervous and hormonal control and can be altered by injury or drugs.

Refractoriness. The period following the initiation of an action potential during which another action potential cannot be initiated and propagated regardless of stimulus is known as the effective refractory period (ERP; Figure 24-2). A change in the action potential duration is accompanied by a similar change in the duration of the ERP, though the ratio of change may not be 1:1. If the ERP is lengthened with respect to the action potential duration, the cardiac cells will have repolarized more completely before they respond to a stimulus. The larger transmembrane potential at the time of stimulation then results in a faster rate of depolarization

Table 24-1. Cardiovascular drug classes, uses, and effects

Classification	Example drugs	Uses	Mechanisms of action
Cardiac glycosides	Digoxin, digitoxin	Congestive heart failure	↑ Cardiac contractility
		Antiarrhythmic	↓ A-V conduction velocity
β-Adrenergic blocking drugs	Propranolol, metoprolol, timolol	Antiarrhythmic	↓ Cardiac automaticity
		Antianginal	↓ Cardiac oxygen consumption
		Prevent reinfarction	↓ Cardiac oxygen consumption
		Antihypertensive	↓ Cardiac output, renin release
		Migraine prophylaxis	↑ Cerebral vasoconstriction
		Anti–stage fright	↓ Autonomic signs of anxiety (tachycardia, palpitations)
		Hypertrophic cardiomyopathies	↓ Cardiac oxygen consumption
Diuretics	Chlorothiazide, furosemide, triamterene	Antihypertensive	↓ Peripheral vascular tone, ↓ extracellular fluid volume
		Congestive heart failure	↓ Extracellular fluid volume
		Ascites	↓ Edema
		Renal disease	↓ Edema
		Diabetes insipidus	↓ Glomerular filtration load
Centrally acting adrenergic drugs	Clonidine	Antihypertensive	↓ Peripheral vascular tone
		Menopausal flushing	↓ Cardiac output
		Migraine prophylaxis	?
		Relief of narcotic withdrawal symptoms	Central α-receptor agonist
α-Adrenergic and neuronal blocking drugs	Prazosin, guanethidine	Antihypertensive	↓ Peripheral vascular tone, ↓ cardiac output
Direct-acting peripheral vasodilators	Hydralazine, minoxidil	Antihypertensive	↓ Peripheral vascular tone
		Peripheral vascular disease	↓ Peripheral vascular tone
Calcium entry blockers	Verapamil, nifedipine	Antianginal	↓ Cardiac oxygen consumption, ↓ coronary artery spasm
		Antiarrhythmic	↓ A-V conduction velocity
		Antihypertensive	↓ Peripheral vascular tone
		Hypertrophic cardiomyopathies	?
Angiotensinase inhibitors	Captopril	Antihypertensive	↓ Peripheral vascular tone (reduced angiotensin II)

and improved conduction. Since some drugs increase the duration of the ERP and others decrease it, it is possible for an antagonistic effect to occur.

Responsiveness. Responsiveness describes the relationship between the maximal rate of depolarization (measured as the change in voltage per unit time, or dV/dt) during phase 0 of the action potential and the membrane potential at the time of stimulation. It has been widely accepted that the rate of phase 0 depolarization is the main determinant of conduction velocity.[4] Additionally, other things being equal, the more negative the membrane potential at the beginning of phase 0 depolarization, the greater the maximal dV/dt.[20] This relationship is illustrated by changes in membrane responsiveness curves (Figure 24-3). Thus, if an antiarrhythmic agent causes an increase in responsiveness, the rate of phase 0 depolarization will be increased, and the conduction velocity will likewise be increased. As with refractoriness, specific drugs may have an antagonistic effect on responsiveness and thus, when used in combination, may have inconsistent effects or collectively may have no effect.

Basic cardiovascular biochemistry*

Biochemical events in smooth muscle contraction are not well defined; however, in cardiac mus-

---

*This section on basic cardiovascular biochemistry was written by Dr. Frank Dowd, whose chapter on cardiac glycosides follows.

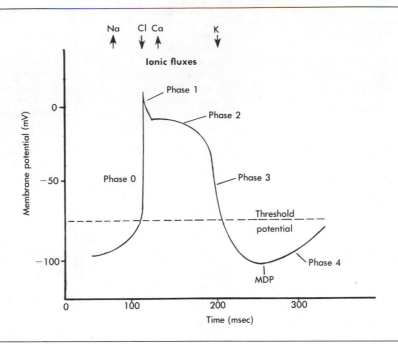

Figure 24-1. Diagrammatic representation of a membrane action potential from a Purkinje fiber. Phase 0 = rapid depolarization beginning when membrane potential reaches threshold potential; phase 1 = early repolarization; phase 2 = plateau phase; phase 3 = late repolarization, which continues until maximum diastolic potential (MDP) is reached; phase 4 = slow spontaneous diastolic depolarization. The times at which the various ionic fluxes begin are shown at the top; ↑ = a depolarizing current; ↓ = a repolarizing current.

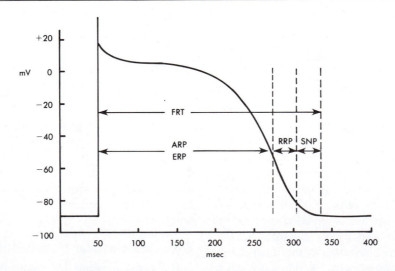

Figure 24-2. Schematic diagram of the usual temporal relationship between transmembrane potential and cathodal excitability in a cardiac muscle cell. FRT = full recovery time, ARP = absolute refractory period, ERP = effective refractory period, RRP = relative refractory period, SNP = supernormal period. (From Hoffman, B.F., and Cranefield, P.F. Electrophysiology of the Heart. New York, McGraw-Hill Book Co., 1960.)

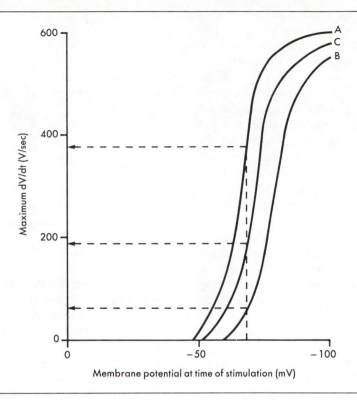

Figure 24-3. Curves of membrane responsiveness. Curve C represents the responsiveness of a control fiber. Small differences in the membrane potential at time of stimulation cause large changes in the rate of phase 0 depolarization as measured by the maximum change in dV/dt. Curves A and B indicate, respectively, an increase and a decrease in membrane responsiveness at a given membrane potential (e.g., arrows at −68 mV) that may result from drug treatment: curve A, Ca^{++} or phenytoin; curve B, quinidine or procainamide. (Adapted from Hoffman, B.F., and Bigger, J.T., Jr. Antiarrhythmic drugs. In DiPalma, J.R., ed. Drill's Pharmacology in Medicine, ed. 4. New York, McGraw-Hill Book Co., 1971.

cle it is known that several ions are involved in the depolarization-contraction sequence. Depolarization is effected by an initial, "fast channel" current of sodium ions in the inward direction (phase 0 of the action potential, Figure 24-1). Another major inward current, carried by calcium ions and conducted through "slow channels," contributes to the plateau phase (phase 2) of the action potential. Outward potassium currents are responsible, at least in part, for repolarizing the muscle fiber in phase 3 and, by slowly deactivating in phase 4, for spontaneous depolarization in those cardiac cells such as Purkinje fibers that display automaticity. Differential effects on these ion fluxes help explain variations in the therapeutic uses and adverse effects of the cardiovascular drugs.

Role of calcium in muscle contraction. In addition to its role in the action potential, calcium is intimately involved in the actomyosin contractile process. Tropomyosin and troponin, which are associated with actin, regulate the interaction between actin and myosin. Troponin consists of three subunits; the binding of calcium to one of these sets off a series of conformational changes in troponin and tropomyosin that result in the exposure of sites on actin that interact with myosin. This process requires energy. ATP is hydrolyzed by a myosin-bound ATPase, at which time an "active" actomyosin complex is formed, and chemical energy is converted into mechanical work.

The source of calcium responsible for cardiac muscle contraction depends ultimately on extracellular calcium entering the cell with the slow inward current or by a sodium-calcium exchange mechanism. Calcium must first traverse the plasma membrane, and a special invagination of the plasma membrane called the T tubule is probably a key entry point. Calcium ions are then thought to pass through the subsarcolemmal cisternae prior to reaching the contractile proteins.[6] This small influx of calcium during the slow inward current is believed to trigger the release of larger amounts of intracellular calcium from the subsarcolemmal cisternae and from the sarcoplasmic reticulum, which is contiguous with the cisternae. The sudden rise in cytoplasmic calcium then stimulates contraction, and the cycle is completed by the active reuptake of calcium ions by the sarcoplasmic reticulum (and mitochondria) and extrusion from the cell via sodium-calcium exchange.[24]

In contrast to the heart, the contraction of smooth muscle depends almost entirely on extracellular calcium and may be initiated by two different mechanisms. Certain calcium channels may be triggered by depolarization, whereas others are receptor operated and do not require depolarization.

Role of cyclic adenosine monophosphate. cAMP, an important mediator of β-adrenergic stimulation (see Chapter 5), plays very different roles in the contraction process of cardiac and smooth muscle. In smooth muscle, cAMP stimulates efflux and inhibits influx of calcium ions into the cytosol and thus promotes relaxation. In contrast, cAMP enhances contraction in cardiac muscle by augmenting Ca^{++} influx across the sarcolemma, by stimulating Ca^{++} release from the sarcoplasmic reticulum, and by increasing the sensitivity of the contractile elements to Ca^{++}.[14]

Conclusion. Although limited in scope, these comments on the physiology and biochemistry of the cardiovascular system will be useful when considering the antiarrhythmic drugs covered in the remainder of this chapter and the cardiac glycoside, antianginal, and antihypertensive drugs described in the chapters that follow. Clinically, the continuing replacement of empirically based therapies with treatments designed to correct particular physiologic and biochemical derangements will pay increasing dividends in the form of improved patient care.

ORIGINS OF ARRHYTHMIAS

Arrhythmias are thought to result from abnormal impulse generation or impulse conduction or a combination of both. Arrhythmias caused by abnormal impulse generation are believed to be due to changes in the rate of diastolic depolarization (slope of phase 4) in pacemaker cells. A change

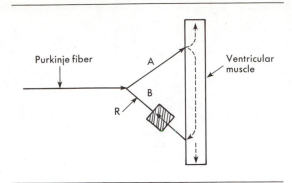

Figure 24-4. Reentry in the presence of unidirectional block. The hatched area in path B indicates a unidirectional block of impulse conduction.

in the slope of phase 4 depolarization can result in alteration of the heart rate or in ectopic impulse formation by latent pacemaker cells. Phase 4 depolarization can be altered by changes in input from the autonomic nervous system, by changes in the concentrations of ions in the extracellular fluid, by hypoxia, by mechanical trauma, or by weak currents arising from areas of myocardial ischemia or infarction.[9]

Two mechanisms have been proposed to explain how alterations in impulse conduction result in arrhythmias. The first is the occurrence of a phenomenon known as reentry, or circus movement.[13,23] The second is a disturbance in the relationship of fast and slow responses of cardiac fibers.[1,22,25]

Figure 24-4 shows how a reentrant rhythm can develop.[8] As illustrated, conduction in branch A is normal, whereas impulses in branch B can proceed in only one direction (unidirectional block). A normally conducted impulse through branch A can then be conducted in a retrograde fashion through branch B to reexcite an area of tissue (point R) that was previously excited by the normal path of conduction. For this phenomenon to occur, the tissue at point R must have repolarized to a point where excitation is possible. Thus, a wave of reexcitation traveling in a circular path through fiber A, the ventricular muscle, and fiber B can result in a self-sustaining arrhythmia.

It can be seen from Figure 24-5 that arrhythmias may also arise because of delay in conduction of an impulse through an area.[8] The area of block, in contrast to that shown in Figure 24-4, prevents retrograde conduction and slows normal conduc-

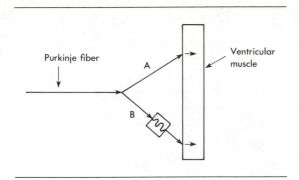

Figure 24-5. Delayed conduction (path B) through a Purkinje fiber, resulting in reexcitation of an area of ventricular muscle.

tion through the Purkinje fiber B, a phenomenon known as delayed conduction. Under the proper conditions, the ventricular muscle will be excited by the normal impulse through fiber A and reexcited by the same impulse, which was delayed by the area of block in fiber B.

Disturbances in the relationship of the fast and slow electrical responses of certain cardiac cells may play an important role in the genesis of arrhythmias.[1,2,25] The fast response refers to the rapid phase 0 depolarization caused by rapid sodium influx (Figure 24-1). This kind of activity is seen in atrial and ventricular muscle fibers and specialized conducting fibers. In addition to the rapid inward current carried by sodium, the fast fibers exhibit a second, slower inward current carried by calcium (Figure 24-1). The slow current does not contribute significantly to phase 0 depolarization but persists after rapid depolarization and is thus thought to be responsible for the prolonged plateau phase characteristic of these fibers. Certain fibers (slow fibers) located in the S-A and A-V nodes, the A-V ring fibers, and the mitral and tricuspid valve leaflets demonstrate only the slow response. Whereas the fast fibers exhibit rapid depolarization and thus remain refractory and conduct impulses safely, the slow fibers exhibit a slow rate of depolarization, low resting potential, and low impulse amplitude, resulting in slow conduction and susceptibility to aberrant stimulation. In addition to slow and fast fibers, there are transitional fibers that convert the slow response seen in S-A nodal fibers to a fast response for conduction to the rest of the heart. In disease states, the fast response may become inactivated, leaving the slow response dominant. These conditions favor genesis of arrhythmias because of the low safety factor associated with the slow response. These findings have led to the proposal that most, if not all, arrhythmias result from either slow conduction or rhythmic activity in a discrete, localized group of cells exhibiting only the slow-type response.[1] It follows from this discussion that there exists in the heart an intricate relationship between conduction velocity, path length, refractory period duration, and impulse generation that, when altered through one or more mechanisms, may result in the development of arrhythmias.

ELECTROCARDIOGRAM AND COMMON ARRHYTHMIAS

Generally, arrhythmias are classified as supraventricular (originating in the atria or conducting system, not in the ventricle) or ventricular. A few of the most common arrhythmias will be described. For comparison, a diagram of the normal electrocardiogram (ECG) with the electrical events in the various regions of the heart is provided in Figure 24-6. In Figure 24-7, representations of ECGs recorded during arrhythmias of ventricular and supraventricular origin are shown.

The first arrhythmia shown is a simple tachycardia caused by rapid impulse generation in the sinus. With higher rates of atrial activity, as in flutter (300 beats/min) or fibrillation (400 to 500 beats/min), heart block, another type of arrhythmia, will intervene. Heart blocks arise from failure of the A-V node to conduct electrical impulses in a normal fashion and are classified as first, second, and third degree. A first-degree A-V block has a prolonged P-R interval. A second-degree block, as illustrated in the atrial fibrillation tracing, is characterized by the occasional dropping of a QRS complex. In a third-degree block (also shown) there is complete dissociation between atrial and ventricular contractions.

The ventricular arrhythmias are caused by development of ectopic foci in the ventricles. The first one shown in Figure 24-7 is paroxysmal ventricular tachycardia, a serious arrhythmia often caused by excessive blood concentrations of digitalis, quinidine, and procainamide. Ventricular flutter is identified by an ECG recording of large waveforms in which P waves cannot be distinguished. In the most serious arrhythmia, ventricular fibrillation, multiple ventricular pacemakers cause erratic depolarization of different areas of the ventricle. The uncoordinated contraction of the heart renders the cardiac pump ineffective, and cardiac

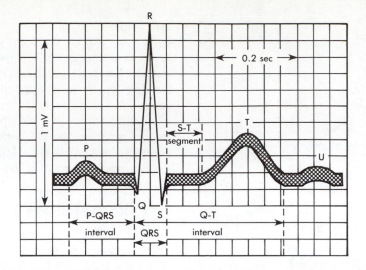

Figure 24-6. Normal electrocardiogram. P = atrial depolarization, QRS = ventricular depolarization, T = ventricular repolarization. (From Milnor, W.R. The electrocardiogram. In Mountcastle, V.B., ed. Medical Physiology, ed. 14. St. Louis, The C. V. Mosby Co., 1980.)

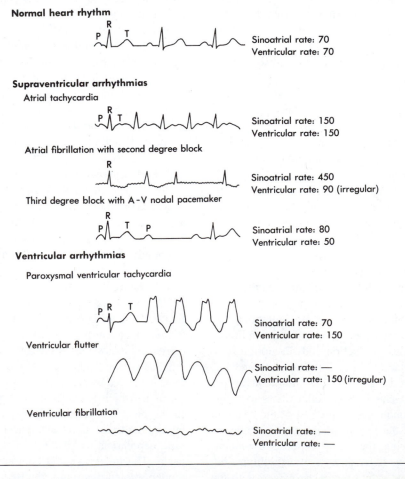

Figure 24-7. Various cardiac rhythms as recorded by ECG. Arrhythmias are classified as supraventricular or ventricular in origin. Rates are given in beats per minute. (Adapted from Shepard, R.S. Human Physiology. Philadelphia, J. B. Lippincott Co., 1971.)

output drops precipitously. In both ventricular flutter and fibrillation, immediate treatment (usually cardioversion and intravenous lidocaine) must be provided to prevent death.

ANTIARRHYTHMIC DRUGS

Antiarrhythmic drugs are used to modify, or restore to normal, aberrant contractions of cardiac muscle. Arrhythmias may result from various disease conditions or drug treatments. However, in all arrhythmias some facet of the normal electrophysiologic system that governs cardiac contractions is behaving abnormally. In practice, cardioversion (precordial DC shock) is the preferred method for acute termination of disorders of the cardiac rhythm.[15] Though some of the drugs classified as antiarrhythmic can bring about the reversal of certain arrhythmias and a return to normal sinus rhythm, their main use is in preventing a recurrence of arrhythmias after normal sinus rhythm has been established by electroconversion.

The drugs used in the treatment of cardiac arrhythmias can be appropriately categorized according to their dominant electrophysiologic or pharmacologic property (Table 24-2).[18] However, it should be noted that in vivo effects, especially at higher doses, may involve additional mechanisms. Agents like quinidine, procainamide, and lidocaine act through depression of the fast or sodium response, whereas drugs like verapamil and nifedipine depress the slow or calcium response. Propranolol and related β-blocking agents inhibit

cardiac stimulation by sympathetic nervous system activity. An additional group of antiarrhythmics, represented by bretylium and amiodarone, prolong the duration of action potentials. The use of cardiac glycosides for certain kinds of arrhythmias is covered in Chapter 25.

Quinidine

Quinidine is an effective agent in the treatment of atrial fibrillation and certain other arrhythmias. It was described and prepared many years before its antiarrhythmic properties were discovered. During treatment with quinine and quinidine of patients suffering from malaria, the reversal of atrial fibrillation was noted in some patients. Although this effect of the alkaloids had been noted earlier, widespread use of quinidine as the drug of choice for patients with supraventricular arrhythmias followed reports from Wenckebach[21] in 1914 and Frey[7] in 1918.

Quinidine, the *d*-isomer of quinine, is found in the bark of the cinchona tree, which is indigenous to certain regions of South America. Synthesis of this compound has been accomplished, but the synthesized drug is expensive, and quinidine is still isolated from the natural source. Its structural formula is shown in Figure 24-8.

Pharmacologic effects. Quinidine is a myocardial depressant. In clinical doses, it reduces automaticity and responsiveness and increases refractoriness. Automaticity is depressed through an increase in the threshold potential and a decrease in

Table 24-2. Classification of antiarrhythmic drugs*

Type I† (depress fast or Na⁺ response)	Type II (inhibit sympathetic activity)	Type III (prolong duration of action potential)	Type IV (depress slow or Ca⁺⁺ response)
Type Ia	Propranolol	Bretylium	Verapamil
Quinidine	Metoprolol‡	Amiodarone‡	Nifedipine‡
Procainamide	Nadolol‡		Diltiazem‡
Disopyramide	Pindolol‡		
Type Ib	Alprenolol‡		
Phenytoin‡	Atenolol‡		
Lidocaine	Sotalol‡		
Lidocaine-like drugs (e.g., tocainide)‡	Oxprenolol‡		

*This classification is based on major in vitro actions. Most of the drugs in all of the groups have depressant actions on pacemaker generation. In vivo actions may vary with the dose.

†Type I drugs are further subdivided on the basis of their differential effects on the action potential duration (APD) and effective refractory period (ERP). Type Ia drugs prolong APD and ERP; type Ib drugs shorten them. All of the type I drugs, however, increase the ratio of ERP to APD.

‡Not officially approved for use as an antiarrhythmic in the United States.

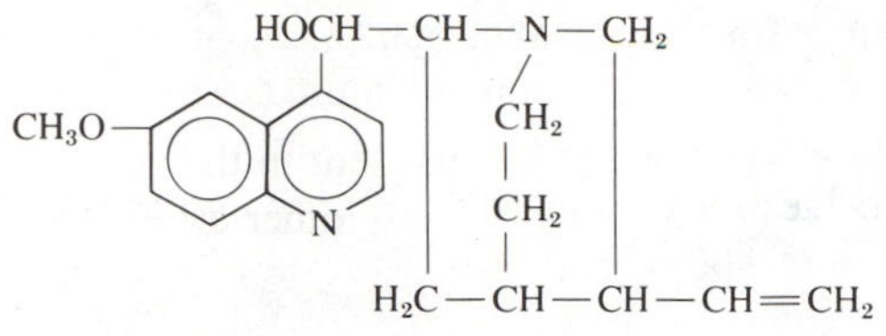

HOCH — CH — N — CH₂

Figure 24-8. Structural formula of quinidine.

the slope of spontaneous diastolic depolarization (phase 4) in pacemaker fibers, particularly in areas other than the S-A node. Thus, quinidine has the potential to slow or abolish tachyarrhythmias. Membrane responsiveness (shown in Figure 24-3 as a sigmoid curve relating maximum depolarization rate during phase 0 to membrane potential) is shifted to the right by quinidine. This shift translates to a decrease in the slope of phase 0 depolarization and a subsequent decrease in conduction velocity. The result is that the cell membrane must be more fully repolarized before another action potential can be initiated and propagated. Through this action, quinidine may prevent premature stimulation arising from an ectopic focus or a reentrant pathway. Refractoriness is increased by therapeutic doses of quinidine through an increase in the length of the ERP, with little accompanying increase in action potential duration. After quinidine treatment, cardiac cells remain refractory for a significant period following full repolarization. This action thus has the potential for preventing or abolishing reentrant rhythms.

In addition to its direct actions on the heart, quinidine has an antimuscarinic action, preventing the bradycardia that follows vagal stimulation or cholinergic drug administration. As a consequence, administration of quinidine normally results in an increased heart rate. Since the ERP is decreased by vagal stimulation, quinidine increases it both directly and indirectly. The anticholinergic action of quinidine on A-V nodal conduction is of special importance. It may result in increased conduction velocity and a decreased refractory period of the A-V node and thus presents a hazard in treating atrial tachyarrhythmias by allowing the rapid atrial impulses to be conducted more readily to the ventricles.

The ECG changes that result from quinidine administration are predictable from the electrophysiologic effects previously discussed. Anticholin-

ergic action produces sinus tachycardia, but with high doses S-A block may result from its direct depressant actions. Increased duration of the QRS complex and the Q-T interval results from the lengthening of the ERP and from a decrease in ventricular conduction velocity. In high doses, quinidine can cause ventricular ectopic rhythms or ventricular fibrillation.

As a result of its depressive effects on electrical activity of the heart, quinidine causes a slight reduction of myocardial contractility that might be important in the management of a patient with heart disease.

In large doses quinidine causes peripheral vasodilation and a concomitant decrease in arterial pressure. Clinically significant decreases in arterial pressure are usually seen only after parenteral use of this compound.

Absorption, fate, and excretion. Absorption of quinidine after oral administration is fairly rapid and nearly 100%. Maximal plasma concentrations are reached in approximately 1 to 2 hours, and the biologic half-life is about 6 hours. Given intramuscularly, peak concentrations occur within 60 minutes. When quinidine is given intravenously, it should be administered slowly because its therapeutic effects are not instantaneous, and overdosage might occur. In therapeutic doses approximately 60% of the circulating drug is bound to plasma albumin. Essentially all of an administered dose of quinidine is excreted in the urine, about 20% being the parent compound and the balance being hydroxylated derivatives formed in the liver.

Toxic reactions and side effects. In addition to the previously mentioned cardiac toxicity of quinidine, the drug causes a group of symptoms collectively referred to as cinchonism: blurred vision, tinnitus, tremor, vertigo, and lightheadedness. Gastrointestinal irritation is a common occurrence with oral administration. Other rare manifestations are urticaria, purpura, and asthma. One absolute contraindication to quinidine is a history of thrombocytopenic purpura on previous administration of the drug.

Procainamide

Procaine was shown by Mautz[12] in 1936 to have an action on the heart similar to that of quinidine. Because its duration of action is short, a systematic study was undertaken to find a congener with similar action and a longer duration.[11] This investi-

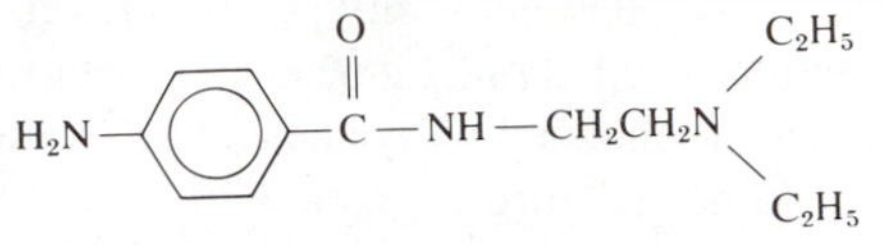

Figure 24-9. Structural formula of procainamide.

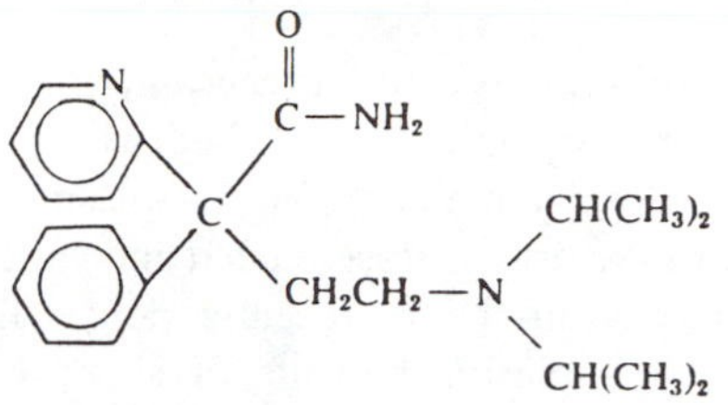

Figure 24-10. Structural formula of disopyramide.

gation led to the introduction in 1951 of procainamide as an antiarrhythmic drug.

Chemically, procainamide differs from procaine by having an amide linkage instead of an ester linkage (Figure 24-9).

Pharmacologic effects. The advantages of procainamide over procaine as an antiarrhythmic are its longer duration of action and its less potent effect on the central nervous system. The actions of procainamide on the heart are essentially the same as those of quinidine. Both automaticity and responsiveness are decreased, whereas refractoriness is increased; therefore, like quinidine, it can be described as a cardiac depressant.

The most frequently observed change induced by procainamide in the ECG is an increase in the duration of the QRS complex. Less frequently, lengthening of the Q-T and P-R intervals is observed.

There are no significant effects on other systems when procainamide is administered orally. Intravenous injection, on the other hand, causes a decrease in blood pressure because of peripheral vasodilation and occasionally causes mental confusion and hallucinations through actions on the central nervous system.

Absorption, fate, and excretion. After oral administration, procainamide is rapidly and essentially completely absorbed, with maximal plasma concentrations being reached in approximately 1 hour. Peak plasma concentrations are reached in 15 minutes to 1 hour after intramuscular administration. A small portion (15% to 20%) of the circulating procainamide is bound to plasma constituents. About 60% of an administered dose of this compound is excreted unchanged in the urine.

The major metabolite of procainamide, N-acetylprocainamide (NAPA), is formed in the liver. Normally, 25% of an administered dose of procainamide is acetylated to yield NAPA, but rapid acetylators or patients with renal disease will convert more of the drug to this form. NAPA has antiarrhythmic properties and is currently undergoing clinical trial. It has a plasma half-time of 6 hours and is eliminated by renal excretion.

Toxic reactions and side effects. Like quinidine, procainamide may allow a dangerous ventricular tachycardia to develop when used to treat atrial tachyarrhythmias. Also, like quinidine, it can in high doses cause ventricular arrhythmias.

The most frequent side effects after oral administration are nausea, vomiting, and anorexia. Other, more rarely seen effects are diarrhea, weakness, flushing, a bitter taste, and CNS manifestations such as hallucinations and depression. Allergic reactions, such as skin rashes, have been reported, and cross-sensitivity to procaine and other structurally similar compounds should be expected. Long-term administration has led to fatal occurrences of agranulocytosis. Thus, frequent blood tests should accompany therapy with this drug. Procainamide may also produce a syndrome resembling lupus erythematosus.

Disopyramide

Although structurally unrelated to either agent (Figure 24-10), disopyramide has actions similar to those of quinidine and procainamide. Its effectiveness in the treatment of premature extrasystoles and tachycardias of both supraventricular and ventricular origin has been established[5,10]; nevertheless, in the United States it is approved only for the treatment of ventricular arrhythmias.

Pharmacologic effects. Like quinidine, disopyramide decreases the rate of diastolic depolarization (phase 4), particularly in ectopic pacemaker cells; it also decreases the upstroke velocity of the action potential (phase 0) in cardiac fibers and increases the action potential duration and the effective refractory period.[2,3] Disopyramide thus tends to lessen automaticity and conduction velocity. One difference between disopyramide and the other type

Ia agents is that the P-R interval and QRS complex are less affected.

Absorption, fate, and excretion. Disopyramide is almost completely absorbed within several hours after oral administration. The plasma protein binding of the drug is dose related and varies from 20% to 60% in the therapeutic range. Disopyramide has a plasma half-life of about 7 hours; elimination of the parent drug and metabolites is largely via renal excretion.

Toxic reactions and side effects. The most common side effects of disopyramide are dose dependent and largely result from its anticholinergic action. These include urinary retention; dryness of the mouth, nose, throat, or eyes; blurred vision; constipation; nausea; and skin rashes. Rarely, acute psychosis, cholestatic jaundice, hypoglycemia, and agranulocytosis have occurred, but these disappear on drug withdrawal. As with other type I antiarrhythmic drugs, cardiovascular depression and a variety of arrhythmias may develop with overdosage.

Lidocaine

Lidocaine, like procaine, is widely used as a local anesthetic and has antiarrhythmic properties. Unlike procaine, it has become firmly established as an agent of choice for arresting and preventing certain arrhythmias in emergency situations. For a discussion of its chemistry, see Chapter 17.

Pharmacologic effects. Lidocaine has direct effects on the heart similar to those of quinidine and procainamide. This compound causes decreases in both automaticity and responsiveness and an increase in refractoriness. Its effect on automaticity is thought to be due to increased potassium conductance. In contrast to the action of quinidine and procainamide, lidocaine shortens the action potential duration and, to a lesser degree, the ERP. However, the end result is the same with all these agents: an increase in refractoriness. Although the actions of quinidine, procainamide, and lidocaine are generally similar, lidocaine seems preferentially to affect ventricular function. Lidocaine is usually administered intravenously for the treatment of ventricular ectopic rhythms and has a more rapid onset of action than quinidine or procainamide. Since lidocaine must be administered parenterally (IV or IM), it is most frequently used in emergency situations. Its use is contraindicated in supraventricular arrhythmias because it is ineffective against atrial arrhythmias and excessive ventricular rates may result.

Absorption, fate, and excretion. As an antiarrhythmic, lidocaine is usually given intravenously by injection or infusion. Lidocaine is metabolized by the liver to monoethylglycine and 2,6-xylidine. The xylidine is further metabolized to 4-hydroxy-2,6-xylidine and largely excreted in the urine.

Toxic reactions and side effects. Arterial pressure is not depressed by lidocaine as much as it is by procainamide. After acute high dosages or prolonged infusion, lidocaine has been shown to cause convulsions. (This reaction, however, occurs only very rarely with dosages and routes of administration used in dentistry.)

Phenytoin

For a general discussion of phenytoin and its chemistry, see Chapter 15.

Pharmacologic effects. Phenytoin (diphenylhydantoin) has been used for many years in the treatment of seizure disorders. It generally has the same effects on the electrophysiologic functions of the heart as the antiarrhythmic drugs previously discussed. Automaticity and responsiveness are depressed, whereas refractoriness is increased. Automaticity is reduced by a decrease in the slope of phase 4 spontaneous diastolic depolarization in pacemaker cells. This compound affects refractoriness in the same manner as lidocaine; that is, the action potential duration is abbreviated and the ERP reduced to a lesser degree. Although there is some controversy concerning this matter, it is likely that phenytoin decreases responsiveness by decreasing the rate of phase 0 depolarization. Like lidocaine, phenytoin seems to have a profound effect on ventricular ectopic rhythms, especially those resulting from digitalis intoxication.

As compared with quinidine, phenytoin has less of a depressant effect on myocardial contractility. Hypotension is less likely to occur with phenytoin than with quinidine or procainamide but has been seen with rapid intravenous administration.

Absorption, fate, and excretion. Phenytoin can be administered orally or parenterally. Intravenous injection leads to a rapid onset of action (10 to 15 minutes), and oral dosage can then be used for maintenance. The plasma half-life of this compound is about 24 hours. Phenytoin is bound to plasma proteins to the extent of 85% to 95%. Only a very small amount of phenytoin is excreted unchanged in the urine, the majority being metabolized by the hepatic microsomal enzyme system. The parahydroxyphenyl derivative is the major metabolite. It is excreted in the bile and subsequently in the urine as a glucuronide conjugate.

Toxic reactions and side effects. Phenytoin must be used cautiously in patients in whom S-A nodal depression exists, because cardiac arrest may follow intravenous use. Caution should also be exercised in the presence of advanced A-V blockage. CNS toxicity is the most frequently encountered adverse effect. About 20% of patients medicated with phenytoin on a long-term basis develop gingival hyperplasia, which may or may not be minimized by good oral hygiene and disappears on discontinuation of medication.

β-Adrenergic receptor blocking drugs

Since the introduction of propranolol in 1968 for clinical use in the United States, several similar agents have been approved. All of the β-adrenergic blocking drugs have essentially the same basic action, but, as shown in Tables 7-1 and 28-4, they vary in their cardioselectivity (i.e., the ratio of β_1 to β_2 blockade), in the intensity of their intrinsic agonist activity, in their local anesthetic action, and in their duration of effect. (The β-adrenergic blocking drugs are covered in Chapters 7, 26, and 28.) These drugs, like many other cardioactive drugs, are useful in such cardiovascular disease states as angina pectoris and hypertension.

In this chapter, the pharmacology of propranolol alone will be discussed in detail, but it should be born in mind that other β-blockers, with slightly different properties, may be useful in the treatment of arrhythmias.

Pharmacologic effects. Propranolol has two types of actions on the heart: indirect actions as a consequence of blockade of β-adrenergic receptors, and direct actions similar to those of quinidine. In general, this compound has the same overall effects on the heart as the drugs previously discussed, that is, decreased automaticity and responsiveness and increased refractoriness. However, the relative magnitude of effects is somewhat different; for example, propranolol has a comparatively greater effect on S-A nodal automaticity and a lesser effect on membrane responsiveness.

Stimulation of the sympathetic nervous system leading to β-receptor activation causes increased automaticity by increasing the slope of phase 4 depolarization, causes increased responsiveness by increasing conduction velocity, and causes decreased refractoriness by shortening the refractory period (especially in the A-V node). Thus, propranolol can cause opposite effects by blocking β

receptors, provided there is significant sympathetic input to the heart at the time of administration. Additionally, propranolol exhibits direct quinidine-like actions by decreasing the slope of phase 4 depolarization, decreasing the slope of phase 0 depolarization, and prolonging the refractory period with respect to the action potential duration. These direct actions lead to decreases in automaticity and responsiveness and an increase in refractoriness. Propranolol has been shown to be effective in treating supraventricular, ventricular, and cardiac glycoside–induced arrhythmias. However, phenytoin is probably a more useful agent for treatment of rhythm disturbances induced by cardiac glycosides.

Absorption, fate, and excretion. Propranolol is readily absorbed after oral administration, with peak plasma concentrations being reached in 1 to 2 hours. The rate of metabolism of this drug in the liver varies considerably among individuals, so plasma titers may differ markedly. After oral administration the plasma half-life is about 4 to 6 hours. Propranolol can be administered intravenously to obtain a rapid effect and by this route has a plasma half-life of about 3 hours. A high percentage (90%) of circulating propranolol is bound to plasma proteins, and after metabolism (hydroxylation or deamination) it is excreted largely in the urine, with part as the glucuronide conjugate.

Toxic reactions and side effects. The important adverse effects of propranolol can be explained by its blocking action on β-adrenergic receptors. Heart rate, myocardial contractility, and blood pressure are all reduced. After large doses, severe bradycardia or even asystole may occur. Bronchoconstriction occurs and may be significant in susceptible individuals, such as asthmatics. Propranolol inhibits the glycogenolytic and lipolytic actions of endogenous catecholamines released in response to hypoglycemia and thus may prevent the usual response to insulin-induced hypoglycemia in diabetic patients or to hypoglycemia in other patients. For this reason, caution must be exercised when this drug is used in these patients.

Bretylium

Bretylium tosylate, like propranolol, interferes with sympathetic control of the heart and has direct actions on cardiac function (see Chapter 7 for a discussion of its chemistry). Whereas propranolol blocks β-adrenergic receptors, bretylium prevents the release of the adrenergic neurotransmitter norepinephrine from adrenergic neurons. It can thus be called an adrenergic neuron blocking agent, because although it initially induces release of norepinephrine, it causes a prolonged blockade of the release of this transmitter from sympathetic nerve endings, which may be related to its local anesthetic properties. Other adrenergic neuron blockers, however, do not exhibit the pronounced antiarrhythmic properties of bretylium, and it is likely that the direct effects of the drug, some of which are incompletely understood, account for a major portion of its therapeutic efficacy.

Pharmacologic effects. The neuron-blocking action of bretylium decreases automaticity dependent on sympathetic outflow. Through its direct actions, bretylium causes an increase in refractoriness by increasing the action potential duration in ventricular tissue and lengthening the refractory period. In contrast to the previously described agents, bretylium increases conduction velocity and thus responsiveness.

Absorption, fate, and excretion. Bretylium can be administered orally, intramuscularly, or intravenously. It is, however, unpredictably absorbed from the gastrointestinal tract. Bretylium is not metabolized and is excreted unchanged in the urine and feces.

Toxic reactions and side effects. The side effects of bretylium can in most cases be explained by its adrenergic neuron blocking actions and therefore resemble the side effects of other drugs, such as reserpine and guanethidine, that affect the adrenergic neuron terminal. Because of its tendency to produce hypotension, bretylium is reserved for use in ventricular tachyarrhythmias that are not responsive to other therapeutic measures.

Calcium entry blockers

The calcium entry (slow calcium channel) blockers (CEBs), represented by nifedipine, diltiazem, and verapamil, have been marketed for oral use in the treatment of angina pectoris. They are being investigated, however, for their efficacy in the treatment of various arrhythmias. This application of these drugs can be attributed to their depressant effects on cardiac excitability and conduction. Their pharmacology and side effects are discussed in Chapter 26.

Verapamil, which has the greatest influence on cardiac electrophysiology of the three drugs mentioned above, has already been approved for the treatment of several arrhythmias. By interfering with the slow inward calcium current in pacemaker cells, verapamil depresses automaticity and greatly retards conduction through the A-V node.[19] It is particularly useful in supraventricular tachyarrhythmias and has been employed with success in terminating attacks of paroxysmal atrial tachycardia not responsive to vagal stimulation.[17]

New antiarrhythmics

A number of compounds with antiarrhythmic activity are in various stages of drug development. Some of these agents, such as tocainide, aprindine, encainide, and mexiletine, are closely related pharmacologically to lidocaine but are resistant to rapid first-pass degradation in the liver and are therefore effective on oral administration.[16,26] Structural formulas for two of these drugs are shown in Figure 24-11.

Some investigational drugs are broad-spectrum. Like quinidine, they are effective against supraventricular as well as ventricular arrhythmias. Amiodarone and ethmozin are two examples. Ethmozin is notable because it is a phenothiazine derivative,[5] amiodarone because it is a benzofuranyl relative of thyroxine and has some unique antiarrhythmic properties.[26]

It is not clear at this time which of these drugs, if any, will emerge as major antiarrhythmics clinically. However, inasmuch as 30% of patients given quinidine must discontinue therapy because of adverse reactions to the drug and other patients are refractory to current pharmacotherapy, it is evident that there is a need for new antiarrhythmic medications.

Drugs of choice for specific arrhythmias

Table 24-3 reflects the general usefulness of the various agents discussed in this chapter in treating some of the most commonly encountered arrhythmias. It is not intended to be a comprehensive listing of applications of these drugs, nor does it purport to order the agents in any meaningful way. Agents administered orally, such as quinidine often is, are largely used to prevent the recurrence of arrhythmias, whereas drugs administered parenterally, such as verapamil and lidocaine, are mostly used to treat existing disorders.

Implications for dentistry

Patients who are being treated on a long-term basis with antiarrhythmic drugs, if under adequate control, should not present a management problem

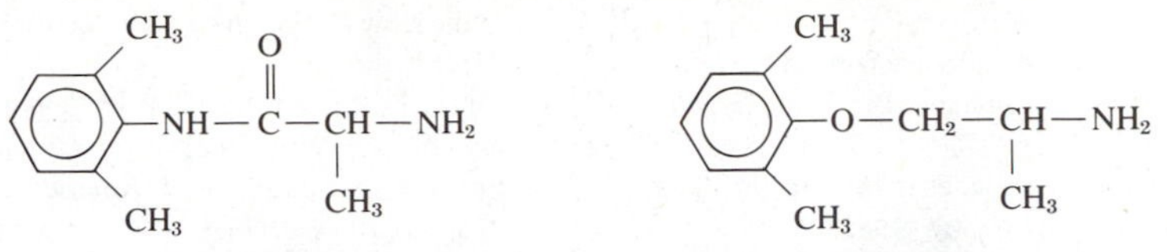

Figure 24-11. Structural formulas of tocainide and mexiletine.

Table 24-3. Indications for antiarrhythmic agents

Arrhythmia	Most effective agents
Supraventricular	
Atrial premature depolarizations, flutter, or fibrillation; paroxysmal atrial or A-V junctional tachycardia	Quinidine, procainamide, disopyramide, propranolol, verapamil
Ventricular	
Ventricular premature depolarizations, tachycardia	Lidocaine, phenytoin, procainamide, bretylium, disopyramide
Glycoside-induced	
Supraventricular and ventricular arrhythmias	Phenytoin, lidocaine

for the dentist. Because some antiarrhythmic agents may depress cardiovascular function, the potential for an increased incidence of orthostatic hypotension and hypotensive syncope exists. There is also a greater probability that arrhythmias will develop in a patient with a previous history of arrhythmias who is undergoing dental treatment.

It is important to remember that long-term administration of phenytoin can cause gingival hyperplasia. This disorder disappears after withdrawal of the medication and may or may not be controlled by good oral hygiene practices.

Antiarrhythmic drugs

Nonproprietary name	Proprietary name
acecainide (N-acetyl-procainamide)	—
amiodarone*	Cordarone
aprindine*	Fibocil

*Not currently approved for use in the United States.
†Several different salts are available for parenteral and oral administration.

Antiarrhythmic drugs—cont'd

Nonproprietary name	Proprietary name
bretylium	Bretylol
disopyramide	Norpace
lidocaine	Xylocaine
mexiletine*	Mexitil
phenytoin	Dilantin
procainamide	Pronestyl, Procan
propranolol	Inderal
quinidine†	Quinaglute Dura-Tabs, Cardioquin, Quinidex Extentabs
tocainide*	—
verapamil	Calan, Isoptin

CITED REFERENCES

1. Cranefield, P.F. Conduction of the Cardiac Impulse. Mount Kisco, N.Y., Futura Publishing Co., Inc., 1975.
2. Danilo, P., Jr., Hordoff, A.J., and Rosen, M.R. Effects of disopyramide on electrophysiologic properties of canine cardiac Purkinje fibers. Journal of Pharmacology and Experimental Therapeutics **201**:701-710, 1977.
3. Dean, R.R. The pharmacology of Norpace. Angiology **26**(suppl. 1):67-84, 1975.
4. Dreifus, L.S., de Azevedo, I.M., and Watanabe, Y. Electrolyte and antiarrhythmic drug interaction. American Heart Journal **88**:95 -107, 1974.
5. Duchene-Marullaz, P. New trends in antiarrhythmic drugs. Trends in Pharmacological Science **10**:407-409, 1980.
6. Fabiato, A., and Fabiato, F. Calcium and cardiac excitation-contraction coupling. Annual Review of Physiology **41**:473-484, 1979.
7. Frey, W. Weitere Erfahrungen mit Chinidin bei absoluter Herzenregelmassigkeit. Weiner Klinische Wochenschrift **55**:849-853, 1918.
8. Hoffman, B.F. The genesis of cardiac arrhythmias. Progress in Cardiovascular Disease **8**:319-329, 1966.
9. Hoffman, B.F., and Cranefield, P.F. The physiologic basis of cardiac arrhythmias. American Journal of Medicine **37**:670-684, 1964.
10. Koch-Weser, J. Drug therapy: disopyramide. New England Journal of Medicine **300**:957-962, 1979.
11. Mark, L.C., Kayden, H.J., Steele, J.M., Cooper, J.R., Berlin, I., Rovenstine, E.A., and Brodie, B.B. The physiological disposition and cardiac effects of procaine amide. Journal of Pharmacology and Experimental Therapeutics **102**:5-15, 1951.
12. Mautz, F.R. Reduction of cardiac irritability by the epicardial and systemic administration of drugs as a protection

in cardiac surgery. Journal of Thoracic Surgery **5:**612-628, 1936.

13. Moe, G.K. Evidence for reentry as a mechanism of cardiac arrhythmias. Reviews of Physiology, Biochemistry, and Pharmacology **72:**55-81, 1975.

14. Opie, L.H. Role of cyclic nucleotides in heart metabolism. Cardiovascular Research **16:**483-507, 1982.

15. Resnekov, L. Drug therapy before and after the electroconversion of cardiac dysrhythmias. Progress in Cardiovascular Disease **16:**531-538, 1974.

16. Roden, D.M., Reele, S.B., Higgens, S.B., Mayol, R.F., Gammans, R.E., Oates, J.A., and Woosley, R.L. Total suppression of ventricular arrhythmias by encainide. Pharmacokinetic and electrocardiographic characteristics. New England Journal of Medicine **302:**877-882, 1980.

17. Smith, W.M., and Gallagher, J.J. Management of arrhythmias and conduction abnormalities. In Hurst, J.W., ed. The Heart, Arteries and Veins, ed. 5. New York, McGraw-Hill Book Co., 1982.

18. Vaughan Williams, E.M. Classification of antidysrhythmic drugs. Pharmacology and Therapeutics. Part B. General and Systemic Pharmacology **1:**115-138, 1975.

19. Vohra, J.K. Clinical use of verapamil. Drugs **13:**219-224, 1977.

20. Weidmann, S. Elektrophysiologie der Herzmuskelfasen. Bern, Switzerland, Hans Huber Medical Publisher, 1956.

21. Wenckebach, K.F. Die Unregelmassige Herztätigkeit und Ihre Klinische Bedeutung. Leipzig, Germany, W. Engelmann, 1914.

22. Wit, A.L., Rosen, M.R., and Hoffman, B.F. Electrophysiology and pharmacology of cardiac arrhythmias. II. Relationship of normal and abnormal electrical activity of cardiac fibers to the genesis of arrhythmias. A. Automaticity. American Heart Journal **88:**515-524, 1974.

23. Wit, A.L., Rosen, M.R., and Hoffman, B.F. Electrophysiology and pharmacology of cardiac arrhythmias. II. Relationship of normal and abnormal electrical activity of cardiac fibers to the genesis of arrhythmias. B. Re-entry. Section II. American Heart Journal **88:**798-806, 1974.

24. Wohlfart, B., and Noble, M.I.M. The cardiac excitation contraction cycle. Pharmacology and Therapeutics **16:**1-43, 1982.

25. Zipes, D.P., Besch, H.R., Jr., and Watanabe, A.M. Role of the slow current in cardiac electrophysiology. Circulation **51:**761-766, 1975.

26. Zipes, D.P., and Troup, P.J. New antiarrhythmic agents: amiodarone, aprindine, disopyramide, ethmozin, mexiletine, tocainide, verapamil. American Journal of Cardiology **41:**1005-1024, 1978.

GENERAL REFERENCES

Awalt, C.H. Antiarrhythmic drugs. Clinical Anesthesia **10:**167-183, 1974.

Benchimol, A., and Desser, K.B. New drugs for treating cardiac arrhythmias. Postgraduate Medicine **69:**77-84, 1981.

Bigger, J.T., Jr., and Hoffman, B.F. Antiarrhythmic drugs. In Gilman, A.G., Goodman, L.S., and Gilman, A., eds. Goodman and Gilman's The Pharmacological Basis of Therapeutics, ed. 6. New York, Macmillan, Inc., 1980.

Hauswirth, O., and Singh, B.N. Ionic mechanisms in heart muscle in relation to genesis and the pharmacological control of cardiac arrhythmias. Pharmacological Reviews **30:**5-63, 1979.

Mason, D.T., De Maria, A.N., Amsterdam, E.A., Zelis, R., and Massumi, R.A. Antiarrhythmic agents. I. Mechanisms of action and clinical pharmacology. Drugs **5:**261-291, 1973.

Mason, D.T., De Maria, A.N., Amsterdam, E.A., Zelis, R., and Massumi, R.A. Antiarrhythmic agents. II. Therapeutic considerations. Drugs **5:**292-317, 1973.

Morgan, P.H., and Mathison, I.W. Arrhythmias and antiarrhythmic drugs: mechanism of action and structure-activity relationships. II. Journal of Pharmaceutical Sciences **65:**635-648, 1976.

Moses, J.W., and Yu, P.N. Antiarrhythmic drugs. Journal of Clinical Pharmacology **20:**598-618, 1980.

Sasyniuk, B.I., and Ogilvie, R.I. Antiarrhythmic drugs: electrophysiological and pharmacokinetic considerations. Annual Review of Pharmacology and Toxicology **15:**131-155, 1975.

Singh, B.N., and Hauswirth, O. Comparative mechanisms of action of antiarrhythmic drugs. American Heart Journal **87:**367-382, 1974.

25 Cardiac glycosides

Frank Dowd

Cardiac glycosides, most notably digitalis, have been used for centuries to treat a number of ailments. The history of their use is marked by an awareness of their therapeutic efficacy, as well as their toxic potential. Today these drugs are the mainstay of the treatment of congestive heart failure and are useful in treating certain cardiac arrhythmias.

Ancient Egyptians used cardiotonic components from the sea onion, or squill. The Romans used these drugs as diuretics and heart tonics. Dried toad skin, which contains substances with cardiotonic activity, was used by the Chinese for dropsy and related illnesses. The cardiac glycoside ouabain, from *Strophanthus gratus,* was used by Africans as poison for arrows.[14]

Fuchs in 1542 gave the name *digitalis* to the foxglove plant, which was used for a variety of medicinal purposes. The first detailed scientific study of digitalis on record was made by Sir William Withering[46] of Shropshire, England in 1785. In his book, ''An Account of the Foxglove, and Some of Its Medical Uses; With Practical Remarks on Dropsy, and Other Diseases,'' Withering detailed clinical uses for the leaf of the *Digitalis purpurea* (purple foxglove) plant and described its effects on the heart. His recognition of the potential usefulness of digitalis plant derivatives was occasioned by their extensive use in local folk medicines. Withering ascribed the beneficial effects of digitalis in treating dropsy to a direct diuretic effect, even though he was aware of beneficial effects on the heart as well. He also detailed many toxic effects of the plant.

The history of the use of digitalis since Withering's time has been characterized by a realization of its potential therapeutic benefits on the one hand and its low margin of safety on the other. Advances in digitalis research and clinical use up to the present day have contributed greatly to our knowledge of this drug class.

CHEMISTRY AND CLASSIFICATION

The term *digitalis* is often used interchangeably with the term *cardiac glycoside*. Both refer to many compounds, naturally occurring or semisynthetic, that have similar cardiotonic effects. For this reason, the terms will also be used interchangeably in this chapter. Strictly speaking, however, the term *digitalis* is reserved for compounds derived from the botanical sources *Digitalis purpurea* and *Digitalis lanata,* from which are derived the glycosides used clinically (digoxin, digitoxin, digitalis leaf, deslanoside, and gitalin). Another compound of experimental importance is ouabain. In addition, other plant sources and at least one animal source (certain toads, e.g., *Bufo marinus*) have cardioactive components similar in structure and activity to digitalis. These are mainly of historic and toxicologic interest, although drugs from some of these sources are used in countries other than the United States. Table 25-1 lists some of the principal cardiac glycoside preparations as well as their main botanical sources.

The basic chemical structure of clinically useful cardiac glycosides can be discussed with reference to the structure of digitoxin, shown in Figure 25-1. The molecule is composed of a steroid ring structure (cyclopentanoperhydrophenanthrene; A, B, C, and D in the figure) that in two dimensions resembles the adrenal or nonestrogenic sex steroids. The three-dimensional structure is quite different from these hormones, however, in that the relationship of the C and D ring in cardiac glycosides is the *cis* rather than the *trans* configuration, as is the case for the steroid hormones.[37,42] Other distinguishing molecular characteristics include an α,β-unsaturated lactone ring, usually five-membered, at carbon 17 (C_{17}), a hydroxyl group at C_{14}, and a carbohydrate moiety in glycosidic linkage at C_3. The presence of a sugar in glycosidic linkage accounts for the name *glycoside*. These sugars are usually deoxysugars.[14,42]

Structural differences among clinically useful cardiac glycosides primarily involve differences in the sugar substituent and a difference in the number of hydroxyl groups on the steroid nucleus. The structure of digoxin, for instance, differs from that of digitoxin only in that digoxin contains a hydroxyl group at C_{12}.

Sugar substituents at C_3 can be removed by acid hydrolysis. The products of these reactions are carbohydrates and the appropriate steroids with attached lactone. A steroid lacking the sugar group is generically called a genin or aglycone. The names of particular genins are derived from the parent compounds, for example, digoxin—digoxigenin.[10]

STRUCTURE-ACTIVITY RELATIONSHIPS

The following structural characteristics are required for full cardiac activity: *cis* fusion of rings

Table 25-1. Some clinically useful cardiac glycosides

Drug	Plant source
Digoxin	*Digitalis lanata* (leaf)
Digitoxin	*Digitalis lanata* (leaf), *Digitalis purpurea* (leaf)
Digitalis leaf	*Digitalis purpurea*
Ouabain	*Strophanthus gratus* (seed)
Deslanoside	*Digitalis lanata* (leaf)

C and D, an α,β-unsaturated lactone ring in β-configuration on C_{17}, a hydroxyl group at C_{14}, and a sugar in glycosidic linkage at C_3.[10,14] The bond between C_3 and the oxygen must be in the β-configuration for significant activity to be present. Saturation of the lactone results in about a tenfold loss in activity, whereas cleavage of the lactone ring abolishes activity. Removal of the sugar substituent has interesting effects. The resulting genins are less potent and have a more transient effect than their parent compounds.[14] Nevertheless, toxicity of the genins seems to be quantitatively similar to the corresponding glycoside.

Hydroxyl groups increase aqueous solubility. Ouabain, for instance, which has five free hydroxyl groups on the steroid ring structure and adjoining carbons, is more water soluble than digitoxin, which has only one hydroxyl group attached to the steroid nucleus. Such structural differences also account for large differences in duration of action of the drugs, extent of biotransformation, degree of gastrointestinal absorption, and other clinical characteristics.

PHARMACOLOGIC EFFECTS
Cardiac effects

Contractility. The experiments of Cattell and Gold[9] clearly showed that cardiac glycosides have direct effects on the isolated heart. In isolated heart preparations, the drugs increase the force of contraction of the myocardium (positive inotropic effect). Maximum tension developed and rate of tension development (dP/dt) are both increased, whereas time from onset of contraction to peak contraction is decreased. The duration of the contractile process during systole is abbreviated because of an increase in the rate at which tension is

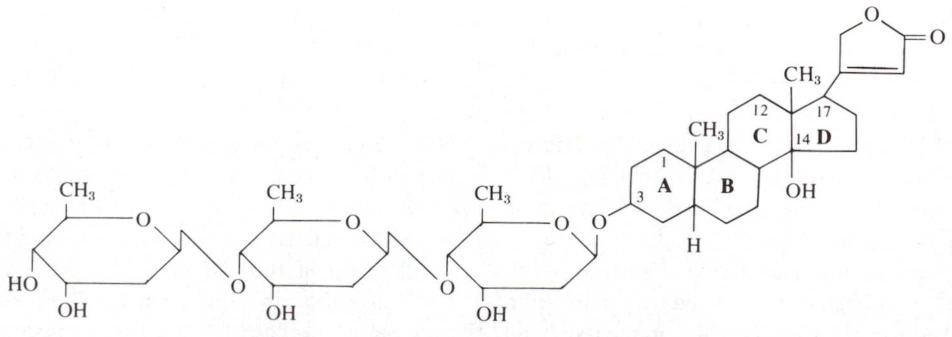

Figure 25-1. Structural formula of digitoxin.

developed. These effects, demonstrated on the cat papillary muscle, are shown in Figure 25-2. The overall cardiodynamic effect of cardiac glycosides on the isolated heart therefore can be summarized as an increased force of contraction of the myocardium caused by an increased rate of force development by the myocardium, resulting in a systolic phase of shorter duration but greater effectiveness.[9,27,39]

In vivo, many factors complicate the effects of cardiac glycosides on contractility. In the normal intact individual, cardiac glycosides directly increase the force of contraction of the heart, but this effect is more than negated by compensatory autonomic reflexes. Cardiac glycosides, in addition to their cardiac effects, constrict peripheral blood vessels by a direct action on vascular smooth muscle and by an indirect effect mediated via the central and peripheral nervous systems. The outcome of such vasoconstriction is an increase in blood pressure and a reduction in myocardial contractile force and cardiac output because of reflex mechanisms.[6] The net effect in normal individuals is that reflex mechanisms cancel out the positive effects of digitalis on heart contractility.[27,37]

In patients with failing hearts, a different situation prevails. Vasoconstriction, a physiologic response to reduced cardiac output, is already significant in peripheral vessels, and digitalis has little additive effect on vascular tone. Therefore, in patients with heart failure, compensatory mechanisms do not cancel out the cardiac effects of digitalis. Cardiac glycosides increase cardiac output, thus reducing the need for high sympathetic tone in the blood vessels. Sympathetic tone is therefore decreased in the vasculature when these patients receive digitalis, and vasodilation may even result. The effect of digitalis in vivo therefore depends on the state of cardiac function at the time of administration. Since in isolated heart preparations autonomic influences are avoided, digitalis increases cardiac contractility. It follows then that in the failing heart in vivo the effects of digitalis resemble those in the isolated heart preparation.[27]

According to Starling's law of the heart, cardiac output, or more precisely the ventricular stroke volume, increases as ventricular filling pressure increases. Stated simply, the heart pumps whatever is supplied to it by way of venous return, maintaining a near optimal heart size. As ventricular

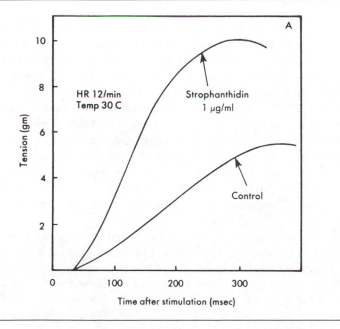
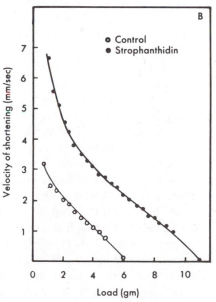

Figure 25-2. Effects of the digitalis glycoside strophanthidin on the course of isometric contraction, **A,** and the force-velocity relation, **B,** of the cat papillary muscle. (Adapted from Sonnenblick, E.H., Williams, J.F., Jr., Glick, G., Mason, D.T., and Braunwald, E. Studies on digitalis. XV. Effects of cardiac glycosides on myocardial force-velocity relations in the nonfailing human heart. Circulation **34:**532-539, 1966. By permission of the American Heart Association, Inc.)

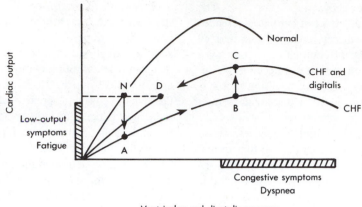

Figure 25-3. Operation of the Frank-Starling mechanism in the preload compensation for heart failure. The three curves represent ventricular function curves in the normal state, in congestive heart failure (CHF), and in heart failure after treatment with digitalis. Points N through D indicate, in sequence, normal cardiac status (N), depression of contractility with decompensated heart failure (A), Frank-Starling compensation (B), increase in contractility with digitalis (C), and reduction in use of Frank-Starling preload compensation that digitalis allows (D). Points N, D, and B indicate the same cardiac output on the vertical axis, but each point is at a different end-diastolic pressure on the horizontal axis. The excessive end-diastolic pressures causing congestive symptoms and the lowered levels of cardiac performance resulting in low-output symptoms are shown by the hatched areas. (From Mason, D.T. American Journal of Cardiology **32:**437-448, 1973.)

end-diastolic pressure increases, ventricular stroke work and stroke volume increase. Normal heart function is within well-defined limits and is described by a single curve (Figure 25-3).

When cardiac contractility is reduced in heart failure, three mechanisms are available by which the heart can compensate for the defect: (1) an increase in ventricular end-diastolic pressure, which enhances cardiac output (Frank-Starling preload mechanism), (2) an increase in number of contractile units (hypertrophy), and (3) employment of chronotropic and inotropic reserves of the heart through reflex mechanisms (adrenergic activity).[26] If these mechanisms are sufficient to produce normal cardiac output, the heart failure is said to be compensated. In this condition a new ventricular function curve is generated (Figure 25-3). For any given ventricular end-diastolic pressure, therefore, ventricular stroke work, stroke volume, and cardiac output are lower in the failing heart than in the normal heart. Consequently, the heart enlarges to maintain cardiac output, and heart rate increases to help compensate for poor cardiac function. In decompensated heart failure, the situation is more acute. Here, compensatory mechanisms are unable to maintain cardiac output. In both compensated

and decompensated heart failure, digitalis can improve cardiac function so that normal cardiac output can be achieved without as much reliance on compensatory mechanisms. Figure 25-3 shows that a new ventricular function curve is generated as a result of digitalis. This curve more closely approximates the normal situation.

Heart failure can occur when the work load placed on the heart exceeds the ability of the heart to perform. Heart failure may arise from an unknown cause or from known causes such as myocardial infarction or hypertension. Myocardial infarction can lead to heart failure as a result of a reduction in the heart's ability to perform work (pump failure).

An increase in total peripheral vascular resistance, as is seen in hypertension or as a reflex reaction in congestive heart failure, can contribute to heart failure because of increased outflow resistance on cardiac contraction. The first reaction of the heart to an increase in outflow resistance is often enlargement resulting in temporary higher efficiency in cardiac function. This is followed, however, by progressive signs of cardiac failure characterized by decreased stroke volume and stroke work as indicated above.

Cardiac size and rate of contraction. Congestive heart failure is accompanied by an increase in heart size. As the heart begins to fail, it is unable to eject as much blood per stroke as the normal heart, and the size of the heart increases, compensating for loss of contractility. The right or left side of the heart, or both, may be affected.

Digitalis, by increasing the force of contraction, reduces the size of the heart. Digitalis enables the heart to pump with greater force at any given filling pressure. This increased force leads in turn to a reduction in diastolic pressure, and the heart returns to a near normal size.[26]

The reduction in heart size accounts for a greater efficiency of the heart. It can be shown, for instance, that cardiac glycosides can reduce the ratio of oxygen consumption to contractile force in cardiac muscle. The effect is largely caused by decreased fiber length of cardiac muscle and diastolic wall tension. (Oxygen consumption is highly dependent on wall tension.) The net result of digitalis on the failing heart, therefore, is to increase contractility without a commensurate increase in oxygen consumption—in other words, to improve efficiency.[27,37]

In the clinical management of congestive heart failure, the administration of digitalis is most often associated with reduction in heart rate. This reduction is due to both a vagal and a direct effect on the heart by digitalis. The cardiac glycoside stimulates the vagus nerve, probably indirectly by an effect on baroreceptors, afferent nerve pathways, and central vagal nuclei, and at therapeutic doses reduces the sympathetic tone of the heart indirectly by improving cardiac function.[26] Both effects account for a reduction in heart rate. The effect of digitalis on heart rate during the treatment of certain cardiac arrhythmias is discussed below.

Electrophysiology. The effects of digitalis on the electrical properties of the heart can be divided into at least four interrelated categories: automaticity, ERP, excitability, and conduction velocity. Because digitalis has both vagal and nonvagal effects on the heart and since the areas of the heart affected by the vagus include only the S-A node, the atrial myocardium, and the upper portions of the A-V node, a discussion of discrete regions of the heart is necessary.

Unspecialized atrial myocardium. Digitalis at therapeutic doses shortens the atrial refractory period. This effect is due to vagal influences of the drug, since it can be reversed by atropine. The vagal effects of digitalis on the atria are more in evidence than the nonvagal, an important distinction since the nonvagal effects of digitalis are quite different. Digitalis, for instance, prolongs the atrial refractory period when the vagus nerve has been blocked.

The effect on atrial excitability is variable, but at higher therapeutic and toxic doses digitalis decreases excitability. This decrease in excitability is accompanied by a decrease in conduction velocity.

Sinoatrial node. The effect of therapeutic doses of digitalis is a reduction in S-A node automaticity caused by a slowing of the diastolic depolarization in the cells of the node. As in the atrial myocardium, this effect is largely vagal. In the presence of atropine, digitalis may actually increase the automaticity of the S-A node.

Atrioventricular node. One of the most important and characteristic effects of digitalis is its effect on the A-V node. Under the influence of digitalis, the duration of the ERP is increased and conduction velocity decreased. Mechanistically, as the resting membrane potential is reduced as a result of Na,K-pump inhibition (see Mechanism of Action), the action potential spike is slowed, leading to delayed A-V conduction. This is a direct or nonvagal effect of digitalis. However, both vagal and nonvagal effects of digitalis account for the slowing of A-V conduction. Generally, vagal effects predominate with lower doses of digitalis. Digitalis therapy can lead to various degrees of heart block because of effects on the A-V node.[28]

Purkinje fibers. The automaticity of the Purkinje fibers is increased by digitalis. Automaticity can be enhanced by an increase in the rate of phase 4 depolarization (see Chapter 24). This effect is heightened if extracellular potassium is lowered. Digitalis can also increase automaticity by inducing oscillatory afterpotentials. These afterpotentials are thought to be caused by fluctuations in intracellular calcium ion concentrations resulting in increased sodium conductance in the membranes. If the amplitude of these afterpotentials is sufficiently great, they may lead to an action potential. At lower doses of digitalis, excitability is increased, whereas at higher, toxic doses excitability is reduced. Because of the increase in automaticity at these sites, subsidiary pacemaker activity can lead to arrhythmias, especially in the presence of a slow sinus rhythm or heart block.[21] Conduction velocity is reduced, and the duration of the ERP is increased in most cases by digitalis, similar to the effects on the

Table 25-2. Electrophysiologic effects of digitalis

Site	Automaticity	Duration of effective refractory period	Excitability	Conduction velocity
Atrial myocardium		↓, ↑ A	↑,* ↓ T	↑,* ↓ T
S-A node	↓, ↑ A or T			
A-V node		Ⓤ↑		Ⓓ↓
Purkinje fibers	Ⓤ↑	↑,* ↓ T	↑,* ↓ T	↓
Ventricular myocardium		Ⓓ↓	↑,* ↓ T	↑,* ↓ T

Key: ○ = most important effects, A = after atropine, T = at toxic doses.
*Lower therapeutic doses only.

A-V node. Unlike the situation in the A-V node, high or toxic concentrations of digitalis can decrease the duration of the ERP of the Purkinje fibers. The duration of the action potential is likewise shortened, and reentrant arrhythmias are more likely to occur, leading to extrasystoles.[19]

Unspecialized ventricular myocardium. In the ventricle, the duration of the ERP is shortened by digitalis. Conduction velocity changes are dependent on dose. At lower doses digitalis increases conduction velocity, whereas at higher and toxic doses digitalis decreases conduction velocity. Excitability is reduced by digitalis, but only at high concentrations. Lower concentrations may actually increase excitability. The ventricular myocardium is more resistant to reduction in excitability than are the specialized conductive tissues.

Summary. The most important effects of digitalis on the electrophysiology of the heart can be summarized as follows: reduced conduction velocity and increased duration of the ERP in the A-V node, increased automaticity of subsidiary pacemaker activity in the conductive tissues of the ventricle, and decreased duration of the ERP of the ventricular myocardium. Cardiac vagal effects of digitalis are limited to effects on the atria, the S-A node, and the A-V node. They consist of a decrease in the duration of the ERP of the atrial myocardium, a decrease in the automaticity of the S-A node, and an increase in the duration of the ERP and a decrease in the conduction velocity of the A-V node. These are shown in Table 25-2.

Electrocardiography. Therapeutic and toxic effects of digitalis are associated with changes on the ECG that are a reflection of the electrophysiologic effects shown in Table 25-2. They include alterations in the shape of the T wave, the configuration of the S-T segment, and the length of the Q-T and P-R intervals, atrioventricular dissociation, and the presence of extrasystoles.

At therapeutic doses, changes often occur in the T wave and the S-T segment configuration. The T wave may be inverted or distorted, whereas the S-T segment may appear "sunken." These changes are due to alterations in the sequence of repolarization of various ventricular myocardial cells. Also at therapeutic doses, the P-R interval is lengthened by digitalis as a result of a decreased conduction velocity in the A-V node. The Q-T interval, on the other hand, is shortened because of the shortened ventricular systole.[37]

Although several effects of digitalis are observed at toxic doses, two effects are most ominous. The first is heart block caused by excessive reduction in A-V nodal conduction; the second is ventricular arrhythmias caused by ectopic pacemaker activity.[21,37]

Effects on systemic vasculature

Vasoconstriction by digitalis is usually not observed in patients with congestive heart failure because sympathetic vascular tone is already elevated. In fact, vasodilation often results from digitalis administration because of the improvement in cardiac function.[6,27]

Diuretic effects

Digitalis was for years thought to act primarily on the kidney, because diuresis is such a prominent feature of its use in congestive heart failure. However, the diuretic effect is due primarily to improved cardiac function, which results in reduced peripheral sympathetic tone and increased blood flow to the kidney. Thus, glomerular filtration is increased, renin secretion in most cases is lowered, and aldosterone secretion is indirectly reduced. Sodium and water retention are thereby reduced. Digitalis also promotes fluid mobilization by lowering venous pressure, which increases return of edema fluid to the vascular space and indirectly increases renal excretion.

It is possible that some of the diuretic effect of digitalis may result from its direct action on the sodium-potassium pump in the kidney, but this is of secondary importance to the diuresis based on improved cardiovascular dynamics.

Miscellaneous effects

Although the crude preparation, digitalis leaf, quite commonly causes gastrointestinal upset as a result of local gastrointestinal irritation, the purified cardiac glycosides can also cause anorexia, nausea, and vomiting, especially at toxic doses. Excessive salivation often accompanies these effects.[11] Significant neurologic effects of digitalis usually seen in toxic situations are listed in the discussion on digitalis toxicity and in Table 25-3. Although digitalis does contain a steroid ring structure, digitalis drugs rarely show effects associated with steroid hormones. Perhaps the only endocrine effect of any importance is a weak estrogen effect or an affinity for estrogen receptors.[37] Digitalis is not an aldosterone antagonist.

MECHANISM OF ACTION

The precise molecular mechanism of action of digitalis is not known; nevertheless, a great deal of research has been devoted to the elucidation of this mechanism, particularly with regard to how the force of the heart's contraction is increased. This research has led to plausible theories that could explain the in vivo effects of digitalis. The inotropic action of digitalis does not depend on release of endogenous catecholamines, since a reserpinized heart will respond to digitalis. Rather, digitalis has a direct action on heart cells.

Cardiac glycosides are known to be specific inhibitors of the sodium-potassium pump and Na,K-ATPase, an integral component of the sodium-potassium pump.[33,36] This is the only enzymatic process of the cell known to be specifically affected by low concentrations of cardiac glycosides. The enzyme is located in plasma membranes, and both in vivo and in vitro studies strongly suggest that the site of action of digitalis is the plasma membrane, more specifically the Na,K-ATPase.[30,35]

It is widely agreed that digitalis increases the force of contraction of the myocardium by increasing the calcium concentration at a critical intracellular site. This critical site is often called the "activator pool" of calcium, and the degree of cardiac contractility appears to depend on the calcium concentration in this activator pool, which acts as a trigger for contraction.[35] Therefore, it is accepted that if the mechanism of action of digitalis involves inhibition of Na,K-ATPase, this inhibition must result in a change, at least indirectly, in calcium dynamics.[3] Indeed, digitalis at therapeutic levels increases myocardial intracellular calcium concentrations[20] and appears to be affecting a superficial calcium pool that is rapidly turning over.[19]

Several theories linking inhibition of Na,K-ATPase with calcium distribution have been proposed.[33,35] These theories relate inhibition of Na,K-ATPase to an increased cellular influx of calcium, resulting in an increase in activator calcium. For instance, inhibition of the sodium-potassium pump could promote an increase in a sodium-calcium exchange reaction (insensitive to digitalis), providing an increase in the activator pool of calcium. Sodium efflux from the cell would be coupled with calcium influx.[30,33] Alternatively, the consequence of increased intracellular sodium (from inhibition of Na,K-ATPase) may be the displacement of calcium from an intracellular site. Finally, binding of digitalis to Na,K-ATPase may result in a change in affinity of adjacent membrane phospholipids for calcium that would increase the supply of calcium entering the cell with each beat.[19] This last hypothesis is consistent with findings that ouabain can alter the affinity of membrane phospholipids for calcium. It is also consistent with evidence that there may be more than one state of Na,K-ATPase to which cardiac glycosides bind. The existence of two states of Na,K-ATPase permits a mechanism for an inotropic effect to occur prior to the loss of Na,K-ATPase activity, despite the fact that both events result from binding of the cardiac glycoside to Na,K-ATPase.[45] Membrane phospholipids may mediate this inotropic effect brought about by digitalis binding to, but not necessarily inhibiting, Na,K-ATPase. Furthermore, inhibition of catecholamine uptake by cardiac glycosides may account for a cardiac inotropic action at very low concentrations of the cardiac glycosides.[19]

It should be emphasized that certain findings have led to doubts about the involvement of Na,K-ATPase in the inotropic effects of digitalis, even though there is general agreement that toxic effects of digitalis are associated with demonstrable inhibition of the enzyme.[31] The possible role of phospholipids in the inotropic action of digitalis and the existence of more than one state of Na,K-ATPase may help clarify the discrepancies between Na,K-ATPase inhibition and inotropic effect of digitalis. With the complexity of events associated with the interaction of digitalis and Na,K-ATPase, it is perhaps not surprising that a unifying hypothesis on the mechanism of action of digitalis is still not complete.

ABSORPTION, FATE, AND EXCRETION

The discussion that follows is limited to digoxin and digitoxin, because they are the most widely prescribed cardiac glycosides. Both drugs are commonly administered by the oral route. The amount of absorption of digitoxin from the gastrointestinal tract is nearly 100%, whereas absorption of digoxin ranges from 60% to 85%. Absorption is chiefly from the small intestine.[12,37] The cardiac glycosides may be given parenterally in emergencies; the route of choice is intravenous. It should be emphasized that parenteral administration carries with it added risks.

A comparison of various oral digoxin preparations has shown marked variability in drug bioavailability, the difference being due apparently to dissolution rates of the tablets.[24] A greater bioavailability of digoxin has been noted with the use of a solution of digoxin in soft gelatin capsules.

The degree to which digoxin binds to plasma protein is significantly different from that of digitoxin. Digitoxin is almost totally bound to plasma albumin, whereas digoxin is largely in the free form in the plasma (approximately 75%). This fact accounts for the higher total plasma concentration of digitoxin at therapeutic levels and in part for its longer duration of action. Digoxin and digitoxin plasma half-lives are approximately 36 hours and 4 to 7 days, respectively.[12]

Significant differences also exist in the biotransformation of digoxin and digitoxin. The metabolism of digoxin is in most circumstances minor in importance, whereas digitoxin undergoes substantial metabolism in the hepatic microsomal enzyme system. The rate of metabolism is stimulated by phenobarbital and other inducers, whereas reduction in liver function prolongs the effect of digitoxin. Liver function has little effect on digoxin kinetics, except in a small minority of patients who

metabolize digoxin rapidly. These people are very resistant to the therapeutic effects of digoxin. In rare cases a patient will form antibodies to digoxin, thereby preventing its therapeutic effects.

The metabolism of digitoxin chiefly involves the removal of the sugar portion of the molecule, leading to formation of digitoxigenin; then epimerization of the free hydroxyl group at C_3 leads to inactivation of the drug. Glucuronide conjugation may also occur. Finally, hydroxylation at C_{12}, leading to formation of digoxin, may also take place, but this route appears to be a minor pathway in humans.[37]

Digoxin is excreted by the kidney largely in the active form. The mechanism involves glomerular filtration and tubular secretion and accounts for almost all of the excretion of the drug. The metabolites of digitoxin are excreted chiefly, but not entirely, by the kidney.[12]

TOXIC REACTIONS AND SIDE EFFECTS
Signs and symptoms

Although allergic reactions to digitalis are rare, toxic reactions are not. Withering himself was well aware of many toxic effects of digitalis when for instance he wrote:

In the year 1775 my opinion was asked concerning a family recipe for the cure of dropsy. I was told that it had long been kept a secret by an old woman in Shropshire who had sometimes made cures after the more regular practitioners had failed. I was informed also that the effects produced were violent vomiting and purging; for the diuretic effects seemed to have been overlooked. This medicine was composed of twenty or more different herbs; but it was not very difficult for one conversant in these subjects to perceive that the active herb could be no other than foxglove.[46]

Digitalis toxicity represents a significant clinical problem even today. Recent estimates show that approximately 20% of hospitalized patients receiving digitalis are in toxic states. The toxicity of the various cardiac glycosides is in proportion to their relative potency for therapeutic effects. Therefore, the therapeutic index for clinically useful cardiac glycosides is similar and very low. Toxic signs are often seen at roughly twice the minimum effective dose. In practice, toxicity usually results from cumulation of the drug. The duration of action of digitoxin is much longer than that of digoxin, and this factor may compound the problem of toxicity. Individual differences in patient response do exist and may account for unexpected clinical results;

Table 25-3. Common signs
of digitalis toxicity

Gastrointestinal	Salivation
	Anorexia
	Nausea
	Vomiting
	Diarrhea
	Abdominal pain
Central nervous system	Headache
	Visual disturbances
	Fatigue
	Drowsiness
Cardiac	Atrioventricular block
	Excessive slowing of the heart
	Ventricular extrasystoles
	Other arrhythmias
Miscellaneous	Excessive urination

therefore, dosages have to be tailored for each patient. The more common toxic effects of digitalis are outlined in Table 25-3.

Extracardiac toxic effects include anorexia, nausea, diarrhea, and vomiting, although gastrointestinal symptoms may occur at nontoxic levels. The mechanism involves stimulation of the chemoreceptor trigger zone of the medulla.[31] Excessive salivation, as well as headache, fatigue, drowsiness, and abdominal pain often accompany these toxic symptoms. Visual disturbances, such as the appearance of halos and distortions in color perception, can also occur, perhaps caused by a direct effect of digitalis on the visual cortex. Objects often appear yellow or green. Giddiness and trigeminal neuralgia are sometimes observed; excessive urination often occurs with digitalis intoxication. Gynecomastia may occasionally develop in men. This side effect is of little value in determining toxicity, however, because it seldom occurs. The drugs may also suppress follicle-stimulating hormone (FSH), as well as lead to vaginal cornification. Such effects are probably caused by an interaction with estrogen receptors.

In about half the cases of digitalis toxicity, extracardiac signs of toxicity precede the cardiac signs. A typical pattern would be the development of anorexia, followed in 1 or 2 days by nausea and vomiting and other signs. Nevertheless, the absence of extracardiac signs is no guarantee that cardiac toxicity is not occurring.

Cardiac toxicity is the most serious consequence of digitalis therapy. Although it is difficult to spe-

cifically characterize cardiac toxicity caused by digitalis, two effects stand out as the most typical—A-V nodal block and ventricular extrasystoles.[21] Complete A-V dissociation can occur at toxic levels of digitalis. This effect is an extension of a therapeutic effect of the drug, mediated by a reduction in A-V nodal conduction rate. Dropped ventricular beats caused by partial heart block are also a sign of toxicity. The effect of A-V conduction accounts in great measure for the excessive slowing of the heart seen in some toxic situations. Thus, excessive cardiac slowing may be an important sign of toxicity in many patients.

Digitalis also produces arrhythmias in toxic situations. Increased activity in secondary, ectopic pacemakers as a result of increased automaticity accounts for these effects.[21] This activity can result in extrasystoles of ventricular origin, which often take the form of bigeminy (a sinus beat followed by a premature beat) or trigeminy (heart beat grouped in trios, usually one sinus beat followed by two extrasystoles). The occurrence of these patterns of extrasystoles is very important because it often signals impending ventricular fibrillation. Other arrhythmias both of atrial and ventricular origin may occur. Examples of toxic effects on A-V conduction and ventricular automaticity are diagrammed in Figure 25-4.

It has been postulated that cardiac arrhythmic effects of digitalis are due to inhibition of Na,K-ATPase. Furthermore, vagal effects of digitalis can contribute to certain cardiac effects, such as heart block. However, in addition, digitalis may have significant stimulatory effects on the sympathetic nervous system, and these actions may account for such toxic effects as arrhythmias. Proposed sites of action of digitalis have included peripheral afferent pathways, the central nervous system, peripheral efferent nerve endings, the adrenal medulla, and ganglia.[17,43]

Drug monitoring

Attempts have been made to correlate blood concentrations of cardiac glycosides with signs of toxicity. These attempts offer a technical problem, since digoxin at therapeutic levels is on the order of 0.7 to 1.2 ng/ml of serum, and toxic effects may start to appear around 2.3 ng/ml.[30,38]

Bioassay, isotope labeling, ATPase inhibition, and physicochemical techniques have been described for measuring cardiac glycosides, but they are not used extensively in clinical practice. A re-

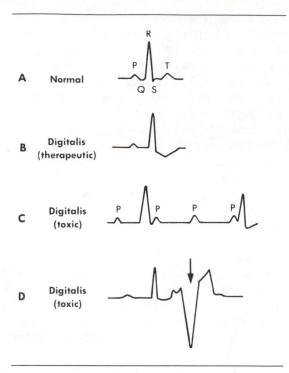

Figure 25-4. Some effects of digitalis on the electrocardiogram (lead II). **A,** Normal ECG. **B,** Typical changes at therapeutic concentrations include depression of the S-T segment and lengthening of the P-R interval. **C,** Toxic effect of digitalis on A-V conduction involves A-V dissociation, such as complete A-V block. Notice the lack of relationship between P and QRS complexes. **D,** Toxic effect of digitalis on ventricular automaticity results in ectopic ventricular beats. An example of bigeminy is shown, with the ectopic beat marked by an arrow.

cent development has been the competitive protein-binding assays for cardiac glycosides, most notably the radioimmunoassay.[38] This assay is of limited usefulness in confirming toxic states of patients. Monitoring of drug toxicity can best be accomplished by both clinical examination and measurement of drug blood concentrations, the more important being careful clinical examination. Patient education is a necessary prerequisite for the early detection and prevention of digitalis toxicity.

A method of determining digitalis toxicity from saliva electrolyte concentrations has been described.[41,47] It has been shown that the product of the potassium and calcium concentrations in whole saliva is significantly higher in states of digitalis toxicity than at therapeutic concentrations of the drug. This finding has been viewed with some optimism as a possible diagnostic tool for detection and confirmation of digitalis toxicity. It may have

signfiicant value in the diagnosis of early and subclinical toxic states.

Treatment

When digitalis toxicity is diagnosed, the drug is temporarily discontinued, along with diuretics that may have exacerbated the problem. If digitalis has to be readministered before signs of toxicity have abated, small doses are given with constant monitoring. Potassium chloride can be administered intravenously to replace lost potassium but generally is not used if A-V conduction is significantly impaired, since potassium will worsen this condition. Atropine can be helpful in controlling A-V block, S-A arrest, and sinus bradycardia.

Several antiarrhythmic drugs are useful in treating digitalis toxicity. They are given in these situations by the intravenous route, at least initially. The use of phenytoin is advantageous because it suppresses both digitalis-induced ectopic pacemaker activity and A-V block. Lidocaine is also useful in that it suppresses ectopic pacemaker activity; however, it has little effect on A-V conduction. Propranolol is effective in treating ventricular and supraventricular arrhythmias, but since it retards the A-V conduction rate, its usefulness is limited in those situations involving A-V block.

Cholestyramine, an anion exchange resin, has been used experimentally to bind digitoxin in the intestine during its enterohepatic circulation. This shortens the half-life of digitoxin but is of little value in reducing the half-life of digoxin. Antidigitalis antibodies have also been the subject of experimentation but as yet have not been routinely employed clinically.

GENERAL THERAPEUTIC USES
Congestive heart failure

In the United States the most widely used cardiac glycoside is digoxin. Digitoxin is a distant second. The primary use for digitalis is in the treatment of congestive heart failure. The direct effect of digitalis on the heart in most cases enables the heart in congestive failure to increase its contractile force and output. Some patients with congestive heart failure accompanied by normal sinus rhythm may only need temporary digitalis therapy; many other patients require treatment indefinitely.[40]

Digitalis is, unfortunately, not very effective when heart failure is due to some obstructive cause such as constrictive pericarditis and is contraindicated in hypertrophic subaortic stenosis. Digitalis is most efficacious in those patients with chronic, continuous heart failure in which the ventricle is enlarged at rest, early ventricular filling is rapid, and the compliance of the heart wall has not been reduced because of a condition such as hypertrophy or amyloid infiltration.[40] Furthermore, the best candidates for digitalis have enlarged hearts despite diuretic therapy. It has been shown that patients with a third heart sound, presumably caused by the enlarged heart striking the chest wall, often experience improved cardiac function from digitalis whereas those without this heart sound gain little benefit.[23] Symptoms such as the third heart sound may help indicate the condition of the heart and predict with greater accuracy the value of using digitalis. At present, however, further work needs to be done to establish the precise predictive criteria for digitalis therapy in various conditions of heart failure.

Cardiac arrhythmias

Initial treatment of paroxysms of tachycardia caused by atrial or A-V node activity usually involves reflex vagal stimulation by mechanical means, such as application of pressure to the carotid sinus. If these attempts fail, one of several drugs, including digitalis, can be used. Since digitalis has vagal effects, it reduces automaticity at the origin of the tachycardia. A low dose may be all that is required, since a combination of low doses of digitalis with mechanical measures may be effective.

Digitalis is quite effective in reducing increased ventricular rate caused by atrial fibrillation. Vagal and nonvagal effects of the drug account for a decrease in conduction rate in the A-V node and therefore protect the ventricle from atrial electrical impulses arriving in rapid succession. The dosage can be adjusted to "titrate" the drug to a given ventricular rate. On occasion, atrial fibrillation reverts to normal sinus rhythm during therapy. However, it must be emphasized that this is not the main goal of digitalis therapy, which is to protect the ventricles from the rapid rate of the atria.

Atrial flutter may be defined as an atrial rate of approximately 250 to 350 contractions per minute. The reasons for using digitalis here and in treating atrial fibrillation are similar. Even in untreated patients, partial heart block (for instance, 2:1 block) usually keeps the ventricular rate below the atrial rate, but digitalis can be used to increase the block and lower the ventricular rate to acceptable levels.

Of perhaps greater importance, digitalis tends to prevent large fluctuations in ventricular rate caused by moment-to-moment changes in sympathetic and vagal tone. In addition, atrial flutter is often converted to atrial fibrillation during digitalis therapy. This conversion is actually considered beneficial, since ventricular rate is more easily "titrated" in atrial fibrillation than in atrial flutter.

PREPARATIONS AND DOSAGE SCHEDULES

Only general statements will be made regarding dosages for the cardiac glycosides. More detailed information is available from other sources.[37] (See also general references.) Dose schedules are extremely important for digitalis because attaining a therapeutic effect without toxicity requires precise regulation of the amount of drug administered. Children by and large are less sensitive than adults to digitalis and usually require proportionally larger doses on the basis of weight. Dosages of the cardiac glycosides can be discussed from two aspects: loading, or digitalizing, dose and maintenance dose.

The purpose of the loading dose, as in therapy with other drugs, is to build up to a steady-state (plateau) drug concentration faster than would occur using maintenance doses. Maintenance doses, on the other hand, are meant to replace daily losses of a drug during the steady state. Digitalis dosages depend on the preparation used, disease state, concurrent drug therapy, and electrolyte balance. In all cases, patients must be continually monitored, and final judgment on optimal dosages depends on clinical observations. Pharmacokinetic data on major cardiac glycoside preparations are shown in Table 25-4.

CONDITIONS AFFECTING DIGITALIS THERAPY
Disease state

Because of the pharmacokinetic properties of digoxin and digitoxin, patients with liver or kidney hypofunction will require downward dosage adjustments for these drugs.[37]

Thyroid status has important implications for digitalis therapy. Hypothyroidism increases and hyperthyroidism reduces the sensitivity of the patient to digitalis.[4,22] The half-lives of ouabain and digoxin are reduced in thyrotoxicosis, in part as a result of increased excretion of the drugs.[37] Increased volume of distribution and decreased intestinal absorption of digoxin in hyperthyroid states

Table 25-4. Cardiac glycosides and clinical data

Drug	Trade name(s)	Gastro-intestinal absorption	Peak drug effect	Average plasma half-life	Main route of elimination	Approximate daily adult oral maintenance dose
Digoxin	Lanoxin	60%-85%	1-5 hr	36 hr	Kidney excretion	0.25-0.5 mg
Digitoxin	Crystodigin, Purodigin	90%-100%	4-12 hr	4-7 days	Liver metabolism	0.1 mg
Digitalis (leaf)	Digifortis	Approx. 40%	—	4-7 days	Liver metabolism	0.1 gm
Ouabain	—	Unreliable	½-2 hr	21 hr	Kidney excretion	—
Deslanoside	Cedilanid-D	Unreliable	1-3 hr	33 hr	Kidney excretion	—

have also been reported.[22] In addition, sensitivity of the heart itself to cardiac glycosides appears to be a function of thyroid status. This sensitivity may relate to the fact that the number of Na,K-ATPase active sites appears to increase with thyroid function.

Patients with chronic lung disease and cor pulmonale tend to be very susceptible to the toxic effects of cardiac glycosides. This undue susceptibility is the result of hypoxemia and disturbances in acid-base balance in these patients.

Since the mechanism of action of digitalis in all likelihood involves an increase in a critical calcium "pool" in the heart, it is not surprising that high plasma calcium concentrations can worsen digitalis toxicity. Magnesium, on the other hand, inhibits many calcium-induced events; it too has a predictable influence on digitalis toxicity, that is, magnesium deficiency can increase susceptibility to digitalis toxicity.

Hypokalemia can also predispose a patient to digitalis toxicity. Low plasma potassium concentrations allow greater uptake of digitalis in the heart and alter myocardial membrane properties.[29] In addition, potassium has been shown to inhibit the rate of binding of digitalis to Na,K-ATPase.[33] Together these factors may account for increased digitalis toxicity at low plasma potassium concentrations.[29] (For drugs that lower plasma potassium, see the section on drug interactions.) Loss of intracellular potassium also plays an important role in digitalis toxicity. When digitalis is administered, intracellular potassium concentrations will gradually decrease, reducing the ratio of intracellular to extracellular potassium. This ratio change and the membrane potential alterations that follow make the heart more sensitive to digitalis toxicity. Reduced intracellular potassium may be present without a significant reduction in plasma potassium concentrations.[5] The effect of major electrolyte changes on digitalis toxicity is shown in Table 25-5.

Table 25-5. Effects of plasma electrolyte concentration on digitalis toxicity

	Normal total plasma concentration (millimolar)	Digitalis toxicity more likely if plasma electrolyte concentration is:
Potassium	3.8-5.4	Lowered
Calcium	2.2-2.8	Raised
Magnesium	0.8-1.1	Lowered

Drug interactions

Drugs affect digitalis therapy mainly by reducing its absorption, by altering the rate of its metabolism, by changing plasma and intracellular potassium concentrations, or by directly influencing the myocardium.

Kaolin-pectin and oral antacids reduce intestinal absorption of digoxin by forming a complex with the drug.[1,7] Sulfasalazine, neomycin, phenytoin, *p*-aminosalicylic acid, and metoclopramide have also been reported to reduce intestinal absorption of digoxin.[1]

Cholestyramine is used to bind bile acids in the gastrointestinal tract and thereby lower plasma concentrations of cholesterol. It is also able to bind certain drugs in the intestine, including digitalis. Digitalis preparations given concurrently by mouth will therefore be prevented from being absorbed. Furthermore, since digitoxin circulates in an enterohepatic cycle, it can be bound by cholestyramine after its initial absorption. The half-life of digitoxin will be shortened and the therapeutic effect reduced.

Since digitoxin is the only cardiac glycoside enjoying extensive clinical use that is subject to significant liver metabolism, drugs that induce the hepatic microsomal enzyme system will reduce the half-life of digitoxin but not of the other pure digitalis preparations. (Digitalis leaf contains primarily digitoxin and is similarly affected.) The most important example in this regard is phenobarbital.[1] When phenobarbital is administered, especially on a long-term basis, digitoxin dosages generally have to be increased. When a patient is taking one of the inducing drugs together with digitoxin and the inducer is removed from therapy, digitoxin dosages may have to be adjusted downward.

A number of drugs can predispose a patient to digitalis toxicity by lowering plasma potassium concentrations. These include amphotericin B, corticosteroids, and diuretics (except the potassium-sparing diuretics).[1,37] The most notable example is the benzothiadiazide (thiazide) class of diuretics, the most commonly used class. The clinical problem is a significant one, since the thiazide diuretics are often used in conjunction with digitalis to help reduce edema associated with congestive heart failure or to reduce blood pressure. Thus, regulation of potassium concentration is important. Thiazide diuretics may also increase plasma pH, resulting in increased digitalis toxicity.

Several reports have indicated a substantial interaction between quinidine and digitalis.[13] The most important clinical results of concurrent therapy are enhanced digitalis toxicity and enhanced quinidine toxicity. This effect is particularly significant since cardiac glycosides have a low therapeutic index and the two drugs have significant overlapping side effects and toxicities, such as A-V block and gastrointestinal effects. Adverse reactions can occur, therefore, at normal therapeutic dosages. Quinidine increases plasma digoxin concentrations by two mechanisms: first, renal clearance of digoxin is decreased, and , second, digoxin is displaced from tissue stores as a result of quinidine administration.[13] Because of the interaction with digoxin, concurrent therapy usually requires a reduction, typically 50%, in dose of both drugs. It should be remembered, however, that this interaction is highly variable from patient to patient. Quinine, the levo stereoisomer of quinidine, also increases plasma digoxin concentrations. An interaction between digitoxin and quinidine is apparently less significant.

Sympathomimetic amines interact with digitalis, since both classes of drugs increase the possibility of ectopic cardiac pacemaker activity.[37] Cardiac arrhythmias are more likely to occur when β-adrenergic agonists are used concurrently with digitalis.

Both cholinergic and anticholinergic drugs will interact with digitalis. The cholinergic agents en-

hance, whereas the anticholinergic drugs antagonize, atrial, S-A nodal, and A-V nodal effects of digitalis. Succinylcholine, by increasing vagal tone and altering potassium distribution, may also increase digitalis toxicity.

Verapamil, nifedipine, and diltiazem, agents that block the plasma membrane calcium channels (slow channels), are newer drugs for the treatment of angina pectoris. Since these agents reduce calcium entry into the cell, it is to be expected that they would have some influence on the effects of digitalis. Furthermore these agents may penetrate the plasma membrane and alter calcium metabolism at intracellular sites. In addition, verapamil is used to treat certain cardiac arrhythmias and nifedipine has been shown to be effective in treating hypertension. Although there are indications that these drugs may reduce some arrhythmic effects of digitalis, and sometimes may be administered with digitalis in the absence of toxicity, at least one of the calcium antagonists, verapamil, is contraindicated in digitalis toxicity because it may lead to sinus arrest and A-V block. On the other hand, the cardiac glycosides tend to reverse the cardiodepressant effect of verapamil.[34] The interaction and combined use of the calcium entry blockers with digitalis is still a subject of investigation.[44]

Canrenone is a metabolite of spironolactone. Canrenone partially inhibits Na,K-ATPase and antagonizes the binding of cardiac glycosides to Na,K-ATPase.[15] This accounts for some complex interactions between digitalis, spironolactone and congestive heart disease. Some evidence supports the fact that canrenone will also antagonize digitalis toxicity.

In about 10% of patients, gut bacteria can metabolize a significant portion of digoxin.[25] In these patients, antibiotics, by reducing certain bacteria, can increase the amount of digoxin absorbed and thereby increase the potential for digoxin toxicity. This interaction between antibiotics and digoxin has in some cases resulted in a twofold increase in serum digoxin concentrations.

INVESTIGATIONAL CARDIOSTIMULANTS
Amrinone

Amrinone is a bipyridine drug that has a positive inotropic action on the heart. The cardiac effects of amrinone cannot be attributed to an action on Na,K-ATPase, the β-adrenergic receptor, or adenylate cyclase. It has been proposed that amrinone acts directly on the contractile mechanism of cardiac muscle or on calcium distribution. The drug has some promise clinically, especially in cases where the heart is refractory to other cardiotonic drugs.

Endogenous digitalis-like compounds

Endogenous digitalis-like compounds, sometimes called *endodigins,* have been isolated from various tissues. There is a tendency to draw an analogy between these substances and the enkephalins and endorphins with their action on the opioid receptors. It is in this context that investigators are examining chemical substances present in the body that can act like digitalis. Substances that may serve this role include a low molecular weight substance isolated from guinea pig brain[16] and peptides with digitalis-like activity in volume-expanded dogs.[18] These substances inhibit Na-K pump activity or Na,K-ATPase as well as the binding of digitalis to Na,K-ATPase. Agents exhibiting the latter reaction also bind with antibodies specific for digoxin. An endogenous rat brain cyclic dipeptide, histidyl-proline diketopiperazine, which is a metabolite of thyrotropin-releasing hormone, has been shown to inhibit brain plasma membrane Na,K-ATPase.[2] This peptide does not block the binding of digitalis to Na,K-ATPase and therefore must inhibit the enzyme at a site distinct from that of the cardaic glycosides.

Vanadate (VO_4^{-3}) is a potent inhibitor of Na,K-ATPase.[8] Since vanadium is present in mammalian tissues at 10^{-7} to 10^{-6} M concentrations,[32] it is possible that vanadate modulates endogenous Na,K-ATPase activity in vivo. Inotropic activity of cardiac glycosides can be enhanced by vanadate. Vanadate can also promote the binding of cardiac glycosides to Na,K-ATPase under certain conditions.[32] Therefore, vanadate may alter the therapeutic effect of cardiac glycosides and could explain, in part, individual variations in response to digitalis. Vanadate also affects enzyme systems other than Na,K-ATPase and has been shown to activate adenylate cyclase.

IMPLICATIONS FOR DENTISTRY
Stress factors

The practitioner should strive to eliminate needless stress for cardiac patients, especially anxiety or pain associated with dental procedures. It must be emphasized that patients taking digitalis still possess an underlying cardiac defect. Therefore, patients receiving digitalis pose a risk in stressful situations, because the stress puts a greater work load on the heart in addition to stimulating the release of endogenous catecholamines. By increasing the possibility of ectopic pacemaker activity of the heart, catecholamines increase the risk of digitalis-induced arrhythmias. Fear and apprehension may also increase the likelihood of adverse CNS reactions to digitalis. One practical conclusion is that antianxiety agents or analgesics should be used if emotional stress or pain is likely.

Drug interactions

The use of catecholamines in local anesthetic injections in patients taking digitalis is not contraindicated but should be approached with special precautions. Proper injection technique, with the avoidance of intravascular injection, should be followed. Many factors will influence the decision to use vasoconstrictors in local anesthetic solutions, including the preference of the clinician, the ability to achieve adequate anesthesia without vasoconstrictors, and the volume of anesthetic solution required. The chief danger of sympathomimetic vasoconstrictors to patients taking digitalis is that the combination of both drugs increases the risk of cardiac arrhythmias.

The use of gingival retraction cords impregnated with epinephrine is definitely not recommended in digitalized patients. In fact, cardiac disease in general is a contraindication for their use. Considerable amounts of vasoconstrictor may be absorbed systemically from these retraction cords, and the possibility of cardiac arrhythmias developing is significant. If hemostatic retraction cords are to be used in digitalized patients, they should be impregnated with some other agent such as alum or zinc chloride.

Long-term barbiturate therapy (for example, of several days) is a rarity in dentistry. Nevertheless, it should be noted the barbiturates and other drugs that induce liver microsomal enzymes can increase the rate of biotransformation of digitoxin. (Other major pure cardiac glycosides are not affected, since they are not metabolized to a significant degree in the liver.) In the barbiturate group, induction is primarily observed with long-acting drugs, for instance phenobarbital. Multiple doses of barbiturates and other inducing drugs should be instituted only after arrangements for dosage adjustment of digitoxin are made. This decision necessitates close cooperation with the physician.

The effects of digitalis on the S-A node and the

atria are mediated primarily by the vagus nerve. Effects on the A-V node are both vagal and nonvagal. Many beneficial effects of digitalis depend on vagal influences. This is especially true in the treatment of supraventricular arrhythmias. Hence, cholinergic and anticholinergic drugs can influence digitalis therapy. Of these agents, only the anticholinergics are used with any regularity in dentistry. Antisialagogues, such as atropine and methantheline, should not be used in digitalized patients since they tend to reduce digitalis's effects.

Antibiotic therapy may alter the intestinal flora and, in so doing, increase the absorption of digoxin in those patients whose gastrointestinal flora metabolizes digoxin. Erythromycin, an antibiotic widely used in dentistry, has been shown to have this effect. When the need arises, concurrent antibiotic therapy, especially with erythromycin or a broad-spectrum antibiotic, should be undertaken with sufficient cognizance given to its possible interaction with digitalis.

Cardiac glycosides

Nonproprietary name	Proprietary name
deslanoside	Cedilanid-D
digitalis*	Digifortis
digitalis glycosides mixture	Digiglusin
digitoxin	Crystodigin, Purodigin
digoxin	Lanoxin
gitalin	Gitaligin
lanatoside C†	Cedilanid
ouabain†	—

*A mixture of cardiac glycosides.
†Not available in the United States.

CITED REFERENCES

1. Adverse interactions of drugs. Medical Letter on Drugs and Therapeutics **23**:17-27, 1981.
2. Battaini, F., and Peterkofsky, A. Histidyl-proline diketopiperazine, an endogenous brain peptide that inhibits (Na$^+$, K$^+$)-ATPase. Biochemical and Biophysical Research Communications **94**:240-247, 1980.
3. Biedert, S., Barry, W.H., and Smith, T.W. Inotropic effects and changes in sodium and calcium contents associated with inhibition of monovalent cation active transport by ouabain in cultured myocardial cells. Journal of General Physiology **72**:479-494, 1979.
4. Bonelli, J., Haydl, H., Hruby, K., and Kaid, G. The pharmacokinetics of digoxin in patients with manifest hyperthyroidism and after normalization of thyroid function. International Journal of Clinical Pharmacology and Biopharmacy **16**:302-306, 1978.
5. Brater, D.C., and Morrelli, H.F. Digoxin toxicity in patients with normokalemic potassium depletion. Clinical Pharmacology and Therapeutics **22**:21-33, 1977.
6. Braunwald, E., Bloodwell, R.D., Goldberg, L.I., and Morrow, A.G. Studies on digitalis. IV. Observations in man on the effects of digitalis preparations on the contractility of the non-failing heart and on total vascular resistance. Journal of Clinical Investigation **40**:52-59, 1961.
7. Brown, D.D., and Juhl, R.P. Decreased bioavailability of digoxin due to antacids and kaolin-pectin. New England Journal of Medicine **295**:1034-1037, 1976.
8. Cantley, L.C., Jr., Cantley, L.G., and Josephson, L. A characterization of vanadate interactions with the (Na$^+$, K$^+$)-ATPase. Mechanistic and regulatory implications. Journal of Biological Chemistry **253**:7361-7368, 1978.
9. Cattell, M., and Gold, H. The influence of digitalis glucosides on the force of contraction of mammalian cardiac muscle. Journal of Pharmacology and Experimental Therapeutics **62**:116-125, 1938.
10. Chen, K.K. Possibilities of further developments in the glycoside field by modifying the glycoside structure. In Wilbrandt, W., and Lindgren, P., eds. Proceedings of the First International Pharmacology Meeting, vol. 3. New Aspects of Cardiac Glycosides. New York, Macmillan, Inc., 1963.
11. Chung, E.K. Digitalis Intoxication. Baltimore, The Williams & Wilkins Co., 1969.
12. Doherty, J.E. Digitalis glycosides: pharmacokinetics and their clinical implications. Annals of Internal Medicine **79**:229-238, 1973.
13. Doherty, J.E. The digoxin-quinidine interaction. Annual Review of Medicine **33**:163-170, 1982.
14. Fieser, L.F., and Fieser, M. Steroids. New York, Reinhold Publishing Corp., 1959.
15. Finotti, P., and Palatini, P. Canrenone as a partial agonist at the digitalis receptor site of sodium-potassium-activated adenosine triphosphatase. Journal of Pharmacology and Experimental Therapeutics **217**:784-790, 1981.
16. Fishman, M.C. Endogenous digitalis-like activity in mammalian brain. Proceedings of the National Academy of Science, U.S.A. **76**:4661-4663, 1979.
17. Gaitondé, B.B., and Joglekar, S.N. Mechanism of neurotoxicity of cardiotonic glycosides. British Journal of Pharmacology **59**:223-229, 1977.
18. Gruber, K.A., Whitaker, J.M., and Buckalew, V.M., Jr. Endogenous digitalis-like substance in plasma of volume expanded dogs. Nature **287**:743-745, 1980.
19. Langer, G.A. Mechanism of action of the cardiac glycosides on the heart. Biochemical Pharmacology **30**:3261-3264, 1981.
20. Langer, G.A., and Serena, S.D. Effects of strophanthidin upon contraction and ionic exchange in rabbit ventricular myocardium: relation to control of active state. Journal of Molecular and Cellular Cardiology **1**:65-90, 1970.
21. Lathers, C.M., and Roberts, J. Digitalis cardiotoxicity revisited. Life Sciences **27**:1713-1733, 1980.
22. Lawrence, J.R., Sumner, D.J., Kalk, W.J., Ratcliffe, W.A., Whiting, B., Gray, K., and Lindsay, M. Digoxin kinetics in patients with thyroid dysfunction. Clinical Pharmacology and Therapeutics **22**:7-13, 1977.
23. Lee, D.C., Johnson, R.A., Bingham, J.B., Leahy, M., Dinsmore, R.E., Goroll, A.H., Newell, J.B., Strauss, H.W., and Haber, E. Heart failure in outpatients: a ran-

domized trial of digoxin versus placebo. New England Journal of Medicine **306**:699-705, 1982.

24. Lindenbaum, J. Bioavailability of digoxin tablets. Pharmacological Reviews **25**:229-237, 1973.

25. Lindebaum, J., Rund, D.G., Butler, V.P., Jr., Tse-Eng, D., and Saha, J.R. Inactivation of digoxin by the gut flora. New England Journal of Medicine **305**:789-794, 1981.

26. Mason, D.T. Regulation of cardiac performance in clinical heart disease: interactions between contractile state mechanical abnormalities and ventricular compensatory mechanisms. American Journal of Cardiology **32**:437-448, 1973.

27. Mason, D.T. Digitalis pharmacology and therapeutics: recent advances. Annals of Internal Medicine **80**:520-530, 1974.

28. Moe, G.K., and Mendez, R. The action of several cardiac glycosides on conduction velocity and ventricular excitability in the dog heart. Circulation **4**:729-734, 1951.

29. Murthy, R.V., Kidwai, A.M., and Daniel, E.E. The uptake of cardiac glycosides by rabbit and rat myometrium. Journal of Pharmacology and Experimental Therapeutics **182**:166-178, 1972.

30. Noble, D. Review: Mechanism of action of therapeutic levels of cardiac glycosides. Cardiovascular Research **14**:495-514, 1980.

31. Okita, G.T. Dissociation of Na$^+$, K$^+$-ATPase inhibition from digitalis inotropy. Federation Proceedings **36**:2225-2230, 1977.

32. Ramasarma, T., and Crane, F.L. Does vanadium play a role in cellular regulation? In Horecker, B.L., and Stadtman, E.R., eds. Current Topics in Cellular Regulation, vol. 20. New York, Academic Press, Inc., 1981.

33. Schwartz, A., and Collins, J.H. Na$^+$,K$^+$-ATPase. Structure of the enzyme and mechanism of action of digitalis. In Martonosi, A., ed. Membranes and Transport. New York, Plenum Press, 1982.

34. Schwartz, A., Grupp, G., Millard, R.W., Grupp, I., Lathrop, D., Matlib, M.A., Vaghy, P.L., and Valle, R. Calcium channel blockers: possible mechanisms of protective effects on the ischemic myocardium. In Weiss, G.B., ed. New Perspectives on Calcium Antagonists. Bethesda, Md., American Physiological Society, 1981.

35. Schwartz, A., Lindenmayer, G.E., and Allen, J.C. The sodium-potassium adenosine triphosphatase: pharmacological, physiological, and biochemical aspects. Pharmacological Reviews **27**:3-134, 1975.

36. Skou, J.C. Effect of digitalis glycosides on membrane transport of sodium and potassium. In Marks, B.H., and Weissler, A.M., eds. Basic and Clinical Pharmacology of Digitalis. Springfield, Ill., Charles C Thomas, Publisher, 1972.

37. Smith, T.W. Drug therapy: digitalis glycosides (first of two parts). New England Journal of Medicine **288**:719-722, 1973.

38. Smith, T.W., and Haber, E. Clinical value of the radioimmunoassay of the digitalis glycosides. Pharmacological Reviews **25**:219-228, 1973.

39. Sonnenblick, E.H., Williams, J.F., Jr., Glick, G., Mason, D.T., and Braunwald, E. Studies on digitalis. XV. Effects of cardiac glycosides on myocardial force-velocity relations in the nonfailing human heart. Circulation **34**:532-539, 1966.

40. Spector, R. Digitalis therapy in heart failure: a rational approach. Journal of Clinical Pharmacology **19**:692-696, 1979.

41. Swanson, M., Cacace, L., Chun, G., and Itano, M. Saliva calcium and potassium concentrations in the detection of digitalis toxicity. Circulation **47**:736-743, 1973.

42. Tamm, C. The stereochemistry of the glycosides in relation to biological activity. In Wilbrandt, W., and Lindgren, P., eds. Proceedings of the First International Pharmacology Meeting, vol. 3. New Aspects of Cardiac Glycosides. New York, Macmillan, Inc., 1963.

43. Weaver, L.C., Akera, T., and Brody, T.M. Digoxin toxicity: primary sites of drug action on the sympathetic nervous system. Journal of Pharmacology and Experimental Therapeutics **197**:1-9, 1976.

44. Weiss, G.B., ed. New Perspectives on Calcium Antagonists. Bethesda, Md., American Physiological Society, 1981.

45. Wellsmith, N.V., and Lindenmayer, G.E. Two receptor forms for ouabain in sarcolemma-enriched preparations from canine ventricle. Circulation Research **47**:710-720, 1980.

46. Withering, W. An Account of the Foxglove, and Some of Its Medical Uses; With Practical Remarks on Dropsy, and Other Diseases. London, C. G. J. and J. Robinson, 1785. (Reprinted in Medical Classics **2**:305-443, 1937.)

47. Wotman, S., Bigger, J.T., Jr., Mandel, I.D., and Bartelstone, H.J. Salivary electrolytes in the detection of digitalis toxicity. New England Journal of Medicine **285**:817-876, 1971.

GENERAL REFERENCES

Ewy, G.A., and Bressler, R., eds. Cardiovascular Drugs and the Management of Heart Disease. New York, Raven Press, 1982.

Greeff, K., ed. Cardiac Glycosides, Parts I and II. New York, Springer-Verlag Publishers, 1981.

Hoffman, B.F., and Bigger, J.T., Jr. Digitalis and allied cardiac glycosides. In Gilman, A.G., Goodman, L.S., and Gilman, A., eds. Goodman and Gilman's The Pharmacological Basis of Therapeutics, ed. 6. New York, Macmillan, Inc., 1980.

Katz, A. Physiology of the Heart. New York, Raven Press, 1977.

26 Antianginal drugs

James L. Matheny

Angina pectoris (from the Latin, literally meaning pain in the chest) is characterized by periodic episodes of severe oppressive substernal pain. The pain and associated changes in the ECG (e.g., depressed S-T segment) result from ischemia (hypoxia) of some area of the myocardium, probably a subendocardial area.[7] The most frequent pathologic cause of angina is coronary artery sclerosis leading to compromised blood flow and oxygen supply to a prescribed region of the myocardium.

As represented in Figure 26-1, the normal response to increased myocardial oxygen demand is satisfied by coronary vasodilation, increased blood flow, and thus increased oxygen supply. In contrast, in the classic anginal patient, coronary artery sclerosis precludes vasodilation, and the increased demand for oxygen cannot be compensated for by increased blood flow. Cardiac determinants of oxygen consumption and factors that can precipitate changes in these determinants are also shown in Figure 26-1.

Systolic intraventricular pressure is important in determining flow in subendocardial regions because of compression of blood vessels in the involved area. Alterations of ventricular size cause concurrent changes in ventricular work. Increased heart rate, of course, requires increased oxygen supply because of the increased rate of metabolism. Finally, the inotropic state of the myocardium is also a factor in determining oxygen consumption. One of the more important controls of heart rate is exerted by the sympathetic nervous system through catecholamine release.

It is beyond the scope of this chapter to consider in detail the specific changes in the cardiac determinants of myocardial oxygen consumption caused by each of the factors that may precipitate an anginal attack. It is sufficient to say that any factor that compromises the balance between oxygen demand and oxygen supply may precipitate an attack of angina. Thus, an anginal attack may follow exercise, emotional upset, or exposure to cold or may occur after meals or smoking. Certain individuals experience nocturnal attacks of angina, probably as a result of the effects of posture on cardiac performance. Anginal attacks may also result from self-medication with various drugs, such as cold remedies that contain sympathomimetic agents.

There are basically three types of angina pectoris: chronic stable exertional angina (classic angina), Prinzmetal's, or variant, angina, and unstable angina (also known as preinfarction angina, intermediate coronary syndrome, acute coronary insufficiency, and accelerated angina). Chronic stable exertional angina occurs in patients who have fixed atherosclerotic coronary artery disease. Pain in these individuals occurs when the myocardial oxygen requirement exceeds the supply. Prinzmetal's, or variant, angina occurs as a result of coronary artery spasm and a subsequent decrease in coronary blood flow and oxygen supply. It is believed that α-adrenergic receptor stimulation may play a role in this vasospasm. These patients usually also exhibit coronary atherosclerosis, although in some it may be minimal. Variant angina is characterized by chest pain occurring at rest and, frequently, during sleep. The third type, unstable angina, refers to a new onset of pain at rest or a sudden worsening of pain in a patient with previously stable exertional angina. The majority of these patients have severe coronary artery disease; coronary spasm may also be involved.[11]

There are three classes of drugs used extensively in the treatment of angina pectoris. The first class contains drugs of well-established value (nitroglycerin, amyl nitrite) in providing immediate relief from anginal symptoms or acute prophylaxis

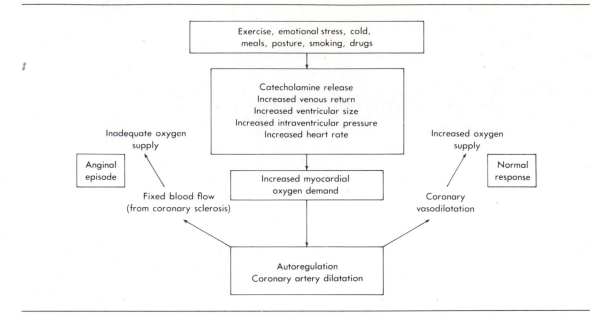

Figure 26-1. Pathophysiology and precipitating causes of classic angina pectoris.

of an attack, as well as other drugs (isosorbide dinitrate, pentaerythritol tetranitrate) that are promoted for long-term protection from anginal episodes.

The second class contains the β-adrenergic receptor blocking agents, and these are administered on a long-term basis, frequently in conjunction with the nitrites, to decrease the frequency and severity of anginal attacks.

The third class of drugs useful in the management of angina are the calcium entry blockers (calcium antagonists). This class includes nifedipine, diltiazem, verapamil, and perhexiline. These agents, like the β-adrenergic blockers, are useful prophylactically in angina therapy.[1]

NITRITES AND NITRATES

Nitroglycerin (glyceryl trinitrate) has been for many years and still is considered to be the drug of choice for the relief of the acute symptoms of angina pectoris. Amyl nitrite was introduced for use in angina in 1867, and nitroglycerin was introduced in 1879. Nitroglycerin is administered sublingually, amyl nitrite by inhalation, and both have a short duration of action. In more recent years, various organic nitrates and sustained-release forms of nitroglycerin have been developed in attempts to find a suitable, long-lasting preparation for the control of anginal pain.

Chemistry

Nitroglycerin is chemically a simple compound. Figure 26-2 shows its structure and, for comparison, that of one of the organic nitrates marketed for oral administration.

Pharmacologic effects

The pharmacologic effects of all the members of this class are similar and are thought to be due to actions of a reduced intermediate formed by denitration reactions in the tissues.

The most important action of nitrates and nitrites is the direct relaxation (not mediated through other receptor systems, such as adrenergic or cholinergic) of vascular smooth muscle, resulting in vasodilation in nearly all vascular beds. Nitroglycerin has been shown to cause varying degrees of change in coronary flow in normal and diseased mammalian hearts.[4] Its efficacy in angina is attributed in part, to a preferentially increased oxygen supply to ischemic areas, with variable actions on total coronary blood flow.[6] More importantly, through a reduction in venous tone there is a reduction in venous pressure, pulmonary and systemic arterial pressure, and intraventricular pressure. These actions lead to a decrease in ventricular volume, producing a fall in intramyocardial tension and thus a drop in myocardial oxygen demand.

The nitrates and nitrites relax almost all smooth muscle and are largely devoid of actions on tissues

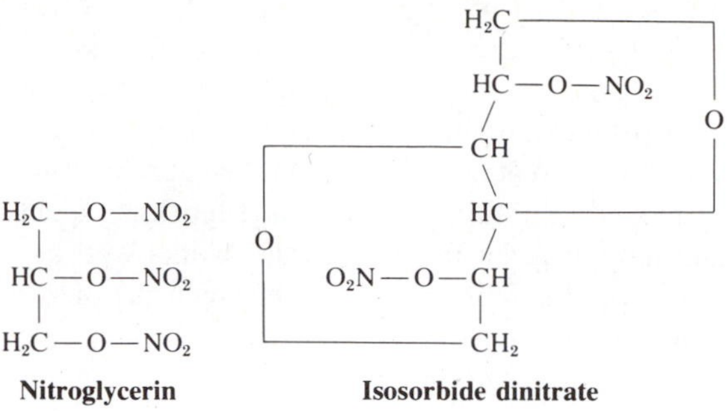

Figure 26-2. Structural formulas of nitroglycerin and isosorbide dinitrate.

other than smooth muscle. Bronchial, biliary, and gastrointestinal smooth muscles are relaxed. As noted in the discussion of toxicity, these actions are of little importance in comparison with their cardiovascular actions.

Absorption, fate, and excretion

Nitroglycerin is rapidly absorbed after sublingual administration (onset 1 to 3 minutes, duration 30 to 60 minutes). It has a much slower onset when applied topically but enjoys a comparably longer duration of action. Although organic nitrates administered orally are readily absorbed, they are extensively metabolized during the first pass through the liver.

In addition to undergoing denitration reactions in tissues, nitrates are metabolized in the liver by gluthathione–organic nitrate reductase. The products of hepatic biotransformation, including the released nitrite ions, are much less effective than the parent compound; they are subsequently excreted in the urine, at least in part, in the form of glucuronide conjugates.

Long-acting agents

Although sublingual nitroglycerin is highly effective for the treatment of acute anginal episodes, its short duration of action makes it ill-suited for long-term prophylaxis. Several nitrates formulated for oral administration have been marketed for many years for the prevention of anginal attacks. When administered sublingually, one of the most promising long-lasting agents, isosorbide dinitrate, was shown to be similar but not superior to nitroglycerin.[3] Unfortunately, when administered orally in recommended dosages, this compound offered no protection against exercise-induced angina. This finding led to the conclusion that there was no rationale for the use of these newer nitrates in the treatment of angina pectoris.[9,10] More recent investigations have shown, however, that large doses of isosorbide dinitrate (and nitroglycerin also) do, in fact, improve exercise tolerance in patients with angina.[8] There is, of course, a concomitantly increased possibility of drug overdose, and the role of orally administered organic nitrates remains unsettled.

In order to avoid the first-pass phenomenon that plagues the orally administered nitrates, nitroglycerin has been prepared in several forms. The first of these, nitroglycerin ointment, is effective prophylactically, but it must be administered every 3 to 4 hours. A further development is the nitroglycerin transdermal system, which comes in the form of an adhesive patch. When applied to the skin, the transdermal patch slowly releases nitroglycerin over a 24-hour period. Not only does this system minimize the potential for toxicity inherent in large-dose oral administration, it overcomes the mess and frequency of application associated with the ointment.

One problem shared by all of the long-acting preparations is the development of tolerance. In vitro studies suggest that a diminished capacity of peripheral tissues to reduce the nitrates is responsible. Such tolerance is not observed with the intermittent administration of sublingual nitroglycerin.

Toxic reactions and side effects

Almost all side effects of these drugs are direct results of their effects on the cardiovascular system. Headache is the most common untoward response and can be very severe. Tolerance to this effect may develop in some patients before tolerance to other cardiovascular effects occurs. Orthostatic hypotension resulting in cerebral ischemia, weakness, dizziness, and syncope may follow drug administration. Syncope is very likely to occur if the patient is standing and immobile while taking medication or has drunk alcoholic beverages. Nitrite ions readily oxidize hemoglobin to methemoglobin, and formation of large amounts of methemoglobin can seriously impair the oxygen-carrying capacity of the blood, resulting in anemic hypoxia. Severe poisoning and even death may result from the ingestion of nitrates by infants. Occasionally, drug rash may occur and appears most frequently with pentaerythritol tetranitrate and topical nitroglycerin.

β-ADRENERGIC BLOCKING AGENTS

The history and chemistry of β-adrenergic blocking agents have been previously discussed (Chapters 5 and 7). In addition, the use of these compounds in the treatment of cardiac arrhythmias and hypertension is covered in Chapters 24 and 28, respectively. Propranolol is a β_1 and β_2 antagonist; metoprolol is an antagonist selective for the β_1 receptor. Several other β-blocking agents are approved for use in the United States, and others are marketed outside of this country. It is safe to say that more of these drugs will become available in the next few years.

Pharmacologic effects

As indicated by the listing of exercise and emotional stress as possible precipitating factors in angina (Figure 26-1), increases in sympathetic nervous system activity can bring on attacks of angina in susceptible individuals. Thus, the blockade of adrenergic responses can be of benefit in the treatment of this condition. The effects of β-adrenergic blocking drugs that are of benefit in treating angina are protection from reflexes, decreased heart rate, depressed myocardial contractility, decreased cardiac output, and, in some cases, reduced blood pressure. These effects are, as would be expected, more prominent when sympathetic activity is elevated, such as during exercise or emotional stress. Total coronary blood flow may actually be reduced after β blockade, but this reduction in flow seems to be in well-perfused areas and thus is not detrimental in classic angina. Drug-induced vasoconstriction (from unopposed α-receptor activity), however, may be detrimental in patients with variant angina. Propranolol has several other effects that are not of benefit in treating angina, such as an increase in ventricular volume and end-diastolic pressure and an increase in the duration of mechanical systole. In most patients taking blocking agents, there is an overall decrease in myocardial oxygen requirements.

Absorption, fate, and excretion

The absorption, fate, and excretion of β-adrenergic blocking agents are discussed in Chapter 7.

Use in treatment of angina

Both propranolol and nadolol are approved for use as prophylactic agents in the treatment of angina pectoris; there has been a great deal more clinical experience with propranolol, however, since it has been available for a longer time. Long-term administration of these drugs does not usually prevent attacks of angina but makes their occurrence less frequent and individual attacks less severe. Thus, patients receiving long-term treatment with β-blocking agents usually still require nitroglycerin for treatment of acute anginal attacks. This combined-drug therapy, using a β-blocking agent and nitroglycerin or related drug, works well because the drugs have different mechanisms of action.

Although not officially approved for use in angina at this time, selective β_1 antagonists such as metoprolol appear to be as effective as propranolol and may be advantageous in some patients (see below).

Toxic reactions and side effects

As is mentioned in Chapter 7, nonselective blockade of β-receptors may cause bronchoconstriction or prevent the normal response to insulin-produced hypoglycemia in susceptible patients, or both. These reactions can occur with propranolol, which blocks β_1 and β_2 receptors. It may be less of a problem with the more selective drug metoprolol, which does not block β_2 receptors as effectively and has been used without adverse effects on patients with bronchospastic disease. It is not yet established that metoprolol spares the adrenergic receptor that modulates insulin secretion. A problem encountered with both drugs and related to their ability to block cardiac β_1 receptors is that severe myocardial depression and heart failure may occur if initial dosages are too high or if there is concomitant myocardial incompetence. For this reason, dosages should be gradually increased until levels offering therapeutic effects in the management of angina are reached. The sudden discontinuance of propranolol has been implicated in rebound overstimulation of the heart, worsening of angina, and myocardial infarction.

CALCIUM ENTRY BLOCKERS

Calcium entry blockers are also referred to as calcium antagonists (for structures see Figure 26-3). This class of drugs includes nifedipine, diltiazem, verapamil, and several other agents. These compounds have been shown to be effective in the prophylactic treatment of chronic stable exertional angina, variant angina, and unstable, or preinfarction, angina. They have also proved useful in the treatment of other cardiovascular disorders, such as atrial arrhythmias and hypertension.

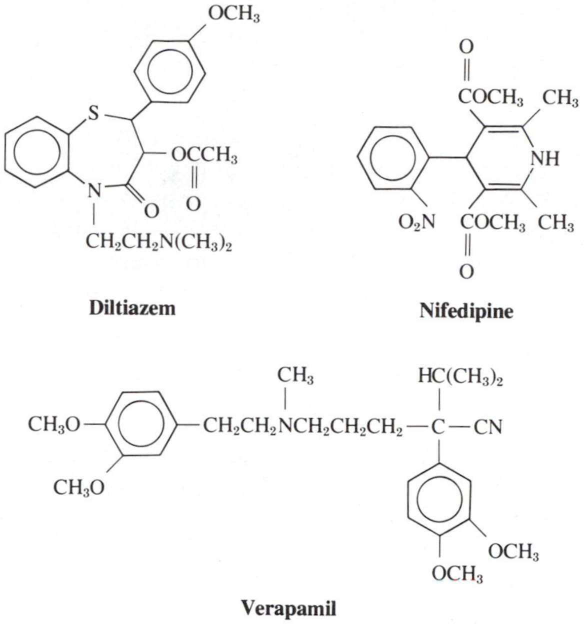

Figure 26-3. Structural formulas of some calcium entry blockers.

Pharmacologic effects

Calcium entry blockers are believed to exert their primary action on calcium channels that carry the slow inward calcium flux. Calcium entry blockers differ from fast channel blockers, such as local anesthetics, which depress the rapid inward flux of sodium. Although the primary action of the calcium antagonists is on the slow current, they may also act through other mechanisms. For example, diltiazem, especially at higher doses, has been shown to affect the sodium or fast channels.

Some of the diverse actions of calcium entry blockers can be explained by the roles that calcium and slow channels have in different cell types. For instance, in the sinus and A-V nodes, slow channels may be the primary conduit for the generation and propagation of action potentials. They may also be involved in regulating sinus node automaticity by altering diastolic depolarization. These actions may explain the effectiveness of the calcium entry blockers as antiarrhythmics. The full role of calcium antagonists in smooth muscle, in which membrane depolarization may not always involve the movement of calcium, is not well defined. Despite the lack of detailed information regarding mechanisms, these agents have clearly been shown to dilate both coronary and peripheral blood vessels. The vasodilator action probably explains their use as antianginals and antihypertensives. Other uses for calcium entry blockers include acute congestive heart failure, hypertrophic cardiomyopathy, and possibly cerebral vasospasm.[5]

Absorption, fate, and excretion

All of the calcium entry blockers are rapidly and almost completely absorbed following oral administration. Most of these agents undergo extensive hepatic metabolism, some to active metabolites (verapamil, diltiazem) and others to inactive compounds (nifedipine). Most are also highly protein bound, especially to serum albumin. Excretion is primarily via the urine.

Use in treatment of angina

The calcium entry blockers have been shown to be effective in the treatment of all types of angina whether or not coronary spasm is involved. Diltiazem and verapamil seem to be especially effective in preventing coronary vasospasm, though laboratory studies indicate they may act through different mechanisms to decrease intracellular calcium. In chronic stable exertional angina, calcium entry blockers may afford relief of pain through one or more mechanisms: coronary and peripheral vasodilation, attenuation of increased heart rate caused by exercise, or a negative inotropic effect on the heart.[2]

Toxic reactions and side effects

The toxicity of the calcium entry blockers varies with the individual agent; however, there are some side effects common to this class of drugs. These side effects include dizziness, headache, and nausea and those related to systemic vasodilation: sensation of heat, facial flushing, hypotension, reflex tachycardia (palpitations), and peripheral edema. Verapamil is the most, and diltiazem the least, likely to reduce myocardial contractility. On the other hand, both drugs decrease conduction through the A-V node. Fortunately, myocardial depression and reduction of atrioventricular conduction are rarely a problem clinically with these agents.[2] Coadministration with a β-adrenergic antagonist, though, may lead to a deterioration in cardiac performance; in this situation nifedipine, which spares atrioventricular conduction, might be the calcium entry blocker of choice.

Perhexiline therapy has been associated with severe adverse reactions, including hepatotoxicity, peripheral neuropathy, ataxia, and papilledema. Thus this drug will probably not achieve widespread clinical acceptance.

IMPLICATIONS FOR DENTISTRY

It has been stated that anginal attacks can be precipitated by physical or emotional stress. Since these situations often arise in the dental operatory, the dentist should be aware of the symptoms and treatment of angina. A complete medical history will reveal whether a patient is being treated for angina. If so, the dentist should be sure that the patient has medication (nitrate) available before a procedure is performed. The patient will know when an attack is imminent; for ready access, the patient's medication should be placed on a nearby tray or counter. Also, nitroglycerin or amyl nitrite should be included on the emergency tray. The patient should be medicated in a sitting or supine position, because standing may lead to hypotension and syncope. In most cases, anginal pain will subside rapidly (2 to 3 minutes), and the patient will probably experience headache. As a precaution, patients should be handled carefully and be fully informed about the procedure and, if they feel it necessary, be given prophylactic medication. Preoperative sedation may be helpful and is not contraindicated if significant cardiovascular depression is avoided.

Because the β-adrenergic blocking drugs are cardiac depressants, any drugs that might cause further depression of cardiac function should be used with caution. Conversely, epinephrine in gingival retraction cord is contraindicated because the unopposed α-vasoconstriction may lead to hypertension, and the cardiostimulatory properties may partially overcome the β blockade. Similar considerations dictate prudence in, though not necessarily avoidance of, the use of local anesthetics with vasoconstrictors. In reference to the calcium entry blockers, orthostatic hypotension might be a problem, but cardiac depression is not usually clinically significant. Sensations of heat or facial flushing may be evident in these patients.

Drugs used in treatment of angina pectoris

Nonproprietary name	*Proprietary name*
Nitrates and nitrites	
amyl nitrite	—
erythrityl tetranitrate	Cardilate
isosorbide dinitrate	Isordil, Sorbitrate
mannitol hexanitrate*	Nitranitol
nitroglycerin	Nitrobid, Nitrostat, Nitrol, Transderm-Nitro
pentaerythritol tetranitrate	Peritrate
β-adrenergic blocking agents	
alprenolol*	Aptine
atenolol	Tenormin
metoprolol	Lopressor
nadolol	Corgard
oxprenolol*	Trasicor
pindolol	Visken
propranolol	Inderal
sotalol*	Sotacor
timolol	Blocadren
Calcium entry blockers	
diltiazem	Cardizem
flunarizine*	Sibelium
lidoflazine*	Clinium
nifedipine	Procardia
perhexiline*	Pexid
verapamil	Isoptin, Calan

*Not currently available in the United States.

CITED REFERENCES

1. Drugs for prophylaxis of angina pectoris. Medical Letter on Drugs and Therapeutics **17:**57-58, 1975.
2. Flaim, S.F., and Zelis, R. Clinical use of calcium entry blockers. Federation Proceedings **40:**2877-2881, 1981.
3. Goldstein, R.E., Rosing, D.R., Redwood, D.R., Beiser, G.D., and Epstein, S.E. Clinical and circulatory effects of isosorbide dinitrate: comparison with nitroglycerin. Circulation **43:**629-640, 1971.
4. Goldstein, R.E., Stinson, E.B., Scherer, J.L., Seningen, R.P., Grehl, T.M., and Epstein, S.E. Intraoperative coronary collateral function in patients with coronary occlusive disease. Circulation **49:**298-308, 1974.
5. Hope, R.R., and Lazzara, R. The clinical uses of calcium antagonists. Advances in Internal Medicine **27:**435-452, 1982.
6. Kay, H.B. Angina pectoris: getting the most from drug therapy. Drugs **13:**276-287, 1977.
7. Moir, T.W. Subendocardial distribution of coronary blood flow and the effect of antianginal drugs. Circulation Research **30:**621-627, 1972.
8. Oral isosorbide dinitrate for angina. Medical Letter on Drugs and Therapeutics **21:**88, 1979.
9. Riseman, J.E.F., Koretsky, S., and Altman, G.E. Stereoisomeric nitrates in the treatment of angina pectoris. American Journal of Cardiology **15:**220-229, 1965.
10. Russek, H.I. The therapeutic role of coronary vasodilators: glyceryl trinitrate, isosorbide dinitrate, and pentaerythritol tetranitrate. American Journal of the Medical Sciences **252:**9-20, 1966.
11. Zelis, R. Calcium-blocker therapy for unstable angina pectoris. New England Journal of Medicine **306:**923-928, 1982.

GENERAL REFERENCES

Godfraind, T. Mechanisms of action of calcium entry blockers. Federation Proceedings **40:**2866-2871, 1981.

Goldstein, R.E., and Epstein, S.E. Medical management of patients with angina pectoris. Progress in Cardiovascular Disease **14:**360-398, 1972.

Goldstein, R.E., and Epstein, S.E. Nitrates in the prophylactic treatment of angina pectoris. Circulation **48:**917-920, 1973.

Lambert, D.M. Effect of propranolol on mortality in patients with angina. Postgraduate Medical Journal **52**(suppl. 4):57-60, 1976.

Needleman, P., and Johnson, E.M., Jr. Mechanism of tolerance development to organic nitrates. Journal of Pharmacology and Experimental Therapeutics **184:**709-715, 1973.

Needleman, P., Lang, S., and Johnson, E.M., Jr. Organic nitrates: relationship between biotransformation and rational angina pectoris therapy. Journal of Pharmacology and Experimental Therapeutics **181:**489-497, 1972.

Prichard, B.N.C. β-Adrenergic receptor blocking drugs in angina pectoris. Drugs **7:**55-84, 1974.

Prichard, B.N.C. Propranolol in the treatment of angina: a review. Postgraduate Medical Journal **52**(suppl. 4):35-41, 1976.

Robinson, B.F. Mechanism of action of beta-blocking drugs in angina pectoris: a review. Postgraduate Medical Journal **52**(suppl. 4):43-45, 1976.

Stipe, A.A., and Fink, G.B. Prophylactic therapy of angina pectoris with organic nitrates: relationship of drug efficacy and clinical experimental design. Journal of Clinical Pharmacology **13:**244-250, 1973.

Thadani, U., Sharma, B., Meeran, M.K., Majid, P.A., Whitaker, W., and Taylor, S.H. Comparison of adrenergic beta-receptor antagonists in angina pectoris. British Medical Journal **1:**138-142, 1973.

27 Diuretic drugs

James L. Matheny

Although juniper berries, hops, and many natural products containing irritant materials were known to increase urine flow, the first drugs found to be clinically useful in the control of renal function were the mercurial diuretics. Calomel (mercurous chloride) was first used as a diuretic (as well as a cathartic) in the sixteenth century, but this use was soon forgotten. Organic mercurials were originally synthesized for use as antisyphilitics, and in 1919 a medical student at the University of Vienna discovered that one of these compounds had a marked diuretic effect. In the succeeding 30 years, thousands of mercurials were synthesized for use as diuretics and some enjoyed clinical popularity. They are no longer widely used, however, because most had to be injected, they are relatively toxic, and they lose their effectiveness with continued use. The first nonmercurial diuretic, acetazolamide, was discovered in the 1950s and is an inhibitor of carbonic anhydrase. Since then, many structurally similar diuretics have been developed that are more potent and less toxic then the mercurial diuretics and more effective than acetazolamide.

Some diuretics exhibit actions on the cardiovascular system that are beneficial in the management of essential hypertension. Along with the adrenoceptor blocking drugs, diuretics are currently the agents of choice for the initial treatment of mild to moderate hypertension and are generally included in any combination of drugs used to treat more severe hypertension. The basic role of diuretics in the therapy of hypertension and the high incidence of this disease in the population make the diuretics one of the most frequently prescribed groups of drugs.

Diuretics can be classified according to their structure, efficacy, or mode of action. In the classification adhered to in this chapter, a combination of these criteria is used.

The major sites of action of specific diuretics on the nephron are shown in Figure 27-1, and their mechanisms of action are summarized in Table 27-1. As illustrated in Figure 27-1, diuretics may be referred to by their primary site of action, for example, loop diuretics (high-efficacy drugs) and distal tubular agents (potassium-sparing drugs).

Diuretics that act through three basic mechanisms will be discussed. Osmotic drugs cause the retention of water in the tubular fluid and are capable of inducing a water diuresis. Xanthines increase cardiac output, and thus glomerular filtration rate, and also produce more of a water diuresis. In addition, these agents have some direct tubular effects to induce natriuresis, a rather specific excretion of sodium ions. The remaining groups, including the most important diuretics clinically, act on ion-transport mechanisms to increase sodium excretion and have differing actions on potassium.

OSMOTIC NONELECTROLYTES

Mannitol, urea, isosorbide, and glycerol are osmotic nonelectrolytes that, in the presence of normal cardiorenal function, induce a water diuresis rather than the natriuresis seen with the thiazides. The therapeutic indications for these agents are totally different from those for other diuretics. Mannitol is the most frequently used agent in this category and will be discussed here as a prototype.

Mannitol is freely filtered by the glomerulus. It is not reabsorbed by the renal tubular cells and therefore retains water osmotically in the tubular fluid, increasing urine volume. High urine flows can be maintained using mannitol without extraction of excessive body fluids or production of electrolyte disturbances.[12,25] This agent can also have

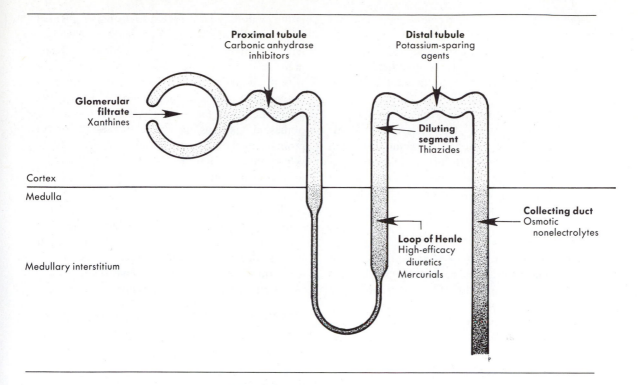

Figure 27-1. Primary sites of action of diuretics on the nephron.

Table 27-1. Summary of urinary properties during treatment and mechanisms of action of diuretic drugs*

	Volume (ml/min)	pH	Na^+	K^+	Cl^-	HCO_3^-	Mechanism of action
Control	1	6	50	15	60	1	
Mercurials	7	6	150	8	160	1	Decreases reabsorption of Na^+ and Cl^- in ascending loop of Henle
Thiazides (benzothiadiazides)	3	7.4	150	25	150	25	Decreases reabsorption of Na^+ and Cl^- in distal tubule
Ethacrynic acid, furosemide	8	6	140	10	155	1	Decreased Cl^- reabsorption leads to decreased Na^+ transport in ascending loop of Henle and proximal tubule
Triamterene	3	7.2	130	5	120	15	Decreases Na^+ reabsorption in distal tubule with increased K^+ retention
Spironolactone	3	7.2	125	5	120	15	Inhibits aldosterone; blocks Na^+ exchange for K^+ and H^+ in distal tubule
Acetozolamide	3	8.2	70	60	15	120	Carbonic anhydrase inhibition; decreases H^+ for Na^+ exchange and HCO_3^- reabsorption
Mannitol	10	6.5	90	15	110	4	Osmotic diuresis; H_2O retained in tubules; urine volume increases
Theophylline	3	6	150	15	160	1	Increased cardiac output leads to increased glomerular filtration rate and urine volume; also decreases Na^+ and Cl^- reabsorption

*These values represent peak diuretic responses in humans with a normal water and electrolyte balance. Electrolyte concentrations are given in mEq/L.

a dehydrating effect on body fluid chambers into which it does not penetrate, thus causing water to leave these areas in response to the greater tonicity of the circulation. Examples of structures that respond in this manner are the brain and the anterior chamber of the eye.

Mannitol is inactive pharmacologically and produces no direct toxicity. However, the acute administration of large volumes of mannitol solution can produce vascular overfilling, which may cause further decompensation in patients with congestive heart failure or precipitate congestive heart failure in patients with renal disease.

XANTHINES

Xanthines are the principle active ingredients of common beverages: caffeine and theophylline are found in tea; caffeine in coffee; and theobromine in cocoa. A complexed salt of theophylline, aminophylline, is widely used for the treatment of asthma. Other aspects of xanthine pharmacology are covered in Chapters 14 and 32.

Of the three xanthines, theophylline is the most potent diuretic. However, even in maximal therapeutic doses, theophylline produces significantly less diuresis than do the thiazides. It is generally reserved for diuretic use when other therapeutic measures fail.

Theophylline has effects on renal and cardiovascular function that, in combination, account for its diuretic efficacy. The rates of Na^+ and Cl^- excretion by the renal tubules are increased as a consequence of a direct tubular effect of the xanthines. In addition, cardiac output is increased. Thus, diuresis is in part attributable to an increase in renal blood flow and a higher glomerular filtration rate.[22]

Adverse reactions to theophylline result from extensions of its effect on the cardiovascular system and its stimulatory effects on the central nervous system. Cardiovascular responses include palpitations, hypotension, and circulatory collapse. CNS effects range from dizziness and headache to convulsions and are dose related and reversible.

ORGANOMERCURIAL DIURETICS

As discussed earlier, the mercurial diuretics were introduced as diuretics many years ago. Though historically important, these agents are rarely used today.

The major effect of mercurial diuretics is exerted through the inhibition of Na^+ and Cl^- reabsorption in the medullary and cortical segments of the thick ascending limb of the loop of Henle.[5,14] Also they have a minor inhibitory action on cationic exchange in the distal tubule; thus less kaliuresis is seen than with more potent diuretics, such as furosemide. It appears that mercuric ions released in response to the acidic pH of the urine account for the activity of these drugs. Inasmuch as the mercurial diuretics promote metabolic alkalosis by causing a disproportionate excretion of chloride over bicarbonate, they tend to inhibit their own effectiveness with time.

The use of mercurial diuretics is very limited. This is partially because of the development of refractoriness and the need to administer them intramuscularly. Moreover, mercuric poisoning in the form of renal failure and hemorrhagic cystitis can occur with continued administration.

CARBONIC ANHYDRASE INHIBITORS

The carbonic anhydrase inhibitors acetazolamide, dichlorphenamide, and methazolamide are weak diuretic agents with limited applications since the introduction of the thiazides. Because acetazolamide has the most indications for use, it will be discussed in detail.

Pharmacologic effects

The diuresis induced by acetazolamide is caused by inhibition of the enzyme carbonic anhydrase in the proximal and, to a lesser extent, distal segments of the renal tubule. The carbonic anhydrase inhibitors block the catalysis of the following reaction.

$$CO_2 + H_2O \underset{\text{anhydrase}}{\overset{\text{Carbonic}}{\rightleftharpoons}} H_2CO_3 \underset{\text{dissociation}}{\overset{\text{Nonenzymatic}}{\rightleftharpoons}} H^+ + HCO_3^-$$

Carbonic anhydrase thus allows conversion of carbon dioxide to bicarbonate, which can be excreted by the kidney. As seen in the above reaction the hydrogen ion concentration is also affected by this process.

Even though carbonic anhydrase is distributed throughout the body, therapeutic doses of acetazolamide exert their most prominent effect on the kidney. Effects on other systems, with the exception of the eye and brain, are seen only with large doses. After administration of acetazolamide, sufficient hydrogen ions cannot be produced for the normal absorption of bicarbonate and hydrogen exchange with sodium. Chloride ions are retained in the blood to offset the anionic bicarbonate loss; potassium is excreted in exchange for the increased

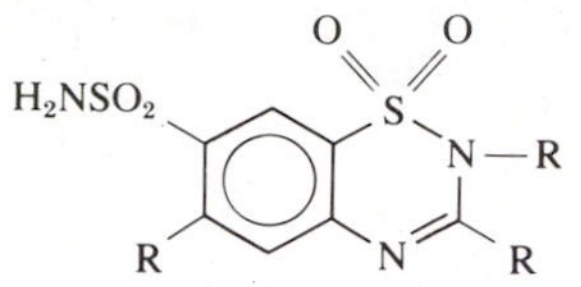

Figure 27-2. Structural formula of the parent compound of thiazide diuretics.

sodium present in the distal tubule.[16] Consequently, the urine of patients treated with acetazolamide contains increased amounts of Na^+, K^+, and HCO_3^-, with only a moderate increase in water output. The diuretic effect of the carbonic anhydrase inhibitors is self-limiting; the resultant metabolic acidosis eventually provides enough hydrogen ions for renal function to return toward normal.

Absorption, fate, and excretion

Acetazolamide is readily absorbed from the gastrointestinal tract. After oral administration, peak plasma concentrations are reached in 2 hours and the duration of action is 8 to 12 hours.

Toxic reactions and side effects

As mentioned, prolonged use of these compounds can result in systemic metabolic acidosis because of the decreased plasma bicarbonate concentrations. Minor CNS side effects, including drowsiness and disorientation, have been reported; however, a reduction of dosage usually reverses these symptoms.

THIAZIDE DIURETICS

Thiazide (benzothiadiazide) diuretics are derivatives of 1,2,4-benzothiadiazine-7-sulfonamide 1,1-dioxide. The basic structure of this parent compound is shown in Figure 27-2. The activity of the different derivatives varies, depending on the substituents present at the R positions. Chlorothiazide, hydrochlorothiazide, and cyclothiazide are examples of this group of diuretics. Although they differ structurally, chlorthalidone and several other agents are identical pharmacologically to the thiazide diuretics and are thus included in this class of drugs.[17] The thiazides are sometimes referred to as "ceiling" diuretics because larger than normal doses produce little if any further diuresis.

Pharmacologic effects

Thiazide diuretics increase the excretion of Na^+, Cl^-, and water by interfering with the transport of sodium ions across the renal tubular epithelium. The exact mechanism of action of the thiazides is unknown; however, evidence indicates that they alter the metabolism of the tubular cells. The primary site of action of these diuretics appears to be in the cortical diluting segment of the ascending limb of the loop of Henle and the early portion of the distal tubule.[23] All thiazides inhibit carbonic anhydrase, but the extent of this effect varies among the different derivatives[9] and does not account for their major diuretic action. Other effects of the thiazides on renal function include a decreased rate of glomerular filtration, increased K^+ excretion, and decreased uric acid excretion.

In addition to their actions on renal function, thiazides exhibit a direct action on vascular smooth muscle. Thus, direct arteriolar dilation[3,8] probably accounts for part of the antihypertensive action of thiazide diuretics. On initiation of therapy, thiazides cause decreases in extracellular fluid volume, plasma volume, and cardiac output, which probably account for the early drop in blood pressure. However, after a few weeks of therapy, extracellular fluid and plasma volume remain only slightly below normal.[24] Cardiac output returns to normal, but peripheral resistance remains decreased.[3]

Plasma renin activity is elevated by thiazide treatment, possibly as a result of the change in plasma volume.[24] Aldosterone secretion is increased by thiazide therapy and augments the direct hypokalemic effect of these drugs.

Absorption, fate, and excretion

Absorption of thiazides from the gastrointestinal tract varies with the particular agent. Peak diuretic activity occurs 3 to 6 hours after oral administration, with the onset of action at about 2 hours. The different durations of action of these agents reflect their rates of excretion and range from 6 to 12 hours for chlorothiazide to 24 to 72 hours for chlorthalidone.

The hypotensive action of thiazides is apparent only after 3 to 4 days of therapy and disappears slowly (1 week) after cessation of treatment. Excretion of the thiazides in the urine is accomplished through glomerular filtration and active secretion in the proximal tubule.

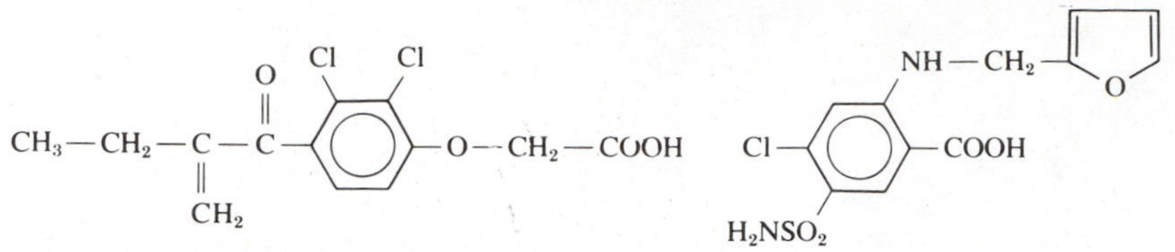

Figure 27-3. Structural formulas of ethacrynic acid and furosemide.

Toxic reactions and side effects

Electrolyte imbalances are the most common side effects of thiazide therapy. Potassium depletion occurs frequently but only rarely causes symptoms. In patients receiving cardiac glycosides, potassium depletion by thiazides can be particularly detrimental because hypokalemia potentiates the toxicity of these drugs. Other symptoms secondary to electrolyte disturbances include dryness of mouth, thirst, weakness, lethargy, drowsiness, restlessness, oliguria, and muscle cramps. Uric acid excretion is decreased by the thiazides and may lead to hyperuricemia in many patients. This action is clinically significant in patients who have a history of gout or chronic renal failure. The induction of gout in a patient being treated with thiazide diuretics is a good example of an iatrogenic disease, that is, a disease caused by medical treatment. Hyperglycemia and glucosuria may also result from thiazide administration to diabetic patients but can be overcome by an increased dosage of insulin or oral hypoglycemic agent.[2]

HIGH-EFFICACY DIURETICS

Furosemide, ethacrynic acid, and bumetanide are categorized as high-efficacy or high-ceiling diuretics because they can produce a much greater dose-dependent diuresis than can the thiazides even though they act through a similar mechanism.

Furosemide and ethacrynic acid are chemically unrelated, as shown by their structural formulas (Figure 27-3). Ethacrynic acid is an unsaturated ketonic derivative of aryloxyacetic acid, whereas furosemide is a derivative of anthranilic acid.

Pharmacologic effects

The high-efficacy diuretics inhibit sodium and chloride reabsorption in the ascending limb of the loop of Henle. In addition to increasing sodium and chloride excretion, these drugs enhance the excretion of potassium, magnesium, and calcium. As with the thiazides, the high-efficacy diuretics may cause hyperuricemia and gout in susceptible individuals.

The hypotensive effect of the high-efficacy agents, as with the thiazides, results from their diuretic action and direct influences on vascular reactivity. These drugs are preferred in certain hypertensive situations because they can induce a more profound and rapid decrease in blood pressure than is seen with the thiazides.

Absorption, fate, and excretion

These agents are readily absorbed from the gastrointestinal tract and are bound to plasma proteins to a considerable extent. They are rapidly excreted in the urine through glomerular filtration and tubular secretion. After oral administration, diuresis occurs within 1 hour. After intravenous injection, diuresis ensues in 2 to 10 minutes.[19] About 70% of an administered dose appears as either the parent compound or metabolites in the urine, with the remaining portion being excreted by the liver.[4]

Toxic reactions and side effects

Fluid and electrolyte imbalances are the most common forms of toxicity associated with high-efficacy diuretics. The electrolyte disturbances, such as hypokalemia and hyperuricemia, are similar to those seen with the thiazides, but the high-efficacy diuretics are less diabetogenic.[20] Deafness, either transient or permanent, is a rare but serious complication of long-term use of ethacrynic acid. Transient deafness has also been reported to occur with furosemide therapy. This ototoxic effect is thought to result from changes in the electrolyte composition of the endolymph because of inhibition of ATPase.[6] The long-term use of ethacrynic acid is further limited by a relatively steep dose-response curve that increases the possibility of drug overdose.

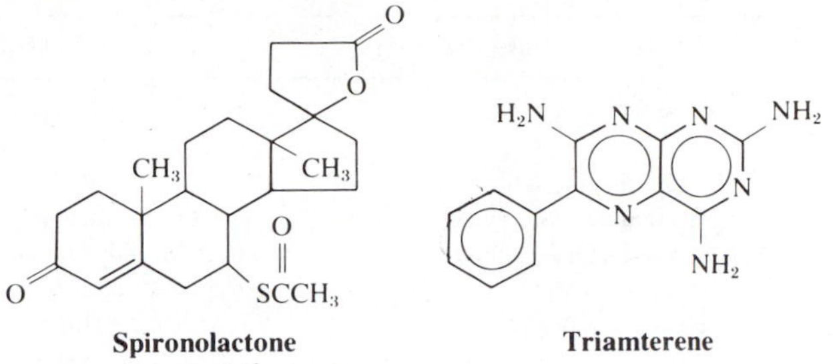

Figure 27-4. Structural formulas of spironolactone and triamterene.

POTASSIUM-SPARING DIURETICS

Spironolactone, triamterene, and amiloride are classed together not because their structures or mechanisms of diuretic action are similar but because they have a potassium-sparing effect accompanying their diuresis. Spironolactone is an aldosterone antagonist,[10] whereas the natriuretic effect of triameterene and amiloride results from a direct inhibition of tubular transport.[13,21]

The structural formulas of spironolactone and triamterene are shown in Figure 27-4. Spironolactone is a 17-spirolactone steroid, and triamterene is a pteridine compound chemically similar to folic acid.

Pharmacologic effects

Spironolactone exerts its diuretic action through competitive antagonism of the endogenous mineralocorticoid aldosterone. Aldosterone normally stimulates the renal tubular reabsorption of Na^+ and Cl^- and increases the excretion of K^+ by facilitating Na^+-K^+ exchange. Thus, antagonism of aldosterone by spironolactone causes a mild natriuresis and a decrease in potassium excretion.

Triamterene and amiloride cause mild diuresis by interfering directly with the distal tubular transport of Na^+. This effect is accompanied by little or no change in K^+ because the ionic driving force for K^+ secretion is eliminated. The potassium-sparing action of these drugs is greatly enhanced in the presence of other diuretics, such as the thiazides.

Absorption, fate, and excretion

Spironolactone is readily absorbed after oral administration. Its onset of action is very slow, and 2 weeks or longer may be required before an adequate response is obtained. Spironolactone is ex-

creted principally as the glucuronide conjugate in the urine.

Triamterene is absorbed rapidly from the gastrointestinal tract. About 70% of plasma triamterene is bound to plasma proteins. Its onset of action is fairly rapid (1 hour), and it is rapidly excreted in the urine as hydroxylated derivatives by filtration and tubular secretion.

Amiloride is partially absorbed when given orally. Its diuretic effect begins within 2 hours after ingestion and lasts for 1 day. The drug appears to be excreted unchanged in the urine.

Toxic reactions and side effects

Toxicity from spironolactone is rare. The most frequent disorder is hyperkalemia, seen usually when this drug is given in combination with potassium supplements. Triamterene and amiloride also produce few side effects other than hyperkalemia. When they do occur, they are usually mild and include nausea, vomiting, dizziness, and muscle cramps.

GENERAL THERAPEUTIC USES

The clinical uses of the diuretic drugs vary considerably according to their mechanism of action, route of administration, and diuretic efficacy (Table 27-2). The xanthines, for instance, are rarely used for their diuretic effects, although they may be of benefit in some patients with congestive heart failure. Because of their unique properties, the osmotic nonelectrolytes have special, though limited, applications. The osmotically active agents are generally used to reduce fluid or pressure in body cavities into which they do not penetrate. A good example of this is the administration of mannitol to reduce cerebrospinal fluid volume and intracranial pressure in patients with traumatic head injuries.

Table 27-2. Therapeutic uses of diuretic drugs

Classification	Representative drugs	Therapeutic uses
Mercurials	Mersalyl	Congestive heart failure, nephrotic syndrome (rarely used)
Thiazides	Chlorothiazide, chlorthalidone	Congestive heart failure, renal disease, hypertension
High-efficacy diuretics	Furosemide, ethacrynic acid	Same as thiazides, hypertensive crisis
Potassium-sparing agents	Spironolactone, triamterene	Alone for mild diuresis, with thiazides to maintain K^+ balance
Inhibitors of carbonic anhydrase	Acetazolamide, methazolamine	Weak diuretic (limited use), intraocular pressure reduction, anticonvulsant treatment
Osmotic nonelectrolytes	Mannitol, urea	Treatment of oliguria and anuria, intraocular and intracranial pressure reduction
Xanthines	Theophylline	Congestive heart failure, bronchial asthma

Several osmotic agents find similar use in ophthalmology. Perhaps the most important use of mannitol, however, is for the preservation of urine flow in acute renal failure. Osmotic diuresis can prevent tubular necrosis caused by the build-up of toxic drugs (e.g., barbiturates and salicylates) or substances (e.g., blood breakdown products).

Most of the diuretics that directly affect ion transport have similar indications for use. These are discussed below; where appropriate, differences between the various diuretics are noted.

Hypertension

The increased urinary output that follows the administration of the diuretics that alter ion transport is a result of their actions on the renal tubular handling of electrolytes, particularly sodium. In general, Na^+ excretion is increased and is accompanied by an increase in excretion of water. The mechanism by which this occurs varies with the particular type of diuretic. The importance of natriuresis in the treatment of hypertension lies initially in the decrease in blood volume and the subsequent decline in blood pressure. In addition to their diuretic action, both the thiazides and the high-efficacy agents have been shown to decrease venous reactivity and arterial resistance.[1,7,18] These effects are thought to be caused by a direct depressant action on the smooth muscle of the vascular beds. Neither the reduction of blood volume nor the decrease in venous tone and arterial resistance are of great magnitude, but together they result in an amelioration of blood pressure sufficient to control mild to moderate hypertension.

The thiazides are often the drugs of choice for the initial treatment of all degrees of hypertension, except in certain cases of severe hypertension where prompt, aggressive therapy is indicated.[8] In mild or moderate hypertension, a thiazide may be the only drug required. In moderate to severe hypertension, one or more antihypertensive agents of another class may be needed in addition to the thiazide to lower blood pressure to an acceptable level. The high-efficacy diuretics are indicated only when the thiazides are ineffective or when prompt diuresis is deemed advisable. The potassium-sparing diuretics are too weak for general use as the sole agent in treating hypertension. They are often added, however, to counteract the potassium-depleting effect of the other diuretic groups. Combined drug therapy for hypertension is discussed more fully in Chapter 28.

Congestive heart failure

The rationale for the use of diuretics in congestive heart failure is to relieve edema and symptoms of dyspnea arising from pulmonary congestion.[11] Diuretics increase venous capacitance and lower arterial blood pressure, thus improving cardiac hemodynamics by decreasing ventricular preload and afterload. Overadministration of diuretics may result in unwanted actions, such as excessively reduced plasma volume, decreased cardiac output, and diminished peripheral perfusion. Although a thiazide is often the diuretic of choice, a high-ceiling agent is most appropriate in cases of acute pulmonary edema. The primary therapy for congestive heart failure should include cardiac glycosides, which are discussed in Chapter 25.

Cirrhosis of the liver

Sodium retention and ascites with pooling of blood in the splanchnic circulation, peripheral edema, and portal hypertension usually accompany

Table 27-3. Drug interactions of diuretic agents

Diuretic	Interacting drug	Effect
Spironolactone	Aspirin	Blocks natriuresis by competing for distal tubular receptor sites
Thiazides, high-efficacy diuretics	Digitalis glycosides	Hypokalemia increases digitalis toxicity—may cause arrhythmias
Thiazides, high-efficacy diuretics	Sympathetic blocking agents	Summation of antihypertensive effects
Thiazides, high-efficacy diuretics	Oral hypoglycemics or insulin	Hypokalemia-induced hyperglycemia
Thiazides, high-efficacy diuretics	Uricosuric drugs	Inhibition of secretion or enhancement of reabsorption of uric acid, leading to gout
Thiazides, high efficacy diuretics	Alcohol, barbiturates, opioids	Increased postural hypotension caused by CNS depression

cirrhosis. Diuretics may be of some use in providing patient comfort; however, they have little effect on portal pressure and may reduce cardiac output and peripheral perfusion, thus causing orthostatic hypotension.[11] Management should be directed toward improvement of hepatic function by nutritional control and abstinence from alcohol.

Idiopathic cyclic edema

This disorder, often called premenstrual edema, represents a relatively common complaint from women who exhibit no evidence of cardiac, hepatic, or renal disease. This edematous state can be treated with drugs; unfortunately, some women with idiopathic edema become diuretic abusers. Evidence indicates that an exaggerated antinatriuresis may develop when therapy is discontinued.[15] Hypokalemia with high plasma renin titers may occur; thus, diuretic therapy for this condition should be instituted cautiously.

Edema of pregnancy

Peripheral edema is a common development late in pregnancy. Fluid retention occurs in response to compression by the gravid uterus on the inferior vena cava, increased venous capacitance, and decreased colloid osmotic pressure. If blood pressure does not increase, the edema is usually benign. However, if toxemia develops, blood pressure rises as a result of a decreased venous capacitance and increased salt retention. When this occurs, diuretics are an appropriate therapy.[11]

Nephrogenic diabetes insipidus and idiopathic hypercalciuria

Diuretics in conjunction with low-salt diets are useful in the treatment of idiopathic hypercalciuria and nephrogenic diabetes insipidus. Therapy is directed toward producing extracellular volume depletion, thereby increasing the relative proximal tubular reabsorption of sodium and water with consequent delivery of less filtrate to distal tubular reabsorptive sites.[11] Decreased urine formation occurs in nephrogenic diabetes insipidus; in idiopathic hypercalciuria, calcium reabsorption is improved.

Miscellaneous uses

The carbonic anhydrase inhibitors are used in the treatment of glaucoma and to reduce intraocular pressure for eye surgery. These benefits accrue because carbonic anhydrase is involved in the formation of aqueous humor. Acetazolamide is also employed as an anticonvulsant, and it is given to prevent acute altitude sickness and to treat familial periodic paralysis. With proper salt and water intake, furosemide may be used in the management of hypercalcemia.

IMPLICATIONS FOR DENTISTRY

The major drug interactions of the diuretic agents are summarized in Table 27-3. The only drug interactions of importance in dentistry are (1) the possibility that aspirin therapy might block the natriuretic action of spironolactone, and (2) the increased likelihood of orthostatic hypotension when sedative and opioid analgesics are administered.[26] Otherwise, diuretic therapy does not influence dental practice except when used as an indicator of the underlying disease state for which it has been prescribed. The majority of patients taking diuretics are receiving treatment for essential hypertension. For a complete coverage of the dental implications of this disease and the drugs used to treat it, see Chapter 28.

Diuretic drugs

Nonproprietary name	Proprietary name
Osmotic nonelectrolytes	
glycerin	Glyrol
isosorbide	Ismotic
mannitol	Osmitrol
urea	Ureaphil
Xanthine	
aminophylline (theophylline ethylenediamine)	Aminophylline, Aminodur Dura-tabs
Organomercurials	
mercaptomerin*	Thiomerin
merethoxylline procaine	Dicurin Procaine
mersalyl with theophylline	Mersalyl & Theophylline
Carbonic anhydrase inhibitors	
acetazolamide	Diamox
dichlorphenamide	Daranide
methazolamide	Neptazane
Thiazides and related derivatives	
bendroflumethiazide	Naturetin
benzthiazide	Exna
chlorothiazide	Diuril
chlorthalidone	Hygroton
cyclothiazide	Anhydron
hydrochlorothiazide	Esidrix, HydroDiuril, Oretic
hydroflumethiazide	Diucardin, Saluron
indapamide	Lozol
methyclothiazide	Aquatensen, Enduron
metolazone	Zaroxolyn
polythiazide	Renese
quinethazone	Hydromox
trichlormethiazide	Metahydrin, Naqua
High-efficacy agents	
bumetanide	Bumex
ethacrynic acid	Edecrin
furosemide	Lasix
Potassium-sparing agents	
amiloride	Midamor
spironolactone	Aldactone
triamterene	Dyrenium

*Not available in the United States.

CITED REFERENCES

1. Anderson, J., Godfrey, B.E., Hill, D.M., Munro-Faure, A.D., and Sheldon, J. A comparison of the effects of hydrochlorothiazide and of furosemide in the treatment of hypertensive patients. Quarterly Journal of Medicine **40:**541-560, 1971.
2. Anderson, P.O., and Kepler, J.A. Current drug therapy—thiazide diuretics. American Journal of Hospital Pharmacy **32:**473-480, 1980.
3. Anderton, J.L., and Kincaid-Smith, P. Diuretics. II. Clinical considerations. Drugs **1:**141-165, 1971.
4. Beyer, K.H., Baer, J.E., Michaelson, J.K., and Russo, H.F. Renotropic characteristics of ethacrynic acid: a phenoxyacetic saluretic-diuretic agent. Journal of Pharmacology and Experimental Therapeutics **147:**1-22, 1965.
5. Burg, M., and Green, N. Effect of mersalyl on the thick ascending limb of Henle's loop. Kidney International **4:**245-251, 1973.
6. Cohn, E.S., Gordes, E.H., and Brusilow, S.W. Ethacrynic acid effect on the composition of cochlear fluids. Science **171:**910-911, 1971.
7. Dikshit, K., Vyden, J.K., Forrester, J.S., Chatterjee, K., Prakash, R., and Swan, H.J.C. Renal and extrarenal hemodynamic effects of furosemide in congestive heart failure after acute myocardial infarction. New England Journal of Medicine **288:**1087-1090, 1973.
8. Dustan, H.R., Tarazi, R.C., and Barvo, E.L. Diuretic and diet treatment of hypertension. Archives of Internal Medicine **133:**1007-1013, 1974.
9. Earley, L.E., and Orloff, J. Thiazide diuretics. Annual Review of Medicine **15:**149-166, 1964.
10. Edelman, I.S. The initiation mechanism in the action of aldosterone on sodium transport. Journal of Steroid Biochemistry **3:**167-172, 1972.
11. Francisco, L.L., and Ferris, T.F. The use and abuse of diuretics. Archives of Internal Medicine **142:**28-32, 1982.
12. Goldberg, M., and Ramirez, M.A. Effects of saline and mannitol diuresis on the renal concentrating mechanism in dogs: alterations in renal tissue solutes and water. Clinical Science and Molecular Medicine **32:**475-493, 1967.
13. Gross, J.B., and Kokko, J.P. Effect of D-aldosterone and triamterene on the cortical collecting tubule (CCT) and the distal convoluted tubule (DCT). Clinical Research **23:**363, 1975.
14. Levitt, M.F., Goldstein, M.H., Lenz, P.R., and Wedeen, R. Mercurial diuretics. Annals of the New York Academy of Sciences **139:**375-387, 1966.
15. MacGregor, G.A., Tasher, P.R., and de Wardener, H.E. Diuretic-induced edema. Lancet **1:**489-492, 1975.
16. Maren, T.H. Carbonic anhydrase: chemistry, physiology, and inhibition. Physiological Reviews **47:**595-781, 1967.
17. Mudge, G.H. Agents affecting volume and composition of body fluids. In Gilman, A.G., Goodman, L.S., and Gilman, A., eds. Goodman and Gilman's The Pharmacological Basis of Therapeutics, ed 6. New York, Macmillan, Inc., 1980.
18. Ogilvie, R.I., and Schlieper, E. The effect of hydrochlorothiazide on venous reactivity in hypertensive man. Clinical Pharmacology and Therapeutics **11:**589-594, 1970.
19. Østergaard, E.H., Magnussen, M.P., Nielsen, C.K., Eibertsen, E., and Frey, H.H. Pharmacological properties of

3-n-butylamino-4-phenoxy-5-sulfamylbenzoic acid (bumetanide), a new potent diuretic. Arzneimittel Forschung **22:**66-72, 1972.

20. Riddiough, M.A. Preventing, detecting, and managing adverse reactions of antihypertensive agents in the ambulant patient with essential hypertension. American Journal of Hospital Pharmacy **34:**465-479, 1977.

21. Stoner, L.C., Burg, M.B., and Orloff, J. Ion transport in cortical collecting tubule: effect of amiloride. American Journal of Physiology **227:**453-459, 1974.

22. Strewler, G.J., and Orloff, J. The role of cyclic nucleotides in the transport of water and electrolytes. Advances in Cyclic Nucleotide Research **8:**311-361, 1977.

23. Suki, W.N., Eknoyan, G., and Martinez-Maldonado, M. Tubular sites and mechanisms of diuretic action. Annual Review of Pharmacology and Toxicology **13:**91-106, 1973.

24. Tarazi, R.C., Dustan, H.P., and Frohlich, E.D. Long-term thiazide therapy in essential hypertension: evidence for persistent alteration in plasma volume and renin activity. Circulation **41:**709-717, 1970.

25. Velasquez, M.T., Natargiacomo, A.V., and Cohn, J.N. Comparative effects of saline and mannitol on renal cortical blood flow and volume in the dog. American Journal of Physiology **224:**322-327, 1973.

26. Vidt, D.G. Diuretics: use and misuse. Postgraduate Medicine **59:**143-151, 1976.

GENERAL REFERENCES

Blaschke, T.F., and Melmon, K.L. Antihypertensive agents and the drug therapy of hypertension. In Gilman, A.G., Goodman, L.S., and Gilman, A., eds. Goodman and Gilman's The Pharmacological Basis of Therapeutics, ed. 6. New York, Macmillan, Inc. 1980.

Ferguson, R.K., and Vlasses, P.H. Systematic approach to therapy and special therapeutic problems. In Brunner, H.R., and Gavras, H., eds. Clinical Hypertension and Hypotension, vol. 2. New York, Marcel Dekker, Inc., 1982.

Francisco, L.L., and Ferris, T.F. The use and abuse of diuretics. Archives of Internal Medicine **142:**28-32, 1982.

Haeusler, G.W. A catalog of available antihypertensive agents. In Brunner, H.R., and Gavras, H., eds. Clinical Hypertension and Hypotension, vol. 2. New York, Marcel Dekker, Inc., 1982.

Hays, R.M. Agents affecting the renal conservation of water. In Gilman, A.G., Goodman, L.S., and Gilman, A. eds. Goodman and Gilman's The Pharmacological Basis of Therapeutics, ed. 6. New York, Macmillan, Inc., 1980.

Morgan, T.O. Diuretics: basic clinical pharmacology and therapeutic use. Drugs **15:**151-158, 1978.

Wilhelm, M., and DeStevens, G. Antihypertensive agents. Fortschritte der Arzneimettelforschung **20:**197-259, 1976.

28 Antihypertensive drugs

James L. Matheny

Hypertension affects approximately 15% of the American population. The percentage increases dramatically with age; 40% of whites and 50% of blacks over 65 years old are hypertensive. Although widespread screening and treatment programs have accomplished much, many hypertensives remain unaware that they have the disorder, and many others who are aware of their condition are receiving either no treatment or inadequate treatment.[8] The reason for this situation is that in its early stages hypertension is largely an asymptomatic disease. Readily recognizable symptoms occur only as a result of long-term exposure of the cardiovascular system, central nervous system, and kidneys to the abnormal pressure levels. Thus, screening programs are absolutely essential to detect hypertension early so that treatment can be instituted before major complications ensue. Education of the patient is also essential to ensure compliance with recommended therapy because of the asymptomatic nature of this disease in its early stages and because the unpleasant side effects of the drugs may sometimes make the patient feel better when not receiving medication.

CLINICAL ASPECTS
Classification

Hypertension is an age-related disorder, but blood pressure above 140/90 or 150/90 mm Hg is generally considered hypertension in the average patient. Although a classification of hypertension according to a blood pressure reading is necessarily imprecise, one is presented in Table 28-1 as a reference for discussion of the antihypertensive drugs.

Hypertension can be classified according to its cause into two broad categories—essential and secondary. Essential hypertension is of unknown etiology and represents the majority (80% to 90%) of the cases of hypertension. Though much is known

Table 28-1. Classification of severity of hypertension according to blood pressure elevation

	Diastolic pressure (mm Hg)
Mild	90-114
Moderate	115-129
Severe	130+

about the cardiovascular changes that occur in essential hypertension, no single pathologic change can be cited as the primary cause. Most likely there is a combination of factors responsible for the initiation and progression of this disease, ranging broadly from structural changes in the cardiovascular system to alterations of cardiovascular control by emotional factors.[31]

Secondary hypertension, on the other hand, results from a known disorder, such as renal malfunction or pheochromocytoma. Treatment of this type of hypertension is designed to eliminate the cause, in contrast to treatment of essential hypertension, which is purely symptomatic therapy designed to lower blood pressure.

Because essential hypertension is by far the most frequently encountered form of hypertension, this chapter will consider only those drugs used to treat this disorder. In another form of hypertension, known as hypertensive crisis or emergency, there is a sudden excessive elevation of blood pressure that requires immediate treatment because of life-threatening complications involving the heart, kidneys, and central nervous system. The treatment of hypertensive crisis will be considered separately, because both the aims of therapy and the drugs used differ from those for essential hypertension.

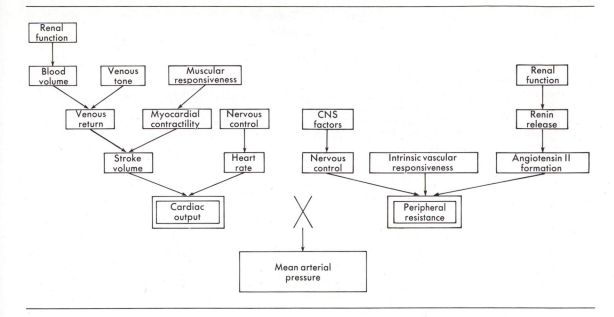

Figure 28-1. Factors that govern the mean arterial pressure.

Pathophysiology of essential hypertension

Blood pressure in the normal individual is maintained and controlled through a variety of mechanisms (Figure 28-1). Ultimately, mean arterial pressure reflects the product of cardiac output and peripheral resistance. Cardiac output is determined by both the load presented to the heart (venous return) and the inotropic and chronotropic state of the myocardium at a given time. Peripheral resistance depends on the direct responsiveness of the vasculature, vasoactive substances in the bloodstream, and the degree of nervous control at any given time. Normally, blood pressure remains within set limits as a result of physiologic feedback mechanisms, such as the arterial baroreceptor reflexes. For some unknown reason, this control range becomes higher early in essential hypertension (that is, blood pressure is still regulated within limits but the limits are higher).[21] Whether this change in regulation is a cause or an effect is equivocal. During this initial stage, the vasculature seems to be structurally and functionally normal. However, after prolonged hypertension, irreversible changes in vascular structure and function occur that progress and result in damage to many organs.

The role played by renin, an enzyme secreted by the kidney, in hypertension has received much attention over the past several years. Renin splits angiotensinogen, a protein found in the blood, to form angiotensin I, a peptide with ten amino acid residues. Angiotensin I is converted into angiotensin II, an octapeptide, by the removal of two of these amino acid residues. In turn, angiotensin II is metabolized to yield the slightly less active and shorter-lived heptapeptide, angiotensin III. Increased renin activity thus leads to overproduction of angiotensins II and III, vasoconstrictors of peripheral arterioles, and to an elevation of blood pressure.[10,32] Moreover, angiotensin peptides stimulate thirst and the secretion of aldosterone and antidiuretic hormone; the resultant increase in extracellular fluid and electrolytes augments the direct pressor effects.

Patients with essential hypertension can be divided into three groups according to their renin-sodium index (i.e., plasma activity relative to sodium excretion). Approximately 15% of the patients have renin concentrations that are higher than normal, 25% have renin concentrations lower than normal, and the remaining 60% show normal renin titers. Renin titers tend to decrease with age. Blacks tend to have a higher incidence of low-renin hypertension.

The percentage of hypertensive patients with a "normal" renin activity may be misleadingly high since renin release is normally depressed as the result of increased blood pressure.[15] Although renin

Table 28-2. Clinical disorders resulting from hypertension and atherosclerosis

Hypertension	Atherosclerosis
Congestive heart failure	Coronary artery disease
Cerebral hemorrhage	Angina pectoris
Renal failure	Myocardial infarction
Retinopathy	Secondary renovascular hypertension
Dissecting aneurysms	Peripheral vascular insufficiency
Hypertensive crisis	Cerebral thrombosis—stroke

Table 28-3. Risk factors for cardiovascular complications in hypertensives

Age	Obesity
Race	Salt intake
Sex	Previous cardiovascular disease
Hyperlipoproteinemia	Family history of
Diabetes mellitus	cardiovascular disease
Cigarette smoking	

and thus angiotensin II may be the main causative agent in high-renin hypertension and may be a factor in the normal-renin hypertension group, other influences have been implicated in low-renin hypertension, and these may contribute to normal-renin hypertension as well.

Evidence exists to support roles for vasopressin and adrenergic mechanisms in low-renin and normal-renin hypertension. The adrenergic system has been specifically implicated in the early phase of essential hypertension in certain young patients. The initial symptoms that these individuals display are tachycardia, increased cardiac output, and elevated blood catecholamines.[13] In addition, the relationship between blood catecholamine concentrations and vascular responsiveness to these agents may be important. In normotensive subjects, there is an inverse relationship between plasma norepinephrine concentrations and reactivity to exogenous norepinephrine, whereas essential hypertensives show a significant positive correlation between these two factors.[33]

From the previous discussion it follows that treatment of essential hypertension can be more appropriately designed if blood renin and catecholamine concentrations are known. Certainly, it would seem rational to select drugs that interfere with the renin-angiotensin-aldosterone axis in patients with high-renin hypertension.[6] It is also obvious that agents such as the neuronal and adrenergic receptor blocking drugs and the centrally acting adrenergic antihypertensives would be the drugs of choice if clinical findings demonstrate involvement of catecholamines.

For a more thorough treatment of the physiologic and psychologic factors in the early pathophysiology of essential hypertension the reader is referred to other sources.[21,23]

Although the etiology of essential hypertension has not been determined, it is well established that high blood pressure leads to cardiovascular and renal disease. Disorders associated with high blood pressure can be divided into two groups: those caused directly by hypertension and those caused by atherosclerotic vascular disease secondary to hypertension (Table 28-2).[9] Disorders in the first category result directly from the effect of increased pressure on the vasculature or the heart. Those in the second category result from atherosclerotic vascular disease but are classed as complications of hypertension because high blood pressure along with other factors promotes atherosclerosis.

It is evident from Table 28-2 that the consequences of uncontrolled hypertension are severe, and it should be clear why early detection and treatment of this disorder are essential. Epidemiologic studies of the incidence of hypertension have yielded much information, including the facts that high blood pressure increases the risk of premature death and that it increases the morbidity from cardiovascular and renal disease.[34] Except in certain undeveloped communities,[38] blood pressure increases gradually with age regardless of sex or race. Men tend to show higher pressures than women, at least until middle age, and blacks in the United States exhibit higher systolic pressures than whites regardless of age or sex. It is clear that the clinical disorders that result from hypertension and atherosclerosis are predominantly cardiovascular (Table 28-2). Furthermore, as is shown in Table 28-3, the risk of cardiovascular complications is increased in certain kinds of hypertensives, for instance those with diabetes.

It should be emphasized that essential hypertension is a progressive disease if not treated. The higher blood pressure initiates a whole sequence of events damaging to the entire cardiovascular system. A lowering of blood pressure causes all these disease processes to proceed more slowly and some, such as cardiac hypertrophy, to regress.

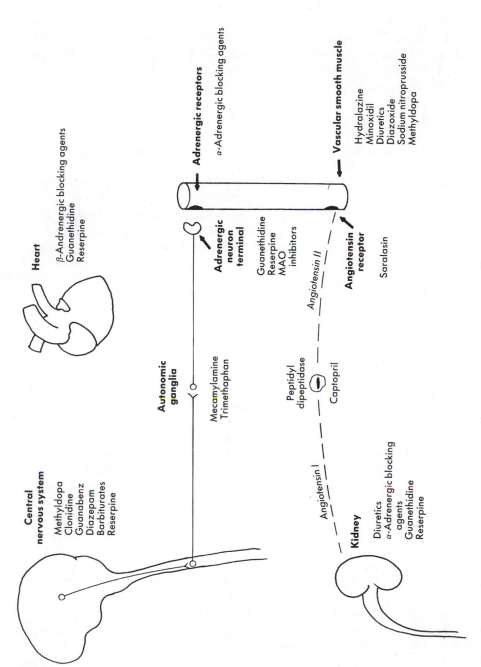

Heart

β-Andrenergic blocking agents
Guanethidine
Reserpine

Adrenergic receptors

α-Adrenergic blocking agents

Vascular smooth muscle

Hydralazine
Minoxidil
Diuretics
Diazoxide
Sodium nitroprusside
Methyldopa

Adrenergic neuron terminal

Guanethidine
Reserpine
MAO inhibitors

Angiotensin II

Angiotensin receptor

Saralasin

Autonomic ganglia

Mecamylamine
Trimethaphan

Peptidyl dipeptidase

Captopril

Angiotensin I

Central nervous system

Methyldopa
Clonidine
Guanabenz
Diazepam
Barbiturates
Reserpine

Kidney

Diuretics
α-Adrenergic blocking agents
Guanethidine
Reserpine

Figure 28-2. Sites of action of antihypertensive drugs.

General aims of antihypertensive drug therapy

Treatment of essential hypertension consists of symptomatic therapy aimed at reducing the blood pressure into the normal range. As shown in Figure 28-1, many factors play a role in the determination of blood pressure, and as a consequence pharmacologic agents with diverse mechanisms of action can be used singly or in combination in the treatment of essential hypertension. Antihypertensive agents can be divided into categories according to their mechanisms of action and therapeutic use: diuretics, agents affecting adrenergic function, direct vasodilators, drugs affecting the renin-angiotensin system, and drugs useful in hypertensive crisis. Because the basic pharmacologic properties of many of the drugs useful in treating hypertension have been discussed in previous chapters, only those actions and side effects pertinent to the treatment of hypertension will be discussed in detail in this chapter. A representation of the antihypertensive agents and their sites of action is shown in Figure 28-2.

DIURETICS

The thiazide diuretics are currently among the initial drugs of choice for the management of essential hypertension. The potassium-sparing diuretics are also commonly used for their additive effect and to prevent thiazide-induced hypokalemia. A high-efficacy agent, such as furosemide, may be indicated when prompt mobilization of fluid is desired. For a complete coverage of diuretics used in the treatment of hypertension, see Chapter 27.

AGENTS AFFECTING ADRENERGIC FUNCTION

One of the major homeostatic roles of the autonomic nervous system is control of cardiovascular function. Thus, it follows that drugs that can alter autonomic activity might be useful in the symptomatic control of blood pressure in essential hypertension. This section describes those agents that exert their antihypertensive action on the adrenergic division of the autonomic nervous system. These drugs can conveniently be divided into four groups according to their site of action: (1) agents altering adrenergic transmission, (2) selective α-adrenergic blocking agents, (3) β-adrenergic blocking agents, and (4) agents acting on the central nervous system. It should be pointed out that other drugs that alter adrenergic function, such as

MAO inhibitors and nonselective α-adrenergic receptor blocking agents, have been used in treating hypertension, but their use has been largely superseded by other drugs with somewhat less toxicity and greater effectiveness. Only those actions and side effects pertinent to the current use of these drugs in the treatment of hypertension will be described here. For discussion of other uses and actions of these drugs, see Chapter 7.

Agents altering adrenergic transmission

Guanethidine, guanadrel, and the rauwolfia alkaloids (reserpine, deserpidine, and rescinnamine) exert their primary antihypertensive action on peripheral postganglionic adrenergic nerve endings and are thus classified as adrenergic neuron blocking drugs. A detailed discussion of the chemistry of these drugs is found in Chapter 7.

Pharmacologic effects. The ultimate effect of reserpine, guanethidine, and guanadrel is depletion of norepinephrine from adrenergic nerve endings, although the mechanisms by which depletion occurs differ with each drug. The final result of the actions of these compounds on norepinephrine uptake, storage, and release is a decrease in sympathetic activity. The cardiovascular manifestations that result from these actions and make these agents useful in treating hypertension are decreases in both cardiac output and peripheral resistance.[14] Reserpine enters the central nervous system, and some of its antihypertensive action may be due to effects at this site. Guanethidine and guanadrel do not readily cross the blood-brain barrier and thus exert their actions solely on peripheral postganglionic neurons.

Absorption, fate, and excretion. Reserpine is available for oral or parenteral use. Other rauwolfia derivatives are limited to the oral route. Reserpine is readily absorbed after oral administration but exhibits a slow onset of antihypertensive action (up to 3 weeks for maximum effect). Its duration is long, probably owing to its strong binding to amine storage sites. It is excreted as the parent compound and as various metabolites.

Available for oral or parenteral use, guanethidine is poorly absorbed from the gastrointestinal tract. Although absorption varies among individuals from 3% to 30%, it is usually consistent in a given patient. Guanethidine and its metabolites are rapidly excreted in the urine, but small amounts remain in the tissues for prolonged periods (2 weeks). Guanadrel is available in oral dosage form only.

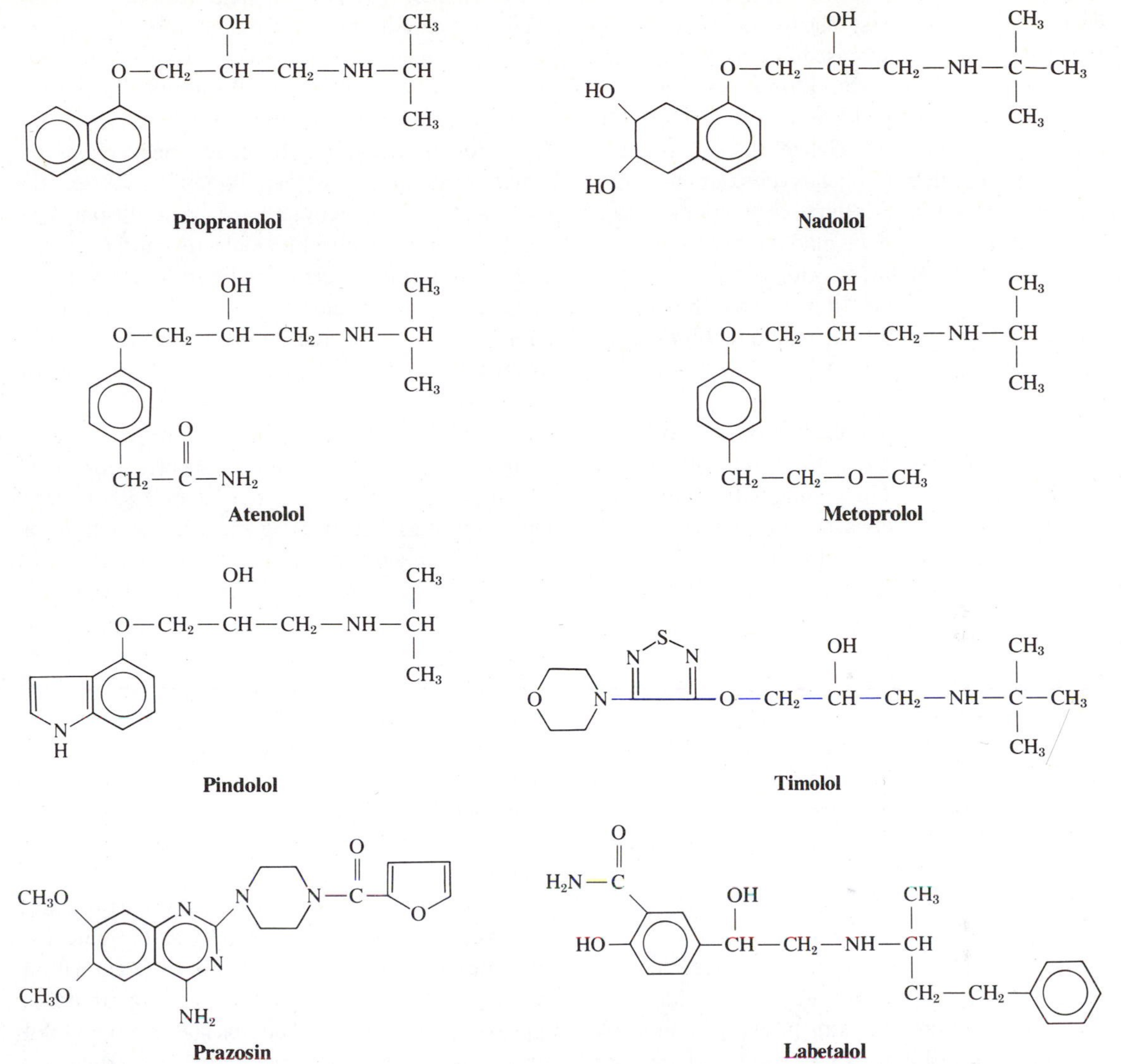

Figure 28-3. Structures of some α- and β-adrenergic receptor blocking drugs.

Toxic reactions and side effects. The most frequent untoward actions of the rauwolfia alkaloids are results of actions on either the central nervous system or the gastrointestinal tract. Although sedation caused by reserpine may be beneficial in hypertension, nightmares and psychic depression leading to suicidal tendencies are clearly undesirable. Abdominal cramps and diarrhea result because reserpine places the gastrointestinal tract under the sole control of the parasympathetic nervous system. Another annoying, but not serious, side effect of reserpine is nasal congestion.[35] In addition, several studies have indicated that long-term rauwolfia therapy may increase the incidence of carcinoma of the breast in women.[1,3,20] This claim has been questioned, however.[29]

The major troublesome side effect of guanethidine and guanadrel is orthostatic hypotension. This effect is an extension of the antihypertensive action of these compounds and occurs in nearly all patients treated. Other side effects include difficulty in ejaculation, nocturia, and intestinal cramps.

Selective α-adrenergic blocking agents

Prazosin is the first of a group of selective α-adrenergic blocking agents used for the treatment of hypertension. Other drugs with similar actions include trimazosin and tiodazosin. The chemical structure of prazosin is shown in Figure 28-3.

Pharmacologic effects. The hypotensive effect of prazosin is ascribed to vasodilation of arterioles and capacitance veins. This action is thought to occur as a result of blockade of α_1 receptors on vascular smooth muscle.[37] Unlike older, nonselective α blockers such as phenoxybenzamine, prazosin does not strongly inhibit α_2 receptors. This compound can be used in mild to moderate hypertension, either alone or with diuretics or β-receptor blocking agents. An increase in heart rate is seen with prazosin, but not as frequently as with hydralazine. For a complete description of prazosin see Chapter 7.

Absorption, fate, and excretion. Prazosin is absorbed from the gastrointestinal tract and is available only for oral use. The plasma half-life of prazosin (about 2 hours) does not correlate with the hypotensive action because of tissue binding. It is excreted principally as glucuronide conjugates, with approximately 90% appearing in the feces and 10% in the urine.[22]

Toxic reactions and side effects. Prazosin produces less reflex tachycardia than do direct vasodilators or other α-adrenergic blockers,[28] but it has been reported to precipitate anginal attacks.[26] Although orthostatic hypotension is rarely seen, postural dizziness has been reported, suggesting some orthostasis.

β-Adrenergic blocking drugs

An increasing number of drugs that specifically block β-adrenergic receptors are now available in the United States, and the structures of several of these are shown in Figure 28-3. The prototype for the β-adrenergic receptor blocking drugs is propranolol. It and the other drugs in its class are not only used as antihypertensives but are employed in other disorders, such as cardiac arrhythmias, angina pectoris, and migraine headache. As indicated in Chapter 7, some of these agents such as propranolol competitively block β_1 and β_2 receptors, whereas others such as metoprolol appear to have a selective effect on the β_1 receptors of the heart (cardioselective) and less affinity for β_2 receptors (Table 28-4). β-Adrenergic blocking drugs may also have a partial adrenergic agonistic action and exert a membrane stabilizing effect analogous to that of the local anesthetics (Table 28-4). Since the local anesthetic action of the β-blocking agents occurs at doses higher than those used clinically, it may not be clinically relevant.[17]

Pharmacologic effects. The various β-adrenergic blocking drugs are about equally effective in the management of hypertension. They can be used alone or in combination with diuretics and other antihypertensive medications. Although much information is available, the exact mechanisms by which these drugs decrease blood pressure remain equivocal.[17] Their actions have been attributed to the following effects: blockade of cardiac β_1 receptors resulting in decreased cardiac output and resetting of baroceptors; decreased central sympathetic outflow; decreased renin secretion; sensitization of vascular adenylate cyclase to activation by nonadrenergic stimuli; and blockade of prejunctional β receptors on adrenergic nerve endings. Some investigators believe that hypertension characterized by high cardiac output or high plasma renin activities represents a specific indication for adrenergic antagonist therapy.[5] Individual β antagonists that exhibit some intrinsic agonist action produce less bradycardia (Table 28-4). Cardioselective β antagonists, having less affinity for bronchial β_2 adrenoreceptors, are less likely to precipitate asthmatic attacks in prone individuals. The same could be expected for those agents with intrinsic sympathomimetic activity.

Absorption, fate, and excretion. Propranolol is readily absorbed from the gastrointestinal tract; it is also available for injection. About 90% of circulating propranolol is bound to plasma proteins. It is excreted in the urine partially as the glucuronide conjugate after hydroxylation or deamination in the liver. The plasma half-life of propranolol is approximately 4 hours. The dosage of propranolol for use in different disease states (hypertension, angina, arrhythmias) and among individuals varies markedly.

Metoprolol is available only in oral dosage form and is readily and rapidly absorbed from the gastrointestinal tract. Because of a significant liver first-pass elimination, only about 50% of the administered dose reaches the circulation, where about 11% is bound to plasma proteins. It is extensively biotransformed, with only 3% being excreted unchanged by the kidney. It has a half-life of 3 to 4 hours.

Other β blockers vary as to protein binding, plasma half-life, and excretion. Unique among the currently available agents is nadolol, which has a plasma half-life of 20 to 24 hours. Its extended duration of action permits single daily dosing (Table 28-4).

Toxic reactions and side effects. β-Adrenocep-

Table 28-4. Comparison of β-adrenergic receptor blocking drugs

Nonproprietary name	Cardioselective	Intrinsic β-agonist action	Local anesthetic action	Dosing frequency (times/day)
Acebutolol*	+ +	+ +	+ +	2-3
Atenolol	+ +	—	—	1-2
Labetalol*	α and β	—	—	2-3
Metoprolol	+ +	—	—	2-3
Nadolol	—	—	—	1
Oxprenolol*	—	+ +	+ +	2-3
Pindolol	—	+ +	—	1-2
Propranolol	—	—	+ +	2-3
Timolol	—	—	—	1-2

*Not currently available for use in the United States.

tor antagonists cause a variety of side effects; tolerance may develop to some of these but not to others. Those side effects to which early tolerance may develop include nausea, vomiting, anorexia, dizziness, and bradycardia. Other CNS effects include confusion, vivid dreams, nightmares, insomnia, and depression. One of the major toxic actions of the β antagonists is the aggravation of an existing defect in myocardial contractility or atrioventricular conduction. Nonselective β blockers inhibit the glycogenolytic and lipolytic actions of endogenous catecholamines and therefore should be used with caution in patients prone to hypoglycemia or those being treated with insulin or sulfonylureas for diabetes. Blockade of β-adrenoceptor-mediated vasodilation may exacerbate peripheral arterial insufficiency, intermittent claudication, and Raynaud's phenomenon.

Abrupt withdrawal of β-adrenoceptor antagonists in patients with coronary heart disease increases the likelihood of severe ischemic events such as a myocardial infarction, an anginal attack, or an arrhythmia. Abrupt withdrawal in hypertensives may result in increased blood pressure and heart rate, palpitations, tremors, and sweating. It is important, therefore, that dosages be decreased gradually.

Salt retention, which has been a problem with some antihypertensives, has not been reported with the β-adrenergic blocking drugs. Postural hypotension is also not generally encountered, except in the case of labetalol, which has both α and β antagonistic properties.

Agents acting on the central nervous system

Methyldopa, clonidine, and guanabenz are drugs that have been shown to exert their antihypertensive effect through actions on the central nervous system. These agents alter the central control of blood pressure through effects on the cardioregulatory and vasomotor centers of the brain. The structures of methyldopa, clonidine, and guanabenz are shown in Figure 28-4. The structural similarity of methyldopa to the catecholamine transmitter norepinephrine is obvious. Clonidine and guanabenz are not chemically related to norepinephrine but are very similar in structure to tolazoline, an α-adrenergic receptor blocking agent.

Pharmacologic effects. Methyldopa appears to act as a result of its biotransformation in the brain to α-methyldopamine and then to α-methylnorepinephrine. The latter probably stimulates important α_2-adrenoceptor sites in the lower brain stem, resulting in inhibition of sympathetic outflow. In addition, there is evidence that vagal activity to the heart is increased. Clonidine and guanabenz appear to act directly as central α_2-adrenoceptor agonists. With all three drugs, the reduction in central sympathetic outflow and increased vagal activity lead to reduced peripheral vascular resistance and cardiac output.[40] Although agreement exists that these agents act through central α-agonist action, there is controversy as to whether the receptors are presynaptic or postsynaptic.

Absorption, fate, and excretion. Methyldopa can be given orally or parenterally. About 50% of an administered dose of methyldopa is absorbed from the gastrointestinal tract. Although methyldopa and its metabolites appear rapidly in the urine, significant concentrations remain in the body for longer periods. It has a relatively long duration of action (up to 24 hours), probably because α-methylnorepinephrine is not metabolized by MAO but is stored in synaptic vesicles in central adrenergic nerve terminals.

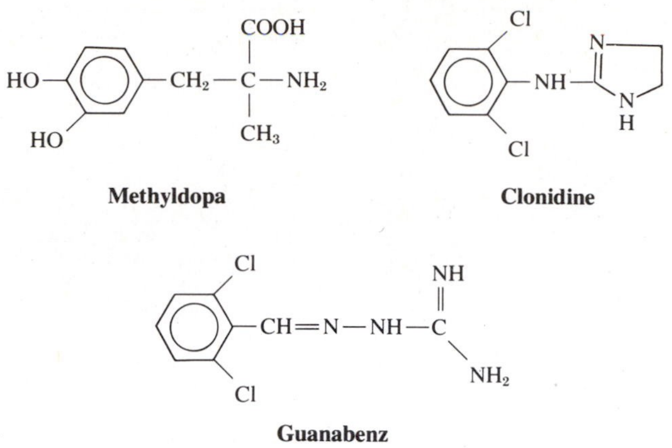

Figure 28-4. Structural formulas of centrally acting antihypertensive drugs.

Clonidine is available for both oral and parenteral use and is well absorbed after oral administration. Peak plasma concentrations are achieved in 3 to 5 hours, and its half-life is 12 to 16 hours. Clonidine is primarily excreted in the urine after metabolism.

Approximately 75% of an oral dose of guanabenz is absorbed, with peak plasma concentrations appearing between 2 and 5 hours after administration. The exact metabolic disposition of guanabenz has not been established.

Toxic reactions and side effects. Untoward effects of methyldopa include drowsiness, depression, nightmares, dry mouth, and nasal stuffiness. The drowsiness caused by this agent, though usually transient, may be particularly bothersome to patients required to do mental work. Orthostatic hypotension may occur but is less frequent than with guanethidine.

The most common side effects of clonidine are dry mouth and sedation. The incidence and severity of these effects are high, but some tolerance may develop during long-term therapy. Constipation and impotence occur in a significant number of patients treated with clonidine. Other, less frequent, side effects are allergic manifestations and orthostatic hypotension. Rebound hypertension has been observed on withdrawal of clonidine therapy.

Guanabenz has not been found to cause postural hypotension. Adverse side effects, listed in decreasing order of frequency, are drowsiness, dry mouth, dizziness, weakness, and headache.

DIRECT VASODILATORS

Hydralazine and minoxidil are considered together in this section because they exert their primary antihypertensive action through a direct effect on vascular smooth muscle. This similarity does not imply that these agents do not act through other mechanisms but only that their major action is direct vasodilation. Vascular relaxation is thought to occur through interference with calcium transport across smooth muscle cell membranes, resulting in depression of the active state of contraction.[16] Prizidilol is an antihypertensive with properties similar to hydralazine but which also exhibits nonselective β-blocking activity. It is currently under investigation.

Hydralazine

Hydralazine is one of a series of phthalazine derivatives that have been shown to reduce blood pressure and is the only agent of this series available in the United States. The chemical structure of this compound is shown in Figure 28-5.

Pharmacologic effects. Hydralazine exerts a preferential effect on arterioles as compared with veins. The resulting changes are decreased peripheral resistance, decreased blood pressure, and increased heart rate, stroke volume, and cardiac output. The preferential effect on arterioles results in a low incidence of orthostatic hypotension with this agent. The reflex inotropic and chronotropic effects that accompany hydralazine vasodilation may cause exacerbation of existing angina pectoris. Hy-

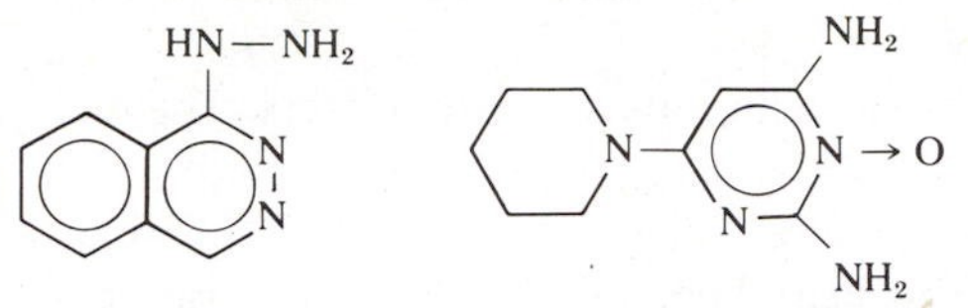

Figure 28-5. Structural formulas of hydralazine and minoxidil.

dralazine has no important actions on systems other than the cardiovascular system.

Absorption, fate, and excretion. Hydralazine is available for parenteral and oral use. It is readily absorbed from the gastrointestinal tract, and peak blood concentrations are reached in 3 to 4 hours. This drug exhibits a high affinity for vascular muscle[30] and is slowly removed from these sites. Only a small percentage of hydralazine is excreted unchanged, with the major portion undergoing ring acetylation.

Toxic reactions and side effects. A high incidence of side effects is associated with hydralazine therapy. The more common untoward effects are palpitation, headache, anorexia, nausea, dizziness, and sweating. Less frequently encountered effects include nasal congestion, flushing, tremors, and cramps. Tolerance to these effects may develop, especially if the initial dosage is increased gradually. Long-term administration of hydralazine in large doses may cause a syndrome resembling lupus erythematosus, particularly in patients who are "slow acetylators."

Minoxidil

Minoxidil is another antihypertensive drug that acts through peripheral vasodilation. The chemical structure of this piperidinopyrimidine compound is shown in Figure 28-5. Minoxidil is a potent antihypertensive agent and at this time is reserved for use in hypertension refractory to other therapy.

Pharmacologic effects. Minoxidil, like other peripheral vasodilators, reduces blood pressure by decreasing total peripheral resistance. The decrease in blood pressure is accompanied by reflex increases in both cardiac rate and output and substantial retention of fluid. These may be corrected by use of β-adrenergic blocking agents and diuretics. Minoxidil has no central depressant effects.

This compound may also impair peripheral adrenergic function, an action that appears to enhance its hypotensive effect.[12] Studies have shown minoxidil to be more effective than hydralazine in lowering blood pressure.

Absorption, fate, and excretion. The onset of action of minoxidil after oral administration is rapid, and its hypotensive action is of long duration. This compound is primarily excreted in the urine as the glucuronide conjugate, along with small amounts of the parent compound and hydroxylated derivatives.[39]

Toxic reactions and side effects. The marked fluid retention caused by minoxidil can lead to congestive heart failure. There are reports of pericardial effusion and cardiac tamponade, sometimes with fatal outcomes. As with other vasodilators, the reflex tachycardia may initiate or intensify angina. Finally, abnormal hair growth, or hypertrichosis, is very common and limits the use of this drug.

AGENTS AFFECTING THE RENIN-ANGIOTENSIN SYSTEM

As discussed earlier, the renin-angiotensin system may be etiologically involved in certain cases of hypertension. Pharmacologic intervention to reduce blood pressure can theoretically be made anywhere along the system, that is, from the release of renin by the kidney juxtaglomerular cells to the formation of angiotensin peptides to the union of angiotensins II and III with receptors in vascular smooth muscle. In the discussion that follows, attention will be limited to those agents whose primary mechanism of action is interference with this series of events. It should be recognized, however, that other antihypertensive drugs also affect the renin-angiotensin system. In general, drugs that inhibit adrenergic function also inhibit renin release, whereas diuretics and direct vasodilators stimulate renin release. Studies indicate that, regardless of the specific drug regimen, treatment of hypertension tends to restore renin to normal whether it was initially high or low.[4,25]

Saralasin

The octapeptide saralasin (1-sar-8-ala-angiotensin II) is a competitive inhibitor of vascular receptors for angiotensin II. It has been shown experimentally to lower blood pressure in patients with renin-dependent hypertension and is used clinically

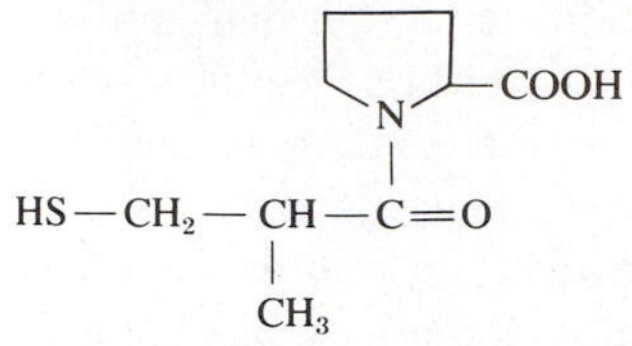

Figure 28-6. Structural formula of captopril.

to diagnose such patients. Although saralasin is limited by a lack of oral efficacy, a partial agonistic action, and a short duration of effect, it did illustrate the potential for specific therapeutic control of renovascular hypertension.[27]

Captopril

Captopril was the first clinically useful drug specifically tailored to disrupt the renin-angiotensin mechanism. Captopril is an inhibitor of peptidyl dipeptidase (the angiotensin-converting enzyme) and thus blocks the activation of angiotensin I to angiotensin II. Unlike saralasin, captopril is orally active and has a reasonable duration of action. Its structure is shown in Figure 28-6.

Pharmacologic effects. Angiotensin-converting enzyme inhibitors such as captopril markedly decrease blood concentrations of angiotensin II and induce an immediate fall in blood pressure. They may also act to maintain the lowered blood pressure by elevating bradykinin (a potent vasodilator) in the blood. (It should be noted that angiotensin-converting enzyme is also known as bradykininase II, an enzyme responsible for the breakdown of bradykinin.) Interestingly, captopril may have an antihypertensive effect even in patients without signs of major activation of the renin-angiotensin system.[17] Blood pressure is reduced mainly through decreased peripheral resistance, with little effect on cardiac output or renal blood flow. Sodium and water retention are not induced nor is orthostatic hypotension or bradycardia a problem. The efficacy of captopril appears to be equal to or greater than that of the β-adrenergic blocking agents used alone or in combination with a diuretic.[7]

Absorption, fate, and excretion. The onset of action of captopril is rapid, and the duration of effect is relatively short, requiring administration 3 times daily. Because food in the gastrointestinal tract significantly reduces the absorption of cap-

topril, the drug should be taken 1 hour before meals.

Toxic reactions and side effects. The most frequent side effects of captopril are skin rashes and loss of taste. These may disappear following continued use. The significance of reported cases of proteinuria and neutropenia is not established at this time.[17] Angioedema of the face, mucous membranes of the mouth, or extremities, and flushing, pallor, and hypotension have been documented. A few reports have indicated that angina pectoris or Raynaud's phenomenon may be precipitated.[19]

MISCELLANEOUS AGENTS

A number of drugs have limited application in the treatment of hypertension. Some of these agents, such as the ganglionic blocking drugs (e.g., mecamylamine) and the MAO inhibitors (e.g., pargyline) were once widely used but have been largely replaced by more effective or less toxic compounds. The veratrum alkaloids are unique in that they lower blood pressure by stimulating baroreceptor reflexes to decrease peripheral resistance and heart rate. Unfortunately, they induce a high incidence of nausea and vomiting in conventional doses and so are considered drugs of last refuge.

Metyrosine (α-methyltyrosine) is an inhibitor of tyrosine hydroxylase, the rate-limiting enzyme in the formation of epinephrine. Although not recommended for essential hypertension, metyrosine is useful, often in combination with a nonselective α-adrenergic blocker such as phenoxybenzamine, in the treatment of hypertension associated with pheochromocytoma.

The calcium entry blockers, represented by nifedipine, diltiazem, and verapamil, are approved for use in the United States for the treatment of angina pectoris. These agents are also being used to treat essential hypertension although they are not officially approved for this therapeutic application. This use takes advantage of their peripheral vasodilator action, which results from the prevention of calcium entry into smooth muscle fibers. Untoward effects most frequently seen are dizziness, headache, facial flushing, and nausea. The side effect that might most importantly influence dental treatment is the tendency of these agents to cause postural hypotension. It should be noted that some agents in this class are relatively safe, although others may cause severe toxic reactions (see Chapter 26).

Table 28-5. Combination antihypertensive preparations

Combined agents	Proprietary name
Amiloride, hydrochlorothiazide	Moduretic
Clonidine, chlorthalidone	Combipres
Chlorthalidone, reserpine	Regroton
Guanethidine, hydrochlorothiazide	Esimil
Hydralazine, hydrochlorothiazide	Apresazide, Apresoline-Esidrix
Methyldopa, hydrochlorothiazide	Aldoril
Prazosin, polythiazide	Minizide
Propranolol, hydrochlorothiazide	Inderide
Reserpine, hydralazine, hydrochlorothiazide	Ser-Ap-Es
Spironolactone, hydrochlorothiazide	Aldactazide
Triamterene, hydrochlorothiazide	Dyazide

Table 28-6. Drugs used in hypertensive emergencies

Classification	Nonproprietary name	Proprietary name
Peripheral vasodilators	Diazoxide	Hyperstat
	Sodium nitroprusside	Nipride
α-Adrenergic blocking agent	Phentolamine	Regitine
Ganglionic blocking agent	Trimethaphan	Arfonad

COMBINED-DRUG THERAPY FOR ESSENTIAL HYPERTENSION

Two major reasons can be given for the use of combinations of two or more drugs in the management of essential hypertension. First, agents that act through different mechanisms may have additive hypotensive effects, and, second, unwanted effects of one drug can be reduced by using it in smaller doses in combination with other agents to obtain an adequate hypotensive effect. Separate preparations of the different agents can be prescribed: there are also several fixed-dose combinations available (Table 28-5). Fixed-dose combinations are not generally recommended because they do not offer the flexibility of adjusting the dose of each agent to the patient's needs. However, in certain cases their use is justified by their convenience and by the likelihood of greater patient compliance when fewer drugs have to be taken.

Diuretics are currently the agents of choice for the initial treatment of essential hypertension. Other drugs are subsequently used in combination with diuretics, as required, to obtain an adequate hypotensive effect. Diuretics have been shown to increase the magnitude of the fall in blood pressure with almost all other antihypertensive drugs in use.[11] This effect probably occurs because most agents, other than diuretics, cause retention of salt and water.

Some other drug combinations and reasons for their use include β-receptor blocking agents used with peripheral vasodilators to minimize reflex tachycardia, centrally acting drugs used with agents that act peripherally to cause an additive hypotensive action, and potassium-sparing diuretics used with other diuretics.

DRUGS USED IN HYPERTENSIVE EMERGENCIES

In contrast to the gradual increase in blood pressure seen in essential hypertension, a sudden elevation of blood pressure to severely hypertensive levels (i.e., diastolic pressure greater than 130 mm Hg) may sometimes occur. Hypertensive emergencies may arise in the course of any hypertensive disease, including renal hypertension, toxemia of pregnancy, or pheochromocytoma. These situations, regardless of etiology, are life-threatening and require prompt treatment. It is beyond the scope of this presentation to discuss in detail the etiology of hypertensive emergencies or the pharmacologic management of these conditions. Only the agents used will be mentioned, along with a brief statement concerning their mechanism of action.

Some drugs discussed earlier in this chapter are used in hypertensive emergencies, in addition to their use in long-term therapy for essential hypertension. These include hydralazine, methyldopa, and reserpine. Other drugs used specifically in managing hypertensive emergencies are diazoxide, sodium nitroprusside, trimethaphan, and phentolamine (Table 28-6). Diazoxide is a benzothiadiazide derivative chemically related to the thiazide diuretics. It has no diuretic actions but exerts its hypotensive action through peripheral arteriolar dilation.[18] Sodium nitroprusside is another potent hypotensive agent that causes direct dilation of arteries and veins.[36] The onset of its action is rapid, and its action subsides rapidly on termination of an infusion.

Trimethaphan lowers blood pressure by competitive blockade of ACh at autonomic ganglia[14] (see Chapter 10). Like many of the other agents used in hypertensive emergencies, this compound is rapidly effective; it is usually given by infusion because of its short duration of action. Phentolamine competitively blocks the action of catecholamines at α-adrenergic receptors (see Chapter 7), leading to vasodilation and decreased blood pressure. This agent is especially useful in hypertensive emergencies associated with excess circulating levels of catecholamines such as would occur in pheochromocytoma.

ANTIHYPERTENSIVE DRUG WITHDRAWAL SYNDROME

Withdrawal of antihypertensive drug therapy has been shown to be associated wtih several signs and symptoms, depending on the abruptness of the withdrawal, the degree of hypertension, and the drugs involved. The classes of drugs reported to be involved in withdrawal reactions include centrally acting agents, β-adrenoceptor blocking drugs, neuronal blocking agents, and some vasodilators (e.g., minoxidil and sodium nitroprusside).

The symptoms of antihypertensive drug withdrawal are somewhat vague and include nervousness, agitation, tremors, palpitations, insomnia, headache, sweating, facial flushing, nausea, and vomiting; however, the clinical signs are more characteristic and include tachycardia, hypertension, diaphoresis with occasional elevation of plasma catecholamines, and rarely malignant hypertension, accelerated angina, myocardial infarction, ventricular arrhythmias, or ventricular failure. The mechanisms through which these adverse withdrawal symptoms occur seem to involve enhanced activity or supersensitivity of the physiologic systems involved (i.e., the sympathoadrenal, renin-angiotensin, or thyroid).

Recommendations for managing hypertensive patients on drug therapy include encouraging patient compliance and avoiding excessive dosage. Also the dentist can advise against abrupt withdrawal and inform the patient of the possible hazards of such action. Patients at highest risk for such problems are patients with severe hypertension who are receiving multiple drug therapy over long periods. To avoid these complications, antihypertensive drugs should be withdrawn slowly, and patients should be carefully monitored, especially those with coronary artery or cerebrovascular disease.

IMPLICATIONS FOR DENTISTRY
Drug interactions

Since there are several categories of antihypertensive drugs (each class having a different mechanism of action), there are numerous possibilities of drug interactions. Of primary significance to the dentist is the category of centrally acting agents that have a sedative side effect. When dealing with patients taking these drugs, the dentist must proceed cautiously with agents that depress the central nervous system. In combination with antihypertensives with sedative side effects, these agents may lead to excessive sedation or inability to function mentally. Use of a smaller dose is mandated in the premedication of a patient taking methyldopa, clonidine, guanabenz, or an antianxiety agent for hypertension.

The use of vasoconstrictors is *not* contraindicated in the hypertensive patient.[24] According to the American Heart Association and the American Dental Association, the use of up to 0.2 mg of epinephrine does not endanger the patient. The rationale is that if the combination of local anesthetic and vasoconstrictor is properly injected and excessive doses avoided, less catecholamine would reach the circulation than if adrenal release were stimulated because of pain in the presence of poor anesthesia. A possible exception to this statement, however, is the patient receiving an adrenergic neuron blocking drug like guanethidine. Use of guanethidine on a long-term basis produces a supersensitivity to the actions of exogenously administered catecholamines. Injudicious use of sympathomimetic amine vasoconstrictors in local anesthetic solutions or in gingival retraction cord could lead to possibly serious disturbances of blood pressure and cardiac rhythm.

Side effects

One side effect related to antihypertensive medication of significance to the dentist is orthostatic, or postural, hypotension. After being in a supine position, many patients receiving antihypertensive therapy may be unable to compensate adequately for a sudden change in position. Such patients should be observed carefully at the end of dental appointments. Drugs affecting peripheral adrenergic transmission are most likely to cause orthostatic hypotension, although other agents may also have this action.

Another side effect that may have implications in dentistry is central salivary inhibition, leading to dry mouth in patients medicated with the centrally acting antihypertensive agents methyldopa, clonidine, and guanabenz.

Hypertension detection

The American Heart Association has stressed the need for more effective hypertension detection, and dentists are encouraged to include blood pressure determinations as a part of routine office visits. Studies indicate that many patients identified by dentists as being hypertensive were unaware of their condition.[2] A majority of those identified sought medical attention in an attempt to treat the hypertension.

Screening for hypertension in the dental office is a simple procedure that can be carried out effectively by auxiliary personnel. Because hypertension is a dangerous but asymptomatic disease in its early stages, the dentist's efforts to identify and aid these patients by its detection will be worthwhile.

Antihypertensive drugs

Nonproprietary name	Proprietary name
Diuretics	
see Chapter 27	
Agents affecting adrenergic function	
Transmitter synthesis inhibiting	
metyrosine	Demser
Neuronal blocking	
alseroxylon	Rauwiloid
deserpidine	Harmonyl
guanadrel	Hylorel
guanethidine	Ismelin
pargyline	Eutonyl Filmtabs
rescinnamine	Moderil
reserpine	Serpasil
whole root rauwolfia	Rauwolfia
α-*Adrenergic blocking*	
phenoxybenzamine	Dibenzyline
phentolamine	Regitine
prazosin	Minipress
tolazoline	Prescoline
β-*Adrenergic blocking*	
acebutolol*	—
atenolol	Tenormin
metoprolol	Lopressor
nadolol	Corgard
oxprenolol*	Trasicor
pindolol	Visken
propranolol	Inderal
timolol	Blocadren
α- *and* β-*adrenergic blocking*	
labetalol*	Trandate

Nonproprietary name	Proprietary name
Ganglionic blocking	
mecamylamine	Inversine
trimethaphan	Arfonad
Centrally acting	
clonidine	Catapres
guanabenz	Wytensin
methyldopa	Aldomet
Direct vasodilators	
diazoxide	Hyperstat IV
hydralazine	Apresoline
minoxidil	Loniten
nitroprusside	Nipride
Inhibitors of the renin-angiotensin system	
captopril	Capoten
enalapril*	—
saralasin	Sarenin
Miscellaneous	
cryptenamine	Unitensen
veratrum viride alkaloids	Vera-67

*Not currently available in the United States.

CITED REFERENCES

1. Armstrong, B., Stevens, N., and Doll, R. Retrospective study of the association between use of rauwolfia derivatives and breast cancer in English women. Lancet **2:**672-675, 1974.
2. Berman, C.L., Guarino, M.A., and Giovannoli, S.M. High blood pressure detection by dentists. Journal of the American Dental Association **87:**359-363, 1973.
3. Boston Collaborative Drug Surveillance Program. Reserpine and breast cancer. Lancet **2:**669-671, 1974.
4. Brown, T.C., Lever, A.F., and Robertson, J.I.S. Plasma renin concentration in human hypertension. American Heart Journal **74:**413-418, 1967.
5. Bühler, F.R., Laragh, J.H., Baer, L., Vaughan, E.D., Jr., and Brunner, H.R. Propranolol inhibition of renin secretion: a specific approach to diagnosis and treatment of renin-dependent hypertensive diseases. New England Journal of Medicine **287:**1209-1214, 1972.
6. Brunner, H.R., Gavras, H., Waeber, B., Kershaw, G.R., Turini, G.A., Vukovich, R.A., McKinstry, D.N., and Gavras, I. Oral angiotensin-converting enzyme inhibitor in long-term treatment of hypertensive patients. Annals of Internal Medicine **90:**19-23, 1979.
7. Brunner, H.R., Gavras, H., Waeber, B., Turini, G.A., McKinstry, D.N., Vukovich, R.A., and Gavras, I. Orally active angiotensin-converting enzyme inhibitor (SQ14, 225) as a treatment for essential hypertension. British Journal of Clinical Pharmacology **7:**205S-211S, 1979.
8. Caldwell, J.R. Perspectives in hypertension—1976. Geriatrics **31:**46-47, 1976.
9. Chobanian, A.V. Hypertension: major risk factor for cardiovascular complications. Geriatrics **31:**87-95, 1976.
10. Davis, J.O., and Freeman, R.H. Mechanisms regulating renin release. Physiological Reviews **56:**1-56, 1976.
11. Dollery, C.T. Pharmacological basis for combination ther-

apy of hypertension. Annual Review of Pharmacology and Toxicology **17:**311-323, 1977.

12. DuCharme, D.W., Freyburger, W.A., Graham, B.E., and Carlson, R.G. Pharmacologic properties of minoxidil: a new hypotensive agent. Journal of Pharmacology and Experimental Therapeutics **184:**662-670, 1973.

13. Esler, M., Julius, S., Zweifler, A., Randall, O., Harburg, E., Gardiner, H., and DeQuattro, V. Mild high-renin essential hypertension. Neurogenic human hypertension? New England Journal of Medicine **296:**405-411, 1977.

14. Frohlich, E.D. Inhibition of adrenergic function in the treatment of hypertension. Archives of Internal Medicine **133:**1033-1048, 1974.

15. Gavras, H., and Brunner, H.R. Essential hypertension. In Brunner, H.R., and Gavras, H., eds. Clinical Hypertension and Hypotension, vol 2. New York, Marcel Dekker, Inc., 1982.

16. Gottlieb, T.B., and Chidsey, C.A. The clinician's guide to pharmacology of antihypertensive agents. Geriatrics **31:**99-110, 1976.

17. Haeusler, G.W. A catalog of available antihypertensive agents. In Brunner, H.R., and Gavras, H., eds. Clinical Hypertension and Hypotension, vol. 2. New York, Marcel Dekker, Inc., 1982.

18. Hamby, W.M., Jankowski, G.J., Pouget, J.M., Dunea, G., and Gantt, C.L. Intravenous use of diazoxide in the treatment of severe hypertension. Circulation **37:**169-174, 1968.

19. Hayes, A.H., Jr., and Novitch, M. Captopril approved for hypertension. FDA Drug Bulletin **11:**10-11, 1981.

20. Heinonen, O.P., Shapiro, S., Tuominen, L., and Turunen, M.I. Reserpine use in relation to breast cancer. Lancet **2:**675-677, 1974.

21. Henry, J.P. Understanding the early pathophysiology of essential hypertension. Geriatrics **31:**59-72, 1976.

22. Hess, H. Prazosin: biochemistry and structure-activity studies. Postgraduate Medicine **58**(suppl.):9-17, 1975.

23. Hollander, W. Role of hypertension in atherosclerosis and cardiovascular disease. American Journal of Cardiology **38:**786-800, 1976.

24. Jastak, J.T., and Yagiela, J.A. Vasoconstrictors and local anesthesia: a review and rationale for use. The Journal of the American Dental Association **107:**623-630, 1983.

25. Johnston, C.I. Effect of antihypertensive drugs on the renin-angiotensin system. Drugs **12:**274-291, 1976.

26. Kellaway, G.S.M. Adverse drug reactions during treatment of hypertension. Drugs **11**(suppl. 1):91-99, 1976.

27. Laragh, J.H., Sealey, J.E., Bühler, F.R., Vaughan, E.D., Jr., Brunner, H.R., Gavras, H., and Baer, L. The renin axis and vasoconstriction volume analysis for understanding and treating renovascular and renal hypertension. American Journal of Medicine **58:**4-13, 1975.

28. Lund-Johansen, P. Hemodynamic changes at rest and during exercise in long-term prazosin therapy of essential hypertension. In Cotton, D.W.K., ed. Prazosin—evaluation of a new antihypertensive agent. Excerpta Medica Foundation International Congress Series **331:**43-51, 1974.

29. Mack, T.M., Henderson, B.E., Gerkins, V.R., Arthur, M., Babtista, J., and Pike, M.C. Reserpine and breast cancer in a retirement community. New England Journal of Medicine **292:**1366-1371, 1975.

30. Moore-Jones, D., and Perry, H.M., Jr. Radioautographic localization of hydralazine-1-C_{14} in arterial walls. Pro-

ceedings of the Society for Experimental Biology and Medicine **122:**576-579, 1966.

31. Page, I.H. Arterial hypertension in retrospect. Circulation Research **34:**133-142, 1974.

32. Peach, M.J. Renin-angiotensin system: biochemistry and mechanism of action. Physiological Reviews **57:**313-370, 1977.

33. Philipp, T., Distler, A., and Cordes, U. Sympathetic nervous system and blood pressure control in essential hypertension. Lancet **2:**959-963, 1978.

34. Remington, R.D. Blood pressure: the population burden. Geriatrics **31:**48-54, 1976.

35. Riddiough, M.A. Preventing, detecting, and managing adverse reactions of antihypertensive agents in the ambulant patient with essential hypertension. American Journal of Hospital Pharmacy **34:**465-479, 1977.

36. Rowe, G.G., and Henderson, R.H. Systemic and coronary hemodynamic effects of sodium nitroprusside. American Heart Journal **87:**83-87, 1974.

37. Schirger, A., and Sheps, S.G. Prazosin—new hypertensive agent. Journal of the American Medical Association **237:**989-991, 1977.

38. Shaper, A.G. Communities without hypertension. In Shaper, A.G., Hutt, M.S.R., and Fejfar, J., eds. Cardiovascular Disease in the Tropics. London, British Medical Association, 1974.

39. Thomas, R.C., and Harpootlian, H. Metabolism of minoxidil, a new hypotensive agent. II. Biotransformation following oral administration to rats, dogs, and monkeys. Journal of Pharmaceutical Sciences **64:**1366-1371, 1975.

40. Walker, B.R., Deitch, M.W., Schneider, B.E., and Hare, L.E. Comparative antihypertensive effects of guanabenz and methyldopa. Clinical Therapeutics **4:**275-284, 1981.

GENERAL REFERENCES

A.M.A. Drug Evaluations, ed. 5. Chicago, American Medical Association, 1983.

Blaschke, T.F., and Melmon, K.L. Antihypertensive agents and the drug therapy of hypertension. In Gilman, A.G., Goodman, L.S., and Gilman, A., eds. Goodman and Gilman's The Pharmacological Basis of Therapeutics, ed. 6. New York, Macmillan, Inc., 1980.

Brater, D.C., and Morrelli, H.F. Cardiovascular drug interactions. Annual Review of Pharmacology and Toxicology **17:**293-309, 1977.

Brogden, R.N., Heel, R.C., Speight, T.M., and Avery, G.S. Metoprolol: a review of its pharmacological properties and therapeutic efficacy in hypertension and angina pectoris. Drugs **14:**321-348, 1977.

Brunner, H.R., and Gavras, H., eds. Clinical Hypertension and Hypotension, vol. 2. New York, Marcel Dekker, Inc., 1982.

Caldwell, J.R. Drug regimens for long-term therapy of hypertension. Geriatrics **31:**115-119, 1976.

Cohen, L.A. Synopsis of Medicine in Dentistry. Philadelphia, Lea & Febiger, 1977.

Cummings, D.M., and Vlasses, P.H. Antihypertensive drug withdrawal syndrome. Drug Intelligence and Clinical Pharmacy **16:**817-822, 1982.

Davies, D.S., and Reid, J.L. Central Action of Drugs in Blood Pressure Regulation. Baltimore, University Park Press, 1975.

Frishman, W.H. Drug therapy: β-adrenoceptor antagonists: new drugs and new indications. New England Journal of Medicine **305:**500-506, 1981.

Hansson, L. The use of propranolol in hypertension: a review. Postgraduate Medical Journal **52**(suppl. 4):77-80, 1976.

Koch-Weser, J. Drug therapy: metoprolol. New England Journal of Medicine **301:**698-703, 1979.

Messerli, F.H. Individualization of antihypertensive therapy: an approach based on hemodynamics and age. Journal of Clinical Pharmacology **21:**517-58, 1981.

Onesti, G., Fernandes, M., and Kim, K.E. Regulation of Blood Pressure by the Central Nervous System. New York, Grune & Stratton, Inc., 1975.

Pascual, A.V. How to manage hypertensive emergencies and urgencies. Geriatrics **31:**123-130, 1976.

Perloff, D. Diagnostic assessment of the patient with hypertension. Geriatrics **31:**77-83, 1976.

Romankiewicz, J.A. Pharmacology and clinical use of drugs in hypertensive emergencies. American Journal of Hospital Pharmacy **34:**185-193, 1977.

29 Lipid-lowering drugs

James L. Matheny

Atherosclerosis is probably the leading cause of death in the United States. The major clinical sequelae of this disorder of the circulatory system are coronary heart disease, cerebral vascular disease, and peripheral vascular disease.

PATHOPHYSIOLOGY OF ATHEROSCLEROSIS

Atherosclerosis is characterized by the occurrence of atheromatous plaques in large- and medium-sized arteries. These plaques are lesions found in the intimal wall of the vessels and have been shown to contain deposits of lipid. The particular clinical manifestation of atherosclerosis depends on the degree to which the lesions have progressed in a particular part of the vasculature, that is, the aorta or the coronary, peripheral (especially of the legs), cerebral, or renal arteries. The presence of atheromatous lesions can have several effects on the circulation to a prescribed area: (1) blood flow may actually be obstructed, (2) vascular reactivity, and thus control of blood flow, may be lost, or (3) vessels become weakened and may be more likely to rupture. It is believed by some that this disease begins at an early age and progresses gradually, with clinical symptoms appearing much later.[24]

Role of lipids in atherosclerosis

The presence of lipid deposits as integral components of arterial plaque formations has been known for many years, and many studies have been carried out to determine whether the concentrations of circulating lipids are involved in the origin or progress of plaque formation. These studies have shown that plasma cholesterol,[11] triglyceride,[1] and low-density lipoprotein (LDL)[12] concentrations are higher in patients with coronary artery disease than in normal patients.[15] Although there is controversy at this time about the importance of the different classes of lipids in the pathogenesis of atherosclerosis, evidence strongly indicates a major pathologic role for lipids as a group in this disease process.

Most lipids present in plasma are found as lipoprotein complexes. In hyperlipidemia, the concentration of one or more lipoproteins is elevated. Hyperlipidemia may be genetic in origin or may result from diet or some unknown cause. Classification of plasma lipoproteins is based on the ratio of lipid to protein and thus density, with the lower density indicating higher lipid content. A summary of the various types of hyperlipidemias is provided in Table 29-1. It is beyond the scope of this chapter to discuss in detail the relationships between the different lipoproteins, cholesterol, and triglycerides. The reader is referred to other sources for more complete coverage of this topic.[14,17,18] It can be stated, however, that hypercholesteremia can result from elevation of any of the lipoprotein families, whereas hypertriglyceridemia can result from increased concentrations of chylomicrons, very low density lipoproteins (VLDL), or intermediate low density lipoproteins (ILDL), alone or in various combinations. The lipid-lowering drugs will be discussed in terms of their effects on the five main lipoprotein classes: chylomicrons, VLDL, LDL, ILDL, and high density lipoproteins (HDL).

Chylomicrons originate in the intestine and are primarily composed of recently absorbed dietary triglycerides. Chylomicrons serve to transport dietary lipids to the sites of use and storage. On reaching the capillary endothelium of tissues such as fat and muscle, the chylomicron triglycerides are rapidly degraded to fatty acids, glycerol, and monoglycerides by the enzyme lipoprotein lipase.

Table 29-1. Hyperlipoproteinemias: types and characteristics

	Lipoprotein increased*	Incidence	Genetics	Age of onset	Clinical manifestations	Therapy†
Type I	Chylomicrons, VLDL‡	Rare	Autosomal recessive	Childhood	Eruptive xanthomas, hepatosplenomegaly, lipemia retinalis, abdominal pain, low incidence of cardiovascular disease	Low fat diet
Type II	LDL,§ sometimes VLDL	Very common	Simple mendelian dominant	Childhood or adulthood	Xanthomas, arcus cornea, xanthelasma, early, severe atherosclerosis	Low cholesterol and saturated fat diet, lipid-lowering drugs
Type III	ILDL‖	Uncommon	Autosomal recessive	Adulthood	Xanthomas, high incidence of coronary and peripheral atherosclerosis	Weight reduction, low cholesterol and carbohydrate diet, lipid-lowering drugs
Type IV	VLDL	Most common	?	Adulthood	Obesity, abdominal pain, arcus cornea, coronary atherosclerosis	Weight reduction, low carbohydrate diet, lipid-lowering drugs
Type V	Chylomicrons, VLDL	Uncommon	?	Early adulthood	Obesity, abdominal pain, lipemia retinalis, xanthomas, hepatosplenomegaly, infrequent cardiovascular disease	Weight reduction, low fat and carbohydrate diet, lipid-lowering drugs

*Cholesterol and triglyceride concentrations are increased to variable degrees among the types of hyperlipoproteinemias.
†See Table 29-2 for specific lipid-lowering agents used in different hyperlipoproteinemias.
‡Very low density lipoproteins.
§Low density lipoproteins.
‖Intermediate low density lipoproteins.

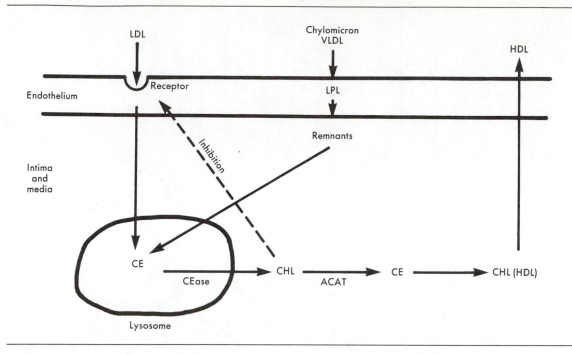

Figure 29-1. Vascular lipoprotein metabolism and cholesterol regulation. LDL is absorbed through a receptor-assisted mechanism and is metabolized to yield cholesteryl esters (CE). Chylomicrons and VLDL may also contribute to intracellular CE stores. Under the influence of lysosomal acid cholesterol esterase (CEase), cholesterol (CHL) is made available to the cell. Cholesterol limits its own intracellular concentration by inhibiting LDL-receptor synthesis, by stimulating its reconversion to CE via the enzyme acyl CoA cholesterol acyl transferase (ACAT), and by blocking its endogenous synthesis. Cholesterol products may also leave the cell to re-enter the bloodstream in the form of HDL.

The remaining chylomicron remnants are then removed by the liver. VLDL originates in the liver and small intestine and, like chylomicrons, is primarily triglyceride in composition and is metabolized by lipoprotein lipase. ILDL is essentially a transitional form in the catabolism of VLDL and has a short plasma half-life. LDL is the final product of the intravascular metabolism of VLDL. An increase in LDL may be caused either by overproduction of its VLDL precursor or, more likely, by retarded clearance of LDL from the blood. The plasma half-life of LDL is much longer than that of VLDL and ILDL. LDL is removed by a wide variety of cells from the extracellular space through receptor- and non-receptor-mediated pinocytosis. Although receptor-dependent uptake predominates normally, receptor-independent catabolism is the only route available in patients with severe familial hypercholesterolemia who congenitally lack LDL receptors. LDL contains about 50% cholesterol; thus, a subject with excess LDL will usually have elevated cholesterol concentrations. LDL is also the lipoprotein group most directly associated with coronary heart disease.[17] HDL is formed in both the liver and intestine and may represent in part a chylomicron remnant form. The role of HDL in lipid transport and its sites of degradation are not clear. HDL may serve to remove cholesterol from tissues or to accept cholesterol during VLDL metabolism (Figure 29-1). HDL plasma concentrations are *inversely* related to the risk of coronary heart disease.

Studies of the protein moieties of lipoproteins, apoproteins, have shown that they play key roles in both normal and abnormal lipoprotein metabolism. The findings of these investigations will allow a more specific classification of lipoprotein disorders in the future.

Risk factors in atherosclerosis

In addition to high plasma lipid titers, there are several other risk factors that have been identified with increased incidence of atherosclerosis. Among these are hypertension, cigarette smoking, sedentary habits, obesity, and a family history of this disease or diabetes. As shown in Table 29-1, the clinical manifestations of the genetic or familial hyperlipoproteinemias are severe. The lipid-lowering agents to be discussed have proved quite useful in treating these disorders.

GOALS OF THERAPY AND DRUG TYPES

Therapy with drugs that lower plasma lipid concentrations is an attempt to delay or reverse the progression of atherosclerotic vascular disease and thus decrease the morbidity from the associated clinical manifestations of this disease.[13] All of the drugs discussed in this section have been shown to lower plasma lipid concentrations, but the classes of lipids affected by them differ. The major question of whether therapy of this type reduces morbidity caused by atherosclerosis has not been adequately answered at this time.[7,10,25]

Although the lowering of plasma lipids is of questionable benefit in avoiding the long-term complications of ischemic disease, enough clinical and experimental evidence supports the idea that correction or lowering of plasma lipid concentrations may be beneficial in some patients. These drugs are definitely helpful in treating familial lipid abnormalities, and they are also recommended for use in patients with hyperlipidemias of unknown etiology that cannot be corrected by diet alone. The goal of therapy is to reduce lipid titers as much as possible without producing hypolipidemia or adverse effects of the drugs. Since lipid concentrations, even in the broad normal range, correlate with the incidence of ischemic heart disease, treatment of individuals with hyperlipidemias of familial or unknown origin may be indicated. Altering the diet is the initial therapeutic measure. Then, depending on other factors such as age, sex, presence of ischemic vascular disease, or coexistence of other risk factors (see above), drugs may be prescribed. Obviously, no simple answer can be given as to when therapy should be recommended. For this question, the reader is referred to other sources.[3,9]

The hypolipidemic drugs most frequently used can be grouped in six major categories: (1) clofibrate, (2) gemfibrozil, (3) nicotinic acid or esters of nicotinic acid, (4) bile acid sequestrants, (5) probucol, and (6) thyroid-active substances. The effects of these drugs on the various classes of lipoproteins are shown in Table 29-2.

Clofibrate

Clofibrate is the ethyl ester of p-chlorophenoxyisobutyric acid. Its structural formula is shown in Figure 29-2. Clofibrate treatment lowers elevated plasma cholesterol and triglyceride concentrations in a majority of patients.[21,22] It also has been shown to lower the plasma free fatty acid concentration[19] and inhibit lipolysis in adipose tissue.[5] Thus, its hypolipidemic effect results from alterations of lipid metabolism. In general, clofibrate reduces plasma ILDL, VLDL, and LDL, but there are some differences in effect depending on the lipid abnormality being treated.[3] Clofibrate is the drug of choice for type III hyperlipoproteinemia. Infrequent side effects of clofibrate therapy are nausea, diarrhea, muscle cramps, and cholelithiasis. Clofibrate potentiates the effects of coumarin anticoagulants, perhaps by displacing them from protein binding sites, and it may have similar effects on other protein-bound drugs, such as phenytoin. An association with increased risk of cardiovascular complications (e.g., angina pectoris, arrhythmias, and peripheral vascular disease) and other disorders (e.g., pancreatitis) has restricted the use of clofibrate to patients with severe hyperlipoproteinemia.

Gemfibrozil

Gemfibrozil is a new antihyperlipidemic agent related in some respects to clofibrate (Figure 29-3). The drug has been shown to lower triglycerides, cholesterol, VLDL, and LDL in patients with types IV and V hyperlipoproteinemias. It may also increase HDL in these patients. Gemfibrozil inhibits peripheral lipolysis and decreases the hepatic extraction of free fatty acids, thus reducing hepatic triglyceride production. In addition, it inhibits synthesis of VLDL and may act through other mechanisms as well. Principal side effects of gemfibrozil include abdominal pain, diarrhea, nausea, epigastric pain, rash, and vomiting. Less frequent adverse effects are headache, dizziness, anemia, eosinophilia, and leukopenia. Like clofibrate, gemfibrozil enhances the action of oral anticoagulants and may cause cholelithiasis.

Nicotinic acid

In large doses (>1 gm) nicotinic acid (niacin or vitamin B_3) reduces plasma cholesterol and triglyceride concentrations.[2,4] Nicotinamide, on the other hand, does not, nor do other B vitamins. At least initially, nicotinic acid, like clofibrate, lowers the free fatty acid concentration and thus exerts its

Table 29-2. Properties of lipid-lowering drugs

	Lipoprotein concentrations	Plasma cholesterol concentrations	Plasma triglyceride concentrations	Indications for use	Toxicity	Drug interactions
Clofibrate	↓ILDL, ↓VLDL, ↓LDL	↓	↓	Type III, IV, V	Nausea, diarrhea, myositis, abnormal liver function tests, ventricular ectopy	Enhanced effect of coumarin anticoagulants
Gemfibrozil	↓LDL, ↓VLDL, ↑HDL	↓	↓	Type IV, V	Abdominal pain, epigastric pain, diarrhea, nausea, vomiting, flatulence, dermatitis, headache, dizziness, anemia, eosinophilia, leukopenia	Enhanced effect of coumarin anticoagulants
Cholestyramine	↓LDL, possible ↑ VLDL	↓	May increase modestly in some patients	Type II	Constipation, nausea, hyperchloremic acidosis, biliary-tract calcification, steatorrhea	Decreased absorption of phenylbutazone, thiazides, tetracycline, phenobarbital, thyroxine, digitalis, coumarins
Nicotinic acid	↓VLDL, ↑HDL, ↓LDL, ↓chylomicrons	↓	↓	Type II, III, IV, V	Flushing, pruritus, nausea, diarrhea, glucose intolerance, hyperuricemia, hepatotoxicity	Increased antihypertensive action of ganglionic blocking agents
Dextro-thyroxine	↓LDL, ↓ILDL	↓		Type II	Increased metabolic rate, increased incidence of angina and cardiac irritability in patients with heart disease, glucose intolerance, neutropenia	Enhanced effect of coumarin anticoagulants, catecholamines
Probucol	↓LDL	↓		Type II	Diarrhea, flatulence, abdominal pain, nausea, excess perspiration, angioedema	

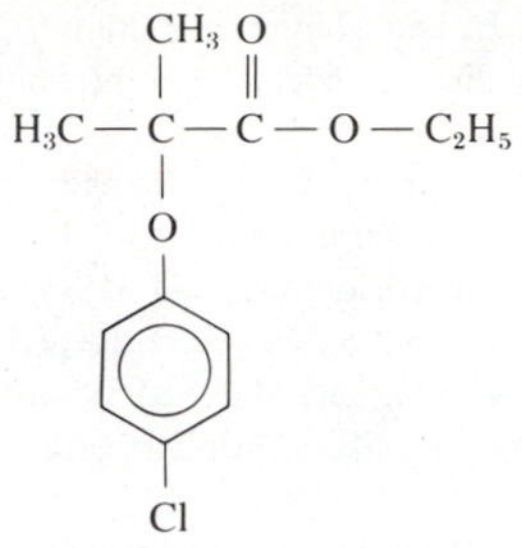

Figure 29-2. Structural formula of clofibrate.

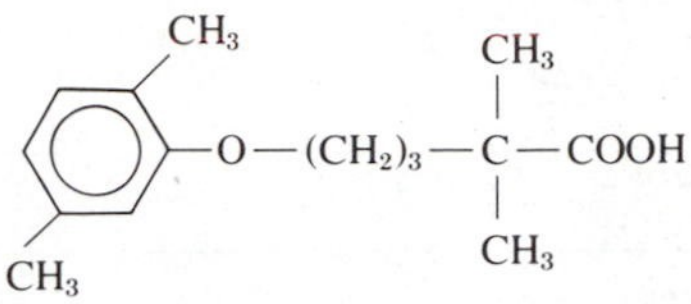

Figure 29-3. Structural formula of gemfibrozil.

hypolipidemic effect through alterations in fat metabolism. In contrast to clofibrate, the lipid-lowering effect of nicotinic acid is more dose dependent, allowing better control of therapy.[3] Nicotinic acid reduces the plasma concentrations of VLDL, LDL, and chylomicrons. The major disadvantages of nicotinic acid, compared with clofibrate, are its side effects: cutaneous flushing, pruritus, and gastrointestinal distress. If treatment is instituted slowly, with gradually increasing dosage, tolerance to the cutaneous flushing occurs, and therapy can be continued. Withdrawal of therapy is most frequently necessitated by gastric disturbances. Other side effects are hyperuricemia, decreased glucose tolerance, and abnormal liver function tests.

Bile acid sequestrants

Bile acid sequestrants are anion exchange resins that exchange chloride ions for bile acids in the intestinal lumen, and by binding the bile acids they prevent their reabsorption and promote their excretion in the feces. Since bile acids are synthesized in the liver from cholesterol, cholesterol catabolism is accelerated, and plasma cholesterol concentrations are decreased. Cholestyramine is one of the more widely used drugs in this category. Its structural formula is shown in Figure 29-4. Plasma LDL concentrations are decreased by cholestyramine, whereas VLDL may be unchanged or may increase.[16] The adverse effects of this drug are primarily gastrointestinal and include nausea, vomiting, abdominal distension, and sometimes long-term constipation. All drugs in this category may bind, decrease the absorption, and thus decrease the therapeutic effect of other drugs, especially acidic agents such as warfarin, thyroxine, digitalis, thiazides, and tetracycline. This interaction

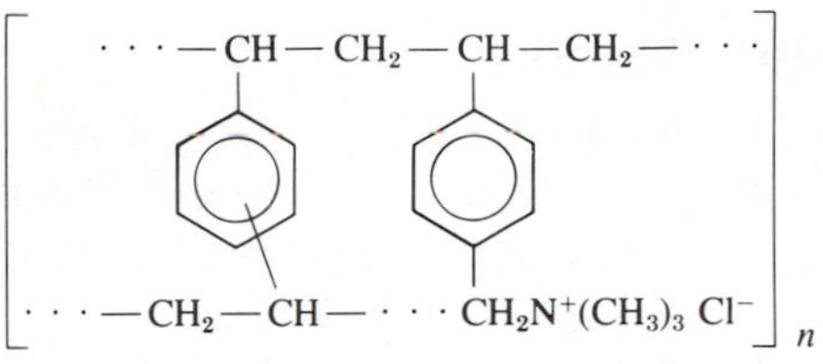

Figure 29-4. Structural formula of cholestyramine.

can be partially overcome by proper timing of dosage.

Probucol

The chemical structure of probucol (Figure 29-5) differs from that of other lipid-lowering agents. Probucol acts through several mechanisms to lower elevated serum cholesterol and LDL concentrations and has no consistent effect on triglyceride concentrations.[20] It is poorly absorbed from the gastrointestinal tract, and there is no correlation between blood level and hypocholesterolemic effect. The most frequently encountered side effects of this compound are diarrhea, flatulence, abdominal pain, and nausea. Other more rarely seen adverse effects include excessive perspiration and angioedema.

Thyroid-active substances

Early animal experiments indicated that the dextroisomers of thyroxine and liothyronine (triiodothyronine) decrease plasma lipids with no increase of oxygen consumption, an effect that might be useful in treating hyperlipidemias.[23] However, these compounds have been shown to increase the incidence of angina pectoris and increase the death

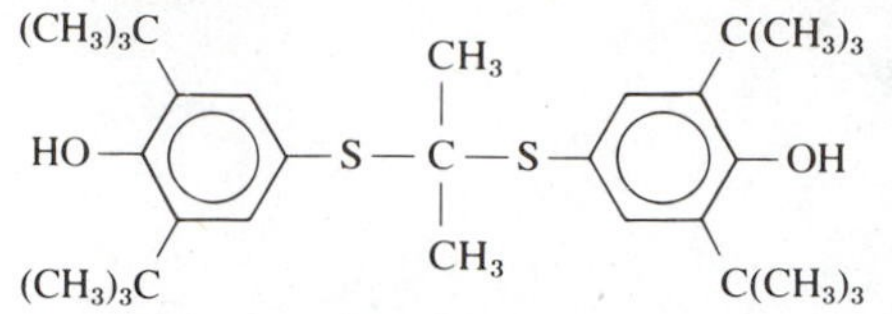

Figure 29-5. Structural formula of probucol.

rate in patients with coronary artery disease.[6] These findings restrict the use of these drugs as lipid-lowering agents and indicate that they should be employed with extreme caution, if at all, in patients with heart disease.

COMBINED-DRUG THERAPY

Lipid-lowering drugs from the different categories are used in combination for two reasons. First, combined-drug therapy may result in a more profound reduction of lipids than can be achieved by single-drug therapy. Second, as stated previously, some drugs may actually elevate certain lipids; thus, combined therapy with a drug of another category can be used to overcome this unwanted effect.

GENERAL THERAPEUTIC USES

Lipid-lowering agents are used to treat patients with familial hyperlipidemias, patients who exhibit high plasma lipid levels, and patients who have disorders believed to be secondary to sclerotic vascular disease. These compounds are most frequently administered to patients with a history of ischemic heart disease in an attempt to avoid future fatal episodes of ischemia. Although these agents are capable of lowering plasma lipid concentrations, their usefulness in decreasing deaths caused by ischemic heart disease is equivocal.[8] Dietary control of plasma lipid concentrations is preferred; if this fails, then the drugs should be considered.

Lipid-lowering drugs

Nonproprietary name	Proprietary name
cholestyramine	Questran
clofibrate	Atromid-S
colestipol	Colestid
dextrothyroxine	Choloxin
gemfibrozil	Lopid
nicotinic acid (niacin)	Nicolar
probucol	Lorelco

CITED REFERENCES

1. Albrink, M.J., and Man, E.B. Serum triglycerides in coronary artery disease. Archives of Internal Medicine **103**:4-8, 1959.
2. Altschul, R., Hoffer, A., and Stephen, J.D. Influence of nicotinic acid on serum cholesterol in man. Archives of Biochemistry and Biophysics **54**:558-559, 1955.
3. Carlson, L.A., and Olsson, A.G. Hyperlipidaemia and its management. In Oliver, M.F., ed. Modern Trends in Cardiology. Woburn, Mass., Butterworth (Publishers) Inc., 1975.
4. Carlson, L.A., Orö, L., and Östman, J. Effect of nicotinic acid on plasma lipids in patients with hyperlipoproteinemia during the first week of treatment. Journal of Atherosclerosis Research **8**:667-677, 1968.
5. Carlson, L.A., Walldius, G., and Butcher, R.W. Effect of chlorophenoxyisobutyric acid (CPIB) on fat-mobilizing lipolysis and cyclic AMP levels in rat epididymal fat. Atherosclerosis **16**:349-357, 1972.
6. Coronary Drug Project Research Group. The coronary drug project: initial findings leading to modifications of its research protocol. Journal of the American Medical Association **214**:1303-1313, 1970.
7. Coronary Drug Project Research Group. The coronary drug project: findings leading to further modifications of its protocol with respect to dextrothyroxine. Journal of the American Medical Association **220**:996-1008, 1972.
8. Coronary Drug Project Research Group. The coronary drug project: clofibrate and niacin in coronary heart disease. Journal of the American Medical Association **231**:360-381, 1975.
9. Fejfar, Z. Prevention against ischaemic heart disease: a critical review. In Oliver, M.F., ed. Modern Trends in Cardiology. Woburn, Mass., Butterworth (Publishers) Inc., 1975.
10. Friedewald, W.T., and Halperin, M. Clofibrate in ischemic heart disease. Annals of Internal Medicine **76**:821-823, 1972.
11. Gertler, M.M., Garn, S.M., and Lerman, J. The interrelationships of serum cholesterol, cholesterol esters, and phospholipids in health and in coronary artery disease. Circulation **2**:205-214, 1950.
12. Gofman, J.W., Jones, H.B., Lindgren, F.T., Lyon, T.P., Elliott, H.A., and Strisower, B. Blood lipids and human atherosclerosis. Circulation **2**:161-178, 1950.
13. Gresham, G.A. Is atheroma a reversible lesion? Atherosclerosis **23**:379-391, 1976.
14. Hayashi, E., and Tomita, T. How does hypertension accelerate atherosclerosis? A possible mechanism from changes in aortic enzymes. Trends in Pharmacological Sciences **3**:31-38, 1982.
15. Kannel, W.B., Castelli, W.P., and McNamara, P.M. The coronary profile: 12-year follow-up in the Framingham study. Journal of Occupational Medicine **9**:611-619, 1967.
16. Levy, R.I., Frederickson, D.S., Shulman, R., Bilheimer, D.W., Breslow, J.L., Stone, N.J., Lux, S.E., Sloan, H.R., Krauss, R.M., and Herbert, P.N. Dietary and drug treatment of primary hyperlipoproteinemia. Annals of Internal Medicine **77**:267-294, 1972.
17. Levy, R.I. Hypercholesterolemia: genetic, dietary, and pharmacologic interrelationships. In Selvey, N., and White, P.L., eds. Nutrition in the 1980's—The Constraints in Our Knowledge. New York, Alan R. Liss, Inc., 1981.

18. Levy, R.I., Morganroth, J., and Rifkind, B.M. Treatment of hyperlipidemia. New England Journal of Medicine **290:**1295-1301, 1974.

19. McMillan, D.C., Oliver, M.F., Simpson, J.D., and Tothill, P. Effect of ethylchlorophenoxyisobutyrate on weight, plasma volume, total body water, and free fatty acids. Lancet **2:**924-926, 1965.

20. Murphy, B.F. Probucol (Lorelco) in treatment of hyperlipidemia. Journal of the American Medical Association **238:**2537-2538, 1977.

21. Oliver, M.F. Further observations on the effects of Atromid and of ethyl chlorophenoxyisobutyrate on serum lipid levels. Journal of Atherosclerosis Research **3:**427-444, 1963.

22. Oliver, M.F. Current therapeutics. CXCV. Atromid-S and Atromid. Practitioner **192:**424-430, 1964.

23. Oliver, M.F., and Boyd, G.S. Reduction of serum cholesterol by dextrothyroxine in men with coronary heart disease. Lancet **1:**783-785, 1961.

24. Oster, K.A. Evaluation of serum cholesterol reduction and xanthine oxidase inhibition in the treatment of atherosclerosis. Recent Advanced Studies in Cardiac Structure and Metabolism **3:**73-80, 1973.

25. Veterans Administration Drug Lipid Cooperative Study Group. Failure of cholesterol-lowering drugs to influence coronary mortality: a double blind 5-year secondary prevention study. Annals of Internal Medicine **76:**868, 1972.

GENERAL REFERENCES

Benditt, E.P. The origin of atherosclerosis. Scientific American **236:**74-85, 1977.

Havel, R.J. Symposium on Lipid Disorders. Medical Clinics of North America **66:**2, 1982.

Jackson, R.L., Morrisett, J.D., and Gotto, A.M., Jr. Lipoprotein structure and metabolism. Physiological Reviews **56:**259-316, 1976.

Kritchevsky, D. Newer hypolipidemic compounds. Advances in Experimental Biology **63:**135-150, 1975.

Levy, R.I. The effect of hypolipidemic drugs on plasma lipoproteins. Annual Review of Pharmacology and Toxicology **17:**499-510, 1977.

Oliver, M.F., ed. Modern Trends in Cardiology. Woburn, Mass., Butterworth (Publishers) Inc., 1975.

Silber, E.N., and Katz, L.N. Metabolic diseases of the heart. In Silber, E.N., and Katz, L.N., eds. Heart Disease. New York, Macmillan, Inc., 1975.

30 Antianemic drugs

Thomas E. Nelson, Jr.

Hematopoiesis involves the germination and development of all the formed elements of the blood. This includes not only erythrocytes and leukocytes (neutrophils, eosinophils, basophils, monocytes, and lymphocytes) but also megakaryocytes and platelets (thrombocytes). With the exception of the lymphocytes and monocytes, which originate from lymphoid tissue including spleen, thymus, lymph glands, and tonsils, all the other blood cells are referred to as myelogenous cells because they are derived from bone marrow. Hematopoietically active bone marrow retains essentially the same mass throughout life, and although this includes practically all bones through adolescence, the active mass becomes restricted to vertebrae, sternum, and ribs after about age 20. The white cells, like the red blood cells, are dependent on the adequate intake of certain vitamins, amino acids, and other nutrients and are notably sensitive to folic acid deficiency. A deficiency in certain vital dietary constituents (e.g., iron, copper, cobalt, vitamin B_{12}, pyridoxine, and riboflavin) is often first recognized by specific anemias and accompanying neuropathies.

The blood cells are frequently the earliest biologic indicators of drug toxicity, which may take the form of granulocytopenia, hemolytic or aplastic anemia, or thrombocytopenia. Probably the most sensitive indicator of glucose-6-phosphate dehydrogenase deficiency is the blood platelet and its less readily observed precursor cell, the megakaryocyte. In addition, hemoglobin may be converted to abnormal oxidation forms that are no longer functional oxygen carriers, for example, cyanohemoglobin and methemoglobin. Table 30-1 lists some of the many drugs and common chemicals that have caused thrombocytopenia in humans. The consequences of thrombocytopenia are defective hemostasis, spontaneous hemorrhage, and purpura.

ANEMIA

Anemia is a generic term indicating a lower than normal concentration of hemoglobin per unit volume of whole blood (normally 16 gm/100 ml for men and 14 gm/100 ml for women). In clinical application, however, there are several distinct anemias that fall into the general categories of microcytic and macrocytic anemias. The term *hypochromic* implies the presence of less hemoglobin than normal in each red cell, a condition rarely occurring in the presence of normocytic (normalsized) erythrocytes but generally associated with microcytic anemias. Microcytic hypochromic anemia is usually the result of defective or inadequate iron absorption. In contrast to the iron deficiency anemias, the macrocytic (usually megaloblastic) anemias are associated with depressed DNA synthesis. Megaloblastic anemia, characterized by the presence of bone marrow germ cells, generally occurs as the result of a deficiency of vitamin B_{12} or folic acid or both, whereas normoblastic, normocytic (rarely macrocytic) anemia results from a hypoplastic or aplastic bone marrow.

Whether the anemia is microcytic-hypochromic (small cells with insufficient hemoglobin) or macrocytic, the early signs of the disease often include a sore tongue with progressive epithelial loss that gives a smooth, red appearance to the dorsal surface. The dentist may thus be able to diagnose the disease before it has caused symptoms warranting medical attention. In fact, since the oral signs frequently precede a drop in hemoglobin below the normal range, the dentist, faced with these signs, should actively encourage the patient to consult a physician. If the condition is allowed to persist, the patient may develop a serious infection, such as disseminated *Candida albicans,* or other serious systemic conditions, including thrombocytopenia and hemorrhage.

Since intuitive treatment of any disease state that

Table 30-1. Partial listing of drugs and other chemicals known to cause thrombocytopenia in humans

Acetazolamide	Meprobamate
Benzene	Phenylbutazone
Carbutamide	Quinidine
Chloramphenicol	Quinine
Chlordane	Ristocetin
Chlorothiazide	Streptomycin
Chlorpropamide	Sulfisoxazole
Colchicine	Tolbutamide
Gold salts	Trimethadione

is accompanied by extreme fatigue, weakness, and loss of color includes increased dietary intake, it is not surprising that the ancient Greeks, Hindus, and other early peoples turned to iron in many forms simply because it represented "strength." Although Sydenham is generally credited with the first rational use of iron (iron filings in wine) for treating anemia in 1681, it was not known that iron was actually present in blood until 30 years later, when Lemery and Goeffry demonstrated its presence. Shortly thereafter it was shown by an Italian physician, Menghini, that foods with iron actually increase blood iron, but it was not until about 1830 that a pill containing iron (ferrous sulfate and potassium carbonate, 1:1) was introduced into medicine by Pierre Blaud,[2] an event that marked the beginning of modern treatment of iron deficiency anemia. An excellent history is presented by Fairbanks and colleagues.[5]

As spectacular as iron therapy often appeared, some anemic patients failed to respond to Blaud's pills or other iron remedies, and their disease was described as pernicious (fatal) anemia. Although pernicious anemia was described by Addison[1] and others in the early 1800s, it remained for Minot and Murphy[9] in 1926 to demonstrate the value of raw liver in the treatment of the disease and for Castle[3] in 1927 to show that a factor in the gastric juice, intrinsic factor, plays a critical role in reversing the lethal course of pernicious anemia. The isolation of vitamin B_{12}[12,13] two decades later led to the conception that a factor in food, extrinsic factor or vitamin B_{12}, is normally bound in the stomach to intrinsic factor (a glycoprotein secreted by parietal cells). The intact complex is carried to the ileum, from which vitamin B_{12} is absorbed into the circulation, ultimately entering many tissues, particularly the liver, where it is a factor in the

production of various cells and functions as an antianemic principle. The pernicious anemia patient either lacks intrinsic factor or has antibodies to it.

In the course of an attempt to isolate extrinsic factor and to treat another form of macrocytic anemia peculiar to Hindu women, a different hematopoietic factor, folic acid (folacin or pteroylglutamic acid) was recognized and isolated.[10,15] Since the hematologic picture produced by vitamin B_{12} deficiency is almost indistinguishable from that of folic acid deficiency, it is not surprising that the paths of discovery of these two essential antianemic factors were so entwined. Both deficiencies cause an arrest of DNA synthesis. Because the nuclear DNA can no longer replicate and permit nuclear division, RNA builds up and the cells increase in size, leading to an accumulation in the bone marrow of oversized (megaloblastic) erythrocyte precursors, giant myeloid cells, and platelet precursors. The result is a slow release of abnormally large erythrocytic, leukocytic, and platelet progeny.

A combined deficiency of iron, folic acid, and vitamin B_{12} is not uncommon clinically, and in such cases the microcytic effect of iron deficiency may obscure the macrocytic nature of folate and B_{12} deficiency. Depending on the relative severity of each deficiency, there are subtle gradations between microcytic and macrocytic anemias.[7] In megaloblastic anemia, in contrast to iron deficiency disease, there is full myelogenous involvement, and the resulting leukopenia and thrombocytopenia predispose the patient to systemic infection (particularly in the urinary tract) and spontaneous hemorrhage. Another sign of B_{12} deficiency is anorexia, which of course minimizes the likelihood of proper dietary compensation.

IRON
Nutrition and physiology

Iron deficiency anemia may occur for many reasons: inadequate nutrition (qualitative or quantitative); defective absorption, transport, or storage (e.g., congenital atransferrinemia or inability to release iron from transferrin to the red blood cells and their precursors); or hemorrhage, menstruation, or pregnancy concomitant with inadequate diet. However, the iron reserves and recycling in a normal, healthy man are so effective that even extreme reduction of iron intake may be insufficient to cause severe anemia. There are continuous losses of iron through exfoliation of cells (chiefly from the gastrointestinal tract and skin) and through excretion (urine and sweat), and these total about 0.5 to 1.0 mg per day. During menstruation an extra 0.5 to 1.0 mg per day is lost, and during a normal pregnancy a woman may require as much as 1000 mg of additional iron.

Foods considered high in iron (over 0.5% by weight) are liver, heart, oysters, egg yolks, and yeast. Other meats and green vegetables have somewhat less iron. Absorption of iron from dietary sources is ordinarily 10% efficient or less, and since the normal diet contains 5 to 7 μg of iron per calorie, the need for iron supplementation in menstruating or pregnant women is not uncommon. According to a 1970 World Health Organization technical report,[6] however, women who have sufficient iron reserves to support the increase in hemoglobin production during pregnancy and who breast-feed their infants generally can maintain their iron needs by diet alone.

Iron absorption occurs along the entire length of the intestine, but maximum absorption occurs in the duodenum. This is not surprising since iron is absorbed primarily as the ferrous ion (Fe^{++}) and conversion of ferric to ferrous iron is favored by an acid medium. In the duodenum and lower portions of the gastrointestinal tract, there is a trend toward increasing alkalinity, which favors the formation of less soluble iron salts and complexes. Iron absorption is hindered by antacids, particularly calcium carbonate and aluminum or magnesium hydroxides.

Control of absorption appears to be related directly to the capacity of the intestinal mucosa to transport iron into the bloodstream, where it is bound immediately to transferrin. Although high dietary intake may cause some passive diffusion, excess iron in the mucosal epithelium is oxidized to Fe^{+++} and bound to apoferritin, thus yielding ferritin. Ferritin subsequently is excreted via the intestine when the mucosal cells are replaced by new epithelium. This binding process can control only small overloads, and high dosages of iron will increase absorption, albeit with decreased efficiency.

Attached to transferrin, iron is delivered to the bone marrow, where it is stored temporarily in reticulum cells. Without this intermediary storage in the marrow, there may be no exchange of iron from transferrin to developing erythrocytes.

The concentration of iron in the plasma at any one time represents a balance between absorption rate, storage capacity, rate of hemoglobin formation, and rate of iron excretion. Plasma iron is higher in men than in women, regardless of menstruation; it is low in iron deficiency anemia and high in pernicious anemia and folate deficiency. Total body iron constitutes only $\frac{1}{20,000}$ (3.5 gm) of body weight. About two thirds of this is in the form of hemoglobin; the rest is in myoglobin, ferritin, transferrin, and heme enzymes or is attached to ferritin and hemosiderin and sequestered in the reticuloendothelial cells of the liver, bone marrow, and spleen (Figure 30-1). Stored iron varies with intake and demand, averaging about 400 mg in women and 1000 mg in men. Excessive blood loss depletes heme iron, whereas excessive turnover of erythrocytes releases it. The normal person can lose as much as a quarter to a third of the erythrocyte mass through hemorrhage without need for iron therapy. This amounts to a loss of 200 to 250 gm of hemoglobin and thus about 600 to 800 mg of iron in a 70 kg man.

Therapeutic use

Iron therapy is indicated in iron deficiency anemia; it is contraindicated in anemia of any other etiology. Although parenteral iron preparations are available, they are not generally used because of the simplicity of oral medication. Iron should be administered parenterally if the oral preparations are inadequately absorbed or poorly tolerated, as in patients with enteritis or colitis, or if it is necessary to quickly replace a serious iron deficit. The greatest drawbacks to parenteral administration are the discomfort (intramuscular injection can cause prolonged pain), the risk, and the expense.

Iron is available in the form of ferrous salts (sulfate, gluconate, and fumarate), which are well absorbed, and ferric compounds, which are not as well absorbed. The most commonly used ferrous preparation, and the agent of choice for uncomplicated iron deficiency anemia, is ferrous sulfate. It is normally given in doses much larger than should theoretically be needed because of its limited absorption (no more than 15%). The response to oral iron preparations is usually evident in 5 to 10 days and is first manifested as an increase in reticulocytes.

Adverse effects associated with orally administered iron are gastrointestinal symptoms, chiefly nausea and vomiting, because of the direct irritation of the stomach. Although the drug is unquestionably best absorbed when taken between meals,

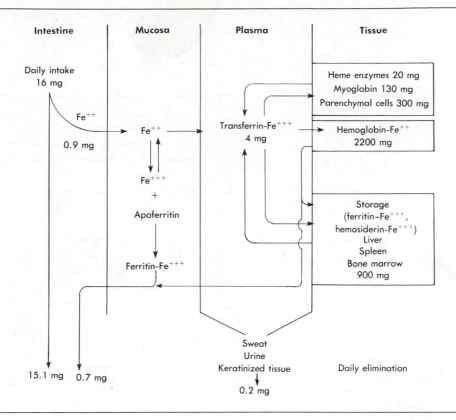

Figure 30-1. Absorption, excretion, and storage of iron within the body of a 70 kg man. The amounts of iron absorbed, excreted, and stored in the three major compartments are expressed in milligrams. Note the balance between daily absorption and excretion.

gastrointestinal distress is lessened if the medication is taken with meals.

Iron dextran is a sterile colloidal solution of ferric hydroxide and low molecular weight dextran and is administered by intramuscular or intravenous injection only when parenteral iron therapy is absolutely needed. Severe, even fatal, anaphylactic reactions have occurred after the use of this preparation. Other adverse reactions include pain and staining at the site of injection (intramuscular), urticaria, fever, arthralgia, lymphadenopathy, nausea, and vomiting.

It should be emphasized that adverse effects associated with iron therapy occur most often in patients who are taking iron by both the oral and parenteral routes. This reaction occurs because the transferrin becomes saturated, and iron enters the blood in excess. It is this portion of the iron that is toxic.

Acute iron poisoning is not uncommon, particularly since many of the iron formulations are brightly colored and attractive to children. Ingestion of large doses of iron has caused severe gastrointestinal disturbances and circulatory collapse. Chelating agents have been used in the treatment of acute iron toxicity; deferoxamine, a potent and specific iron chelating compound, is capable of removing iron from both ferritin and transferrin but not from hemoblobin. It is, however, no substitute for other measures, such as induced vomiting, gastric lavage, and fluid administration, that should be carried out in the event of iron poisoning.

VITAMIN B_{12} AND FOLIC ACID
Deficiency syndromes

Anemias resulting from vitamin B_{12} or folate deficiency are characterized by large and often oval or irregularly shaped erythrocytes and bone marrow precursors (megaloblastic germ cells). Both vitamin B_{12} and folate are essential for the synthesis of DNA throughout the body, but this need is most evident in rapidly growing tissues. In the absence

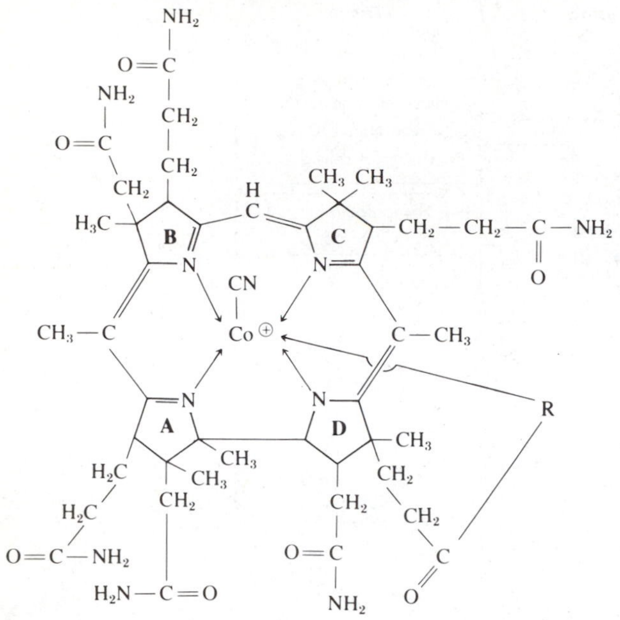

Figure 30-2. Heme structure of cyanocobalamin (vitamin B_{12}). Substitution of other groups, such as — OH, — H_2O, and — NO_2, for — CN produces, respectively, hydroxocobalamin, aquocobalamin, and nitritocobalamin. R indicates the nonheme portion of the molecule. Replacement of — CN by — 5'-deoxyadenosyl and — CH_3 groups in vivo yields the active coenzymes deoxyadenosylcobalamin and methylcobalamin.

of B_{12} and folic acid, division of the blood cells is arrested, thereby resulting in larger cells with immature nuclei but mature cytoplasm. Whether the deficiency stems from insufficient dietary intake, decreased absorption, decreased utilization, or increased destruction of these essential components, the net result will be a bone marrow characterized by megaloblastic erythrocytic precursors and large myeloid cells and megakaryocytes. The cells released into the bloodstream are macroovalocytes, hypersegmented polymorphonuclear leukocytes, and oversized platelets. Since the cell membranes are substandard, the life span of these cells is shortened. Thus, the resulting anemia is also hemolytic in nature. In addition to several chemical agents that interfere with purine metabolism, an intestinal parasite, the fish tapeworm (*Diphyllobothrium latum*), competes rather successfully with the host for available vitamin B_{12}, and this ultimately leads to megaloblastic anemia.

Because all of the formed elements of the blood are affected, patients with megaloblastic anemia are leukopenic and therefore more susceptible to infection, are thrombocytopenic and thus more prone to hemorrhage, and may suffer from fatigue caused by erythropoietic depression. Both vitamin B_{12} and folate deficiencies result in megaloblastic anemia, but the deficiency of one does not resemble the deficiency of the other. Folate deficiency alone is characterized by pallor, anemia, fatigue, and glossitis, but there is no neurologic involvement. On the other hand, vitamin B_{12} deficiency, which is most often the result of a lack of intrinsic factor, results in inadequate hematopoiesis, myelin synthesis, and epithelial replacement in the gastrointestinal tract. Symptoms of vitamin B_{12} deficiency include gastrointestinal disturbances, glossitis, weight loss, hepatomegaly and splenomegaly, and prominent neurologic disturbances. In fact, the neurologic symptoms may be present even in the absence of anemia. Thus, the treatment of a megaloblastic anemia with folic acid alone could be very detrimental, because although the hematologic picture will be quickly reversed, the neurologic symptoms will not be affected at all.

Vitamin B_{12}

In a general sense, the term vitamin B_{12} represents a group of cobalamins in which the cobalt atom is covalently linked to several different groups (Figure 30-2). Pharmacologically, however, it represents only cyanocobalamin, which is a stable, man-made congener of cobalamin. The sole natural source of cobalamin is synthesis by microorganisms. Although many animals can use vitamin B_{12} produced by their own enteric bacteria, microbial synthesis in humans is limited to the large intestine, a site from which the vitamin cannot be absorbed. Foods rich in vitamin B_{12} include liver, kidney, and heart of mammals and shellfish, such as oysters and clams (greater than 10 $\mu g/100$ gm tissue). Hydroxocobalamin, vitamin B_{12a}, is closely related to cyanocobalamin and is hematopoietically equivalent.

Cyanocobalamin is rapidly absorbed from parenteral routes of administration; hydroxocobalamin is less rapidly absorbed because it is more strongly bound to local tissue proteins. Vitamin B_{12} is poorly absorbed from the gastrointestinal tract, and an effective oral dose is 100 times larger than the parenteral dose. Cyanocobalamin is distributed to all tissues, where it is converted to active coenzyme forms (Figure 30-2), but at least 50% of the body's stores of vitamin B_{12} are concentrated in the liver, where it exists principally as the desoxyadenosyl coenzyme. Vitamin B_{12} is not biotransformed, so any loss from the body stores is the result of excretion into the bile and by the kidney. The recommended daily allowance for B_{12} is 3 μg, and the liver can store substantial quantities of it. This permits long intervals between injections of vitamin B_{12} in the pernicious anemia patient (once the blood picture has been restored to normal) and explains the delayed onset of pernicious anemia after cessation of secretion of gastric intrinsic factor or after switching to a strict vegetarian diet.

A variety of preparations are available for vitamin B_{12} therapy. The agents of choice are cyanocobalamin and hydroxocobalamin; both are given by intramuscular or deep subcutaneous injection. The use of liver injections has been largely abandoned because of allergic reactions, and oral preparations, such as vitamin B_{12} with intrinsic factor concentrate, liver extract, or cyanocobalamin alone, are not widely used because they are relatively ineffective and often needlessly expensive.

Initial treatment of pernicious anemia involves twice weekly intramuscular injections of B_{12} for several months. Such treatment will bring about a change in the bone marrow from megaloblastic to normoblastic erythropoiesis and will relieve the glossitis, neuritis, and spinal cord degeneration. As the blood picture improves, the interval between doses can be increased to 2 or 3 weeks. Eventually, the patient will be put on maintenance therapy involving an injection every 2 months for life. Neurologic damage that is not reversed after 1 or 1½ years of therapy must be considered permanent.

There have been no reports of toxic effects from cyanocobalamin or hydroxocobalamin other than occasional allergic responses to impurities in the preparations.

Folic acid

Folic acid occurs widely in nature as folates. Folic acid itself is pteroylglutamic acid, a compound formed from glutamic acid, *p*-aminobenzoic acid, and pterin, as is shown in Figure 30-3. Fresh green vegetables are an excellent source of folic acid (although prolonged cooking can destroy it), as are yeast and liver. In the body, folic acid is reduced to tetrahydrofolic acid and conjugated with a one-carbon moiety to yield several active coenzyme forms. As such, it acts in the transfer of single carbon units in purine and pyrimidine synthesis. Tetrahydrofolate is also involved in conversion reactions of several amino acids.

The daily folate requirement for humans is approximately 50 μg, and because of less than complete absorption, a daily intake of 400 μg of free folate is recommended. Deficiency of folates may occur during pregnancy and infancy, as a result of various malabsorption syndromes, and in individuals taking certain medications, such as antiepileptic drugs, contraceptives, and antimalarials. As was pointed out earlier, folic acid deficiency causes a megaloblastic anemia without neurologic manifestations.

Folate deficiency can often be treated with simple dietary supplements such as an additional piece of fresh fruit daily. Folic acid can be administered either orally or, in rare cases, by injection. Leucovorin (folinic acid, Figure 30-3) has been used to counteract the effects of folic acid antagonists used in cancer chemotherapy. The response to oral folic acid therapy is rapid, and an improvement in the blood picture is seen in 5 to 10 days after the daily administration of folic acid has begun. Adverse effects directly attributable to folic acid have not been reported.

SYNTHETIC OXYGEN-TRANSPORT FLUIDS AND PLASMA EXTENDERS

The agents described in this section differ from those previously discussed in that they are used to replace blood temporarily rather than to support its endogenous production.

Perfluorochemicals

Surgical procedures in severely anemic patients are usually delayed until the anemia is reversed by appropriate therapy or compensated by blood transfusion. As neither approach may be practical in an emergency or in patients whose religious beliefs preclude blood transfusion, the search for synthetic oxygen-transport materials has been of great interest to the medical profession. Since the demonstration by Clark and Gollan[4] in 1966 that a fluid containing oxygenated fluorocarbon could support respiration of mice totally immersed in it, stable inert aqueous solutions have been developed. One such product, Fluosol-DA, has now been used successfully in human trials. Fluosol-DA consists of two perfluorochemicals: 14% perfluorodecalin and 6% perfluorotripropylamine. Oxygen is highly soluble (45 to 48 ml of oxygen/100 ml solution) in

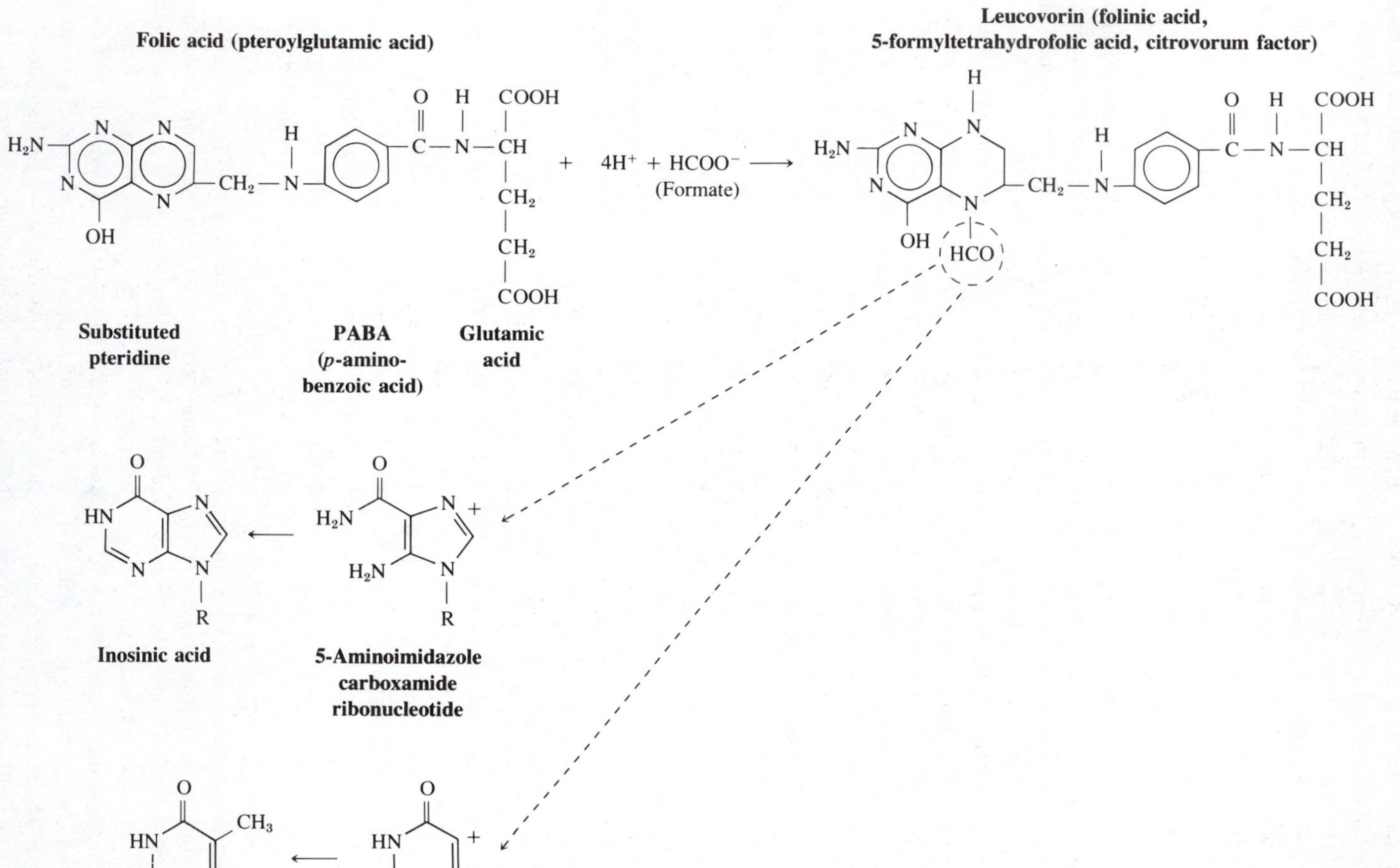

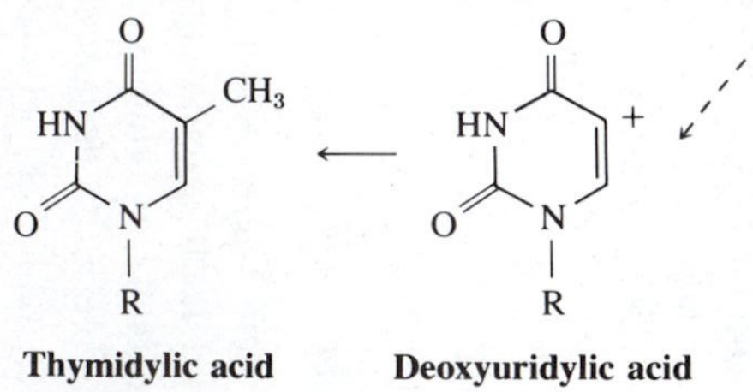

Figure 30-3. Folic acid metabolism showing its origin and conversion to leucovorin, which can serve as a source for the transfer of carbon units during purine and pyrimidine synthesis. R = ribose monophosphate.

both substances. In one report of seven volunteer patients with seriously depleted hemoglobin titers (ranging from 1.9 to 7.2 gm/100 ml) who received a total infusion of 20 ml solution per kg, the perfluorochemical combination served primarily as a plasma extender at ambient oxygen tensions.[14] However, when the patients breathed pure oxygen, the perfluorochemicals accounted for approximately one quarter of their oxygen consumption. It has been suggested that other applications might include treatment of carbon monoxide poisoning, acute myocardial infarction, cerebral vasospasm, and sickle-cell crisis. As yet there are no extensive toxicologic data in humans, and much more clinical experience is needed before release of this drug for general use.

Synthetic plasma extenders

There are no true substitutes for whole blood loss except whole blood, but within fairly wide limits of total hemoglobin one can substitute various colloidal solutions in order to sustain an acceptable blood pressure. Whole plasma is obviously the most effective replacement; however, individual units of plasma have a hepatitis B risk equal to that of individual whole blood units. Five percent plasma protein solution (pooled plasma heated to 60° C for 10 hours to minimize the risk of hepatitis) or 5% human albumin is a suitable alternative. Unfortunately, the former preparation may cause hypotension through the presence of Hageman factor prekallikrein activators, and both are expensive and unacceptable to certain religious groups because of their human origins.

In theory, the development of a synthetic substitute to fulfill the oncotic functions of plasma proteins would be an ideal approach. To be of more value than isotonic saline as an oncotic substitute, a substance must be relatively inert, nontoxic, nonallergic, and have a molecular size and weight in excess of that which can be easily filtered across the glomerulus. Of the many materials that have been tested, the most suitable have proved to be polysaccharide derivatives, namely dextran and hetastarch.[11]

Dextran. A branched polysaccharide, dextran is produced by certain bacteria and consists of as many as 200,000 glucose molecules interconnected by glucosidic linkages to produce a molecular weight of about 4×10^7. Controlled hydrolysis of this material can yield a wide range of molecules that are then fractionated according to size. Available dextrans for injection include two forms: high molecular weight dextran, a 6% solution of dextran with a mean molecular weight of approximately 70,000 or 75,000, depending on manufacturer, and low molecular weight dextran having a weight of about 40,000. The main advantage of the smaller material, which of course can escape more readily across the glomerular membranes, is the fact that it seems to improve the microcirculation by reducing the rouleau formation and red cell sludging that usually accompany hemorrhagic and other forms of shock. Dextran-induced rouleau formation interferes with blood typing, which therefore must precede dextran injection, and dextran impairs platelet function, resulting in an iatrogenic form of von Willebrand's disease. Fibrin formation is also impaired. The major disadvantage of the dextrans is their antigenic potential. Enteric bacteria produce dextran, and a small percentage of the population have precipitins for dextran in their blood. Fortunately, when used as a plasma extender a massive dose is usually given that overwhelms the immune response (immunologic paralysis), and anaphylactic risk is as low as, or lower than, that of blood transfusion.

Hetastarch. Hetastarch is a hydroxyethylated derivative of amylopectin, with a mean molecular weight of 69,000 and a range of 10,000 to 1 million.[8] The lower weight molecules (under 50,000) are excreted via glomerular filtration within 24 hours. Remaining molecules are metabolized slowly over a 2- to 3-week period to smaller products by serum α-amylase activity. The volume expansion produced by this agent lasts approximately 24 to 36 hours. Hematologically, there appears to be no obvious advantage of this material over dextran; however, it has an extremely low incidence of anaphylaxis (less than 0.006%) and may have less of an effect on blood clotting. Besides being effective as a volume expander, hetastarch has been found useful in leukapheresis (the harvesting of granulocytes for patient use) and as a priming fluid for extracorporeal pumps used in coronary surgery.

Antianemic drugs

Nonproprietary name	Proprietary name	Route of administration
Iron preparations		
ferrous fumarate	Feostat	Oral
ferrous gluconate	Fergon	Oral
ferrous sulfate	Feosol, Fer-In-Sol	Oral
iron dextran	Imferon	IM, IV
iron-polysaccharide	Hytinic	Oral
Iron chelating agent		
deferoxamine	Desferal	IM, IV
Vitamin B_{12} preparations		
cyanocobalamin	Betalin 12	IM, SC
hydroxocobalamin	AlphaRedisol	IM

Nonproprietary name	Proprietary name	Route of administration
Folic acid preparations		
folate sodium	Folvite Solution	IM, IV, SC
folic acid	Folvite	Oral
leucovorin calcium (folinic acid)	Wellcovorin	IM
Oxygen transport fluid		
perfluorochemicals*	Fluosol-DA, 20%	IV
Plasma volume extenders		
dextran, high molecular weight	Dextran 70, Macrodex, Gentran 75	IV
dextran, low molecular weight	Dextran 40, Rheomacrodex	IV
hetastarch	Hespan	IV

*Not currently available in the United States.

CITED REFERENCES

1. Addison, T. Anemia—disease of the supra-renal capsules. London Medical Gazette **43**:517, 1849. Cited by Kass, L. Pernicious Anemia. Philadelphia, W. B. Saunders Co., 1976.
2. Blaud, P. Sur les maladies chlorotiques, et sur un môde de traitement spécifiques dans ces affections. Revue Médical Française et Etrangère **45**:341-367, 1832.
3. Castle, W. B. Observations on the etiologic relationship of achylia gastrica to pernicious anemia. I. Effect of administration to patients with pernicious anemia of contents of normal human stomach recovered after ingestion of beef muscle. American Journal of Medical Sciences **178**:748-764, 1929.
4. Clark, L.C., Jr., and Gollan, F. Survival of mammals breathing organic liquids equilibrated with oxygen at atmospheric pressure. Science **152**:1755-1756, 1966.
5. Fairbanks, V.F., Fahey, J.L., and Beutler, E. Clinical Disorders of Iron Metabolism, ed. 2. New York, Grune & Stratton, Inc., 1971.
6. FAO-WHO Expert Group. Requirements of ascorbic acid, vitamin D, vitamin B_{12}, folate, and iron. World Health Organization Report. Geneva, Switzerland, World Health Organization, 1970.
7. Herbert, V. Megaloblastic anemias. In Beeson, P.B., and McDermott, W., eds. Cecil-Loeb Textbook of Medicine, ed. 14. Philadelphia, W. B. Saunders Co., 1975.
8. Hulse, J.D., and Yacobi, A. Hetastarch: an overview of the colloid and its metabolism. Drug Intelligence and Clinical Pharmacy **17**:334-341, 1983.
9. Minot, G.R., and Murphy, W.P. Treatment of pernicious anemia by a special diet. Journal of the American Medical Association **87**:470-476, 1926.
10. Mitchell, H.K., Snell, E.E., and Williams, R.J. The concentration of "folic acid." Journal of the American Chemical Society **63**:2284, 1941.
11. Mudge, G.H. Agents affecting volume and composition of body fluids. In Gilman, A.G., Goodman, L.S., and Gilman, A., eds. Goodman and Gilman's The Pharmacological Basis of Therapeutics, ed. 6. New York, Macmillan, Inc., 1980.
12. Rickes, E.L., Brink, N.G., Koniuszy, F.R., Wood, T.R., and Folkers, K. Crystalline vitamin B_{12}. Science **107**:396-397, 1948.
13. Smith, E.L. Purification of anti–pernicious anemia factors from liver. Nature **161**:638-639, 1948.
14. Tremper, K.K., Friedman, A.E., Levine, E.M., Lapin, R., and Camarillo, D. The preoperative treatment of severely anemic patients with a perfluorochemical oxygen-transport fluid, Fluosol-DA. New England Journal of Medicine **307**:277-283, 1982.
15. Wills, L., Clutterbuck, P.W., and Evans, B.D.F. A new factor in the production and cure of macrocytic anaemias and its relation to other haemopoietic principles curative in pernicious anemia. Biochemical Journal **31**:2136-2147, 1937.

GENERAL REFERENCES

Hardesty, R.M., and Weatherall, D.J. Blood and Its Disorders. Oxford, England, Blackwell Scientific Publications, 1974.
Williams, W.J., Beutler, E., Erslev, A.J., and Rundles, R.W. Hematology, New York, McGraw-Hill Book Co., 1972.
Wintrobe, M.M., Lee, G.R., Boggs, D.R., Bithell, T.C., Athens, J.W., and Foerster, J. Clinical Hematology, ed. 7. Philadelphia, Lea & Febiger, 1974.

31 Hemostasis, hemostatics, and anticoagulants

Thomas E. Nelson, Jr.

Rational pharmacologic control of blood clotting demands an appreciation of the total hemostatic process, which involves enzymatic interactions of blood components and the responses of damaged tissue. Blood coagulation is an essential mechanism in the defense of vascular integrity. Nevertheless, it is at times necessary to compromise normal hemostasis in order to reduce the likelihood of life-threatening intravascular coagulation. Of more immediate importance to dentistry, however, are the several means of initiating or promoting hemostasis (Table 31-1). The clinician should also be aware of physiologic factors normally present that may need to be supplemented in deficiency states, as well as pharmacologic agents, particularly anticoagulants, whose dose may have to be adjusted to normalize clotting activity before surgery. The mechanisms of hemostasis and blood clotting are reviewed in the following sections.

HEMOSTASIS

Large or intermediate arteries and veins are generally not severed intentionally without prior ligation, but it is common for extraction of impacted teeth and for other oral surgical procedures to disrupt small arteriolar, venous, and capillary vessels, from which extensive blood loss may occur if hemostasis is delayed. The actual physical response of these vessels to injury occurs in a stepwise fashion, as described in detail by Zucker.[33] In the laboratory animal, transection of small arteries and arterioles that contain smooth muscle has revealed several patterns of hemorrhagic flow.[24,33] Generally, after a sudden surge of blood there is a moderate to severe reduction in flow, apparently caused by contraction of vascular smooth muscle initiated directly by the trauma. This initial hemostasis is independent of blood coagulation and platelet agglutination, since it occurs in heparinized animals.

Furthermore, it appears to be maintained only for short periods (i.e., 5 to 20 minutes).

The next event is the aggregation of platelets at the severed edges of the vessel.[33] In normal, untraumatized blood vessels, platelets show little tendency to adhere to the endothelium, but injury to the intima, even if the vessel wall remains intact, leads to a rapid localization of platelets and the formation of a platelet plug or thrombus. If nonmuscular vessels are severed, the immediate hemostatic action of the platelet plug is especially important. Indeed, the true significance of the platelet in hemostasis becomes evident in the management of the thrombocytopenic patient.

In addition to forming a physical plug in the open end of the vessel, the agglutinated platelets release several humoral agents that participate both directly and indirectly in hemostasis. Among these are 5-HT (serotonin), which helps to prolong smooth muscle contraction in the immediate area,[24] and several factors that promote the blood clotting reaction. Platelets are also essential in clot retraction, a process that facilitates wound healing by bringing the severed ends of small blood vessels into closer apposition. Clot retraction, or syneresis, occurs when pseudopodia, which are produced by platelets during clotting, attach to fibrin strands and contract. A contractile, actomyosin-like protein (thrombosthenin) has been described in platelets.[4] ATP, which is freed from platelets during coagulation,[1] may serve to facilitate contraction much as it does in muscle.

BLOOD COAGULATION

Although it is possible to single out the events of hemostasis (e.g., platelet agglutination and formation of fibrin), it must be realized that the whole process occurs synergistically. The fundamental clotting interactions were known at the turn of the

Table 31-1. Methods of controlling bleeding

Desired result	Physiologic methods	Physical procedures	Chemical agents
Hemostasis	Vasoconstriction, platelet plugs, clot retraction	Cooling, pressure, cautery	Epinephrine, astringents-styptics*
Clotting	Procoagulants: thrombin, platelets, other clotting factors	Cautery, physical matrices (gelatin or cellulose sponge)	Topical thrombin, astringents-styptics*

*Chemicals that denature protein: Al^{+++}, Zn^{++}, Fe^{++}, Ag^+, alcohol, tannic acid, cellulosic acid.

Table 31-2. Blood clotting factors

International number*	Plasma factor and alternate names	Cause or incidence of deficiency
I	Fibrinogen	Liver disease
II	Prothrombin	Liver disease or vitamin K deficiency
III	Thromboplastin, tissue factor	Deficiency of tissue thromboplastin probably does not occur
IV	Ca^{++}	Never deficient without tetany
V	Proaccelerin, accelerator globulin (AcG)	Parahemophilia, rare
VII	Proconvertin, autoprothrombin I, SPCA	Liver disease or vitamin K deficiency
VIII	Antihemophilic globulin (AHG), AHF A, platelet cofactor I	True hemophilia, 75% of "hemophiliacs"
IX	Plasma thromboplastin component (PTC), Christmas factor, autoprothrombin II, AHF B, platelet cofactor II	Hemophilia B, 20% of "hemophiliacs" (Christmas disease); depressed with vitamin K deficiency
X	Stuart-Prower factor, autoprothrombin III	Liver disease or vitamin K deficiency
XI	Plasma thromboplastin antecedent (PTA), AHF C	Hemophilia C, 5% of "hemophiliacs"
XII	Hageman factor (HF)	No clinical symptoms, rare
XIII	Fibrin stabilizing factor (FSF), Laki-Lorand factor, fibrinase	Defective healing, rare

*Roman numerals were assigned in 1958 by the International Committee on Blood Clotting Factors, Number VI, originally assigned to "prothrombin converting principle" (prothrombinase), has since been abandoned. Clotting factors (e.g., prekallikrein) without an international number are not listed.

century, primarily through the discovery of thrombin by Schmidt in 1872[27] and formulation of the basic clotting scheme by Morawitz in 1905.[20] This simple scheme, in which thromboplastin, in the presence of calcium ions, promotes the conversion of prothrombin to thrombin, which in turn produces fibrin from fibrinogen, is the backbone of current concepts of the clotting mechanism (Figure 31-1). Many refinements in our understanding of blood coagulation have come about through study of "experiments of Nature" in which discrete defects of the clotting process are identified in patients with a bleeding diathesis, as illustrated by the factors and deficiency states listed in Table 31-2.

Initiation of coagulation after injury is a complex process involving two pathways of thromboplastin generation and activation: *extrinsic* and *intrinsic*. Although once considered to be entirely separate, it is now recognized that the two are intertwined and that both must function correctly for normal hemostasis.[23]

Plasma thromboplastin can be generated in the test tube through a process initiated by the surface activation of the Hageman factor (XII). Surface activation of a similar type occurs with injured tissue. In normal individuals, surface-activated factor XII is believed to work in conjunction with the three "antihemophilic" factors (VIII, IX, XI) and phospholipid (largely platelet factor 3 released during platelet agglutination) to form plasma (intrinsic) thromboplastin, which has actions comparable to those of activated tissue thromboplastin. Tissue thromboplastin, or factor III, is a lipoprotein substance released from injured tissue that forms an active complex with factor VII and Ca^{++}. (Figure 31-1 describes the formational interdependence of the plasma and tissue thromboplastins.) Regardless of origin, thromboplastin activates Stuart-Prower factor (X), which in turn splits the prothrombin molecule, thereby releasing the active proteolytic enzyme, thrombin. Calcium ions are also required for this process.

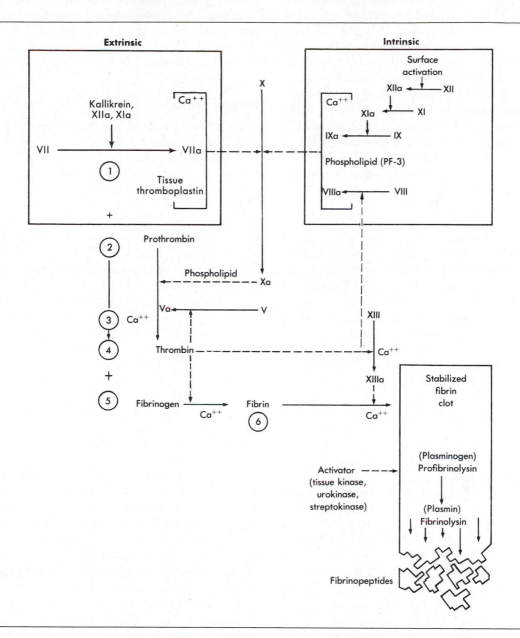

Figure 31-1. Schematic flow diagram of blood coagulation. The original Schmidt-Morawitz scheme is represented by Arabic numerals on the left (i.e., thromboplastin + prothrombin and Ca^{++} → thrombin + fibrinogen → fibrin). Now two separate thromboplastin systems are recognized: *extrinsic,* in which tissue
thromboplastin with factor VII and Ca^{++} form an activating complex for factor X, and *intrinsic,* in which a
plasma activating complex of IXa, VIIIa, platelet factor 3, and Ca^{++} forms the activator. A functional interdependence of the two systems has been demonstrated, with extrinsic factor VII being activated by factors
associated with the intrinsic cascade and (not shown) tissue thromboplastin, once activated, being able to replace
XIa in the intrinsic pathway. Conversion of prothrombin to thrombin is the result of a third complex composed
of factor Xa, phospholipid, Va, and Ca^{++}. Fibrin, once it is formed by the proteolytic action of thrombin, is
stabilized by thrombin-activating factor XIII. Fibrinolysis occurs normally by the activation of the proteolytic
enzyme precursor profibrinolysin either by an endogenous activator system or by one of several kinases.

The conversion of prothrombin to thrombin is slow in its early stages; however, an accelerator mechanism exists that is capable of greatly increasing the rate of thrombin generation. The initial formation of a small amount of thrombin catalyzes the activation of proaccelerin (V), which then acts autocatalytically to accelerate thrombin formation. Thrombin further augments its own formation by stimulating thromboplastin generation (Figure 31-1). It also is significant that thrombin labilizes platelets, thereby releasing several active substances, one of which (platelet factor 1) resembles proaccelerin in function.

The final phase of blood clotting consists of the proteolytic splitting, by thrombin, of arginyl-glycine bonds of the fibrinogen molecules to release active fibrin monomers, which then readily combine with each other to form long fibrillar strands tying the clot together.[5] This reaction is accelerated by a platelet material (platelet factor 2). The initial clot is not very stable, being held together primarily by hydrogen bonds. With time, however, the fibrin strands become cross-linked with covalent bonds by the action of a transglutaminase, fibrin stabilizing factor (XIII). Stabilized clots can be broken down only by proteolysis.

Entrapped in this coagulum are blood cells, including many intact platelets, which then promote clot retraction as previously described. These events are followed by inflammatory processes of organization and wound healing, requiring, among other things, an effective proteolytic (fibrinolytic) mechanism described later in this chapter.

LOCALLY AND SYSTEMICALLY ACTIVE HEMOSTATIC AGENTS

In medical and dental practice it is essential that maximum precautions be taken to avoid serious hemorrhage. This is particularly true for patients receiving anticoagulants or for those requiring antihemophilic globulin or other therapy known to affect hemostasis. Conservative precautions, which may include hospitalization, are prudent in these cases. In contrast, the normal patient requires no more than temporary hemostatic assistance, for example, pressure packs, hemostatic forceps, ligation, or other means to permit hemostasis and clotting to take place.

A most perplexing hemostatic problem may arise from continued, slow oozing of blood from small arterioles, veins, and capillaries. These vessels obviously cannot be ligated, and one must resort to pressure packs, vasoconstrictor agents, and procoagulants. Styptics or astringents, once extensively used, are no longer viewed as rational procedures for routine hemostasis. However, some astringents are used commonly for gingival retraction.

Pressure packs

Simple cotton packing may be inadequate to provide hemostasis and can be replaced by the hydrophilic colloidal material carboxymethylcellulose, a substance that expands readily when moistened, thereby exerting needed pressure for physical stasis in enclosed areas. For open areas, which are more difficult to control, a gelatinous dressing is available as an oral adhesive powder, to which thrombin may be added if desired.

Several other spongy materials also make effective packing, some of which can serve as a synthetic fibrin net. These include a fairly delicate sponge of gelatin, which can absorb 40 to 50 times its own weight in blood. Gelatin sponge also facilitates platelet disruption, which aids in blood coagulation. Unlike other synthetic packing, it is absorbed in 4 to 6 weeks, which is usually rapid enough to avoid scar formation. Since it is a gelatin, it must be applied dry. Unfortunately, its affinity for moisture makes it difficult to handle, and for this reason many practitioners prefer to use denatured cellulose preparations.

Denatured cellulose sponge or gauze serves as a physical plug as well as a chemical hemostatic. The apparent coagulation-promoting action stems from the release of cellulosic acid, which denatures (coagulates) hemoglobin. Cellulosic acid, like tannic acid, inactivates thrombin; thus, the use of cellulose sponge in conjunction with the procoagulant is ineffective. Two forms of cellulose sponge, oxidized cellulose and oxidized regenerated cellulose, are available. Both of these materials cause delayed healing, particularly the oxidized cellulose, which notably interferes with bone regeneration and epithelialization. Although regenerated cellulose is said to have less inhibitory action, neither dressing should be left permanently in the wound.

A novel hemostatic agent, microfibrillar collagen (Avitene), made from purified bovine skin collagen has been approved for topical use only in arresting certain hemorrhagic conditions. Collagen accelerates the aggregation of platelets, and therefore it may have limited effectiveness in platelet disorders or hemophilia.[2] Whether microfibrillar collagen will prove useful in dental surgical situations has not yet been fully assessed.

Astringents and styptics

The terms *astringents* and *styptics* are interchangeable, referring to different concentrations of the same drugs. Many chemicals have vasoconstrictive or protein-denaturing ability, but relatively few are appropriate for dentistry. The suitable preparations are primarily salts of several metals, particularly zinc, silver, and aluminum. Aluminum and iron salts are quite acidic and therefore irritating. Furthermore, iron causes annoying, though temporary, surface staining of the enamel, whereas silver stains may be quite permanent.

Currently, astringents are not looked on with as much favor as they were in the past, when 20% ferric subsulfate (Monsel's solution) and 8% zinc chloride were among the best agents available. Unfortunately, denaturation of blood and tissue proteins inhibits normal coagulation and retards healing, leading to complications such as the distressful "dry socket." Tannic acid (0.5 to 1%) is an effective astringent; it therefore also precipitates proteins, including thrombin, and is often incompatible with other drugs and metal salts used therapeutically.

Vasoconstrictors

Temporary hemostasis may be obtained with adrenergic vasoconstrictor agents, generally epinephrine. Obviously, such vasoconstrictors should be applied only topically for restricted local effects and for very short periods to avoid prolonged ischemia and tissue necrosis. Unfortunately, some systemic absorption does occur, particularly in inflamed tissue, which may cause severe cardiovascular responses. Epinephrine solutions from 0.1% (1:1000) to 8% and dry cotton pellets impregnated with racemic epinephrine are available for topical application.

Procoagulants

The most physiologic hemostatic aids are the blood clotting factors themselves. Assuming an otherwise normal clotting system, however, the only procoagulant with any clinical utility is topical thrombin. *If given intravenously, thrombin causes extensive thrombosis and death*. Topically applied thrombin (particularly in conjunction with a compatible matrix such as gelatin sponge) operates as a hemostatic, particularly if the patient has a coagulation deficiency or is receiving oral anticoagulants, since all that is required for clotting is a normal supply of fibrinogen in the plasma. In the event that blood flows too freely, temporary physical hemostasis must be attained before topical thrombin can be of practical value.

Patients with bleeding disorders usually suffer from deficiencies in platelet number or function or from faulty or missing clotting factors. Bleeding may develop several hours after trauma or surgery. Although bleeding does not generally appear with superficial abrasions, hemarthrosis and deep hemorrhage are common. Although platelet deficiency (thrombocytopenia) is frequently drug induced or associated with other myelogenous diseases, the hemophilias are generally inherited. In either case, with proper evaluation and supportive therapy (Table 31-3), extensive surgery can usually be accomplished without serious incident. Patients with a platelet count of less than $50,000/mm^3$ are at risk of surgical or other trauma but generally do not demonstrate spontaneous hemorrhage until the count drops to $20,000/mm^3$ or less. Platelet transfusion should be reserved for acute situations, since alloimmunization to injected platelets occurs readily. One unit of platelet concentrate elevates the platelet count in adults anywhere from 4000 to $10,000/mm^3$. Drug-induced disease generally is alleviated by withdrawal of the offending drug. Idiopathic forms may benefit from corticosteroid administration, splenectomy, or injections of the vinca alkaloid vincristine, an immunosuppressive agent effective also in acute leukemia.

In addition to disorders related directly to the quantitative or qualitative deficiency of platelets or hypovitaminosis K, several other coagulation disorders must be recognized. These are the hemophilias A, B, and C and von Willebrand's disease.

Hemophilia A and von Willebrand's disease are both caused by a deficiency in the large globular protein complex commonly referred to as factor VIII or antihemophilic globulin (AHG). Factor VIII consists of two separable protein components: (1) the antihemophilic procoagulant factor (VIII:C), and (2) the factor VIII-related protein (VIIIR or von Willebrand factor). Normally, VIII:C and VIIIR are held in close (but noncovalent) association in the plasma in a ratio of approximately 1 VIII:C to 100 VIIIR.[13] Although VIII:C and VIIIR are found together in plasma (which is necessary for the preservation of VIII:C activity),

Table 31-3. Procoagulant preparations used in the management of

Hemostatic disease	Blood component preparation	Content	Dosage for surgery or severe hemorrhage		Major complications
			Initial	Maintenance	
Thrombocytopenia (platelet deficiency)	Whole blood	1 unit (450-500 ml)	Variable, 1 unit increases platelet count by 4000 to 10,000	Variable	Hepatitis, circulatory overload, allergic reactions
	Platelet-rich plasma	1 unit from 1 unit of blood (200-250 ml)	Variable, 1 unit increases platelet count by 4000 to 10,000	Variable	Hepatitis, circulatory overload, allergic reactions, development of platelet antibodies
	Platelet concentrate	1 unit from 1 unit of plasma (10-30 ml)	Variable, 1 unit increases platelet count by 4000 to 10,000	Variable	Hepatitis, allergic reactions, development of platelet antibodies
Hemophilia A (factor VIII deficiency)	Fresh plasma (single units)	1 unit from 1 unit of blood (200-250 ml)	30 ml/kg	15 ml/kg every 8-12 hours	Hepatitis (least risk of factor VIII preparations), allergic reactions
	Cryoprecipitate (single units, bags)	1 bag = 60-120 units factor VIII	4 bags/10 kg	2 bags/10 kg every 8-12 hours	Hepatitis risk similar to plasma but less expensive
	Lyophilized factor VIII concentrate, multiple donor	250 factor VIII units/vial	30 units/kg	15 units/kg every 8-12 hours	Hepatitis risk high but high potency (assayed for each vial)
Hemophilia B (factor IX deficiency)	Fresh or frozen plasma (single units)	1 unit from 1 unit of blood (200-250 ml)	60 ml/kg	10 ml/kg every 8-12 hours	Hepatitis (least risk of factor IX preparations), allergic reactions
	Lyophilized purified factor IX complex	500 factor IX units/vial	60 units/kg	10 units/kg every 12 hours	Hepatitis risk very high, contains factors II, VII, and X in addition to IX

they appear to be synthesized by different organs. The procoagulant factor VIII:C is thought to be produced in the liver and probably some extrahepatic sites as well, but the cell type is not known. The genetic code for VIII:C resides on the X chromosome. On the other hand, von Willebrand factor, associated wtih an autosomal gene, has been synthesized by vascular endothelial cells in tissue culture.

Factor VIII:C generally is believed to accelerate blood coagulation by serving as a cofactor along with phospholipid and Ca^{++} in the enzymatic activation of factor X by factor IX_a, a mechanism likened to that of factor V in prothrombin activation (Figure 31-1). Both factor VIII:C and proaccelerin (V) in the inactive state are asymmetric protein molecules of similar size and both cofactors must be activated by thrombin proteolysis. Thrombin activation involves cleavage of protein chains of VIII:C, with a decrease in molecular weight of more than 50%. In the absence of factor IX_a, VIII:C_a has no intrinsic ability to activate factor X, just as IX_a is inadequate in the absence of VIII:C_a.

In contrast to the cofactor role of VIII:C in factor X activation, the function of von Willebrand factor VIIIR appears to be one of surface interaction with platelets. Purified radiolabeled VIIIR binds specifically to platelet membranes, suggesting a specialized receptor site. A little-used antibacterial drug, ristocetin, reputed to cause thrombocytopenia (Table 30-1), also binds to platelet membranes and enhances the binding of VIIIR. A positive correlation can be shown between VIIIR-platelet binding and ristocetin-induced platelet aggregation.

The hemostatic disorder of von Willebrand's disease can affect both the structure and the concentration of VIIIR, and it may occur in several forms. In severe von Willebrand's disease, the patient suffers not only from extensive VIIIR deficiency but also from a lack of VIII:C. This fortunately is an unusual syndrome, usually occurring in homozygous offspring of parents with mild or asymptomatic von Willebrand's disease. Since the normal association of VIII:C with VIIIR is known to protect the labile VIII:C from rapid inactivation, it is not surprising that VIII:C also is missing in the severe form of this disease.

Treatment of either hemophilia A or von Willebrand's disease requires the restoration of factor VIII complex activity by infusion of fresh plasma (if deficiency is mild) or a cryoprecipitate of plasma (if hypervolemia presents a problem). In severe cases, factor VIII concentrate (which unlike the other preparations is made from blood of several donors and carries an increased risk of hepatitis) may be the drug of choice. The relationship between factor VIII concentration and hemorrhagic risk begins at 50% of normal concentration of factor VIII. Below this value, excessive bleeding from surgery may result, the risk becoming increasingly severe as blood concentrations fall below 25%. Spontaneous bleeding regularly occurs when the factor VIII concentration is less than 1% of normal. Since the half-life of factor VIII is about 8 to 12 hours, the patient must be reinfused with at least half the original dose every 12 hours. A small percentage of patients with hemophilia A do not respond to conventional therapy. They produce an immunoglobulin inhibitor to factor VIII and may require either larger than normal doses of factor VIII or the administration of anti-inhibitor coagulant complex. The latter is a preparation from pooled human plasma that contains activated as well as precursor clotting factors. It bypasses the factor VIII defect but carries a risk of disseminated intravascular coagulation if used unwisely.

In contrast to the more labile factor VIII, factor IX deficiency, or Christmas disease (hemophilia B), may be treated with stored plasma. Factor IX also enjoys a longer biologic half-life. As with factor VIII concentrate, however, the use of factor IX concentrate increases the risk of hepatitis. Since factor IX preparations also contain prothrombin and factors VII and X, some preparations are stabilized with heparin to reduce thrombin generation during storage.

AGENTS THAT PROMOTE OR INHIBIT FIBRINOLYSIS

Therapeutic measures designed to induce or facilitate fibrinolysis are available for use in relieving certain types of peripheral thromboses. A globulin precursor of an enzyme capable of lysing both fibrin clots and fibrinogen is present in circulating plasma. This proenzyme, profibrinolysin (plasminogen), appears to be physically associated with fibrinogen and is therefore incorporated in the clot (Figure 31-1). To initiate lysis, it is necessary to activate the proenzyme, a procedure best accomplished immediately, since aging thrombi become increasingly refractory to treatment.

Normal physiologic activation of profibrinolysin is not well understood. Release of endogenous activators may be induced by stress, dilation of blood vessels, autonomic stimulation, drugs such as salicylates, and certain proteolytic enzymes, for example, chymotrypsin and trypsin. One natural activator, urokinase, is excreted in normal urine. Streptokinase, an exotoxin from hemolytic streptococci, may also serve as an activator of profibrinolysin. Both streptokinase and urokinase may be of value in patients with life-threatening pulmonary emboli or deep venous thrombosis.[29] An endogenous substance, urokinase, is non-antigenic and avoids the allergic reactions that are often seen with streptokinase. It is significant that an inhibitor of fibrinolysis is present in plasma. The concentration of this inhibitor may increase during the third trimester of pregnancy, thereby reducing the fibrinolytic potential during this period.

Streptokinase and urokinase are finding increasing use in the treatment of myocardial infarctions. They are infused via an intracoronary catheter to digest fibrin clots in the coronary arteries shortly after the interruption of blood flow to the myocardium has occurred. The treatment is effective in reducing the ischemic myonecrosis if given within 5 or 6 hours of the onset of chest pain. Because intracoronary injection is not simple, the intravenous route for administration of these agents is being evaluated.[7]

In some circumstances it is advantageous to limit fibrinolytic activity, as for example after intraurethral surgery of the prostate where the wound is constantly bathed by urokinase and thus is prevented from healing. The drug used for this purpose is aminocaproic acid, which selectively inhibits profibrinolysin activators.

ANTICOAGULANTS

Though dentists are unlikely to ever prescribe an anticoagulant agent, it is essential that they be aware of any hemostatic deficiency in the patient, whether it be pathologic in origin or the result of therapeutic manipulation. Quite simply, there are two kinds of anticoagulants in clinical use: *direct-acting* agents, which are capable of acting in the test tube and which have direct-acting antagonists, and *indirect-acting* agents, which interfere with the synthesis of coagulation system proteins and can be blocked only by indirect measures. Dentists should be familiar with the pharmacology of each class and understand how their effects can be modified.

Direct-acting anticoagulants

First extracted by McLean[12] in 1916, heparin is at present the only systemically effective direct-acting anticoagulant. Certainly the development of a nontoxic synthetic alternative capable of heparin-like activity would be of tremendous value, but to date those drugs (heparinoids) that have been tested have invariably produced unacceptable side effects. Moreover, although salts of EDTA (ethylenediaminetetraacetic acid), citrate, and oxalate are useful calcium chelators and are used routinely in vitro to prevent clotting of blood samples taken for clinical testing, they cannot be used as systemic anticoagulants. The binding of free Ca^{++} necessary for muscle and nerve activity causes tetany to intervene before any anticoagulant action is realized.

Heparin is a linear mucopolysaccharide primarily composed of repeating units of D-glucosamine in 1,4 glucosidic linkage with D-glucuronic and L-iduronic acid. These disaccharide residues, which are partially esterified (up to 40%) with sulfuric acid, make heparin the strongest organic acid normally occurring in the body. Figure 31-2 depicts a pentasaccharide segment of heparin that is believed to constitute an important functional site for anticoagulant activity.[30] Actually, the term *heparin* describes a heterogeneous mixture of molecules (with molecular weights ranging from 6000 to 20,000), none of which has been completely synthesized. At present, commercial preparations are made from extracts of bovine and porcine intestinal mucosa. Heparin must be administered parenterally since it is rapidly hydrolyzed in the gastrointestinal tract. It has a dose-dependent biologic half-life of 1 to 3 hours when given intravenously, and it is removed primarily by the liver.

Heparin is produced endogenously in mast cells, where it is stored in a large macromolecular form complexed with histamine. Both heparin and histamine are released together, providing a physiologic example of a fixed-drug combination, the significance of which is not yet fully understood.

Ever since heparin was first discovered, many investigators have attempted to explain the in vivo maintenance of blood fluidity by its presence in plasma. Although Howell introduced this concept shortly after McLean's successful isolation of the anticoagulant, suitable assay techniques were not available until 1949, when Jaques and co-workers[14] found human blood to contain approximately 10

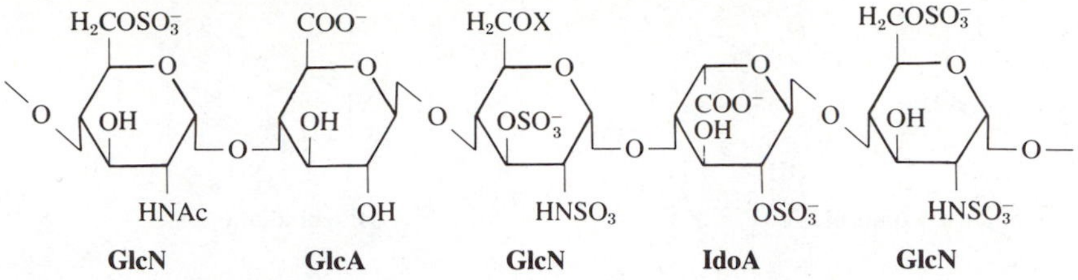

Figure 31-2. Pentasaccharide sequence of heparin. This sequence, unique in its high affinity for antithrombin III, nevertheless reflects the general structure of heparin: repeating units of sulfate-substituted glucosamine (GlcN), glucuronic acid (GlcA), and iduronic acid (IdoA) residues. Ac = an acetyl group; X = H or SO_3^-.

µg of heparin per 100 ml of blood; that is, only 10% to 20% of the concentration required to delay blood clotting significantly.[32] The Howell concept has received renewed support from the work of Engelberg and others, who were able to measure protein-bound as well as free heparin and arrived at a concentration of 150 to 180 µg/100 ml, well within the effective anticoagulant range.[8] However, this issue is by no means laid to rest, since it is not proved that protein-bound drug is functional as an in vivo anticoagulant. Heparin was described by Hahn[10] in 1943 to be the lipemia-clearing factor. In this capacity it releases and stabilizes lipoprotein lipase, which hydrolyzes the triglycerides of chylomicrons. (The free fatty acids are then rapidly taken up by tissue cells.) Since this effect occurs at low, physiologic blood concentrations, it is more likely that this or some other undiscovered action may be heparin's normal role within the blood and that the anticoagulant effect, though pharmacologically fortuitous, is only a secondary function. This idea has received recent support through the work of Bengtsson and associates,[3] who confirmed that only a fraction of the total mammalian heparin is anticoagulant, whereas all of it is capable of activating lipoprotein lipase. The anticoagulant properties of heparin, as well as its antilipemic action, depend on the presence of an α-globulin cofactor, antithrombin III, normally present in the plasma. Therefore, heparin cannot act as an anticoagulant in a system composed of isolated clotting factors alone, nor can it function as a lipemia-clearing agent in the absence of cofactor.

Mechanism of action. Heparin, by increasing the activity of antithrombin III, interferes with blood coagulation in at least two ways: it inhibits the prothrombin-thrombin conversion, and it

blocks the proteolytic action of thrombin on fibrinogen. Prevention of thrombin formation is more readily accomplished, however, than is inhibition of thrombin's enzymatic action. Since thrombin is not formed or is rendered inactive, platelet agglutination and lysis are also reduced. Heparin activity may best be measured by the partial thromboplastin time (PTT) assay, which is sensitive even to low doses of heparin. The normal PTT is 30 to 35 seconds, and it should not exceed a sustained level of twice this value. The one-stage prothrombin time, routinely used to monitor the oral (indirect) anticoagulants, is of little value for heparin assay primarily because the heparin is diluted out in that procedure.

Antidotes. The action of heparin can be readily terminated by intravenous injection of one of several highly positively charged compounds, including protamine sulfate, toluidine blue dye, or a synthetic compound, hexadimethrine bromide.[22] Only protamine, however, is currently recommended for this purpose. Since protamine is itself anticoagulant (antithromboplastic), only enough drug should be given to neutralize the heparin (approximately 1 mg protamine/100 units heparin). The drug should be given intravenously but very slowly (5 mg/min) to avoid depression of the myocardium and vascular smooth muscle.

Indirect-acting anticoagulants

Discovery of the prothrombin-depressant action of spoiled sweet clover by Roderick[25] in 1929 led to the isolation and synthesis of dicumarol (bishydroxycoumarin) by Campbell and Link[6] in the 1940s. These advances introduced a new era of relatively inexpensive, self-administered oral anticoagulant therapy. Since then, several other cou-

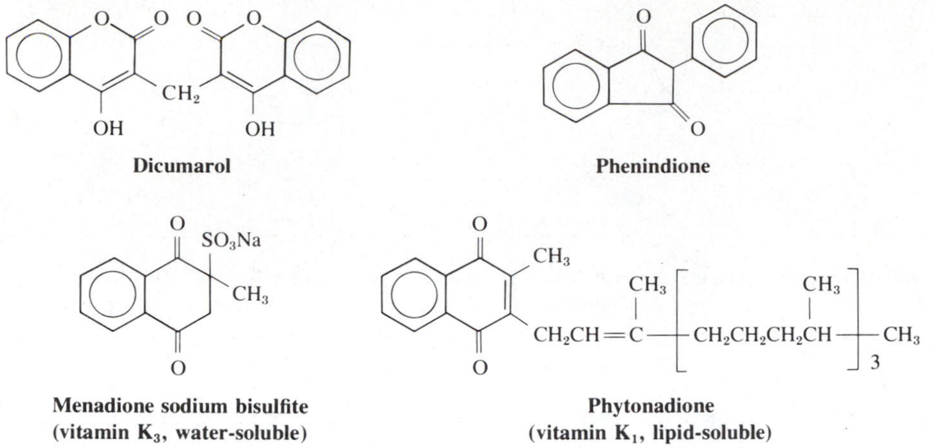

Figure 31-3. Structural formulas of several indirect-acting anticoagulants and analogues of vitamin K.

marin compounds have been introduced, as have drugs of a related group, the indanediones. Because there is little qualitative difference in the action of any of these agents, they are referred to here as a single group, the coumarin-indanediones. The indanediones, however, are generally more toxic.

Mechanism of action. The indirect anticoagulants act by competitively inhibiting vitamin K, which is essential for the synthesis of certain coagulation factors by the liver. (Note the structural similarity between these drugs and vitamin K, as shown in Figure 31-3.) Vitamin K serves as a cofactor in the γ-carboxylation of glutamic acid residues of several proteins, including the clotting factors II, VII, IX, and X. The novel carboxyglutamic acid moieties formed are able to chelate Ca^{++}, which is necessary for activation of those macromolecules. Vitamin K is oxidized in the carboxylation process and must be reduced enzymatically to regain cofactor activity. The coumarin-indanediones inhibit this reduction.

The most sensitive indicator of hypovitaminosis K, or of dicumarol anticoagulation, is the depression of factor VII, proconvertin. Prothrombin (II) is the most resistant of the factors affected. This apparent ordering of sensitivity is a reflection of the plasma half-lives of the clotting factors. Proconvertin is initially depressed because its half-life is only 6 hours. Prothrombin, with a half-life 10 times longer, is the last to be diminished.

Because of the close relationship between hypovitaminosis K and spontaneous hemorrhaging in patients and animals receiving coumarin-indanedione drugs, it is generally assumed that there is a direct causal relationship between coagulation impairment and hemorrhage. This has never been proved, however, and there is reason to doubt that the incoagulability of blood per se is sufficient to cause leaky vessels.[21] It appears, in fact, that vitamin K may have physiologic functions not yet fully realized, including an important role in carboxylation of bone proteins[11] necessary for calcium binding.

Toxic reactions and side effects. The indirect anticoagulants notably produce adverse reactions in the presence of certain drugs and medical conditions. These effects most often arise from interference with vitamin K absorption or metabolism, competition for the drug binding sites of proteins, or competition for, or activation of, the hepatic microsomal enzymes responsible for biotransformation. By far the most important toxic effect of the coumarin-indanediones is hemorrhage.

Any change in the absorption or availability of vitamin K from the intestine will obviously affect the balance between the anticoagulant and vitamin K in the liver and be reflected in the prothrombin time. A fall in vitamin K uptake may result from a disease such as sprue (biliary stasis with concomitant loss of fat-emulsifying bile salts) or from the use of mineral oil for laxation, or, in patients with marginal amounts of vitamin K, in the diet it can reflect the depressed bacterial synthesis of vitamin K in the intestine resulting from administration of a wide range of antimicrobial agents. Thus, sensitivity to the coumarin-indanedione drugs may be increased by sulfisoxazole, chloramphenicol, tetracycline, neomycin, and other bacteriostatic or bactericidal drugs. A great deal of attention has been directed in recent years toward the effects of oral contraceptive agents on the blood coagulation mechanism. In this regard, it is interesting to note that oral estrogen, such as that used in contraceptive preparations, greatly increases vitamin K_1 absorption in experimental animals.[15] It is also noteworthy that estrogen promotes prothrombin synthesis in animals with experimentally induced hypovitaminosis K.[16]

The coumarin compounds are exceptionally highly protein bound in the plasma (dicumarol approximately 99%, warfarin 97%). This constitutes a tremendous reserve of drug in the bloodstream, a very small displacement of which could easily increase the concentration of active free drug by 100%. Many unrelated compounds that are highly protein bound serve to displace the coumarins and potentiate their action. Some antiinflammatory agents, such as phenylbutazone, the antiepileptic agent phenytoin, and clofibrate, a drug capable of lowering blood cholesterol, have been reported to successfully compete with indirect anticoagulants for albumin binding sites. It has been suggested that part of the salicylate potentiation of dicumarol may also result from this kind of mechanism.

A measurable amount (about 1%) of the coumarin-type anticoagulants is excreted unchanged, but the major disposal involves biotransformation pathways used in common with many other chemical compounds. Certain of these agents, particularly the barbiturates (including phenobarbital, which is only partially metabolized and is excreted mostly intact), are capable of hepatic microsomal enzyme induction, which in turn tends to "desensitize" the patient to the coumarin compounds. Microsomal enzyme induction may also be demonstrated with such drugs as chloral hydrate, glutethimide, meprobamate, griseofulvin, haloperidol, and steroids like testosterone.[17] In some instances, a reverse "sensitization" may be demonstrated in which the coumarin compounds potentiate these and other drugs by inhibiting their

metabolism through competition for microsomal enzymes, but usually the most insidious effect is the generalized hemorrhaging caused by overaccumulation of the anticoagulant.

A number of other drug interactions involving the anticoagulant agents have not always been explained on the basis of vitamin K absorption, carrier protein displacement, or biotransformation. For example, drugs such as quinine, aspirin, dextrothyroxine, and norethandrolone have sensitized patients to oral anticoagulants, but the mechanisms are not always clear. Solomon and Schrogie[28] suggested a change in receptor-site affinity to explain the effects of dextrothyroxine. Much of the antihemostatic effect of aspirin analgesics has been ascribed to platelet acetylation and interference with collagen aggregation[26] or to inhibition of platelet thromboxane A_2 (a proaggregatory material related to prostaglandins) resulting in decreased platelet agglutination.[19] However, there are many still unexplained interactions, such as the lethal hemorrhagic effects of ACTH, reserpine, and various stress situations.[31]

Antidotes. Except where an emergency demands the replacement of whole blood or plasma, the usual antidote for coumarin-indanedione toxicity is some form of vitamin K administered parenterally in fairly high concentrations. Unfortunately, this therapy depends on the synthesis of clotting factors, and significant shortening of the prothrombin time cannot be expected to occur for several hours. Of the two major congeners available, vitamin K_1 (naturally occurring, lipid-soluble phytonadione) and vitamin K_3 (water-soluble menadione), the more efficient drug is vitamin K_1. As it occurs naturally, vitamin K_1 is not water soluble, but it is now available in solubilized form (with a polyoxyethylated fatty acid derivative), thus avoiding both the hazard of injecting an emulsion intravenously and the added delay of oral administration.

General pharmacology and therapeutic uses

The principal pharmacologic action of both the direct- and indirect-acting anticoagulants is interference with some step in the blood coagulation process. Beyond this, neither type has outstanding effects on the cardiovascular, respiratory, or other systems except through competition with other drugs for protein binding sites and drug-metabolizing enzymes.

There are many indications in medicine for the use of anticoagulants, including myocardial infarction, cerebrovascular thrombosis, pulmonary embolism, venous thrombosis, rheumatic heart disease, and disseminated intravascular coagulation. Both heparin and oral anticoagulants are useful in the treatment and prevention of these disorders. Heparin, although it is costly and requires parenteral administration, acts immediately and is more effective than coumarin-indanediones in arterial thrombosis. The oral anticoagulants, most commonly warfarin, provide a less expensive, more easily administered, and more readily controlled form of sustained therapy.

IMPLICATIONS FOR DENTISTRY

There are no accepted reasons for the use of anticoagulants in the practice of dentistry. However, many patients requiring dental treatment receive some form of anticoagulant therapy for the reasons cited above. Such patients present two kinds of problems to the dentist: they may have a tendency to bleed excessively, which of course will compromise oral surgery, and they present a real danger of drug interaction between the anticoagulants and agents commonly employed in dental practice, such as chloral hydrate, barbiturates, and salicylates. It is essential that the dentist have a complete and thorough knowledge of the patient's drug history, particularly when anticoagulant therapy is involved. Oral surgery requires some degree of preliminary planning and consultation with the patient's physician. It is the physician's prerogative to adjust the anticoagulant activity to within a safe range for surgical procedures. For coumarin-indanedione anticoagulants this is generally agreed to be within 1½ times the control (normal) one-stage prothrombin time.[18] Thus, if the control prothrombin time were 14 seconds, it would be desirable to return the patient's prothrombin time to 21 seconds or less. This may take several days to

a week to accomplish. Some physicians may elect to supplement the patient with vitamin K_1 in addition to withdrawal of the coumarin anticoagulant. In situations where the surgical intervention is considered minimal, however, prothrombin times up to twice normal may be acceptable. If the anticoagulant is heparin, the drug may be totally withheld or a coumarin agent may be gradually substituted prior to surgery.

Managing the patient with special bleeding problems has received considerable attention in recent years. Patients with hemophilia and other coagulopathic diseases who were once considered inoperable are now being treated routinely in many hospitals. The availability of cryoprecipitates of factor VIII, platelet concentrates, and other specific fractions from single donors decreases the incidence but does not eliminate the ever present danger of hepatitis. Evans and Aledort[9] believe that the dentist is capable of performing dental and periodontal examinations for hemophiliacs in the office, although many dentists prefer to operate in a hospital under the supervision of a hematologist. For oral surgery, including extraction, the only difference between the normal patient and the hemophiliac is the need for a preoperative infusion of cryoprecipitate (as many as 25 bags for an adult) followed by the administration of a normal maintenance dose after surgery. This regimen is sometimes supplemented with aminocaproic acid administered postoperatively: 100 mg/kg every 6 hours for children and 6 gm every 6 hours for adults for 10 days.[9] Aminocaproic acid is a very active inhibitor of urokinase, and the reduction of normal fibrinolytic activity can effectively potentiate the less than efficient hemostatic mechanism. Avitene, a microfibrillar collagen preparation, has been used as an adjunct in packing the apical third of the socket in these patients.[9] An alternative is the use of oxidized regenerated cellulose (neutralized with sodium bicarbonate) and topical thrombin

Agents that affect coagulation and hemostasis

Nonproprietary name	Proprietary name
Astringents-styptics	
aluminum chloride	Hemodent
negatol	Negatan
tannic acid compound	Amertan
Vasoconstrictors	
epinephrine	Adrenalin
Topical procoagulants	
absorbable gelatin film	Gelfilm
absorbable gelatin sponge	Gelfoam
carboxymethylcellulose	in Orabase
microfibrillar collagen	Avitene
oxidized cellulose	Oxycel
oxidized regenerated cellulose	Surgicel
thrombin	Thrombostat
Systemic procoagulants	
antihemophilic factor, human	Hemofil
antiinhibitor coagulant complex	Autoplex
factor IX complex, human	Konyne
Fibrinolytics	
fibrinolysin, human	in Elase
streptokinase	Streptase
urokinase	Abbokinase
Fibrinolytic inhibitors	
aminocaproic acid (EACA)	Amicar
Direct-acting anticoagulants	
heparin*	Liquaemin, Calciparine
Indirect-acting anticoagulants	
acenocoumarol†	Sintrom
anisindione	Miradon
dicumarol (bishydroxycoumarin)	—
diphenadione†	Dipaxin
phenprocoumon	Liquamar
phenindione	Hedulin
warfarin*	Coumadin, Athrombin-K
Antidotes for anticoagulants	
phytonadione (vitamin K_1)	AquaMEPHYTON
protamine sulfate	—

*Available in several salt forms.
†Not currently available in the United States.

CITED REFERENCES

1. Adelstein, R.S., Pollard, T.D., and Kuehl, W.M. Isolation and characterization of myosin and two myosin fragments from human blood platelets. Proceedings of the National Academy of Sciences of the United States of America **68:**2703-2707, 1971.
2. Avitene—a new topical hemostatic agent. Medical Letter on Drugs and Therapeutics **19:**28, 1977.
3. Bengtsson, G., Olivecrona, T., Höök, M., and Lindahl, U. Interaction of heparin with proteins: demonstration of different binding sites for antithrombin and lipoprotein lipase. FEBS Letters: Federation of European Biochemical Societies **79:**59-63, 1977.
4. Bettex-Galland, M., and Lüscher, E.F. Thrombosthenin—a contractile protein from thrombocytes: its extraction from human blood platelets and some of its properties. Biochimica et Biophysica Acta **49:**536-547, 1961.
5. Blombäck, M., Blombäck, B., Gröndahl, N.J., Gardlund, B., Hessel, B., Kowalska-Loth, B., and Reuterby, J. On the molecular structure of fibrinogen. In Thrombosis: Mechanisms and Control. Transactions of the Third Congress of the International Society of Thrombosis and Haemostasis. Stuttgart, Germany, F. K. Schattauer Verlag, 1973.
6. Campbell, H.A., and Link, K.P. Studies on the hemorrhagic sweet clover disease. IV. The isolation and crystallization of the hemorrhagic agent. Journal of Biological Chemistry **138:**21-33, 1941.
7. Connors, C.S. Intravenous streptokinase in acute myocardial infarction. Drug Intelligence and Clinical Pharmacy **17:**367-368, 1983.
8. Engelberg, H. Probable physiologic functions of heparin. Federation Proceedings **36:**70-72, 1977.
9. Evans, B.E., and Aledort, L.M. Hemophilia and dental treatment. Journal of the American Dental Association **96:**827-834, 1978.
10. Hahn, P.F. Abolishment of alimentary lipemia following injection of heparin. Science **98:**19-20, 1943.
11. Hauschka, P.V., Lian, J.B., and Gallop, P.M. Vitamin K and mineralization. Trends in Biological Sciences **3:**75-78, 1978.
12. Howell, W.H., and Holt, E. Two new factors in blood coagulation: heparin and antithrombin. American Journal of Physiology **47:**328-341, 1918.
13. Hoyer, L.W. The factor VIII complex: structure and function. Blood **58:**1-13, 1981.
14. Jacques, L.B., Monkhouse, F.C., and Stewart, M. A method for the determination of heparin in blood. Journal of Physiology **109:**41-48, 1949.
15. Jolly, D.W., Craig, C., and Nelson, T.E., Jr. Estrogen and prothrombin synthesis: effect of estrogen on absorption of vitamin K_1. American Journal of Physiology **232:**H12-H17, 1977.
16. Jolly, D.W., Kadis, B.M., and Nelson, T.E., Jr. Estrogen and prothrombin synthesis: the prothrombinogenic action of estrogen. Biochemical and Biophysical Research Communications **74:**41-49, 1977.
17. Kato, R. Sex-related differences in drug metabolism. Drug Metabolism Reviews **3:**1-32, 1974.
18. Little, J.W., and Falace, D.A. Dental Management of the Medically Compromised Patient. St. Louis, The C.V. Mosby Co., 1980.

19. Moncada, S., and Vane, J.R. Unstable metabolites of arachidonic acid and their role in haemostasis and thrombosis. British Medical Bulletin **34:**129-135, 1978.
20. Morawitz, P. Die Chemie der Blutgerinnung. Ergebnisse der Physiologie, Biologischen Chemie, und Experimentellen Pharmakologie **4:**307-422, 1905.
21. Nelson, T.E., Jr., and Cooper, W.N. Lack of relationship between hypoprothrombinemia and transvascular protein exchange. American Journal of Physiology **211:**105-116, 1966.
22. Preston, F.W., and Parker, R.P. New antiheparin agent (''Polybrene''): effect in peptone shock and in experimental radiation injury. Archives of Surgery **66:**545-551, 1953.
23. Ratnoff, O.D. The role of haemostatic mechanisms. In Prentice, C.R.M., ed. Clinics in Haemotology, vol. 10, Thrombosis. London, W.B. Saunders, 1981.
24. Rius, R., del Castillo, J., and Nelson, T.E., Jr. Patterns of spontaneous hemostasis in the blood vessels of the rabbit's ear. Archives Internationales de Physiologie et de Biochimie **71:**471-498, 1963.
25. Roderick, L.M. A problem in the coagulation of the blood: ''sweet clover disease of cattle,'' American Journal of Physiology **96:**413-425, 1931.
26. Rosenberg, F.J., Gimber-Phillips, P.E., Groblewski, G.E., Davison, C., Phillips, D.K., Goralnick, S.J., and Cahill, E.D. Acetylsalicylic acid: inhibition of platelet aggregation in the rabbit. Journal of Pharmacology and Experimental Therapeutics **179:**410-418, 1971.
27. Schmidt, A. Neue Untersuchung über die Faserstoffgerinnung. Pfluegers Archiv fur die Gesamte Physiologie des Menschen und der Tiere **6:**413-420, 1872.
28. Solomon, H.M., and Schrogie, J.J. Change in receptor site affinity: a proposed explanation for the potentiating effect of D-thyroxin on anticoagulant response to warfarin. Clinical Pharmacology and Therapeutics **8:**797-799, 1967.
29. Streptokinase and urokinase. Medical Letter on Drugs and Therapeutics **20:**37-38, 1978.
30. Thunberg, L., Bäckström, G., and Lindahl, U. Further characterization of the antithrombin-binding sequence in heparin. Carbohydrate Research **100:**393-410, 1982.
31. van Cauwenberge, H., and Jaques, L.B. Haemorrhagic effect of ACTH with anticoagulants. Canadian Medical Association Journal **79:**536-540, 1958.
32. Ware, A.G. Blood coagulation. University of Southern California Medical Bulletin **2:**20-31, 1950.
33. Zucker, M.B. Platelet agglutination and vasoconstriction as factors in spontaneous hemostasis in normal, thrombocytopenic, heparinized, and hypoprothrombinemic rats. American Journal of Physiology **148:**275-288, 1947.

GENERAL REFERENCES

Gilbert M.S., and Aledort, L.M., eds. Comprehensive care in hemophilia: a team approach. Mount Sinai Journal of Medicine **44:**313-479, 1977.

Modell W., ed. Drugs of Choice, 1984-1985. St. Louis, The C.V. Mosby Co., 1984.

Orten, J.M., and Neuhaus, O.W. Human Biochemistry, ed. 10. St. Louis, The C.V. Mosby Co., 1982.

O'Reilly, R.A. Anticoagulant, antithrombotic, and thrombolytic drugs. In Gilman, A.G., Goodman, L.S., and Gilman, A., eds. Goodman and Gilman's The Pharmacological Basis of Therapeutics, ed. 6. New York, Macmillan, Inc., 1980.

Wintrobe, M.M., Lee, G.R., Boggs, D.R., Bithell, T.C., Athens, J.W., and Foerster, J. Clinical Hematology, ed. 7. Philadelphia, Lea & Febiger, 1974.

32 Drugs acting on the respiratory system

Glenn T. Housholder

Because the number of drugs that act directly or indirectly on the respiratory system is large, this chapter will be limited to those drugs used for support and stimulation of respiration in emergency situations, those prescribed for the asthmatic patient, and those that improve ventilation or provide symptomatic relief from respiratory infections. Since the pharmacology of some drugs referred to here has been presented in other chapters, appropriate references will be made to those chapters.

DRUGS USED IN RESPIRATORY EMERGENCIES
Oxygen

Oxygen is a colorless, odorless, and tasteless gas. Although it is not flammable, it vigorously supports combustion. Oxygen is an essential emergency drug in the dental office and is indicated in all emergencies other than hyperventilation. The deprivation of oxygen by any mechanism is termed *hypoxia*.

A reduction of both arterial blood oxygen tension (Pa_{O_2}) and total oxygen content (hypoxic hypoxia) can occur by several mechanisms. One mechanism is the inadequate oxygenation of normal lung tissue, which can occur as a result of (1) airway obstruction by a foreign body, edema, or bronchial constriction, (2) insufficient pulmonary ventilation as a complication of disease or depression of respiration by morphine or similar drugs, or (3) deficiency of oxygen in the inspired air, as at high altitudes. Hypoxic hypoxia can also be a consequence of inadequate oxygenation caused by abnormal pulmonary function (pulmonary edema or fibrosis, emphysema) or anatomical arteriovenous shunts (congenital heart disease). This type of hypoxia is the most common form seen clinically.

Administration of oxygen is most effective when the hypoxia is a result of insufficient pulmonary ventilation. It is of benefit as an adjunctive agent in the support of the cardiovascular system when hypoxia is a result of impaired circulation.

The central nervous system is particularly vulnerable to the effects of hypoxia. As the arterial oxygen tension decreases, mental aberrations, impaired judgment, disorientation, loss of visual acuity and sense of time, and impaired muscular coordination occur. Loss of consciousness ensues when the oxygen saturation of hemoglobin decreases to about 65%, at which point cyanosis may be present.

Cerebral hypoxia, produced in animals by the arrest of cerebral circulation, causes unconsciousness within seconds. Arrest for even 2 minutes has been shown experimentally to produce histologic changes in the cerebral cortex and blood vessels. Some return of function occurred in those animals surviving 6 minutes of cephalic stasis, but in those surviving 8 minutes, irreversible damage resulted and consciousness was never restored.[8]

Toxic reactions and side effects. There are situations, more likely to be encountered in the hospital than in the dental office, when the administration of oxygen can produce untoward effects. Respiratory tract irritation can occur after inhalation of 80% to 100% oxygen at atmospheric pressure for 12 to 24 hours. A progressive decrease in vital capacity is accompanied by a sore throat, coughing, nasal congestion, and substernal pain. Continued administration of oxygen at high concentrations is likely to produce even more severe pulmonary complications. On the other hand, long-term administration of oxygen at a concentration of 50% or less does not produce these effects.

There are some clinical situations in which the response of the respiratory centers to carbon dioxide is so depressed that respiration is maintained by the reflex hypoxic stimulus, mediated by the carotid body and aortic arch chemoreceptors. Chronic pulmonary disease or severe barbiturate overdosage could present such a situation. The administration of oxygen here could eliminate the hypoxic drive to respiration and produce apnea and respiratory acidosis. These problems can be circumvented by provision of artificial ventilation along with oxygen therapy.

Premature infants who require oxygen supplementation for any substantial length of time are usually not exposed to oxygen concentrations greater than 40%. Oxygen is administered only to those infants who need it and for the shortest time possible, because high concentrations of oxygen can cause retrolental fibroplasia and ultimately blindness. Retinal damage can also occur in adults if 100% oxygen is inhaled at an ambient pressure of 2 to 3 atmospheres. The patient with compromised retinal circulation is particularly susceptible.

Long-term low-flow oxygen therapy. Long-term low-flow oxygen therapy has emerged as a useful tool in the care of selected patients with chronic obstructive lung disease.[3,19] A major advance in long-term oxygen therapy began in 1967 with the development and use of a portable, continuous, low-flow liquid oxygen system.[15] Using a nasal cannula, which replaced bulky tents or uncomfortable masks, this system allows for storage and transportation of liquid oxygen under low pressure and administration of oxygen to ambulatory outpatients in a safe and practical manner. Using this system, the patient can be away from the large conventional oxygen reservoir for as long as 8 hours. Patients selected for long-term low-flow oxygen therapy require oxygen in the range of 1 to 3 L per minute, a flow rate adequate to provide the benefits of oxygen therapy without significant risk of respiratory depression from abolition of the hypoxic stimulus to breathe. Although patients receiving this therapy must remain under close medical supervision, complications appear to be negligible.

Preparation. Oxygen U.S.P. is available as a compressed gas at about 2000 psi. As with other therapeutic gases, oxygen is marketed in steel cylinders that, for safety's sake, have a unique color code (green for oxygen) and a pin-indexed or otherwise noninterchangeable connector system. A two-stage, grease-free regulator is usually employed to provide oxygen at flow rates and pressures commensurate with therapeutic needs.

Aromatic ammonia spirit

Aromatic ammonia spirit is a pungent aromatic solution containing ammonium hydroxide and ammonium carbonate in alcohol. It acts as a reflex stimulant and has a very brief duration of action. It is available in 0.4 ml gauze-wrapped glass ampules, which can be crushed with the fingers and then held under the patient's nose. Such medication should be on every dental emergency tray for use in syncope. Caution must be taken not to confuse aromatic ammonia spirit with amyl nitrite, which comes in similar ampules.

Doxapram

Doxapram is one of a class of general CNS stimulants known as analeptics, which collectively have had very limited usefulness as adjuncts in the treatment of ventilatory arrest or insufficiency. The margin between the analeptic and convulsant doses of the older analeptic drugs is narrow, and their use is now discouraged in such clinical situations as drug-induced coma, overdose of inhalation anesthetics, shock, hypoxemia, increased intracranial pressure, and acute or chronic lung disease. In the rare cases in which analeptic therapy is elected, doxapram is the safest drug in this category.

Doxapram stimulates ventilation by increasing tidal volume and ventilatory rate. There is some evidence that it may prevent or reverse narcotic-induced and anesthetic-induced ventilatory depression. Doxapram hastens arousal when administered immediately after surgery, but the clinical usefulness of the drug remains to be established. The pharmacology of doxapram and the hazards associated with its use are discussed more fully in Chapter 14.

DRUGS USED TO TREAT ASTHMA

Bronchial asthma is a disease caused by excessive irritability of the respiratory tree. Whether induced by an extrinsic allergen or chemical irritant or by an intrinsic factor such as emotional distress, an asthmatic attack is characterized by a diffuse airway obstruction related to bronchial and bronchiolar constriction coupled with hypersecretion of viscous mucus. The condition is characterized pathologically by hypertrophy of the bronchial smooth muscle and by the presence of intralumenal mucous plugs and submucosal edema. These alterations are believed to reflect the actions of various chemical mediators, such as histamine and slow reacting substance of anaphylaxis (SRS-A, leukotriene C), on target tissues of the lung. Bronchial asthma is unique in that the airway obstruction is largely reversible by certain drugs and therapeutic measures.

The rationale of drug therapy for bronchial asthma can be explained in part by advances in the understanding of the cyclic adenosine monophosphate–guanosine monophosphate (AMP-GMP) system. The release of mediators (e.g., histamine, SRS-A) from mast cells and basophils is regulated by the autonomic nervous system.[28] The mast cell has, among other things, β-adrenergic receptors that respond to β-receptor agonists by increasing the intracellular concentration of cAMP. The catalysis by adenylate cyclase of adenosine triphosphate (ATP) to cAMP is discussed in detail in Chapter 5. The accumulation of cAMP leads to bronchial smooth muscle relaxation and inhibition of mast cell release of mediators. Therefore, one approach to drug therapy is to increase the concentration of cAMP, either by stimulating its formation by β-adrenergic drugs or by preventing its degradation by the enzyme cyclic nucleotide phosphodiesterase. Theophylline is an example of a drug administered to inhibit the action of phosphodiesterase, and it has been a mainstay of bronchodilator therapy for many years.

Another approach might be to inhibit the release of chemical mediators from the mast cell. Cromolyn sodium was introduced for clinical trial in the United States in 1973 for this purpose. It plays no part in the treatment of acute asthma but is of value in the management of the patient with chronic symptoms. One of the more significant aspects of cromolyn prophylaxis has been its ability to reduce the requirement for corticosteroids in patients receiving long-term therapy with these drugs.

The mechanism of action of corticosteroids in allergic diseases remains obscure, and controversy still exists about their precise role in the treatment of asthma. When conventional drugs fail to produce remission, the short-term use of corticosteroids can cause rapid improvement. It is imperative, however, that these agents be used judiciously.

Various other therapeutic measures may also be used. The prompt administration of antibiotics is indicated for respiratory infections of nonviral origin. Sedatives may be used to minimize emotional stress; expectorants may aid in the removal of secretions. Finally, avoiding tobacco and environmental irritants or allergens may help prevent episodes of asthma.

Table 32-1. Common theophylline formulations and their theophylline equivalents

Nonproprietary name	Proprietary name	Theophylline equivalent (%)
Theophylline	Elixophyllin, Marax,* Quibron*	100
Aminophylline (theophylline ethylenediamine)	Aminodur Duratabs, Amesec*	79–86
Oxtriphylline (choline theophyllinate)	Choledyl, Brondecon*	64
Dyphylline (dihydroxypropyl theophylline)	Dilor, Lufyllin, Neothylline	70†
Theophylline sodium glycinate	Synophylate, Asbron G*	49

*Combination drug.
†Does not release free theophylline; therapeutic equivalent is only about 10%.

Xanthines

Theophylline. Theophylline (1,3-dimethylxanthine) is a naturally occurring plant alkaloid closely related to caffeine and theobromine. It is very insoluble in aqueous solutions and is prepared as a salt to increase its solubility and absorption. Aminophylline (theophylline ethylenediamine) is the most widely used of the soluble salts. The clinical efficacy of theophylline salts depends on the amount of anhydrous theophylline equivalent that they contain (Table 32-1).

Theophylline has widespread pharmacologic actions. These include stimulation of respiration, augmentation of cardiac rate and force of contraction, diuresis, and relaxation of smooth muscle, particularly in the bronchi and in blood vessels other than cerebral vessels. These actions of theophylline were believed to be mediated through inhibition of the enzyme cyclic nucleotide phosphodiesterase, thus increasing the intracellular concentration of cAMP.[24] However, it is now recognized that significant inhibition of phosphodiesterase requires concentrations several times higher than those achieved clinically and that other mechanisms of action (e.g., blockade of adenosine receptors, alteration of prostaglandin synthesis or function, and effects on calcium metabolism) may be more important. Currently, there is no consensus on how theophylline acts to relieve asthma.[10,18]

Theophylline is a versatile drug because its preparation in the form of various salts allows for several modes of administration. The rate of absorption of theophylline depends on the preparation used and its route of administration. Oral absorption of the alkaloid alone was once thought to be poor and variable because of its low aqueous solubility, but, in fact, theophylline is well absorbed. The salt aminophylline, which contains about 85% theophylline by weight, is also readily absorbed. It is the only preparation used for intravenous injection. The rectal administration of theophylline, in the form of a retention enema, is an effective way to achieve rapid action in acute asthma. Rectal suppositories, however, are unreliably absorbed and frequently irritating.

Theophylline undergoes hepatic biotransformation and is excreted in the urine as 1,3-dimethyluric acid, 1-methyluric acid, and 3-methylxanthine.[26] Less than 10% is excreted unchanged. Biliary excretion has not been demonstrated in humans.[2] At therapeutic doses, about 60% of the drug is bound to plasma proteins.[13]

The half-life of theophylline averages 3.5 hours in children and 8 hours in adults. The plasma concentrations of theophylline can be reduced and the half-life shortened by cigarette smoking. Increased plasma concentrations and prolonged half-lives are seen in alcoholism, in reduced liver or renal function, in congestive heart failure, and in patients receiving cimetidine or certain antibiotics (e.g., erythromycin or clindamycin).[27]

Oral theophylline has long been the basic therapy for bronchial asthma. Used correctly, it is a safe and effective agent for both chronic and acute asthma in children and adults, but because of the variations in the absorption and metabolism of theophylline preparations, the dose should be individualized by using clinical response and serum concentration as guides.[26] Optimal effects are observed at a serum concentration of 10 to 20 μg/ml. Failure of therapy is often associated with failure to achieve therapeutic plasma levels.

The theophylline regimen that is chosen depends on the frequency of asthma attacks. For example, the patient who experiences attacks only rarely may require treatment for the episode and for a week or so thereafter. Some asthmatic patients have marked airway obstruction between attacks, even while they are apparently asymptomatic, and for these cases the long-term use of theophylline at 6-hour intervals has proved advantageous.[20] Mild exacerbations are treated with the addition of β-ad-

renergic agonists to the regimen. For the rapid relief of acute symptoms, an intravenous loading dose of aminophylline is recommended, followed by maintenance infusion. Other therapy, with antibiotics or steroids, can be added if required.

Theophylline toxicity is related to dose and plasma concentration. The adverse effects associated with long-term use are anorexia, nausea, vomiting, and abdominal discomfort. Serious toxicity, which is infrequent, is more likely to follow rapid intravenous injection of the drug. Exposure of vital organs to an excessive concentration of theophylline can result in convulsions, cardiac arrhythmias, or respiratory and cardiac arrest.

There are numerous oral formulations of theophylline available. Some of the theophylline salts are combined with other agents, such as adrenergic drugs, expectorants, or sedatives. Table 32-1 identifies some of the common formulations and their anhydrous theophylline equivalents.

Adrenergic agents

The pharmacology and structure-activity relationships of the adrenergic drugs are discussed in Chapter 6. These agents have long provided an effective means of obtaining symptomatic relief in the treatment of asthma.

Epinephrine. Epinephrine is administered parenterally in acute episodes of asthma requiring immediate relief. In such cases, 0.2 to 0.5 ml of a 1:1000 aqueous solution is injected subcutaneously to produce bronchodilation. Since epinephrine possesses both α- and β-receptor activity, it can also improve respiration by relieving congestion of the bronchial mucosa.

Epinephrine may be administered by oral inhalation of a nebulized form of the drug. Although this technique has become quite popular because of its efficacy and convenience, absorption of the drug from the respiratory tract can occur, causing systemic side effects. Too frequent administration can result in drying and irritation of the bronchial mucosa, and in certain patients this technique may induce an asthmatic attack.

Ephedrine. Ephedrine stimulates both α and β receptors, partially by a direct action and partially through the release of endogenous catecholamines. Its actions are thus similar to those of epinephrine. Ephedrine has been useful in treating mild to moderate acute asthma because of its long duration of action. It is not as effective as epinephrine in severe attacks because its bronchodilator action is weaker. The drug is frequently administered at bedtime to prevent nocturnal wheezing. The tendency of ephedrine to produce tachyphylaxis when used for long periods may limit its use in chronic asthma.

Ephedrine is marketed as a single-entity drug and as a component in numerous fixed-dose combination products. It is often combined with aminophylline, sedatives, or expectorants.

The adverse reactions are similar to those of epinephrine. In addition, there may be CNS stimulation, the most common signs of which are nervousness, excitability, and insomnia.

Isoproterenol. Isoproterenol is the prototypical β-receptor agonist. It acts on β_1 receptors to increase the rate and force of cardiac contractions and on β_2 receptors located in the smooth muscle of the bronchi, blood vessels, and other locations. Oral inhalation is recommended for the treatment of asthmatic attacks, but excessive use of the nebulized drug can produce adverse effects, such as nervousness, headaches, severe arrhythmias, including fibrillation, as well as tolerance and refractoriness. In susceptible patients, oral inhalation of isoproterenol may precipitate an asthmatic attack. The short duration of action is another disadvantage of isoproterenol.

Metaproterenol. Metaproterenol is a derivative of isoproterenol in which the hydroxyl group is moved from C_4 to C_5 of the benzene nucleus in the molecule (Figure 32-1). This structural change produces a predominant β_2 stimulant action, with little activity on β_1 receptors. It also protects metaproterenol from enzymatic degradation, thus prolonging the drug's duration of action.

An effective clinical response is obtained after inhalation or oral administration of metaproterenol.[14] Inhalation produces a peak effect in 30 to 60 minutes, and there is sustained improvement in pulmonary function tests for up to 5 hours. The incidence and severity of cardiac reactions following metaproterenol inhalation are less than with isoproterenol.

Terbutaline. Terbutaline, a modification of metaproterenol, was introduced for the treatment of asthma in 1970.[1,7] It is of clinical interest because of its long duration of action and because it has equivalent or fewer side effects than metaproterenol. For patients with spontaneous asthma, it is reported to provide greater protection against bronchoconstriction than an equivalent dose of metaproterenol.[1] The most common side effect

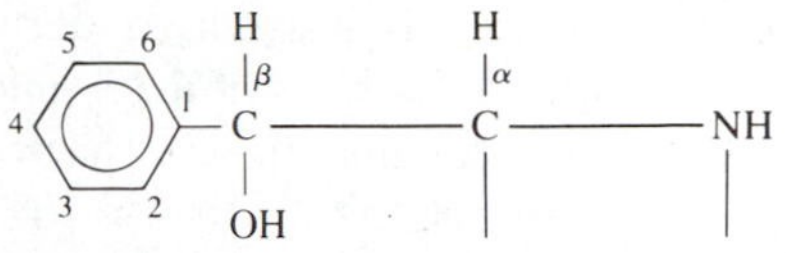

Isoproterenol	3-OH, 4-OH	H	$CH(CH_3)_2$
Metaproterenol	3-OH, 5-OH	H	$CH(CH_3)_2$
Terbutaline	3-OH, 5-OH	H	$C(CH_3)_3$
Albuterol	3-CH_2OH, 4-OH	H	$C(CH_3)_3$
Isoetharine	3-OH, 4-OH	CH_2CH_3	$CH(CH_3)_2$

Figure 32-1. β-Adrenergic drugs that can suppress bronchoconstriction in the asthmatic patient.

seen at therapeutic levels is a slight tremor. Other side effects, typical of isoproterenol and epinephrine, are few.

Albuterol. Albuterol is a β_2-adrenergic bronchodilator that has received extensive clinical testing outside the United States.[12,22] It is available in the United States in tablet form and as a metered-dose pressurized aerosol providing 0.09 mg of the drug with each inhalation. The recommended dosage is two inhalations (0.18 mg) every 4 to 6 hours. In a comparison of drugs administered by metered-dose inhalers, 0.2 mg of albuterol was more effective and longer lasting than 1.0 mg of isoproterenol or 1.5 mg of metaproterenol.[22] Adverse reactions to albuterol are similar to those of other adrenergic drugs, but they occur less frequently than with isoproterenol.

Isoetharine. Isoetharine, an agent with modest selectivity for β_2 receptors, is available only for inhalation. Reportedly, it produces less cardiac stimulation than inhaled metaproterenol.

New drugs. There are several investigational β_2-stimulating drugs that show promise in the treatment of reversible airway obstruction. Fenoterol, another derivative of metaproterenol, is now being evaluated in the United States. The drug is effective orally and by inhalation and has minimal side effects. The onset of bronchodilation after inhalation is comparable to that obtained with isoproterenol, but the effect from fenoterol lasts much longer (8 hours).[17] It has been rated superior to albuterol in some reports.[16] Fenoterol may emerge as a valuable drug in the treatment of reversible airway obstruction. Other selective β_2 agonists include carbuterol, salmefamol, soterenol, and tretoquinol.

Cromolyn sodium

Cromolyn sodium is a synthetic derivative of khellin, the agent in extracts of the *Ammi visnaga* plant that produces smooth muscle relaxation. Cromolyn is available as a powder, which is inhaled via a spinhaler device, or as an aqueous solution for administration via a power-operated nebulizer and face mask. The drug is poorly absorbed when given orally. Approximately 8% of the inhaled drug is absorbed from the lung and is rapidly excreted in the urine and bile. The remainder is either exhaled or swallowed and excreted via the gastrointestinal tract. The amount of cromolyn absorbed after inhalation of 20 mg does not appear to exert any general pharmacologic effects. Apparently no major metabolism of the drug occurs in humans.

Cromolyn is a unique drug for the control of chronic asthma since it has no bronchodilating or antiinflammatory actions. Instead, it appears to inhibit the degranulation of mast cells and the release of histamine and other spasmogens after immunologic (antigen-antibody) challenge,[5] thus blocking bronchospasm. The drug also blocks bronchospasm of nonimmunologic origin, such as from exercise or hyperventilation. The mechanism by which cromolyn suppresses mediator release is under investigation. At the present time, the data suggest that cromolyn inhibits calcium influx into the mast cell, which is a required step in the release process.[11] Cromolyn also inhibits phosphodiesterase and so may have an additional mechanism of action.

Clinically, cromolyn is ineffective in the treatment of acute attacks of asthma, including status asthmaticus. It functions exclusively as a prophylactic agent in the management of chronic symptoms. Both long-term and short-term studies have documented clinical improvement in patients taking cromolyn, with a low incidence of toxic side effects. Most adverse reactions have been mild and have consisted mainly of wheezing, coughing, and dryness of the throat. There have been rare reports, however, of eosinophilia with pulmonary infiltration, pulmonary granulomatosis, and the development of subacute and acute allergic reactions. Generally, any patient who demonstrates a reaction other than a transitory irritative response is removed from cromolyn therapy.

During cromolyn therapy, patients are maintained on regular medication, such as oral bronchodilators. In cromolyn-treated patients receiving corticosteroids, there have been reports of a decreased corticosteroid requirement, which permitted many patients to convert from a daily steroid schedule to an alternate day program or to discontinue steroids completely.[21] A decreased requirement for sympathomimetic and xanthine bronchodilators has also been noted. This medication-sparing effect is one of the major advantages of cromolyn therapy.

Ketotifen

Ketotifen is a recently developed oral agent for the prophylaxis of bronchial asthma. It has strong antihistaminic (H_1) actions, but additionally it has powerful antianaphylactic properties.[6] The drug intervenes in several biologic systems and causes (1) inhibition of the release of leukotriene mediators of anaphylaxis, (2) inhibition of the bronchospasm provoked by SRS-A in vivo, and (3) antagonism of calcium uptake by mast cells and of the effect of Ca^{++} on depolarized smooth muscle.

Treatment with ketotifen consistently inhibits the immediate and delayed reactions of asthmatic patients to inhaled allergens. The drug also blocks exaggerated responses to histamine and protects against drug-induced asthma (e.g., aspirin).[29] This increased resistance to bronchospasm-inducing stimuli has been ascribed to a progressive reduction in overall bronchial hyperreactivity.

Clinical studies have shown that the oral administration of ketotifen and the inhalation of cromolyn have a similar prophylactic efficacy. As with cromolyn, an important benefit of ketotifen treatment is that dosages of bronchodilators and corticosteroids can be reduced during therapy.

The major side effect of ketotifen is sedation, which is experienced by 10% to 15% of patients during the first week of treatment. Drowsiness diminishes with time. The drug is well tolerated, and the oral route of administration promotes patient compliance.

Corticosteroids

The corticosteroids have been of major importance for more than 25 years in the clinical management of patients with bronchial asthma. The mechanisms by which their beneficial actions are achieved in this disease are still not fully understood, although they are believed to be a consequence of the common pattern of corticosteroid action, as described in Chapter 22. The ultimate expression of the corticosteroid effect occurs as a result of new protein synthesis within the target cell, and several hours are required for the completion of this process. Consequently, an immediate therapeutic response cannot be expected to follow the administration of a corticosteroid, and these agents cannot be used as a substitute for adrenergic or xanthine bronchodilators in acute asthma. The corticosteroids may, in part, prevent bronchoconstriction by facilitating the stimulation of adenyl cyclase by catecholamines. In conjunction with an increased formation of cAMP, there is a decrease in the rate of its degradation. Corticosteroids decrease the activity of ATPase and phosphodiesterase in various tissues. There is a possibility too that corticosteroids may have effects on the synthesis of chemical mediators of allergic reactions. SRS-A precursors have been reported to be reduced by these drugs, and high doses of cortisone have been shown to decrease histamine titers in lung tissue. Corticosteroids also prevent the reappearance of histamine granules in mast cells following depletion by chemical histamine-releasers. The relevance of these observations with regard to the beneficial effects of corticosteroids in asthma is unclear at this time.

The continued use of corticosteroids in pharmacologic doses can cause adrenal suppression and hyperadrenocorticism. The risk of adrenal suppression depends on the dosage as well as the duration of action of the specific drug and on the length of treatment. Prednisone and prednisolone, for example, produce fewer complications than do the longer-acting preparations, such as betamethasone and dexamethasone. In fact, the administration of a short-acting drug for a brief time (7 to 10 days) is generally not associated with significant toxicity.

An alternate-day regimen for oral administration of corticosteroids has been developed for patients with chronic asthma.[9] Patients suffer fewer adverse reactions on this regimen, and the short-acting compounds cause the least adrenal suppression. Nevertheless, patients receiving long-term corticosteroid therapy should be continually monitored by the physician.

There are other specific clinical situations for which corticosteroid therapy is justified. One example is the hospitalized patient who remains in status asthmaticus longer than 12 to 18 hours after intensive treatment with intravenous fluids and sympathomimetic and xanthine bronchodilators. The intravenous administration of hydrocortisone hemisuccinate has proved effective in this situa-

tion, with no adverse reactions when given for 2 to 4 days.[4] Usually the corticosteroid can be quickly discontinued, and most of these patients can be discharged without steroid medication. Another candidate for corticosteroid therapy is the patient who, despite a 24-hour regimen of bronchodilators, still continues to have symptoms requiring medical attention.

Aerosols. Aerosol corticosteroids have been intensively investigated in an attempt to minimize potential adverse effects of the drugs. This technique allows the drug to be deposited directly into the lung, where it might be expected to exert a local action at much lower doses than are needed orally. Cortisone, hydrocortisone, prednisone, and prednisolone in aerosol form have been evaluated, but they are all absorbed into the circulation and consequently can produce systemic side effects. Extensive use of dexamethasone has indicated that although this drug has a significant therapeutic action and can replace oral steroids in the majority of patients, the therapeutic effect is associated with features of Cushing's syndrome as well as with adrenal suppression in many patients.

The most promising corticosteroid to date for inhalation is beclomethasone dipropionate, which was developed and extensively evaluated in Europe before becoming available in the United States. It is a chlorinated analogue of betamethasone and holds great promise in the management of intractable asthma.

After inhalation of an aerosolized suspension of beclomethasone dipropionate, the drug is deposited in the mouth, nasal passages, trachea, principal bronchi, and lungs. A considerable amount is swallowed. The drug is rapidly absorbed from the respiratory and gastrointestinal tissues. It is rapidly metabolized in the lung to beclomethasone-17-monopropionate and more slowly to free beclomethasone. The drug and its metabolites are excreted principally in the feces, with less than 10% appearing in the urine.

At the recommended dosage, beclomethasone does not appear to produce adrenal suppression and does achieve reasonable control in adult and child asthmatic patients. Impaired adrenal function has been reported in patients maintained on 5 times the recommended daily dose. The major side effects associated with the inhalation of beclomethasone are dryness of the mouth and an increased incidence of transient oral candidiasis, which responds readily to local therapy.

It is imperative that the patient understand that these drugs are preventive agents that must be taken regularly. They are not suitable for the treatment of an attack. In fact, if a severe attack of asthma occurs, the patient may not be able to inhale the drug or it may fail to reach the bronchioles.

Implications for dentistry

To provide the most effective and the safest dental care for the asthmatic patient, it is important that the dentist be knowledgeable about the patient's history of asthma and how this medical problem is being managed. One important question the dentist should ask is whether the patient is being maintained on corticosteroids; another is whether the patient has received this therapy in the last 6 to 12 months. The answers to these questions will determine, at least to some extent, whether the patient will require antibiotic therapy before or during dental treatment and whether the patient will manifest signs of adrenal hypofunction under the stress of dental procedures.

Another consideration is how the patient reacts to dental appointments. Many persons become apprehensive and anxious about impending visits to the dental office, and it is known that emotional factors play an active role in precipitating or exacerbating asthmatic symptoms. For this reason, the asthmatic patient should be questioned about the medication the physician has prescribed for acute attacks and should be requested to bring antiasthmatic medication to the dental office should it be needed during the appointment.

If the patient is a candidate for preoperative or postoperative sedation, hydroxyzine is a good choice; chloral hydrate, diazepam, or meprobamate are reasonable alternatives. Unusually large doses of sedative drugs may be required if the patient is receiving continuous treatment with CNS stimulants, such as aminophylline and ephedrine.

Another consideration is the choice of an analgesic for the asthmatic patient. Aspirin and aspirin-containing compounds should be avoided, because asthmatic episodes can be precipitated in some patients in minutes to hours after ingestion of these drugs. Asthmatic patients unable to tolerate aspirin may also react adversely to indomethacin, mefenamic acid, phenylbutazone, and the fenamate analgesics.[25] Large doses of morphine and meperidine can produce bronchial constriction, although this is not often observed after therapeutic doses. Inasmuch as these drugs have been reported to pre-cipitate asthmatic attacks in anesthetized patients, they should certainly be avoided during an asthmatic attack. Their ultimate action is to decrease the respiratory drive, a dangerous liability to the patient whose airway resistance may be many times greater than normal.

If a severe asthmatic attack does occur in the dental office, drug therapy is indicated. A subcutaneous injection of 0.2 to 0.5 ml of 1:1000 epinephrine (equivalent to 0.2 to 0.5 mg of epinephrine) should relax the bronchioles and relieve the bronchospasm.

DRUGS USED TO IMPROVE VENTILATION

Numerous drugs are used to improve ventilation or to provide symptomatic relief of some uncomfortable symptoms of respiratory infection. These include bronchodilators (discussed in previous sections), antitussives, nasal decongestants, expectorants, and mucolytic agents.

Antitussives

Coughing is a protective reflex that clears the respiratory tract of accumulated secretions or noxious substances. A productive cough, with the elimination of excessive secretions, is beneficial, but a nonproductive cough may impair rest and increase discomfort. An ideal antitussive agent should decrease the frequency and intensity of coughing but still allow adequate elimination of excessive secretions from the respiratory tract.

Opioids. The ability of opioids to suppress coughing parallels their analgesic effect and their abuse potential. Because of their side effects and addicting liability, the more potent drugs, such as morphine and hydromorphone, are not commonly used as antitussives.

Codeine is the most useful narcotic for cough suppression. At therapeutic doses and for short-term use, its addicting potential is minimal and depressed ventilation is infrequent. Overdosage results in respiratory depression, convulsions, hypotension, and tachycardia.

Hydrocodone, like codeine, acts centrally on the medullary cough center. On the basis of weight, hydrocodone appears to be about three times greater in antitussive activity that codeine. It also has a greater addiction liability than codeine. At therapeutic doses, the most common side effects include nausea, constipation, and dizziness.

Nonopioids. Nonopioid drugs that act centrally on the medullary cough center include benzonatate, chlophedianol, dextromethorphan, and noscapine. These agents generally produce fewer adverse reactions than the opioid drugs.

Benzonatate is an antitussive structurally related to tetracaine. Although the primary action of benzonatate is apparently depression of the central cough mechanism, it may also act by inhibiting the stretch receptors of the respiratory mucosa. The most common adverse reactions include nausea, constipation, headache, drowsiness, and vertigo. Nasal congestion, as well as numbness of the tongue, mouth, and pharynx, has been noted if the capsules are chewed before swallowing.

Chlophedianol is an antitussive prepared in a syrup. Adverse reactions include nausea, vomiting, and dry mouth. In addition, nightmares, hallucinations, visual disturbances, and excitability have been reported after its use.

Dextromethorphan, the methyl ester of the dextroisomer of levorphanol, appears to be the most popular cough suppressant. In OTC mixtures, it is often used in combination with other agents, such as bronchodilators, antihistamines, and expectorants. It has no addiction liability or analgesic properties. At recommended doses, side effects are minimal.

Noscapine is one of the isoquinoline series of opium alkaloids. It has no analgesic effect or addiction liability but possesses effective antitussive activity, with few adverse reactions. At high doses, nausea, headache, and drowsiness have been reported. Noscapine is occasionally included in multientity OTC preparations.

Nasal decongestants

The most commonly used nasal decongestants are adrenergic agents. These drugs act by stimulating the excitatory α receptors of vascular smooth muscle, thereby constricting the dilated arterioles within the nasal mucosa. This constriction reduces blood flow in the edematous area and opens obstructed nasal passages.

Most of these drugs are used topically. Topical application may cause temporary stinging, burning, or drying of the mucosa. A rebound congestion occurs after the use of many of these agents, often causing misuse of the drugs. Prolonged topical use may be irritating enough to induce a chronic swelling of the nasal mucosa, but discontinuing the drug will remedy this situation.

Phenylephrine, an α-adrenergic receptor agonist, is a widely used decongestant. It is less potent than some of the older agents, but its duration of action is longer. The side effects include those typical of epinephrine and ephedrine.

Both ephedrine and epinephrine are effective decongestants, but they are seldom used in this capacity today. Ephedrine can produce a swelling of the nasal mucosa and tachyphylaxis, as well as CNS stimulation, palpitations, and transient hypertension. Epinephrine frequently produces rebound nasal congestion and the typical symptoms of CNS stimulation such as anxiety, palpitations, restlessness, dizziness, and headache. The adverse reactions produced by either drug disappear rapidly after the medication is discontinued.

Propylhexedrine is administered by nasal inhalation. It has essentially no toxic effects, and it can even be used for those patients in whom the pressor effect of ephedrine is to be avoided.

Oxymetazoline is an effective decongestant with a long duration of action. It is available as a solution and as a spray. The adverse reactions associated with its use are mild and include stinging or drying of the nasal mucosa, headache, palpitations, and insomnia.

Expectorants and mucolytic agents

Agents administered to stimulate the flow of respiratory tract secretions are termed *expectorants*. Mucolytic agents are used to reduce the viscosity of respiratory tract secretions. Both of these enhance the movement of secretions upward and outward by ciliary movement and coughing.

Expectorants are believed to act by stimulating receptors in the gastric mucosa, thus initiating the reflex secretion of respiratory tract fluid. This action is assumed to increase the volume and decrease the viscosity of the fluid. There is little clinical evidence of the efficacy of these agents.

Potassium iodide is an example of a drug used traditionally as an expectorant and for which there is little proof of effectiveness. It is readily absorbed and produces untoward reactions on prolonged use. Iodism, characterized by skin rash, fever, parotitis, and lacrimal gland enlargement, can be produced. Thyroid enlargement or decreased thyroid function can also occur. Sensitivity reactions can develop, and anaphylaxis has occasionally been reported.

Ammonium chloride is another example of a drug used traditionally to stimulate the flow of respiratory secretions. It is used most frequently in multientity mixtures. It is readily absorbed and can produce metabolic acidosis if large doses are administered.

Guaifenesin (glyceryl guaiacolate) is available as an ingredient in various tablets and syrups. In clinical evaluations,[23] it reportedly increased sputum volume, facilitated raising of sputum, and reduced cough frequency, cough intensity, and chest discomfort when compared with a matching vehicle. Occasionally, nausea and gastrointestinal upset may occur, but no serious adverse reactions have been reported.

Syrup of ipecac is a traditional expectorant and is used widely in combination with other drugs in OTC mixtures. At higher doses, it is an effective emetic.

Acetylcysteine is used in the hospital setting to reduce the viscosity of respiratory tract secretions. It must be administered by inhalation techniques, such as nebulization, or by direct instillation into the trachea. The drug may cause gastrointestinal disturbances, including nausea and vomiting. It can produce bronchospasm in asthmatic patients. Acetylcysteine should be used only where suction apparatus is available, since it produces large amounts of secretions that must be removed.

Drugs acting on the respiratory system

Nonproprietary name	Proprietary name
Emergency drugs	
aromatic ammonia spirit	Aromatic Ammonia Aspirols
doxapram	Dopram
oxygen	—
Xanthines	
see Table 32-1	
Adrenergic bronchodilators	
albuterol	Ventolin, Proventil
ephedrine	—
epinephrine	Sus-Phrine, Primatene Mist
ethylnorepinephrine	Bronkephrine
fenoterol*	Berotec
isoetharine	Bronkometer, Bronkosol
isoproterenol	Isuprel
metaproterenol	Alupent, Metaprel
terbutaline	Brethine, Bricanyl
Corticosteroids	
beclomethasone	Vanceril
dexamethasone	Decadron Phosphate Respihaler
see also Table 22-6	

Agents limited to prophylaxis of asthma	
cromolyn	Intal
ketotifen*	Zaditen
Antitussives	
benzonatate	Tessalon Perles
chlophedianol	Ulo
codeine	—
dextromethorphan	Romilar
diphenhydramine	Diphen Cough
hydrocodone	Dicodid
levopropoxyphene	Novrad
noscapine	Tusscapine
Nasal decongestants	
ephedrine	Efedron Nasal
epinephrine	Adrenalin
1-desoxyephedrine	Vicks inhaler
naphazone	Privine
oxymetazoline	Afrin
phenylephrine	Neo-Synephrine
phenylpropanolamine	Propadrine
propylhexedrine	Benzedrex
pseudoephedrine	Sudafed
tetrahydrozoline	Tyzine
xylometazoline	Otrivin
Expectorants and mucolytics	
acetylcysteine	Mucomyst
ammonum chloride	in Endotussin-NN
guaifenesin	Robitussin
iodinated glycerol	Organidin
potassium iodide	Pima
syrup of ipecac	—

*Not currently available in the United States.

CITED REFERENCES

1. Arner, B. A comparative clinical trial of different subcutaneous doses of terbutaline and orciprenaline in bronchial asthma. Acta Medica Scandinavica Supplement **512:**45-48, 1970.
2. Barnhart, J.L., and Combes, B. Effect of theophylline on hepatic excretory function. American Journal of Physiology **227:**194-199, 1974.
3. Bone, R.C. Acute respiratory failure and chronic obstructive lung disease: recent advances. Medical Clinics of North America **65:**563-578, 1981.
4. Collins, J.V., Clark, T.J.H., Harris, P.W.R., and Townsend, J. Intravenous corticosteroids in treatment of acute bronchial asthma. Lancet **2:**1047-1049, 1970.
5. Cox, J.S.G. Disodium cromoglycate (FPL 670) ("Intal"): a specific inhibitor of reaginic antibody-antigen mechanisms. Nature **216:**1328-1329, 1967.
6. Craps, L. Ketotifen in the oral prophylaxis of bronchial asthma: a review. Pharmacotherapeutics **3:**18-35, 1981.
7. Formgren, H. Clinical comparison of inhaled terbutaline and orciprenaline in asthmatic patients. Scandinavian Journal of Respiratory Diseases **51:**203-211, 1970.
8. Grenell, R.G. Central nervous system resistance. I. The

effects of temporary arrest of cerebral circulation for periods of two to ten minutes. Journal of Neuropathology and Experimental Neurology **5:**131-154, 1946.

9. Harter, J.G., Reddy, W.J., and Thorn, G.W. Studies on an intermittent corticosteroid dosage regimen. New England Journal of Medicine **269:**591-596, 1963.

10. Isles, A.F., MacLeod, S.M., and Levison, H. Theophylline: new thoughts about an old drug. Chest **82** (suppl.):49S-54S, 1982.

11. Johnson, H.G., and Bach, M.K. Prevention of calcium iontophore-induced release of histamine in rat mast cells by disodium cromoglycate. Journal of Immunology **114:**514-516, 1975.

12. Kennedy, M.C., and Simpson, W.T. Human pharmacological and clinical studies on salbutamol: a specific beta-adrenergic bronchodilator. British Journal of Diseases of the Chest **63:**165-174, 1969.

13. Koysooko, R., Ellis, E.F., and Levy, G. Relationship between theophylline concentration in plasma and saliva of man. Clinical Pharmacology and Therapeutics **15:**454-460, 1974.

14. Leifer, K.N., and Wittig, J.Z. The beta-2 sympathomimetic aerosols in the treatment of asthma. Annals of Allergy **35:**69-80, 1975.

15. Levine, B.E., Bigelow, D.B., Hamstra, R.D., Beckwitt, H.J., Mitchell, R.S., Nett, L.M., Stephen, T.A., and Petty, T.L. The role of long-term continuous oxygen administration in patients with chronic airway obstruction with hypoxemia. Annals of Internal Medicine **66:**639-660, 1967.

16. Minnette, A. Ventilatory results and side effects of salbutamol given by different routes in coal miners with reversible bronchoobstruction. Postgraduate Medical Journal **47**(suppl.):55-61, 1971.

17. Pennock, B.E., Rogers, R.M., Ryan, B.R., and Ayers, L.N. Aerosol administration of fenoterol hydrobromide (Th 1165a) in subjects with reversible obstructive airway disease. Chest **72:**731-736, 1977.

18. Persson, C.G.A. Universal adenosine receptor antagonism is neither necessary nor desirable with xanthine antiasthmatics. Medical Hypotheses **8:**515-526, 1982.

19. Petty, T.L. Home oxygen in advanced chronic obstructive pulmonary disease. Medical Clinics of North America **65:**615-627, 1981.

20. Piafsky, K.M., and Ogilvie, R.I. Dosage of theophylline in bronchial asthma. New England Journal of Medicine **292:**1218-1222, 1975.

21. Read, J., and Rebuck, A.S. Steroid-sparing effect of disodium cromoglycate (''Intal'') in chronic asthma. Medical Journal of Australia **1:**566-569, 1969.

22. Riding, W.D., Dinda, P., and Chatterjee, S.S. The bronchodilator and cardiac effects of five pressure-packed aerosols in asthma. British Journal of Diseases of the Chest **64:**37-45, 1970.

23. Robinson, R.E., Cummings, W.B., and Deffenbaugh, E.R. Effectiveness of guaifenesin as an expectorant: a cooperative double-blind study. Current Therapeutic Research **22:**284-296, 1977.

24. Sutherland, E.W., Robison, G.A., and Butcher, R.W. Some aspects of the biological role of adenosine 3',5'-monophosphate (cyclic AMP). Circulation **37:**279-306, 1968.

25. Szczeklik, A., Gryglewski, R.J., and Czerniawska-Mysik, G. Relationship of inhibition of prostaglandin biosynthesis by analgesics to asthma attacks in aspirin-sensitive patients. British Medical Journal **1:**67-69, 1975.

26. Thompson, R.D., Nagasawa, H.T., and Jenne, J.W. Determination of theophylline and its metabolites in human urine and serum by high-pressure liquid chromatography. Journal of Laboratory and Clinical Medicine **84:**584-593, 1974.

27. Weinberger, M., Hendeles, L., and Ahrens, R. Pharmacologic management of reversible obstructive airways disease. Medical Clinics of North America **65:**579-613, 1981.

28. Wilson, A.F., and Galant, S.P. Recent advances in the pathophysiology of asthma. Western Journal of Medicine **120:**463-470, 1974.

29. Wuethrich, B., Radielovic, P., and Debelic, M. The protective effect of a new oral anti-asthma agent (ketotifen, HC20-511) against experimentally induced bronchospasm (5 different models). International Journal of Clinical Pharmacology **16:**424-429, 1978.

GENERAL REFERENCES

Chakrin, L.W., and Krell, R.D. Pathophysiology and pharmacotherapy of asthma; an overview. Journal of Pharmaceutical Sciences **69:**236-238, 1980.

Middleton, E.A., Jr. Rational approach to asthma therapy. Postgraduate Medicine **67:**107-116, 120-122, 1980.

Middleton, E.A., Jr. Antiasthmatic drug therapy and calcium ions: review of pathogenesis and role of calcium. Journal of Pharmaceutical Sciences **69:**243-251, 1980.

Pierce, A.K. Recent advances in the therapy of asthma. Part 2. Hospital Formulary **14:**154-167, 1979.

Plummer, A.L. Choosing a drug for obstructive pulmonary disease. 1. Agents to achieve bronchodilatation. Postgraduate Medicine **63:**36-41, 44-46, 48, 1978.

Plummer, A.L. Choosing a drug for obstructive pulmonary disease. 2. Agents other than bronchodilators. Postgraduate Medicine **63:**113-119, 1978.

Smith, T.C., Cooperman, L.H., and Wollman, H. The therapeutic gases. In Gilman, A.G., Goodman, L.S., and Gilman, A., eds. Goodman and Gilman's The Pharmacological Basis of Therapeutics, ed. 6. New York, Macmillan, Inc., 1980.

Svedmyr, K. beta 2-Adrenoceptor stimulants and theophylline in asthma therapy. European Journal of Respiratory Diseases **62**(suppl.116):1-48, 1981.

33 Drugs acting on the gastrointestinal tract

Glenn T. Housholder

Numerous drugs exert an effect, sometimes therapeutic, on the gastrointestinal tract, and a patient coming to the dental office may be on a regimen of one or more of these agents. These drugs can include anticholinergics, antacids, antiemetics, laxatives, antidiarrheal or antispasmodic drugs, and spasmodic drugs. Some of these are sold over the counter without prescription and may be used at the whim of the patient. Knowing that these drugs are being used may influence the dentist's choice of a therapeutic agent. Furthermore, should gastrointestinal disturbance arise during the course of therapy, it would be important to determine if one of these agents was responsible.

Many of the drugs discussed here are described in detail in other parts of the book. This chapter will focus attention on those drugs that are used exclusively for their effect on the gastrointestinal tract, as well as those drugs with a wider spectrum of activity that have application to gastrointestinal disorders. Some drugs that act on the gastrointestinal tract and are likely to be used in dentistry are listed in Table 33-1.

DRUGS USED IN ULCER THERAPY

Traditionally, therapy for duodenal ulcer has been directed at neutralizing gastric acids and inhibiting their secretion. Elevation of gastric pH suppresses in turn the proteolytic activity of pepsin. The cornerstone of treatment currently is the administration of H_2-receptor antihistamines but a variety of therapeutic regimens using acid-neutralizing salts on different schedules and with anticholinergic or other drugs have been developed. Therapy for gastric ulcer is essentially similar; however, the control of pain may be more difficult to achieve.

Gastric antacids

For many years the use of gastric antacids was the primary method for relieving the pain of peptic ulceration. Although their importance has declined since the introduction of cimetidine, they remain useful drugs, especially in patients who cannot successfully be treated with H_2 antagonists. There are a number of metallic salts marketed as antacids, either alone or in combination; the discussion that follows includes some of the more commonly used preparations.

Sodium bicarbonate. Sodium bicarbonate is an antacid that is widely used by the public. It is very effective in neutralizing gastric acid, the pH of which is normally 1 to 2. When complete neutralization is effected, pepsin becomes irreversibly inactivated, the stomach empties rapidly, and a rebound of gastric acid secretion occurs. If the pH is maintained between 4 and 5, the rebound does not develop. There are serious drawbacks to the repeated use of large doses of sodium bicarbonate, one of which is that it may cause sodium overload and systemic alkalosis. Sodium bicarbonate is contraindicated in patients on a low salt diet.

Magnesium hydroxide and magnesium-aluminum mixtures. Milk of magnesia (magnesium hydroxide) has a rapid onset of action and high neutralizing capacity that can elevate the pH of gastric contents to greater than 7. A disadvantage is its laxative effect, and few ulcer patients can tolerate it as the sole antacid for any length of time. Its combination with aluminum hydroxide offers certain advantages, including the fact that the combination has different buffering characteristics, which produce a gastric pH of less than 5, and a diminished laxative effect since aluminum hydroxide is in itself constipating.

Table 33-1. Preparations used in dentistry to affect the gastrointestinal tract

Therapeutic use	Nonproprietary name	Proprietary name	Dose*
Antisialagogue	Atropine sulfate	Atropine Sulfate	0.25-1.0 mg
	Propantheline bromide	Pro-Banthine	15-30 mg
	Methantheline bromide	Banthine	50-100 mg
Antiemetic	Promethazine hydrochloride	Phenergan	25 mg; 12.5-25 mg (children)
	Hydroxyzine hydrochloride	Vistaril, Atarax	25-100 mg; 12.5-25 mg (children)
	Trimethobenzamide hydrochloride	Tigan	250 mg; 100-200 mg (children)
	Dimenhydrinate	Dramamine	50-100 mg; 25-50 mg (children)

*Dose is for the oral route only.

Magnesium trisilicate. Magnesium trisilicate is much weaker than magnesium hydroxide, and therefore substantially more of the drug is required for the same degree of neutralization. Its onset of action is slow, and it reacts with gastric acid to form silicon dioxide in the stomach. Silicate kidney stones have been reported after its prolonged use. It is generally used in combination with other antacids, such as aluminum hydroxide and calcium and magnesium carbonates.

Aluminum hydroxide. Aluminum hydroxide gel usually brings gastric pH to about 4. The drug is poorly absorbed, and liquid preparations are more effective than solid dosage forms. Systemic toxicity, other than occasional nausea and vomiting, has not been reported. Its most common side effect is constipation, which is minimized when the drug is taken with magnesium hydroxide. Because the aluminum ion can combine with phosphate in the intestine to form insoluble aluminum phosphate, which is then excreted, prolonged use of large doses of aluminum hydroxide gel may result in phosphate depletion, particularly when phosphate intake is low. Anorexia, malaise, and muscle weakness are characteristic of phosphate depletion. The combination of aluminum and phosphate has been used by nephrologists to prevent the formation of renal phosphatic calculi.

Calcium carbonate. Calcium carbonate is a potent antacid capable of raising gastric pH to about 9 in a short period and producing a rebound hypersecretion. Its ingestion is associated with increased serum gastrin concentrations and evidence of gastric hypersecretion. Also, striking increases in serum calcium and phosphorus levels, accompanied by a decline in renal function, have been reported in ulcer patients. These effects, as well as its chalky taste and constipating effect, limit the use of calcium carbonate in routine antacid therapy.

H₂-receptor antihistamines

Histamine is a primary mediator of gastric acid secretion. As discussed in Chapter 23, H_2 receptors are located on the acid-secreting cells of the stomach. These cells release acid when they bind histamine and so contribute to ulcer formation. The H_2-receptor antihistamines interfere with this binding, thus blocking acid secretion. Cimetidine, the first of these drugs to enjoy widespread use, has revolutionized the treatment of duodenal ulcers.

Cimetidine. Cimetidine suppresses daytime and nocturnal basal gastric acid secretion, as well as secretion induced by food, histamine, pentagastrin, caffeine, and insulin. It is more effective than anticholinergic drugs in inhibiting acid secretion.[10] The therapeutic efficacy of cimetidine in severe duodenal ulceration was demonstrated in an early double-blind study that showed a good correlation between symptomatic relief and ulcer healing as judged endoscopically.[14] In one clinical trial, the incidence of ulcer healing averaged 59% after 4 weeks and 76% after 6 weeks of cimetidine therapy.[3]

Most patients tolerate cimetidine well, but, with widespread use of the drug, some serious adverse effects have been reported. For example, cimetidine inhibits oxidative microsomal biotransformation of several drugs, including diazepam.[2] It has been shown that just one day of pretreatment with cimetidine causes much higher plasma concentrations of diazepam, a more pronounced sedative effect, and slowed elimination of the drug.[16] If diazepam is prescribed for a patient on cimetidine therapy, the dose of the antianxiety agent should be appropriately reduced. Other adverse effects include fever, leukopenia, and an antiandrogenic effect, as well as CNS symptoms (confusion, delirium, hallucinations), especially with high doses, in elderly patients and in those with renal impairment.[26] Sudden discontinuance of the drug can lead to perforation of unhealed ulcers. Inasmuch as indiscriminate use increases the risk of side effects and drug interactions, cimetidine should be administered only for approved and literature-supported indications.

Ranitidine. Ranitidine, the second H_2 antihistamine approved for use in the United States, is similar to cimetidine in therapeutic efficacy and may have fewer side effects. The drug is at least 5 times as potent as cimetidine. Although it has a similar plasma half-life (of about 2 hours), ranitidine depresses gastric acid secretion for a much longer period after a single dose, thus permitting twice daily dosing. Ranitidine is less lipid soluble than cimetidine, is largely excluded by the blood-brain barrier, and has fewer CNS effects. Ranitidine does not appear to have any antiandrogenic properties nor does it inhibit the microsomal oxidation of other drugs.[26] (For more information on ranitidine and H_2-receptor blockade, the reader is referred to Chapter 23.)

Sucralfate

Sucralfate, a complex of aluminum hydroxide and sulfated sucrose, is used in the treatment of duodenal ulcer.[21] The drug has been shown to bind preferentially to the ulcer site, producing an adherent, cytoprotective barrier against further attack by acid, pepsin, or bile salts. Sucralfate also directly inhibits the action of pepsin and absorbs bile salts. It possesses no antacid properties. Since it is minimally absorbed from the gastrointestinal tract, sucralfate is considered a nonsystemic agent.

In clinical trials sucralfate has been shown to be significantly more effective than placebo[19] and as effective as cimetidine in the treatment of peptic ulceration.[20] Adverse side effects have been minor, constipation being the most frequent complaint, occurring in about 2% of the patients.

Implications for dentistry

Whether a patient is on a regimen of cimetidine or antacids or has a history of gastric or duodenal ulcer is important for a dentist to know and can influence a dentist's choice of therapeutic agent. The use of aspirin as an analgesic is contraindicated because of its irritating effect on gastric mucosa. An alternative analgesic such as acetaminophen could be used, based on evidence that it produces minimal damage to gastric mucosa as compared with aspirin.[15] All antiinflammatory drugs share the ulcerogenic property of the salicylates. Topical steroids are sometimes used in the management of oral ulcerations, but because of the possibility that absorption through the mucosa will occur, use of these agents, topically or systemically, is to be avoided in the ulcer patient.[9]

The choice of a preoperative or postoperative sedative is particularly important for the ulcer patient. Although chloral hydrate is not widely used today, it should be noted that the drug is quite irritating, and gastrointestinal side effects such as nausea and vomiting can occur. Diazepam would be appropriate for selected patients since, in addition to producing sedation, it can also suppress the nocturnal secretion of gastric acid.[4] Furthermore, it has been shown that absorption of orally administered diazepam is increased by the use of aluminum hydroxide.[23] For the patient being treated with cimetidine, however, a prudent choice would be to prescribe lorazepam or oxazepam, drugs not dependent on hepatic oxidative biotransformation. They are eliminated in the urine as glucuronide conjugates, and cimetidine does not impair their elimination.[25]

Sucralfate, aluminum hydroxide gels, antacids containing calcium and magnesium, and sodium bicarbonate impair the absorption of the tetracyclines. This action is shared by milk and milk products and appears to result from chelation and an increased gastric pH.

ANTISIALAGOGUES

The pharmacology of the anticholinergic drugs is presented in Chapter 9. These drugs block the action of ACh on the receptor site of effector cells innervated by postganglionic cholinergic fibers. Their use in dentistry is limited to the control of excessive salivation and as a preanesthetic medication. In medicine, they are widely used as antispasmodics.

Salivary secretion is readily inhibited by anticholinergic drugs. The prototype for this class is atropine, but scopolamine is a more potent antisialagogue. These drugs, some of which are listed in Table 33-1, can be used to control salivation, but many patients experience unpleasant side effects. The decision to use an antisialagogue will depend in part on the patient's medical history. Atropine is contraindicated in patients with prostatic hypertrophy or narrow-angle glaucoma, and the topical use of atropine is absolutely contraindicated in all forms of glaucoma. It should be administered with caution in patients with cardiovascular disease, since it can increase the pulse rate without increasing cardiac output. It may also antagonize the vagal effects of digitalis. Toxic effects are not uncommon, particularly in children.

The synthetic anticholinergic drugs propantheline and methantheline have also been used before in dental procedures to control excessive salivation. They are quaternary amines, which are always ionized at the pH of the body, and thus are unable to cross the blood-brain barrier. Therefore, they do not have the CNS effects that atropine and scopolamine have, and this property constitutes a distinct advantage. In comparison with atropine and scopolamine, these compounds are, unfortunately, poorly absorbed and less selective at controlling salivation. Precautions for their use in dentistry are similar to those for atropine.

EMETICS

Emergency occasions may arise that require an agent to induce a forceful emptying of the stomach. The drugs apomorphine and ipecac are the most commonly used emetics.

Apomorphine is produced by treating morphine with strong acids. It lacks the analgesic properties of morphine but does produce a combination of CNS excitation and depression. It stimulates the medullary chemoreceptor trigger zone (CTZ), and this is the basis for its therapeutic emetic properties. Large doses can cause respiratory depression, so it should not be administered at too frequent intervals or to patients who already show respiration depression. Naloxone can reverse the emetic and respiratory effects of apomorphine. Syrup of ipecac is a nonprescription emetic that has been recommended by many pediatricians in case of accidental poisoning in the home. A mixture of plant alkaloids (principally emetine), ipecac acts centrally on the CTZ and perhaps locally by irritation of the stomach and duodenum.

ANTIEMETICS

In contrast to the limited number of emetic agents, there are numerous agents that have a demonstrated antiemetic action. Vomiting is a complex process, and there are several sites, including the CTZ, cerebral cortex, vestibular apparatus, and the vomiting center in the medulla, at which antiemetic drugs may act to prevent or relieve nausea and vomiting.

As a class, the most effective antiemetics are the phenothiazines. These drugs are dopamine antagonists and inhibit stimulation of the CTZ. Most of the phenothiazines are not effective for motion sickness, but they are often used successfully for the nausea of pregnancy, postoperative emesis, or vomiting induced by radiation or cancer chemotherapy. Among the most commonly used agents are chlorpromazine, prochlorperazine, and promethazine. Promethazine, unlike the other phenothiazines, has little effect on vomiting caused by stimulation of the CTZ but is effective in preventing motion sickness. Its sedative action is advantageous in the treatment of postoperative nausea and vomiting. Promethazine enjoys fairly wide use in dentistry, principally for its sedative, antiemetic, and antisialagogic properties.

As is pointed out in Chapter 23, certain antihistamines are also effective antiemetics. Diphenhydramine, dimenhydrinate, meclizine, and cyclizine are especially useful in the treatment of the nausea and vomiting associated with motion sickness, pregnancy, and the postoperative state; but it should be emphasized that these drugs should not be used during pregnancy unless absolutely necessary. The antihistamines are not of value in relieving the nausea associated with administration of cytotoxic drugs.

Hydroxyzine, an antianxiety drug mentioned in Chapter 13, has antiemetic activity as well as antihistaminic and anticholinergic properties. It is contraindicated in early pregnancy, however, because high doses have produced fetal abnormalities in experimental animals. Scopolamine is a very effective antiemetic, but its use is limited by its unpleasant side effects. Trimethobenzamide, a nonphenothiazine antiemetic, also inhibits the CTZ and has the same range of actions as the phenothiazines.

Nausea and vomiting, sometimes very marked, are almost universal sequelae of cancer chemotherapy. The protracted bouts of drug-induced retching and vomiting, which may be only slightly relieved by standard antiemetic therapy, have led to the failure of some patients to complete courses of potentially curative treatment. Well-controlled clinical trials have now demonstrated the antiemetic efficacy of the dopamine antagonist metoclopramide in patients with advanced cancer who were receiving anticancer drugs.[13] Compared to other antiemetics and placebo, there were significantly fewer episodes of vomiting, decreased volume of vomitus, and shortened duration of nausea and vomiting in metoclopramide-treated patients. Metoclopramide acts both peripherally and centrally. Peripherally, the drug stimulates the release of ACh and sensitizes gastric smooth muscle to ACh. It also blocks the CTZ. Central antagonism of dopamine is probably an important part of its antiemetic action. Sedation is the most common side effect. A procainamide derivative, metoclopramide lacks significant cardiac effects. Extrapyramidal reactions occur infrequently with large doses and are rarely persistent.

Delta-9-tetrahydrocannabinol (Δ^9-THC), which is discussed in Chapter 46, is another agent that is being clinically evaluated as an antiemetic in patients undergoing cancer chemotherapy. These studies were undertaken following anecdotal reports that marijuana smokers suffered less nausea and vomiting in association with cytotoxic agents than other patients. Oral Δ^9-THC has been shown to be significantly better than placebo[5] and comparable to metoclopramide[29] in reducing chemotherapy-induced vomiting in some patients. However, Δ^9-THC can at times produce acute, and often intolerable, mental disturbances, particularly in older patients who are unaccustomed to its effects. Further investigation is indicated for Δ^9-THC and other cannabinoid derivatives, alone and in combination with other approaches to the control of vomiting in patients receiving cancer chemotherapy.

Domperidone, a drug that blocks dopamine receptors both in the gastrointestinal tract and in the CTZ, has recently been introduced for the control of cytotoxic chemotherapy-induced nausea and vomiting. Studies have shown it to be an effective alternative to metoclopramide, without significant side effects or toxicities.

LAXATIVES

Of all the drugs exerting a therapeutic effect on the gastrointestinal tract, the laxative drugs are the best known and the most overused by the public. Over $130 million are spent each year for OTC laxative preparations, of which there are hundreds. Traditionally, these drugs have been classified as stimulants (or irritants), wetting agents, saline cathartics, bulk-forming agents, and lubricants. The use of such arbitrary categories, which do not reflect the pathophysiologic principles of altered intestinal fluid and electrolyte transport, has come under criticism.[31]

Stimulants

The largest number of laxatives belong to the stimulant category. These drugs promote peristalsis presumably through irritation of the colonic mucosa.

Castor oil. Castor oil is obtained from the seeds of *Ricinus communis* and is composed primarily of the triglyceride of ricinoleic acid. In vivo, it is hydrolyzed by intestinal lipases to glycerol and ricinoleic acid, an unsaturated hydroxy fatty acid that is the active ingredient. Castor oil acts on the small intestine to produce a very prompt cathartic effect.

Phenolphthalein. Phenolphthalein is a widely used stimulant laxative and is an ingredient in numerous OTC preparations. It is believed to exert its pharmacologic action on the colon, producing laxation in 6 to 8 hours. Approximately 15% of an oral dose is absorbed, and the majority of this is excreted in the urine, primarily as conjugated metabolites. Both the urine and feces can become colored pink to red if the pH of either becomes alkaline. The major toxicity associated with its use is due to overdosage, with resultant fluid and electrolyte deficits. It has also been associated with allergic reactions.

Bisacodyl. Bisacodyl is structurally related to phenolphthalein and has similar pharmacologic actions. After oral administration, about 5% of a therapeutic dose is absorbed from the digestive tract, with no apparent systemic effects. The laxative effect is obtained in about 6 to 8 hours but can be accelerated by use of the drug in suppository form. The major toxicity is diarrhea with overdosage.

Anthraquinone cathartics. The most useful drugs in this group are senna and cascara sagrada, or their derivatives. These contain emodine (or anthracene) alkaloids in an inactive glycoside form. The glycosides are hydrolyzed within the lumen of the large intestine to liberate the active principle. The laxative action is produced in 6 to 8 hours. Cascara sagrada is considered to be the milder of these two drugs. In addition to senna and cascara sagrada, a synthetic anthraquinone derivative, danthron, is available. In general, adverse reactions to these agents relate to excessive catharsis.

Wetting agents

Docusate sodium and docusate calcium (dioctyl sodium sulfosuccinate and dioctyl calcium sulfosuccinate, respectively) are drugs that are used to soften the stool when it is desirable to lessen the discomfort or the strain of defecation. They are anionic surface-active agents that probably produce their effect by lowering the surface tension and allowing intestinal fluids to penetrate the fecal mass. They may require several days to exert their full effect if used alone, but they are combined with other laxatives in many OTC preparations. Diarrhea is the only adverse effect reported.

Mineral oil (liquid petrolatum) may be considered together with the surface-active agents since it also softens the stool. Its use is attended by several potential hazards not associated with the other agents. Prolonged oral use or administration with meals can reduce the absorption of the fat-soluble vitamins (A, D, E, K). Lipid pneumonia can result from the accidental aspiration of the oil. It is absorbed to a limited extent from the intestinal tract; therefore, its use with wetting agents, which could increase its absorption, is contraindicated. The seepage of oil through the anal sphincter is another disadvantage.

Saline cathartics

The saline cathartics are salt solutions containing one or more ions that are only poorly absorbed. Typical examples include magnesium salts, such as the hydroxide, sulfate, or citrate, and various other sulfates, phosphates, and tartrates. The salt solutions osmotically increase the fluid volume in the intestinal lumen, and peristalsis is stimulated indirectly. It has also been postulated that magnesium sulfate increases colonic motility by causing the release of cholecystokinin. Administration of these agents generally results in the production of a fluid to semifluid stool within 2 to 6 hours. Some absorption of the saline cathartics does occur, and consequently systemic effects may be noted. For this reason, the sodium salts are contraindicated in patients on a low salt diet and in patients with edema or congestive heart failure. Magnesium and potassium salts are contraindicated in patients with impaired renal function. Magnesium sulfate (Epsom salt), which is an effective and frequently used cathartic, may cause serious loss of body water with repeated use. Milk of magnesia, a suspension of magnesium hydroxide, is a widely used OTC preparation.

Bulk-forming agents

This family of agents is composed of a variety of natural and semisynthetic polysaccharides and cellulose derivatives that have the property of absorbing water and expanding, thereby increasing the bulk of the intestinal contents. The elevated luminal pressure stimulates reflex peristalsis, and the increased water content serves to soften the stool. Two or three days of medication may be required to achieve the full therapeutic benefit of these agents, but they have the advantage of having few systemic effects and being least likely to produce laxative abuse.

Plantago preparations. Plantago (psyllium) seeds are rich in a hemicellulose that forms a gelatinous mass with water. The refined hydrophilic colloid from the seeds is the most widely used form of this agent.

Semisynthetic cellulose derivatives. Methylcellulose and carboxymethylcellulose are marketed in combination with other laxatives. They are indigestible and not absorbed systemically.

Bran. Bran contains about 20% indigestible cellulose, which makes it a good source of intestinal bulk. It is easily supplied as breakfast cereal and has been used to relieve the symptoms of diverticular disease.

Miscellaneous agents

Several preparations, notably glycerin and lactulose, do not readily fit into the categories of laxatives described above. Glycerin is used in suppository form to promote defecation. It osmotically dehydrates exposed rectal tissue; the resultant irritation promotes evacuation of the lower bowel within 30 minutes. Lactulose, a relatively new laxative, is a semisynthetic disaccharide. In the large intestine, lactulose is metabolized by enteric bacteria to various acids and carbon dioxide. The acidification and increased osmolarity of the bowel contents causes fecal softening and a more normal bowel movement. Up to 2 days may be required for a therapeutic effect to occur.

ANTIDIARRHEAL AGENTS

One out of every six illnesses of adults and children involves the digestive system, and one of the more common complaints is diarrhea. The antidiarrheal agents generally available in the past lacked gastrointestinal specificity or demonstrated efficacy, often produced undesirable side effects, and some even possessed abuse potential.

Traditional opioid preparations

The opioids are effective and prompt-acting antidiarrheal agents. As is pointed out in Chapter 20, they enhance tone in segments of the longitudinal muscle of the gastrointestinal tract and inhibit propulsive contraction of circular and longitudinal muscle.

Paregoric. Paregoric (camphorated tincture of opium) is one of the most commonly used opioid antidiarrheal agents. At therapeutic doses, minimal side effects are seen, consisting chiefly of nausea and gastrointestinal disturbances. Because euphoria and analgesia are not produced, there is little risk of addiction, but prolonged usage has produced physical dependence. Paregoric is classified as a schedule III drug and contains 40 mg of morphine equivalent per 100 ml. Its unpleasant taste deters most people from abusing the drug.

Opium tincture. Tincture of opium (laudanum) is a schedule II drug containing 1 gm of morphine equivalent per 100 ml. It is therefore 25 times as strong as paregoric. It does not have the unpleasant taste of paregoric.

Diphenoxylate

Diphenoxylate, a congener of meperidine, was synthesized in the search for compounds similar to the opioid analgesics in actions on the gastrointestinal tract but devoid of their analgesic effects. The efficacy of diphenoxylate was found to be approximately equal to that of camphorated tincture of opium in patients with diarrhea of various causes.[1] It has been suggested that this drug inhibits mucosal receptors and abolishes the mucosal peristaltic reflex. Inasmuch as it is structurally related to meperidine, its addiction potential has been studied. Single therapeutic doses produced no opioid-like effects, but high doses produced euphoria and prevented withdrawal signs when administered to narcotic addicts.[11] The abrupt withdrawal of diphenoxylate or a challenge with nalorphine during long-term clinical trials has established a very low incidence of physical dependence at therapeutic levels.[22,32] The addiction potential has been compared with that of codeine, and it has been diminished by the incorporation of atropine (as in Lomotil) and by the low water solubility of diphenoxylate salts, which prevents parenteral administration.

A variety of minor side effects have been reported. These include abdominal cramps, nausea, weakness, drowsiness, xerostomia, gingival swelling, partial intestinal obstruction, and urinary retention. In patients with inflammatory bowel disease, diphenoxylate has caused toxic megacolon and, in patients with severe liver disease, hepatic

coma. Toxic doses have produced respiratory depression and unconsciousness, which can be effectively antagonized by the opioid antagonists. Although clinical studies have indicated only minimal, if any, drug interactions during diphenoxylate therapy,[33] it should be emphasized that the drug may potentially augment the actions of barbiturates, alcohol, opioids, and antianxiety and antipsychotic drugs.

Loperamide

Loperamide is a recently developed, long-acting, and specific antidiarrheal. It is a derivative of both haloperidol and diphenoxylate, but when loperamide is administered orally at therapeutic doses, there is essentially complete dissociation of the gastrointestinal effect from any central narcotic effect.[24] This is in part caused by the large amounts of the drug that become concentrated in target tissues along the gastrointestinal tract. One hour after oral administration, most of the drug (85%) is distributed to the gastrointestinal tract, 5% to the liver, and less than 0.04% to the brain. The drug has been shown to bind to brain and intestinal opioid receptors. However, bioavailability studies have indicated that only parenteral administration, preferably by the intravenous route, makes the drug available to central opioid receptors in a concentration sufficient to produce central opioid effects in vivo.

Some aspects of loperamide action are comparable to those of morphine. For example, the in vitro inhibitory effects of loperamide on gastrointestinal motility can be reversed to some extent, but not completely, by naloxone. When administered intravenously at near-lethal doses to rodents, loperamide produces analgesia and other behavioral effects.

At least part of the action of loperamide is attributed to nonopioid effects, and this is supported by the above-mentioned incomplete naloxone antagonism of loperamide action on intestinal motility and by the fact that studies have revealed some qualitative and quantitative differences in activity between morphine and loperamide. Loperamide has been found to inhibit hypersecretion of water and sodium elicited by a wide variety of intestinal stimuli, thus suggesting that the drug may interfere with basic mechanisms of fluid loss. Such an action might be more important in controlling diarrhea than the inhibition of propulsion through the intestinal tract. Regardless of mechanism, an impressive body of clinical data demonstrates that loperamide is at least as effective as codeine, diphenoxylate, or other treatments in a variety of acute and chronic diarrheal illnesses.

The most frequent adverse effect of loperamide is constipation. Occasional reports have been made of abdominal pain, nausea, xerostomia, drowsiness, and dizziness. Physical dependence has not been observed in humans; however, the repeated administration of high doses of loperamide has produced dose-related withdrawal symptoms in rodents[17]. It does not appear to potentiate the actions of barbiturates, antianxiety drugs, or alcohol when it is used in the treatment of chronic diarrhea.[12]

Loperamide is classified as a schedule V drug. Acute overdosage can cause depression of the central nervous system and should be treated with gastric lavage, activated charcoal and repeated doses of the narcotic antagonist naloxone.

Kaolin-pectin mixtures

Kaolin is a hydrated aluminum silicate claimed to have adsorbent properties. Its use in the treatment of diarrhea is based on its purported ability to adsorb bacteria and toxins. It also decreases the absorption of several drugs, including the tetracyclines and anticholinergics. Pectin is the purified carbohydrate product obtained from an acid extract of apple peel or the inner rind of citrus fruit. It forms an opalescent, viscous, colloidal solution with water. In the colon it may act as an adsorbent or protective. These two substances are customarily used together. They may also be combined with other drugs, such as opium and anticholinergic drugs. Controlled clinical studies demonstrating the efficacy of these preparations are lacking.

Agents used for the prevention of travelers' diarrhea

Diarrheal disease occurring among travelers to foreign countries results from infection with one of a variety of enteropathogens, the most common of which are the enterotoxigenic *Escherichia coli* (ETEC). ETEC infection is also an important cause of childhood diarrhea in many countries and is spread by contaminated food or water.

Several approaches to the prevention of travelers' diarrhea have been evaluated. Large doses of an OTC suspension of bismuth subsalicylate not only prevented diarrhea[7] but, when taken after the onset of diarrhea, diminished the number of loose bowel movements and relieved abdominal cramps.[6] The dosage (60 ml 4 times a day) was arbitrarily chosen, and it is not known whether smaller doses would be effective. The protective effect became apparent a few days after initiation of therapy and became more obvious as the time of treatment and period at risk continued. The drug was well tolerated, and constipation was not a problem. The method of action of bismuth subsalicylate on ETEC is unknown.

Prophylactic doxycycline treatment has been effective in preventing travelers' diarrhea.[27,28] One recommended regimen is a single dose of doxycycline (200 mg) on the day of travel, followed by 100 mg daily for 3 weeks. This regimen provides protection for about 1 additional week. Doxycycline was chosen to be evaluated in travelers' diarrhea because of the high sensitivity of ETEC to tetracycline and the long experience in the use of tetracycline drugs in the treatment and prevention of cholera, a disease with a similar pathophysiology. The long half-life of doxycycline allows it to be administered in a single daily dose. The drug also has a unique mode of excretion in that it diffuses across the small bowel mucosa into the lumen of the gut,[34] which places the drug at the site of infection.

Trimethoprim-sulfamethoxazole (TMP-SMZ) is currently considered the most active antimicrobial preparation against the broad range of bacterial enteropathogens known to be implicated in travelers' diarrhea.[8] TMP-SMZ taken twice daily for 3 weeks has been shown to reduce the occurrence of diarrheal illness by 70% and to decrease the incidence of milder forms of diarrhea. Although resistance to TMP-SMZ has apparently occurred among strains of ETEC, it is unusual. Advantages of TMP-SMZ are a low potential for the development of resistance among enteric flora during therapy and activity against enteropathogens such as *Shigella* and *Salmonella*.

In countries where travelers' diarrhea is common, what one eats or does not eat may be as important as chemoprophylaxis in reducing the risk. Common sense is an important preventive measure.

GASTROINTESTINAL STIMULANTS

Drugs that stimulate smooth muscle of the gastrointestinal and urinary tracts are used in the treatment of nonobstructive urinary retention, paralytic ileus, gastrointestinal atony, and postoperative abdominal distension. The drug of choice for oral administration in these situations is the cholinergic drug bethanechol (see Chapter 8). Bethanechol is a useful agent because it is relatively insusceptible to the cholinesterases, its actions are essentially muscarinic, and its effects on the gastrointestinal tract are much more pronounced than those on the cardiovascular system. The side effects of bethanechol are those typical of other cholinergic drugs, but serious adverse reactions are rare with therapeutic doses. This drug is contraindicated in patients with obstructive ileus or urinary retention, peptic ulcer, bronchial asthma, hyperthyroidism, or serious cardiac disease.

Gastroparesis is a common disorder that leads to debilitation in patients with diabetes mellitus. Clinically, it is characterized by intractable nausea, vomiting, anorexia, abdominal distension, and delayed gastric emptying.[18] Clinical trials have indicated that metoclopramide, cited earlier for its antiemetic activity, may be useful in this syndrome, since the drug stimulates the motility of the upper gastrointestinal tract.[18,30] Metoclopramide augments esophageal peristalsis, gastric antral contractions, and small intestinal transit time. Additionally, metoclopramide increases resting pressures of the lower esophageal and pyloric sphincters. It does not stimulate gastric, biliary, or pancreatic secretions and has little effect on colonic motor activity. Oral administration of metoclopramide is indicated for relief of symptoms associated with diabetic gastroparesis. The usual duration of therapy is 2 to 8 weeks, depending on the response. An injectable form of metoclopramide is also approved for use in facilitating intubation of the small intestine and the passage of barium into the intestine for radiographic procedures. Of particular concern to the dentist is that the dental use of opioids or anticholinergic drugs will antagonize the gastrointestinal effects of metoclopramide.

ANTISPASMODICS

Naturally occurring belladonna alkaloids and their derivatives, including propantheline and methantheline, may be useful as adjuncts in the management of selected patients with peptic ulcer. Their anticholinergic effects on smooth muscle and secretory glands, as discussed above and in Chapter 9, reduce the gastric motility and secretion of hydrochloric acid.

ADVERSE REACTIONS OF THE GASTROINTESTINAL SYSTEM TO DRUGS

The gastrointestinal tract must also be considered to be a target for the adverse side effects of many drug groups, some important to dentistry. For example, the opioid analgesics may produce constipation, nausea, and vomiting. Aspirin and aspirin-containing mixtures, such as propoxyphene compounds, are associated with gastric distress, fecal blood loss, and ulceration. All antiinflammatory agents, in fact, share the ulcerogenic action of aspirin. Diarrhea and enterocolitis have followed the use of the tetracyclines. Clindamycin and lincomycin have produced diarrhea as well as ulcerative and pseudomembranous colitis. Chloral hydrate is frequently prescribed by the dentist for the child or elderly patient. A major complaint against its use is the gastric irritation it produces.

Other drugs not directly related to dentistry cause a wide spectrum of gastrointestinal effects. These include mercurial diuretics, antineoplastic drugs, digitalis glycosides, and oral contraceptives.

Drugs acting on the gastrointestinal tract

Nonproprietary name	Proprietary name	Nonproprietary name	Proprietary name
Antacids		**Laxatives**	
aluminum carbonate gel	Basaljel	bisacodyl	Dulcolax
aluminum hydroxide gel	Amphojel	carboxymethylcellulose sodium	in Disoplex
aluminum phosphate gel	Phosphaljel	cascara sagrada	—
calcium carbonate	Dicarbosil	castor oil	Purge
calcium carbonate with glycine	Titralac	danthron	Dorbane, Modane
dihydroxyaluminum aminoacetate	Robalate	docusate calcium	Surfak
dihydroxyaluminum sodium carbonate	Rolaids	docusate potassium	Dialose
		docusate sodium	Colace, Doxinate
magaldrate	Riopan	glycerin	Fleet Babylax
magnesium carbonate	—	lactulose	Chronulac
magnesium hydroxide–aluminum hydroxide mixture	Maalox, in Gelusil, in Mylanta	magnesium citrate	Citroma
		magnesium sulfate	Epsom Salt
magnesium oxide	Par-Mag	methylcellulose sodium	Cologel
magnesium trisilicate	—	milk of magnesia (magnesium hydroxide)	—
magnesium trisilicate with aluminum hydroxide	Neutracomp		
		mineral oil	Nujol
magnesium trisilicate with aluminum and magnesium hydroxide	Magnatril	phenolphthalein	Phenolax, Ex-Lax
		poloxamer 188	Alaxin
milk of magnesia (magnesium hydroxide)	—	polycarbophil	Mitrolan
		psyllium	Konsyl, Metamucil
sodium bicarbonate	Soda Mint	senna	Senokot
		sodium phosphate	—
Histamine₂-receptor antagonists			
cimetidine	Tagamet	**Antidiarrheal agents**	
ranitidine	Zantac	bismuth subsalicylate	Pepto-Bismol
		diphenoxylate with atropine	Lomotil
Ulcer adherent complex		doxycycline	Vibramycin
aluminum salt	—	kaolin mixture with pectin	Kaopectate
sucralfate	Carafate	loperamide	Imodium
		opium tincture	in Parelixir
Antisialagogues		paregoric (camphorated opium tincture)	in Corrective Mixture with Paregoric
see Table 33-1 and Chapter 9			
		polycarbophil	Mitrolan
Emetics		trimethoprim-sulfamethoxazole	Bactrim, Septra
apomorphine	—		
ipecac syrup	—	**Gastrointestinal stimulants**	
		bethanechol	Urecholine
Antiemetics		dexpanthenol	Panol
benzquinamide	Emete-Con	metoclopramide	Reglan
buclizine	Bucladin-S Softabs		
chlorpromazine	Thorazine	**Antispasmodics**	
cyclizine	Marezine	see Chapter 9	
diphenhydramine	Benadryl		
diphenidol	Vontrol		
meclizine	Bonine		
metoclopramide	Reglan		
perphenazine	Trilafon		
prochlorperazine	Compazine		
scopolamine	Triptone		
thiethylperazine	Torecan		
triflupromazine	Vesprin		
see also Table 33-1			

CITED REFERENCES

1. Barowsky, H., and Schwartz, S.A. Method for evaluating diphenoxylate hydrochloride: comparison of its antidiarrheal effect with that of camphorated tincture of opium. Journal of the American Medical Association **180:**1058-1061, 1962.

2. Bauman, J.H., and Kimelblatt, B.J. Cimetidine as an inhibitor of drug metabolism: therapeutic implications and review of the literature. Drug Intelligence and Clinical Pharmacy **16:**380-386, 1982.

3. Binder, H.J., Cocco, A., Crossley, R.J., Finkelstein, W., Font, R., Friedman, G., Groarke, J., Hughes, W., Johnson, A.F., McGuigan, J.E., Summers, R., Vlahcevic, R., Wilson, E.C., and Winship, D.H. Cimetidine in the treatment of duodenal ulcer: a multicenter double-blind study. Gastroenterology **74:**380-388, 1978.

4. Birnbaum, D., Karmeli, F., and Tefera, M. The effect of diazepam on human gastric secretion. Gut **12:**616-618, 1971.

5. Colls, B.M., Ferry, D.G., Gray, A.J., Harvey, V.J., and McQueen, E.G. The antiemetic activity of tetrahydrocannabinol versus metoclopramide and thiethylperazine in patients undergoing cancer chemotherapy. New Zealand Medical Journal **91:**449-451, 1980.

6. DuPont, H.L., Sullivan, P., Pickering, L.K., Haynes, G., and Ackerman, P.B. Symptomatic treatment of diarrhea with bismuth subsalicylate among students attending a Mexican university. Gastroenterology **73:**715-718, 1977.

7. DuPont, H.L., Sullivan, P., Evans, D.G., Pickering, L.K., Evans, D.J., Jr., Vallet, J.J., Ericsson, C.D., Ackerman, P.B., and Tjoa, W.S. Prevention of traveler's diarrhea (emporiatric enteritis). Prophylactic administration of subsalicylate bismuth. Journal of the American Medical Association **243:**237-241, 1980.

8. DuPont, H.L., Evans, D.G., Rios, N., Cabada, F.J., Evans, D.J., Jr., and DuPont, M.W. Prevention of travelers' diarrhea with trimethoprim-sulfamethoxazole. Reviews of Infectious Diseases **4:**533-539, 1982.

9. Eggleston, D.J., and Nally, F. Hazards of systemic corticosteroid therapy. Oral Surgery, Oral Medicine, and Oral Pathology **31:**590-594, 1971.

10. Feldman, M., Richardson, C.T., Peterson, W.L., Walsh, J.H., and Fordtran, J.S. Effect of low-dose propantheline on food-stimulated gastric acid secretion. Comparison with an "optimal effective dose" and interaction with cimetidine. New England Journal of Medicine **297:**1427-1430, 1977.

11. Fraser, H.F., and Isbell, H. Human pharmacology and addictiveness of ethyl-1-(3-cyano-3,3-phenyl-propyl)-4-phenyl-4-piperidine carboxylate hydrochloride (R-1132, Diphenoxylate). Bulletin on Narcotics **13:**29-43, 1961.

12. Galambos, J.T., Hersh, T., Schroder, S., and Wegner, J. Loperamide: a new antidiarrheal agent in the treatment of chronic diarrhea. Gastroenterology **70:**1026-1029, 1976.

13. Gralla, R.J., Itri, L.M., Pisko, S.E., Squillante, A.E., Kelsen, D.P., Braun, D.W., Jr., Bordin, L.A., Braun, T.J., and Young, C.W. Antiemetic efficacy of high-dose metoclopramide: randomized trials with placebo and prochlorperazine in patients with chemotherapy-induced nausea and vomiting. New England Journal of Medicine **305:**905-909, 1981.

14. Gray, G.R., Smith, I.S., McKenzie, I., Crean, G.P., and Gillespie, G. Oral cimetidine in severe duodenal ulceration: a double-blind controlled trial. Lancet **1:**4-7, 1977.

15. Ivey, K.J., Settree, P., and Gemmell, R. Comparison of acetaminophen and aspirin on gastric mucosal barrier in man: correlation with ultrastructural changes. Gastroenterology **68:**918, 1975.

16. Klotz, U., and Reimann, I. Delayed clearance of diazepam due to cimetidine. New England Journal of Medicine **302:**1012-1014, 1980.

17. Mackerer, C.R., Broughham, L.R., East, P.F., Bloss, J.L., Dajani, E.Z., and Clay, G.A. Antidiarrheal and central nervous system activities of SC-27166 (2-[3-5-methyl-1,3,4-oxadiazol-2-yl)-3,3-diphenylpropyl]-2-azabicyclo [2.2.2]octane), a new antidiarrheal agent, resulting from binding to opiate receptor sites of brain and myenteric plexus. Journal of Pharmacology and Experimental Therapeutics **203:**527-538, 1977.

18. Malagelada, J.R., Rees, W.D.W., Mazzotta, L.F., and Go, V.L.W. Gastric motor abnormalities in diabetic and postvagotomy gastroparesis: effect of metoclopramide and bethanechol. Gastroenterology **78:**286-293, 1980.

19. Marks, I.N., Wright, J.P., Denzer, M., Garisch, J.A.M., and Lucke, W. Comparison of sucralfate with cimetidine in the short-term treatment of chronic peptic ulcers. South African Medical Journal **57:**567-573, 1980.

20. Martin, F., Farley, A., Gagnon, M., and Bensemana, D. Comparison of the healing capacities of sucralfate and cimetidine in the short-term treatment of duodenal ulcer: a double-blind randomized trial. Gastroenterology **82:**401-405, 1982.

21. McGraw, B.F., and Caldwell, E.G. Sucralfate. Drug Intelligence and Clinical Pharmacy **15:**578-580, 1981.

22. Merlo, M., and Brown, C.H. The effect of diphenoxylate hydrochloride on diarrhea. American Journal of Gastroenterology **34:**625-630, 1960.

23. Nair, S.G., Gamble, J.A.S., Dundee, J.W., and Howard, P.J. The influence of three antacids on the absorption and clinical action of oral diazepam. British Journal of Anaesthesia **48:**1175-1180, 1976.

24. Niemegeers, C.J.E., Colpaert, F.C., and Awouters, F.H.L. Pharmacology and antidiarrheal effect of loperamide. Drug Development Research **1:**1-20, 1981.

25. Patwardhan, R.V., Yarborough, G.W., Desmond, P.V., Johnson, R.F., Schenker, S., and Speeg, K.V., Jr. Cimetidine spares the glucuronidation of lorazepam and oxazepam. Gastroenterology **79:**912-916, 1980.

26. Ranitidine (Zantac). Medical Letter on Drugs and Therapeutics **24:**111-113, 1982.

27. Sack, D.A., Kaminsky, D.C., Sack, R.B., Itotia, J.N., Arthur, R.R., Kapikian, A.Z., Ørskov, F., and Ørskov, I. Prophylactic doxycycline for travelers' diarrhea. Results of a double-blind study of Peace Corps volunteers in Kenya. New England Journal of Medicine **298:**758-763, 1978.

28. Sack, R.B., Froehlich, J.L., Zulick, A.W., Hidi, D.S., Kapikian, A.Z., Ørskov, F., Ørskov, I., and Greenberg, H.B. Prophylactic doxycycline for travelers' diarrhea. Results of a prospective double-blind study of peace corps volunteers in Morocco. Gastroenterology **76:**1368-1373, 1979.

29. Sallan, S.E., Zinberg, N.E., and Frei, E., III. Antiemetic effect of delta-9-tetrahydrocannabinol in patients receiving cancer chemotherapy. New England Journal of Medicine **293:**795-797, 1975.

30. Snape, W.J., Jr., Battle, W.M., Schwartz, S.S., Braunstein, S.N., Goldstein, H.A., and Alavi, A. Metoclopramide to treat gastroparesis due to diabetes mellitus: a double-blind controlled trial. Annals of Internal Medicine **96:**444-446, 1982.

31. Stewart, J.J., Gaginella, T.S., Olsen, W.A., and Bass, P. Inhibitory actions of laxatives on motility and water and electrolyte transport in the gastrointestinal tract. Journal of Pharmacology and Experimental Therapeutics **192:**458-467, 1975.

32. Van Derstappen, G., Vantrappen, G., and Vandenbroucke, J. Long-term studies with R 1132, a new constipating drug. Gastroenterology **39:**725-729, 1960.

33. Weingarten, B., Weiss, J., and Simon, M. A clinical evaluation of a new antidiarrheal agent. American Journal of Gastroenterology **35:**628-633, 1961.

34. Whelton, A., von Wittenau, M.S., Twomey, T.M., Walker, W.G., and Bianchine, J.R. Doxycycline pharmacokinetics in the absence of renal function. Kidney International **5:**365-371, 1974.

GENERAL REFERENCES

Binder, H.J. Pharmacology of laxatives. Annual Review of Pharmacology and Toxicology **17:**355-367, 1977.

Chapman, M.L. Peptic ulcer. A medical perspective. Medical Clinics of North America. **62:**39-51, 1978.

Ewe, K. The physiological basis of laxative action. Pharmacology **20**(suppl. 1):2-20, 1980.

Hirschowitz, B.I. Controls of gastric secretion. A roadmap to the choice of treatment for duodenal ulcer. American Journal of Gastroenterology **77:**281-293, 1982.

Morrissey, J.F., and Barreras, R.F. Antacid therapy. New England Journal of Medicine **290:**550-554, 1974.

Ponte, C.D., and Nappi, J.M. Review of a new gastrointestinal drug—metoclopramide. American Journal of Hospital Pharmacy **38:**829-833, 1981.

Seigel, L.J., and Longo, D.L. The control of chemotherapy-induced emesis. Annals of Internal Medicine **95:**352-359, 1981.

Sucralfate for peptic ulcer—a reappraisal. Medical Letter on Drugs and Therapeutics **26:**43-44, 1984.

Villeneuve, J.P., and Branch, R.A. Clinicopharmacologic perspective of duodenal ulcer therapy. Southern Medical Journal **71:**1115-1120, 1978.

34 Hormones of homeostasis

William Warner

The two major integrating and modulating systems of the body are the nervous system and the endocrine system. The influence of the latter is mediated by chemical substances called hormones that are produced by ductless glands. Three criteria for hormones are that they be produced by ductless glands, be transported by body fluids to target cells, and interact with specific receptor sites. These sites may be precisely limited to a select tissue or organ target or may have wide distribution on different cell types and organs.

Many chemicals produced by the body share some, but not all, of these characteristics and therefore are not hormones in the strict sense. For example, neurosecretory products such as ACh, norepinephrine, and dopamine are passed, like endocrines, from the cells in which they originate through body fluids to receptor sites, but they do not originate in ductless glands. Other chemicals, the so-called local hormones, are produced in the wall of the gastrointestinal tract, pass through body fluids, and affect specific target cells. Products such as secretin and cholecystokinin, which influence pancreatic secretion and gallbladder contraction, respectively, are examples of such local hormones, as are the products of neurons. Although they do not originate in ductless glands, certain chemical products of neurons that are secreted directly into the posterior lobe of the pituitary are considered hormones (i.e., oxytocin and antidiuretic hormone). In this and the next chapter, which deal with the pharmacology of the endocrine system, only those hormones that meet the three criteria will be considered.

MECHANISMS FOR CONTROL OF ENDOCRINE SECRETIONS

The endocrine system is in large part regulated by the pituitary gland, which has both glandular and glandular (adenohypophyseal) and neural (neurohypophyseal) components. The cells of the adenohypophysis produce and release *tropic* hormones that regulate the activity of other endocrine glands, such as the adrenal cortex, which is influenced by adrenocorticotropic hormone (ACTH), and the thyroid gland, which is regulated by thyroid-stimulating hormone (TSH). The production and release of tropic hormones are in turn controlled by so-called *releasing* hormones, which are produced by cells in the hypothalamus and are secreted into the hypothalamic-hypophyseal portal circulation, which traverses the adenohypophysis. Secretion of releasing factors from the hypothalamus is critically influenced by the concentration in the hypothalamic circulation of hormones from target glands (e.g., adrenal cortex and thyroid). Thus, a complex feedback, or regulatory, loop exists in which the titers of endocrine secretions, releasing factors, and tropic hormones provide a precise regulation of hormone levels. For example, a decrease in the concentration of thyroxine in the blood perfusing the hypothalamus will provide a stimulus to the hypothalamic cells to secrete thyrotropin-releasing hormone (TRH). TRH passes through the portal system, causing the release of TSH, which enters the general circulation and is carried to the thyroid gland, where it stimulates production of thyroxine. As the titer of thyroxine in the circulation to the hypothalamus rises, the stimulus to production of TRH is diminished, and TSH production drops.

The neurohypophysis stores and releases hormones that originate, as neurosecretory products, in neurons located in distinct nuclei of the hypothalamus. The neurosecretory substances antidiuretic hormone (ADH) and oxytocin are transported to the posterior lobe of the pituitary by the hypothalamic axons that terminate there. Although

496

$$H^\# \quad + \quad Ab \quad \rightleftharpoons \quad H^\# — Ab$$

(Free labeled hormone)   (Specific antibody)   (Bound labeled hormone)

$$+$$

$$H \qquad \text{(Unlabeled hormone in plasma or in standard solution)}$$
$$\updownarrow$$
$$H — Ab$$

Figure 34-1. Representation of the reactions that form the basis of radioimmunoassays. A hormone-specific antibody (Ab) is exposed to a known amount of free radioactive hormone ($H^\#$) and to a quantity of nonradioactive hormone (H) to be assayed. The radioactive bound hormone ($H^\#$-Ab) is physically separated from the free labeled hormone of the assay mixture and is then quantified.

less is known about the factors controlling their secretion and release than about the hormones of the anterior pituitary, it is probable that a regulatory loop with other substances, like the one described earlier for thyroid hormone, exists for products of the neurohypophysis.

The parathyroid glands, the calcitonin-secreting cells of the thyroid, and the islet cells of the pancreas are all independent of direct tropic control of the pituitary. Nevertheless, since circulating levels of other hormones influence their actions, the pituitary may have a secondary regulating influence. In the case of the parathyroid and the thyroid calcitonin-secreting cells, the concentration of calcium ions in the blood has a significant regulatory influence, whereas the islet cell secretion of glucagon and insulin is closely related to plasma and intracellular glucose concentrations. In the case of islet cells, it is clear that factors influencing glucose metabolism, such as epinephrine and glucocorticoid concentrations in the blood, have secondary influence on their control systems.

DETECTION OF PROTEIN HORMONES

One technical advance that has had a major impact on the fields of endocrinology and pharmacology has been development of the radioimmunoassay (RIA). This procedure allows the direct measurement of circulating hormones, the concentrations of which are often in the picomolar (10^{-12} molar) range. The ability to measure minute quantities of these substances has greatly expanded the understanding of the mechanisms of hormone action and the control of their release from endocrine glands.

Because proteins can be used as antigenic substances, it has been possible to produce and isolate antibodies to a number of peptide hormones. These hormone antibodies often demonstrate exquisite stereospecificity and sensitivity, that is, high affinity for the hormone. Using a radioisotopically tagged hormone makes it possible to quantitate antibody-hormone complexes by the RIA technique. The basic scheme for this procedure is represented by the equation in Figure 34-1.

The binding of radiolabeled hormone is quantitatively inhibited in proportion to the concentration of unlabeled hormone present. The concentration of unlabeled hormone in unknown samples is determined by comparison of the degree of inhibition observed in the sample with that produced by standard solutions of hormone. The simple procedure for assessing radioactivity after incubation of reactants and physical separation of the free and bound hormone makes RIA an excellent diagnostic and research tool.

TARGET CELL RECEPTOR SITE ACTION

Recently, great strides have been made in the identification of hormone receptors and the cells with which they are associated.[7,25] Using hormones and hormone antagonists to obtain dose-response data on different cell types, investigators have determined the specific target cells for individual hormones. Another major advance has been the synthesis of radioactive hormones of high specific activity that still retain a considerable level of biologic activity. The technology now exists to measure the binding of radioactive hormones to isolated cells, to purified plasma membranes from cell homogenates, and, in the case of steroids, to purified receptor proteins. By measuring the binding of radioactive hormones to these cellular preparations in the absence and presence of nonradioactive forms of the same substances, the binding characteristics of the natural hormone can be studied.[25] In addition, it is now possible to identify genetic and pathologic alterations in the number of hormone receptors and in the affinity of these receptors for their hormones.

PANCREATIC HORMONES AND AGENTS AFFECTING BLOOD GLUCOSE

The islets of Langerhans, part of the endocrine system located in the pancreas, secrete two hormones, insulin and glucagon. Insulin is produced by β cells of the islets and glucagon by α cells. δ cells, also in the islets, contain somatostatin, but the function of these cells is speculative.[2]

Insulin is a small protein consisting of two chains of amino acids coupled by disulfide bonds and has a total molecular weight of about 6000. The substitution of only a few amino acids accounts for the variations among species in the structure of this peptide hormone. Insulin is synthesized in the endoplasmic reticulum of β cells as a pre-prohormone, which is rapidly converted to proinsulin. Subsequently, proinsulin is packaged into vesicles and partially digested to yield both insulin and a protein called C-peptide.[26] The insulin-containing vesicles are then stored in a complex relationship with microtubules until their contents are released in response to any of the insulin secretagogues (e.g., glucose or amino acids). Although the exact mechanism of release is a matter of great controversy, it appears to be a calcium-dependent process in which contractile proteins (associated with the microtubules) transport the hormone vesicles to the cell membrane in preparation for exocytosis.[22]

Glucagon has a molecular weight of 3500 and consists of a chain of 29 amino acids. Like insulin, glucagon acts on receptors that are located on the surfaces of target cells and modulates the activity of target cell adenylate cyclase. Here, however, the similarities between the two peptide hormones end. Glucagon activates adenylate cyclase, whereas insulin appears to inhibit the activity of this enzyme.[17] As would be expected, both hormones demonstrate many different actions.

Both insulin and glucagon secretions are regulated by blood glucose content. High glucose concentrations stimulate the release of insulin, whereas low concentrations stimulate the release of glucagon. The ratio of insulin to glucagon secretion directly controls the blood glucose concentration, maintaining it at approximately 100 mg/dl, and significantly influences cell glucose metabolism.

Insulin

The role of glucose as an insulin secretagogue has already been mentioned, but many other substances can in varying degrees stimulate the release of this hormone. For example, amino acids, fatty acids, gastrin, secretin, pancreozymin, β-adrenergic agonists, and muscarinic agonists all enhance insulin release.[21,23] α-Adrenergic agonists appear to depress insulin release, and α-adrenergic antagonists may disinhibit secretion of the hormone.

Pharmacologic effects. Insulin lowers the blood concentration of glucose by (1) enhancing facilitated diffusion of glucose through cell membranes, (2) increasing the rate of glucose utilization, (3) increasing the rate of glycogen deposition, and (4) inhibiting hepatic gluconeogenesis. In the process of lowering this concentration, however, not all cells are equally affected. The effect of insulin on glucose metabolism at different tissue sites is summarized in Table 34-1. As demonstrated here, glucose uptake and glycogen storage in muscle and fat cells are greatly dependent on insulin. However, brain cells are relatively insensitive to the action of insulin and are dependent on circulating glucose concentrations for an adequate supply of carbohydrate.

When the β cells produce an insufficient supply of insulin, plasma glucose concentrations rise because of enhanced gluconeogenesis and depressed glucose uptake. Furthermore, the activity of lipase in adipocytes is increased, whereas the activity of triglyceride synthetase is decreased. The result is an excess of circulating unesterified fatty acids, which are metabolized to acetyl coenzyme A. The subsequent overproduction of ketone bodies (condensation products of acetyl coenzyme A) is a prime factor in the development of metabolic acidosis, which sometimes accompanies diabetic hyperglycemia. Also, the consequent elevation of blood solutes contributes to the polyuria and dehydration of diabetes mellitus.

General therapeutic uses. Diabetes mellitus is the pathologic condition associated with a deficiency of insulin activity, even though in some cases the insulin concentration may actually be normal. The underlying cause may be an absolute de-

Table 34-1. Effect of insulin on glucose metabolism in different tissues

	Liver	Heart	Muscle	Fat	Brain
Glucose transport into cells	0	+ +	+ +	+ +	0
Glycogen stores	0	+	+	+	0
Glucose metabolism	+	+ +	+ +	+ +	0
Amino acid transport into cells	+	+	+	+	0

Key: + = increase, 0 = no change.

ficiency of insulin, a defective response to insulin, or possibly hyperglucagonemia. Hyperglucagonemia was considered when it was demonstrated that the insulin requirements of some diabetics could be lowered by the simultaneous administration of somatostatin, a hormone that inhibits glucagon release.

The major therapeutic use of insulin is as a replacement or supplement for endogenous insulin in diabetic patients. Insulin injection may also be administered intravenously and is also used for the emergency treatment of ketoacidosis and nonketotic diabetic coma.

Preparations. A variety of insulin preparations are available for use in the treatment of diabetes mellitus. These preparations, which differ with respect to formulation, species of origin, and degree of purity, provide some flexibility in matching the treatment to the needs of the patient.

Alterations in the physical form of the hormone change its speed of onset and its duration of action (Table 34-2). Insulin injection, which is a solution of the hormone, has the most rapid onset and the shortest duration of action of all insulin preparations. Although its rapidity makes it valuable in situations where speed is desirable, insulin injection is too short-acting to provide the diabetic patient with an adequate supply of insulin throughout the day. Consequently, most patients use a combination of a rapid-acting insulin preparation and one or more slowly absorbed insulin suspensions.

Suspensions of insulin can be prepared by using one of two techniques. In the first, the hormone is precipitated with zinc to form crystals of differing sizes. By varying the chemical conditions, it is possible to form small, rapidly dissolving crystals (as in prompt insulin zinc injection) or larger crystals that dissolve more slowly (as in insulin zinc suspension and extended insulin zinc suspension). With the second method the hormone is allowed to react with another protein (as in protamine zinc insulin suspension and isophane insulin suspension).

Table 34-2. Insulin preparations

	Time of onset (hours)	Duration of action (hours)
Fast-acting insulins		
Insulin injection	1	6
Prompt insulin zinc suspension (Semilente insulin)	1	14
Intermediate-acting insulins		
Isophane insulin suspension (NPH insulin)	2	24
Insulin zinc suspension (Lente insulin)	2	24
Long-acting insulins		
Protamine zinc insulin suspension	7	36
Extended insulin zinc suspension (Ultralente insulin)	7	36

Whether a solution or a suspension, most of the insulin that is used in the United States is a beef-pork mixture. Neither peptide is identical to human insulin. Pork insulin differs from the human hormone by one terminal amino acid, whereas beef insulin differs at three positions. As might be expected, the use of beef-pork insulin frequently results in the production of antibodies. For patients who experience an allergic reaction to the mixture, beef-only insulin is available, as well as the less allergenic pork-only insulin.

Insulin that is indistinguishable from the human hormone has recently been approved for marketing. The hormone subunits are synthesized individually by two nonpathogenic strains of *Escherichia coli* that have been created by gene-splicing techniques. The subunits are then chemically joined. Use of the human hormone in diabetic patients will eliminate one major source of antibodies that often complicate insulin therapy.

Antibodies to chemical impurities in commercial insulin preparations may also be produced. However, in recent years the severity of this problem has been significantly reduced. Insulin is now purified by chromatographic techniques that remove contaminants of differing molecular size. Currently, all insulin preparations available in the United States are 99% pure, a level of purity that was not achievable in the past. Insulin may be further purified by ion-exchange techniques to produce "single component" preparations. Such highly purified hormones have been used in fast-acting, intermediate-, and long-lasting preparations of beef-only and pork-only insulin.

Absorption, fate, and excretion. The diabetic patient requires a steady supply of insulin throughout the day and higher concentrations of the hormone at mealtimes. These needs can be met by administering insulin preparations of differing absorption characteristics. In a typical regimen, a mixture of rapid-acting insulin preparation and a longer-acting suspension is injected subcutaneously. Some insulin is quickly absorbed, thereby providing coverage for the first meal of the day. The dissolution and absorption of insulin from the longer-acting suspension provides a slowly rising hormone concentration that peaks later in the day. The midday meal must be taken at the time when this peak of insulin activity is expected. Later in the day, another subcutaneous injection of both a rapid-acting and a long-lasting preparation may be made to provide coverage for an evening meal and to supply insulin for the night.

Effective insulin therapy requires discipline on the part of the patient. Extra meals or missed meals will result in inadequate control of the disease. The importance of keeping to a daily routine may, in the future, be minimized by portable insulin pumps.[9] These devices, which are currently under investigation, are programmed to provide a continuous infusion of insulin throughout the day. At mealtimes, the pumps can be manually triggered to administer an additional quantity of hormone. The portable pump is small enough to fit on a belt and can be set up to administer the hormone by subcutaneous, intravenous, or intraperitoneal routes. Work is in progress on subcutaneously implanted insulin pumps.

Once in the blood, insulin has a short half-life (approximately 10 minutes in humans). Insulin is degraded by both the liver and the kidney into smaller, inactive peptides. Renal excretion of the intact insulin is not a major route of elimination, but failure of the renal enzymatic inactivating system may significantly prolong the half-life of the hormone.

Toxic reactions and side effects. Even after the maintenance dose of insulin has been determined and the patient's condition has stabilized, many factors, such as exercise, fever, and diet, may modify the need for the hormone. Thus, there exists the possibility of insulin overdose, the most serious consequence of which is hypoglycemia. Mild hypoglycemia is characterized by drowsiness, irritability, and sometimes confusion caused by reduced glucose supply to the brain. More severe reactions may involve motor symptoms, such as clonic spasms or seizures. Intravenous glucose, or orally administered glucose if the patient is conscious, may be used to correct the situation.

In view of the need for diabetic patients to constantly monitor their insulin requirements, the use of propranolol by diabetics may result in a clinically significant problem. Propranolol masks the tachycardia that serves as a warning to the patient of developing hypoglycemia and may also block the glucose release initiated by an increase in sympathoadrenal activity.

Another problem associated with long-term use of exogenous insulin is the development of insulin antibodies. The immunoproteins may reduce the effective concentration of circulating insulin, necessitating the administration of unusually large doses of the hormone to compensate. In a small percentage of patients, allergic reactions to insulin injections have occurred. As previously discussed, however, this problem has been reduced in recent years by the development of very pure insulin preparations, including the human form.

The frequent subcutaneous administration of insulin may also result in atrophy of underlying adipose tissue, but this can be circumvented by varying the site of injection. The use of purified insulin may also reduce the severity of lipoatrophy.

Glucagon

Glucagon, another peptide produced by the pancreas, is also involved in the regulation of plasma glucose. Glucagon is released from α cells in response to hypoglycemia and α-adrenergic agonists. Its release is inhibited by hyperglycemia.

Pharmacologic effects. Glucagon stimulates hepatic gluconeogenesis and glycogenolysis. In adipose tissue, the hormone accelerates the breakdown of triglycerides, resulting in the release of free fatty acids into the blood.

General therapeutic uses. Glucagon is indicated only in the emergency treatment of insulin-induced hypoglycemia. Since glucose is considered the treatment of choice, glucagon is administered only when glucose is unavailable. In such circumstances, glucagon is often given intravenously.

Oral hypoglycemic agents

As an outgrowth of sulfonamide therapy, a series of compounds classified as sulfonylureas were found to be effective as oral hypoglycemic agents. Because of their potential as replacements for parenterally administered insulin, sulfonylureas, such as tolbutamide, acetohexamide, and chlorpropamide achieved a high level of popularity. More recently, concerns about their efficacy and safety have dampened enthusiasm for their use. Another class of oral hypoglycemic agents, the biguanides, was formerly widely used but has been removed from the market in the United States and is currently only available for investigational purposes. A second generation of sulfonylureas (glyburide and glipizide) has recently been approved. They differ from the older agents primarily with respect to their pharmacokinetics.

Pharmacologic effects. The sulfonylureas enhance the secretion of endogenous insulin from pancreatic islet cells and may also depress glucagon release.[31] Obviously, the activity of these drugs requires that significant quantities of insulin be available for release. Only in adult-onset diabetes is this criterion met. As a secondary mechanism, these agents appear to enhance the antilipolytic activity of endogenous insulin.[4]

The biguanides reduce blood glucose concentrations by interfering with glucose absorption from the intestine, by inhibiting gluconeogenesis, and by enhancing carbohydrate metabolism, particularly anaerobic glycolysis.

General therapeutic uses. The sulfonylureas are currently used, along with dietary restrictions, for the control of adult-onset (insulin-independent), nonketotic diabetes. The advantage of these drugs over dietary restrictions alone is a matter of great controversy at the present time. As would be expected, the sulfonylureas are useless in the treatment of diabetes mellitus that is associated with the complete loss of β-cell activity (termed juvenile-onset or insulin-dependent diabetes).

Toxic reactions and side effects. An area of major concern with the sulfonylureas is the problem of potential drug interactions. The sulfonylureas may cause an intolerance to ethanol and may alter the patient's response to oral anticoagulants. For example, tolbutamide and dicumarol appear to compete for binding sites on plasma proteins. The sulfonylureas are also capable of producing blood dyscrasias and may be teratogenic. Recent studies have suggested that regimens of oral hypoglycemic agents, including the sulfonylureas, may increase the risk of myocardial infarction and ventricular tachycardia and fibrillation.[30] The significance of these studies is currently being debated, and new studies are being carried out.

The biguanides were removed from the market because of the occurrence of a number of cases of fatal lactic acidosis, apparently a direct consequence of their mechanism of action.

THYROID HORMONES

The thyroid gland, controlled by the pituitary peptide hormone TSH, secretes an iodinated peptide hormone called thyroxine. The iodine required for the synthesis of this hormone is concentrated in thyroid cells by an energy-dependent process. The degree of iodine trapping depends on the concentration of TSH, but under optimal conditions thyroid iodide titers may be 300 times higher than plasma concentrations. Inside the thyroid cell, the iodide ion is oxidized to a reactive form (iodine), which in turn combines with the tyrosine moieties of a previously synthesized protein, thyroglobulin. Once this neutral, high molecular weight protein is iodinated, its tyrosine residues are coupled. Each tyrosine molecule can be iodinated at a maximum of two sites. The degree of iodination determines which of two biologically active molecules is formed by this coupling reaction: thyroxine (tetraiodothyronine, T_4) or liothyronine (triiodothyronine, T_3) (Fig. 34-2). Thyronine molecules (formed by coupling two tyrosine molecules) may also be iodinated to a lesser degree or not at all, but these compounds have no known biologic importance.

Iodination and coupling appear to take place at the apical microvilli of thyroid cells. Once these reactions are completed, the finished iodinated thyroglobulin is stored in the thyroid colloid. This amorphous mass of prohormone is surrounded by a single layer of thyroid cells. The transcellular colloid and its associated cells compose the thyroid follicle.

When the thyroid is stimulated by TSH, varying amounts of thyroglobulin are taken back into the

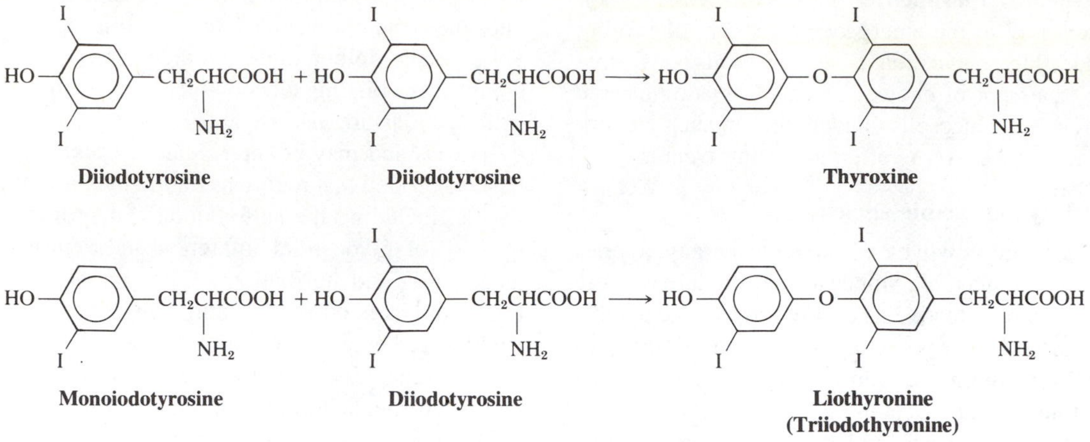

Figure 34-2. Coupling reactions in the synthesis of the two principal thyroid hormones, thyroxine and liothyronine (triiodothyronine).

cell by endocytosis and are digested by lysosomal enzymes. The T_4 and T_3 that are released in this manner then pass into the general circulation.

Thyroxine represents the major secretory product of the thyroid gland, although T_3 is also normally released in small amounts. Once released from the thyroid, both T_4 and T_3 bind to plasma proteins, principally thyroxine-binding globulin (TBG) and thyroxine-binding prealbumin. These transport proteins not only help solubilize the hormones but also serve as a depot to replace those free hormone molecules that have been metabolized or excreted.

During a state of iodine deficiency, the proportion of T_3 that is released from the gland is increased because of the presence of many tyrosine moieties iodinated at only one site. Liothyronine demonstrates a greater potency than T_4 and a more rapid onset of action, the speed of which is due in part to its lower affinity for TBG and therefore the relatively large amounts of hormone that remain unbound and thus active. As a result, during iodine deficiency, secretion of the more potent thyroid hormone, T_3, reduces the physiologic impact of thyroxine deficiency.

The steps in the thyroxine biosynthetic pathway, as well as the size of the thyroid gland itself, are controlled by TSH from the anterior pituitary gland. As described earlier, negative feedback mechanisms involving T_4 and T_3 control the release of TSH from the pituitary and of TSH-releasing hormone from the hypothalamus. The combination of positive control from the hypothalamic-pituitary axis and negative control from the thyroid serves to finely regulate the circulating concentrations of thyroid hormone.

Pharmacologic effects

The most prominent effect of thyroxine is its ability to stimulate the basal metabolic rate (the number of kcal of heat produced by a resting individual during a 24-hour period). This effect on heat production requires many hours to develop and persists for days after removal of the hormone. Early studies suggested that the elevation in heat production by thyroxine was a result of an uncoupling of oxidative phosphorylation in mitochondria, but more recently an increase in the activity of sodium pump enzymes has been proposed as the principal source of heat.[16]

In addition to its effect on heat production, thyroxine has long been known to be essential for normal growth. This role is best demonstrated by considering the characteristics of cretinism (hypothyroidism of very early onset). Children with this disease have severely depressed physical growth, including poor and late dentition, abnormalities in neuron myelinization, and severe mental retardation. Hypothyroidism of adult onset is not as devastating. This disease, known as myxedema, is characterized by intolerance to cold, deposition of a hydrophilic mucopolysaccharide beneath the skin, lethargy, sleepiness, and diminished mental capacity. Of particular interest is a decreased responsiveness to catecholamines, which often results in bradycardia.

In recent years, numerous studies have attempted to demonstrate the biochemical correlates of these effects. While thyroid hormones have been found to alter the activities of many enzymes, no general mechanism of thyroxine activity has emerged to date.

General therapeutic uses. Various thyroid preparations, both glandular extracts and purified hormones, are used in the treatment of thyroid deficiency. Thyroid insufficiencies may be caused by functional abnormalities of the thyroid, pituitary, or hypothalamus. The problem may be caused by physical damage, such as an infarct, or by infectious diseases or genetic abnormalities. Myxedema may be successfully treated with thyroid hormone supplements, but cretinism requires very prompt diagnosis if thyroid hormone treatment is to have any effect on the catastrophic course of this disorder. Thyroid hormones may also be used in the treatment of nontoxic goiter and chronic thyroiditis. The use of these hormone preparations for dysmenorrhea and weight reduction is of questionable value and probably should be discontinued.

Toxic reactions and side effects

The use of thyroid supplements in normal individuals, or an overdose in hypothyroid patients, may cause nervousness, palpitations, and precordial pain.[8,27] Combination of these hormones and sympathomimetic amines for weight reduction has resulted in a number of fatal cardiac arrhythmias.[19] The elderly and those with preexisting heart disease are particularly susceptible to cardiac toxicity.

ANTITHYROID DRUGS

A number of compounds have been found to be goitrogenic,[20] that is, capable of causing an enlargement of the thyroid gland. By inhibiting one or more steps in the synthesis of thyroxine, these drugs disrupt the feedback control of the hypothalamic-pituitary-thyroid axis, which in turn results in a hyperplastic and highly vascularized gland. Some drugs of this type are useful in the treatment of hyperthyroidism.

Antithyroid drugs display a wide variety of chemical structures. Anions such as thiocyanate, nitrate, and perchlorate diminish iodide accumulation by thyroid cells. Aniline derivatives, most notably *p*-aminosalicylic acid (PAS) and the sulfonamides, also inhibit thyroid function. In the case of PAS, thyroid suppression once caused a significant clinical problem because the drug was widely used in the treatment of tuberculosis. A group of drugs that may indirectly depress thyroid function is the nonsteroidal antiinflammatory agents (e.g., phenylbutazone). These drugs displace thyroid hormones from their transport proteins, and the resulting increase in hormone activities decreases TSH release. Currently, the only drugs that are therapeutically useful in the treatment of hyperthyroidism are the thioamides and radioactive isotopes of iodine.

Pharmacologic effects

In vitro studies suggest that the thioamides (propylthiouracil and methimazole) inhibit the oxidation-iodination step in the synthesis of thyroid hormone,[29] although other sites of action cannot be ruled out.

Paradoxically, iodine has been used in the treatment of hyperthyroidism. After approximately 2 weeks of iodine therapy, the vascularity of the gland is reduced, and there is a marked decline in the basal metabolic rate. Although nonradioactive iodine is no longer used in the control of hyperthyroidism because of its incomplete and transient action, it may be employed to prepare the thyroid gland for surgery and (along with antiadrenergic drugs) to treat thyrotoxic emergencies.

Sodium iodide I 131 ($Na^{131}I$) is used in the diagnosis and treatment of hyperthyroidism. When radioactive iodine is administered in low concentrations, radioactive scanning can determine the size and shape of the thyroid gland. At higher concentrations, the radioactivity of the compound destroys thyroid cells and thyroid carcinomas. Indeed, use of this agent commonly results in iatrogenic myxedema.

Absorption, fate, and excretion

Thioamides are rapidly absorbed from the gastrointestinal tract and are widely distributed throughout the body. Their rapid rate of metabolism necessitates frequent administration. Radioactive iodide is also effective orally, but this compound is concentrated in normal thyroid cells and in thyroid carcinomas that, after metastasizing, might be located anywhere in the body.

General therapeutic uses

Thioamides and $Na^{131}I$ are currently used for the treatment of hyperthyroidism. Thioamides are also used to control a hyperactive thyroid gland before surgery. Radioactive iodide may also be used to treat thyroid carcinoma.

Toxic reactions and side effects

Thioamides may cause blood dyscrasias and allergic reactions in sensitive individuals. When taken during pregnancy, these drugs can cross the placenta and cause fetal hypothyroidism. The use of Na[131]I is also contraindicated during pregnancy.

PARATHYROID HORMONE

The parathyroid glands are located within the capsule of the thyroid. Usually, there are two superior and two inferior parathyroid glands, although variation in number and position is common. These glands have two major parenchymal cell types—chief, or principal, cells and oxyphil cells. The principal cells are the source of parathyroid hormone (PTH). This hormone consists of a chain of 84 amino acids, but a larger protein, a prohormone, is initially synthesized. The prohormone loses six amino acids from its N-terminal end, and the remaining peptide chain is secreted into adjacent blood vessels.

The principal factor in the control of PTH release is the plasma calcium concentration. High calcium concentrations depress PTH secretion, whereas low calcium concentrations enhance release of the hormone.

Pharmacologic effects

The major effects of PTH are to produce an increase in plasma calcium concentration and a fall in plasma phosphate concentration. The mechanisms by which these effects are accomplished are complex. PTH increases calcium and phosphate reabsorption from stable, mature bone. Both the number of osteoclasts and the metabolic activity of bone-resorbing cells (including osteocytes) are increased. The hormone also inhibits the synthesis of collagen and the glycoprotein ground substance of bone. In the kidney, PTH promotes the reabsorption of calcium by the renal tubule and increases the excretion of phosphate.[1,5] Both of these effects may be mediated by cAMP-dependent mechanisms. PTH does not have a direct effect on intestinal absorption of calcium, but because the hormone does enhance the activation of vitamin D, it may indirectly stimulate calcium absorption.

General therapeutic uses

The sole therapeutic use of PTH is as a replacement for the endogenous hormone. Even this use, however, is rare. Because individual response to the hormone varies and allergic reactions may occur, hypocalcemia is most commonly treated with vitamin D or calcium supplements or both. PTH is most useful as an aid in the diagnosis of pseudohypoparathyroidism. In this disease, renal and osseous tissues become unresponsive to PTH. Infusion of the hormone into these patients fails to bring about the expected increases in plasma calcium and urinary cAMP.

CALCITONIN

The discovery of calcitonin completed a hormonal system in which PTH elevates and calcitonin, also called thyrocalcitonin, lowers plasma calcium concentration. The calcitonin molecule consists of a chain of 32 amino acids, but it shows considerable species variation. Indeed, immunologic heterogeneity has been found among patients with calcitonin-secreting tumors. Calcitonin release is enhanced by elevated extracellular calcium concentrations and by several gastrointestinal hormones (pancreozymin and gastrin).

Pharmacologic effects

Calcitonin lowers plasma calcium and phosphate concentrations by enhancing mineral deposition in bone and by inhibiting bone resorption. However, with long-term administration bone formation is also inhibited. Calcitonin also brings about an increase in the urinary excretion of calcium and phosphate. In the intestine, there does not appear to be a direct effect of calcitonin on calcium absorption, but it may indirectly inhibit the process by increasing the formation of a less active form of vitamin D (24,25-dihydroxycholecalciferol). The increase in calcitonin secretion elicited by gastrointestinal hormones suggests that one function of calcitonin may be to protect against the hypercalcemia that would normally occur after the ingestion of, for example, a meal rich in dairy products.

General therapeutic uses

Calcitonin has been successfully used in correcting hypercalcemia resulting from a variety of etiologies, including hypervitaminosis D and some malignancies. The hormone is also useful in the treatment of Paget's disease. Individuals with this disease often suffer from numerous fractures and spinal cord injuries as a result of excessive, disorganized bone remodeling. Paget's disease may also be treated with etidronate disodium, a pyrophosphate analogue. This compound slows the processes of hydroxyapatite dissolution and crystallization. Unlike calcitonin, resistance does not develop to the actions of etidronate.

VITAMIN D

Vitamin D refers collectively to cholecalciferol (vitamin D_3) and its vegetable counterpart, ergocalciferol (vitamin D_2). In humans, both forms are equally active in preventing the respective deficiency diseases of children and adults, rickets and osteomalacia. Although cholecalciferol is commonly called a vitamin, in the form of active metabolites it meets the criteria for a hormone.

The skin of normal individuals synthesizes a vitamin D precursor compound, 7-dehydrocholesterol, and when exposed to ultraviolet radiation, this precursor is converted to cholecalciferol. The activation of cholecalciferol involves two further reactions, both hydroxylations, which take place at two different sites. Though not discussed, ergocalciferol undergoes essentially identical transformations.

In the liver, cholecalciferol is hydroxylated to 25-hydroxycholecalciferol. This agent is marketed under the nonproprietary name of calcifediol. The reaction appears to be inhibited by excessive concentrations of vitamin D. Final activation occurs in the kidney, where either of two reactions may take place, depending on the calcium needs of the individual. Hydroxylation at C_1, facilitated by PTH, low calcium concentrations, and possibly estrogen and prolactin, yields 1,25-dihydroxycholecalciferol (Figure 34-3), which is the major active form of vitamin D. Given the nonproprietary designation of calcitriol, this agent is about 1000 times more potent than calcifediol in binding to its receptor. In the presence of high concentrations of calcium, calcitriol, and perhaps calcitonin, C_{24} is hydroxylated instead of C_1. The resulting compound and its C_1-hydroxylated metabolite are relatively inactive.

Once fully activated, vitamin D binds to cytoplasmic receptors in target organs. The hormone-receptor complex then attaches to the chromatin of the cell nucleus. This sequence of events, which is similar to that known to occur with other steroid hormones, results in an increased synthesis of proteins that may be involved with calcium transport.[3]

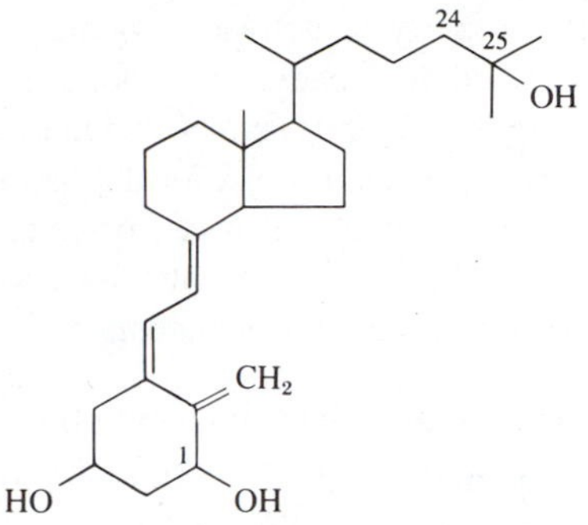

Figure 34-3. Structural formula of the primary active form of vitamin D, 1,25-dihydroxycholecalciferol (calcitriol).

Pharmacologic effects

The principal effect of calcitriol is to enhance the absorption of calcium from the intestine. The exact mechanism is unknown, but the compound apparently increases the activity of the calcium transport system in the brush border of intestinal epithelial cells.[14] Physiologically, activated vitamin D acts in concert with PTH to mobilize bone calcium, and a lack of either agent inhibits the effects of the other. Pharmacologic doses of calcitriol, however, will act even in the absence of PTH. In the kidney, vitamin D metabolites slightly increase calcium reabsorption.[24]

General therapeutic uses

Vitamin D is employed in the prevention and treatment of nutritional rickets and metabolic rickets (disorders associated with a reduced ability to activate vitamin D or to respond to its metabolites) and in the control of hypoparathyroidism. Vitamin D has also been used to treat osteoporosis, but this use is controversial.

Dihydrotachysterol is a vitamin D derivative with several therapeutic advantages over the parent compound. Activation of dihydrotachysterol requires hydroxylation only at C_{25}, and the drug does not inhibit its own activation.[13] By not requiring hydroxylation at C_1, dihydrotachysterol bypasses renal regulation. It is commonly used to treat hypoparathyroidism and is indicated for the management of postoperative and idiopathic tetany.

Calcitriol and calcifediol are generally reserved for the treatment of metabolic bone disease or hypocalcemia in patients on long-term renal dialysis.

Calcitriol is advantageous because these patients are unable properly to activate vitamin D. Calcifediol is effective because it is administered in much higher doses. Then, either residual renal hydroxylase activity is sufficient for the formation of physiologic amounts of calcitriol, or calcifediol is present in high enough concentrations to act directly in restoring calcium homeostasis.

Toxic reactions and drug interactions

Excessive administration of vitamin D or its derivatives leads to a condition known as hypervitaminosis D, which is characterized by hypercalcemia, osteoporosis, and calcium deposition in soft tissues. Despite the fact that the activation of dihydrotachysterol bypasses two regulatory steps, overdose with this agent is less of a problem than is overdose with the other forms of vitamin D. This is because the duration of action of dihydrotachysterol is much shorter than that of vitamin D. Consequently, if the overdose is recognized by monitoring plasma calcium concentrations, withdrawal of the drug will prevent the onset of serious toxicities. Because of its high potency and rapid onset, calcitriol is more likely than other vitamin D preparations to produce acute hypercalcemia on accidental overdosage. Removal of the drug by gastric lavage, induction of emesis, or use of mineral oil may be indicated.

Long-term administration of barbiturates or phenytoin may reduce the activity of these hypercalcemic agents by inducing the enzymes responsible for their inactivation.[12]

ANTIDIURETIC HORMONE

ADH, officially called vasopressin after its vasoconstrictive activity at relatively high concentrations, is one of the peptide hormones synthesized in the supraoptic nucleus of the hypothalamus and released into the general circulation from the posterior pituitary gland. The other posterior pituitary hormone, oxytocin, shares some of the properties of ADH. This pharmacologic overlap is due to structural similarities between the two hormones. Both are made up of nine peptide units differing in only two amino acids.

Release of ADH is controlled by the activity of hypothalamic neurons, which serve as osmoreceptors. For example, high osmolarity of extracellular fluid causes an enhancement of ADH release. Water retention, resulting from the activity of ADH, reduces the osmolarity of the hypothalamic extracellular fluid, which in turn inhibits further ADH release. The release of ADH is also influenced by other neuronal signals and pharmacologic stimuli, including alcohol, nicotine, meperidine, and some barbiturates (but not thiopental).

Pharmacologic effects

The principal action of ADH is on the tubular reabsorption of water by the nephron, particularly the distal tubule and the collecting ducts. ADH binds to its receptor and, by means of a cAMP-dependent mechanism, brings about an increase in the passage of water from the lumen of the tubules through the epithelial cells into the peritubular capillaries. This water-sparing effect is termed *antidiuresis*. Inadequate release of ADH results in a condition called diabetes insipidus.

General therapeutic uses

The use of vasopressin in the treatment of diabetes insipidus superseded that of crude pituitary extracts. Vasopressin may be used subcutaneously for acute control of the disease, but intramuscular injections of vasopressin tannate in oil offer more prolonged activity. Lypressin, a lysine analogue of vasopressin, may be used as a substitute for the parent compound. Unfortunately, the short duration of action of lypressin limits its usefulness. A more promising analogue has recently been introduced. Desmopressin is a peptide that does not demonstrate the overlap of antidiuretic and pressor activities exhibited by vasopressin. Furthermore, the effect of desmopressin is prompt and long lasting.

Nonhormonal agents may also be used to produce antidiuresis. The antihyperlipidemic drug clofibrate brings about an increase in the release of ADH from the pituitary, and the sensitivity of renal tubular cells to ADH may be enhanced by the hypoglycemic agent chlorpropamide. The benzothiadiazide diuretics paradoxically reduce urine production in individuals with ADH-resistant (nephrogenic) diabetes insipidus (see Chapter 27).

Toxic reactions and side effects

The major adverse effect associated with the therapeutic use of vasopressin results from the vasoconstrictor properties of the hormone. Vasopressin increases peripheral vascular resistance and may cause constriction of coronary blood vessels. Other smooth muscles may be stimulated as well, particularly those of the intestinal tract and uterus.

OXYTOCIN

Oxytocin is synthesized in cell bodies that are located predominantly in the paraventricular nucleus of the hypothalamus. Biochemical studies indicate that oxytocin (as well as vasopressin) is synthesized as a pre-prohormone. Shortly after synthesis, a portion of the peptide chain is cleaved off, leaving the prohormone, which is packaged into vesicles. Before release, the prohormone is split into two peptide chains, the hormone and another peptide called a neurophysin. Both the hormone and the corresponding neurophysin are released into the general circulation. Release of oxytocin is elicited by suckling of the breast and by uterine stretching.

Pharmacologic effects

Oxytocin appears to bind to receptors that are located on the smooth muscle of the uterus and oviducts and on the myoepithelial cells of the mammary glands. Binding to the receptors in the mammary glands mediates the process of milk ejection whereby contraction of myoepithelial cells forces milk into the mammary ducts. Oxytocin also brings about rhythmic contractions of the uterus. This effect is enhanced by estrogen but antagonized by progesterone. It is widely believed that the rising oxytocin concentrations in late pregnancy may play a key role in normal parturition. According to this theory, the high progesterone concentrations that are present up until the time of parturition inhibit the stimulatory effects of oxytocin. When this inhibition is released parturition is initiated.

General therapeutic uses

Oxytocin may be used intravenously to induce labor in patients with preexisting disease for whom a pregnancy of normal duration would be dangerous. In recent years, however, the use of oxytocin to induce labor has diminished significantly. Additionally, oxytocin may be administered after delivery to prevent or reduce postpartum hemorrhage.

Toxic reactions and side effects

The principal toxicities of oxytocin include allergic reactions to the drug and overstimulation of the uterus. The possible consequences of excessive uterine contractions include impairment of placental blood flow, cervical laceration, uterine rupture, and fetal hypoxia. The use of the hormone may also result in fetal cardiac arrhythmias.

IMPLICATIONS FOR DENTISTRY

The principal impact of the endocrine systems discussed in this chapter on dentition is indirect. It represents the consequence of improper control of hormone release, such as a deficiency or overproduction syndrome, and is usually not the result of an adverse effect of hormonal therapy.

Inadequate thyroid hormone release during childhood, for example, will adversely affect tooth development. The dentition of cretins has been described as both late and abnormal and corresponds with the delayed bone development that is characteristic of the disease. The tongue is often enlarged in these children, and they have an unusual facial appearance because of underdevelopment of the chin, maxillary prognathism, and failure of the mandibles to fuse.

Diabetes mellitus may also have oral manifestations. Gingivitis is common in diabetic patients and is more likely to progress to periodontitis.[6,15,28] Abscesses and polyps of the gingiva have also been reported, as well as a greater prevalence of gingival vascular abnormalities.[11] Diabetic patients often develop atrophic lesions of the tongue, most commonly central papillary atrophy.[10]

Although diabetic patients are quite susceptible to infection, careful operative technique should circumvent the need for prophylactic antibiotic therapy. Care should also be taken, when adjusting dentures, to avoid conditions that will lead to the development of tissue and bone necrosis. The patient should be given the opportunity to schedule his appointments for times that will coincide with expected peaks of insulin activity.

Dental problems secondary to bone abnormalities may result from altered calcium metabolism. The mineral of alveolar bone, like that of other bones, is subject to rapid exchange. As a result, incomplete mineralization and excessive mineral resorption may have indirect dental implications.

Hypoparathyroidism may have dental manifestations. Delayed eruption, blunted root apices, and hypoplastic enamel have been reported in hypoparathyroid patients.[18] These problems can be prevented if a diagnosis is made early in life and if treatment with vitamin D is initiated. Similarly, the hypoplastic enamel associated with some cases of childhood rickets can be prevented with vitamin D therapy.

Drugs mimicking or affecting hormones of homeostasis

Nonproprietary name	Proprietary name	Route of administration*
Hypoglycemic agents		
acetohexamide	Dymelor	Oral
chlorpropamide	Diabinese	Oral
glipizide	Glucotrol	Oral
glyburide	Micronase	Oral
insulin (see Table 34-2)		
tolazamide	Tolinase	Oral
tolbutamide	Orinase	Oral
Hyperglycemic agents		
diazoxide	Proglycem	Oral
glucagon	—	SC, IM, IV
glucose	Monojel	Oral, IV
Thyroid hormones		
levothyroxine	Synthroid	Oral, IM, IV
liothyronine	Cytomel	Oral
liotrix	Thyrolar	Oral
thyroglobulin	Proloid	Oral
thyroid	Thyrar	Oral
Antithyroid agents		
methimazole	Tapazole	Oral
propylthiouracil	—	Oral
sodium iodide	—	Oral, IV
sodium iodide I131	Iodotope	Oral
Posterior pituitary hormones		
desmopressin	DDAVP	IN
lypressin	Diapid	IN
oxytocin	Pitocin	IN, IM, IV
posterior pituitary	Pituitrin	IN, SC, IM
vasopressin	Pitressin	IN, SC, IM
Agents for ADH-resistant diabetes insipidus		
chlorpropamide	Diabenese	Oral
clofibrate	Atromid-S	Oral
thiazide diuretics (see Chapter 27)		
Agents altering calcium metabolism		
calcifediol	Calderol	Oral
calcitonin (salmon)	Calcimar	SC, IM
calcitriol	Rocaltrol	Oral
cholecalciferol	—	Oral
dihydrotachysterol	Hytakerol	Oral
ergocalciferol	Drisdol	Oral, IM
etidronate disodium	Didronel	Oral

*IN = intranasal, SC = subcutaneous, IM = intramuscular, IV = intravenous.

CITED REFERENCES

1. Agus, Z.S., Gardner, L.B., Beek, L.H., and Goldberg, M. Effects of parathyroid hormone on renal tubular reabsorption of calcium, sodium, and phosphate. American Journal of Physiology **224:**1143-1148, 1973.

2. Basabe, J.C., Cresto, J.C., and Aparicio, N. Studies on the mode of action of somatostatin on insulin secretion. Endocrinology **101:**1436-1443, 1977.

3. Bikle, D.D., Zolock, D.T., Morrissey, R.L., and Herman, R.H. Independence of 1,25-dihydroxyvitamin D₃-mediated calcium transport from de novo RNA and protein synthesis. Journal of Biological Chemistry **253:**484-488, 1978.

4. Brown, J.D., Steele, A.A., Stone, D.B., and Steele, F.A. The effect of tolbutamide on lipolysis and cyclic AMP concentration in white fat cells. Endocrinology **90:**47-59, 1972.

5. Brunette, M.G., Taleb, L., and Carriere, S. Effect of parathyroid hormone on phosphate reabsorption along the nephron of the rat. American Journal of Physiology **225:**1076-1081, 1973.

6. Cohen, D.W., Friedman, A.A., Shapiro, J., and Kyle, G.C. Diabetes mellitus and periodontal disease: two-year longitudinal observations. Part I. Journal of Periodontology **40:**709-712, 1970.

7. Cuatrecasas, P., Hollenberg, M.D., and Chang, K.J. Hormone receptor complexes and their modulation of membrane function. Recent Progress in Hormone Research **31:**37-94, 1975.

8. De Groot, L.J. Thyroid and the heart. Mayo Clinic Proceedings **47:**864-871, 1972.

9. Eaton, R.P. Portable insulin infusion pumps: what is their role in therapy? Drugs **23:**245-249, 1982.

10. Farman, A.G. Atrophic lesions of the tongue: a prevalence study among 175 diabetic patients. Journal of Oral Pathology **5:**255-264, 1976.

11. Frantzis, T.G., Reeve, C.M., and Brown, A.L., Jr. The ultrastructure of capillary basement membranes in attached gingiva of diabetic and nondiabetic patients with periodontal disease. Journal of Periodontology **42:**406-411, 1971.

12. Hahn, T.J., Birge, S.J., Scharp, C.R., and Avioli, L.V. Phenobarbital-induced alterations of vitamin D metabolism. Journal of Clinical Investigation **51:**741-748, 1972.

13. Hallick, R.B., and DeLuca, H.F. Metabolites of dihydrotachysterol₃ in target tissues. Journal of Biological Chemistry **247:**91-97, 1972.

14. Haussler, M.R., Nagode, L.A., and Rasmussen, H. Induction of intestinal brush border alkaline phosphatase by vitamin D and identity with Ca-ATPase. Nature **228:**1199-1201, 1970.

15. Hove, K.A., and Stallard, R.E. Diabetes and the periodontal patient. Journal of Periodontology **41:**713-718, 1970.

16. Ismail-Beigi, F., and Edelman, I.S. Mechanism of thyroid calorigenesis: role of active sodium transport. Proceedings of the National Academy of Sciences of the United States of America **67:**1071-1078, 1970.

17. Jefferson, L.S., Exton, J.H., Butcher, R.W., Sutherland, E.W., and Park, C.R. Role of cyclic AMP in the effects of insulin and anti-insulin serum on liver metabolism. Journal of Biological Chemistry **243:**1031-1038, 1968.

18. Jensen, S.B., Illum, F., and Dupont, E. Nature and frequency of dental changes in idiopathic hypoparathyroidism and pseudohypoparathyroidism. Scandinavian Journal of Dental Research **89**:26-37, 1981.

19. Levey, G.S. Catecholamine sensitivity, thyroid hormone, and the heart: a reevaluation. American Journal of Medicine **50**:413-420, 1971.

20. Liberti, P., and Stanbury, J.B. The pharmacology of substances affecting the thyroid gland. Annual Review of Pharmacology and Toxicology **11**:113-142, 1971.

21. Malaisse, W., Malaisse-Lagae, F., Wright, P.H., and Ashmore, J. Effects of adrenergic and cholinergic agents upon insulin secretion in vitro. Endocrinology **80**:975-978, 1967.

22. Ostlund, R.E. Contractile proteins and pancreatic beta cell secretion. Diabetes **26**:245-252, 1977.

23. Porte, D., Jr., and Robertson, R.P. Control of insulin secretion by catecholamines, stress, and the sympathetic nervous system. Federation Proceedings **32**:1792-1796, 1973.

24. Puschett, J.B., Moranz, J., and Kurnick, W.S. Evidence for a direct action of cholecalciferol and 25-hydroxycholecalciferol on renal transport of phosphate, sodium, and calcium. Journal of Clinical Investigation **51**:373-385, 1972.

25. Roth, J., Kahn, C.R., and Lesniak, M.A. Receptor for insulin, NSILA-s, and growth hormone: applications to disease states in man. Recent Progress in Hormone Research **31**:95-139, 1975.

26. Rubenstein, A.H., Block, M.B., Starr, J., Melani, F., and Steiner, D.F. Proinsulin and C-peptide in blood. Diabetes **21**(suppl. 2):661-672, 1972.

27. Shanks, R.G., Hadden, D.R., Lowe, D.C., McDevitt, D.G., and Montgomery, D.A.D. Controlled trial of propranolol in thyrotoxicosis. Lancet **1**:993-994, 1961.

28. Sznajder, N., Carraro, J.J., Rugna, S., and Sereday, M. Periodontal findings in diabetic and nondiabetic patients. Journal of Periodontology **49**:445-448, 1978.

29. Taurog, A. Thyroid preoxidase and thyroxine biosynthesis. Recent Progress in Hormone Research **26**:189-241, 1970.

30. University Group Diabetes Program. A study of the effects of hypoglycemic agents on vascular complications in patients with adult onset diabetes. Diabetes **19**(suppl. 2):747-830, 1970.

31. Widstrom, A., and Cerasi, E. On the action of tolbutamide in man. I. Role of adrenergic mechanism in tolbutamide-induced insulin release during normoglycemia and induced hypoglycemia. Acta Endocrinologica (Kobenhavn) **72**:506-518, 1973.

GENERAL REFERENCES

Czech, M.P. Molecular basis of insulin action. Annual Review of Biochemistry **46**:359-384, 1977.

DeLuca, H.F. Vitamin D: metabolism and function. In Gross, F., Grumbach, M.M., Labhart, A., Lipsett, M.B., Mann, T., Samuels, L.T., and Zander, J., eds. Monographs on Endocrinology, vol. 13. Springer-Verlag, Berlin, 1979.

Raisz, L.G., and Kream, B.E. Hormonal control of skeletal growth. Annual Review of Physiology **43**:225-238, 1981.

Rasmussen, H., and Bordier, P. The Physiological and Cellular Basis of Metabolic Bone Disease. Baltimore, The Williams & Wilkins Co., 1974.

Stern, P.H. The D vitamins and bone. Pharmacological Reviews **32**:47-80, 1980.

Williams, R.J. Textbook of Endocrinology, ed. 6. Philadelphia, W.B. Saunders Co., 1981.

35 Hormones of reproduction and sexual development

William Warner

The endocrine functions of the various reproductive tissues have been studied since the nineteenth century. Despite this early work, insight into the biochemical mechanisms of the reproductive hormones has been achieved only in the last 3 decades and has been the result of intensive interdisciplinary research. The most notable fruit of these cooperative endeavors has been the beginnings of an understanding of the maintenance of fertility and its pharmacologic control.

The use of sex hormones in therapy has similarly undergone radical change in the last few decades. Before the isolation and identification of estrogen in the early 1930s and progesterone in the mid 1930s, dried ovary and corpus luteum enjoyed official drug status, which continued until 1950. Within 15 years of the elucidation of the chemical structure of estrogen and progesterone, purified drug preparations from biologic sources of both estrogen and progesterone were included in official compendia, followed shortly by the synthetic hormones. Forms of testosterone were first admitted to *The United States Pharmacopeia* in 1947. These agents were not, however, preceded by official androgen-containing tissue extracts. More recently, peptide hormones of pituitary origin have become available for the treatment of a limited number of conditions.

Perhaps more so than with most drugs in current use, the pharmacology of the sex hormones is closely intertwined with their physiologic actions. For this reason, an understanding of the therapeutic application of exogenous sex steroids and peptides is most readily achieved after a review of basic reproductive physiology.

FEMALE SEX HORMONES

Maturation of ovarian follicles and the synthesis and secretion of female sex hormones are under the control of the two gonadotropic hormones of the adenohypophysis: FSH and LH. The release of each of these glycoprotein hormones is cyclic in nature, being under the positive control of a hypothalamic releasing hormone (RH) and under the negative control of a feedback mechanism. In both females and males, one protein serves as the releasing hormone for both FSH and LH.

Under the influence of the pituitary gonadotropins, the two female sex steroids—estrogen and progesterone—are secreted by the ovary. Since gonadotropin release is cyclic, so is the synthesis and release of the steroid hormones. The result of this cyclic pattern is a characteristic series of ovarian and uterine changes defined as the menstrual cycle.

Menstrual cycle

The ovary has a limited number of ova that develop from primitive germ cells, each of which is in a primary follicle. After puberty, the increase in FSH release that occurs at the beginning of each 28-day menstrual cycle results in the growth of a small fraction of these follicles and their contained ova and the secretion of estrogen. After 14 days have elapsed (the midpoint of the cycle), the high concentration of estrogen gradually depresses FSH release and greatly enhances the secretion of LH. The result of this surge of LH is ovulation. Of the approximately 30 follicles that begin maturation each month, usually only one attains full maturity and releases its ovum from the ovary. The remainder degenerate into atretic follicles.

After ovulation, in which the ovum and its associated follicular cells are expelled from the ovarian surface, the remaining cells of the follicle form the corpus luteum. This ovarian structure secretes progesterone for approximately 8 days and then begins to degenerate unless stimulated by a placental hormone, chorionic gonadotropin (CGH). The secretory activity of the follicle, followed by that of the corpus luteum, forms the basis of a sequential secretion of estrogen and progesterone. This sequence of steroid secretion in turn mediates the cyclic proliferative and secretory changes in the uterus that favor fertilization and implantation and that are the basis of the menstrual cycle. The initial portion of the cycle, during which estrogen levels rise, is called the proliferative phase, and it is characterized by an increase in the size and vascularity of the myometrium and endometrium. The portion of the cycle during which the corpus luteum exists is called the secretory phase, and it is characterized by secretory activity of endometrial glands and by an increase in the blood flow to this tissue.

If the corpus luteum is allowed to degenerate, the resulting decline in progesterone in conjunction with already declining estrogen produces a regression of the endometrium. The ensuing loss of blood and cells makes up the menstrual flow. The appearance of blood marks the end of one, and the beginning of the next, 28-day menstrual cycle.

If the secretory function of the corpus luteum is maintained, as it is when implantation occurs, menstruation is avoided, and the pregnancy is maintained. Eventually the corpus luteum becomes refractory to further hormonal stimulation, but by that time the placenta is able to secrete sufficient quantities of estrogen and progesterone to maintain the uterus in a condition that is supportive of pregnancy.

Hormonal changes in pregnancy

As mentioned previously, CGH, originating in the placental cytotrophoblastic cells, first appears shortly after implantation. The circulating concentrations of this hormone rise quickly at about the fourth week of pregnancy, remain high for about 12 weeks, and then decline slowly. CGH replaces LH and to a degree FSH, which are normally inhibited by estrogen and progesterone, both of which are present in increasing amounts until parturition.

During pregnancy, titers of prolactin, a hormone of anterior pituitary origin, are elevated, altering the morphology of the mammary glands and re-sulting in characteristic changes in the ducts and alveoli of breast tissue. The ability of prolactin to initiate milk production, however, is not manifest until steroid levels decline after parturition. After the termination of pregnancy lactation is maintained by prolactin release elicited by the suckling reflex. This same reflex mediates oxytocin release from the posterior pituitary, bringing about ejection of milk into the mammary ducts.

Pregnancy is also associated with increases in the activity of other portions of the endocrine system. For example, the concentrations of thyroxine, glucocorticoids, insulin, and growth hormone are usually elevated.

Estrogen

Three natural estrogens are produced in physiologically effective amounts during the menstrual cycle: 17β-estradiol, estrone, and estriol. Therapeutically, the most important of these is estradiol, the chemical structure of which is presented in Figure 35-1. In addition to these naturally occurring steroids, a number of synthetic estrogenic compounds have been developed that have the great advantage of being active after oral administration. The structure of one such compound, diethylstilbestrol (DES), is shown in Figure 35-2. As can be seen, estrogenic activity can be demonstrated by compounds with widely differing structures.

Progesterone

Progesterone (Figure 35-3) is quite similar structurally to 17β-estradiol. The hormone is available for therapeutic application, but its use has been largely superseded by orally effective progestins. Progestins are chemical analogues of progesterone, but they frequently demonstrate estrogenic and androgenic activity. Consequently, the pharmacologic activity of the various progestins displays subtle variations that cannot be considered in a chapter of this scope.

Mechanism of action

In recent years, estrogen-receptor proteins have been found in the cytoplasm of estrogen-sensitive cells,[16] including gingival tissue.[26] This is in contrast to most other hormone receptor proteins, which are located in the plasma membrane. The association of estrogen with its receptor brings about a conformational change in the protein and a migration of the hormone-receptor complex into the cell nucleus. Studies suggest that the complex

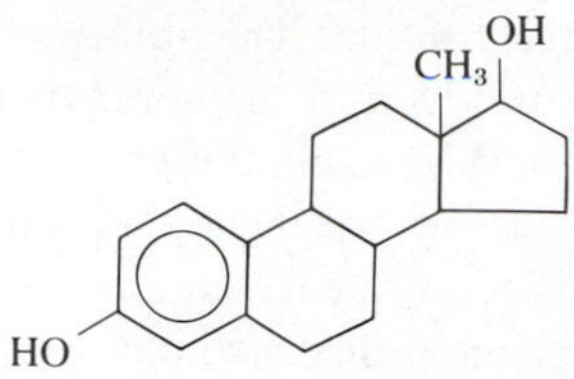

Figure 35-1. Structural formula of 17β-estradiol.

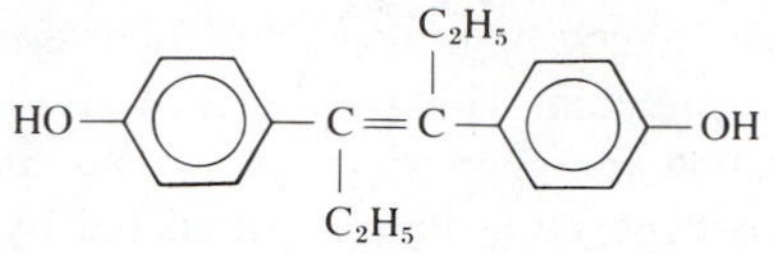

Figure 35-2. Structural formula of diethylstilbestrol.

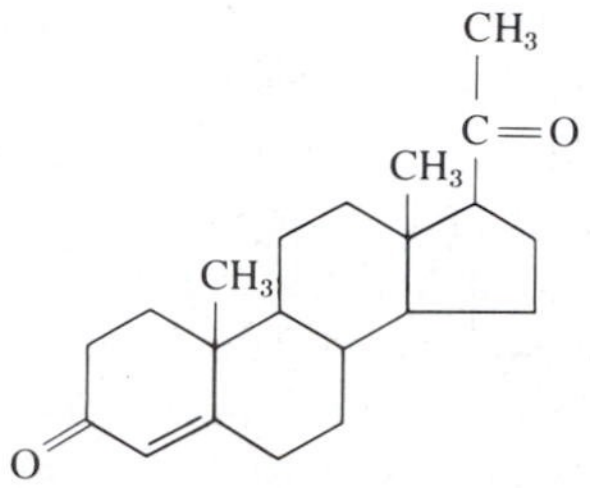

then binds to various nonhistone proteins that are themselves normally bound to chromosomal DNA. By an unknown mechanism, the interaction of the receptor-steroid complex with the chromosomal DNA facilitates the transcription of discrete sections of the DNA strand. The resulting increased synthesis of enzymes and structural proteins represents the biochemical basis of estrogen action. A similar series of events appears to mediate the activities of progesterone and testosterone.

Figure 35-3. Structural formula of progesterone.

Pharmacologic effects

Anabolic effects. The development of female sex characteristics and mediation of the pubertal growth spurt are both manifestations of the mild anabolic activity of estrogen. An anabolic mechanism is also invoked to explain the apparent ability of estrogen to stimulate hepatic synthesis of a variety of proteins.

Blood chemistry. Administration of estrogen may increase the concentrations of a number of circulating plasma proteins, for example, corticosteroid-binding globulin and some of the clotting factors. The latter effect may explain, in part, the ability of estrogen to hasten clot formation. Complex alterations of plasma lipids, including an increase in circulating triglycerides, have also been noted during estrogen therapy. In addition, estrogens cause salt and water retention, which at times may result in clinically significant edema.

Skeletal system. The skeletal system is particularly sensitive to estrogens. The trabeculae of cancellous bone in egg-laying hens are remarkably labile, and they grow and resorb cyclically in response to oscillating hormone concentrations. This effect on bone is not as dramatic in humans, but closure of epiphyseal growth plates does occur. At very high hormone titers, bone resorption may actually take place. Osteoporosis in postmenopausal women may be at least partly a result of reduced

estrogen concentrations. The role of estrogen in alveolar bone loss in postmenopausal women is not clear. The dentist may observe changes in the oral mucosa as a consequence of pregnancy or of taking contraceptive medications.

Endocrine and reproductive systems. The endocrine and reproductive systems are by far the most sensitive to the influences of estrogen and progesterone. In the uterus, the development of endometrial glands, the proliferation of connective tissue, and the increase of cellular glycogen storage are mediated by rising estrogen levels. In addition, cornification of vaginal epithelium occurs.

The actions of progesterone and estrogen at the site of target tissues are often complementary. For example, estrogen brings about proliferation of the uterine endothelium, whereas progesterone promotes its secretory activity. Similarly, progesterone increases blood flow to the endometrium after the vascular proliferation mediated by estrogen has occurred. However, in other tissues the two steroids have antagonistic effects. Muscular and ciliary activity of the oviducts is increased by estrogen and decreased by progesterone. Furthermore, secretions of the uterine cervix are made more viscous by progesterone and less viscous by estrogen.

In addition to these actions, the sex steroids show complex interactions with other segments of the endocrine system. Estrogen enhances the release of prolactin during pregnancy, but it inhibits milk production until after parturition, when its concentration declines. The sensitivity of the uterus to oxytocin stimulation is increased by estrogen but decreased by progesterone.[1] Estrogen, and testosterone in men, also increases the sensitivity of the anterior pituitary gland to growth hormone releasing factor.

Absorption, fate, and excretion

Although 17β-estradiol and progesterone are readily absorbed from the gastrointestinal tract, their effectiveness after oral administration is limited by rapid inactivation in the liver. All of these natural steroids are converted to inactive sulfates and glucuronides. Synthetic forms of these hormones are generally inactivated more slowly and may therefore be given orally.

Once absorbed, the sex steroids are extensively protein bound. Although these compounds may bind to many plasma proteins, the most important seems to be sex steroid–binding globulin, which is synthesized in the liver and has a high affinity for 17β-estradiol, progesterone, and testosterone. Steroid metabolites are excreted primarily in the urine, but significant amounts may also be excreted in milk. To date, however, toxicities involving breast-fed newborns have not been reported.

General therapeutic uses

Estrogen and progesterone, or compounds with activities similar to these hormones, may be used in replacement therapy for a number of natural and iatrogenic hormone deficiencies. For example, estrogen may be used to partially relieve endocrine inbalances in girls with hypopituitarism and in women whose ovaries failed to develop, grew abnormally, or were surgically removed. Similarly, it has been known for many years that some of the symptoms of menopause, particularly those with vasomotor components, may be alleviated by estrogen. This particular use of estrogen has, in the opinion of some authorities, been abused. Progesterone has limited usefulness in replacement therapy. Progesterone, not progestins, which may have some androgenic activity, has been used in cases of luteal phase defect, a condition in which the capacity of the corpus luteum to synthesize progesterone is diminished.

Table 35-1. Some oral contraceptives

	Progestin	Estrogen
Combination		
Ortho-Novum 2 mg	Norethindrone 2 mg	Mestranol 100 μg
Ovcon-35	Norethindrone 0.4 mg	Ethinyl estradiol 35 μg
Enovid 5 mg	Norethynodrel 5 mg	Mestranol 75 μg
Enovid-E	Norethynodrel 2.5 mg	Mestranol 100 μg
Lo/Ovral	Norgestrel 0.3 mg	Ethinyl estradiol 30 μg
Ovulen	Ethynodiol 1 mg	Mestranol 100 μg
Demulen	Ethynodiol 1 mg	Ethinyl estradiol 50 μg
Single-entity		
Micronor	Norethindrone 0.35 mg	
Ovrette	Norgestrel 0.075 mg	

As an outgrowth of the pioneering work of Pincus and his co-workers,[19] estrogens and progestins have been successfully used to suppress conception. Since 1958, estrogens and progestins alone, in combination, or in sequence have been used as oral contraceptives. At present, two basic regimens are used: administration of estrogen and progestin combinations for approximately 20 days per month or continuous administration of low doses of a progestin. The inclusion of a progestin in the first regimen primarily serves to induce a regular menstrual flow. Table 35-1 lists several oral contraceptive preparations.

The mechanism by which conception is prevented is not completely understood. In the first regimen, ovulation is prevented by an estrogen-mediated suppression of FSH and LH release.[15,24] The mechanism of the second regimen might be to impair sperm transport as a result of enhanced viscosity of cervical secretions or aberrant secretion and motility of the oviducts or to produce an endometrium that is unsuitable for implantation.

DES has been approved for use as a postcoital contraceptive. The drug is given in high doses for 5 days, starting no later than 72 hours after coitus and after determining that the patient is not already pregnant. This regimen is believed to prevent implantation. Because of the severe side effects caused by the high doses of DES, this treatment is reserved for emergencies.

Before their use as contraceptives, the principal therapeutic application of the female sex hormones was in the treatment of various menstrual disorders. For example, dysmenorrhea can be relieved by estrogens, and functional uterine bleeding can be controlled by using a progestin to bring about normal menstrual flow. Endometriosis also responds favorably to progestin therapy.

An interesting use of estrogen takes advantage of its anabolic activity. Osteoporosis can be partially, albeit perhaps transiently, alleviated by estrogen therapy. The hormone is most effective if the condition is secondary to menopause,[11,21] especially when caused by surgical removal of the ovaries before the age of menopause. By increasing the production of bone matrix, estrogen strengthens osteoporotic bones and minimizes the risk of fracture. The use of estrogen requires the careful monitoring of the patient, because of the association of postmenopausal estrogen treatment with endometrial cancer.[21]

Sex steroids have also been used in the treatment of certain neoplastic states. DES and ethinyl estradiol have been used in the treatment of prostate carcinoma and of mammary cancer in postmenopausal women, and progestins have shown promise in the treatment of endometrial carcinomas (see Chapter 40).

Toxic reactions and side effects

The numerous side effects associated with estrogen therapy have precipitated a reduction in the dosages of this steroid in contraceptive medications. The most common side effects of oral contraceptives are mild and usually transient. These include headache, nausea, weight gain, and mood changes. Irregular menstrual bleeding sometimes occurs, and several months may be required for normal menstrual cycles to become reestablished after cessation of therapy.

Alterations of blood chemistry may result in several problems. For example, a slight increase in the incidence of thromboembolic disease has been reported for individuals on contraceptive regimens as compared with nonpregnant women in the control group. An exact measure of the risk of thromboembolic disorders related to the use of oral contraceptives would require large-scale double-blind studies. For ethical reasons, these studies will probably never be performed. During the 1960s, retrospective studies were conducted, but the results were conflicting. More recently, prospective studies were conducted that demonstrated an increased risk of thromboembolic disease associated with

contraceptive medications, but these results have also been criticized. The current consensus is that women taking oral contraceptives do assume a greater risk of heart attack and stroke and that the risk is highest among women who are over 35 years of age and are heavy smokers.[8,18,25] Interestingly, the therapeutic response to anticoagulants is diminished by contraceptive agents. Laboratory studies have demonstrated estrogen-induced alterations in the circulating concentrations of clotting factors as well as changes in platelet function, but these effects may not correlate with the enhanced incidence of thromboembolic problems that has been reported. Estrogen-induced changes in blood lipids may result in hyperlipidemia and pancreatitis.

A number of other potential adverse effects of estrogen and progesterone have been reported. For example, hypertension occasionally develops in women who take oral contraceptives.[12] Estrogens are also known to alter liver function, but they do not appear to produce irreversible liver damage. However, the use of the hormone in patients with a history of cholestatic hepatic and biliary abnormalities requires caution. In addition, neuroophthalmic disorders have been observed in patients taking oral contraceptives, including several types of retinal disorders and an intolerance to contact lenses. Also, animal experiments suggest that estrogens may be carcinogenic, and clinical studies have revealed an association between endometrial carcinoma and estrogen therapy for menopausal and postmenopausal women.[10] One link between an estrogenic agent and cancer is the well-documented increased incidence of vaginal and cervical carcinomas in young women who have experienced in utero exposure to DES. Estrogens have also been shown to be teratogenic,[9] causing fetal limb abnormalities. Although similar problems have not arisen with progesterone, the slight androgenic activity of some progestins has caused fetal virilization. In any event, pregnancy must be considered a contraindication to the use of sex steroids.

These toxicities may be summarized with a list of contraindications. Women with a history of breast or sex organ cancer, thromboembolic disease, stroke, heart attack, angina pectoris, or suspected pregnancy should not take oral contraceptives. Although these contraindications underscore the risks implicit in contraceptive medications, the other side of the therapeutic equation must also be considered. Pregnancy itself carries substantial risks that must be weighed before a decision is made concerning the propriety of contraceptive medication.

Implications for dentistry

During the last 10 years it has become clear that the sex steroids alter dental structures. Pregnancy and the onset of puberty are associated with gingival inflammation[17] (which is diminished by good dental hygiene) and an increase in tooth mobility[20] and pocket depth.[4] Desquamative gingivitis has also been reported to occur with increasing frequency after menopause.[6]

The use of oral contraceptives is associated with increased gingival exudation[13] and an increased incidence of radiopacities of the mandible.[5] There also appears to be a greater risk of developing dry socket after mandibular third molar extractions in women who are taking estrogen-containing contraceptives.[23] One study demonstrated, however, that this risk was significantly reduced if the surgery was performed during the time of the month when a contraceptive is not taken (specifically, several days after the last dose of estrogen was ingested).[3]

The sex steroids have also been used to treat recurrent, menstrually related aphthous ulcers in women. Improvement was noted in women who were treated with oral contraceptives[2] or with medroxyprogesterone.[7] The potential adverse effects associated with these regimens have already been mentioned.

ANTIESTROGENS

Both progestins and androgens may be considered physiologic antagonists of estrogen. One drug in current use, however, may be classified as a pharmacologic estrogen antagonist. This drug is clomiphene. Recent studies have demonstrated that clomiphene binds to cytoplasmic estrogen receptors. The drug-receptor complex then migrates into the target cell nucleus, but it does not elicit a response.

The principal therapeutic use of clomiphene is the stimulation of ovulation in infertile women.[14] It is presumed that the drug's mechanism of action is to block the normal inhibitory effect of endogenous estrogen on gonadotropin release. Although clomiphene has not been used extensively, several adverse effects have come to light. The use of clomiphene to enhance fertility often results in multiple births and may cause the formation of ovarian cysts.

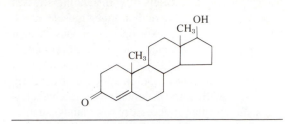

Figure 35-4. Structural formula of testosterone.

MALE SEX HORMONES

The male sex hormones are primarily produced in the Leydig cells (interstitial cells) of the testis and, to a smaller degree, in the adrenal cortex. The major hormone produced by the testis is the steroid testosterone, the structure of which is shown in Figure 35-4. This hormone is metabolized in the liver to two much less active forms, androsterone and etiocholanolone. All compounds with testosterone-like activity, regardless of origin, are called androgens.

Control of testosterone production is effected by the gonadotropic hormones LH and FSH. As in women, secretion of gonadotropins in men is governed by the appropriate hypothalamic releasing hormone, whose release is in turn controlled by a feedback mechanism involving testosterone. Thus, although fluctuations occur, testosterone release is self-regulating and noncyclic.

LH exerts its influence on the Leydig cells, and FSH appears to exert a proliferative stimulus on the spermatogonia-spermatocyte population. Final maturation of spermatozoa requires other localized processes that are beyond the scope of this chapter.

Mechanism of action

As with estrogen and progesterone, testosterone activity appears to be mediated by cytoplasmic receptors that, on entering target cell nuclei, enhance the synthesis of specific proteins.

Pharmacologic effects

Development of the male gonads, descent of the testes in the fetal stage, and development of the secondary male sex characteristics are all functions of the androgens. An anabolic effect results in pronounced development during adolescence of both the muscular and skeletal systems. Enhanced bone matrix production is followed by normal deposition of hydroxyapatite such that thicker cortical bone is made, providing a means of withstanding stresses imposed by the larger and stronger muscle mass.

Deficiencies in gonadotropic hormones in men are frequently associated with underdevelopment of the testes or, if the deficiency is congenital, with cryptorchidism. These abnormalities are frequently associated with loss of definitive male characteristics and atrophy of accessory sex glands, such as the prostate gland and seminal vesicles.

On the other hand, oversecretion of androgens, caused by tumors either of the pituitary, Leydig, or Sertoli cells or of the adrenal cortex (which may occur in men or women), often results in marked exaggeration of secondary sex characteristics in men or virilization in women.

Absorption, fate, and excretion

The characteristics of testosterone with respect to absorption, distribution, and excretion are similar to those already described for estrogen and progesterone. As with these steroid hormones, orally effective androgens are available.

General therapeutic uses

The principal medicinal use of testosterone is in replacement therapy. Oligospermia, various androgen deficiencies, and male climacteric have been treated with testosterone. Other indications for this drug have also been found. For example, androgens have been used to control metastatic carcinomas of female reproductive tissues (see Chapter 40).

Androgens with anabolic activity have been used along with a high protein diet to counteract the catabolism frequently associated with surgery, physical trauma, and debilitating diseases. A somewhat related, although often discouraged, use of androgens is found in sports.[22] The administration of anabolic steroids along with a high-protein diet has been claimed to increase the rate of muscle development. Similar reasoning has led to the use of androgens to stimulate erythropoiesis in anemic patients.

Toxic reactions and side effects

The therapeutic application of androgens is often difficult to evaluate and is not without hazard. The virilizing effects of these drugs must be taken into consideration when they are to be used in children or women. Administration of androgens to pregnant women may cause irreparable harm to the developing fetus. When given to children, premature epiphyseal closure will result in short adult stature.

As with the female sex steroids, androgens may alter liver function, but these effects are usually reversible. Although significant alterations in the blood clotting mechanism have not been reported, testosterone may enhance the therapeutic response to anticoagulants. Testosterone has been reported to cause retention of salt and water and possibly hyperglycemia.

PITUITARY GONADOTROPINS

Two of the gonadotropins currently available for therapeutic use are of human origin. Menotropin is derived from the urine of postmenopausal women and CGH from the urine of pregnant women. Purified pituitary gonadotropins are available only for investigational use.

Pituitary gonadotropins have been used primarily to bring about ovulation in infertile women. Because of the expense involved in the long-term use of these agents and the time required for sperm to mature, they have not been used to stimulate spermatogenesis in infertile men. However, CGH has been used to treat cryptorchidism.

Because they are proteins subject to gastrointestinal digestion, gonadotropins must be administered parenterally. Significant amounts of gonadotropins, especially CGH, are excreted in the urine in unchanged form, but large amounts are also degraded to inactive proteins. As with clomiphene, another agent used to treat infertility, multiple births have occurred after gonadotropin therapy.

BROMOCRIPTINE

Bromocriptine is a nonhormonal agent that has proved useful in the treatment of some cases of female infertility associated with hyperprolactinemia. The release of prolactin from the anterior pituitary is normally inhibited by the activity of dopaminergic neurons. Bromocriptine, a dopamine receptor agonist, inhibits the release of prolactin. Once the circulating concentration of prolactin is reduced, the inhibition exerted by the hormone on gonadotropin release is relieved.

Hormones of reproduction and sexual development

Nonproprietary name	Proprietary name
Estrogens	
chlorotrianisene	TACE
combined estrogens	Gynogen R.P.
conjugated estrogens	Premarin
diethylstilbestrol (DES)	—
esterified estrogens	Estratab
estradiol	Estrace
estrogenic substance	Gravigen
estrone	Bestrone
estropipate	Ogen
ethinyl estradiol	Estinyl
quinestrol	Estrovis
Progestins	
hydroxyprogesterone	Delalutin
medroxyprogesterone	Provera
norethindrone	Norlutin
progesterone	Progelan
Oral contraceptives	
see Table 35-1	
Androgens	
fluoxymesterone	Halotestin
methyltestosterone	Metandren
testosterone	Delatestryl
Anabolic steroids	
ethylestrenol	Maxibolin
methandriol	Anabol
nandrolone	Durabolin
oxandrolone	Anavar
oxymetholone	Anadrol-50
stanozolol	Winstrol
Gonadotropins	
chorionic gonadotropin (human)	Follutein
menotropins	Pergonal
Antiestrogen	
clomiphene	Clomid
Dopamine agonist	
bromocriptine	Parlodel

CITED REFERENCES

1. Caldeyro-Barcia, R., and Posiero, J.J. Oxytocin and the human uterus. Annals of the New York Academy of Sciences **75**:813-830, 1959.
2. Carruthers, R. Recurrent aphthous ulcers. Lancet **2**:259, 1979.
3. Catellani, J.E., Harvey, S., Erickson, S.H., and Cherkin, D. Effect of oral contraceptive cycle on dry socket (localized alveolar osteitis). Journal of the American Dental Association **101**:777-780, 1980.
4. Cohen, D.W., Friedman, L., Shapiro, J., and Kyle, G.C. A longitudinal investigation of the periodontal changes during pregnancy. Journal of Periodontology **40**:563-570, 1969.
5. Darzenta, N.C., and Giunta, J.L. Radiographic changes of the mandible related to oral contraceptives. Oral Surgery, Oral Medicine, Oral Pathology **43**:478-481, 1977.
6. Engel, M.B., Ray, H.G., and Orban, B. The pathogenesis of desquamative gingivitis: disturbance of connective tissue ground substance. Journal of Dental Research **29**:410-418, 1950.
7. Ferguson, M.M., McKay, H.D., Lindsay, R., and Stephen, K.W. Progeston therapy for menstrually related aphthae. International Journal of Oral Surgery **7**:463-470, 1978.
8. Jain, A.K. Mortality risk associated with the use of oral contraceptives. Studies in Family Planning **8**:50-54, 1977.
9. Janerich, D.T., Piper, J.M., and Glebatis, D.M. Oral contraceptives and congenital limb-reduction defects. New England Journal of Medicine **291**:697-700, 1974.
10. Jick, H., Watkins, R.N., Hunter, J.R., Dinan, B.J., Madsen, S., Rothman, K.J., and Walker, A.M. Replacement estrogens and endometrial cancer. New England Journal of Medicine **300**:218-222, 1979.
11. Lafferty, F.W., Spencer, G.E., and Pearson, O.H. Effects of androgens, estrogens, and high calcium intakes on bone formation and resorption in osteoporosis. American Journal of Medicine **36**:514-528, 1964.
12. Laragh, J.H. Oral contraceptive-induced hypertension—nine years later. American Journal of Obstetrics and Gynecology **126**:141-147, 1976.
13. Lindhe, J., and Bjorn, A.L. Influence of hormonal contraceptives on the gingiva of women. Journal of Periodontal Research **2**:1-6, 1967.
14. Macgregor, A.H., Johnson, J.E., and Bunde, C.A. Further clinical experience with clomiphene citrate. Fertility and Sterility **19**:616-622, 1968.
15. Minaguchi, H., and Meites, J. Effects of norethynodrel-mestranol combination (Enovid) on hypothalamic and pituitary hormones in rats. Endocrinology **81**:826-834, 1967.
16. O'Malley, B.W., and Means, A.R. Female steroid hormones and target cell nuclei. Science **183**:610-620, 1974.
17. O'Neil, T.C.A. Maternal T-lymphocyte response and gingivitis in pregnancy. Journal of Periodontology **50**:178-184, 1979.
18. Oral contraceptives: new drug requirement for labeling directed to the patient. Federal Register **43**:4214-4222, 1978.
19. Pincus, G. Clinical effects of new progestational compounds. In Astwood, E.B., ed. Clinical Endocrinology, vol. 1. New York, Grune & Stratton, Inc., 1960.
20. Rateitschak, K.H. Tooth mobility changes in pregnancy. Journal of Periodontal Research **2**:199-206, 1967.

21. Riggs, B.L., Jowsey, J., Goldsmith, R.S., Kelly, P.J., Hoffman, D.L., and Arnaud, C.D. Short- and long-term effects of estrogen and synthetic anabolic hormone in post-menopausal osteoporosis. Journal of Clinical Investigation **51:**1659-1663, 1972.

22. Ryan, A.J. Anabolic steroids are fool's gold. Federation Proceedings **40:**2682-2688, 1981.

23. Schow, S.R. Evaluation of postoperative localized osteitis in mandibular third molar surgery. Oral Surgery, Oral Medicine, Oral Pathology **38:**352-358, 1974.

24. Swerdloff, R.S., and Odell, W.D. Serum luteinizing and follicle stimulating hormone levels during sequential and nonsequential contraceptive treatment of eugonadal women. Journal of Clinical Endocrinology and Metabolism **29:**157-163, 1969.

25. Tietze, C. New estimates of mortality associated with fertility control. Family Planning Perspectives **9:**74-76, 1977.

26. Vittek, J., Hernandez, M.R., Wenk, E.J., Rappaport, S.C., and Southren, A.L. Specific estrogen receptors in human gingiva. Journal of Clinical Endocrinology and Metabolism **54:**608-612, 1980.

GENERAL REFERENCES

Blackwell, R.E., and Guillemin, R. Hypothalamic control of adenohypophyseal secretions. Annual Review of Physiology **35:**357-390, 1973.

Emmens, C.W., Cox, R.I., and Martin, L. Antiestrogens. Recent Progress in Hormone Research **18:**415-560, 1962.

Fink, G. Feedback actions of target hormones on hypothalamus and pituitary, with special reference to gonadal steroids. Annual Review of Physiology **41:**571-586, 1979.

Means, A.R., and Ghafouleas, J.G. Calmodulin in endocrine cells. Annual Review of Physiology **44:**667-682, 1982.

Richards, J.S. Maturation of ovarian follicles: actions and interactions of pituitary and ovarian hormones on follicular cell differentiation. Physiological Reviews **60:**51-89, 1980.

Williams, R.J. Textbook of Endocrinology, ed. 6. Philadelphia, W.B. Saunders Co., 1981.

36 Principles and mechanisms of antibiotic therapy

Edward H. Montgomery

Initiation of the therapeutic use of sulfonamides in the late 1930s and penicillin shortly thereafter represents one of the highlights in the history of medicine. Indeed, there is no development that has had a greater impact on the treatment of disease than the discovery and clinical introduction of the antimicrobial agents. The concept of chemotherapy was originally formulated by Paul Ehrlich in 1906, but the use of agents effective specifically in the treatment of infectious diseases actually dates back to ancient China. Although the Chinese physicians who about 2500 years ago employed such materials as moldy soybean curd, soil and mud packs, and various plant derivatives did not recognize them as antibiotics, their antiinfectious properties were noted and used in the treatment of carbuncles and similar infections. It is interesting that many of the newer antibiotics were discovered in soil samples; no doubt the ancient physicians' mud packs also contained antibiotic-producing molds and bacteria.

Chemotherapy may be defined as the use of synthetic, semisynthetic, and naturally occurring chemicals that selectively inhibit specific organisms causing infectious diseases or that exhibit effectiveness in the treatment of cancer. Thus, any chemical that can be used in the control of infections or neoplasms can be considered a chemotherapeutic agent. The term *antibiotic* literally means "against life" (from the Greek *anti*, against, and *biosis*, life) and may be defined as a substance produced by microbes, or a semisynthetic derivative of a naturally occurring substance, that inhibits the growth or causes the death of other microbes. However, some antibiotics are used solely in the treatment of neoplastic disease rather than microbial infections, and a number of synthetic agents, generally not classified as antibiotics, are highly effective antimicrobial drugs. Since distinctions between chemotherapeutic agents based on their origin make little pharmacologic sense and are also becoming outmoded by advances in pharmaceutical chemistry, the terms *antibiotics* and *antimicrobial agents* will be used here interchangeably.

The modern era of specific chemotherapy for microbial diseases began with the introduction of the sulfonamides into medicine in the middle 1930s. In 1932, Domagk[11,12] discovered that prontosil, an azo dye containing a sulfonamide moiety, possessed antibacterial properties when injected into mice with streptococcal infections. Shortly thereafter, it was established that the sulfanilamide portion of the molecule, which was released in vivo by cleavage of the azo bond of prontosil, was responsible for the antibacterial action of the dye.[17,42] By 1936, the clinical effectiveness of sulfanilamide had been established. The "golden age" of antimicrobial therapy began with the first clinical use of penicillin in 1941. Although Fleming had discovered this substance in 1929, the techniques for production of sufficient quantities for widespread clinical use did not become available until 12 years later, when the deep fermentation process for biosynthesis of penicillin was perfected.[5]

The therapeutic significance of these discoveries cannot be overemphasized. It is exemplified by the drastic reduction in infection and mortality through the use of sulfonamides early in World War II and the use of penicillin toward the end of the war. Diseases such as syphilis, gonorrhea, tuberculosis, pneumococcal pneumonia, typhoid fever, diphtheria, scarlet fever, and meningococcal meningitis have been successfully treated or eradicated with antibiotics. As newer chemotherapeutic drugs have been developed, an increasing number of diseases that were once debilitating or even fatal have become manageable, so that today almost every disease of bacterial etiology can be treated, with varying degrees of success, with antimicrobial agents.

During the past 40 years, a large number of antibiotics have been developed, and approximately 70 are currently employed therapeutically. The development of new antibiotics is in part necessitated by the increasing incidence of acquired bacterial resistance. Because of widespread and often indiscriminate use of penicillin G, particularly in the early days of its history, microorganisms that were initially sensitive to penicillin are no longer affected by the drug. Although newer antibiotics have proved effective against some of these resistant microorganisms, they are also often more toxic to the host. At present, the development and therapeutic application of new antibiotics is barely keeping pace with the growing problem of bacterial resistance.

PRINCIPLES OF EFFECTIVE CHEMOTHERAPY

Chemical agents must possess certain properties if they are to be effective as chemotherapeutic drugs, and the way they are used depends on their mechanisms of action. These properties of antimicrobial agents will be explored in this section.

Selective toxicity

Selective toxicity is an essential property of chemotherapeutic agents. The fundamental concept of selective toxicity is that these agents must be toxic, or preferably lethal, to the invading microorganisms but have no effect on host cells. Many of the antibiotics discovered in recent years have been quickly discarded because they have not exhibited sufficient selectivity; those in current use show varying degrees of selective toxicity.

The extent to which antibiotics are selectively toxic is determined primarily by their mechanism of action. Selective toxicity is achieved in two major ways: (1) the antibiotic blocks a reaction that is vital to the invading microorganism but not to the host or (2) the antibiotic blocks a reaction that is vital to both the host and the microbe, but because of differences in the pathways involved, the effects are exerted predominantly on the microbial cells. The first mechanism is exemplified by antibiotics that block a reaction occurring only in the microorganism, such as synthesis of cell wall material. Penicillin and several other antibiotics inhibit cell wall synthesis at specific stages in the overall process. This action is specific for bacteria and does not apply to fungi, viruses, or protozoal parasites. Other antimicrobial drugs achieve maximum se-

lective toxicity by altering the formation of a product that may be used by both the host and the invading microorganisms but is acquired through different mechanisms. For example, the sulfonamides inhibit the synthesis of folic acid, which, after reduction to tetrahydrofolic acid, serves as a coenzyme in intermediary metabolism. The coenzyme is vital to both host and microbial cells, but the method of obtaining the product is different. Mammalian cells use preformed folic acid, which is obtained from the diet or as a by-product from the normal intestinal flora, whereas microorganisms susceptible to sulfonamides lack an enzyme that allows passage of folic acid across their cell membranes and must therefore synthesize folic acid. Obviously, bacteria that have the ability to use preformed folic acid are resistant to the effects of sulfonamides.[52]

A lesser degree of selective toxicity is achieved when the chemotherapeutic agent blocks a reaction that is vital to both the host and the microbe or parasite. Such a reaction is protein synthesis, but subtle differences in the number and structure of ribosomes between microbial and mammalian cells provide an accessible point of inhibition for antibiotics. Structural differences in bacterial ribosomes result in a greater affinity of these organelles for antibiotics than is exhibited by mammalian ribosomes.[44] In addition, protein synthesis in microbial cells occurs at a much faster rate than in the more slowly dividing mammalian cells. Therefore, concentrations and exposure times of antibiotics that are insufficient to significantly affect protein synthesis in mammalian cells can have profound effects on bacterial protein synthesis.

Another means of achieving selective toxicity through subtle differences between microbial and mammalian cells is illustrated by trimethoprim. Trimethoprim inhibits dihydrofolate reductase, the enzyme that catalyzes the conversion of dihydrofolic acid to the active coenzyme tetrahydrofolic acid. The dihydrofolate reductase of bacterial origin has 40,000 times the affinity for trimethoprim as does the mammalian liver enzyme,[16] so concentrations of trimethoprim that effectively inhibit bacterial coenzyme synthesis do not affect mammalian cells. In all cases in which the chemotherapeutic agent blocks a reaction vital to both the host and the microorganism, the in vivo concentration of antibiotic becomes an important factor in determining its selective toxicity.

In summary, effective chemotherapy is based on

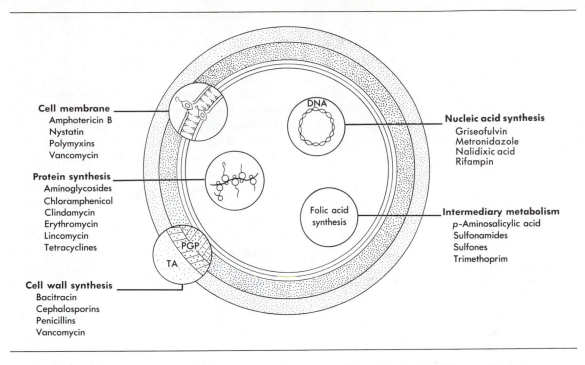

Cell membrane
Amphotericin B
Nystatin
Polymyxins
Vancomycin

Protein synthesis
Aminoglycosides
Chloramphenicol
Clindamycin
Erythromycin
Lincomycin
Tetracyclines

Cell wall synthesis
Bacitracin
Cephalosporins
Penicillins
Vancomycin

DNA

Nucleic acid synthesis
Griseofulvin
Metronidazole
Nalidixic acid
Rifampin

Folic acid
synthesis

Intermediary metabolism
p-Aminosalicylic acid
Sulfonamides
Sulfones
Trimethoprim

PGP

TA

Figure 36-1. Site and mechanism of action of antimicrobial agents. TA = teichoic acid; PGP = peptidoglycan polymer.

selective toxicity, which can be achieved to varying degrees, provided that the affected biochemical processes differ sufficiently between mammalian cells and microbial or parasite cells. When the cellular processes are basically similar, it is difficult to attain an effective degree of selective toxicity. This problem is encountered with the chemotherapeutic agents used in the treatment of neoplastic disease. Because the basic processes of normal and neoplastic cells lack any significant differences, there is no specific process that can be selectively affected in the cancer cell. A small degree of selective toxicity is achieved on the basis of the more rapid growth (division) of the cancer cells. Most antineoplastic drugs affect DNA replication or transcription, which occurs at a higher rate in cancer cells than in normal cells. Therefore, toxic effects are most pronounced in the rapidly growing neoplastic cells. They are also prominent in normal cells that exhibit a high rate of mitosis (e.g., gastrointestinal mucosal and bone marrow cells).

Mechanism of action of antimicrobial drugs

Antibiotics are frequently classified according to their mechanism of action, as shown in Figure 36-1. Antibacterial and antifungal antibiotics may act as antimetabolites, inhibitors of cell wall synthesis, inhibitors of protein synthesis, agents affecting cell membranes, and inhibitors of nucleic acid synthesis. Enzymatic reactions within the bacterial cell are a major target; however, binding to ribosomes and physical and chemical alterations of microbial cell components also are involved. The following discussion is applicable to agents affecting true bacteria, chlamydiae, rickettsiae, mycoplasma, and fungi. Chemotherapy for viral infections is discussed in Chapter 38, and neoplastic agents are presented in Chapter 40.

Antimetabolites. An antimetabolite may be defined as a false substrate. Because of its structural similarity to the normal substrate, it competes with this substrate for binding to a specific enzyme involved in a given metabolic pathway. The false substrate–enzyme complex is nonfunctional in producing the end product, and the metabolic pathway is inhibited at that point. As a group, the sulfonamides serve as a prototype of those agents that act as antimetabolites. PAS, an antituberculosis agent, and the sulfones, agents used in the treatment of leprosy, act in a similar manner. Also, several agents used in cancer chemotherapy (e.g., methotrexate) are antimetabolites.

Specifically, the sulfonamides inhibit the syn-

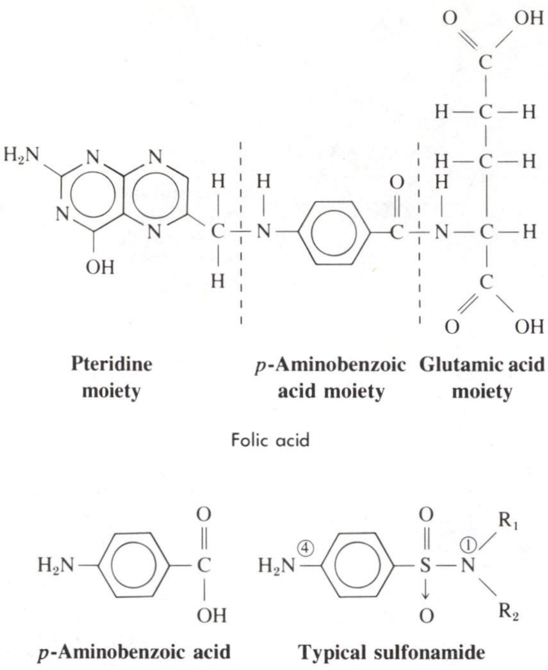

Figure 36-2. Structural formulas of folic acid, a sulfonamide, and *p*-aminobenzoic acid.

thesis of folic acid within the bacterial cell. Folic acid is synthesized from precursor molecules—a pteridine nucleus, *p*-aminobenzoic acid (PABA), and glutamic acid (Figure 36-2). The first step in this synthetic pathway is the covalent bonding of PABA to the pteridine moiety, a reaction that is catalyzed by dihydropteroate synthetase. The structural resemblance between the sulfonamides and PABA results in competition between these two substances for binding to this enzyme. Generally, the sulfonamide–dihydropteroate synthetase complex is inactive, and folic acid is not synthesized. However, in some bacteria a sulfonamide-containing analogue of dihydropteroic acid is synthesized and may exhibit inhibitory effects.[4] In either case, the bacterial cell is deprived of folic acid. Since the binding of the sulfonamide to this enzyme is reversible and follows the law of mass action, excessive amounts of PABA, such as occur in infected tissue exudates (pus), may antagonize the antibacterial effects of the sulfonamides. Similarly, substances that are biotransformed to PABA, such as some ester-type local anesthetics, can antagonize the sulfonamides.

Inhibitors of cell wall synthesis. Several antibiotics exert their effects by inhibition of cell wall synthesis. These agents are effective only during that phase in the bacterial cell cycle in which new cell wall material is being produced; they exhibit maximum selective toxicity because mammalian cells do not possess cell walls. Those antibiotics that affect cell wall formation act at specific points in the synthetic pathway (Table 36-1).[1,38]

The result of interference with cell wall synthesis is a bacterium with a defective cell wall. The intracellular osmolarity of an actively metabolizing bacterial cell is highly hypertonic with respect to mammalian body fluids. This high osmotic content within bacterial cells in contact with body fluids will result in the diffusion of water into the cell. Normally, bacterial cells can withstand very high internal pressures; gram-positive cocci, for instance, can sustain internal pressures as high as 20 atmospheres.[35] But if the wall has been damaged by an antibiotic, the movement of water into the cell will be followed by swelling, extrusion of the cellular contents through weak areas of the wall, and lysis.

If bacteria with damaged cell walls are grown or placed in media that are isotonic to the bacteria (highly hypertonic in comparison with mammalian body fluids), they survive in the form of spheroblasts or protoplasts rather than undergoing lysis. Ultimate destruction of the bacterial cells resulting from the action of inhibitors of cell wall synthesis, then, is dependent on two requirements: the bacterial cells must be growing (i.e., synthesizing new cell wall material), and there must be an osmotic difference between the bacterial cytoplasm and the extracellular milieu.[51] Concomitant administration of an agent that blocks bacterial metabolism and growth, such as an inhibitor of protein synthesis, will negate the first requirement and render the cell wall inhibitor ineffective. (Antagonisms between bacteriostatic and bactericidal antibiotics are explored further in the section on combinations of antibiotics.) In reference to the second requirement, bacteria present in an environment that is unusually hypertonic, such as that of the renal medulla, may not undergo lysis in the presence of an antibiotic that interferes with cell wall synthesis. In such cases, the action of the antibiotic may cease at spheroblast formation, and if the spheroblasts are not removed by host defense mechanisms, they may revert to the original form of the bacteria fol-

Table 36-1. Stages in bacterial cell wall synthesis and sites of action of antimicrobial agents

Stage and site of action	Process inhibited	Antimicrobial agent
Stage I (cytoplasm)	Synthesis of cell wall subunits	Cycloserine
	↓	
Stage II (cell membrane)	Linear polymerization of subunits	Ristocetin, bacitracin, vancomycin
	↓	
Stage III (cell wall)	Cross-linking of polymers	Penicillins, cephalosporins

lowing antibiotic withdrawal, and the infection may recur.

Inhibitors of protein synthesis. A number of commonly used antibiotics act as inhibitors of protein synthesis by binding to a bacterial ribosome. The bacterial ribosome has a sedimentation coefficient of 70 Svedberg units (S) and may be dissociated into a 30 S and a 50 S subunit, to each of which various antibiotics that inhibit protein synthesis preferentially bind. The process of translation in bacteria is divided into three phases: (1) formation of an initiation complex, (2) peptide chain elongation, and (3) termination and release of the newly synthesized protein.[24] The aminoglycosides (e.g., streptomycin and neomycin) bind to a ribosomal protein present in the 30 S subunit of the bacterial ribosome,[31] resulting in a distortion of ribosomal conformation that inhibits protein synthesis at the first phase.[25] Although this effect normally occurs in vivo with therapeutic doses, lower concentrations of aminoglycosides may not totally inhibit protein synthesis but lead to a misreading of the genetic code.[9] In this case, defective proteins are formed that are nonfunctional biochemically. In either case, the result is the same—deprivation of proteins necessary for cell growth and survival.

Chloramphenicol, erythromycin, lincomycin, and clindamycin bind to the 50 S subunit of the bacterial ribosome and inhibit growth of the amino acid chain by acting at specific steps in the process of peptide chain elongation. Chloramphenicol, lincomycin, and clindamycin specifically inhibit peptide bond formation, whereas erythromycin inhibits a translocation reaction that is necessary for incorporation of new amino acids into the peptide chain.[48] Generally, antibiotics that prevent protein synthesis exhibit bacteriostatic activity, but the aminoglycosides and occasionally some of the other antibiotics are bactericidal at concentrations that can be achieved clinically.

Agents affecting cell membranes. An intact cell membrane performs a number of functions that maintain the internal environment of the cell in a state conducive to life and growth. Disruption of the cell membrane or alteration of membrane permeability leads to inhibition of growth or even death of the cell. The polymyxins are polypeptide antibiotics containing both lipophobic and lipophilic groups. They interact with phospholipid components of the cell membrane, thus distorting membrane structure.[34] The cell membrane no longer functions as an osmotic barrier, and cellular contents, such as nucleosides, metabolites, ions, and proteins, escape from the cell. Depending on the severity of the damage, these antibiotics may inhibit the growth of the bacterial cell or cause cell death, usually the latter.

Nystatin and amphotericin B are polyene antibiotics that exhibit antifungal activity. They combine with sterols present in the fungal cell membrane and produce permeability changes that result in inhibition of growth and sometimes in death of the fungal cell.[49] Because bacterial cell membranes do not contain this sterol moiety, the action of these agents is selective for fungi. Inasmuch as the polymyxin and polyene antibiotics act on cell membranes, their microbicidal effect is not totally dependent on cell growth, but they do appear to be more active against growing cells. This is in contrast to those agents that inhibit cell wall synthesis and absolutely require cell growth for activity.

Because differences between mammalian and microbial cell membranes are subtle, antibiotics affecting these structures exhibit a low order of selective toxicity and are potentially destructive to mammalian cells. The antifungal agents do exhibit some selective toxicity, because the sterol/phospholipid ratios are different in mammalian and fungal cells. Nevertheless, all of these agents cause a number of serious side effects (some of which are probably unrelated to their action on cell membranes) that preclude their systemic use in all but those serious infections that are refractory to less toxic antibiotics.

Inhibitors of nucleic acid synthesis. Rifampin, a bacteriostatic antibiotic used mainly in the treatment of tuberculosis, inhibits RNA synthesis by binding to the DNA-dependent RNA polymerase in microorganisms (but not in human cells).[23] Nalidixic acid, griseofulvin, metronidazole, and several antineoplastic drugs also act by inhibiting nucleic acid synthesis.[23,35]

Factors determining bactericidal activity

One factor that determines whether an antimicrobial agent will be bacteriostatic or bactericidal is the mechanism of action. Two additional important factors are the concentration of drug to which the bacteria are exposed and the type of microorganisms involved. The generalization can be made that a bactericidal antibiotic will exhibit only bacteriostatic activity at doses that provide less than the minimum lethal concentration (MLC) for a given microorganism. In contrast, increasing the dose of a chemotherapeutic agent that is characterized as bacteriostatic does not necessarily result in bactericidal activity; sulfonamides, for example, are always bacteriostatic, regardless of the concentration to which the microbes are exposed.

Because of differences in susceptibility to antibiotics, the type of microorganism involved in an infection may determine whether inhibition of cell growth or cell death will be the predominant clinical effect. Penicillin G at doses normally used in the treatment of gram-positive infections has little effect on many gram-negative organisms. However, with relatively huge intravenous doses of this antibiotic, bacteriostatic and even bactericidal activity against these microorganisms can be achieved. Some microorganisms that are highly susceptible to a bacteriostatic antibiotic may be killed in the presence of higher concentrations of the drug. In contrast, many other microorganisms may only be inhibited, even at the maximum concentrations of the antibiotic that can be achieved clinically.

The three factors discussed above—mechanism of action, concentration, and type of microorganism—all contribute to the final clinical effect obtained with a particular antibiotic in the treatment of a specific infection.

VARIABLES INFLUENCING THE EFFECTIVENESS OF ANTIMICROBIAL THERAPY

The success of antimicrobial therapy depends on a number of variables involving the host, the bacteria, and the drug. These factors are discussed below.

Diagnosis and choice of antibiotic

Clinical effectiveness in treating an infection is based on the correct diagnosis of the infecting microorganism (or microorganisms) and the choice of the most specific and effective chemotherapeutic drug. The most effective antibiotic cannot be selected without first determining the antibiotic susceptibility of the infecting organism. Ideally, bacteriologic assessment should be completed before treatment is started, but certain conditions may prevent this. Obviously, in an acutely ill patient treatment cannot be delayed for the 48 hours or more required for the results of bacteriologic tests. In this situation, the choice of antibiotic must be initially based on a knowledge of the usual causative microorganisms in a specific disease entity and the antibiotic to which these organisms are normally susceptible. This empirical approach usually results in clinical effectiveness. Although previous studies using aerobic culture techniques indicated that gram-positive aerobic microorganisms were major etiologic factors in dental infections, recent investigations using anaerobic techniques indicate that many dental infections (e.g., alveolar abscesses, infection in intact pulp chambers after traumatic injury, periodontal abscesses, advanced chronic periodontitis, periodontosis, Vincent's stomatitis) are associated with anaerobic microorganisms (mainly gram-negative anaerobes).* This is not a surprising finding since more than three fourths of the oral microflora is known to consist of anaerobes.[20,29,40] Obviously, in the treatment of an acute dental infection it would be reasonable to start with an antibiotic to which the probable organisms (gram-positive aerobes and intraoral anaerobes) are susceptible, namely a penicillin. But if it fails to be effective, another antibiotic must be chosen at a time when the refractory infection has been fulminating for 48 hours or more since the initiation of treatment. If samples had been obtained before the start of antibiotic therapy and then assessed

---

*References 14, 18, 20-21, 30, 32, 35, 43, and 50.

microbiologically, the choice of a second antibiotic (after failure of the first) would be relatively simple.

Bactericidal versus bacteriostatic antibiotics

Although either a bacteriostatic or a bactericidal antibiotic may be effective in treating an infection, there are four reasons why bactericidal agents are preferred. First, antibiotics do not eradicate an infection but cause a reduction in the number of viable organisms, either by inhibiting their proliferation or by producing cell death. The final eradication of the infection is the result of the powerful role played by the immune processes and the leukocytes and macrophages. Since bactericidal antibiotics effect a reduction in the number of microorganisms present rather than merely preventing an increase in their number, there is less reliance on host defense mechanisms when such an agent is employed. Therefore, a microbicidal drug is always chosen, if possible, for treating an infection in a patient with impaired host defense mechanisms.

Second, bactericidal agents are preferable because bacteriostatic agents may take longer to resolve the infection. Again, the clinical outcome of therapy is strongly influenced by the state of the host defense mechanisms.

Third, bactericidal antibiotics that affect cell wall synthesis produce irreversible damage to the cell walls of growing (dividing) microorganisms. Therapeutically, this means that bactericidal concentrations of the drug do not have to be maintained at all times during the treatment of an infection. Clinical effectiveness is obtained when penicillin V is given every 6 hours, even though most of the drug is excreted within 3 hours.[26] Those microorganisms that make new cell wall material in the presence of the penicillin, and therefore have damaged cell walls, will eventually undergo lysis whether or not penicillin continues to be present. This continued effect during penicillin-free periods provides the basis for the success of the 6-hour dosage interval, but it must be emphasized that effective concentrations must be achieved at the site of infection at least intermittently and then for an adequate length of time. In contrast, bacteriostatic agents that block protein synthesis must be given according to a schedule that maintains inhibitory levels throughout the entire course of treatment. If drug administration is interrupted so that the concentration of antibiotic falls below the minimum inhibitory concentration (MIC) for a given microorganism, sufficient bacteria may survive and multiply, resulting in recurrence of the infection. Also, since less susceptible strains of bacteria will be selected, the resulting relapse may prove considerably less responsive to the antibiotic. This problem is particularly evident when the duration of therapy is inadequate or when subinhibitory concentrations are obtained at the site of infection.

Finally, and this is a matter of paramount importance, with the usual short-term clinical treatment of most infections, antibiotic therapy, even with a bactericidal agent, does not result in death of all of the pathogens. Rather, clinical effectiveness is due to the final elimination of the infection by host defense processes. However, in the case of bacterial endocarditis and some other life-threatening infections, the object of clinical treatment is to kill *all* the pathogens, for otherwise a recurrence is inevitable.[35] Therefore, in the treatment of this disease, septicemia, or any serious infection in a patient with impaired host defense mechanisms, a bactericidal drug or combination of bactericidal drugs would be the agents of choice.

Specificity and spectrum of antibacterial activity

Chemotherapeutic agents are broadly categorized according to their spectrum of activity (Table 36-2). A narrow-spectrum antibiotic is one that is effective mainly against either gram-positive or gram-negative microorganisms but is not effective generally against both. Broad-spectrum antibiotics inhibit both gram-positive and gram-negative bacteria and frequently other microorganisms as well. The choice of an optimally effective antibiotic must be based on knowledge of the type of infecting microorganism. Although the susceptibility of a given pathogen may fall within the spectrum of activity of several antibiotics, the most effective and rational treatment will use the most specific narrow-spectrum antibiotic to which the microorganism is susceptible. There are two reasons for this: (1) narrow-spectrum antibiotics frequently are more effective against specific groups of susceptible microorganisms than are broad-spectrum agents, and (2) narrow-spectrum antibiotics produce less alteration of the normal microflora, there-

Table 36-2. Spectrum of antibacterial activity of certain antimicrobial agents

Narrow	Extended	Broad
Bacitracin	Aminoglycosides	Chloramphenicol
Clindamycin	Cephalosporins	Sulfonamides
Erythromycin	Extended-spectrum	Tetracyclines
Lincomycin	penicillins	Trimethoprim
Metronidazole		
Penicillin G, V		
Penicillinase-		
resistant		
penicillins		
Polymyxins		
Vancomycin		

by reducing the incidence of superinfection. As has been pointed out, the normal microflora of the oral cavity and the bacteria that cause most dental infections are gram-positive aerobes and gram-positive and gram-negative anaerobes. These bacteria are generally susceptible to penicillin V, an agent that does not disturb the normally gram-negative flora of the lower gastrointestinal tract. Ampicillin, which has a somewhat more extended spectrum of efficacy than penicillin V, causes unnecessary alterations in the flora of the gastrointestinal tract that may result in serious fungal or bacterial superinfections refractory to this and possibly other antibiotics. However, in a dental infection involving a mixed bacterial population, both gram-positive and gram-negative bacteria as well as spirochetes, ampicillin may be the drug of choice.[13,36]

Concentration of antibiotic at site of infection

To be effective, an antibiotic must reach the site of infection in amounts above the MLC or MIC for the infecting microorganisms. A number of factors influence the concentration of antibiotic achieved at the site of infection.

Route and time of administration. The route and time of administration are major factors in determining ultimate concentration at the site of the infection. With few exceptions, the absorption of antibiotics given orally is decreased in the presence of food. Some antibiotics are acid-unstable (e.g., penicillin G), and inactivation of such a drug will occur if it is taken at a time when gastric acid secretion is high, that is, just before and after meals. Therefore, in general, antibiotics should be taken no sooner than 1 hour before or at least 2

hours after a meal. Unless there is strict patient compliance, absorption of the drug may be erratic, and therapeutic failure may result. In addition, disease states or interactions with other orally administered drugs can decrease the enteral absorption of some antibiotics. For example, the absorption of the tetracycline antibiotics is decreased by milk, by antacids containing Ca^{++}, Mg^{++}, or Al^{+++}, and by medications containing iron salts. Finally, if predictable and high systemic concentrations of an antibiotic are required, it should be administered parenterally.

Dose, dosage schedule, and duration of therapy. Improper dosing may take three forms: inadequate dosage leading to ineffective concentration of antibiotic at the site of infection, inadequate duration of therapy, and excessive dosage, which may result in toxic effects in the host. Many cases of failure in antibiotic therapy are the result of the first two. Inadequate concentration of antibiotic encourages the development of resistant infections, as described in the section on bacterial resistance. Similarly, inadequate duration of therapy encourages recurrence of infections and also the development of resistant strains. Overdosage with antibiotics is a source of a variety of toxic side effects. This is not a severe problem with relatively nontoxic agents such as penicillin G, but it may be of great importance with relatively toxic drugs such as the aminoglycosides and chloramphenicol. In some instances, the dosages of antimicrobial drugs must be adjusted downward because of alterations in hepatic or renal function that could affect the biotransformation or excretion of the drug.

An understanding of the pharmacokinetics of antibiotics has provided the necessary information for scheduling doses so as to obtain consistent in vivo therapeutic concentrations of drug. For many antibiotics, oral doses repeated at 6-hour intervals maintain effective concentrations. Other antibiotics that are highly bound to serum proteins (this reversible binding site acting as a drug reservoir in equilibrium with the free drug concentrations) or that are slowly excreted have a longer half-life and require less frequent administration. Examples are amoxicillin, which is administered at 8-hour intervals, and doxycycline, which is given once or twice daily.

Inadequate duration of therapy is a frequent cause of failure of chemotherapy. The rule of thumb is that antibiotic coverage should last for at least 48 hours after complete remission of clinical symptoms. The duration varies with the type of infection, the status of the patient's defense mechanisms, and several other factors. Some infections require only a few days for clinical remission, whereas other infections, such as endocarditis, require several weeks of antibiotic therapy. Treatment of the usual oral infections of bacterial origin requires an average of 5 to 7 days of antibiotic therapy; treatment of severe oral infections or infections in patients with lowered resistance may take longer.

Patient compliance. Clinicians must be aware of problems involving patient compliance. A patient may decide not to have a prescription filled, particularly if it is very expensive. The importance of taking the drug exactly as prescribed is not always understood. Doses may be missed, particularly when clinical symptoms of the infection begin to subside, and a patient may choose to discontinue therapy as soon as overt symptoms are absent. Another common reason for discontinuing a course of drug therapy is the occurrence of unpleasant, although possibly innocuous, side effects. In any case, premature termination of drug therapy will favor selection of microorganisms that are more resistant, or only marginally susceptible, to the drug. These first- and second-step mutants, with less susceptibility to the antibiotic, can flourish and cause a recurrence of the infection. Particularly with bacteriostatic agents, patient compliance is a requisite for a successful clinical outcome.

Distribution of antibiotic in the body. The active antibiotic must be distributed to the site of infection in antibacterial concentrations if therapy is to be successful. Chemotherapeutic drugs differ in their ability to penetrate certain body compartments, and this difference must be considered when an antimicrobial agent is chosen. For infections of the central nervous system, such as meningitis, the antibiotic must be able to penetrate the blood-brain barrier and enter the cerebrospinal fluid in adequate concentrations. Infections in areas with relatively poor blood supply, as would be characteristic of well-established abscesses, necrotic areas, and infections of the inner ear and sinuses, are difficult to treat because less antibiotic is distributed to these areas. Most antibiotics exhibit good distribution in soft tissue, as is involved with oral infections. However, penetration into bone constitutes another problem. A few antibiotics (e.g., lincomycin and clindamycin) exhibit such excellent penetration into bone that bone concentrations may even exceed plasma concentrations.[7] These antibiotics would be excellent choices for the treatment of dental infections were it not for their potentially serious side effects. Other agents, such as the tetracyclines, form complexes with bone and are therefore inactive at these sites.[15]

Metabolism and excretion of antibiotics. The time during which an antibiotic is present in effective concentrations at the site of infection depends on the rate of inactivation of the drug through metabolism or excretion, or both. Based on the normal rate of biotransformation and excretion, the dose is repeated at specific intervals so that antibacterial blood concentrations are maintained. Thus, the effectiveness of antibiotic therapy may be altered if the mechanisms for metabolism or excretion are altered. These same mechanisms determine, to a large extent, the toxic effects of many of the antimicrobial drugs. An antibiotic that is excreted mainly by the kidney may be contraindicated in the presence of renal failure, or at least require a reduction in dosage, since the drug may accumulate to toxic systemic concentrations. Similarly, an antibiotic that is inactivated mainly in the liver would be contraindicated in patients with severe hepatic dysfunction. The penicillins, cephalosporins, aminoglycosides, and polymyxins are excreted mainly via the kidney; other antibiotics undergo varying degrees of biotransformation in the liver.

Dosage formulation and quality control. Therapeutic failure with antibiotics will result if the active ingredient has become degraded, if the solid oral dosage form does not dissolve in the gastrointestinal tract, if the active ingredient is not present in the amount stated, or if a number of other inadequacies exist that are directly related to the pharmaceutical manufacturer's level of quality control. Even among drugs manufactured by reputable pharmaceutical companies, there are some differences in bioavailability that can be significant. The recent requirement by the FDA that bioavailability data be provided for drug formulations has minimized many earlier problems of variable absorption associated with some pharmaceutical products.[10]

Age, type, and extent of infection

The length of time an infection has been present plays a significant part in determining the effectiveness of antibiotic therapy. Bactericidal antibiotics require multiplying cells in order to be effective; bacteriostatic agents will not show any activity against a culture that is quiescent. Older, well-established infections grow slowly, and thus both bactericidal and bacteriostatic antibiotics are less effective than they would be in new infections. Abscesses frequently present such a problem when the infection is contained by the body's defense mechanisms and the bacteria multiply at an extremely slow rate.[51]

The larger the size or extent of the infection, the less effective the antibiotic therapy will be, because the increased number of bacteria generally requires that a higher concentration of antibiotic be present at the site of infection. This relationship emphasizes the importance of treating an infection as quickly as possible, since a smaller number of bacteria are present in its early stages, and antibiotic therapy will usually be more effective.

Antibiotics by themselves cannot be relied on to eradicate some infections. Appreciable quantities of pus, necrotic tissue, a foreign body mechanical obstruction, and abscessed areas that are relatively avascular require prompt surgical management in addition to adequate doses of antimicrobial agents. Periodontal and periapical abscesses and most other oral infections require surgical intervention as well.

Host factors of antibiotic effectiveness

A number of host-related factors alter the effectiveness of antibiotic therapy. The pathophysiologic state of the host, the status of the host defense system, age, alterations in biotransformation and excretion of drugs, pregnancy, susceptibility to allergic responses, and genetic factors are all determinants of the host response to antibiotic therapy.[46] Several of these will be discussed.

Host defense mechanisms. It has already been pointed out that antibiotics, whether bactericidal or bacteriostatic, do not by themselves eradicate infection. By decreasing or preventing an increase in the number of viable microorganisms, they allow normal phagocytosis to keep up with the reduced rate of bacterial multiplication and remove the infecting microorganisms.

Impairment of host defense mechanisms may occur as a result of disease (leukemia, agranulocytosis, diabetes mellitus, Addison's disease, certain immune deficiency states, leukopenia) or therapy with drugs that suppress the immune mechanisms (adrenal corticosteroids, antineoplastic drugs). For patients with impaired host defense mechanisms, prophylactic use of antibiotics may be necessary for dental or other procedures that cause bactere-

mia. Obviously, a bactericidal antibiotic should be used in these circumstances.

Age. Age has a significant effect on the rate of elimination of antimicrobial drugs and is therefore a factor in both the effectiveness and toxicity of these drugs. In infants under 1 year of age, the processes for drug biotransformation and complete renal function are not fully developed. Unless the antibiotic dose is reduced, toxic amounts of the drug accumulate and result in a number of untoward effects, such as the "gray syndrome," which is associated with the use of chloramphenicol in neonates.[33] Other adverse effects of antibiotics that are unique to the young patient are kernicterus, resulting from the displacement of bilirubin from its binding sites on albumin by the sulfonamides, and the enamel hypoplasia and discoloration of the dentition produced by the tetracyclines during tooth development (last half of pregnancy through 8 years of age). The elderly patient may also react differently to antibiotics. Because of disease states or the normal process of aging, the rates of glomerular filtration and of metabolic inactivation of drugs are decreased in many patients above the age of 50. Such patients may require lower doses of those antibiotics that exhibit toxic effects at high systemic concentrations, such as the aminoglycosides. The effectiveness of antibiotic therapy may also be altered because of age-related changes in host defense processes.

Pregnancy. The use of drugs during pregnancy is associated with varying degrees of risk, antimicrobial agents being no exception. The clinician must consider carefully the benefit to risk ratio when antibiotics are indicated for the pregnant patient. Streptomycin has been associated with damage to the eighth cranial nerve and with skeletal defects in the fetus; tetracyclines used during the last half of pregnancy cause hypoplasia of teeth and bones of the fetus and have been associated with the occurrence of congenital cataracts.[39] Several other antibiotics that cross the placenta are contraindicated when the mother is close to term, and these include the sulfonamides and chloramphenicol for the reasons described earlier. Finally, some antibiotics are secreted into milk and may present problems for the nursing infant.[2]

Susceptibility to allergic responses. Patients with a history of allergy have a greater than normal probability of exhibiting an allergic reaction to antimicrobial drugs, particularly drugs with a high allergenic potential. Therefore, a history of aller-

Table 36-3. Classification of antimicrobial drugs as bactericidal or bacteriostatic

Bactericidal	Bacteriostatic
Penicillins	Erythromycin
Cephalosporins	Tetracyclines
Vancomycin	Sulfonamides
Aminoglycosides	Chloramphenicol
Bacitracin	Clindamycin
Polymyxins	Lincomycin
Metronidazole	Trimethoprim

gies to such things as foods, pollen, and drugs should alert the clinician to the possibility of an allergic reaction to antibiotics.

THERAPY WITH COMBINATIONS OF ANTIMICROBIAL DRUGS

The rationale for the use of two or more antimicrobial drugs together is to minimize the emergence of antibiotic-resistant microorganisms and to increase the certainty of a successful clinical outcome. Although this approach may seem rational, there are relatively few infections for which combined therapy is indicated. Furthermore, certain combinations of antibiotics can result in antagonism. The antimicrobial agents may be divided into two major groups as shown in Table 36-3.[19] Group I includes bactericidal drugs such as the penicillins and aminoglycosides. Group II antibiotics are bacteriostatic and include chloramphenicol and the tetracyclines.

Combinations of antibiotics within group I generally exhibit additive or synergistic bactericidal activity. Combinations of antibiotics within group II may show additive bacteriostatic effects but never true synergism. The combination of an antibiotic from group I with one from group II often results in antagonism (loss of group I drug's effect) for reasons that were described earlier.

There are only a few infections for which combined antibiotic therapy has been shown to be more effective than treatment with a single drug. Several examples of such combinations, and the diseases for which they have proved useful, include (1) the use of two drugs (isoniazid and rifampin or ethambutol) in the treatment of initial, uncomplicated tuberculosis, (2) the use of carbenicillin and gentamicin for septicemia or pneumonia caused by *Pseudomonas aeruginosa,* (3) the combination of clindamycin or an extended-spectrum penicillin

such as ticarcillin with an aminoglycoside for mixed infections (e.g., sepsis caused by intestinal perforation), (4) the combination of penicillin G and streptomycin for endocarditis caused by *Streptococcus faecalis,* (5) tetracycline and streptomycin for treatment of brucellosis, and (6) chloramphenicol plus streptomycin or gentamicin for the treatment of pneumonia caused by *Klebsiella pneumoniae.*[33,35,41] With one exception, combinations of antibiotics are not used in the dental office. The exception is the prophylactic use of a penicillin plus an aminoglycoside before dental procedures in patients at high risk of developing bacterial endocarditis (such as those with valve prostheses). In all other cases, dental infections are most effectively treated by using the most specific and effective antibiotic to which the infecting microorganisms have been shown, by appropriate tests, to be susceptible.

BACTERIAL RESISTANCE

Bacterial resistance occurs as a result of stable alterations in the genetic composition of the bacterial cell; that is, the alterations are transferable from generation to generation. There are two major types of bacterial resistance—natural resistance and acquired resistance. Natural resistance simply means that some bacterial species are not susceptible to a given antibiotic; for example, many gram-negative microorganisms have always been naturally resistant to penicillin G. Natural resistance is that form of resistance that existed before antibiotic therapy. Acquired resistance occurs as a consequence of antibiotic therapy and is the result of the selection of resistant organisms. In many cases, these resistant mutants were present before antibiotic therapy; in other cases, a resistant strain of bacteria has emerged from the environment. Antibiotic therapy does not cause the development of resistance but merely exerts a genetic selection pressure, inhibiting or killing the more susceptible microorganisms and allowing the less susceptible to grow. In hospital environments or in communities where there is widespread use of antibiotics, the resistant forms become the predominant bacterial strains in that environment. Although the existence of natural or acquired resistance results in failure of chemotherapy, acquired resistance is more important clinically because it is not necessarily suspected at the beginning of antibiotic therapy and becomes a problem only during the course of treatment. In practice, the line of distinction between these two kinds of resistance may be slight, since some bacterial species may acquire such uniform resistance to an antibiotic that they may be automatically considered to be naturally resistant to an antibiotic (e.g., strains of *Staphylococcus aureus* resistant to penicillin G or V).

Because bacterial resistance occurs as the result of genetic alterations of the bacterial cell, any of the processes by which genetic composition of bacteria is altered may be involved. In bacteria, such alterations occur by spontaneous chromosomal mutation, transformation, transduction, and conjugation.

Chromosomal resistance

Resistance resulting from spontaneous changes in the bacterial chromosome is called chromosomal resistance and normally occurs in a stepwise fashion. Full phenotypic expression of resistance usually requires multiple genetic alterations, each additional genetic change resulting in a greater degree of resistance to the antimicrobial agent. The antibiotic acts to select each increasingly resistant mutant, allowing it to multiply and exhibit more mutational changes in its progeny. Ultimately, a highly resistant form is developed that predominates during drug exposure. Low concentrations of antibiotics at the site of infection favor this selection process, but higher concentrations may inhibit the still susceptible first- and second-step mutants before they can grow and produce progeny containing additional mutations. Whether this process occurs rapidly or slowly is dependent on the kind of antibiotic being used. Resistance to the penicillins occurs in a slow, stepwise manner, whereas resistance to erythromycin occurs rapidly, with only a few steps or spontaneous mutations being required for exhibition of a high order of resistance. With streptomycin, resistance can develop in a single step.

For most microorganisms, spontaneous or random mutation occurs at the rate of one gene mutation per 10^5 to 10^9 cell divisions. Although this might appear to be a low rate of mutation, the rapidity of bacterial growth is such that spontaneous mutants resistant to one or more antibiotics may easily be present in a bacterial population otherwise susceptible to the antibiotic. Normally, the growth of these few mutants is suppressed by the large number of "normal" bacterial cells. However, when an antibiotic is given, the normal bacteria are inhibited or killed, and the resistant mutant bacteria can then multiply and become the predominant strains causing the infection.

Infective drug resistance

Until several years ago, the major problems of bacterial resistance encountered in hospitals were associated with penicillin G–resistant strains of staphylococci. Recently, however, gram-negative septicemias have become the major clinical problem of infection in hospital environments.[37] Strains of these microorganisms have been isolated that exhibit resistance to four or more different groups of antibiotics. Multiple antibiotic resistance is believed to occur by the passage of genetic material, coding for resistance to one or more antimicrobial drugs, from one bacterial cell into another, thus, the term *infective drug resistance*. Four mechanisms are involved in infective drug resistance. Conjugation is the transfer of genetic material between two mating cells through a conjugation bridge. Transformation is the uptake of fragments of DNA liberated from ruptured cells and incorporated into the recipient cell's chromosome at a region with a similar base sequence. Transduction is the transfer of genetic material between cells by means of infecting the bacterial cell with bacteriophages that contain within their coat fragments of DNA from other bacterial cells. Finally, transposition refers to the incorporation of DNA in the form of transposons, genetic determinants that create their own sites of insertion without the need for homology between the donor and recipient DNA.

Of these mechanisms, conjugation has the greatest clinical significance. In conjugation, the genetic material transferred is an extrachromosomal, self-replicating segment of DNA that is similar to other bacterial plasmids or episomes and is known as a resistance (R) factor. R factors can replicate independently of the chromosomal DNA, and they contain a variable number of genetic markers or codes for drug resistance. Another unit of DNA, the resistance transfer (RT) factor, exists in combination with the R factor and is responsible for the transfer of R factors between the bacterial cells during conjugation.[33] Of major clinical significance is the fact that R factors can code for high levels of resistance to multiple drugs, that they can be transferred from nonpathogenic to pathogenic microorganisms, and that through conjugation multiple drug resistance can be acquired by formerly

Table 36-4. Mechanisms involved in the development of resistance to certain antimicrobial agents

Drug	Mechanism
Penicillins	β-Lactamase production (penicillinase)
Cephalosporins	β-Lactamase production (cephalosporinase)
Tetracyclines	Decreased uptake; active elimination
Aminoglycosides	Phosphorylation; adenylation; acetylation; decreased uptake; decreased binding to bacterial ribosome
Sulfonamides	Increased production of *p*-aminobenzoic acid; resistant dihydropteroate synthetase
Chloramphenicol	Acetylation
Erythromycin, lincomycin, and clindamycin	Decreased binding to bacterial ribosome

susceptible microorganisms in a single event.

The transfer of resistance to antimicrobial agents during conjugation appears to be confined to gram-negative bacteria.[26,33,35] It should be noted, though, that R factor transfer can occur between different groups of bacteria, (e.g., between *Shigella* and *Escherichia coli*). There are an increasing number of reports from around the world of infections caused by bacteria resistant to many antimicrobial agents. In fact, resistance exists to so many of the commonly used antibiotics that difficulty is sometimes encountered in finding an agent that will be effective in treating a given infection.

The mechanism by which bacteria become resistant to the antimicrobial agents often involves the synthesis of enzymes (the code for which is in the R factor) that inactivate the antibiotic or involves alterations in the permeability of the bacterial cell to antimicrobial drugs.[28] Several examples of these mechanisms and the antibiotics frequently affected are listed in Table 36-4. With enzymes that inactivate the antibiotics, the degree of resistance increases as a function of the microbial population (i.e., more bacteria can produce more enzyme).

The problem of bacterial resistance is far-reaching in that development of resistance to one antibiotic frequently results in cross-resistance to all other drugs within that group. For example, all clinical isolates of penicillin G–resistant strains of *Staphylococcus aureus* produce penicillinase, an enzyme that inactivates penicillin G. This enzyme also inactivates all the other penicillin derivatives, except those few that have been designed to be penicillinase-resistant, (e.g., methicillin and oxacillin). Recently, isolates of staphylococcal infections have exhibited resistance even to the methi-cillin-type penicillins, and cross-resistance frequently exists for several other commonly used antibiotics.

The development of bacterial resistance may be minimized by (1) using antibiotics only when there is a well-established need for such therapy, (2) selecting antibiotics on the basis of bacterial susceptibility tests, (3) administering antibiotics systemically instead of topically, and (4) using adequate concentrations (doses) of the antibiotic for an adequate duration to prevent the growth of first- and second-step mutants. With some bacteria (e.g., *Mycobacterium tuberculosis*), multiple drug therapy is also necessary to minimize the emergence of resistant strains.

ADVERSE EFFECTS OF ANTIMICROBIAL DRUGS

Soon after the development of the sulfonamides and penicillin G it became clear that the antimicrobial agents, like any other drug, could produce a variety of untoward responses as well as superinfection, an effect uniquely associated with antimicrobial therapy. Adverse reactions produced by these agents range from mild to severe and even fatal. They can be divided into three groups: direct toxicities, indirect toxicities, and consequences of disturbances in host microflora.[47]

Direct toxicity

Direct toxicity of antimicrobial agents derives from the innate ability of certain antimicrobial agents directly to affect the cellular processes of the host. Although all antimicrobial drugs possess some toxic potential, the frequency and severity of such reactions vary considerably with the drug, its concentration achieved at target and nontarget sites, and the individual receiving the drug. Toxic reactions may be extremely mild, such as the local discomfort occurring with the intramuscular injection of the penicillins, or they may be more severe, such as the ototoxicity and nephrotoxicity associated with the aminoglycoside antibiotics. Generally, the direct toxicities of antibiotics involve the gastrointestinal tract, liver, kidney, nervous system, and blood and blood-forming organs. Although specific antibiotic-induced toxicities are considered in the discussions of individual agents, an overall view of toxic effects on particular ogran systems is included here.

Gastrointestinal toxicity. Most of the orally administered agents can affect the gastrointestinal tract adversely, the effects varying from nausea and vomiting, which can occur with most of the agents, to severe and sometimes fatal pseudomembranous colitis. These untoward effects may occur as a result of (1) irritation of the gastrointestinal mucosa (commonly associated with erythromycin, tetracyclines, griseofulvin, and even the penicillins), (2) direct anatomical injury leading to damage of gastrointestinal cells, as occurs with orally administered neomycin, or (3) alterations in the microbial ecology of the mouth and gastrointestinal tract (discussed in the section on disturbances of host microflora).

Hepatotoxicity. Many commonly used antimicrobial agents are excreted unchanged by the kidney. However, some drugs are metabolized, to varying degrees, by hepatic mechanisms and appear in the urine as both the parent molecule and its metabolic derivatives. A second route of excretion for several of the antimicrobial agents is via biliary secretion into the gastrointestinal tract. The drug may or may not have been biotransformed in the liver before its excretion into the gastrointestinal tract. If it possesses innate toxicity, the primary manifestation of this toxicity will involve the liver. The antibiotics that are excreted by the biliary system and cause hepatic damage are the tetracyclines, amphotericin B, and isoniazid.

Nephrotoxicity. The antimicrobial agents that exhibit nephrotoxicity use the kidney as their major excretory pathway. Thus, toxic effects on the renal system produced by these drugs cause the accumulation of these agents and further damage to the kidneys. The nephrotoxic manifestations may be the result of direct toxic effects on renal tissue or renal cellular processes or of hypersensitivity reactions involving this organ system. Antimicrobial agents associated with adverse effects on the renal system include the sulfonamides, aminoglycosides, and outdated tetracyclines.

Neurotoxicity. Toxic effects of the antimicrobials on the central or peripheral nervous systems occur as a result of either their irritative properties or their inherent neurotoxicity. Massive doses of penicillin G may produce neurotoxic manifestations because of nonspecific irritation; on the other hand, griseofulvin, the aminoglycosides, and the tetracyclines (when administered to infants) are examples of agents with selective neurotoxicity.

Toxicity to blood and blood-forming organs. A number of the antimicrobial agents can produce hematologic changes of varying degrees of severity. The dose-related toxic effects of chloramphenicol on the bone marrow are an example. An idiosyncratic reaction, exhibited as hemolysis of red blood cells, occurs when sulfonamides, chloramphenicol, or nitrofurantoin are administered to patients with a deficiency of glucose-6-phosphate dehydrogenase.

Indirect toxicity

Indirect toxicity refers to the toxic effects occurring by means other than those involving direct actions on cellular processes. The prime example of an indirect toxicity is the allergic reaction, in which adverse responses are precipitated by immune mechanisms. Although all of the commonly used antimicrobial agents can produce drug allergy, some are more antigenic than others. Thus, although the penicillins as a class are the least toxic of the antibiotics, they are also one of the most allergenic. Because of their widespread use, the penicillins cause more allergic reactions than do other antibiotics and, for that matter, any other drug in widespread use. Topical use of antimicrobial drugs is particularly likely to cause patient sensitization and subsequent allergic reactions.

Since most antimicrobial agents are small molecules, they rarely serve directly as antigens. Rather, they act as haptens by reacting with endogenous proteins to form complete antigens. Degradation products of antimicrobial drugs may also combine with proteins and serve as haptenic determinants. Occasionally, degradation products of a drug polymerize and form molecules of sufficient size to act as direct antigens.[47]

Cross-sensitivity within a given class of antibiotics is common and may occur between classes as well (e.g., between penicillins and cephalosporins). Rarely, a particular salt of an antibiotic may produce allergic responses not associated with other forms of the drug. An example of this is the cholestatic hepatitis elicited in allergic patients by erythromycin estolate.

Disturbances of host microflora

Adverse reactions resulting from disturbances of the patient's microbial ecology are a form of drug toxicity unique to antimicrobials. Symptoms associated with such alterations include superinfection, diarrhea, flatulence, angular stomatitis, black furred tongue, glossodynia, and vitamin deficiencies.

Paramount among these reactions are superinfections, which are new infections that are manifested by bacteriologic and clinical signs and appear during antimicrobial treatment of a primary infection.[45] The organisms are not only resistant to the antimicrobial agent being used but are often difficult to treat with other commonly used antibiotics. Superinfections are frequently caused by *Clostridium, Proteus,* and *Pseudomonas* species, antibiotic-resistant staphylococci, and *Candida* and other fungi. The factors that favor the development of superinfections have been discussed already, but the following characteristics of superinfections are worthy of emphasis. The incidence increases (1) in patients less than 3 years of age or over 50 years, (2) in the presence of acute or chronic pulmonary disease other than tuberculosis, (3) during treatment of prolonged duration, and (4) with the use of agents with a wide range of antibacterial activity.[47] Generally, the broader the spectrum of antibacterial action, the greater the incidence of superinfection. Superinfections are potentially very dangerous, since the causative microorganisms may be highly pathogenic and are notably resistant to the antibiotic used and often to others as well. Since a superinfection may be more devastating or life-threatening than the primary infection for which therapy was initiated, immediate treatment is necessary and includes discontinuance of the antibiotic being given, culture and susceptibility testing of the microorganisms in the infected area, and administration of an antibiotic effective against the organism causing the superinfection.[33]

A serious form of antibiotic-induced superinfection is pseudomembranous colitis, a condition caused by overgrowth of the anaerobic microorganism *Clostridium difficile*.[3,6] This bacterium is normally present in the gastrointestinal tract of 3%

of all patients. It is widely distributed in nature, however, and can be passed from one patient to another by hospital personnel, unsterile instruments, and the like. Normally, the growth of *C. difficile* is prevented by other anaerobes of the gastrointestinal microflora. Suppression of these organisms by an antibiotic permits the resistant *C. difficile* to proliferate and to produce destructive amounts of two potent toxins. Signs and symptoms associated with pseudomembranous colitis include pronounced and persistent diarrhea; severe abdominal cramps; fever; the appearance of blood, neutrophils, and mucus in the stool; and the development of characteristic mucosal lesions in the large intestine. A recent study of the association between the occurrence of pseudomembranous colitis and specific antibiotics showed that 31% of the patients were given a cephalosporin, 27% ampicillin, and 11% clindamycin, with other antibiotics making up the remaining 31%.[3] In addition to the drugs listed above, penicillin G, all of the extended-spectrum penicillins, chloramphenicol, and the tetracyclines have the potential for causing this disease.

Continuation of the offending drug in these circumstances can be fatal. In addition to withdrawal of the antibiotic, treatment of the colitis includes correction of water and electrolyte imbalances, use of resins like cholestyramine and colestipol to bind the toxins, and, in severe cases, administration of antibiotics to eradicate the offending organism. Oral vancomycin has proved highly effective in this regard; other antimicrobials that may be useful include bacitracin and metronidazole. Antiperistaltic agents should not be administered to counteract the diarrhea because they promote retention of the clostridial cytotoxins.

THERAPEUTIC USES IN DENTISTRY

There are three major uses of antimicrobial agents in the practice of dentistry: (1) treatment of an acute dental infection, (2) prophylaxis in patients at risk of developing subacute bacterial endocarditis (SBE, in current nomenclature, bacterial endocarditis) or other problems as the result of bacteremia caused by dental procedures or traumatic injury, and (3) prophylaxis in patients with compromised host defense mechanisms caused by certain diseases or drug therapy. Some of the common acute orodental infections are shown in Table 36-5, along with the antimicrobial drugs of first choice and their alternatives.

Table 36-5. Some common orodental infections and antibiotics for treatment

Infections caused by	Antibiotics	
	First choice	*Alternatives*
Common intraoral pathogens		
Periapical abscess	Penicillin G (IM),	Cephalosporins, clindamycin, erythromy-
Periodontal abscess	penicillin V (PO)	cin, tetracycline, vancomycin
Acute suppurative pulpitis		
Toxic cellulitis		
Postsurgical or posttraumatic infections		
Suppurative infections of major salivary glands		
Ludwig's angina		
Oral-antral or oral-nasal fistulas with sinusitis		
Infections of mucous membranes in patients with pemphigus or impaired host defense mechanisms		
Pericoronitis with cellulitis, fever, and malaise		
Purulent osteitis		
Osteomyelitis		
Specific (unusual) microorganisms		
Localized juvenile periodontitis	Tetracyclines	
Vincent's infection (spirochetes and fusobacteria)	Penicillin G (IM), penicillin V (PO)	Erythromycin, metronidazole, tetracyclines
Penicillinase-producing staphylococci	Penicillinase-resistant penicillins	Cephalosporins, clindamycin, vancomycin
Gram-positive penicillin-resistant penicillinase-negative organisms	Erythromycin	Cephalosporins, clindamycin, sulfonamides, tetracyclines
Mixed gram-positive and gram-negative infection insensitive to penicillin G	Extended-spectrum penicillins	Cephalosporins, sulfonamides, tetracyclines
Gram-positive and gram-negative anaerobes refractory to penicillin G	Clindamycin	Cephalosporins, erythromycin, metronidazole, tetracyclines
Oral candidiasis	Nystatin	Amphotericin B, miconazole

Although the need for an antimicrobial agent in the treatment of an acute infection is usually obvious, the need for prophylactic coverage may not be so clear. Many dental procedures cause a transient bacteremia, and certain categories of patients (Table 36-6) will be placed at risk of developing SBE or other infections as a result. At greatest risk are those with prosthetic cardiac valves, as well as patients with scar tissue in the cardiovascular system, prosthetic devices in any location, indwelling catheters, and some cardiac pacemakers. These factors alter hemodynamics and blood flow characteristics and produce turbulence, which results in the formation of microthrombi. The microthrombi become lodged on scar tissue or foreign material and serve as a growth medium for bacteria that gain access to the bloodstream. Gram-positive cocci, which predominate in the oral aerobic microflora, are implicated in most cases of SBE. Published figures indicate that 16% to 20% of cases

of SBE are caused by dental procedures,[40] but it is reasonable to assume that the actual percentage may be higher.

The American Heart Association has published guidelines for the antibiotic coverage of various kinds of patients who are at risk of developing SBE. Generally, these guidelines may be followed for other groups of patients requiring antibiotic coverage. It is an absolute responsibility of the dental practitioner to be thoroughly familiar with these guidelines and to be aware of any revisions that are made at a later date. Table 36-7 summarizes the latest American Heart Association guidelines.

A few types of cardiovascular defects are not associated with SBE risk and therefore do not usually require antibiotic coverage.[22] An example is a patient who has had coronary artery surgery uncomplicated by other cardiac defects and who is thoroughly recovered. The dental practitioner who is in doubt as to whether a cardiac patient requires

Table 36-6. Some reported indications for the prophylactic use of antibiotics in dentistry

---

Prevention of subacute bacterial endocarditis in patients with:
    Congenital and acquired heart defects
    History of rheumatic fever
    History of endocarditis
    Prosthetic heart valves
    Certain cardiac pacemakers, implanted shunts, indwelling catheters
    Mitral valve prolapse with mitral regurgitation
Treatment of patients with artificial or transplanted organs:
    Orthopedic prostheses (hip, elbow, knee)
    Renal transplants
Treatment of hydrocephalic patients with implanted shunts
Treatment of patients with a history of nephritis syndrome after streptococcal pharyngitis
Treatment of patients with decreased host defense mechanisms because of:
    Disease:
        Aplastic anemia
        Lupus erythematosus
        Uncontrolled Addison's disease
        Uncontrolled diabetes mellitus
        Agammaglobulinemia
        Agranulocytosis
    Drugs and other therapy:
        Antineoplastic drugs
        Immunosuppressant drugs
        Adrenal corticosteroids
        X-radiation
Treatment of patients with certain orofacial traumatic wounds or compound mandibular fractures

---

antibiotic coverage during and after dental procedures should consult with the patient's cardiologist.

Some patients without cardiovascular problems also should receive prophylactic antibiotic coverage, since problems can still occur as a result of the bacteremia caused by dental procedures. Such patients include those with a history of nephritis resulting from a streptococcal infection. Patients with hip or other joint prosthesis may also require prophylaxis, as these devices can serve as a nidus for bacteria, and an ensuing infection at the site may result in rejection of the prosthesis.[27,53] However, patient selection and the choice of antibiotics are controversial at the present time.

Some practitioners advocate prophylactic coverage prior to bacteremia-inducing dental procedures for hydrocephalic patients with implanted ventriculovenous or ventriculoperitoneal shunts, even though no shunt infection as so far been directly related to dental procedures. The ventriculovenous shunt is susceptible to infection following bacteremia because of its communication with the circulatory system.[8] However, since the ventriculoperitoneal shunt is completely extravascular, the need for prophylactic antibiotics in these patients is questionable.

Another category of dental patients who should receive prophylactic antibiotics during and after dental procedures are those with impaired host defense mechanisms. Some of the obvious disease states leading to compromised host defense mechanisms are listed in Table 36-6. A number of pharmacologic agents, including corticosteroids, immunosuppressant drugs used after organ transplantation, and antineoplastic drugs, decrease host defense mechanisms. So also does x-ray therapy.

Several generalizations apply to the prophylactic use of antibiotics. First, as mentioned previously, bactericidal agents are preferred for prophylaxis, because the primary goal is to kill microorganisms before they have a chance to infect susceptible tissue sites. Second, prophylactic antibiotic therapy should be started with a high priming, or loading, dose given shortly before the procedure so as to achieve the maximum blood concentration when the operator-induced bacteremia is most likely to occur. Antibiotic coverage should not be started 2 days, or even 1 day, before the procedure. This practice was once advocated, and some practitioners still erroneously adhere to it. Investigations have shown that the oral microflora can be significantly altered within 24 hours after the initiation of antibiotic therapy, and this means that microorganisms in the oral cavity, the very organisms that will be etiologic factors in the bacteremia produced by the dental procedure, may become resistant to the concentrations of antibiotic in the oral environment. Finally, drug therapy may be significantly abbreviated in duration. Indeed, prophylaxis should be continued only for as long as the bacteremia may be expected to exist.

On occasion, questions have arisen concerning implementation of the American Heart Association guidelines in clinical practice. For example, how should a patient be managed who is scheduled for dental treatment on 2 successive days or who is allergic to penicillins and intolerant to erythromycin? The following suggestions are offered in the absence of official recommendations. Patients requiring two procedures a day apart should initially receive the prophylactic regimen most appropriate to their needs. The initial regimen should be given and another course of the same therapy instituted at the second appointment. If the patient

Table 36-7. Dosage regimens for prophylactic use of antibiotics for dental procedures*

Regimen	Adults	Children†
Use of penicillin is acceptable		
Parenteral-oral		
A	Aqueous crystalline penicillin G (1,000,000 units) IM, plus procaine penicillin G (600,000 units) IM, 30 to 60 minutes before procedure	Aqueous penicillin G (30,000 units/kg) IM, plus procaine penicillin G (600,000 units) IM, 30 to 60 minutes before procedure
	FOLLOWED BY	FOLLOWED BY
	Penicillin V (500 mg) orally every 6 hours for 8 doses	Penicillin V (500 mg) orally every 6 hours for 8 doses for children over 60 pounds; for children under 60 poundts, penicillin V (250 mg) orally every 6 hours for 8 doses
Oral		
	Penicllin V (2 gm) orally 30 to 60 minutes before procedure	For children over 60 pounds, penicillin V (2 gm) orally 30 to 60 minutes before procedure; for children under 60 pounds, penicillin V (1 gm) orally 30 to 60 minutes before procedure
	FOLLOWED BY	FOLLOWED BY
	Penicillin V (500 mg) orally every 6 hours for 8 doses	Penicillin V (250 mg) orally every 6 hours for 8 doses
Parenteral-oral		
B§	Aqueous crystalline penicillin G (1,000,000 units) IM, plus procaine penicillin G (600,000 units) IM, plus streptomycin (1 gm) IM, all given 30 to 60 minutes before procedure	Aqueous crystalline penicillin G (30,000 units/kg) IM, plus procaine penicillin G (600,000 units) IM, plus streptomycin (20 mg/kg) IM, all given 30 to 60 minutes before procedure
	FOLLOWED BY	FOLLOWED BY
	Penicillin V (500 mg) every 6 hours for 8 doses	Penicillin V (500 mg) orally every 6 hours for 8 doses for children over 60 pounds; for children under 60 pounds, penicillin V (250 mg) orally every 6 hours for 8 doses
Use of penicillin is not acceptable because of patient allergy		
Oral		
A	Erythromycin (1 gm) orally 90 to 120 minutes before procedure	Erythromycin (20 mg/kg) orally 90 to 120 minutes before procedure
	FOLLOWED BY	FOLLOWED BY
	Erythromycin (500 mg) every 6 hours for 8 doses	Erythromycin (10 mg/kg) orally every 6 hours for 8 doses
Intravenous-oral		
B§	Vancomycin (1 gm) diluted with 200 ml physiologic saline IV over a 30- to 60-minute period, starting infusion 30 to 60 minutes before procedure	Vancomycin (20 mg/kg) diluted IV over a 30- to 60-minute period using same protocol and timing as for adults‡
	FOLLOWED BY	FOLLOWED BY
	Erythromycin (500 mg) orally every 6 hours for 8 doses	Erythromycin (10 mg/kg) orally every 6 hours for 8 hours

*This information is taken from a statement prepared by the Committee on Prevention of Rheumatic Fever and Bacterial Endocarditis of the American Heart Association. It has been printed in Circulation **56:**139A-143A, 1977 and in the Journal of the American Dental Association **95:**600-605, 1977.
†Doses for children should not exceed recommendations for adults for a single dose or for a 24-hour period.
‡The total dose of vancomycin for children should not exceed 44 mg/kg/24 hours.
§Regimen B is recommended for most patients with prosthetic heart valves.

is experiencing gastrointestinal disturbances as a result of the first course, the parenteral route of administration should be used, at least for the initial, high dose of drug. For patients who are allergic to penicillins and suffer gastric distress from the high doses of erythromycin, several approaches may be tried. Substitution of one form of erythromycin for another (such as an enteric-coated formulation) may limit the gastric upset. Alternatively, parenteral vancomycin can be used to replace the initial dose of erythromycin. It may be appropriate for some patients to be tested for penicillin allergy. Inasmuch as 75% of individuals revert to the nonallergic state within a few years, a penicillin could be used safely in patients with negative skin tests whose prior reaction was not of the immediate type. Finally, cephalosporins and clindamycin have spectrums of activity that overlap that of penicillin V. They may be used in high doses when other remedies are exhausted, with the understanding that such use is not officially sanctioned. In addition to antibiotic therapy, the degree of bacteremia may be reduced by the use of an effective antibacterial mouthwash immediately prior to the dental procedure, since this measure significantly reduces the number of bacteria in the oral cavity for 30 to 60 minutes.[40]

CITED REFERENCES

1. Anderson, J.S., Matsuhashi, M., Haskin, M.A., and Strominger, J.L. Lipid-phosphoacetylmuramyl-pentapeptide and lipid-phosphodisaccharide-pentapeptide: presumed membrane transport intermediates in cell wall synthesis. Proceedings of the National Academy of Sciences of the United States of America **53**:881-889, 1965.
2. Anderson, P.O. Drugs and breast feeding—a review. Drug Intelligence and Clinical Pharmacy **11**:208-223, 1977.
3. Bartlett, J.G. Antimicrobial agents implicated in *Clostridium difficile* toxin-associated diarrhea of colitis. Johns Hopkins Medical Journal **149**:6-9, 1981.
4. Brown, G.M. The biosynthesis of folic acid. II. Inhibition by sulfonamides. Journal of Biological Chemistry **237**:536-540, 1962.
5. Chain, E.B. The development of bacterial chemotherapy. Antibiotics and Chemotherapy **4**:215-241, 1954.
6. Check, W. Colitis following antibiotic therapy due to *Clostridium difficile*. Journal of the American Medical Association **239**:2101-2102, 1978.
7. Cleocin. Compendium. Kalamazoo, Mich., The Upjohn Co., 1970.
8. Croll, T.P., Greiner, D.G., and Schut, L. Antibiotic prophylaxis for the hydrocephalic dental patient with a shunt. Pediatric Dentistry **1**:81-85, 1979.
9. Davies, J., and Davis, B.D. Misreading of ribonucleic acid code words induced by aminoglycoside antibiotics: the effect of drug concentration. Journal of Biological Chemistry **243**:3312-3316, 1968.
10. Dittent, L.W., and Di Santo, A.R., coordinators. The Bioavailability of Drug Products. Washington, D.C., American Pharmaceutical Association, 1975.
11. Domagk, G. Ein Beitrag zur Chemotherapie der bakteriellen Infektionen. Deutsche Medizinische Wochenschrift **61**:250-253, 1935.
12. Domagk, G. Eine neue Klasse von Desinfektionsmitteln. Deutsche Medizinische Wochenschrift **61**:829-832, 1935.
13. Ellison, S.A. Oral bacteria and periodontal disease. Journal of Dental Research **49**:198-202, 1970.
14. Epstein, S., and Scopp, I.W. Antibiotics and the intraoral abscess. Journal of Periodontology **48**:236-238, 1977.
15. Evaskus, D.S., Laskin, D.M., and Kroeger, A.V. Penetration of lincomycin, penicillin, and tetracycline into serum and bone. Proceedings of the Society for Experimental Biology and Medicine **130**:89-91, 1969.
16. Ferone, R., Burchall, J.J., and Hitchings, G.H. *Plasmodium berghei* dihydrofolate reductase: isolation, properties, and inhibition by antifolates. Molecular Pharmacology **5**:49-59, 1969.
17. Fourneau, E., Tréfouël, J., Tréfouël, J., Nitti, F., and Bovet, D. Chimiothérapie des infections streptococciques par les dérivés du *p*-aminophénylsulfamide. Comptes Rendus des Seances de la Societé de Biologie et de Ses Filiales **122**:652-654, 1936.
18. Gabrielson, M.L., and Stroh, E. Antibiotic efficacy in odontogenic infections. Journal of Oral Surgery **33**:607-610, 1975.
19. Jawetz, E., and Gunnison, J.B. Studies on antibiotic synergism and antagonism: the scheme of combined antimicrobial activity. Antibiotics and Chemotherapy **2**:243-248, 1952.
20. Kannangara, D.W., Thadepalli, H., and McQuirter, J.L. Bacteriology and treatment of dental infections. Oral Surgery, Oral Medicine, Oral Pathology **50**:103-109, 1980.
21. Kantz, W.E., and Henry, C.A. Isolation and classification of anaerobic bacteria from intact pulp chambers of nonvital teeth in man. Archives of Oral Biology **19**:91-96, 1974.
22. Kaplan, E.L., Anthony, B.F., Bisno, A., Durack, D., Houser, H., Millard, H.D., Sanford, J., Shulman, S.T., Stillerman, M., Taranta, A., and Wenger, N. Prevention of bacterial endocarditis. American Heart Association Committee Report. Circulation **56**:139A-143A, 1977.
23. Konno, K., Oizumo, K., and Oka, S. Mode of action of rifampin on mycobacteria. II. Biosynthetic studies on the inhibition of ribonucleic acid polymerase of *Mycobacterium bovis* BCG by rifampin and uptake of rifampin-^{14}C by *Mycobacterium phlei*. American Review of Respiratory Disease **107**:1006-1012, 1973.
24. Lipmann, F. Polypeptide chain elongation in protein biosynthesis. Science **164**:1024-1031, 1969.
25. Luzzatto, L., Apirion, D., and Schlessinger, D. Polyribosome depletion and blockage of the ribosome cycle by streptomycin in *Escherichia coli*. Journal of Molecular Biology **42**:315-335, 1969.
26. Mandell, G.L., and Sande, M.A. Antimicrobial agents. Penicillins and cephalosporins. In Gilman, A.G., Goodman, L.S., and Gilman, A., eds. Goodman and Gilman's The Pharmacological Basis of Therapeutics, ed. 6. New York, Macmillan, Inc., 1980.
27. Mulligan, R. Late infections in patients with prostheses for

total replacement of joints: implications for the dental practitioner. Journal of the American Dental Association **101:**44-46, 1980.

28. Neu, H.C. Resistance of gram-negative bacteria to antimicrobial agents. In Lauler, D.P., ed. Gram Negative Sepsis. New York, Medical Communications, Inc., 1971.

29. Olson, R.E., Morello, J.A., and Kieff, E.D. Antibiotic treatment of oral anaerobic infections. Journal of Oral Surgery **33:**619-621, 1975.

30. Owen, R.C., and Kenyon, R. An investigation of erythromycin stearate and erythromycin succinate in the treatment of oral infections. Dental Digest **72:**166-169, 1966.

31. Pratt, W.B. Fundamentals of Chemotherapy. New York, Oxford University Press, 1973.

32. Sabiston, C.B., Jr., and Gold, W.A. Anaerobic bacteria in oral infections. Oral Surgery, Oral Medicine, and Oral Pathology **38:**187-192, 1974.

33. Sande, M.A., and Mandell, G.L. Antimicrobial agents. General considerations. In Gilman, A.G., Goodman, L.S., and Gilman, A. eds. Goodman and Gilman's The Pharmacological Basis of Therapeutics, ed. 6. New York, Macmillan, Inc., 1980.

34. Sebek, O.K. Polymyxins and circulin. In Gottlieb, D., and Shaw, P.D., eds. Antibiotics, vol. 1. Mechanism of Action. Berlin, Springer-Verlag, 1967.

35. Smith, H. Antibiotics in Clinical Practice, ed. 3. Baltimore, University Park Press, 1977.

36. Socransky, S.S. Microbiology of periodontal disease—present status and future considerations. Journal of Periodontology **48:**497-504, 1977.

37. Spink, W.W. Reflections on gram-negative sepsis—a quarter century later. In Lauler, D.P., ed. Gram Negative Sepsis. New York, Medical Communications, Inc., 1971.

38. Strominger, J.L. The action of penicillin and other antibiotics on bacterial wall synthesis. Johns Hopkins Medical Journal **133:**63-81, 1973.

39. Sutherland, J.M., and Light, I.J. The effect of drugs on the developing fetus. Pediatric Clinics of North America **12**(3):781-806, 1965.

40. Sweet, J.B., Gill, V.J., Chusid, M.J., and Elin, R.J. Nitroblue tetrazolium and *Limulus* assays for bacteremia after dental extraction: effect of topical antiseptics. Journal of the American Dental Association **96:**276-281, 1978.

41. Tenenbaum, M.J., and Kaplan, M.H. Antibiotic combinations. Medical Clinics of North America **66:**17-24, 1982.

42. Tréfouël, J., Tréfouël, J., Nitti, F., and Bovet, D. Activité du *p*-aminophénylsulfamide sur les infections streptococcique expérimentale de la souris et du lapin. Comptes Rendus des Seances de la Societé de Biologie et de Ses Filiales **120:**756-758, 1935.

43. Turner, J.E., Moore, D.W., and Shaw, B.S. Prevalence and antibiotic susceptibility of organisms isolated from acute soft-tissue abscesses secondary to dental caries. Oral Surgery, Oral Medicine, and Oral Pathology **39:**848-857, 1975.

44. Vazquez, D. Uptake and binding of chloramphenicol by sensitive and resistant organisms. Nature **203:**257-258, 1964.

45. Weinstein, L. Superinfection: a complication of antimicrobial therapy and prophylaxis. American Journal of Surgery **107:**704-709, 1964.

46. Weinstein, L., and Dalton, A.C. Host determinants of response to antimicrobial agents. New England Journal of Medicine **279:**467-473, 524-531, 580-588, 1968.

47. Weinstein, L., and Weinstein, A.J. The pathophysiology and pathoanatomy of reactions to antimicrobial agents. Advances in Internal Medicine **19:**109-134, 1974.

48. Weisblum, B., and Davies, J. Antibiotic inhibitors of the bacterial ribosome. Bacteriological Reviews **32:**493-528, 1968.

49. Weissman, G., and Sessa, G. The action of polyene antibiotics on phospholipid-cholesterol structures. Journal of Biological Chemistry **242:**616-625, 1967.

50. Wittgow, W.C., and Sabiston, C.B. Microorganisms from pulpal chambers of intact teeth with necrotic pulps. Journal of Endodontics **1:**168-171, 1975.

51. Wood, W.B., and Smith, M.R. An experimental analysis of the curative action of penicillin in acute bacterial infections. The relationship of bacterial growth rates to the antimicrobial effect of penicillin. Journal of Experimental Medicine **103:**487-498, 1956.

52. Woods, D.D. The biochemical mode of action of the sulphonamide drugs. Journal of General Microbiology **29:**687-702, 1962.

53. Zallen, R.D., and Black, S.L. Antibiotic therapy in oral and maxillofacial surgery. Journal of Oral Surgery **34:**349-351, 1976.

GENERAL REFERENCES

Bartlett, J.G. Antibiotic-associated pseudomembranous colitis. Hospital Practice **16**(12):85-88, 93-95, 1982.

Cunha, B.A., ed. Symposium on antimicrobial therapy. The Medical Clinics of North America **66:**1-316, 1982.

Root, R.K., and Hierholzer, W.J., Jr. Infectious disease. In Melmon, K.L., and Morrelli, H.F., eds. Clinical Pharmacology, ed 2. New York, Macmillan, Inc., 1978.

Smith H. Antibiotics in Clinical Practice, ed. 3. Baltimore, University Park Press, 1977.

37 Antibacterial antibiotics

Edward H. Montgomery

Discussed in this chapter are the currently available antimicrobial agents used in the prevention and treatment of bacterial infections. Some of these agents—the penicillins, cephalosporins, erythromycin, and tetracyclines—have enjoyed widespread use in dentistry. Others have specific indications, for example, clindamycin as an alternative to penicillin V for the treatment of anaerobic dental infections. Still others, invaluable to the general practice of medicine, have at best very limited application in the therapy of oral infections. Such drugs include the sulfonamides and trimethoprim, the aminoglycosides, chloramphenicol, antituberculosis agents, and the antibiotics normally reserved for topical use. The antifungal and antiviral agents are considered in Chapter 38.

PENICILLINS

The story of the discovery of penicillin and the realization of Paul Ehrlich's dream that chemicals would be used in the eradication of infectious diseases began in 1928 in a laboratory in London where Alexander Fleming was doing research on vaccines. In one of his experiments he noticed that a culture of staphylococci had undergone lysis as a result of contamination with a mold, but nearly a year passed before he could pursue that observation. Fleming finally isolated the mold, *Penicillium notatum,* and found that the fluid beneath it possessed antibacterial properties and that it was nontoxic when injected into infected mice. In 1929 Fleming reported his discovery of penicillin, and in the years that followed he attempted to extract and purify penicillin from the mold culture medium. Similar efforts were also made by a group of scientists from Oxford University (Florey, Chain, and Heatley). In the early days of 1941, penicillin was still very impure, and 100 L of mold culture media were required to extract enough penicillin for the treatment of one patient for 24 hours. Every available container (even bedpans) was used for culturing the mold that, because of its aerobic nature, grew only on the surface of the media. The first reported patient to receive penicillin was an Oxford policeman who was dying of a mixed staphylococcal and streptococcal infection. After treatment with penicillin, he underwent a remarkable, if temporary, recovery. Because the supply was so limited and since penicillin is primarily excreted by the kidneys as the unchanged molecule, the drug was extracted from his and other patients' urine for reuse. The supply of penicillin was finally exhausted, and the policeman died, but the event established the safety and effectiveness of penicillin in the treatment of human infectious disease. This early experiment prompted an Oxford professor to describe penicillin as a remarkable antibacterial substance that is produced in bedpans, purified by passage through the Oxford police force, and then administered to patients.[63]

The initial clinical trials of penicillin led to a greatly increased demand for the agent, but it was impossible for Great Britain, then engaged in World War II, to devise techniques for its large-scale production. Florey and Heatley came to the United States in 1941 and with the aid of the U.S. Department of Agriculture developed the deep-vat culture technique, which made possible the production of large quantities of penicillin. It was not until 1946 that penicillin became available for treatment of civilians (formerly its use had been reserved for the armed forces of Great Britain and the United States).[63] The dramatic success of penicillin stimulated a search for other antibiotics, a search that still goes on.

Penicillins G and V as prototypes

Although several different types of penicillin were extracted during the 1940s, penicillin G, otherwise known as benzylpenicillin, was the most effective and became the prototype of the penicillin antibiotics. Certain limitations inherent in penicillin G, such as acid instability, narrow antibacterial spectrum, and rapid renal excretion, led to the search for derivatives that might be effective orally, have a somewhat broader spectrum, be less rapidly excreted by the kidney, and be resistant to enzymes (penicillinases) that inactivate the parent drug. The results were penicillin V (which is today the most widely used oral penicillin and the one of greatest importance to the dentist) and a series of penicillinase-resistant and extended-spectrum penicillins. In the discussion that follows, the properties, characteristics, pharmacology, and therapeutic applications of the penicillins in general and penicillins G and V in particular will be presented. At the end of this section, certain distinctive features of the penicillinase-resistant and extended-spectrum penicillins will also be considered.

Chemistry and classification. All of the penicillin derivatives have the same basic nucleus, 6-aminopenicillanic acid (6-APA), which is synthesized by the penicillium mold from two amino acids, L-cysteine and L-valine. Figure 37-1 shows the structure of these amino acids and their conjugation to form the nucleus of the penicillin molecule. This nucleus consists of a β-lactam ring joined by a thiazolidine ring. An intact nucleus is necessary for biologic activity; cleavage of the ring by enzymes known as β-lactamases (such as the penicillinase from *Staphylococcus aureus*) results in various inactive penicilloic acids. Amidase enzymes hydrolyze the amide bond between the acyl side chain and 6-APA. Various side chains can be linked to the 6-APA molecule to produce the semi-synthetic penicillins, as is shown in Table 37-1. These functional groups determine the specific pharmacologic and antibacterial properties exhibited by the penicillin derivatives, for example, acid stability, antibacterial spectrum, and resistance to β-lactamases. Penicillin G is the naturally occurring penicillin, currently produced from a high-yield mutant of *Penicillium chrysogenum*, which was initially obtained from the stem of a moldy cantaloupe. Penicillin V (phenoxymethylpenicillin) was introduced in 1953, when phenylacetic acid was added to the culture medium; phenethicillin followed in 1959 and was the first of many compounds to be synthesized from 6-APA. (Phenethicillin is no longer commercially available in the United States.)

Mechanism of action. All of the penicillins have the same mechanism of action, namely inhibition of enzymes responsible for the cross-linking of peptidoglycan polymers during the last stage of bacterial cell wall synthesis (see Table 36-1). Penicillins also promote the activity of enzymes (autolysins) that normally function in concert with peptidoglycan synthesis to effect cell growth and division. Unopposed activity of these enzymes causes damage to the existing cell wall and promotes lysis. The penicillins are bactericidal against growing bacteria but are ineffective against dormant microbes.

Antibacterial spectrum. Penicillin G, penicillin V, and the penicillinase-resistant penicillin derivatives are considered narrow-spectrum antibiotics in that at usual doses they mainly affect gram-positive aerobic and facultative microorganisms, some anaerobes, and spirochetes. The remaining penicillin derivatives exhibit an extended spectrum of antibacterial activity including many gram-negative bacilli.

Basically, all the penicillins are active in vitro, and at the usual concentrations achieved in vivo, against many gram-positive cocci (streptococci, staphylococci, and pneumococci), gram-positive rods (*Bacillus, Corynebacterium, Clostridium,* and other genera), and spirochetes (e.g., *Treponema pallidum*). Penicillin G is slightly more effective against these organisms than is penicillin V, but this is not a factor of clinical importance in the treatment of most infections of mild or moderate severity. Penicillin G is also active against some gram-negative aerobic cocci, such as the *Neisseria.* Here, however, the oral forms of penicillin (including penicillin V) are not clinically useful because relatively large parenteral doses are generally required. The penicillins are effective against many anaerobic microorganisms, including most of the anaerobes found in the oral cavity that have been associated wtih dental and periodontal diseases, both acute and chronic: diphtheroids, fusobacteria, peptostreptococci, spirochetes, *Actinomyces, Veillonella,* and some *Bacteroides.* In conventional doses, the narrow-spectrum penicillins are not active against gram-negative bacilli, but some of these microorganisms, such as *Escherichia coli, Shigella, Salmonella, Proteus mirabilis,* and *Enterobacter aerogenes,* are affected by very high

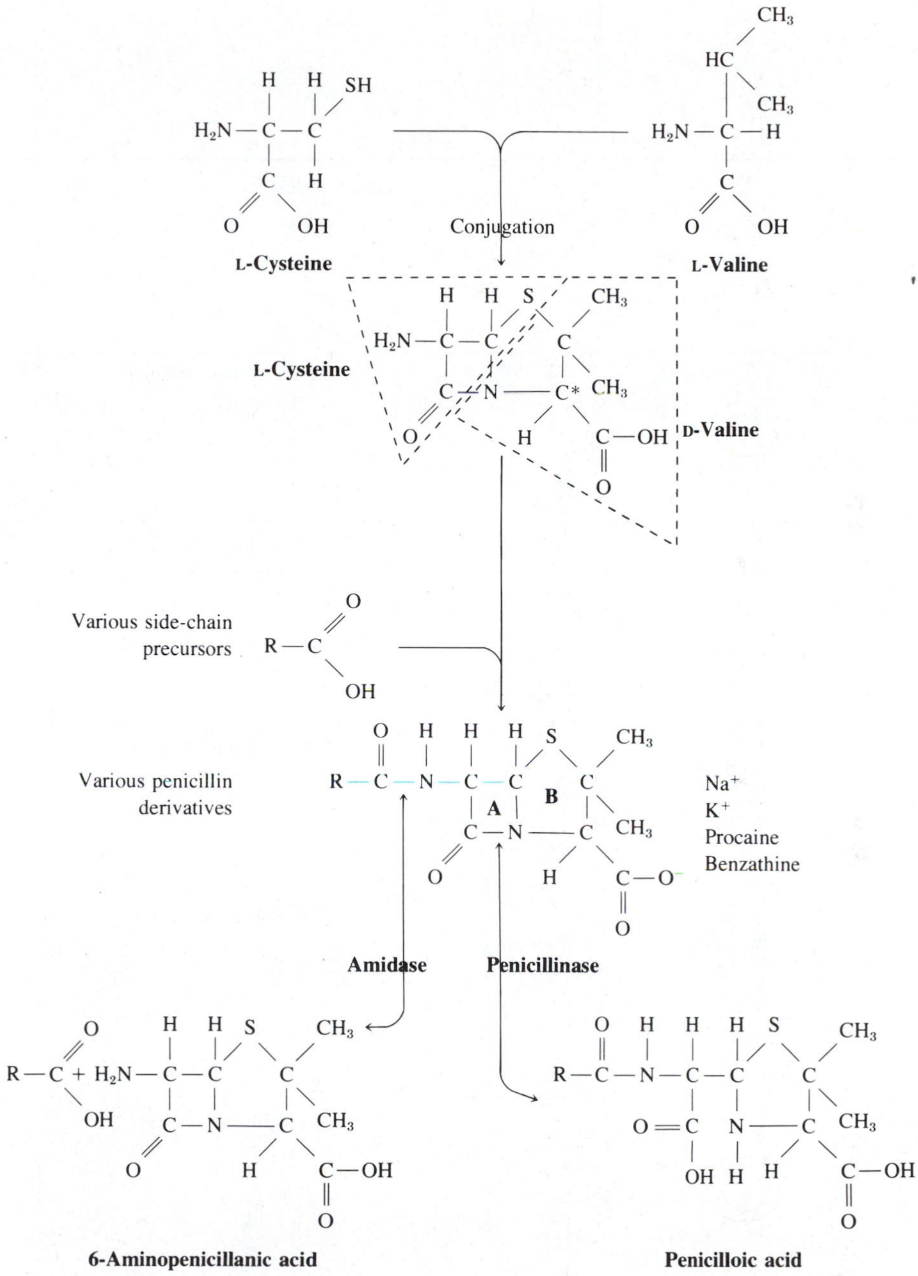

Figure 37-1. Biosynthesis and hydrolysis of penicillins. *Isomeric conversion of L-valine to D-valine during conjugation. **A** = β-lactam ring, **B** = thiazolidine ring.

Table 37-1. Structures and characteristics of the penicillin derivatives

Nonproprietary name	R side chain	Oral absorption*	Special properties
Penicillin G	(phenyl)—CH_2—	Variable	Best for parenteral use
Penicillin V	(phenyl)—O—CH_2—	+ +	
Methicillin	(phenyl with OCH_3, OCH_3)	−	Penicillinase resistant
Nafcillin	(naphthyl with OC_2H_5)	Variable	Penicillinase resistant
Oxacillin	(isoxazole with CH_3)	+	Penicillinase resistant
Cloxacillin	(Cl-phenyl isoxazole with CH_3)	+	Penicillinase resistant
Dicloxacillin	(diCl-phenyl isoxazole with CH_3)	+ +	Penicillinase resistant
Ampicillin	(phenyl)—CH—NH_2	+	Extended spectrum

*−, no absorption after oral route of administration; +, adequate absorption; + +, excellent absorption.

Table 37-1. Structures and characteristics of the penicillin derivatives—cont'd

Nonproprietary name	R side chain	Oral absorption*	Special properties
Hetacillin	Imidazolidinyl derivative of ampicillin	+	Extended spectrum; hydrolyzed to ampicillin in vivo
Bacampicillin	1-Ethoxycarbonyl-oxyethyl ester of ampicillin	+ +	Extended spectrum: hydrolyzed to ampicillin in vivo
Amoxicillin		+ +	Extended spectrum
Cyclacillin		+ +	Extended spectrum
Carbenicillin		−	Extended spectrum; active against *Pseudomonas* and *Proteus;* adequate oral absorption with indanyl salt
Ticarcillin		−	Extended spectrum; active against *Pseudomonas* and *proteus*
Azlocillin		−	Extended spectrum; active against *Pseudomonas* and *Proteus*
Mezlocillin		−	Extended spectrum; active against *Pseudomonas, Proteus, Klebsiella,* and *Bacteroides*
Piperacillin		−	Extended spectrum: active against *Pseudomonas, Proteus, Klebsiella,* and *Bacteroides*

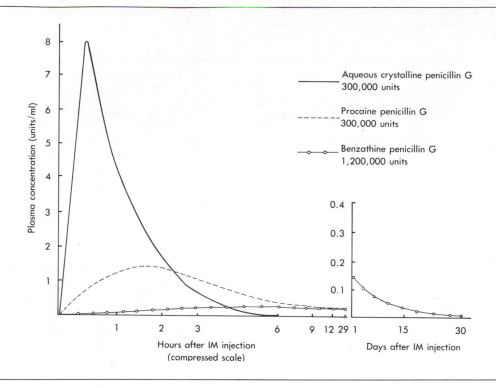

Figure 37-2. Comparative plasma concentrations of penicillin G obtained from soluble versus repository dosage forms.

concentrations of penicillin G achieved with intravenous administration of enormous doses. None of the penicillins directly influences the proliferation of viruses, rickettsiae, fungi, or other nonbacterial parasites.

Bacterial resistance. The problem of bacterial resistance, the mechanisms by which it develops, and its clinical implications are discussed in Chapter 36. Resistance to the penicillins usually appears in a slow, stepwise fashion. A major mechanism by which bacteria, particularly staphylococci, become resistant to the penicillins is through the elaboration of β-lactamases (penicillinases), which inactivate the penicillin by cleavage of the β-lactam ring. At least 60% to 80% of staphylococcal strains found in nonhospitalized patients and up to 95% of those in hospitalized patients are resistant to penicillin G and its nonpenicillinase-resistant congeners. Resistance has developed in some pneumococcal and gonococcal bacteria that were at one time uniformly sensitive.[19,32] Although most of the viridans streptococci found in the oral cavity are sensitive to penicillins G and V, the number of

strains that are resistant or exhibit diminished susceptibility is increasing.[16]

Absorption, fate, and excretion. Penicillin G can be given by all routes of administration. It is inactivated by acid and is therefore susceptible to destruction by gastric juice. At best, only 30% of an orally administered dose is absorbed. Any remaining drug that was not hydrolyzed in the stomach is largely destroyed by bacteria in the colon. Because of its poor efficacy, oral penicillin G has been largely replaced by the acid-stable derivative, penicillin V. When penicillin G is the drug of choice, as it might be for a serious infection, the drug is administered parenterally. Figure 37-2 shows the comparative blood concentrations achieved with intramuscular administration of crystalline penicillin G and includes data on the blood concentrations provided by repository forms of the drug.

Penicillin V is given only orally. Oral administration of penicillin V produces plasma levels 2 to 5 times higher than an equivalent dose of penicillin G. Despite its acid stability, penicillin V is absorbed best when given on an empty stomach.

Repository forms of penicillin G are available, either as procaine penicillin G or as benzathine penicillin G, both of which are water-insoluble salts. These preparations are injected deep into muscle, from which active penicillin G is slowly released into the bloodstream, providing a demonstrable plasma concentration of penicillin G for prolonged periods (Figure 37-2). Because of the lower blood titers provided by the repository preparations, they are used only against organisms of high susceptibility. The major difference between procaine penicillin G and benzathine penicillin G is that the latter is much less soluble in body fluids and provides a considerably slower rate of absorption. The resulting serum concentrations of active penicillin G obtained by injection of benzathine penicillin G are inadequate for treatment of many acute infections. However, this dosage form is quite useful in the prophylactic coverage of patients who have recently had an episode of rheumatic fever.

The penicillins are widely distributed throughout the body, the concentration achieved at a given site being dependent on the vascularity and blood flow to the area. Penicillins gain access to wounds, soft tissue sites, saliva, and even abscesses, but the relatively avascular nature of abscesses limits the concentration of all antibiotics at these sites. The penicillins are reversibly bound in varying amounts to plasma proteins; penicillins G and V are about 60% and 80% bound respectively. Although the penicillins do not readily cross the blood-brain barrier in normal circumstances, inflammation of the meninges may allow therapeutic concentrations to be attained in the cerebrospinal fluid. Concentrations of penicillin in bone are a fraction of those in plasma, but they may be sufficient for effective treatment of certain kinds of bone infections.[57]

Penicillins are rapidly eliminated by the kidney as the intact active molecule; smaller amounts may be metabolized in the liver, excreted in the bile, or both. The elimination half-time for penicillin G is about 30 minutes in normal adults. In severe renal failure, the elimination of penicillin is compromised, and a reduction in daily dosage is required.[2] Tubular secretion accounts for 90% of the excretion of penicillin G and glomerular filtration for the rest. All of the penicillin derivatives are excreted similarly, which means that the active, unaltered drug appears in high concentration in the urine. This accounts for the usefulness of a penicillin derivative such as ampicillin in the treatment of urinary tract infections.

Some acidic drugs actively transported by renal tubules strongly compete with penicillins for the same tubular secretory pathways. In the early days of penicillin use, probenecid, a uricosuric agent now employed in the treatment of gout, was used to interfere with the secretion of penicillin and thus increase its sojourn in the body. This approach is currently used only when high plasma concentrations are required, as in the treatment of a resistant gonococcal infection with penicillin G or a gram-negative septicemia with an extended-spectrum derivative. It should be reemphasized, however, that in normal circumstances adequate plasma concentrations can be achieved safely by increasing the dose of penicillin, that because of the nature of penicillin's effect on bacterial cell walls the drug concentration can actually fall below the MLC between doses without adversely affecting its continuing antimicrobial action, and that, where necessary, repository forms can be used to provide prolonged, if lower, blood concentrations.

General therapeutic uses. The penicillins are among the most widely used antimicrobial agents at the present time because they are relatively safe, are highly effective, and possess a spectrum of activity that includes most common pathogens. Table 37-2 lists the drugs of first choice and alternative drugs for the treatment of infections caused by specific microorganisms; the important role of penicillins in the chemotherapy of microbial disease is self-evident. Unfortunately, some formerly susceptible microorganisms have become resistant, so the therapeutic usefulness of the penicillins (as well as that of most other antibiotics) is not necessarily predictable from a knowledge of the antibacterial spectrum. As has been pointed out repeatedly, sensitivity testing must be carried out when possible to determine whether the infectious organism will respond to a particular antibiotic. Overt symptoms of infection are best used to guide the initial selection of an antimicrobial agent before the results of testing are received. Table 37-3 indicates some clinical conditions in which penicillin G or V is the drug of choice when laboratory findings are not available.

Therapeutic uses in dentistry. Almost all dental infections, with the exception of those of unusual etiology, can be effectively treated with one

Table 37-2. Drugs used to treat infections caused by specific microorganisms

Microorganism	Drug of first choice	Alternative drugs*
Gram-positive cocci		
Staphylococcus aureus		
Penicillinase-negative	Penicillin G or V	Cephalosporin, clindamycin, vancomycin
Penicillinase-positive	Penicillinase-resistant penicillin (e.g., cloxacillin)	Cephalosporin, clindamycin, vancomycin
Methicillin-resistant	Vancomycin	Trimethoprim-sulfamethoxazole
Streptococcus pyogenes	Penicillin G or V	Erythromycin, cephalosporin, vancomycin
Streptococcus, viridans group		
Oral infections	Penicillin G or V	Erythromycin, cephalosporin
Bacteremia or endocarditis	Ampicillin or penicillin G with gentamicin or streptomycin	Cephalosporin, vancomycin
Streptococcus, anaerobic	Penicillin G or V	Erythromycin, cephalosporin, clindamycin
Streptococcus pneumoniae	Penicillin G or V	Erythromycin, cephalosporin, chloramphenicol, vancomycin
Streptococcus, enterococcus group	Ampicillin or amoxicillin	Penicillin or vancomycin with gentamicin or streptomycin
Gram-negative cocci		
Neisseria gonorrhoeae	Penicillin G, tetracycline	Ampicillin or amoxicillin, spectinomycin, cefoxitin
Neisseria meningitidis	Penicillin G	Chloramphenicol, sulfonamide, cefuroxime
Gram-positive bacilli		
Clostridium difficile	Vancomycin	Bacitracin, metronidazole
Clostridium perfringens	Penicillin G	Chloramphenicol, clindamycin, metronidazole, tetracycline
Clostridium tetani	Penicillin G	Tetracycline
Corynebacterium diphtheriae	Erythromycin	Penicillin G
Corynebacterium species (diphtheroids)	Erythromycin	Penicillin G
Gram-negative bacilli		
Bacteroides, oropharyngeal strains	Penicillin G	Clindamycin, cefoxitin, metronidazole, tetracycline
Escherichia coli	Gentamicin or tobramycin	Amikacin, cephalosporin, extended-spectrum penicillin, tetracycline
Klebsiella pneumoniae	Gentamicin or tobramycin	Amikacin, cephalosporin, mezlocillin or piperacillin, tetracycline, trimethoprim-sulfamethoxazole
Haemophilus influenzae	Chloramphenicol, ampicillin or amoxicillin	Cefamandole or cefotaxime, trimethoprim-sulfamethoxazole
Legionella pneumophila (Legionnaire's disease)	Erythromycin with or without rifampin	
Leptotrichia buccalis	Penicillin G	Clindamycin, tetracycline
Proteus mirabilis	Ampicillin or amoxicillin	Aminoglycoside, carbenicillin-like penicillin, cephalosporin
Pseudomonas aeruginosa	Carbenicillin-like penicillin with gentamicin or tobramycin	Carbenicillin-like penicillin with amikacin, cefoperazone
Salmonella typhi	Chloramphenicol	Ampicillin or amoxicillin, trimethoprim-sulfamethoxazole
Shigella	Trimethoprim-sulfamethoxazole	Ampicillin, chloramphenicol, tetracycline

*Listing does not include all alternative drugs.

Table 37-2. Drugs used to treat infections caused by specific microorganisms—cont'd

Microorganism	Drug of first choice	Alternative drugs*
Other microorganisms		
Mycobacterium tuberculosis	Isoniazid with rifampin	*p*-Aminosalicylic acid (PAS), ethambutol, pyrazinamide, streptomycin
Actinomyces israelii	Penicillin G	Tetracycline
Nocardia	Trisulfapyrimidines	Trimethoprim-sulfamethoxazole
Treponema pallidum	Penicillin G	Tetracycline, erythromycin
Chlamydia psittaci	Tetracycline	Chloramphenicol
Rickettsia	Tetracycline	Chloramphenicol
Fusobacterium species	Penicillin G	Chloramphenicol, clindamycin, metronidazole
Candida albicans		
Oral lesions	Nystatin	Amphotericin B, miconazole, ketoconazole
Other infections	Amphotericin B	Clotrimazole, ketoconazole, miconazole, nystatin
Viruses		
Herpes simplex		
Keratitis	Trifluridine	Idoxuridine, vidarabine
Encephalitis	Vidarabine	Acyclovir
Herpes genitalis	Acyclovir	
Influenza A	Amantadine	

Table 37-3. Disease entities for which penicillin G or V is a drug of first choice

Abscesses, including orodental
Bacteremia (gram-positive)
Endocarditis
Gas gangrene
Mastoiditis
Meningitis
Orodental infections
Osteomyelitis
Otitis media
Pericarditis
Periodontal infections
Pharyngitis
Pneumonia
Rat-bite fever
Scarlet fever
Suppurative arthritis
Syphilis
Vincent's stomatitis
Weil's disease
Wound infections

NOTE: These diseases are caused by a variety of gram-positive cocci and bacilli, some gram-negative organisms, spirochetes, and anaerobic microorganisms. Susceptibility testing is essential for some and advisable for all.

of the penicillins. The common dental infections, particularly those occurring as the result of carious lesions, are caused by a variety of aerobic gram-positive cocci and anaerobic microorganisms, and the majority of these are susceptible to penicillin. The agent of choice in these infections is penicillin V, for the obvious reason that the absorption of penicillin G via the oral route is poor. Because the oral route is the safest, most convenient, and least expensive mode of drug administration, it is favored in the treatment of dental patients. Indeed, penicillin V is the most frequently prescribed antibiotic for chemotherapy for infections of dental origin. Penicillin G is largely reserved for severe infections, for some patients requiring prophylactic coverage (see Table 36-7), and for situations in which the oral route is compromised (as in malabsorption syndrome and vomiting).

There are some instances in which penicillins G and V are unsuitable for treating oral infections. Some dental infections are caused by penicillinase-producing organisms; in such cases the appropriate antibiotic would be a penicillinase-resistant penicillin derivative. Furthermore, patients who have been receiving extended prophylactic therapy with penicillin for the prevention of endocarditis will require another antibiotic if they are to undergo a dental procedure. Certain periodontal infections can be caused by both gram-positive and gram-negative organisms for which an antimicrobial agent with a more extended antibacterial spectrum than penicillin V (ampicillin or amoxicillin) might be the agent of choice. In Table 37-4 most of the penicillin preparations that are currently available and their dosage regimens are shown.

Toxic reactions and side effects. The penicillins are among the least toxic drugs known and are certainly among the safest of antibiotics. They exhibit maximum selective toxicity and, unless present in excessive concentrations (when they cause irritation), rarely directly elicit adverse reactions in humans. They are associated, however, with a number of untoward effects. Penicillins can perturb the normal microbial ecology such that gastrointestinal and other disturbances may result. Also, they are the most common cause of drug allergy.

Allergic reactions. The allergic responses caused by penicillins include almost every type of adverse immune reaction known. Although estimates of the incidence of penicillin allergy differ, it is generally reported to occur, with varying degrees of severity, in 2% to 8% of patients treated with these drugs.[64] The frequency and severity of allergic reactions are governed by the route of administration and the type of penicillin derivative used. Topical application is most likely to produce sensitization, and for this reason it is strictly proscribed. Most life-threatening allergic responses are caused by parenteral injection, but oral administration and even the use of minute amounts of drug for intradermal sensitivity testing have caused fatal anaphylaxis. Of all the available penicillin preparations, procaine penicillin G is associated with the highest incidence of drug allergy. Procaine may serve as an adjuvant in promoting the development of antibodies, but the fact that it is allergenic in its own right may also be contributory in this regard. Life-threatening anaphylactoid reactions occur in about 0.02% of patients given some type of penicillin, and about 10% of these victims succumb to respiratory and cardiovascular embarrassment.[50,64,72] It is estimated that between 100 and 300 fatal allergic reactions to penicillin occur annually in the United States.

In order for an allergic reaction to develop, previous exposure to penicillin is necessary. Unfortunately, such exposure can take place subtly and without the individual's knowledge. A patient may have received a sensitizing dose of penicillin in milk, beef, or poultry products, since antibiotics

Table 37-4. Commercially available penicillin preparations

Nonproprietary name	Proprietary name	Usual adult dose	Route*	Preparations
Penicillin G potassium (oral)	Pentids	200,000-800,000 units every 6-8 hours	Oral	Tablets: 200,000, 250,000, 400,000, 500,000, and 800,000 units Powder for solution: 200,000, 250,000, and 400,000 units/5 ml
Penicillin G potassium (injection)	Pfizerpen	1-30 megaunits/day in divided doses	IM, IV	Vials: 0.2, 0.5, 1, 5, 10, and 20 mega units
Procaine penicillin G	Wycillin, Crysticillin A.S.	600,000-1,200,000 units every 24 hours	IM	Vials: 300,000, 500,000, and 600,000 units/ml
Benzathine penicillin G	Bicillin L-A, Permapen	1,200,000 units in a single injection	IM	Vials: 300,000 units/ml Syringes: 600,000 units/ml
Penicillin V potassium	V-Cillin K, Pen-Vee K	250-500 mg every 6 hours	Oral	Tablets: 125, 250, and 500 mg Powder for solution: 125 and 250 mg/5 ml
Methicillin sodium	Staphcillin, Celbenin	1 gm every 4-6 hours	IM, IV	Vials: 1, 4, 6, and 10 gm
Nafcillin sodium	Unipen, Nafcil	250-500 mg every 4-6 hours	IM, IV, oral	Injection: vials of 500 mg, 1, 2, 4, and 10 gm Capsules: 250 mg Tablets: 500 mg Powder for solution: 250 mg/5 ml
Oxacillin sodium	Prostaphlin, Bactocill	250 mg-1 gm every 4-6 hours	IM, IV, oral	Injection: vials of 250 and 500 mg, 1, 2, 4, and 10 gm Capsules: 250 and 500 mg Powder for solution: 250 mg/5 ml

Cloxacillin sodium	Tegopen, Cloxapen	250-500 mg every 6 hours	Oral	Capsules: 250 and 500 mg Powder for solution: 125 mg/5 ml
Dicloxacillin sodium	Dynapen, Pathocil	125-250 mg every 6 hours	Oral	Capsules: 125, 250, and 500 mg Powder for suspension: 62.5 mg/5 ml
Ampicillin	Polycillin, Totacillin	250-500 mg every 6 hours; 150-200 mg/kg/day for septicemia, meningitis	IM, IV, oral	Injection: vials of 125, 250, and 500 mg, 1, 2, and 10 gm Capsules: 250 and 500 mg Powder for suspension: 100, 125, 250, and 500 mg/5 ml
Hetacillin†	Versapen	225-450 mg every 6 hours	Oral	Capsules: 225 mg Powder for suspension: 112.5 and 225 mg/5 ml
Bacampicillin hydrochloride	Spectrobid	400-800 mg every 12 hours	Oral	Tablets: 400 mg Powder for suspension: 125 mg/5 ml
Amoxicillin trihydrate	Amoxil, Larotid	250-500 mg every 8 hours	Oral	Chewable tablets: 125 and 250 mg Capsules: 250 and 500 mg Powder for suspension: 50, 125, and 250 mg/5 ml
Cyclacillin	Cyclapen-W	250-500 mg every 6 hours	Oral	Tablets: 250 and 500 mg Powder for suspension: 125 and 250 mg/5 ml
Carbenicillin disodium	Geopen, Pyopen	200-500 mg/kg/day in divided doses not to exceed 40 gm/day	IM, IV	Vials: 1, 2, 5, 10, 20, and 30 gm
Carbenicillin indanyl sodium	Geocillin	382-764 mg every 6 hours	Oral	Tablets: 382 mg
Ticarcillin disodium	Ticar	150-300 mg/kg/day in 4-8 divided doses by IV infusion or 1-2 gm IM every 6 hours for uncomplicated infections	IM, IV	Vials: 1, 3, 6, and 20 gm
Azlocillin sodium	Azlin	100-300 mg/kg/day in 4-6 divided doses not to exceed 24 gm/day	IV	Vials: 2, 3, and 4 gm
Mezlocillin sodium	Mezlin	100-300 mg/kg/day by IV infusion in 4-6 divided doses not to exceed 24 gm/day, or 1.5-2 gm IM every 6 hours for uncomplicated infections	IM, IV	Vials: 1, 2, 3, and 4 gm
Piperacillin sodium	Pipracil	100-300 mg/kg/day by IV infusion in 2-6 divided doses not to exceed 24 gm/day, or 3-4 gm IM every 12 hours for uncomplicated infections	IM, IV	Vials: 2, 3, and 4 gm

*IM = intramuscular, IV = intravenous.
†Dosages and preparations are listed in ampicillin equivalents.

have been extensively used to increase agricultural productivity. *Penicillium* molds are not uncommon, and sensitization to the natural varieties of penicillin may also occur.

Allergic reactions to the penicillins have been classified into three groups, based on the time of development.[72] *Acute allergic reactions*, such as anaphylactic shock, occur within 30 minutes of penicillin administration. Immediate-onset reactions include the most dangerous responses, which are characterized by urticaria, angioedema, bronchoconstriction, gastrointestinal disturbances, and shock. Death can result in a short time if treatment is not instituted promptly. As described in Chapters 6 and 32, treatment involves the parenteral administration of epinephrine and usually an antihistamine and a corticosteroid as well. *Accelerated allergic reactions* arise 30 minutes to 48 hours after penicillin administration. The manifestations are urticaria, pruritus, wheezing, mild laryngeal edema, and local inflammatory reactions. In general these responses are not life-threatening, but the laryngeal edema is potentially dangerous. *Delayed allergic reactions* take longer than 2 days to develop and are seen after the use of a number of antibiotics. Approximately 80% to 90% of all allergic reactions occurring with penicillin are of this type. These allergic responses are manifested by skin rashes, such as erythema nodosum and bullous eruptions. Generally, they are mild and reversible, although some dangerous reactions, such as exfoliative dermatitis and interstitial nephritis culminating in renal failure, have been reported. Delayed onset reactions to penicillin may also be seen in the oral cavity as acute glossitis, furred tongue, black or brown tongue, cheilosis, and severe stomatitis with loss of the buccal mucosa. Such reactions have generally been the result of the topical use of penicillin in the oral cavity, but they also occur (although much less frequently) when penicillin is given by other routes. Serum sickness is an allergic reaction that also falls into this class, although it may take an accelerated form if the patient has been previously exposed. It usually appears when the duration of penicillin therapy is extended for more than a week, generally takes at least 6 days to develop, and can occur a week or more after discontinuation of therapy. Serum sickness is not a cell-mediated allergy but the result of deposition of antibody complexes (IgG or IgM) plus complement on the walls of arterioles. It is characterized by fever, skin rash (urticaria, mac-

ulopapular eruptions), arthralgia, and lymphadenopathy. Treatment is symptomatic. (For a full discussion of serum sickness, see Chapter 39). The clinician should be aware that an allergic reaction to penicillin may be manifested by fever only and that the persistence of hyperthermia in the face of remission of an infection is evidence that the fever may be caused by a drug allergy. Generally, such febrile conditions disappear within 24 to 36 hours after discontinuance of the drug.

In the development of antibodies to penicillin, it is not the intact penicillin molecule that reacts with protein to form the complete antigen but its degradation products. One of the most reactive penicillin derivatives is penicillenic acid, which reacts with lysine residues to form the major antigenic determinant (Figure 37-3). This penicilloyl determinant composes more than 95% of the hapten-protein conjugates of penicillin[14]; antibodies to it mediate accelerated and late urticarial reactions and some maculopapular and erythematous skin reactions. The remaining 5% of penicillin antigens consist of proteins conjugated by other penicillin moieties (e.g., penicilloic acid) or of nonpenicilloyl derivatives of penicillenic acid. These minor antigenic determinants, so-called because of their lesser abundance, are actually responsible for the majority of immediate-onset allergic reactions. The recurrent arthralgia syndrome associated with penicillin also appears to be mediated by these minor determinants. Since all of the penicillin derivatives possess the same basic nucleus, 6-APA (the breakdown products of which compose the haptenic determinants), cross-reactivity or cross-allergenicity between all the penicillin derivatives is to be expected. Therefore, a patient who exhibits an allergic reaction to one penicillin derivative should be considered allergic to all other penicillins, natural or semisynthetic.

Increased understanding of the mechanisms involved in penicillin allergy has allowed the development of diagnostic skin tests to determine whether an individual is sensitive to penicillin. These skin tests commonly employ benzylpenicilloyl-polylysine as the major determinant and a mixture of penicillin breakdown products as the minor determinant. Although not predictive of delayed allergic responses, a positive reaction to either determinant indicates a significant risk of drug allergy. A negative response to both antigenic determinants indicates that penicillin can be employed with a minimal chance of eliciting an im-

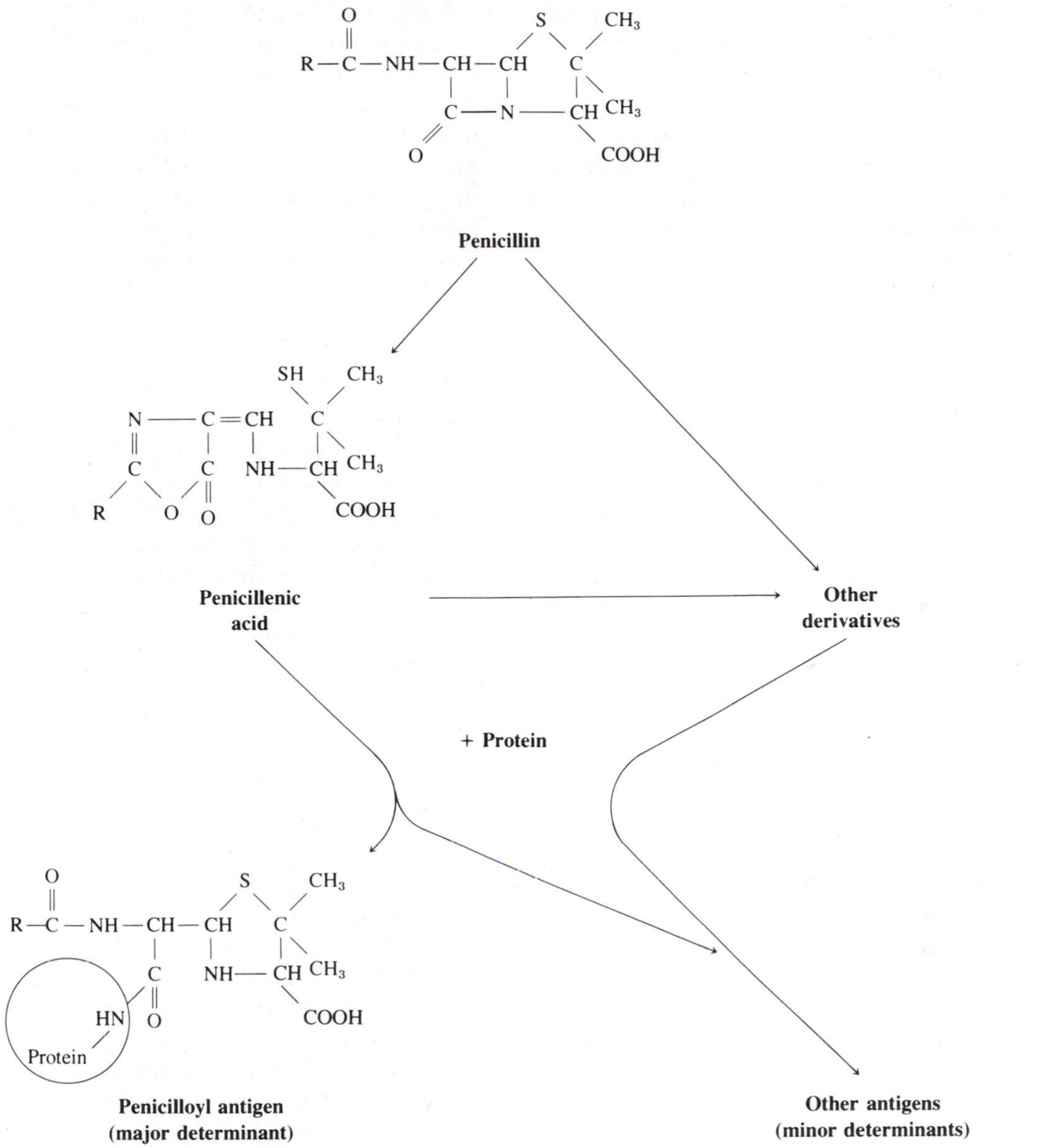

Figure 37-3. Antigenic determinants of penicillin allergy.

mediate or accelerated allergic response. It is not recommended, however, that the dentist employ skin tests to determine allergy to penicillin. Considerable experience is required to give such tests safely and evaluate them properly. Penicillin is not absolutely required for treatment of the vast majority of dental infections, and effective, safe alternatives to penicillin, such as erythromycin, can be used in patients with medical histories suggestive of penicillin allergy.

Allergic reactions to penicillin are relatively unpredictable. Although patients who have experienced an adverse reaction to penicillin should always be considered allergic unless proved otherwise, challenge tests have shown that three fourths of such individuals lose their sensitivity to penicillin with time. On the other hand, patients who have taken penicillin for years without any problems may suddenly develop an allergic reaction, ranging from the mildest forms to the most severe. Patients with a personal or familial history of atopy (allergy to foods, dust, pollens, etc.) exhibit a higher frequency of penicillin allergy than do other individuals. Penicillin should be used with caution and avoided when possible in such patients.

In summary, although penicillin should not be avoided when it is the drug of choice and is not contraindicated, the clinician should be cognizant of the unpredictable nature of penicillin allergy and be prepared to deal intelligently with any reactions that may arise.

Nonallergic responses. Penicillins administered in exceptionally high doses have been associated with direct irritation of tissues. Potentially dangerous is the neurotoxic effect of penicillin, the incidence and severity of which increases directly with the concentration of drug in the cerebrospinal fluid. Signs of neuronal irritation include twitching and localized or generalized epileptiform seizures. Another manifestation of the irritating properties of penicillin may be the nausea, vomiting, and diarrhea that can occur with oral administration of any of the penicillins.

Some direct toxicities are not related to the penicillin molecule per se but to the formulation of drug employed. Thus, when penicillin G salts are administered in heroic doses, sodium may cause congestive heart failure and potassium may produce cardiac toxicity, especially in patients with renal impairment. Also, accidental intravascular injection of repository preparations may result in severe neurovascular damage and pulmonary infarction.

The use of penicillin may lead to superinfections by nonsusceptible bacteria, yeasts, and fungi. The development of superinfection in the course of treatment with penicillin (or other antimicrobial agents) is related to the antibacterial spectrum of the antibiotic, the dose of the agent used, the duration of therapy, and the route of administration. The overall incidence of superinfection associated with the penicillins is approximately 1%. There is a higher rate, however, with the extended-spectrum penicillins (e.g., ampicillin and amoxicillin). The incidence of superinfection is also higher after oral than after parenteral administration. Adverse effects of the penicillins and other antibiotics are outlined in Table 37-5.

Penicillinase-resistant penicillins

Bacteria, particularly staphylococci, develop resistance to the penicillins chiefly through the elaboration of β-lactamase enzymes (penicillinases) that inactivate the penicillins by cleavage of the 6-APA nucleus to yield penicilloic acid derivatives. Methicillin was the first semisynthetic derivative to be introduced that was stable in the presence of β-lactamase. Subsequently, nafcillin and three isoxazolyl derivatives (oxacillin, cloxacillin, and dicloxacillin) were marketed. The structural formulas for these semisynthetic derivatives are shown in Table 37-1.

Mechanism of action and antibacterial spectrum. The mechanism of action of these agents is the same as that of penicillin G. The antibacterial spectrum is also similar except that the penicillinase-resistant derivatives are highly effective against penicillinase-producing *S. aureus,* they are much less active against other gram-positive species, and they have no activity against gram-negative microorganisms. Therefore, their principal use is in the treatment of infections caused by penicillin G–resistant staphylococci.

Bacterial resistance. There have been increasing numbers of reports of methicillin-resistant staphylococci. The exact mechanism by which this resistance develops is not known, but such resistance is of clinical importance because cross-resistance occurs to all other penicillin derivatives, the cephalosporins, and frequently aminoglycosides, tetracyclines, and a variety of other antibiotics.[58,70] Resistance to methicillin is believed to be an infective resistance, but it is not associated with enzyme elaboration.

Absorption, fate, and excretion. Methicillin is acid labile and must be given parenterally. Its distribution in the body is similar to that of penicillin G, and it is excreted unchanged via renal tubular secretion. Nafcillin may be administered orally, but absorption is variable. Nafcillin is unique among the penicillins in that it is primarily excreted via the bile.

The isoxazolyl derivatives have the advantage of relatively good stability in acid media and are the preferred penicillinase-resistant penicillins for oral administration. Dicloxacillin is better absorbed from the gastrointestinal tract than the other derivatives. Although the isoxazolyl derivatives are excreted mainly by renal tubular secretion, there is significant biliary excretion and some hepatic biotransformation. In patients with impaired renal

Table 37-5. Select adverse effects of antimicrobial agents

Antimicrobial agent	Adverse effects*		
	Frequent	*Occasional*	*Rare*
Penicillins	Allergic reactions, skin rash (ampicillin and amoxicillin), diarrhea (ampicillin mainly)	Gastrointestinal disturbances, hemolytic anemia	Anaphylactic shock, seizures (with high doses of penicillin G), pseudomembranous colitis, hepatotoxic reactions, platelet dysfunction (carbenicillin and ticarcillin), granulocytopenia, agranulocytosis, renal damage
Cephalosporins	Thrombophlebitis (IV administration), allergic reactions (serum sickness after prolonged parenteral use and responses in patients allergic to penicillin especially common)	Gastrointestinal disturbances (frequent after oral administration)	Anaphylactic shock, hemolytic anemia, hepatic dysfunction, blood dyscrasias, nephrotoxicity, pseudomembranous colitis
Erythromycin	Gastrointestinal disturbances	Stomatitis, cholestatic hepatitis (primarily with erythromycin estolate)	Allergic reactions, pseudomembranous colitis
Tetracyclines	Gastrointestinal disturbances, hypoplasia and staining of calcifying tissue	Malabsorption, superinfections and pseudomembranous colitis, photosensitivity (demeclocycline usually), vestibular toxicity (minocycline), azotemia and other metabolic disturbances during renal insufficiency (except doxycycline and minocycline), hepatotoxicity during pregnancy or renal dysfunction	Allergic reactions, blood dyscrasias, increased intracranial pressure in infants, diabetes insipidus (demeclocycline), prolonged bleeding time (demeclocycline mainly), fixed-drug eruptions, blurred vision, photoonycholysis
Lincomycin	Diarrhea (particularly when given orally)	Allergic reactions, pseudomembranous colitis	Anaphylaxis, blood dyscrasias, superinfections with yeasts and fungi, nausea and vomiting after oral administration
Clindamycin	Diarrhea, allergic reactions	Pseudomembranous colitis	Blood dyscrasias, superinfections with yeasts and fungi, nausea and vomiting after oral administration
Vancomycin	Thrombophlebitis, chills, fever	Ototoxicity (auditory mainly)	Peripheral neuropathy, allergic reactions including anaphylaxis (mainly skin rashes), superinfections
Metronidazole	Gastrointestinal disturbances, headache, dry mouth	Diarrhea, insomnia, stomatitis, paresthesias	Encephalopathy, ataxia, pseudomembranous colitis
Aminoglycosides	Fever (streptomycin)	Vestibular toxicity (frequent with streptomycin), auditory toxicity, nephrotoxicity, allergic reactions (mainly skin rash, most frequent with topical use, e.g., neomycin)	Neuromuscular blockade, polyneuropathy, neurotoxicity

Modified from Abramowicz, M., ed. The Medical Letter on Drugs and Therapeutics, Handbook of Antimicrobial Therapy, New York, The Medical Letter, Inc., 1982.

*Listing does not include all adverse effects exhibited by these drugs.

Continued.

Table 37-5. Select adverse effects of antimicrobial agents—cont'd

Antimicrobial agent	Adverse effects		
	Frequent	*Occasional*	*Rare*
Sulfonamides	Allergic reactions	Kernicterus in neonates, nephrotoxicity, hepatic damage, Stevens-Johnson syndrome (long-acting sulfonamides), hemolytic anemia and other blood dyscrasias, crystalluria (particularly with older sulfonamides), gastrointestinal disturbances	Superinfections and pseudomembranous colitis, acute myopia
Chloramphenicol		Blood dyscrasias, gastrointestinal disturbances, "gray syndrome" in infants, superinfections	Aplastic anemia, peripheral neuropathy, optic neuritis and other neurotoxicities, blood clotting disorders (mainly after oral use), pseudomembranous colitis
Polymyxins (parenteral)		Nephrotoxicity, peripheral neuropathy, thrombophlebitis with IV use	Allergic reactions, neuromuscular blockade, superinfections
Bacitracin (parenteral)	Nephrotoxicity, gastrointestinal disturbances, pain at injection site	Blood dyscrasias, rash	
Nystatin (topical)		Gastrointestinal disturbances, allergic reactions	
Amphotericin B (parenteral)	Nephrotoxicity, hypokalemia, thrombophlebitis, nausea and vomiting, fever and chills	Anemia, hypomagnesemia	Hemorrhagic gastroenteritis, blood dyscrasias, allergic reactions, neurotoxicity, hepatotoxicity, arrhythmias and cardiac arrest
Ketoconazole	Nausea, vomiting, abdominal pain	Pruritus, headache, dizziness, photophobia, diarrhea, jaundice, chills and fever, gynecomastia, abdominal pain	Hepatotoxicity

function, reduction in the dosage of the isoxazolyl penicillins is not required.[2]

Therapeutic uses. The major indication for the use of penicillinase-resistant penicillin derivatives, in medicine or dentistry, is in the treatment of infections caused by strains of penicillinase-producing *S. aureus.* Because of the high percentage of staphylococcal infections caused by such resistant strains, initial treatment of a known staphylococcal infection, in patients not allergic to penicillin, should be with one of these derivatives until the results of bacteriologic testing have been obtained. If the organism is susceptible to penicillin V, therapy should be changed and treatment continued with penicillin V or G. Occasionally, an oral infection is caused by penicillinase-producing staphylococci, but only if such a bacterial cause is strongly suspected should treatment start with a penicillinase-resistant drug. Because these penicillins can actually induce the elaboration of penicillinase by microorganisms, particularly when subinhibitory concentrations are achieved, and because they have less antibacterial activity than do penicillins G and V, they should never be used routinely and should be restricted to treatment of infections caused by resistant strains of staphylococci. Table 37-4 lists the preparations currently available.

Toxic reactions and side effects. The penicillinase-resistant derivatives can produce the same untoward reactions as penicillins G and V. In addition, methicillin has been associated with the highest incidence of interstitial nephritis occurring during therapy with any of the penicillin derivatives. Apparently this condition is the result of a type II allergic reaction. Methicillin has also been associated, but rarely, with bone marrow depression. High doses of oxacillin have caused hepatitis.

Extended-spectrum penicillins

There are two groups of penicillin derivatives to which the term *extended spectrum* may be applied. One group includes ampicillin, the first extended-spectrum penicillin to be introduced, amoxicillin and cyclacillin, close congeners of ampicillin, and hetacillin and bacampicillin, drugs that are rapidly hydrolyzed in vivo to yield ampicillin (which accounts for their pharmacologic and toxicologic effects).

The second group contains carbenicillin, the first penicillin to demonstrate activity against *Pseudomonas* and indole-positive *Proteus* species, ticarcillin and azlocillin, drugs with improved activity against *Pseudomonas aeruginosa,* and mezlocillin and piperacillin, which enjoy the broadest spectrums of activity of all the penicillins. The molecular structures of these agents are depicted in Table 37-1.

Mechanism of action and antibacterial spectrum. The extended-spectrum penicillins inhibit cell wall synthesis in a manner similar to that of penicillin G. Their enhanced activity against gramnegative organisms may be due to their ability to penetrate the lipid barriers and the more complex cell wall of such microorganisms so that they can ultimately reach their site of action on the enzymes located on the outer side of the lipoprotein bacterial cell membrane.[58]

Ampicillin and related drugs are slightly less active against gram-positive cocci than is penicillin G, with the exception that they are twice as potent against enterococci. In addition to the organisms previously cited as sensitive to conventional doses of penicillin G, ampicillin is effective against the following gram-negative bacilli: *Haemophilus influenzae, E. coli, Proteus mirabilis, Salmonella,* and *Shigella.*

The mechanism of action and antibacterial spectrum of carbenicillin and ticarcillin are similar to those of ampicillin, with the exception that their activity includes *Pseudomonas* and *Proteus* species and some strains of *H. influenzae* and *E. coli* resistant to ampicillin. However, their activity is inferior to that of penicillin G and ampicillin against microorganisms susceptible to these agents.

Mezlocillin and piperacillin have a broader range of activity against gram-negative aerobic and anaerobic organisms than do carbenicillin or ticarcillin. The antibacterial spectrum of these drugs resembles that of the aminoglycosides, with additional activity against *Bacteroides fragilis.* These two agents exhibit excellent activity against *Klebsiella* species and are much more active than carbenicillin against *Pseudomonas,* piperacillin being the most active of all the penicillins against this genus. Their action against enterococci is similar to that of ampicillin.[23,38]

Table 37-2 indicates the various infections against which these agents would be a drug of first choice or an alternate drug.

Bacterial resistance. Many strains of *E. coli* (20% to 40%) have developed resistance to ampicillin. Episome-mediated resistance in *Salmonella* is relatively widespread; a number of strains of *P. mirabilis* and most species of *Shigella* are currently resistant. Also, a small percentage of *H. influenzae* strains are insensitive to ampicillin. Bacterial resistance is said to develop particularly rapidly to carbenicillin if only suboptimal concentrations are achieved. All extended-spectrum penicillins are inactivated by penicillinase. Therefore, penicillinase-producing strains of *E. coli* and *S. aureus* are not susceptible to these agents. Penicillinase-producing strains of *Neisseria gonorrhoeae* do not inactivate piperacillin or mezlocillin and are thus susceptible to these newer penicillin derivatives.[23]

Absorption, fate, and excretion. Ampicillin and related agents are stable in acid media and are well absorbed after oral administration. Although ampicillin and hetacillin are best absorbed on an empty stomach, food does not interfere with the absorption of amoxicillin, bacampicillin, and cyclacillin. Because of its better absorption, the duration of action of amoxicillin is twice as long as for ampicillin.[66] For this reason, amoxicillin is administered only 3 times daily. Orally administered doses of bacampicillin produce higher plasma concentrations than equivalent doses of either ampicillin or amoxicillin, and it is administered twice daily. This agent is completely hydrolyzed to ampicillin after absorption. Cyclacillin produces peak plasma concentrations 4 and 1.5 times higher than ampicillin and amoxicillin, respectively, but it is considerably less bactericidal. The carbenicillin-like penicillins must be given parenterally, since they are not absorbed from the gastrointestinal tract. The indanyl ester of carbenicillin, though, is absorbed after oral administration and is then hydrolyzed in vivo to yield active carbenicillin.

Excretion of the extended spectrum derivatives is similar to that for penicillin G; they have a plasma half-life of about 1½ hours. Ampicillin and some of the other extended-spectrum penicillins are partially eliminated through biliary excretion.

Therapeutic uses. The therapeutic usefulness of ampicillin-like compounds is chiefly in the treatment of susceptible gram-negative infections or mixed infections consisting of susceptible gram-positive and gram-negative microorganisms. Since these drugs are less active than penicillin G and congeners against gram-positive bacteria (with the exception of enterococcci), they should not be used as a substitute for penicillin G or V. Ampicillin and related derivatives have proved to be very useful for the treatment of urinary tract infections caused by susceptible strains of *E. coli, P. mirabilis,* and enterococci, partly because the renal tubular secretion of the penicillins provides very high concentrations of active antibiotic in the urine. These derivatives are also useful for respiratory infections in which *H. influenzae* is one of the etiologic factors and for some infections caused by *Shigella* and *Salmonella.* Because of problems of bacterial resistance, sensitivity testing is, of course, necessary. Ampicillin and amoxicillin are the oral drugs of choice for the treatment of gonococcal infections. They are also useful in orodental infections known to be caused by susceptible gram-negative organisms or involving both gram-negative and gram-positive organisms, especially if the oral route is preferred.

Carbenicillin and related agents are recommended for treatment of urinary tract and other infections caused by susceptible *Pseudomonas* species; they are often used in combination with an aminoglycoside. They have also been used in infections caused by indole-positive *Proteus* and ampicillin-resistant Enterobacteriaceae. They are never used as substitutes for penicillin G or ampicillin when the infecting microorganisms are susceptible to these drugs, and they have essentially no place in the treatment of dental infections.

Toxic reactions and side effects. The toxicity of these derivatives is essentially similar to that of other penicillins. Because greater changes in the oral and intestinal microflora occur with the extended-spectrum penicillins, however, superinfections are more likely to develop. Ampicillin and amoxicillin have been associated with pseudomembranous colitis.

Ampicillin produces the highest incidence of skin rash (about 9%) of any of the penicillin derivatives. The rate may be as high as 20% when it is administered to patients taking allopurinol and almost invariably occurs in patients with lymphatic leukemia or infectious mononucleosis.[58] Such eruptions are presumably caused by direct toxicity and not by allergic phenomena. Ampicillin has also been implicated in agranulocytosis and bone-marrow histiocytosis, both of which are probably caused by direct toxic effects of the drug.

The carbenicillin-like penicillins inhibit platelet aggregation and may produce hemorrhagic manifestions.[28] Carbenicillin and ticarcillin must be given in very large parenteral doses, and, since they are prepared in the form of disodium salts, electrolyte imbalances leading to congestive heart failure may occur. This problem is less likely to occur with piperacillin and the ureidopenicillins (azlocillin and mezlocillin) because they contain less sodium. Ticarcillin has been shown to be teratogenic in mice; this drug is therefore contraindicated in pregnant women.

CEPHALOSPORINS

Although the cephalosporins are used much less in dentistry than are penicillins, they are widely used in medicine and are the antibiotics most frequently administered for prophylaxis in hospital patients undergoing surgery. Currently, more than a dozen cephalosporin derivatives have been marketed in the United States, and more are under investigation. It is likely that some of the newer cephalosporins will be recognized as drugs of first choice for therapy of selected infections as more experience is gained with their use.

Chemistry and classification

Three distinct cephalosporin antibiotics are biosynthesized by the fungus *Cephalosporium acremonium,* which was isolated in 1948 from the sea near a sewer outlet off Sardinia. The currently available cephalosporins are semisynthetic derivatives of the basic nucleus of cephalosporin C, 7-aminocephalosporanic acid, to which side chains are attached at two different positions (Figure 37-4). The intact nucleus is necessary for activity; the different side chains confer certain pharmacologic properties, such as acid stability. The cephalosporin nucleus differs from the penicillin nucleus (6-APA) only in having a six-membered dihydrothiazine ring, rather than the five-membered thiazolidine ring. The structural similarity to the

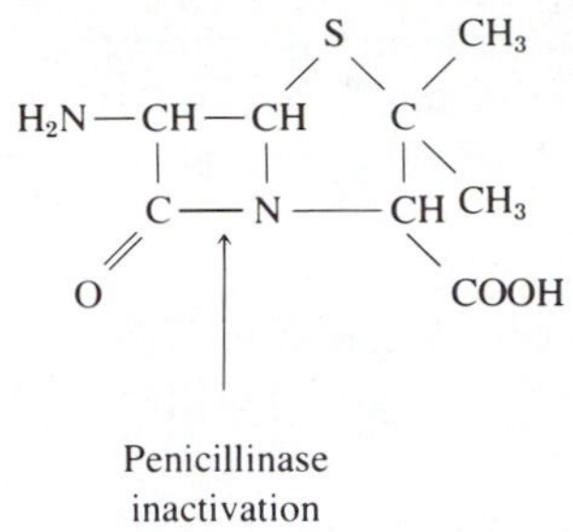

6-Aminopenicillanic acid

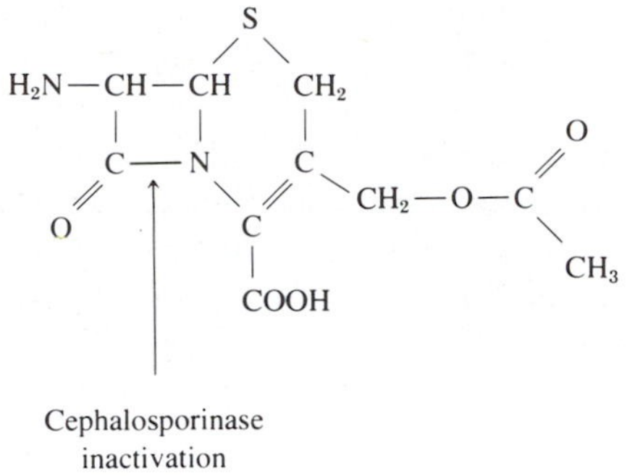

7-Aminocephalosporanic acid

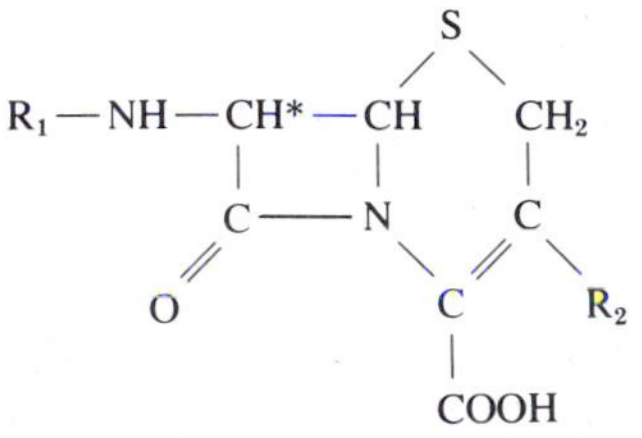

General structure of
cephalosporin derivatives

Figure 37-4. Comparison of basic nuclei of penicillins and cephalosporins. *Hydrogen replaced by a methoxy group in cephamycins.

penicillins accounts for many of the pharmacologic and toxicologic properties shared by these two seemingly different groups of antimicrobial agents. The cephalosporin derivatives, like the methicillin-type penicillins, are not hydrolyzed by penicillinase. However, certain bacteria produce β-lactamases, called cephalosporinases, which hydrolyze the β-lactam ring and inactivate these compounds. Some bacteria produce a single β-lactamase that degrades both penicillins and cephalosporins.

The cephamycins are derived from a natural antibiotic substance, cephamycin C, which is pro-

duced by *Streptomyces lactamdurans*. These compounds contain a methoxy group in the 7-α position of the β-lactam ring that confers a high degree of resistance to inactivation by β-lactamase enzymes such as the penicillinases and cephalosporinases. Cefoxitin, a semisynthetic derivative of cephamycin C, is the only 7-methoxylated cephalosporin derivative in current use. Moxalactam, a β-lactam antibiotic, is similar structurally to the cephalosporins except that the sulfur in the dihydrothiazine ring is replaced by an oxygen and an α-methoxy group is attached to the β-lactam ring.

Mechanism of action and antibacterial spectrum

The cephalosporins, like the penicillins, bind covalently to enzymes involved with the cross-linking of the peptidoglycan strands composing the bacterial cell wall. Also like the penicillins, cephalosporins are bactericidal to susceptible multiplying bacterial cells.

A variety of cephalosporins have appeared, and they are currently classified as first-, second-, or third-generation drugs, based on their spectrum of antibacterial activity as well as the sequence of their development. The first generation, represented by cephalothin, cefazolin, cephapirin, cephradine, cephalexin, and cefadroxil, are active against gram-positive cocci, including most staphylococci and streptococci (but not enterococci), and many strains of gram-negative bacilli, including *E. coli, Klebsiella pneumoniae,* and *P. mirabilis.* Second-generation drugs of this class (cefamandole, cefoxitin, cefaclor, and cefuroxime) exhibit a wider antibacterial spectrum in vitro than do first-generation drugs. As a group, they are slightly less active against gram-positive bacteria[36] but are more effective against bacteria characteristically resistant to earlier cephalosporins, such as indole-positive *Proteus* and *Providencia* and cephalosporin-resistant strains of *E. coli* and *Klebsiella.* The third-generation cephalosporins (cefotaxime, moxalactam, cefoperazone, and ceftizoxime) are generally less active against gram-positive cocci but are highly bactericidal against *H. influenzae* and exhibit better activity than other cephalosporins against enterococci and a number of anaerobes, including *B. fragilis,* a gram-negative rod highly resistant to a number of commonly used antibiotics.[8,44,60] They also are effective against *Serratia, Citrobacter,* and various strains of *Pseudomonas.*[9,60,69] This increased activity is mainly a result of their resistance to inactivation by the β-lactamases.[36,44]

Although the classification of cephalosporins according to generation is generally useful, it must be recognized that there are some important differences within each group. For instance, in the second-generation drugs, cefaclor is less active against gram-negative bacilli than are the other agents. Cefoxitin, but not cefamandole, is effective against *B. fragilis;* the reverse is true with regard to *Enterobacter.*[75] There are also pharmacokinetic dissimilarities among the various drugs that can affect clinical use. Cefaclor, for example, is orally effective, whereas the other drugs are not.

Bacterial resistance

A small but growing percentage of the clinical isolates of *S. aureus* are resistant to the cephalosporins, even though none of these compounds is inactivated by staphylococcal penicillinase. However, as was mentioned above, there are cephalosporinases that inactviate the cephalosporins through cleavage of the β-lactam ring. Bacterial synthesis of cephalosporinases constitutes a major mechanism for acquired resistance to these drugs. Another is decreased permeability of the bacterial cell wall. There appears to be little cross-resistance between the cephalosporins and the penicillins, except with staphylococci that have developed resistance to methicillin-type antibiotics; here, definite cross-resistance occurs between the cephalosporins and the penicillinase-stable penicillin derivatives.

Absorption, fate, and excretion

Some of the first-generation and one of the currently available second-generation cephalosporins are acid stable and are absorbed well enough from the gastrointestinal tract to be orally effective (Table 37-6). All of the third-generation drugs, including those under investigation, are administered parenterally. Intramuscular injection of some of these agents causes intense pain; for this reason the intravenous route is preferred for many of the cephalosporins. Once in the circulation, the cephalosporins are variably bound to plasma proteins (10% to 15% for cephalexin, 82% to 93% for cefoperazone) and well distributed to most body tissues and fluids, with highest concentrations being found in the kidneys and liver. Most of the first- and second-generation cephalosporins do not enter the cerebrospinal fluid, even when the meninges are inflamed;

however, cefuroxime and the third-generation drugs cefotaxime and moxalactam do achieve therapeutic concentrations in inflamed meninges. Cephalexin, cefamandole, and several other cephalosporins may reach therapeutic concentrations in bone after administration of usual doses. In fact, cephalexin may achieve enough concentration in alveolar bone to be bactericidal to certain gram positive aerobic bacteria found in dental infections.[56] The cephalosporins are secreted into the milk of nursing mothers and readily cross the placenta.

Some of the cephalosporins (e.g., cephalothin) are metabolized to less active compounds that are then excreted by the kidneys; the others are mainly eliminated unchanged, either by glomerular filtration or by a combination of filtration and renal tubular secretion. Since concentrations of intact drug or active metabolites in the urine are high, they are useful for treating urinary tract infections caused by susceptible microorganisms. Dosages of the cephalosporins (with the exception of cefaclor and cefoperazone) should be reduced in patients with impaired renal function.

General therapeutic uses

Although the cephalosporins are very popular for prophylactic use in medicine, they are not generally regarded as drugs of first choice for any established infections except perhaps those caused by susceptible *Klebsiella.* They have been used together with an aminoglycoside such as gentamicin for treatment of severe hospital-acquired pneumonia and intraabdominal infections before and, when appropriate, after bacteriologic testing. Most other infections caused by bacteria susceptible to a cephalosporin can be as effectively (and usually much more cheaply) treated with one of the penicillin derivatives. The broader-spectrum cephalosporins should be reserved for situations in which their special properties are needed. These include gram-negative meningitis and septicemia (where *Pseudomonas* is not suspected).

Therapeutics used in dentistry

Several studies indicate that odontogenic infections caused by the genus *Klebsiella* occur in about 4% of patients and that these bacteria compose approximately 2% of all species of microorganisms isolated from various kinds of dental infections.[25,45] A cephalosporin would be an appropriate antibiotic for those rare infections known to be caused by a cephalosporin-susceptible strain of

Table 37-6. Commercially available cephalosporin preparations

Nonproprietary name	Proprietary name	Usual adult dose	Route	Preparations
First generation				
Cephalothin sodium	Keflin	4-12 gm/day	IV	Vials: 1, 2, 4, and 20 gm
		500 mg-1 gm every 4-6 hours	IM	
Cefazolin sodium	Ancef, Kefzol	250 mg-1.5 gm every 6-8 hours	IV, IM	Vials: 250 and 500 mg, 1, 5, and 10 gm
Cephapirin sodium	Cefadyl	500 mg-1 gm every 4-6 hours	IV, IM	Vials: 500 mg, 1, 2, 4, and 20 gm
Cephradine	Anspor, Velosef	250 mg-500 mg every 6 hours	Oral	Capsules: 250 and 500 mg Tablets: 1 gm Oral suspension: 125 and 250 mg/5 ml
		500 mg-1 gm every 6 hours	IV, IM	Vials: 250 and 500 mg, 1 gm Infusion bottles: 2 and 4 gm
Cephalexin	Keflex	250 mg-1 gm every 6 hours	Oral	Capsules: 250 and 500 mg Tablets: 1 gm Oral suspension: 125, 250/5 ml
Cefadroxil	Duricef, Ultracef	1-2 gm every day in 1 or 2 doses	Oral	Capsules: 500 mg Tablets: 1 gm Oral suspension: 125, 250/5 ml
Second generation				
Cefamandole nafate	Mandol	500 mg-1 gm every 4-8 hours (up to 2 gm every 4 hours in life-threatening infections)	IV, IM	Vials: 500 mg, 1 and 2 gm
Cefoxitin sodium	Mefoxin	1-2 gm every 6-8 hours	IV, IM	Vials: 1 and 2 gm
Cefuroxime sodium	Zinacef	750 mg-1.5 gm every 6-8 hours (up to 9 gm every day for meningitis)	IV, IM	Vials: 750 mg and 1.5 gm Infusion bottles: 1.5 gm
Cefaclor	Ceclor	250 mg-1 gm every 8 hours	Oral	Capsules: 250 and 500 mg Oral suspension: 125 and 250 mg/5 ml
Third generation				
Cefotaxime sodium	Claforan	1-2 gm every 6-12 hours (up to 2 gm every 4 hours in life-threatening infections)	IV, IM	Vials: 500 mg, 1 and 2 gm
Moxalactam disodium	Moxam	500 mg-2 gm every 8-12 hours (up to 4 gm every 8 hours in life-threatening infections)	IV, IM	Vials: 1 and 2 gm
Cefoperazone sodium	Cefobid	1-2 gm every 12 hours (up to 4 gm every 8 hours in life-threatening infections)	IV, IM	Vials: 1 and 2 gm
Ceftizoxime sodium	Cefizox	1-2 gm every 8-12 hours (up to 3-4 gm every 8 hours in life-threatening infections)	IV, IM	Vials: 1 and 2 gm

Klebsiella. The cephalosporin derivatives, being broad-spectrum and bactericidal, could also be useful for dental infections in which ampicillin would be used, except for those infections involving spirochetes (e.g., Vincent's stomatitis). They might also be used for treating a penicillinase-producing staphylococcal infection in patients who have a history of allergic responses of the nonimmediate type to penicillin.

Toxic reactions and side effects

Like the penicillins, the cephalosporins are relatively nontoxic antibiotics. The most common systemic adverse effect is drug allergy similar to that associated with the use of penicillins. In fact, there is an increased risk of an allergic reaction to the cephalosporins if the patient has a history of penicillin allergy. It is conservatively estimated that cross-reactions between penicillins and cephalosporins occur at a frequency of about 8%. Although cephalosporins can generally be employed without mishap in patients who exhibited nonacute allergic reactions to penicillin, they should not be administered to patients with a history of immediate-onset allergy to penicillin unless a suitable alternative is not available and the need for medication is great.

Gastrointestinal symptoms, particularly after oral administration, include anorexia, nausea, vomiting, and diarrhea. Pseudomembranous colitis caused by *Clostridium difficile* has also been reported, and its appearance mandates the immediate discontinuance of the drug. It has already been noted that intramuscular injection of some of the cephalosporins causes severe pain; thrombophlebitis has also resulted from intravenous administration. Some less common toxicities include reversible renal impairment (which may require a reduction in dosage for certain patients), hepatic dysfunction, and blood dyscrasias. Cefamandole, cefoperazone, and particularly moxalactam have caused hypoprothrombinemia and prolonged prothrombin time, which can be reversed by vitamin K.[7,44] Interference with platelet function compounds the hemostatic defect. These three agents also may produce alcohol intolerance similar to that caused by disulfiram.

ERYTHROMYCIN

The use of erythromycin for treatment of common orodental infections of bacterial origin is second only to that of the penicillin derivatives. Erythromycin was discovered in 1952 and is produced by a strain of *Streptomyces erythreus* isolated from a soil sample obtained in the Philippine Islands. As its name implies (''erythros,'' red), this species of *Streptomyces* possesses a characteristic red color. Since its introduction, erythromycin has proved valuable in the treatment of a number of infections and has exhibited a relative lack of toxicity.

Chemistry

Erythromycin is one of several ''macrolide'' antibiotics. Structurally, the macrolides contain a many-membered lactone ring to which various deoxy sugars or amino acids or both, are attached

(Figure 37-5). Other macrolide antibiotics that have been employed clinically include spiramycin, oleandomycin, and troleandomycin; only erythromycin and troleandomycin are available at the present time. Spiramycin has been used in Canada and Europe for treatment of plaque diseases such as periodontitis (Chapter 42). Erythromycin is a bitter, yellow-white crystalline substance that is poorly soluble in water but soluble in polar organic solvents. It readily forms salts with various acids and yields esters with organic acids.

Mechanisms of action and antibacterial spectrum

As described in Chapter 36, erythromycin acts by inhibiting protein synthesis in susceptible microorganisms. It binds to the 50 S subunit of the bacterial ribosome at a site presumably the same as, or near to, the binding site for lincomycin, clindamycin, and chloramphenicol, since these antibiotics interfere with its binding.[13] The intracellular concentration of erythromycin that can be achieved in gram-positive bacteria is approximately 100 times that obtained in gram-negative bacteria, which may explain its effectiveness in the former and ineffectiveness in the latter category of microorganisms. Erythromycin usually exhibits bacteriostatic activity against susceptible organisms.

The antibacterial spectrum of erythromycin is similar, but not identical, to that of penicillin G. Although generally considered a narrow-spectrum antibiotic, erythromycin exhibits activity against a number of microorganisms, such as *Mycoplasma, Rickettsia,* and *Chlamydia,* which are not affected by penicillin G. Like other antibacterial drugs, erythromycin does not exhibit activity against yeasts, fungi, or true viruses.

Bacterial resistance

One of the major disadvantages of erythromycin is that bacteria, particularly staphylococci, rapidly develop resistance to this antibiotic. In fact, the rapidity with which staphylococci acquire stepwise resistance to erythromycin is second only to that observed with streptomycin. Resistance has also been shown to occur with strains of *Streptococcus pneumoniae,* the viridans streptococci, enterococci, *Streptococcus pyogenes,* and *H. influenzae.* Half of the strains of *S. aureus* isolated from hospital patients are resistant to erythromycin. Presumably the resistant bacteria have undergone mu-

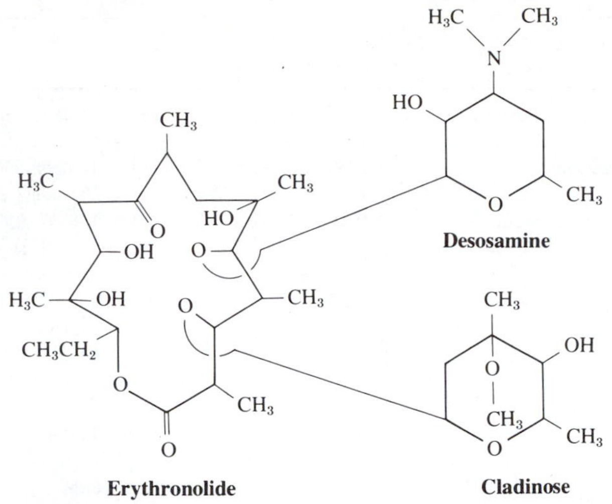

Figure 37-5. Structural formula of erythromycin.

tation so that their ribosomes no longer bind to this drug. Cross-resistance occurs with other macrolide antibiotics. Moreover, certain strains of strepto-cocci (including some viridans streptococci) that have acquired resistance to erythromycin are also resistant to lincomycin and clindamycin.[62] Other-wise there is little cross-resistance between eryth-romycin and other antimicrobial drugs.

Because of the rapidity with which resistance develops, it is necessary that erythromycin be ad-ministered with complete patient compliance and that adequate dosage and duration of therapy be maintained. Since erythromycin is usually bacte-riostatic, it is especially important that effective inhibitory concentrations of the drug be maintained at the site of infection.

Absorption, fate, and excretion

Erythromycin is normally administered orally, but the absorption of active drug is dependent on protection of erythromycin from destruction by the acidity of the gastric contents. The drug is manu-factured in the form of capsules or tablets with acid-insoluble films (enteric-coated preparations) or in the form of water-insoluble salts (stearate) and esters (ethylsuccinate, estolate). Any of these formulations (Table 37-7) can provide adequate amounts of bioavailable drug. Erythromycin in the free base and stearate salt forms is best absorbed on an empty stomach. Occasionally, because of gastrointestinal problems, it is necessary for the patient to take the drug with a small amount of food. In such instances, one of the erythromycin esters or an enteric-coated formulation of the free base is indicated, because absorption of these agents is unimpeded by food.[22]

Erythromycin is well distributed to most soft tissues. It does not readily cross the blood-brain barrier except in the presence of inflammation of the meninges, in which case the concentration of erythromycin in the cerebrospinal fluid may ap-proach 25% of the plasma concentration. Eryth-romycin penetrates well into abscesses, such as those associated with orodental infections, and crosses the placenta, the fetal plasma concentration approaching 20% of the maternal value.

In the presence of normal hepatic function, erythromycin is concentrated in the liver and ex-creted in the bile, mainly in an active form. Fecal concentrations may reach 0.5 mg/gm after the oral administration of large doses. Less than 5% of a dose of erythromycin is excreted unchanged in the urine, and the antibiotic may be used safely in the presence of renal dysfunction.

General therapeutic uses

Erythromycin is an excellent alternative anti-biotic to penicillin G and is a drug of choice for treating many infections for which penicillin is in-dicated but cannot be used because of drug allergy. In this regard, it is principally used as a second line of defense against a number of infections

Table 37-7. Commercially available erythromycin preparations

Nonproprietary name	Proprietary name	Usual adult dose	Route	Preparations
Erythromycin (film-coated)	Erythromycin Base Filmtabs	250-500 mg every 6 hours	Oral	Tablets: 250 and 500 mg
Erythromycin (enteric-coated)	E-Mycin, Ilotycin	250-500 mg every 6 hours	Oral	Tablets: 250, 333, and 500 mg Capsules: 250 mg
Erythromycin stearate	Erythrocin Stearate	250-500 mg every 6 hours	Oral	Tablets: 250 and 500 mg
Erythromycin ethylsuccinate	E.E.S., Pediamycin	400-800 mg every 6 hours	Oral	Chewable tablets: 200 mg Tablets: 400 mg Oral suspension: 200 and 400 mg/5 ml Powder for oral suspension: 100, 200, and 400 mg/5 ml
Erythromycin estolate	Ilosone	250-500 mg every 6 hours	Oral	Chewable tablets: 125 and 250 mg Tablets: 250 and 500 mg Capsules: 125 and 250 mg Oral suspension: 125 and 250 mg/5 ml Powder for oral suspension: 125 mg/5 ml Pediatric drops: 100 mg/ml
Erythromycin lactobionate	Erythrocin Lactobionate-IV	15-20 mg/kg/day, up to 4 gm/day	IV	Vials: 500 mg and 1 gm
Erythromycin gluceptate	Ilotycin Gluceptate	15-20 mg/kg/day, up to 4 gm/day	IV	Vials: 250 and 500 mg, 1 gm

caused by gram-positive organisms. Erythromycin is the drug of first choice for the treatment of infections caused by cell wall–deficient microorganisms (e.g., *Mycoplasma*), which are not affected by the penicillins or other antibiotics that interfere with cell wall synthesis. Erythromycin is also indicated for *Corynebacterium* infections and Legionnaire's disease, and it is useful in the prophylaxis against bacterial endocarditis in penicillin-allergic patients. The drug should not be used for prophylaxis, however, in patients who are undergoing procedures involving the genitourinary tract, because most of the organisms there are not susceptible to erythromycin.

Therapeutic uses in dentistry

Erythromycin is second only to the penicillins for the treatment of dental infections. Although clinical effectiveness in control of orodental infections is generally good with erythromycin, it occupies a secondary position for several reasons: it is usually bacteriostatic rather than bactericidal, resistance can develop rapidly to erythromycin during treatment, and it is slightly inferior to the penicillins in eradicating most orodental infections. However, erythromycin provides an excellent alternative drug for treating infections in patients allergic to penicillin. Erythromycin is effective

against most of the aerobic gram-positive microorganisms that cause orodental infections, and it also exhibits good activity against many oral anaerobic bacteria. The drug has been successfully used for treating oral infections such as pericoronitis, periapical abscesses, periodontal abscesses, cellulitis, infected cysts, purulent osteitis, various forms of infectious stomatitis, and Vincent's stomatitis.

Erythromycin is generally the agent of choice for prophylactic coverage against bacterial endocarditis for a patient who is at risk and is allergic to penicillin. Patients who have prosthetic heart valves, though, should be given vancomycin, as is shown in Table 36-7.

Toxic reactions and side effects

Erythromycin is a remarkably safe antibiotic and causes relatively few adverse effects. Gastrointestinal disturbances caused by the irritative properties of the drug are the most commonly encountered problem. The frequency and severity of gastrointestinal upset are dose related, and symptoms include nausea, vomiting, epigastric distress, and diarrhea. (The latter may also be due to alterations in the intestinal microflora.) These reactions subside on discontinuance of the drug.

The immunogenic potential of erythromycin is

low, and allergic reactions occur infrequently, except with the estolate formulation. Pruritus, skin rashes, fever, and esosinophilia are the usual types of allergic actions encountered. Severe responses are rare but have occurred. There is no cross-allergenicity between erythromycin and other commonly used antibiotics.

A unique form of drug allergy, with a clinical picture consistent with that of cholestatic hepatitis, is produced by erythromycin estolate. The phenomenon is due to sensitization to the propionyl moiety of the estolate rather than to the erythromycin base. Clinical symptoms include malaise, nausea, vomiting, abdominal pain (which may be severe), and fever; jaundice may or may not be a clinical symptom. This reaction usually develops after 10 or more days of treatment with the estolate, but it has been known to occur early during therapy, even in patients without a history of a previous reaction to the agent. The reaction is not dose related, is reversible, subsides after withdrawal of the estolate, and reappears in sensitized patients on subsequent administration of the estolate dosage form.[68] Because this erythromycin preparation has no significant clinical advantage over the others, its use is not recommended. Similar hepatotoxic reactions have occurred rarely with erythromycin ethylsuccinate.[65] Clinically apparent superinfections associated with the use of erythromycin are infrequent, but oral candidiasis and pseudomembranous colitis have been reported.

TETRACYCLINES

The tetracyclines are a group of broad-spectrum, bacteriostatic antibiotics that have been employed extensively in the treatment of infections. Their widespread use, and often misuse, has resulted in the appearance of a number of bacterial strains that are resistant to these drugs, a fact that has curtailed their clinical usefulness. Chlortetracycline, a product of *Streptomyces aureofaciens,* was discovered as a result of the screening of soil samples for antibiotic-elaborating microorganisms and was, in 1948, the first tetracycline drug to be introduced. (It is now limited to topical use in the United States.) Shortly thereafter, oxytetracycline was discovered. After the elucidation of the basic structure of the tetracycline antibiotics, removal of the chlorine atom from chlortetracycline yielded tetracycline, clinically introduced in 1953. Subsequently, demeclocycline and the semisynthetic derivatives methacycline, doxycycline, and min-

ocycline were marketed. Table 37-8 lists the tetracycline preparations currently available.

Chemistry

The structure of tetracycline is shown in Figure 37-6. As is implied by the name ("tetra," four; "cycline," ring), all of the tetracyclines are derivatives of a four-ringed nucleus and differ structurally only with regard to the chemical moieties attached at the 2, 5, 6, and 7 positions of the nucleus. Various derivatives exhibit slightly different pharmacologic properties, such as differences in absorption, protein binding, metabolism, excretion, and degree of activity against susceptible microorganisms.

The tetracyclines form water-soluble sodium or hydrochloride salts. The anhydrous base and salt forms are relatively stable, but solutions of the tetracyclines undergo decomposition quite rapidly at elevated temperature or alkaline pH.

Mechanism of action and antibacterial spectrum

The tetracyclines inhibit protein synthesis by reversibly binding to the 30 S subunit of the bacterial ribosome in susceptible bacteria. These drugs are a prime example of truly broad-spectrum antibiotics (see Table 36-2). Their range of antimicrobial activity includes not only gram-positive and gram-negative bacteria (both aerobes and anaerobes) but also treponemes, *Chlamydia, Rickettsia,* and *Mycoplasma.* The tetracyclines exhibit greater activity against gram-positive microorganisms than against gram-negative, but the appearance of many resistant bacteria has detracted from their clinical usefulness in treating infections caused by gram-positive species. Such infections are usually more effectively treated with one of the penicillins or erythromycin. Some strains of anaerobic bacteria involved with oral infections are inhibited by tetracyclines, but many others show varying degrees of resistance.[46]

Bacterial resistance

Bacterial resistance to the tetracyclines develops in a slow, stepwise fashion similar to that occurring with the penicillin derivatives. Resistance appears to be caused by a decreased uptake of tetracyclines and in some cases by active extrusion of the drug from the bacterial cell. Decreased affinity of bacterial ribosomes for tetracyclines may also be involved. Infective resistance (mediated by R factors)

Table 37-8. Commercially available tetracycline preparations

Nonproprietary name	Proprietary name	Usual adult dose	Route	Preparations
Tetracycline hydro-chloride	Achromycin, Pan-mycin	250-500 mg every 12 hours	IV	Injection—IV: 250 and 500 mg vials
		250 mg every 24 hours	IM	Injection—IM: 100 and 250 mg vials (with procaine)
		250-500 mg every 6-12 hours	Oral	Capsules: 100, 250, and 500 mg Tablets: 250 and 500 mg Syrup: 125 mg/5 ml
Oxytetracycline hy-drochloride	Terramycin, Oxy-mycin	250-500 mg every 12 hours	IV	Injection—IV: 250 and 500 mg vials
		250 mg every 24 hours	IM	Injection—IM: 100 and 250 mg ampules, 500 mg vials (with lidocaine)
		250-500 mg every 6-12 hours	Oral	Capsules: 125 and 250 mg Tablets: 250 mg Syrup: 125 mg/5 ml
Demeclocycline hy-drochloride	Declomycin	150 mg every 6 hours or 300 mg every 12 hours	Oral	Capsules: 150 mg Tablets: 150 and 300 mg
Methacycline hy-drochloride	Rondomycin	150 mg every 6 hours or 300 mg every 12 hours	Oral	Capsules: 150 and 300 mg
Doxycycline hyclate	Vibramycin, Doxy-Tabs	200 mg first day followed by 100-200 mg daily	IV	Injection: 100 and 200 mg vials
		100 mg every 12 hours for first day followed by 100 mg daily	Oral	Capsules: 50 and 100 mg Tablets: 100 mg Suspension: 25 mg/5 ml Syrup: 50 mg/5 ml
Minocycline hydro-chloride	Minocin	200 mg initially followed by 100 mg every 12 hours not to exceed 400 mg/24 hours	IV	Injection: 100 mg vials
		200 mg initially followed by 100 mg every 12 hours	Oral	Capsules: 50 and 100 mg Tablets: 50 and 100 mg Syrup: 50 mg/5 ml

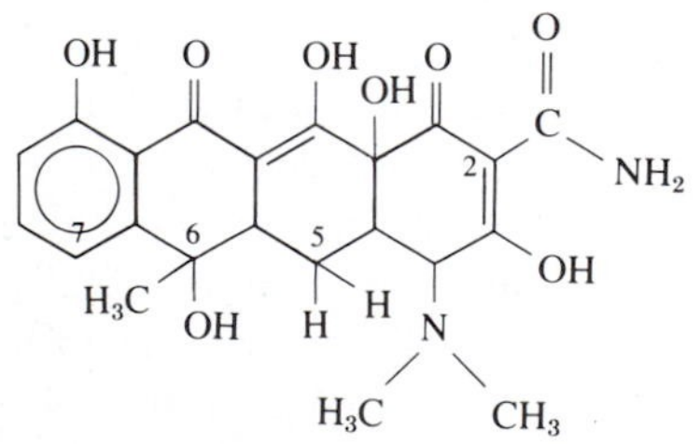

Figure 37-6. Structural formula of tetracycline.

has been shown to occur in some gram-negative bacteria.[21] A number of gram-positive bacteria, including many of those isolated from orodental infections, show varying degrees of resistance to the tetracyclines. Several studies indicate that as many as 14% of the strains of *S. pneumoniae,* 43% of *S. pyogenes,* and a number of *S. aureus* strains are resistant to the tetracyclines.[3,18,30] In three reports

of antibiotic efficacy in the treatment of orodental infections, 19% to 61% of the viridans streptococci were found to be resistant, as were 17% to 44% of strains of *S. aureus.*[25,31,73] The conclusion that can be drawn from the many studies of resistance to the tetracyclines is that the overall efficacy of these drugs for treatment of orodental infections is significantly less than that of the penicillins.

Absorption, fate, and excretion

The tetracyclines are usually administered orally. Absorption from the gastrointestinal tract is incomplete and variable, depending on the derivative, the individual patient, the presence of food in the stomach, concomitant administration of products containing divalent and trivalent cations, and alkalinity of the gastric contents. With the exception of minocycline and doxycycline, food retards the absorption of the tetracyclines. Although absorption is incomplete, in usual circumstances adequate plasma concentrations are obtained after oral administration of recommended doses during the fasting state. Doxycycline and minocycline are absorbed better from the gastrointestinal tract than the other tetracyclines. Because tetracyclines are bacteriostatic, antimicrobial concentrations at the site of infection must be maintained throughout the period of therapy.

The tetracyclines are bound in varying degrees to plasma proteins, with methacycline exhibiting the highest degree of binding (80% to 90%) and oxytetracycline the lowest (20% to 35%). They are well distributed into most body tissues and fluids, including saliva, prostatic fluid, pleural fluid, sweat, semen, and milk (which may contain 50% of the plasma concentration).[58] High concentrations of the tetracyclines are found in the skin. The tetracyclines penetrate, to a limited extent, into the cerebrospinal fluid, but when used for the treatment of meningitis, they must be given parenterally in high doses. These agents form complexes with calcium and are deposited along with calcium during calcification of bone, dentin, and enamel; such tetracyclines are not biologically active. The tetracyclines cross the placenta, and fetal concentrations may be relatively high.

To varying degrees, all of the tetracycline derivatives are removed from the blood by the liver, excreted into the gastrointestinal tract via the bile, and partially reabsorbed. The enterohepatic circulation of these drugs prolongs their blood concentrations for a considerable time after cessation of therapy. With the exception of minocycline, the tetracycline derivatives are essentially not biotransformed. Urinary excretion via glomerular filtration is the primary means of elimination of all the other tetracyclines except doxycycline, which is excreted in the feces (mainly as an inactive conjugate or chelate). In contrast to the other tetracyclines, doxycycline and minocycline may be administered with relative safety to patients with renal dysfunction. The rates of excretion, and therefore plasma half-lives, of the various tetracyclines exhibit significant differences. Tetracycline and oxytetracycline have half-lives ranging from 6 to 10 hours and are thus usually administered every 6 hours to maintain adequate antimicrobial concentrations during therapy. The more lipid soluble doxycycline and minocycline have half lives of 16 to 20 hours and are therefore administered in lower doses and less frequently.

General therapeutic uses

Although the tetracyclines have an unusually broad spectrum of activity, they are agents of first choice for treatment of only a few specific infections (Table 37-2). Many other bacteria nominally within their range of activity should not be treated, at least initially, with a tetracycline because of the large number of resistant strains. However, if susceptibility tests indicate sensitivity to the tetracyclines, they may be used against infections caused by such organisms as *E. coli, N. aerogenes,* and *Shigella* and *Treponema* species, respiratory tract infections caused by *H. influenzae,* and respiratory and urinary tract infections caused by susceptible strains of *Klebsiella* and enterococci.

The tetracyclines have been used in the treatment of severe acne. Although tetracyclines are concentrated in the skin and are effective against *Propionibacterium acne,* there is no definitive proof that any antibiotic therapy per se is beneficial in the treatment of acne. Indeed, benefits obtained with the use of tetracyclines in such conditions are more likely caused by an antiseborrheic action rather than by bacteriostasis. Superinfections and folliculitis may result from prolonged therapy with these agents, and the rationality of their use, at least in the milder forms of acne, is questionable.[40]

Therapeutic uses in dentistry

The usefulness of the tetracyclines in the treatment of acute orodental infections is limited. At best, these agents are third-choice antibiotics, behind the penicillins, erythromycin, the cephalosporins, and clindamycin. Tetracyclines are, however, good alternatives to penicillin for patients with acute necrotizing ulcerative gingivitis (ANUG) who require antibiotic therapy.[59]

An increasing number of reports suggest that the tetracyclines may be very beneficial in the treatment of certain types of periodontal disease. A prime example of this is provided by juvenile periodontitis, a condition that has been linked to the presence of *Capnocytophaga* and *Actinobacillus actinomycetemcomitans.* The tetracyclines are highly effective against these species, and they have been shown to arrest the rapid bone loss associated with this disease. A 2-week course of tetracycline therapy (250 mg every 6 hours) has also been found to be effective in patients with advanced periodontitis unresponsive to conventional therapy alone.[48] An advantage of the tetracyclines over other antibiotics in the treatment of periodontal disease is the fact that they are concentrated severalfold in gingival fluid. This higher concentration may eradicate bacteria resistant to concentrations that can normally be achieved in the plasma. In one study, 350 strains of various organisms isolated from periodontal pockets were determined to be uniformly sensitive to 32 μg/ml tetracycline, a concentration about 8 times higher than in the plasma during optimal therapy.[74] Research is currently under way to develop techniques for the local delivery of tetracycline to periodontal pockets in such a manner that the drug would produce no systemic effects yet provide concentrations in excess of 100 μg/ml for weeks with a single application.[29]

The tetracyclines should not be used as a penicillin substitute for prophylaxis against bacterial endocarditis, since many of the causative organisms are resistant. Nevertheless, the tetracyclines may have a role in preventing endocarditis after dental therapy. Cases of endocarditis have been documented following bacteremias of penicillin-resistant *A. actinomycetemcomitans*. Since 50% of adult periodontitis patients and 90% of juvenile periodontitis patients harbor this organism, it has been recommended that patients at risk be given a full course of tetracycline several weeks before dental treatment to eliminate it.[27] Of course, the American Heart Association Guidelines should also be followed.

Toxic reactions and side effects

Although serious toxicity from tetracycline administration is rare, these agents do produce a large number of adverse effects that may occur as the result of direct toxic effects, allergic reactions, and microfloral disturbances.

The most common adverse effect caused by the tetracyclines is gastrointestinal irritation, which, for the most part, reflects a direct toxic effect of the drugs and is therefore dose related. Symptoms include anorexia, epigastric distress, abdominal distension, nausea, vomiting, diarrhea, soreness of the mouth, and irritation of the perianal region. Some of these symptoms, particularly severe diarrhea, may also be signs of superinfection. The frequency of occurrence of gastrointestinal disturbances is greatest with oxytetracycline and least with demeclocycline.

Tetracyclines produce other adverse effects related to their direct toxicity. Blood-clotting time may be prolonged by an alteration of the physicochemical properties of lipoproteins present in the blood.[54] Demeclocycline is most likely to cause this reaction. (Suppression of microorganisms, normally present in the microflora of the intestine, that synthesize vitamin K may also result in prolonged clotting time.)

Administration of the tetracycline derivatives has been associated with hepatic injury, especially when large doses (above 2 gm/day) are taken or when usual doses are administered in the presence of renal dysfunction. The incidence of tetracycline-induced hepatic injury is increased during pregnancy, particularly if concomitant renal dysfunction exists, and it is worthy of mention that both hepatic and renal function may be decreased during a normal pregnancy. A number of fatalities have occurred after the use of large doses of tetracyclines in pregnant patients with pyelonephritis[37,52]; death has also followed tetracycline-induced liver damage in nonpregnant patients. The use of all tetracycline derivatives except doxycycline and minocycline is contraindicated in the presence of renal impairment. Because of the increased susceptibility to tetracycline-induced hepatic injury and because of potential tetracycline-induced adverse effects on the fetus (see below), *tetracyclines should not be given during pregnancy.*

Although the tetracyclines generally are not considered nephrotoxic per se, they can cause an exaggeration of existing renal insufficiency and produce nephrotoxic symptoms in patients predisposed to renal disease. Administration of outdated tetracyclines that contain toxic degradation products can produce transient renal dysfunction.[11] Tetracyclines that have been exposed to heat, moisture, or increased pH or that are outdated should be destroyed, since toxic substances are formed under these conditions.

Prolonged use of large doses or accumulation in plasma of the tetracyclines can produce significant metabolic alterations. At high concentrations, these agents exhibit antianabolic effects caused by inhibition of protein synthesis in mammalian cells (an extension of their antimicrobial action). In advanced renal failure, administration of a tetracycline (other than doxycycline or minocycline) produces an exaggeration of the uremic state, and hyperkalemia may occur as a result of the increased catabolism.

The tetracyclines are deposited with calcium as a tetracycline–calcium orthophosphate complex in bone and teeth during periods of active calcification. Time and exposure to light result in oxidation of the tetracycline to a brown material that permanently discolors the affected teeth. Deposition of the tetracyclines in the skeleton of human embryos and fetuses may depress bone growth; similarly, hypoplasia of enamel may occur if large amounts of tetracyclines are given during development (calcification) of the deciduous or permanent dentition.[35,78] This results in pitting of enamel, cusp deformation, and a high caries susceptibility. Since the tetracyclines readily cross the placental barrier, use of these drugs during pregnancy is proscribed. Similarly, administration of these drugs to children from birth through 8 years of age should be avoided. After age 8, the crowns of the permanent teeth, with the exception of the third molars, will have been calcified. The degree of discoloration and hypoplasia of the hard tissues is dependent on the total amount of tetracyclines given rather than on the duration of therapy.

The tetracyclines are concentrated in skin and may cause phototoxic reactions. This is especially true of demeclocycline, which may produce photosensitization and severe sunburn in up to 5% of individuals given the drug.[6] The phototoxicity of tetracyclines is not an allergic reaction but rather a direct effect on the skin that results in increased sensitivity of the integument to light waves ranging in length from 2700 to 3200 Å. Light of these wavelengths occurs in summer sunlight in temperate zones and is filtered out by ordinary window glass. If phototoxicity occurs, the drug should be discontinued and the patient instructed to avoid exposure to direct sunlight.

Allergic reactions to the tetracyclines are infrequent; they are exhibited principally as skin eruptions, including maculopapular rash, urticaria, and exfoliative dermatitis. Severe immediate reactions, such as angioneurotic edema and anaphylactic shock, have occurred with both orally and parenterally administered tetracyclines.[24] Some reactions purported to be allergic in nature are manifested in the oral cavity as cheilosis, brown and black coating of the tongue, and soreness of the mouth. Since sensitization develops more frequently with topically administered antibiotics, the tetracyclines should not be administered topically except in the treatment of ophthalmic infections. Cross-allergenicity between all of the tetracycline derivatives is the rule; appearance of an allergic reaction to one derivative interdicts the use of all tetracyclines.

Because the tetracyclines are usually given orally, are incompletely absorbed, are excreted into the bile, and have a broad spectrum of antibacterial activity, they are the most likely of all the antibiotics to cause superinfection. (Because of their biliary excretion, even parenterally administered tetracyclines may be involved.) Superinfections with tetracycline-resistant strains of bacteria, fungi, and yeasts (in particular *Candida albicans* and *S. aureus*) are frequently encountered during therapy, especially in patients with impaired host defense mechanisms. Superinfections may involve the oral cavity, intestine, vagina, and (rarely) internal organs. Pseudomembranous colitis caused by *C. difficile* may also occur. In the event that severe diarrhea develops during tetracycline therapy, it is vital to determine whether the problem is a result of the irritative properties of the drug or of superinfection. All of the tetracyclines can cause superinfections; the incidence is lowest with doxycycline because it is more completely absorbed from the gastrointestinal tract and is excreted in the feces almost entirely as a pharmacologically inactive conjugate.

Drug interactions

Tetracyclines should not be given concomitantly with other antibiotics, unless synergism has been established by microbiologic tests. As is pointed out in Chapter 36, the effectiveness of bactericidal antibiotics is often diminished by bacteriostatic agents.

Absorption of the tetracyclines from the gastrointestinal tract is inhibited by divalent and trivalent cations such as Ca^{++}, Mg^{++}, Fe^{++}, and Al^{+++}. These ions form chelation products with the tetracyclines and thus prevent their absorption. Therefore, tetracyclines should not be given with milk and dairy products, iron-containing vitamins, mineral supplements containing these ions, or antacids. Since tetracyclines are best absorbed in the acidic conditions of the stomach, the increased pH of gastric contents produced by antacids further depresses drug uptake and significantly lowers the resultant blood concentration of antibiotic.

LINCOMYCIN AND CLINDAMYCIN

Lincomycin was introduced into general clinical use in 1965, after its isolation from soil samples obtained near Lincoln, Nebraska. Clindamycin, introduced in 1970, is a semisynthetic derivative of lincomycin.

Although some of the adverse effects produced by lincomycin and clindamycin have limited their

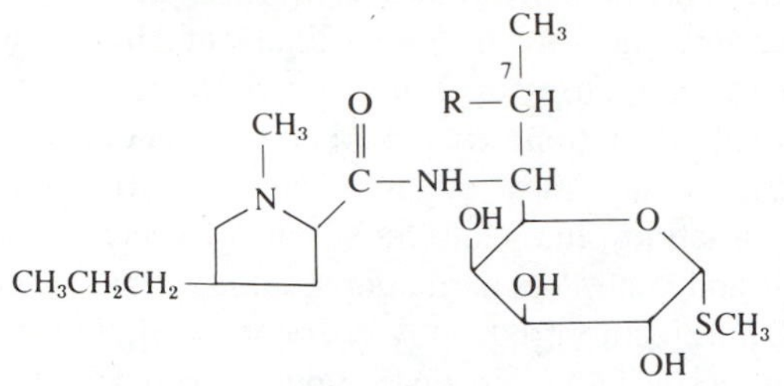

Figure 37-7. Basic structural formula of lincomycin and clindamycin. Substitution of OH at R produces lincomycin; substitution of Cl at R produces clindamycin.

routine use, several unique properties make these drugs, especially clindamycin, excellent agents for a few specific indications encountered in medicine and dentistry. Since their pharmacologic properties are similar, these two antibiotics will be discussed together; it is also helpful to consider lincomycin and clindamycin as pharmacologically similar to erythromycin.

Chemistry

Lincomycin is a derivative of the amino acid trans-L-4-*n*-propylhygrinic acid combined with a sulfur-substituted octose moiety. Clindamycin is produced by exchange of the hydroxyl group with a chlorine atom at C_7 of the lincomycin molecule. The structures of these antibiotics are shown in Figure 37-7.

Mechanism of action and antibacterial spectrum

The mechanism of action of lincomycin and clindamycin is similar to that described for erythromycin and identical with that of chloramphenicol. These drugs bind to the 50 S subunit of bacterial ribosomes, thereby inhibiting protein synthesis. At low concentrations, lincomycin and clindamycin exhibit bacteriostatic activity; however, bactericidal action against a number of susceptible microorganisms occurs at concentrations readily achieved in vivo. The antibacterial spectrums of lincomycin and clindamycin correspond to that of erythromycin, with the following exceptions. Lincomycin and clindamycin (1) have better activity against most strains of *S. aureus,* (2) are more active against most gram-positive and gram-negative anaerobes (clindamycin, in particular, is effective against most strains of *B. fragilis*), and (3)

have a more restricted antibacterial spectrum that does not include *Chlamydia,* spirochetes, *Rickettsia, Mycoplasma,* or most gram-negative aerobes.

As illustrated in Table 37-2, lincomycin is not the first drug of choice for any infection caused by susceptible microorganisms. Clindamycin, however, is 2 to 4 times more active than lincomycin on a weight basis in vitro and is quantitatively more effective in vivo against infections caused by sensitive bacteria. Clindamycin's superior activity against *B. fragilis* makes it the drug of choice for that organism.

Bacterial resistance

Bacterial resistance to lincomycin and clindamycin appears in a slow, stepwise manner reminiscent of penicillin G, but the mechanism involved is similar to that described for erythromycin. Specifically, mutations in the bacterial ribosomes result in decreased affinity and binding capacity for these drugs. About 15% of *S. aureus* strains, some pneumococci, and some strains of Group A streptococci have acquired resistance to lincomycin. Cross-resistance in such microbes has been demonstrated between lincomycin, clindamycin, and, frequently, erythromycin. Some strains of *S. aureus* that have become resistant to methicillin or erythromycin are also resistant to lincomycin and clindamycin. Otherwise, cross-resistance has not been demonstrated between the lincomycin-clindamycin pair and most other antibiotics.

Absorption, fate, and excretion

Both lincomycin and clindamycin are absorbed from the gastrointestinal tract, but the absorption of lincomycin is poor, amounting to only 25% to 30% of an orally administered dose, even in the fasting state. Lincomycin's absorption is markedly inhibited by the presence of food. In contrast, clindamycin is more than 90% absorbed, even when taken with meals. For these reasons, clindamycin can be given orally to achieve plasma titers above the MIC, but lincomycin should be administered parenterally. Lincomycin and clindamycin are well distributed into body tissues and fluids, except the cerebrospinal fluid. The excellent penetration of these antibiotics into bone is of particular interest. Intraosseous concentrations of active drug may approximate those of plasma.[5,57] These antibiotics are therefore excellent agents for treating infections of bone, such as osteomyelitis and purulent osteitis, caused by susceptible microorganisms.

Table 37-9. Miscellaneous antibiotics for dental use: commercially available preparations

Nonproprietary name	Proprietary name	Usual adult dose	Route	Preparations
Lincomycin	Lincocin	600 mg-1 gm every 8 to 12 hours 600 mg every 12-24 hours	IV, IM	Injection: 600 mg and 3 gm vials, 600 mg syringes
		500 mg every 6 to 8 hours	Oral	Capsules: 250 and 500 mg
Clindamycin phosphate	Cleocin Phosphate	600-2700 mg every 24 hours in 2, 3, or 4 equal doses	IV, IM	Injection: 300 and 600 mg ampules
Clindamycin hydrochloride	Cleocin HCl	150-450 mg every 6 hours	Oral	Capsules: 75 and 150 mg
	Cleocin Pediatric	8-12 mg/kg/day in 3 or 4 doses	Oral	Granules for solution (palmitate ester): 75 mg/5 ml
Metronidazole	Flagyl, Metryl	15 mg/kg over 1 hour, then 7.5 mg/kg every 6 hours	IV	Injection: 500 mg vials
		250-750 mg every 8 hours	Oral	Tablets: 250 and 500 mg
Vancomycin hydrochloride	Vancocin	500 mg every 6 hours by IV infusion; for protection against bacterial endocarditis, see Table 36-7	IV	Vials: 500 mg/10 ml
			Oral	Powder: 10 g
Streptomycin sulfate	—	For protection against bacterial endocarditis, see Table 36-7	IM	Vials: 1 and 5 gm

Lincomycin is metabolized by the liver to some degree; clindamycin is biotransformed to a larger extent, the majority of the drug being eliminated in the feces as active and inactive metabolites. Biliary excretion is the major pathway for elimination of these drugs. Hepatic insufficiency will therefore significantly prolong their half-lives, and dosage reduction may be required in patients with liver disease. Because active drug, as well as metabolites, appears in the feces after either oral or parenteral administration, these antibiotics can produce significant alterations in the intestinal microflora, sometimes resulting in superinfection.

General therapeutic uses

Although both lincomycin and clindamycin are effective against gram-positive aerobes and both gram-positive and gram-negative anaerobes, their general use is restricted to the treatment of certain serious infections caused by susceptible strains of streptococci, staphylococci, pneumococci, or anaerobes such as *Bacteroides* that are insensitive to less toxic antimicrobial drugs. These antibiotics may be especially indicated in the treatment of refractory bone infections. For all applications, clindamycin is preferred over lincomycin.

Therapeutic uses in dentistry

In dentistry, as in medicine, clindamycin is generally a reserve agent, and lincomycin is rarely used. Because their use has been associated with severe colitis, lincomycin and clindamycin should be employed when less dangerous antibiotics are contraindicated or ineffective. Currently there are two valid indications for clindamycin in orodental infections: purulent osteitis or other bone infections, and infections caused by anaerobic organisms, such as *Bacteroides* species, or by other pathogens that cannot be eradicated by less toxic antibiotics (e.g., a penicillin or erythromycin). Clindamycin is becoming more widely prescribed as the anaerobic nature of most dental infections is more clearly appreciated and because broad-spectrum penicillin and cephalosporin alternatives to clindamycin generally require parenteral administration. The commercially available preparations of lincomycin and clindamycin are tabulated in Table 37-9 along with several other agents discussed later in this chapter.

Toxic reactions and side effects

Foremost among the adverse effects produced by these antibiotics are gastrointestinal disturbances, which may take the form of severe diarrhea and the potentially fatal pseudomembranous colitis. Although these reactions appear more frequently after oral administration, they may also occur after parenteral administration because of the enterohepatic circulation of drug. It has been estimated that the incidence of severe diarrhea may be as high as 10%

to 20% when lincomycin is administered orally; the incidence drops to about 5% when the drug is given intramuscularly or if clindamycin is used orally.[12,67] Although the relationship between the etiology of diarrhea and antibiotic-associated colitis is not established, severe diarrhea is an early sign of colitis. The pathogenesis and treatment of pseudomembranous colitis is detailed in Chapter 36.

Overgrowth of yeasts and fungi in the oral cavity, intestinal tract, and vagina has occurred with lincomycin and clindamycin, and glossitis, stomatitis, and vaginitis may be the result of such superinfections. Glossitis and stomatitis may also be manifestations of an allergic reaction. These antibiotics can cause gastrointestinal irritation leading to nausea and vomiting.

Lincomycin and clindamycin are less antigenic than penicillin, but allergic reactions of varying severity have been reported. Generally, such reactions are relatively mild, the most common form being a morbilliform rash, which may occur in as many as 10% of patients given clindamycin. More serious dermatologic reactions (Stevens-Johnson syndrome, exfoliative dermatitis, and vesiculobullous eruptions) and immediate allergic responses (urticaria, angioedema, and anaphylaxis) are much less frequently encountered. Cross-allergenicity between lincomycin and clindamycin is to be expected.

These two drugs also produce adverse effects on the hematopoietic system that may be manifested as neutropenia, agranulocytosis, and thrombocytopenia. The intravenous administration of clindamycin has been associated with thrombophlebitis.

Drug interactions

Lincomycin, clindamycin, erythromycin, and chloramphenicol are mutually antagonistic because of their similar, if not identical, binding sites on the 50 S subunit of the bacterial ribosome. Therefore, they should never be given concurrently. Lincomycin and clindamycin exhibit neuromuscular blocking activity; concomitant use of these antibiotics with curare-like drugs should be closely monitored.

METRONIDAZOLE

Metronidazole is a synthetic nitroimidazole (see Figure 37-8) patterned after a naturally occurring antiparasitic substance that was isolated from a

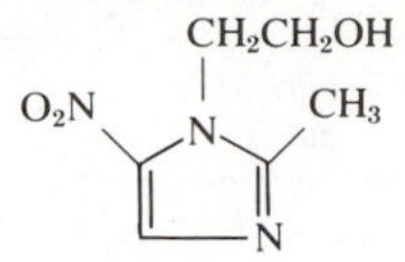

Figure 37-8. Structural formula of metronidazole.

Streptomyces species in 1955. The drug was introduced into medicine in 1959 and was quickly found to possess strong trichomonacidal activity. Since then, metronidazole has become the drug of choice for a variety of protozoal infections. A chance observation that the symptoms of ANUG were relieved in a woman receiving metronidazole for treatment of vaginal trichomoniasis stimulated research on the drug's antibacterial effects, culminating in its approval in 1981 for the treatment of anaerobic bacterial infections.

Mechanism of action and antibacterial spectrum

Metronidazole is active only against obligate anaerobic bacteria, but within this range it is highly efficacious against those groups most responsible for clinical disease: *Bacteroides, Fusobacterium, Veillonella, Campylobacter, Clostridium, Treponema, Peptococcus,* and *Peptostreptococcus.*

Metrondizadole penetrates all bacterial cells equally well. In sensitive anaerobes, however, the nitro moiety of the drug is enzymatically reduced, and it is this metabolite that is believed to be the active form of the drug. Metronidazole is almost always bactericidal. The drug reacts with bacterial DNA, causing inhibition of DNA replication, fragmentation of existing DNA, and, in low doses, mutation of the bacterial genome. To date, there have been few reports of acquired resistance to metronidazole.

Absorption, fate, and excretion

Metronidazole is generally well absorbed after oral administration. Food delays but does not reduce absorption. This effect is not very important, though, because metronidazole has a plasma half-life of about 8 hours. The drug is distributed throughout the total body water; concentrations achieved in bone and in the cerebrospinal fluid are therapeutic. Metronidazole is metabolized in the liver, yielding oxidation products and glucuronide conjugates. These metabolites, some of which are active, are excreted with smaller amounts of the parent drug, chiefly in the urine but also in the bile.

General therapeutic uses

As previously mentioned, metronidazole is a major antiprotozoal drug, effective against *Trichomonas vaginalis, Giardia lamblia,* and *Entamoeba histolytica.* As an antibacterial agent, it is one of the most effective drugs available against *B. fragilis,* particularly for treatment of endocarditis and CNS abscesses. (Metronidazole is bactericidal whereas alternative drugs for these infections are generally bacteriostatic.) Metronidazole has also been used successfully to treat serious anaerobic infections of the abdomen, skeleton, epidermis, and female genital tract. Experimentally, metronidazole has been administered in very high doses to ''sensitize'' hypoxic cancer cells to ionizing radiation.

Therapeutic uses in dentistry

Metronidazole has not been adequately evaluated for use in dentistry. It has been shown to be an effective drug for the treatment of ANUG, but its use in the majority of dental infections will probably be limited by its lack of efficacy against aerobic and facultative bacteria. It would seem to be indicated for *B. fragilis* infections that can occur following mandibular fracture.[33]

Because metronidazole is strongly active against anaerobes. it may be of use in the treatment of advanced periodontitis. In one study, a one-week course of metronidazole produced long-lasting clinical improvement, with alterations in the microflora of the gingival pocket (e.g., large reductions of spirochetes) persisting for 6 months.[41]

Toxic reactions and side effects

Metronidazole is generally well tolerated; nevertheless, some questions about its safety remain unresolved. The most common side effects include nausea, anorexia, epigastric pain, stomatitis, black furred tongue, and a metallic taste in the mouth. Candidal superinfections may account for some of these reactions. Neutropenia that resolves on discontinuation of the drug may also occur. Disulfiram-like reactions contraindicate the ingestion of alcoholic beverages while taking metronidazole. In very high doses, as have been administered experimentally in cancer patients, metronidazole may cause skin rash, peripheral neuropathy, and a variety of CNS derangements.

Questions persist regarding the mutagenic and carcinogenic potential of metronidazole. Human urine contains metabolites of the drug that are mutagenic to some bacteria. Metronidazole may be carcinogenic in some rodent species but not in other mammals. No clinical problems of this nature have been documented for humans; however, prudence currently dictates against the drug's use in the first trimester of pregnancy and at other times when potentially safer drugs are equally efficacious.

VANCOMYCIN

Vancomycin is a glycopeptide antibiotic elab-in medicine only for treatment of infections caused by gram-positive microorganisms susceptible to this agent but resistant to other, more commonly used and less toxic antimicrobial drugs. Vancomycin is also used as prophylaxis for penicillin-allergic patients with prosthetic heart valves (see Table 36-7). Because of its infrequent use, many gram-positive microorganisms that have become resistant to many other antibiotics remain susceptible to vancomycin.

Vancomycin is a glycopeptide antibiotic elaborated by *Streptomyces orientalis,* an actinomycete that was found in soil samples from India and Indonesia. Although it was introduced into clinical use in 1956, its chemical structure was not elucidated until the late 1970s.

Mechanism of action and antibacterial spectrum

Vancomycin has two sites of action: the cell wall in susceptible microorganisms and the bacterial cell membrane (see Figure 36-1). Its action is bactericidal.

The drug has a narrow antibacterial spectrum, being effective mainly against streptococci, pneumococci, staphylococci, and some anaerobes (e.g., clostridia and most intraoral anaerobes). Most strains of *S. aureus,* including methicillin-resistant strains, remain susceptible to vancomycin, as do most strains of viridans streptococci and *S. pyogenes.*[70] Uniquely, bacterial resistance does not appear to occur during treatment, although a few strains of *S. aureus* have been shown to be resistant to vancomycin.

Absorption, fate, and excretion

Vancomycin is not absorbed from the oral mucosa or gastrointestinal tract; therefore, it must be given parenterally for treatment of systemic infections. Because intramuscular injection results in tissue necrosis, and thrombophlebitis occurs with intravenous bolus injection, vancomycin must be given by intravenous infusion (Table 37-9). When administered by this method, vancomycin is well distributed to most tissues (including bone) and body fluids. Penetration into cerebrospinal fluid occurs during periods of meningeal inflammation. The main route of elimination is by renal excretion, with 80% of a parenteral dose appearing in the urine as active vancomycin. Therefore, in the presence of renal dysfunction, the dose of vancomycin must be markedly reduced to avoid accumulation of toxic plasma concentrations of drug.

General therapeutic uses

Vancomycin is reserved for the treatment of those few serious infections caused by gram-positive organisms that are refractory to less toxic antibiotics. Vancomycin is also quite useful for staphylococcal and clostridial enterocolitis; in this instance the drug is given orally, and the poor absorption is helpful in minimizing the risk of adverse reactions.

Therapeutic uses in dentistry

Although vancomycin has been used topically in the past to treat ANUG and in toothpaste to improve the oral hygiene of mentally retarded children,[42,53] such use is extremely controversial. There is only one accepted indication for the use of vancomycin in dentistry and that is for the prophylactic coverage of penicillin-allergic patients with prosthetic heart valves. The use of vancomycin in these circumstances is based on (1) the high risk such patients run of developing endocarditis as a result of a bacteremia of dental origin, (2) the bactericidal activity of vancomycin, (3) the increasing resistance of oral microorganisms to penicillin and erythromycin and their continued susceptibility to vancomycin, (4) the susceptibility to vancomycin of both aerobes and anaerobes found in the oral cavity, and (5) the lack of cross-allergenicity between penicillin derivatives and vancomycin.

Toxic reactions and side effects

Most notable of the adverse effects associated with vancomycin are ototoxicity and nephrotox-icity, but these are not likely to be seen after the short-term prophylactic use of vancomycin in dental procedures. Moreover, renal damage has become much less common since appropriate dosage schedules for patients with oliguria were adopted. Hearing loss and kidney impairment are most likely to develop during prolonged, high-dose therapy; concurrent use of other agents with similar toxicities (e.g., aminoglycosides) increases the risk of damage. Other adverse effects associated wtih vancomycin are pain and tissue necrosis after intramuscular injection, allergic reactions, and occasional superinfections.

AMINOGLYCOSIDES

The aminoglycosides are extremely valuable agents in medicine, being mainstays for the treatment of life-threatening infections caused by certain gram-negative bacteria. Streptomycin, the first of these drugs, was introduced in 1944, shortly after penicillin G. It was the result of a concentrated effort to screen soil samples for antibiotic-producing microorganisms and was the second true antibiotic to be employed in clinical medicine. Although streptomycin remains a drug of choice for selected conditions, it has been largely replaced for most uses by more effective relatives, initially by kanamycin in the late 1950s, and subsequently by gentamicin and other aminoglycosides; tobramycin, amikacin, and netilmicin. Neomycin, the second aminoglycoside to be discovered, is essentially limited to treatment of localized conditions. It is discussed further in the section on topical antibiotics.

Chemistry

Streptomycin is produced by *Streptomyces griseus*. The other aminoglycosides are elaborated by various species of *Streptomyces* and *Micromonospora* or, in the case of amikacin and netilmicin, are semisynthetic derivatives of naturally occurring aminoglycosides. As the name implies, these agents consist of a highly polar amino base attached by glycosidic linkage to one or more sugars. Streptomycin, for example, is composed of three components—streptidine (the amino base) and two sugar moieties, streptose and N-methyl-L-glucosamine (Figure 37-9).

Mechanism of action and antibacterial spectrum

The aminoglycosides inhibit protein synthesis by binding to one or more specific proteins present in

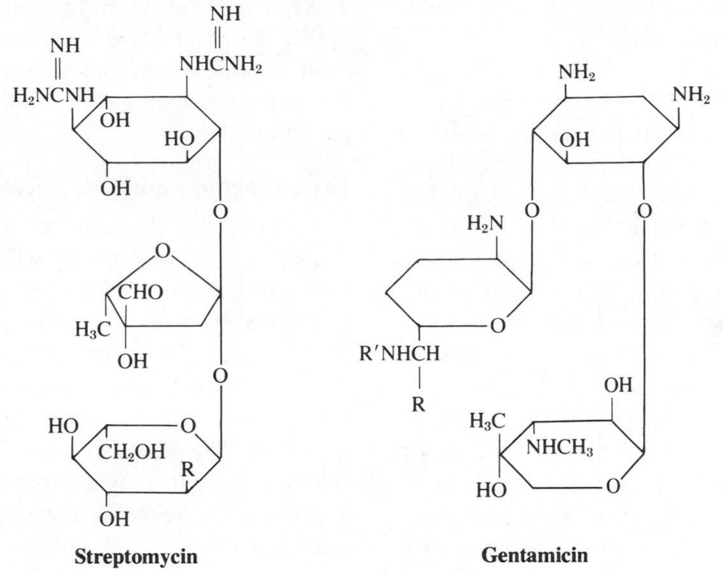

Figure 37-9. Structural formulas of streptomycin and gentamicin. R for streptomycin = CH_3NH. Commercial preparations of gentamicin contain three closely related gentamicins: C_1 (R = CH_3, R' = CH_3), C_{1a} (R = H, R' = H), and C_2 (R = CH_3, R' = H).

the 30 S subunit of the bacterial ribosome. At low concentrations, streptomycin and other aminoglycosides are bacteriostatic, but at concentrations easily achieved clinically they are often rapidly bactericidal. There is as yet no complete explanation why the aminoglycosides, inhibitors of protein synthesis, are strongly bactericidal. It is known that the aminoglycosides cause misreading of messenger RNA by ribosomes and the synthesis of abnormal peptides. This effect and other disturbances of ribosomal function, when coupled with the general inhibition of protein synthesis, may alter cell wall integrity, resulting in cell death.

The aminoglycosides are relatively broad spectrum agents, effective against both gram-positive and gram-negative microorganisms. As a class, their main value is their activity against aerobic gram-negative rods such as *P. aeruginosa*, *E. coli*, and *Klebsiella*, *Enterobacter*, *Serratia*, and *Proteus* species. Quantitative differences occur in the effectiveness of individual aminoglycosides against a particular microorganism.

Bacterial resistance

Streptomycin is unique among antibiotics in the rapidity with which bacterial resistance appears. A single mutation of the bacterial genome can prevent

binding of streptomycin to the ribosome and confer total resistance. In fact, some mutants even require low concentrations of the drug in order to survive (streptomycin-dependent mutants).[61]

Because the aminoglycosides are strongly hydrophilic, uptake by bacteria depends on a carrier-mediated process, which in turn requires oxygen in order to function. Anaerobic bacteria and facultative organisms growing in an anaerobic environment are resistant to these drugs. It also appears that resistance in some bacteria is the result of genetically determined changes in the transport system. The penicillins and other drugs that affect cell wall synthesis may be synergistic with the aminoglycosides because they aid the intracellular penetration of the latter agents.

The most important mechanism of resistance to the aminoglycosides is metabolism of the drugs by bacterial membrane-bound enzymes. Amikacin, specifically designed to resist inactivation by most of these enzymes, has the widest spectrum of all the aminoglycosides.

Although resistance to the aminoglycosides (except streptomycin) generally appears in a slow, stepwise fashion, resistance can be mediated by R factor transfer, particularly with gram-negative bacteria. Because of the presence of resistant strains and the rapidity with which resistance can develop, streptomycin is usually used in combination with other antibiotics.

Absorption, fate, and excretion

The aminoglycosides are negligibly absorbed from the gastrointestinal tract and must be administered parenterally. The drugs are distributed throughout the extracellular space. Penetration into the eye, cerebrospinal fluid, and respiratory secretions is poor; however, these drugs enter bone sufficiently to be effective in the treatment of osteomyelitis caused by susceptible microorganisms. Streptomycin is 30% bound to plasma proteins, which is the highest percentage of the aminoglycosides. These highly polar compounds are mainly excreted as the active drug via glomerular filtration. Plasma half-lives normally range from 1 to 3 hours; in the anephric patient they may be increased 10- to 40-fold. Therefore, doses must be carefully reduced when the agents are used in patients with renal dysfunction.

General therapeutic uses

The major medical use of streptomycin is for the treatment of infections caused by *Mycobacterium tuberculosis,* as described later in this chapter. The drug is also used, usually in combination with other antibiotics, for treatment of bacterial endocarditis caused by viridans streptococci, enterococci such as *Streptococcus faecalis,* or gram-negative bacilli and for chemotherapy of brucellosis, tularemia, plague, peritonitis, and severe urinary tract infections refractory to less toxic antibiotics.

Gentamicin, tobramycin, netilmicin, and to a much lesser extent kanamycin are invaluable for treatment of life-threatening infections caused by gram-negative bacteria and by methicillin-resistant *S. aureus* or group D streptococci (e.g., enterococcal endocarditis.) These drugs are frequently combined with an extended-spectrum penicillin such as carbenicillin for synergistic activity. Amikacin is best reserved for infections refractory to other aminoglycosides.

Therapeutic uses in dentistry

Aminoglycosides, in combination with a parenteral form of penicillin, have only one application in dentistry—the prophylactic protection against bacteremias caused by dental procedures in patients with artificial valves. The schedule for an-

tibiotic administration is provided in Table 36-7. The rationale for use of this combination of drugs is that the agents have a synergistic effect against viridans streptococci and enterococcal transients in the oral cavity that may be relatively insensitive to penicillin alone.

Toxic reactions and side effects

It is unlikely that the prophylactic use of an aminoglycoside in dentistry will result in any notable adverse reactions. That is not to say, however, that these agents are safe antibiotics, for they can produce serious auditory, vestibular, and renal toxicity. Ototoxicity results from destruction of the sensory hair cells of the cochlea and vestibular apparatus. The damage is dose related, associated with prolonged therapy, and often irreversible. Vestibular deficits are most common with streptomycin and gentamicin. Acute clinical symptoms include nausea, vomiting, vertigo, Romberg's sign, inability to perceive cessation of motion, and difficulty in focusing and reading. Fortunately, affected individuals gradually adapt to the loss of vestibular function, although coordination is never fully restored. Tinnitus and pressure in the ears are the first signs of auditory toxicity.[77] Amikacin, kanamycin, and netilmicin preferentially cause hearing loss. Since high-pitched sounds are affected first, the damage may not be recognized unless audiometry is used. Some ototoxicity nearly always occurs during therapy and is clinically significant in about 2% of patients. Renal insufficiency, the need for intensive, protracted medication, and the concomitant administration of other ototoxic drugs (e.g., diuretics) greatly compound the incidence and severity of damage.

The aminoglycosides are destructive to the renal cortex. Gentamicin is the most nephrotoxic of the commonly used drugs, and streptomycin is the least. Coadministration with a cephalosporin or other nephrotoxic substance increases the potential for damage.[10] Other adverse effects include pain at the site of injection, allergic reactions (with skin rash occurring in as many as 5% of patients receiving the drug), neuromuscular blockade, blood dyscrasias, and superinfections.

SULFONAMIDES

The milestone discovery that the antibacterial activity of prontosil resided with the sulfanilamide moiety initiated the era of modern chemotherapy.[15,20,71] Since the first clinical use of sulfanilamide in the 1930s, some 5000 additional sulfonamide compounds have been synthesized. Only a few of these ever reached clinical use, and fewer still have survived to enjoy clinical application today.

Chemistry

All of the sulfonamides are derivatives of *p*-aminobenzenesulfonamide. (See Figure 36-2 for the general structure of these compounds.) For biologic activity, the sulfur must be attached directly to the benzene ring, and the *p*-amino group (N_4) must be free in vivo. Substitutions on the amino group (N_1) of the sulfonamide moiety confer differences in rate of absorption and excretion of these drugs and, to some degree, variations in antibacterial potency. The sulfonamides are weak acids with limited water solubility, particularly in solutions of low pH. This presents problems during the excretion of these drugs in an acidic urine.

Mechanism of action and antibacterial spectrum

As described in Chapter 36, the sulfonamides act as antimetabolites of PABA. By competitively inhibiting the enzyme dihydropteroate synthetase, which catalyzes the linkage of the pteridine moiety and PABA as the initial step in the synthesis of folic acid, the growth of susceptible bacteria is inhibited. The sulfonamides are generally only bacteriostatic.

The sulfonamides are considered broad-spectrum agents since they are effective against gram-positive bacteria (e.g., some streptococci, staphylococci, and pneumococci), some gram-negative microorganisms (e.g., *E. coli*, gonococci, meningococci, and *Haemophilus* species), *Actinomyces*, and "large viruses" belonging to the genus *Chlamydia. Mycoplasma*, rickettsiae, true viruses, and fungi are not affected by these drugs. The sulfonamides are not effective against enterococcal, *Enterobacter, Proteus*, or *Pseudomonas* infections. It is noteworthy that a significant number of strains of viridans streptococci and many anaerobic microorganisms in the oral cavity are insensitive to the sulfonamides.[25] It should also be mentioned that the antibacterial activity of sulfonamides is inhibited in the presence of pus, blood, products from tissue breakdown, and PABA from exogenous or endogenous sources. Moreover, pro-

caine-type local anesthetics may antagonize the antibacterial activity of sulfonamides, since a product of their biotransformation is PABA. Thus, even susceptible bacteria may appear resistant when these materials are present.

Bacterial resistance

Resistance to the sulfonamides usually develops in a slow, stepwise fashion. Spontaneous chromosomal mutation and selection of increasingly resistant mutants occur with gram-positive bacteria; R factor transfer (infective resistance) occurs among gram-negative bacteria. Resistance to one sulfonamide confers resistance to all, but cross-resistance seldom appears between sulfonamides and other antimicrobial agents. One mechanism by which bacteria become resistant to these drugs is via an increased ability to synthesize large quantities of PABA.[79] The occurrence of resistance among a number of microorganisms causing intraoral disturbances is one reason the sulfonamides are not particularly effective in the treatment of most orodental infections.

Absorption, fate, and excretion

The sulfonamides are almost always administered orally, since they are relatively water insoluble and their soluble sodium salts are quite alkaline and irritating. They are adequately absorbed from the gastrointestinal tract and well distributed into various body compartments, including the cerebrospinal fluid. One agent, sulfasalazine, is intended for local effects in the gastrointestinal tract; it releases active sulfonamide (and 5-aminosalicylate) only on hydrolysis by enteric bacteria. Various sulfonamide derivatives are biotransformed to varying extents by acetylation at the N_4 position; such metabolites are inactive but may account for some of the adverse effects associated with these drugs. In some cases the acetylated metabolite is less soluble than the parent compound, resulting in precipitation in the renal tubules unless adequate fluid intake and urine flow are maintained. The major route of excretion of the sulfonamides, both active and inactive forms, is via glomerular filtration.

Since the sulfonamides are bacteriostatic, adequate blood concentrations must be maintained throughout therapy. They are usually prescribed in a loading dose followed by a lower maintenance dose. The various sulfonamide derivatives cur-

Table 37-10. Classification, by use, of selected sulfonamides and trimethoprim preparations

Use	Nonproprietary name	Proprietary name
Systemic infections	Sulfadiazine	Microsulfon
	Sulfamethoxazole	Gantanol
	Sulfisoxazole	Gantrisin
	Trisulfapyrimidines	Terfonyl
	Erythromycin-sulfisoxazole	Pediazole
	Trimethoprim	Proloprim, Trimpex
	Trimethoprim-sulfamethoxazole	Bactrim, Septra
Urinary tract infections	Sulfacytine	Renoquid
	Sulfamethizole	Thiosulfil
Dermatitis herpetiformis	Sulfapyridine	—
Local use in gastrointestinal tract	Sulfasalazine (salicylazosulfapyridine)	Azulfidine
Ophthalmic use	Sulfacetamide sodium	Sodium Sulamyd Ophthalmic
Topical use, burns	Mafenide	Sulfamylon
	Silver sulfadiazine	Silvadene

rently available are listed according to use in Table 37-10.

General therapeutic uses

The need for sulfonamides has been increasingly diminished by the development of more effective antibiotics. Their main indication is in the treatment of urinary tract infections involving gram-positive cocci (other than enterococci) or *E. coli.* The sulfonamides are also employed against infections caused by *Nocardia,* and mafenide and silver sulfadiazine find application in the prevention of skin infections in burn victims. Sulfonamides are seldom agents of first choice but may be useful in the treatment and chemoprophylaxis of infections caused by susceptible strains of *Neisseria meningitidis.* They are beneficial in some patients as prophylactic agents against recurrent attacks of rheumatic fever or other streptococcal infections, but they are not administered for prophylaxis against bacterial endocarditis caused by dental procedures. Topical application of sulfacetamide to the eye is effective in treating trachoma and inclusion conjunctivitis. These agents are used only rarely for treatment of dental infections because of their low degree of effectiveness and the high order of resistance seen among viridans streptococci and other oral microorganisms.

Toxic reactions and side effects

The sulfonamides produce many adverse effects, some of which are severe. The older sulfonamides were poorly soluble in urine, especially at an acid pH, and would cause crystalluria and damage to the renal tubules, renal pelvis, and bladder. Although newer sulfonamides are more soluble, fluid intake should be maintained at a level providing urine flow above 1200 ml per day in adults. Alkalinization of the urine by administration of sodium bicarbonate may be advisable in some patients. Other toxic effects include disturbances such as nausea, vomiting, headaches, dizziness, ataxia, depression, irritability, and restlessness. Adverse effects on the hematopoietic system may occasionally be severe and include aplastic anemia, agranulocytosis, hemolytic anemia, leukopenia, and thrombocytopenia. Allergic reactions of all types and severity may occur with the sulfonamides. For this reason, as well as an enhanced development of resistance, these agents should not be used topically, except in the eye, vaginally, or over burned skin. Concurrent administration of a sulfonamide may exaggerate the effects of warfarin, sulfonylureas, and methotrexate by displacing these drugs from their plasma protein binding sites.

Trimethoprim

In order to increase activity against bacteria, especially those that have developed resistance by increasing production of PABA, sulfonamides have been administered with trimethoprim. Formerly used as an antimalarial drug, trimethoprim binds to dihydrofolate reductase and prevents the conversion of dihydrofolic acid to the active coenzyme tetrahydrofolic acid (see Chapter 36). Thus, trimethoprim depresses the same general pathway affected by the sulfonamides but exhibits activity against those microorganisms that can still synthesize or obtain folic acid despite the presence of the sulfonamides. Because the combination of trimethoprim with sulfamethoxazole is synergistic, bactericidal activity may result. Trimethoprim-sulfamethoxazole is used therapeutically in the treatment of urinary tract infections, otitis media, chronic bronchitis, shigellosis, and pneumonitis caused by *Pneumocystis carinii.* Trimethoprim is also used alone in the control of urinary tract infections caused by susceptible gram-negative microorganisms. Another sulfonamide combination, erythromycin-sulfisoxazole, is indicated for treatment of otitis media caused by susceptible strains of *H. influenzae.*[39] As would be expected, the side effects of these combinations may be attributable to one or both drugs.

CHLORAMPHENICOL

Chloramphenicol was the first truly broad-spectrum antibiotic to be discovered. Initially isolated from *Streptomyces venezuelae* in 1947, the drug is now produced synthetically. By 1950 it was recognized that chloramphenicol could produce serious and even fatal bone marrow aplasia, a fact that has greatly restricted its clinical use. Nevertheless, it is a very valuable drug for treatment of specific infectious diseases not amenable to therapy with less toxic antibiotics.

Chemistry

Chloramphenicol is unique among naturally occurring compounds in that it contains a nitrobenzene group, which is attached to a propanediol moiety linked to a dichloracetamide side chain. Its structure is illustrated in Figure 37-10. Reduction of the nitro group, hydrolysis of the amide linkage, or acetylation of the molecule inactivates the antibiotic.

Mechanism of action and antibacterial spectrum

Chloramphenicol binds to the 50 S subunit of the bacterial ribosome and prevents protein synthesis by inhibition of the enzyme involved in peptide bond formation, a mechanism of action identical to that of lincomycin and clindamycin. Chloramphenicol, lincomycin, clindamycin, and erythromycin bind to the same, or similar, sites on the 50 S subunit and are thereby mutually antag-

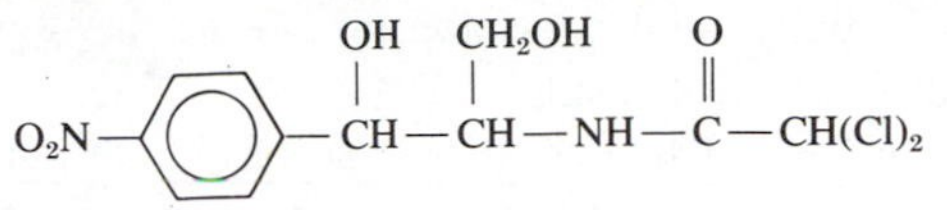

Figure 37-10. Structural formula of chloramphenicol.

onistic. Also, antagonism results from combination of chloramphenicol with aminoglycosides or with antibiotics that inhibit cell wall synthesis. Chloramphenicol is usually bacteriostatic.

Chloramphenicol is a broad-spectrum antibiotic with activity directed against many gram-negative microorganisms, some streptococci and staphylococci, rickettsiae, *Chlamydia,* treponemes, and *Mycoplasma.* Most anaerobes are susceptible to this drug. Its excellent activity against *Salmonella* species is the basis for one of the major indications for use of this antibiotic. It is not effective against most *Pseudomonas* species, fungi, or true viruses.

Bacterial resistance

Although the clinical efficacy exhibited by chloramphenicol is quite consistent, bacterial resistance, particularly among gram-negative bacteria, is an increasing problem. Resistance is acquired in gram-negative bacteria such as *Salmonella, Shigella,* and *E. coli* by R factor transfer during conjugation. Resistance among *S. aureus* is also a problem. Both gram-negative and gram-positive bacteria that have acquired resistance to chloramphenicol inactivate the drug by acetylation via a specific acetyltransferase enzyme.[55]

Absorption, fate, and excretion

Chloramphenicol may be administered orally or parenterally; it is rapidly and adequately absorbed from the gastrointestinal tract after oral administration. It is well distributed throughout the body fluids, including the cerebrospinal fluid. Chloramphenicol is found in bile and in milk, and it readily crosses the placental barrier.

Chloramphenicol is inactivated to the extent of 80% to 90%, mainly by the hepatic formation of a conjugate with glucuronic acid. The immaturity of the glucuronyl transferase system in premature infants and neonates permits the accumulation of toxic plasma concentrations of chloramphenicol when the drug is administered to these infants, and a potentially fatal condition known as the "gray syndrome" may result.

Five percent to 10% of a dose of chloramphenicol is excreted by glomerular filtration as the active drug. Renal tubular secretion accounts for elimination of the glucuronide conjugate. Because the half-life of chloramphenicol is increased in patients with hepatic dysfunction, dosage reduction is necessary.

General therapeutic uses

There are only a few indications for which chloramphenicol is the primary choice; however, in such circumstances this drug is very valuable. One indication for chloramphenicol is the treatment of infections caused by *Salmonella typhi* (typhoid fever) and, to a lesser extent, systemic infections caused by other *Salmonella*. Additional indications are refractory cases of meningitis caused by *H. influenzae* and rickettsial and *Brucella* infections not amenable to therapy with a tetracycline. Finally, rare cases of urinary tract infections caused by microorganisms unresponsive to less toxic antibiotics may require chloramphenicol. Because of the severe and sometimes fatal adverse effects associated with the use of chloramphenicol, the drug should be reserved for treatment of those indicated infections that are life-threatening and resistant to therapy with less toxic antibiotics. There are no indications for the use of this antibiotic in the treatment of orodental infections.

Toxic reactions and side effects

The adverse effects produced by chloramphenicol may be more serious than the original disease entity being treated. Most noteworthy of these are the reactions involving the bone marrow. Two such reactions occur—one is a dose-related toxicity and the other, the more serious of the two, is the result of drug allergy. Dose-related effects on the bone marrow are exhibited as anemia, which frequently appears with prolonged, high plasma concentrations of chloramphenicol. Vacuolization of erythrocyte precursor cells in the bone marrow occurs within several days after initiation of therapy, followed by a decrease in reticulocyte count and progressing hypoproliferative anemia.[49] The major mechanism involved is a decreased uptake of iron (Fe^{++}) by the erythrocyte precursor cells.[76] In a few patients, thrombocytopenia and neutropenia develop; neutropenia may be particularly serious in the presence of infection if it is of sufficient magnitude to prevent effective phagocytosis of bacteria. These effects are reversible after cessation of therapy with chloramphenicol.

The most serious reaction to chloramphenicol is aplasia of the bone marrow and resultant fatal pancytopenia. Complete bone marrow aplasia is nearly always fatal. This reaction is due to an allergic phenomenon and is thus not related to the dose. It is seen most frequently during prolonged or repeated therapy with the drug. The rate of occurrence of this potentially fatal reaction is approximately one in 40,000 courses of therapy with chloramphenicol, and it may appear as late as 6 months after cessation of therapy.[4] Acute leukemia is a common sequel in survivors. Other, less serious allergic reactions include skin rashes, drug fever, hemorrhage of skin and mucous membranes in the oral cavity, atrophic glossitis, black tongue, and Herxheimer reactions.

Additional adverse effects are the previously mentioned "gray syndrome" seen in full-term and premature infants, hemolytic reactions in patients with glucose-6-phosphate dehydrogenase deficiency (an idiosyncratic reaction), gastrointestinal disturbances, and superinfections with bacteria and fungi, including pseudomembranous colitis. Suppression of the normal intestinal flora, an important source of vitamin K, may result in clotting disorders in patients with inadequate dietary intake; these effects are most frequent after oral administration of chloramphenicol.

TOPICAL ANTIBIOTICS

A cardinal rule of antimicrobial therapy is that, with few exceptions, antimicrobial agents should not be used topically. Two major exceptions to this rule are the topical application of nystatin or amphotericin B for treatment of superficial fungal infections of the integument or mucous membranes, and local administration of antibiotics for ophthalmic or otic infections. Topical use of antibiotics for these indications is seldom associated with adverse effects. On the other hand, agents used topically are often ineffective for other conditions, failing to reach inhibitory concentrations at the site of infection. Furthermore, they promote the selection and spread of resistant mutants throughout the environment and significantly increase the incidence of sensitization and resultant allergic reactions during subsequent local or systemic administration of the drugs or, perhaps, even their congeners.[1,47]

Although the efficacy of topical administration of antimicrobial agents is in most instances markedly inferior to systemic administration, these agents have been applied to virtually every external surface of the body and to many internal sites as well. Antibiotic powders and solutions have been instilled into pleural and peritoneal cavities, and numerous antimicrobial ointments and creams have been spread on skin and mucous membranes. In dentistry, antibiotics have been used in periodontal dressings, as ingredients in root canal medicaments, in local treatment of ANUG, in postextraction alveolar sockets, in pulp-capping materials, and for virtually every other conceivable indication. The majority of such uses are invalid and should be condemned.

A principle governing the selection of antibiotics for those few situations where topical administration is appropriate is that agents that have little or no systemic application should be chosen. (An exception to this principle is amphotericin B, largely because the development of resistance during topical use has not been a problem and because systemic administration is so highly toxic.) Common agents falling into this category are neomycin, the polymyxins, and bacitracin. Once reserved for treatment of serious systemic infections, these compounds have been essentially replaced for systemic use by less toxic drugs. The pharmacology of these agents is discussed briefly here; however, there is no valid indication for the use of these drugs, topically or otherwise, in the treatment or prophylaxis of orodental infections.

Neomycin

Neomycin is an aminoglycoside antibiotic pharmacologically similar to streptomycin and gentamicin. The drug exhibits a relatively broad spectrum of antibacterial activity. Although it was once employed parenterally for treatment of infections caused by *Proteus* and certain other species, neomycin is the most toxic of the aminoglycosides and has been replaced by less toxic congeners. The systemic use of neomycin is associated with severe toxicities, including permanent deafness and renal tubular necrosis. The topical use of neomycin may be accompanied by superinfections with resistant microbes and may lead to the spread of neomycin-resistant microorganisms.[1] Bacteria resistant to neomycin are also frequently unresponsive to the other aminoglycosides. Sensitization and allergic reactions (6% to 8% incidence) occur after the topical use of neomycin, and cross-reactivity exists with the other aminoglycosides.[47] Although neomycin is not absorbed from intact, noninflamed skin or mucous membranes, systemic absorption sufficient to cause severe toxicity may occur if excessive amounts of drug are used topically on abraded or otherwise disrupted tissue surfaces. In such instances, permanent deafness has resulted.[34] Topical application of neomycin should therefore be restricted to intact, noninflamed epithelium and should be strictly limited as to dosage and duration of therapy.

Polymyxins

Polymyxin B and polymyxin E (colistin, colistimethate) are polypeptide antibiotics derived from two different species of *Bacillus*. Polymyxin B is the agent usually incorporated into various formulations for topical administration. These agents are surface active and thus alter cell membrane permeability or disrupt the cell membrane to the extent that a bactericidal effect is usually achieved. The antibacterial activity of the polymyxins is exerted mainly against gram-negative bacteria, and they were once the agents of choice for treatment of systemic *Pseudomonas* infections. Systemic use, which requires parenteral administration, is associated with renal tubular necrosis, neurotoxicities, neuromuscular blockade with apnea, infrequent allergic reactions, and superinfections. At present, the polymyxins are rarely used systemically because of the availability of effective, less toxic agents such as gentamicin and carbenicillin.

In contrast to neomycin, polymyxin B is not absorbed to any extent, even from denuded areas of skin or mucous membranes; also, sensitization and allergic reactions occur less frequently. Although polymyxin B is relatively innocuous when employed topically, such use is often ineffective because of lack of penetration of sufficient amounts of drug to achieve adequate antibacterial concentrations at the infected foci. Development of bacterial resistance to the drug and superinfections have also occurred during topical administration of this antibiotic.

Bacitracin

Bacitracin is a polypeptide antibiotic elaborated by a strain of *Bacillus subtilis*. The agent acts by inhibiting cell wall synthesis in susceptible bacteria. Its antibacterial spectrum mainly includes gram-positive cocci, *Neisseria, Haemophilus,* and treponemes, a spectrum somewhat similar to that exhibited by penicillin G. Bacitracin, like other antibiotics, is not active against yeasts, fungi, or viruses. Because of its severe nephrotoxicity, the use of this antibiotic is now confined to topical administration. There are many more reports in the literature of treatment failure after topical use of this and other antibiotics than there are reports of success. Inadequate concentrations reached at the core of the infection after topical administration not only result in treatment failure but also encourage the selection and overgrowth of less susceptible bacteria. Allergic reactions to bacitracin occur rarely with topical application. Except for a few situations, the validity and efficacy of the topical use of this antibiotic, as well as neomycin and polymyxin B, for skin infections and infected wounds or as prophylaxis for wound infections are questionable.

DRUGS RESERVED FOR SPECIFIC INFECTIONS

Some antimicrobial drugs are reserved for the treatment of infections caused by specific microorganisms. Although limited in application, these drugs are nevertheless important because of the impact the diseases they treat have had on humanity.

Drugs used to treat tuberculosis

Successful treatment of tuberculosis, the once widespread disease caused by *Mycobacterium tuberculosis,* became possible only with the advent of chemotherapeutic agents. And yet even though such drugs have been available for some years, 27,000 new cases of this disease were documented in the United States during 1980. Because of the rapid development of antimicrobial resistance in strains of *M. tuberculosis,* a combination of agents is always used for treatment. The primary antituberculosis drugs are isoniazid and rifampin, and, to a lesser extent, ethambutol and streptomycin. For recurrent infections, cases that exhibit microbial resistance, or extrapulmonary infections, a group of secondary drugs are available, including pyrazinamide, aminosalicylic acid, ethionamide,

cycloserine, and others. These agents are generally less active and often more toxic than the primary drugs.

The majority of patients with tuberculosis can be effectively treated with isoniazid and rifampin.[17] In situations where resistance is suspected or documented, or for patients with miliary tuberculosis, including tuberculous meningitis, ethambutol or streptomycin is added to the regimen. The pharmacology of isoniazid, rifampin, and ethambutol is described here. Streptomycin, an aminoglycoside antibiotic, was discussed previously.

Isoniazid. Isoniazid, the name of which derives from its chemical designation, isonicotinic acid hydrazide (INH), is the most important drug for the treatment and prophylaxis of tuberculosis. Its spectrum of activity, however, is limited to *M. tuberculosis* and one species of atypical mycobacteria, *Mycobacterium kansasii.* Although the exact mechanism of action is unknown, it is hypothesized that isoniazid inhibits the synthesis of mycolic acids, unique and necessary components of the cell wall of mycobacteria. The drug is bactericidal to actively growing tubercle bacilli but not to dormant organisms. Resistance to isoniazid occurs by spontaneous mutation of the bacterial chromosome (at a rate of one in 10^6 divisions), which results in the failure of the bacterium to take up the drug. Most established infections can be expected to harbor at least several resistant bacteria. There is no cross-resistance between isoniazid and other antituberculosis drugs.

Isoniazid is well absorbed after either oral or parenteral administration, but the oral route is preferred for reasons of convenience and maximum therapeutic effect. The drug is well distributed into all body fluids, including the caseous material of the tubercle-infected foci. INH is mainly metabolized in the liver and excreted in the urine as metabolites. Genetic differences in the rate of biotransformation are seen, but these appear to have little effect on therapeutic efficacy. The plasma half-life is prolonged in patients with hepatic dysfunction.

One important adverse reaction with isoniazid is peripheral neuritis caused by an isoniazid-induced increase in the excretion of pyridoxine. This reaction and other symptoms of pyridoxine deficiency can be prevented by prophylactic administration of vitamin B_6 (15 to 50 mg daily). Other adverse effects include allergic reactions (fever, rashes, hepatitis), fatal hepatic necrosis (rarely), xerostomia, epigastric distress, hematologic reactions, and convulsions in seizure-prone patients (although administration of isoniazid to patients taking phenytoin has been without problems except for the potential of pharmacokinetic effects on phenytoin metabolism). A nonallergic hepatitis of some severity was reported over a decade ago,[26] and subsequent studies have shown that the incidence of hepatic damage increases with age and in those who drink alcohol regularly.

Isoniazid is the only drug effective for prophylaxis and the only drug approved for single-drug therapy. It is also the most important drug used in tuberculosis therapy for reasons of effectiveness, expense, convenience of administration, and toxicity.

Rifampin. Rifampin is a semisynthetic derivative of one of the rifamycins, a group of macrocyclic antibiotics produced by *Streptomyces mediterranei*. Rifampin is effective against a number of gram-positive and gram-negative bacteria in addition to *M. tuberculosis* and most other species of *Mycobacterium*. Its mechanism of action involves inhibition of DNA-dependent RNA polymerase in susceptible microorganisms. Mammalian RNA polymerase does not bind the drug, and RNA synthesis in host cells is therefore unaffected. Resistance can develop rapidly to rifampin, frequently in a single step, by alteration of the target enzyme.

Rifampin is generally well absorbed from the gastrointestinal tract after oral administration. The drug is distributed throughout the body and imparts an orange-red color to the urine, saliva, sweat, tears, sputum, and feces. It is secreted in the bile and undergoes enterohepatic recirculation, which prolongs its half-life. Elimination occurs by hepatic deacetylation and excretion in the urine and feces.

Rifampin combined with isoniazid is the primary therapeutic regimen for the treatment of most types of tuberculosis. It is also used for prophylaxis of disease in contacts of infected patients and for prophylaxis of tuberculosis in patients intolerant to isoniazid (e.g., patients with hepatic disease). The drug has proved effective in certain diseases refractory to conventional therapy. For example, rifampin combined with a β-lactam antibiotic or vancomycin has been used to treat endocarditis or osteomyelitis caused by methicillin-resistant staphylococci.

The incidence of adverse reactions to rifampin is relatively low (4%). Jaundice, gastrointestinal disturbances, hepatorenal syndrome, suppression of T-lymphocyte function, neurologic disorders, and a variety of allergic reactions, including soreness of the mouth and tongue, have been reported. Decreased effectiveness of oral anticoagulants, oral contraceptives, estrogens, and glucocorticoids has occurred with concomitant administration of rifampin.

Ethambutol. Ethambutol is a synthetic agent with an unknown mechanism of action. It is active against almost all strains of *M. tuberculosis* and *M. kansasii*. Other *Mycobacterium* species show variable sensitivity and other bacteria are not affected by the drug. Ethambutol is tuberculostatic, and resistance develops, although slowly, if it is used alone.

Ethambutol is given orally, since absorption from the gastrointestinal tract is good. Distribution into various body compartments is adequate. The major route of excretion of ethambutol is by renal tubular secretion and glomerular filtration, the drug appearing in the urine as unchanged drug (50%) and two metabolites. Dosage adjustment is required in the presence of renal impairment.

Ethambutol is used along with isoniazid and rifampin for the treatment of severe cases of pulmonary tuberculosis. This practice ensures sensitivity to at least two of the drugs until the results of susceptibility tests are received. A combination of isoniazid, rifampin, and either ethambutol or streptomycin is also used for disseminated tuberculosis.

Adverse reactions to ethambutol are infrequent, the most notable being optic neuritis, with symptoms of decreased visual acuity and loss of the ability to perceive the color green. Other adverse effects include gastrointestinal upset, peripheral neuritis, allergic reactions, usually appearing as skin rashes or drug fever, and increased retention of uric acid.

Drugs used to treat leprosy

Although leprosy is rarely seen in the United States, the World Health Organization estimates that 12 million cases exist throughout the world. Leprosy is a bacterial disease caused by the tubercle bacillus, *Mycobacterium leprae*. Five clinical types of leprosy are recognized, ranging from the skin lesion of tuberculoid leprosy to the neuropathies and spontaneous amputations occurring in disseminated lepromatous disease. Patients may be infectious or noninfectious, depending on the type, duration, and effectiveness of therapy. Generally, this disease can be treated successfully with drugs. Treatment may be as short as 2 to 4 years or extend throughout life, depending on the severity and type of disease.

The sulfones, dapsone in particular, are the major drugs used in the treatment of leprosy. These chemical relatives to the sulfonamides are bacteriostatic against *M. leprae,* with a mechanism of action similar to that of the sulfonamides. These sulfones are used orally. Other drugs, normally used in combination with the sulfones but occasionally alone, are rifampin, clofazimine, and amithiozone.

Drugs used to treat gonorrhea

Gonorrhea is an infection caused by the gram-negative coccus *Neisseria gonorrhoeae.* Traditionally, this microorganism has been susceptible to penicillin G and the ampicillin-like derivatives. However, increased resistance currently requires higher doses of penicillin G, and penicillinase-producing strains totally resistant to penicillin G have emerged. In patients allergic to the penicillins, treatment with a tetracycline has been effective. Erythromycin is a third choice, but relapse rates are high (25%). Alternative antibiotics that have been used with success include several cephalosporins and trimethoprim-sulfamethoxazole.

In the treatment of gonorrhea caused by penicillinase-producing gonococci, spectinomycin has become the drug of choice. This drug may also be used to treat gonorrhea in patients allergic to the penicillins. Spectinomycin is an aminocyclitol antibiotic, similar to the aminoglycosides, with activity against a number of gram-negative bacteria. Spectinomycin is highly active against *N. gonorrhoeae,* however, and its use is largely restricted to this organism. For uncomplicated gonococcal infections, spectinomycin is generally given intramuscularly in a single 2 gm dose.

*Antibacterial antibiotics**

Nonproprietary name	*Proprietary name*
Aminoglycosides	
amikacin	Amikin
gentamicin	Garamycin, Bristagen
kanamycin	Kantrex, Klebcil
neomycin	Mycifradin Sulfate
netilmicin	Netromycin
streptomycin	—
tobramycin	Nebcin
Antituberculosis drugs	
aminosalicylate	Teebacin
capreomycin	Capastat Sulfate
cycloserine	Seromycin Pulvules
ethambutol	Myambutol
ethionamide	Trecator-SC
isoniazid	Nydrazid
pyrazinamide	—
rifampin	Rifadin, Rimactane
Topical antibiotics	
bacitracin	Baciguent
neomycin	Myciguent
polymyxin B	Aerosporin Sterile
bacitracin with neomycin and polymyxin B	Mycitracin, Neosporin, Neo-Polycin
Miscellaneous agents	
chloramphenicol	Chloromycetin
colistimethate	Coly-Mycin M
colistin	Coly-Mycin S
dapsone	—
novobiocin	Albamycin
spectinomycin	Trobicin
troleandomycin	Tao

*Agents not shown here are listed in various tables throughout this chapter.

CITED REFERENCES

1. Alder, V.G., and Gillespie, W.A. Influence of neomycin sprays on the spread of resistant staphylococci. Lancet **2**:1062-1063, 1967.

2. Bennett, W.M., Singer, I., and Coggins, C.J. A guide to drug therapy in renal failure. Journal of the American Medical Association **230**:1544-1553, 1974.

3. Bergner-Rabinowitz, S., and Davies, A.M. Sensitivity of *Streptococcus pyogenes* types to tetracycline and other antibiotics. Israel Journal of Medical Sciences **6**:393-398, 1970.

4. Best, W.R. Chloramphenicol-associated blood dyscrasias. Journal of the American Medical Association **201**:181-188, 1967.

5. Bystedt, H., Dahlback, A., Dornbusch, K., and Nord, C.E. Concentrations of azidocillin, erythromycin, doxycycline and clindamycin in human mandibular bone. International Journal of Oral Surgery **7**:442-449, 1978.

6. Carey, B.W. Photodynamic response of a new tetracycline. Journal of the American Medical Association **172**:1196, 1960.

7. Cefamandole and cefoxitin. Medical Letter on Drugs and Therapeutics **21**:13-15, 1979.

8. Cefotaxime sodium (Claforan). Medical Letter on Drugs and Therapeutics **23**:61-62, 1981.

9. Chabbert, Y.A., and Lutz, A.J. HR-756, the *syn* isomer of a new methoxyimino cephalosporin with unusual antibacterial activity. Antimicrobial Agents and Chemotherapy **14**:749-754, 1978.

10. Chan, R.A., Benner, E.J., and Hoeprich, P.D. Gentamicin therapy in renal failure: a nomogram for dosage. Annals of Internal Medicine **76**:773-778, 1972.

11. Cleveland, W.W., Adams, W.C., Mann, J.B., and Nyhan, W.L. Acquired Fanconi syndrome following degraded tetracycline. Journal of Pediatrics **66**:333-342, 1965.

12. Condon, R.E., and Anderson, M.J. Diarrhea and colitis in clindamycin treated patients. Archives of Surgery **113**:794-797, 1978.

13. Corcoran, J.W., and Hahn, F.E., eds. Mechanism of Action of Antimicrobial and Antitumor Agents. Antibiotics Series, vol. 3. New York, Springer-Verlag, 1974.

14. De Weck, A.L., and Schneider, C.H. Penicillin antigens. In Rose, B., ed. Allergology. Amsterdam, Excerpta Medica Foundation, 1967.

15. Domagk, G. Ein Beitrag zur Chemotherapie der bakteriellen Infektionen. Deutsche Medizinische Wochenschrift **61**:250-253, 1935.

16. Drucker, D.B., and Jolly, M. Sensitivity of oral microorganisms to antibiotics. British Dental Journal **131**:442-444, 1971.

17. Drugs for tuberculosis. Medical Letter on Drugs and Therapeutics **24**:17-19, 1982.

18. Finland, M. Twenty-fifth anniversary of the discovery of Aureomycin: the place of the tetracyclines in antimicrobial therapy. Clinical Pharmacology and Therapeutics **15**:3-8, 1974.

19. Finland, M. And the walls come tumbling down. New England Journal of Medicine **299**:770-771, 1978.

20. Fourneau, E., Tréfouël, J., Tréfouël, J., Nitti, F., and Bovet, D. Chimiothérapie des infections streptococciques par les dérivés du p-aminophénylsulfamide. Comptes Rendus des Seances de la Societé de Biologie et de Ses Filiales **122**:258-259, 1936.

21. Franklin, T.J. Resistance of *Escherichia coli* to tetracyclines: changes in permeability to tetracyclines in *Escherichia coli* bearing transferable resistance factors. Biochemical Journal **105**:371-378, 1967.

22. Fraser, D.G. Selection of an oral erythromycin product. American Journal of Hospital Pharmacy **37**:1199-1205, 1980.

23. Fu, K.P., and Neu, H.C. Azlocillin and mezlocillin: new ureidopenicillins. Antimicrobial Agents and Chemotherapy **13**:930-939, 1978.

24. Furey, W.W., and Tan, C. Anaphylactic shock due to oral demethylchlortetracycline. Annals of Internal Medicine **70**:357-358, 1969.

25. Gabrielson, M.L., and Stroh, E. Antibiotic efficacy in odontogenic infections. Journal of Oral Surgery **33**:607-610, 1975.

26. Garibaldi, R.A., Drusin, R.E., Ferebee, S.H., and Gregg, M.B. Isoniazid-associated hepatitis. Report of an outbreak. American Review of Respiratory Disease **106**:357-365, 1972.

27. Genco, R.J. Antibiotics in the treatment of human periodontal diseases. Journal of Periodontology **52**:545-558, 1981.

28. Gentry, L.O., Jemsek, J.G., and Natelson, E.A. Effects of sodium piperacillin on platelet function in normal volunteers. Antimicrobial Agents and Chemotherapy **19**:532-533, 1981.

29. Goodson, J.M., Holborow, D., Hogan, P., and Dunham, S. Characteristics of monolithic tetracycline containing fibers for periodontal therapy. Journal of Dental Research **61**:274, 1982.

30. Gopalakrishna, K.V., and Lerner, P.I. Tetracycline-resistant pneumococci: increasing incidence and cross resistance to newer tetracyclines. American Review of Respiratory Disease **108**:1007-1010, 1973.

31. Hunt, D.E., King, T.J., and Fuller, G.E. Antibiotic susceptibility of bacteria isolated from oral infections. Journal of Oral Surgery **36**:527-529, 1978.

32. Jacobs, M.R., Koornhof, H.J., Robins-Browne, R.M., Stevenson, C.M., Vermaak, Z.A., Freiman, I., Miller, G.B., Witcomb, M.A., Isaäcson, M., Ward, J.I., and Austrian, R.A. Emergence of multiply resistant pneumococci. New England Journal of Medicine **299**:735-740, 1978.

33. Kannangara, D.W., Thadepalli, H., and McQuirter, J.L. Bacteriology and treatment of dental infections. Oral Surgery **50**:103-109, 1980.

34. Kelly, D.R., Nilo, E.R., and Berggren, R.B. Deafness after topical neomycin wound irrigation. New England Journal of Medicine **280**:1338-1339, 1969.

35. Kline, A.H., Blattner, R.J., and Lunin, M. Transplacental effect of tetracyclines on teeth. Journal of the American Medical Association **188**:178-180, 1964.

36. Kosmidis, J., Hamilton-Miller, J.M.T., Gilchrist, J.N.G., Kerry, D.W., and Brumfitt, W. Cefoxitin, a new semisynthetic cephamycin: an in-vitro and in-vivo comparison with cephalothin. British Medical Journal **4**:653-655, 1973.

37. Kunelis, C.T., Peters, J.L., and Edmondson, H.A. Fatty liver of pregnancy and its relationship to tetracycline therapy. American Journal of Medicine **38**:359-377, 1965.

38. Kurtz, T.O., Winston, D.J., Hindler, J.A., Young, L.S., Hewitt, W.L., and Martin, W.J. Comparative in vitro activity of moxalactam, cefotaxime, cefoperazone, pipera-

cillin, and aminoglycosides against gram-negative bacilli. Antimicrobial Agents and Chemotherapy **18**:645-648, 1980.

39. Lau, W.K., and Young, L.S. Co-trimoxazole treatment of *Pneumocystis carinii* pneumonia in adults. New England Journal of Medicine **295**:716-718, 1976.

40. Leyden, J.J., Marples, R.R., Mills, O.H., Jr., and Kligman, A.M. Gram-negative folliculitis—a complication of antibiotic therapy in acne vulgaris. British Journal of Dermatology **88**:553-538, 1973.

41. Loesche, W.J., Syed, S.A., Morrison, E.C., Laughon, B., and Grossman, N.S. Treatment of periodontal infections due to anaerobic bacteria with short-term treatment with metronidazole. Journal of Clinical Periodontology **8**:29-44, 1981.

42. Mitchell, D.F., and Holmes, L.A. Topical antibiotic control of dentogingival plaque. Journal of Periodontology **36**:202-208, 1965.

43. Moellering, R.C., Jr., and Swartz, M.N. The newer cephalosporins. New England Journal of Medicine **294**:24-28, 1976.

44. Moxalactam disodium *(Moxam)* Medical Letter on Drugs and Therapeutics **24**:13-14, 1982.

45. Owen, R.C., and Kenyon, R. An investigation of erythromycin stearate and erythromycin succinate in the treatment of oral infections. Dental Digest **72**:166-169. 1966.

46. Pien, F.D., Thompson, R.L., and Martin, W.J. Clinical and bacteriologic studies of anaerobic gram-positive cocci. Mayo Clinic Proceedings **47**:251-257, 1972.

47. Pirilä, V., Förström, L., and Rouhunkoski, S. Twelve years of sensitization to neomycin in Finland. Acta Dermato-Venereologica **47**:419-425, 1967.

48. Rams, T.E., and Keyes, P.H. A rationale for the management of periodontal diseases: effects of tetracycline on subgingival bacteria. Journal of the American Dental Association **107**:37-41, 1983.

49. Root, R.K., and Hierholzer, W.J. Infectious disease. In Melmon, K.L., and Morelli, H.F., eds. Clinical Pharmacology, ed. 2, New York, Macmillan, Inc., 1978.

50. Rudolph, A.H., and Price, E.V. Penicillin reactions among patients in venereal disease clinics. A national survey. Journal of the American Medical Association **223**:499-501, 1973.

51. Sabiston, C.B., Jr., and Gold, W.A. Anaerobic bacteria in oral infections. Oral Surgery, Oral Medicine, and Oral Pathology **38**:187-192, 1974.

52. Schultz, J.C., Adamson, J.S., Jr., Workman, W.W., and Norman, T.D. Fatal liver disease after intravenous administration of tetracycline in high dosage. New England Journal of Medicine **269**:999-1004, 1963.

53. Scopp, I.W., Gillette, W., Kumar, V., and Larato, D. Treatment of oral lesions with topically applied vancomycin hydrochloride. Oral Surgery, Oral Medicine, and Oral Pathology **24**:703-706, 1967.

54. Searcy, R.L., Foreman, J.A., Meyers, H.D., and Berquist, L.M. Anticoagulant properties of tetracyclines. In Sylvester, J.C., ed. Antimicrobial Agents and Chemotherapy—1963. Ann Arbor, Mich., American Society for Microbiology, 1964.

55. Shaw, W.V. Comparative enzymology of chloramphenicol resistance. Annals of the New York Academy of Sciences **182**:234-242, 1971.

56. Shuford, G.M. Concentrations of cephalexin in mandibular alveolar bone, blood, and oral fluids. Journal of the American Dental Association **99**:47-50, 1979.

57. Smilack, J.D., Flittie, W.H., and Williams, T.W., Jr. Bone concentrations of antimicrobial agents after parenteral administration. Antimicrobial Agents and Chemotherapy **9**:169-171, 1976.

58. Smith, H., ed. Antibiotics in Clinical Practice, ed. 3. Baltimore, University Park Press, 1977.

59. Socransky, S.S. Microbiology of periodontal disease—present status and future considerations. Journal of Periodontology **48**:497-504, 1977.

60. Sosna, J.P., Murray, P.R., and Medoff, G. Comparison of the in vitro activities of HR756 with cephalothin, cefoxitin, and cefamandole. Antimicrobial Agents and Chemotherapy **14**:876-879, 1978.

61. Spotts, C.R. Physiological and biochemical studies on streptomycin dependence in *Escherichia coli*. Journal of General Microbiology **28**:347-365, 1962.

62. Sprunt, K., Leidy, G., and Redman, W. Cross resistance between lincomycin and erythromycin in viridans streptococci. Pediatrics **46**:84-88, 1970.

63. Stewart, G.T. The Penicillin Group of Drugs. London, Elsevier Publishing Co., 1965.

64. Stilwell, G.A., and Turck, M. Choosing alternatives to penicillin. Drug Therapy **4**:77-87, 1974.

65. Sullivan, D., Csuka, M.E., and Blanchard, B. Erythromycin ethylsuccinate hepatotoxicity. Journal of the American Medical Association **243**:1074, 1980.

66. Sutherland, R., Croydon, E.A.P., and Rolinson, G.N. Amoxycillin: a new semi-synthetic penicillin. British Medical Journal **3**:13-16, 1972.

67. Swartzberg, J.E., Maresca, R.M., and Remington, J.S. Gastrointestinal side effects associated with clindamycin. Archives of Internal Medicine **136**:876-879, 1976.

68. Tolman, K.G., Sannella, J.J., and Freston, J.W. Chemical structure of erythromycin and hepatotoxicity. Annals of Internal Medicine **81**:58-60, 1974.

69. Trager, G.M., White, G.W., Zimelis, V.M., and Panwalker, A.P. LY-127935: a novel beta-lactam antibiotic with unusual antibacterial activity. Antibacterial Agents and Chemotherapy **16**:297-300, 1979.

70. Treatment of methicillin-resistant *Staphylococcus aureus* infections. Medical Letter on Drugs and Therapeutics **24**:107-108, 1982.

71. Tréfouël, J., Tréfouël, J., Nitti, F., and Bovet, D. Activité du p-aminophénylsulfamide sur les infections streptococciques expérimentales de la souris et du lapin. Comptes Rendus des Seances de la Societé de Biologie et de Ses Filiales **120**:756-758, 1935.

72. Turck, M. Alternatives to penicillin. Drug Therapy **6**:8-19, 1976.

73. Turner, J.E., Moore, D.W., and Shaw, B.S. Prevalence and antibiotic susceptibility of organisms isolated from acute soft-tissue abscesses secondary to dental caries. Oral Surgery, Oral Medicine, and Oral Pathology **39**:848-857, 1975.

74. Walker, C.B., Gordon, J.M., McQuilkin, S.J., Niebloom, T.A., and Socransky, S.S. Tetracycline: levels achievable in gingival crevice fluid and in vitro effects on subgingival organisms. Part II. Susceptibilities of periodontal bacteria. Journal of Periodontology **52**:613-616, 1981.

75. Wallick, H., and Hendlin, D. Cefoxitin, a semisynthetic cephamycin antibiotic: susceptibility studies. Antimicrobial Agents and Chemotherapy **5:**25-32, 1974.
76. Ward, H.P. The effect of chloramphenicol on RNA and heme synthesis in bone marrow cultures. Journal of Laboratory and Clinical Medicine **68:**400-410, 1966.
77. Weinstein, L., and Weinstein, A.J. The pathophysiology and pathoanatomy of reactions to antimicrobial agents. Advances in Internal Medicine **19:**109-134, 1974.
78. Weyman, J. Tetracyclines and teeth. Practitioner **195:**661-665, 1965.
79. White, P.J. and Woods, D.D. The synthesis of *p*-aminobenzoic acid and folic acid by staphylococci sensitive and resistant to sulphonamides. Journal of General Microbiology **40:**243-253, 1965.

GENERAL REFERENCES

Kucers, A., and Bennett, N. McK. The Use of Antibiotics: A Comprehensive Review with Clinical Emphasis, ed. 3. Philadelphia, J.B. Lippincott Co., 1979.
Mandell, G.L., and Sande, M.A. Antimicrobial Agents. In Gilman, A.G., Goodman, L.S., and Gilman, A., eds. Goodman and Gilman's The Pharmacological Basis of Therapeutics, ed. 6. New York, Macmillan, Inc., 1980.

38 Antifungal and antiviral agents

Edward H. Montgomery

This chapter will deal with the drugs that are used to combat fungal infections (not including drugs that belong among the antiseptics and disinfectants) and that relatively new and limited group known as the antiviral drugs, whose development has accompanied our growing understanding of viruses.

ANTIFUNGAL AGENTS

Fungal diseases may take the form of superficial or cutaneous infestations or deep mycotic infections involving internal organs of the body (systemic mycotic infections). Some organisms, for example *Candida albicans*, may be involved in both superficial and systemic mycotic afflictions. Predisposing factors to fungal infections include the use of broad-spectrum antibiotics (which frequently lead to superinfections), debilitation of the patient, and disease states or the use of drugs that compromise host defense processes. Patients at risk of developing a fungal infection must be carefully observed during antibiotic therapy, because systemic mycotic diseases can be life-threatening.

A variety of antifungal drugs are currently available. The two antifungal antibiotics of greatest interest to dentistry are nystatin and amphotericin B, because these agents have proved effective in the treatment of oral candidiasis. Flucytosine is used in conjunction with amphotericin B for serious systemic fungal infections refractory to amphotericin B alone. The newer antifungal agents miconazole and ketoconazole are also used for systemic fungal infections and occasionally for certain superficial mycoses refractory to nystatin. A number of other antifungal preparations are available for treatment of superficial fungal infections of the skin (e.g., tolnaftate) or for systemic treatment of dermatophytosis (e.g., griseofulvin).

Nystatin

Nystatin, the first of the antifungal antibiotics, was obtained from *Streptomyces noursei* and was introduced into clinical use in 1954. It is a member of the polyene family, so called because their structure consists of a large lactone (macrolide) ring, with numerous double bonds, attached to amino sugars (Figure 38-1). Nystatin is relatively insoluble in water and unstable except as the dry powder. The antifungal activity of this drug is enhanced at a pH above 6.0 and decreased in an acid environment.

Mechanism of action and antifungal spectrum. At neutral and alkaline pH, nystatin is actively taken up by fungal cells. It binds to sterols present in the fungal cell membrane and induces a change in membrane permeability such that leakage of intracellular ions and other constituents occurs. The drug is most effective during the active growth phase of the fungal cell; it is active against a number of species of *Candida, Histoplasma, Cryptococcus, Blastomyces, Epidermophyton, Trichophyton,* and *Microsporum*. Depending on the concentration of nystatin present and the kind of organism involved, nystatin may be either fungistatic or fungicidal. Since bacteria do not contain the sterol moiety, nystatin has no activity against them or against viruses or protozoa.

Fungal resistance. Although resistance of some species of *Candida* (but not *C. albicans*) can be demonstrated in vitro, resistance does not appear to develop in vivo.

Absorption, fate, and excretion. Nystatin is not appreciably absorbed from the skin, mucous membranes, or gastrointestinal tract. After oral administration, the bulk of the administered dose appears in the feces. Because of its systemic toxicity, nystatin is not used for the treatment of systemic fungal infections.

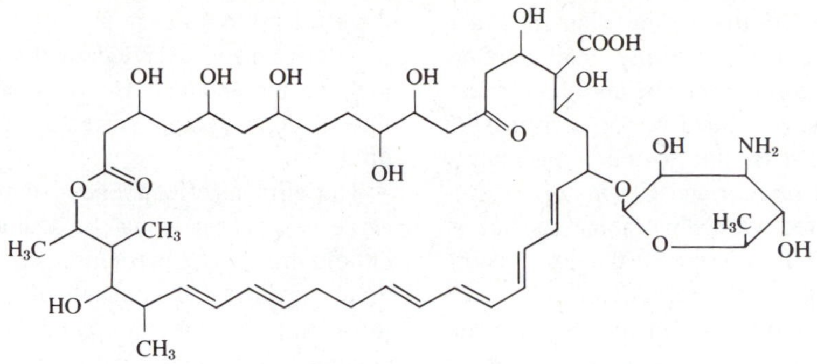

Figure 38-1. Structural formula of nystatin.

Therapeutic uses. Nystatin is used topically for treatment of susceptible fungal infestations involving the skin and the mucous membranes of the mouth, gastrointestinal tract, and vagina. It is the agent of choice for the treatment of candidal infections of the oral cavity (oral moniliasis, thrush, denture stomatitis). For oral candidiasis, nystatin is available in 60 ml bottles containing 100,000 units/ml. Two to 3 ml of the suspension are placed in each side of the mouth, swished, and held for at least 5 minutes before swallowing. This regimen is repeated every 6 hours for at least 10 days or for 48 hours after remission of symptoms. For denture stomatitis, nystatin ointment (100,000 units/gm in 15 and 30 gm tubes) is applied over the tissue side of the dentures every 6 hours and repeated as described above. Though rare, intestinal candidiasis may be present in a patient being treated by a dentist for the oral form of the disease. Severe diarrhea should warn the clinician that the patient may need medical attention and further antifungal therapy.

Toxic reactions and side effects. A few cases of nausea, vomiting, and diarrhea have occurred when nystatin has been used for the treatment of oral or intestinal candidiasis. Otherwise, the use of this drug by topical application is not accompanied by adverse effects.

Amphotericin B

Amphotericin B is a polyene antifungal compound derived from *Streptomyces nodosus*. Amphotericin B is similar chemically and pharmacologically to nystatin; however, it has a wider spectrum of antifungal activity, is slightly less toxic when administered systemically, and may therefore be used parenterally as well as topically. Amphotericin B is the treatment of choice for most systemic mycotic infections.[2]

Amphotericin B is not absorbed from the skin or mucous membranes and may be used for treatment of superficial mycotic infections at these sites. In addition, it can be given intravenously for treatment of systemic mycotic infections. Resistance to this drug is not a clinical problem. The only toxic manifestation accompanying the topical use of amphotericin B is local irritation and mild gastrointestinal disturbances. The systemic use of this drug, however, is associated with a large number of adverse effects, including thrombophlebitis, headache, chills, fever, allergic reactions of all types (including anaphylaxis), neurotoxicity, nephrotoxicity, hepatotoxicity, blood dyscrasias, and cardiodepressant effects. All patients receiving amphotericin B should be hospitalized, at least for the initial period of therapy. Deep-seated mycotic infections are difficult to treat, and drug therapy may have to continue for several months. Currently, no preparation of amphotericin B is marketed for topical application in dentistry, but a 2% concentration of the drug in an adhesive preparation has proved to be effective in the treatment of oral lesions caused by *C. albicans*.

Flucytosine

Chemically, flucytosine is 5-fluorocytosine, a synthetic antimetabolite that was found to have antifungal activity. It is converted within the fungal cell by the enzyme cytosine deaminase to 5-fluorouracil, which is further converted to 5-fluorodeoxyuridylic acid, a competitive inhibitor of thymidylate synthetase. Nucleic acid synthesis is competitively inhibited at this step. Selective toxicity is achieved by the fact that mammalian cells lack cytosine deaminase or convert only small amounts of flucytosine to fluorouracil. The antifungal spectrum of flucytosine is limited in comparison with that of amphotericin B, flucytosine being mainly effective against *Candida* and *Cryptococcus* species. It is also effective against some species of *Cladosporium* and *Phialophora,* the latter being etiologic agents for chromoblastomycosis.

Fungal resistance to flucytosine occurs frequently in vivo, restricting its use as a single agent in the treatment of systemic mycoses. Therefore, it is usually used in combination with amphotericin B. This combination results in supraadditive activity against the above mentioned genera. Flucytosine has, however, been used as a single agent for treatment of chromoblastomycosis.[7]

Fluocytosine is well absorbed from the gastrointestinal tract after oral administration and is distributed throughout the total body water. It attains a concentration in the cerebrospinal fluid of 50% to 90% that of the plasma and even penetrates the aqueous humor. Excretion is mainly by glomerular filtration, and dosage reduction is required in the presence of renal impairment.

Untoward reactions to flucytosine include nausea, vomiting, diarrhea, severe enterocolitis, rash, and bone marrow depression leading to anemia, leukopenia, and thrombocytopenia. Elevation of hepatic enzymes and hepatomegaly have occurred in 5% of the patients treated with flucytosine.

Miconazole

Miconazole is a synthetic antifungal agent. It affects the permeability of the fungal cell membrane and is usually fungicidal. The antifungal spectrum of miconazole is broad and includes species of *Candida, Cryptococcus, Histoplasma, Coccidioides, Paracoccidioides, Aspergillus, Cladosporium, Madurella, Phialophora, Petriellidium, Blastomyces, Microsporum, Epidermophyton,* and *Trichophyton.*

Miconazole must be administered parenterally for treatment of systemic fungal infections. Intravenous infusion of recommended doses produces plasma concentrations exceeding the MIC for most of the pathogenic fungi listed above.[1] The drug is largely excluded from sputum, saliva, and cerebrospinal fluid; treatment of coccidioidal meningitis therefore requires intrathecal administration. Following cutaneous application, miconazole

readily penetrates the stratum corneum and persists there for up to 4 days. The drug is metabolized in the liver and is excreted in the urine, mainly as inactive metabolites. Hence, fungal infections of the bladder require direct irrigation with the drug.

The clinical effectiveness of parenteral miconazole has been adequately demonstrated for coccidioidomycosis, petriellidiosis, and paracoccidioidomycosis.[8] Miconazole also may be of value in treatment of systemic candidiasis, chronic mucocutaneous candidiasis, and cryptococcosis. It should not be used systemically for trivial fungal infections, such as oral candidiasis, tinea pedis (athlete's foot) or vulvovaginal candidiasis, but it may be used topically for these conditions.

Adverse effects of systemically administered miconazole are frequent and include phlebitis, nausea, vomiting, diarrhea, hyponatremia, anemia, thrombocytopenia, severe pruritus, arthralgia, hyperlipidemia, and anaphylaxis.[12] Topically applied miconazole has been associated with burning, irritation, maceration, and urticaria. Intravaginal administration may result in pelvic cramps.

Miconazole must be used cautiously in patients taking coumarin-type anticoagulants, since enhanced anticoagulant activity has been reported after systemic administration. Concomitant administration of miconazole and amphotericin B results in mutual antagonism of antifungal activity.

Ketoconazole

Ketoconazole, released in 1981, is a synthetic imidazole chemically similar to miconazole. The mechanism of action of ketoconazole is the inhibition of the synthesis of ergosterol, an important membrane component of fungal cells but not of mammalian cells. The result is an alteration of fungal cell membrane permeability. The antifungal spectrum of ketoconazole is broad in vitro and includes species of *Candida, Coccidioides, Histoplasma, Cryptococcus, Blastomyces, Paracoccidioides, Phialophora,* and dermatophytes. Fungal resistance to ketoconazole is not a clinical problem at present.

Ketoconazole is readily absorbed from the gastrointestinal tract provided the pH range remains acidic. Peak plasma concentrations are reached in 1 to 4 hours. The drug is distributed into most body compartments, but penetration into the cerebrospinal fluid is poor. The major route of excretion is via the bile, mainly in the form of inactive metabolites. The plasma half-life is sufficiently long to allow once-a-day dosage.

Ketoconazole has been effective in the treatment of coccidioidomycosis, paracoccidioidomycosis, and histoplasmosis.[6] It has been used successfully for treatment of systemic candidiasis, chromomycosis, and dermatophyte infections resistant to other antifungal agents. It appears to be the drug of choice for treatment of chronic mucocutaneous candidiasis even though relapse may occur on discontinuation of therapy.[9] Although ketoconazole has been used for treatment of oral candidiasis, its potential toxicity indicates that it should be reserved for cases refractory to more conventional therapy with topically applied nystatin.

When ketoconazole was first released, adverse effects were thought to be mild and transient, including nausea, vomiting, and pruritus. Wider use of the drug has revealed a number of cases of idiosyncratic hepatocellular dysfunction, some being fatal. Therefore, the use of ketoconazole should be limited to serious systemic fungal infections.

Since ketoconazole requires acidity for dissolution, its absorption is inhibited when used with agents that increase gastrointestinal pH, such as antacids, anticholinergics, and the histamine H_2 blockers.

ANTIVIRAL AGENTS

Advances in the chemotherapy of viral infections have by no means paralleled the achievements in the chemotherapy of other microbial diseases. The reason for this, which applies as well to the chemotherapy of neoplastic disorders, is the inability to achieve an adequate degree of selective toxicity. The intimate relationship between viruses and host cells, viruses being obligate intracellular parasites, leaves the chemotherapeutic agent only a few accessible points of attack on the virus without markedly affecting the invaded cell. In addition, the temporal delay between the infection of cells by the viruses and the onset of clinical symptoms poses problems for chemotherapy. In contrast to bacterial diseases, clinical symptoms of a viral infection usually appear after the processes of viral replication and release of a large number of virons within the body have been completed.[10] Pathologic changes have occurred by this time, and the clinical course of the disease may not be altered significantly even if it were possible to kill only the viruses with chemotherapeutic agents. (Such selective viricidal agents are not available.) Since ac-

cessible points of attack for chemotherapy occur before the onset of clinical symptoms, and treatment must often be initiated at this time in order to be efficacious, antiviral therapy is of necessity largely a prophylactic or preventive measure. The most reliable means of prophylaxis of viral infections is by immunologic mechanisms, that is, the use of vaccines (immunotherapy). Effective chemotherapy of most viral infections remains to be established.

There are a number of antiviral agents, most of which are under investigation. Some are synthetic chemicals, others are naturally occurring antibiotics, and still others are endogenously produced substances (e.g., interferons). Of these agents, amantadine, idoxuridine, vidarabine, trifluridine, and acyclovir are available for general clinical use.

General mechanism of action

There are three events involved in progression of viral infections that can be inhibited by drugs: (1) penetration into the host cell and uncoating of the viral genome (achieved by amantadine), (2) viral nucleic acid replication within the host cell (by acyclovir, idoxuridine, trifluridine, and vidarabine), and (3) synthesis of viral proteins (by interferons).

Idoxuridine

Idoxuridine is a pyrimidine analogue of thymidine. The main effect of the drug results from its conversion to the triphosphate derivative and its incorporation in place of thymidine into DNA. The resultant DNA is defective both structurally and functionally. Idoxuridine is thus active against DNA viruses such as the herpesvirus group, cytomegalovirus, and vaccinia virus. Viral resistance, however, commonly develops during therapy. (Idoxuridine is inactivated by nucleotidases.) The drug has been administered locally for ophthalmic and cutaneous infections caused by susceptible viruses; it is currently marketed in an ophthalmic solution and ointment for the treatment of herpes simplex keratitis. Idoxuridine applied topically has been tried, with some claims of success, for herpes lesions in the mouth. However, such lesions are normally best treated palliatively. Treatment of herpes encephalitis has been disappointing. The systemic use of idoxuridine is associated with severe toxic effects resulting from inhibition of DNA synthesis in mammalian cells. The dose-related adverse reactions include bone marrow depression with thrombocytopenia and leukopenia, stomatitis, nausea, vomiting, gastrointestinal hemorrhage, hepatic damage (jaundice), alopecia, and loss of fingernails. The drug is teratogenic and potentially carcinogenic. The topical use of the drug (e.g., in the eye) may produce local irritation, inflammation, photophobia, and allergic reactions.

Vidarabine

Vidarabine is a purine nucleoside derived from *Streptomyces antibioticus*. It inhibits viral DNA synthesis (by affecting DNA polymerase) and therefore has a similar antiviral spectrum to that of idoxuridine (including herpes simplex types 1 and 2, varicella-zoster, and vaccinia). Topical vidarabine appears to be superior to idoxuridine for the treatment of herpetic keratitis: it is at least as effective as idoxuridine, allergic reactions and viral resistance are less of a problem, and it is less irritating to the eye. Of greater significance is the fact that vidarabine is the first antiviral drug that is curative for a systemic viral infection. Collaborative studies have shown that mortality as a result of herpes simplex encephalitis is reduced from 70% to 28% when vidarabine is administered to noncomatose patients.[13]

Because of the compound's low solubility and poor gastrointestinal absorption, vidarabine must be administered by intravenous infusion. The drug is rapidly deaminated to arabinosyl hypoxanthine, which is then excreted in the urine. Major toxic effects of vidarabine administered systemically include gastrointestinal disturbances (nausea, vomiting, diarrhea), CNS manifestations (dizziness, confusion, ataxia), and hematologic disorders (hyperbilirubinemia, leukopenia, etc.). As with other drugs affecting DNA synthesis, vidarabine is teratogenic and probably carcinogenic.

Trifluridine

Trifluridine is a fluorinated thymidine derivative available for topical use in ophthalmology. As with the previous antiviral agents mentioned, trifluridine is effective in vitro against DNA viruses such as herpes simplex types 1 and 2. Trifluridine is thought to exert several actions: inhibition of thymidine kinase, inhibition of DNA polymerase, and formation of faulty DNA. The drug penetrates into the aqueous humor after topical instillation; the presence of herpetic lesions may enhance local uptake.

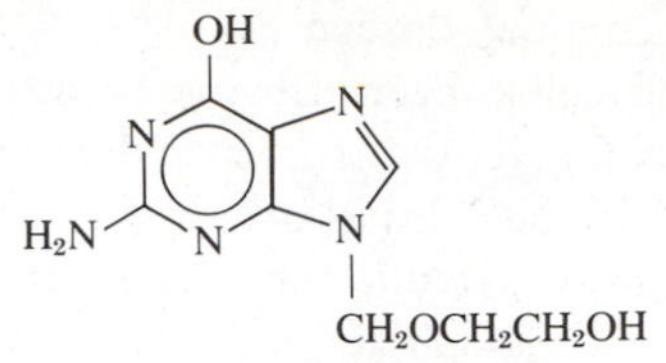

Figure 38-2. Structural formula of acyclovir.

Trifluridine is currently the drug of choice for keratouveitis caused by herpes simplex. It is generally effective in patients who have proved unresponsive or intolerant to idoxuridine or vidarabine. Toxic reactions to trifluridine are infrequent and generally mild, consisting of a burning sensation on instillation and palpebral edema. Allergic reactions are rare. Systemic concentrations of trifluridine are not detectable after topical application. Because trifluridine is mutagenic in vitro, the drug should be used during pregnancy only when clearly indicated.

Acyclovir

Acyclovir is an acyclic analogue of guanosine (Figure 38-2). It is the most potent of the currently available antiviral agents and the only one indicated for genital herpes.

Mechanism of action. The mechanism of action of acyclovir involves its conversion to acyclovir monophosphate by viral thymidine kinase. Acyclovir monophosphate is then converted by cellular enzymes to acyclovir triphosphate, which inhibits viral DNA replication by interfering with viral DNA polymerase. Acyclovir triphosphate is incorporated into growing chains of viral DNA resulting in the termination of replication.[4] Acyclovir appears to have a high degree of selective toxicity because (1) it is preferentially taken up by virus-infected cells, (2) it is not a substrate for human thymidine kinase, although other cellular enzymes may phosphorylate it to a small extent, and (3) cellular DNA polymerase is less sensitive to the action of the active form of the drug than is viral DNA polymerase. Acyclovir exhibits antiviral activity against herpes simplex types 1 and 2, varicella-zoster, Epstein-Barr virus, and cytomegalovirus.

Viral resistance. A potential problem with acyclovir is the development of viral resistance to the drug. Acyclovir-resistant herpes simplex viruses can be produced in vitro, and drug-resistant mutants have been observed during intravenous therapy with acyclovir.[5] Although clinically significant viral resistance has not been associated with topical use of acyclovir ointment thus far, the possibility exists that viral resistance may also develop with this method of administration.

Absorption, fate, and excretion. Topical application of acyclovir ointment to intact skin or to localized viral lesions produces minimal percutaneous absorption. Intravenous infusion of the recommended dosage provides plasma concentrations above those determined to produce 50% inhibition of viral cytopathic effects.[3] The drug is minimally bound to plasma proteins (9% to 33%) and is widely distributed in tissues and body fluids and herpetic vesicular fluid. Cerebrospinal fluid concentrations reach 50% of plasma values. The major route of elimination is by glomerular filtration and renal tubular secretion. Therefore, dosage adjustment of acyclovir is required in the presence of renal impairment and should be adjusted on the basis of creatinine clearance values. Probenecid will increase the half-life of acyclovir by inhibiting tubular secretion of the drug. Acyclovir can be removed from the body by hemodialysis.

Therapeutic uses. Acyclovir is indicated for the treatment of severe initial mucosal and cutaneous herpes simplex infections (herpes labialis and herpes genitalis). Benefit with topical acyclovir is not clinically significant in recurrent forms of these infections, although the duration of viral shedding is decreased if therapy begins within 8 hours of the first symptoms of a lesion. There is no effect on the duration of pain or the time for healing in patients with recurrent herpes labialis.[11] The drug is indicated, however, for both initial and recurrent herpes labialis and herpes genitalis in immunocompromised patients. Intravenous acyclovir has been used experimentally for systemic treatment of herpes simplex encephalitis and varicella-zoster infections in immunocompromised patients.

Toxic reactions and side effects. Adverse effects of topical acyclovir are minimal, consisting mainly of local burning or stinging sensations, pruritus, rash, and vulvitis. Systemic administration of acyclovir has been associated most frequently with inflammation or phlebitis at the site of intravenous infusion, elevation of serum creatinine concentration, rash, and hives. Less frequent adverse effects are diaphoresis, hematuria, hypotension, headache, nausea, and encephalopathic changes (lethargy, tremors, confusion, hallucinations, agitation, seizures, and coma). Slow intravenous infusion (over 1 hour) is required, because bolus injection has been associated with a 10% incidence of renal dysfunction. Infusion lowers this incidence to 4%. This adverse reaction appears to be caused by precipitation of acyclovir crystals in the renal tubules. Preexisting renal disease, use of other nephrotoxic drugs concomitantly, or dehydration increases the chances of further renal impairment after administration of acyclovir. In most cases, altered renal function is transient and reversible with dosage adjustment, withdrawal of the drug, or improved water and electrolyte balance. Bone marrow depression and abnormal hepatic function have been associated with the use of acyclovir in immunocompromised patients. The drug possesses the potential of being mutagenic.

Amantidine

Amantidine is a synthetic agent unrelated to other antiviral drugs. It is effective in the prevention of only one type of viral infection, that caused by strains of influenza A virus. Its major use is in the chemoprophylaxis of this disease; in exposed patients it is frequently used along with vaccines. It may also produce some clinical improvement (shortened febrile period and reduced symptoms) of an established disease if used within 20 hours of the appearance of symptoms. Amantidine is absorbed from the gastrointestinal tract and is administered orally. The major adverse effect associated with its use is CNS excitation, which resembles amphetamine toxicity and may be severe. This adverse effect has limited its clinical use. The use of amantidine in the treatment of Parkinson's disease is discussed in Chapter 16.

Antifungal and antiviral agents

Nonproprietary name	Proprietary name
Antifungal agents	
acrisorcin	Akrinol
amphotericin B	Fungizone
ciclopirox olamine	Loprox
clotrimazole	Lotrimin, Mycelex
econazole	Spectazole
flucytosine	Ancobon
griseofulvin	Grisactin, Grifulvin V
haloprogin	Halotex
ketoconazole	Nizoral
miconazole	Monistat i.v., Monistat-Derm

Antifungal and antiviral agents

Nonproprietary name	Proprietary name
Antifungal agents—cont'd	
natamycin	Natacyn
nystatin	Mycostatin, Nilstat
tolnaftate	Aftate, Tinactin
triacetin	Fungoid, Enzactin
undecylenic acid (and derivatives)	Desenex, Cruex
Antiviral agents	
acyclovir	Zovirax
amantadine	Symmetrel
idoxuridine	Dendrid, Stoxil
trifluridine	Viroptic
vidarabine	Vira-A

CITED REFERENCES

1. Bennett, J.E. Antifungal agents. In Mandell, G.L., Douglas, R.G., Jr., and Bennett, J.E., eds. Principles and Practice of Infectious Diseases. John Wiley & Sons, Inc., New York, 1979.
2. Bindschalder, D.D., and Bennett, J.E. A pharmacologic guide to the clinical use of amphotericin B. Journal of Infectious Diseases 120:427-436, 1969.
3. De Clercq, E., Descamps, J., Verhelst, G., Walker, R.T., Jones, A.S., Torrence, P.F., and Shugar, D. Comparative efficacy of antiherpes drugs against different strains of herpes simplex virus. Journal of Infectious Diseases 141:563-574, 1980.
4. Derse, D., Cheng, Y.-C., Furman, P.A., St. Clair, M.H., and Elion, G.B. Inhibition of purified human and herpes simplex virus-induced DNA polymerases by 9-(2-hydroxyethoxymethyl) guanine triphosphate. Journal of Biological Chemistry 256:11447-11451, 1981.
5. Intravenous acyclovir (Zovirax). Medical Letter on Drugs and Therapeutics 25:34-36, 1983.
6. Ketoconazole (Nizoral): a new antifungal agent. Medical Letter on Drugs and Therapeutics 23:85-87, 1981.
7. Mauceri, A.A., Cullen, S.I., Vandevelde, A.G., and Johnson, J.E. Flucytosine in effective oral treatment for chromomycosis. Archives of Dermatology 109:873-876, 1974.
8. Monistat, i.v. Medical Letter on Drugs and Therapeutics 21:31-32, 1979.
9. Petersen, E.A., Alling, D.W., and Kirkpatrick, C.H. Treatment of chronic mucocutaneous candidiasis with ketoconazole: a controlled clinical trial. Annals of Internal Medicine 93:791-795, 1980.
10. Smith, H., ed. Antibiotics in Clinical Practice, ed. 3. Baltimore, University Park Press, 1977.
11. Spruance, S.L., and Crumpacker, C.S. Topical 5 percent acyclovir in polyethylene glycol for herpes simplex labialis: antiviral effect without clinical benefit. American Journal of Medicine 73(Acyclovir Symposium):315-319, 1982.
12. Stevens, D.A. Miconazole in the treatment of systemic fungal infections. American Review of Respiratory Disease 116:801-806, 1977.
13. Whitley, R.J., Soong, S.J., Dolin, R., Galasso, G.J., Chen, L.T., and Alford, C.A. Adenosine arabinoside therapy of biopsy-proved herpes simplex virus encephalitis. National Institute of Allergy and Infectious Diseases Collaborative Antiviral Study. New England Journal of Medicine 297:289-294, 1977.

GENERAL REFERENCES

Kucers, A., and Bennett, N. McK. The Use of Antibiotics: A Comprehensive Review with Clinical Emphasis, ed. 3. Philadelphia, J.B. Lippincott Co., 1979.

Sande, M.A., and Mandell, G.L. Antimicrobial agents (continued): miscellaneous antibacterial agents; antifungal and antiviral agents. In Gilman, A.G., Goodman, L.S., and Gilman, A., eds. Goodman and Gilman's The Pharmacological Basis of Therapeutics, ed. 6. New York, Macmillan, Inc., 1980.

39 Immunotherapy

Robert R. White

The significance of the immune response in oral medicine has become more apparent with recent discoveries in oral disease processes. It has been increasingly recognized that the immune response is potentially both protective and harmful. The response is commonly described as a two-edged sword, one edge protective, the other injurious. The purpose of immunotherapy is to enhance the former or to suppress the latter. Rapid advances in the fields of immunology and immunochemistry have begun to allow conventional pharmacologic principles, such as structure-activity relationships, receptor interactions, and dose-response curves, to be applied to an increasing number of immunologic agents. These advances have resulted in the development of more sophisticated methods of immunotherapy. Some are directly applicable to oral medicine; others are still in the developmental stage but are potentially of much significance to oral medicine.

IMMUNE RESPONSE

The immune response is a reaction by the body to exposure to certain substances called *antigens*. Antigens are usually molecules of high molecular weight, proteins, polysaccharides, or derivatives thereof that are foreign to the host; that is, they are derived from sources other than the respondent. These outside sources may be animal, plant, microbial, or synthetic.

The immune response is a function of lymphocytes, their progeny, and their products. The response has been divided into two branches: cell-mediated immunity (CMI) and humoral immunity. CMI is mediated by antigen-reactive lymphocytes (also called sensitized lymphocytes) and certain products of these lymphocytes. Humoral immunity is mediated by soluble molecules, antibodies, which are found in plasma and other body fluids. The lymphocytes responsible for each type of immunity develop from different stem cells originating in the bone marrow (Figure 39-1). These stem cells mature and become immunocompetent as a result of activation by different factors in the body.

The lymphocytes responsible for CMI become immunocompetent under the influence of the thymus gland. This maturation process is carried out by a group of thymic factors, possibly hormones, best known by the name *thymosin*. After exposure to an antigen these lymphocytes, called thymus-dependent lymphocytes, or T lymphocytes, are transformed into antigen-reactive cells and produce the various factors associated with CMI.

Humoral immunity is a function of a second group of lymphocytes. This population of cells was first demonstrated in chickens, in which it was shown that the antibody-forming cells matured as a result of a factor or factors originating in an organ called the bursa of Fabricius. These cells are therefore designated as bursa-derived lymphocytes, or B lymphocytes. Mammals do not have a similar organ, but it is thought that the fetal liver or the bone marrow may serve the same function as the bursa of Fabricius. Progeny of B lymphocytes produce antibodies, the mediators of humoral immunity. Immunocompetent T and B lymphocytes populate the spleen, lymph nodes, and other lymphoid tissues, where they await stimulation by antigens.

When an antigen enters the body, it is carried to a lymphoid tissue where it is picked up by a macrophage, processed in some yet unknown manner, and then ''presented'' to the appropriate lymphocyte (Figure 39-2). Presentation to the lymphocyte is not a random event but involves a T cell or B cell that is genetically programmed to respond to that specific antigen. The lymphocyte is stimulated

593

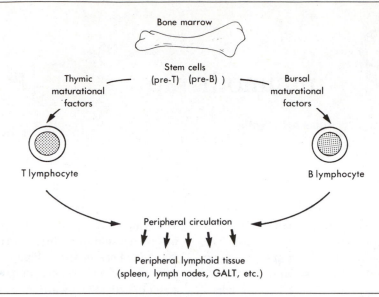

Figure 39-1. Two-component system of immunologic maturation. Stem cells (pre-T and pre-B) from the bone marrow are induced by thymic or bursal factors to become mature T lymphocytes or B lymphocytes, which populate the peripheral lymphoid tissues. (GALT = gut-associated lymphoid tissues.)

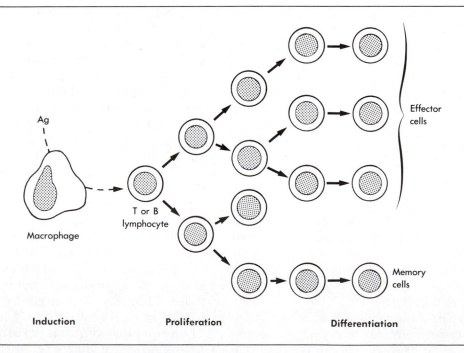

Figure 39-2. Cellular events occurring in the immune response. The macrophage picks up the antigen (Ag), "processes" it, and presents it to the appropriate clone of T lymphocytes or B lymphocytes, which proliferate and differentiate into effector cells. Effector cells in CMI are cytotoxic cells and lymphokine-producing lymphocytes; effector cells in humoral immunity are plasma cells that produce antibody. On subsequent antigenic stimulation, the memory cells repeat the process.

to undergo blast formation, to proliferate, and eventually to differentiate into effector cells and memory cells. Effector cells may either directly mediate the immune reactions or produce molecules that mediate the reactions. The memory cells are responsible for replacing the original clone of reacting lymphocytes. On subsequent exposure to the same antigen, the memory cells will respond as did the original lymphocytes, but their response is usually more rapid and of greater magnitude and duration than the primary response. This memory cell response, called the secondary, booster, or anamnestic response, is unique to immunity and is important in both protective and harmful immunologic reactions. This basic series of events—macrophage processing followed by lymphocyte stimulation, proliferation, and differentiation—occurs in both CMI and humoral immunity. Differences arise in the effector cells, their functions, and their products. The specificity of the reaction between antigen and lymphocyte in the induction of the immune response continues throughout the rest of the response. Thus, an effector cell reacts only with the same antigen, or one very similar to the same antigen, that caused its formation, and antibodies display specificity.

CMI effector cells include *cytotoxic cells* and *antigen-reactive lymphocytes*. The former destroy cells bearing the antigen that stimulated the formation of effector cells. Cytotoxic cells are involved in tumor immunity and in transplant rejection. Antigen-reactive lymphocytes will, on exposure to specific antigen, release biologically active molecules called lymphokines. Lymphokines are vasoactive, chemotactic, mitogenic, and cytotoxic. They also "activate" macrophages. These lymphokine-altered macrophages display enhanced metabolic, phagocytic, and microbicidal properties. Antigen-reactive lymphocytes and lymphokines are especially significant in protection against infectious diseases. Cytotoxic cells and lymphokines also are involved in harmful allergic reactions.

Other subpopulations of activated T cells carry out immunoregulatory functions. *Helper T cells* are necessary adjuncts to the initial proliferative and differentiating stages of the immune response. Without helper cells, the response is absent or incomplete. Another population of T cells, the *suppressor cells,* are thought to limit the immune response to an antigen. It has become apparent that suppressor cells are very important in modulating the immune system. If they are excessively active, the immune response might be totally suppressed; that is, an immunodeficiency may occur. If they are insufficiently active, the body might react to its own tissues, and autoimmunity may ensue. Thus, suppressor cells play a major role in two of the defective immune states most often considered for immunotherapy: immunodeficiency and autoimmunity.[10]

Antigen-stimulated B lymphocytes differentiate into memory cells and plasma cells. The latter produce antibodies, the major effectors of humoral immunity. The antibodies, also called immunoglobulins, are glycoproteins that make up the γ-globulin fraction of blood plasma. They have been divided into five classes (A, G, M, E, and D), based on biologic and physical criteria. Antibodies can neutralize microbial toxins and enzymes, can prevent microbial adherence to and invasion of tissues, and can kill the microbes containing the antigens that caused their production. Antibodies are of extreme importance in protection against infectious diseases, and their total or partial absence usually results in chronic and often fatal infections. Immunoglobulins mediate several allergies, including anaphylaxis, and cytotoxic and immune complex hypersensitivity reactions.

The two branches of the immune response are not as sharply demarcated with respect to derivation and function as may have been suggested. Many activities (e.g., antibody and lymphokine production) are shared or result from cooperation between the two cell types.

Once formed, effector cells and molecules may be found in the lymphoid tissue, in peripheral blood, and at the site of inflammation. The last site may include the periodontium, the endodontium, and the oral mucosa. Within the oral cavity, antibody is found in saliva, whereas all immune components, cellular and molecular, are present in gingival crevicular fluids, their concentration increasing with the degree of gingival inflammation.

IMMUNOPROPHYLAXIS
Active immunization

Historically, the most successful area of immunotherapy has been vaccine prophylaxis. Vaccines have been among the most effective tools in reducing the ravages of infectious diseases since Jenner introduced the smallpox vaccine in the eighteenth century. Active immunization is a means by which the immune system is manipulated to take advantage of a unique phenomenon, the secondary response. On first exposure to the antigens of a pathogenic microbe, there is a slowly developing, low-level primary response. This response is of such limited speed and magnitude that clinical symptoms of the disease occur before immunity develops. However, after recovery, on subsequent exposures to the same microorganisms, the immune response is sufficiently rapid to prevent the disease. The purpose of vaccine prophylaxis is to place the host in an immune state that will allow it to mount a secondary response on the first natural exposure to an infectious microbe. Rather than have the disease act as the primary stimulus, a harmless, or relatively harmless, vaccine is used. The vaccines currently in use encompass the whole spectrum of infectious diseases. They include avirulent live or killed microorganisms, purified antigens from these organisms, and inactivated toxins (toxoids). The composition, recommended dosage, and schedule of administration of these vaccines may be found in several references.[4,8]

Recently, research has focused on two diseases of special interest to dentistry: dental caries and type B viral hepatitis. Vaccines directed against *Streptococcus mutans,* the bacterium suspected of being the major cause of dental caries, are currently under study in several laboratories.[6] Their basic purpose is to induce an immune response that will prevent adherence and subsequent colonization by this bacterium on the tooth surface. Currently, two types of vaccines are being investigated: killed whole bacterial cell preparations and semipure preparations containing enzymes (glucosyl transferases) involved in cell adherence and plaque formation. Whole-cell vaccines have been shown to be anticariogenic in many laboratory animals, including primates.[20] However, the actual antigenic components, dosage, route of administration, and potential adverse effects must be determined before the vaccine can be tested and considered for routine use in humans.

Evidence that the hepatitis B virus is present in the saliva of carriers of the disease and epidemiological studies among practitioners indicate that serum hepatitis poses an even greater threat as a dental occupational hazard than was previously believed. Hepatitis B is potentially catastrophic to the clinician, since contraction of the disease can result in several months suspension of practice, and development of the carrier state could impose even more severe restrictions. Because there is no chemotherapy for this viral disease, development of an effective vaccine has been of the utmost importance to the dental profession. In vitro growth of the virus has been unsuccessful; therefore, a unique method of vaccine production is used.[14] The plasma of chronic hepatitis carriers contains high concentrations of viral particles and antigens. HBsAg, the surface antigen of the virus, is purified from the plasma of carriers and inactivated with urea, pepsin, and formalin. Extensive human testing of the HGsAg vaccine, which contains alum as an adjuvant to potentiate its immunogenicity, has proved the vaccine to be very effective in protecting against hepatitis B, while causing few significant side effects. The efficacy of hepatitis B vaccine, coupled with the high occupational risk to the dentist, makes it imperative that clinicians who are not already immune receive the vaccine.

Passive immunization

A second form of immunization, passive immunization, involves the use of antisera or immunoglobulins either to prevent disease after exposure to an infectious organism or to neutralize circulating toxins, as in tetanus. The injection of antibody obtained from an immune donor into a nonimmune recipient has the advantage of conferring almost instant protection, as opposed to vaccines, which require days or weeks to stimulate a sufficient protective effect. However, the effects of passive immunization last only 4 to 6 weeks.

Serum γ globulins, taken from a large number of adult donors, are pooled and used as a prophylactic treatment in individuals exposed to ubiquitous diseases, such as measles and infectious hepatitis. Pooled immunoglobulins are used because among a large, randomly selected group of adults most individuals will have come into contact with these infectious organisms and will have protective antibodies in their plasma.

In the case of diseases that are not so widespread, sera obtained from recent convalescents are used as sources of immunoglobulins. In addition, either horses or human volunteers may be immunized with appropriate vaccines and their plasma used as a source of antibody. However, the current practice is to avoid the use of equine sera unless there is no other source, because sensitization to the equine antigens may occur. Sensitization causes a more rapid clearance of the antibody and may induce allergic reactions. Allergies are also possible with human globulins, but they may be minimized by using purified or partially purified specific antibody. Immunoglobulins are injected intramuscularly since intravenous injections are more likely to cause anaphylactoid reactions.

Passive immunization is especially effective in the treatment of toxemias, as in diphtheria and tetanus. It is also used, although less effectively, as a prophylactic measure against measles and infectious hepatitis. Immunoglobulins directed against type B viral hepatitis are also available.[8] Finally, as described below, such immunization is used to prevent Rh disease and to treat individuals with a deficiency in antibody formation, such as agammaglobulinemia or hypogammaglobulinemia.

THERAPY FOR IMMUNODEFICIENCY DISEASES

Some individuals cannot respond normally to an antigenic stimulus. They are said to be immunodeficient, a condition that may result in chronic infectious disease or death, depending on the severity of the defect. Chronic candidiasis, juvenile periodontosis, and chronic hepatitis may result, in part, from immunodeficiencies. Immunodeficiency diseases may involve either humoral immunity or CMI or both. The deficiency may occur at the maturation stage, the proliferation stage, or the effector stage of the response, or it may involve a combination of these defects.

Deficiencies in humoral immunity may result from congenital defects in the production of all or selected immunoglobulin classes, or they may be acquired, as occurs with multiple myeloma. Severe deficiencies in humoral immunity, or hypogammaglobulinemias, require replacement therapy if the patient is to survive. This consists of weekly or monthly injections of pooled immunoglobulins, the concentration and frequency depending on the patient's status. The treatments are usually accompanied by antibiotics. Hypogammaglobulinemias involving individual classes of immunoglobulins are usually less severe because the body may compensate by increased production of other immunoglobulin classes. Selective deficiencies also can be treated with immunoglobulins. Secretory immunoglobulin A (IgA), which is locally synthesized and secreted, is an exception (injected γ globulins are not secreted). This fact is of some dental significance, because IgA secreted by the salivary glands may be extremely important in protection against oral diseases, especially dental caries.

Immunotherapy for CMI deficiencies has reached a higher degree of sophistication. Rather than the body simply being furnished with effector components, as with immunoglobulin treatments in humoral immune deficiencies, the emphasis has been on inducing the lymphocytes to carry out their normal activities. Primary CMI deficiencies may result from absence of the thymus or a defect in its function. Treatment has been directed toward inducing maturation of T cells by using thymic tissue or extracts. In several cases, thymus transplants in humans have corrected CMI deficiencies, with subsequent development of immunocompetency. Immunologically immature fetal thymic tissues must be used to prevent a graft-vs.-host reaction in which the lymphocytes present in the transplanted thymus react to the recipient's antigens. Conversely, having become immunocompetent, the recipient's lymphocytes may reject the transplant. These adverse effects can be minimized by histocompatibility matching.

Various thymus extracts have also been used nonspecifically to induce CMI competence.[3] These extracts, which have been given different names, including thymosin, thymopoietin, and thymus factor, are usually extracted from calf thymus glands. The extracts consist of a family of nonimmunogenic polypeptide hormones, several of which have been purified and synthesized in vitro for experimental use in humans.[12] These hormones function at different stages of CMI development. Some transform immature T cells to immunocompetent T lymphocytes; others are responsible for the development of effector cells, such as cytotoxic or suppressor cells. It has been suggested that the former act by increasing intracellular levels of cAMP, while the latter increase cGMP.[9]

Various tumors, chronic mucocutaneous candidiasis, and several other diseases with manifestations of immunodeficiency have responded favorably to thymosin therapy. Thymic extracts usually must be given repeatedly since there are no thymic cells available to produce the hormones. Although it has been found to be of therapeutic benefit, thymosin administration is still experimental, and routine use awaits further development.

CMI deficiencies may be restricted to defects in specific effector cells. Because these diseases do not involve thymic defects, the patients do not respond to treatment with thymic components. For many years, it has been known that lymphocytes from immune individuals can be injected into nonimmune recipients and the recipients will respond to an antigenic stimulus as if immune. This transfer of CMI from one individual to another (called adoptive immunity) is an immunologically specific phenomenon. However, it is of little use in the treatment of immunodeficiencies because the recipient will reject the donor's lymphocytes.

It has been demonstrated that immune lymphocytes contain a factor that can be extracted and used to transfer immunity to a nonimmune recipient.[16] This extract, which is nonantigenic, is known as Lawrence's transfer factor or simply transfer factor (TF). TF has a molecular weight of 5000 to 10,000 and is of uncertain chemical composition. It may be a polynucleotide. Although there is evidence that TF has some nonspecific stimulating effects, it is best known for its ability to transfer CMI without inducing a humoral immune response. The mode of action of TF is not fully understood, but it is possible that the substance, rather than affecting a random lymphocyte, acts on a stem cell that is already committed to respond to the specific antigen.[7]

TF obtained from the lymphocytes of immune individuals has been used with varying degrees of success in treating neonatal herpes, miliary tuberculosis, and chronic mucocutaneous candidiasis, all of which display CMI deficiencies as a part of their symptomatology.[2]

IMMUNOSTIMULANTS

Immunostimulation is the use of various agents to enhance the body's immune response. Immunostimulants may hyperactivate the normal immune response, or they may be used in the treatment of immunodeficient individuals. Immunostimulation may be especially important in cancer therapy, where the purpose is to induce the patient to mount an immune response to tumor antigens and reject the tumor.

The effects of a vaccine may be enhanced by incorporation of adjuvants, substances that increase the immune response. The mechanism of action of some, such as alum, is simply to retard removal of the antigen and to attract lymphoid cells by increasing the inflammatory response in the immediate area of the vaccine. Others also enhance the activity of the responding lymphocytes or macrophages (described below). Many adjuvants that are extremely effective in laboratory animals have not yet been cleared for routine use in humans. Aluminum hydroxide gels are the only adjuvants used routinely with vaccines, such as diphtheria and tetanus toxoids.

Bacillus Calmette-Guérin (BCG) is a live attenuated strain of *Mycobacterium bovis* that has been used as a vaccine against tuberculosis since the early part of this century. Its use as an immunostimulant derived from studies by Landsteiner and Chase,[15] who found that killed *Mycobacterium tuberculosis,* incorporated in an oil suspension, nonspecifically stimulated CMI. Since the protective immune response against tumors has been considered to be CMI, BCG has been evaluated as an antineoplastic agent. The agent has been shown to stimulate specific tumor immunity in experimental animals injected with tumor cells and to inhibit tumor formation. BCG is also a nonspecific stimulator that induces responses in deficient individuals and reverses the effects of several of the immunosuppressive drugs described below. It activates the reticuloendothelial system, particularly macrophages and T lymphocytes. The latter may result from the production by activated macrophages of lymphocyte-activating factor, a substance that induces proliferation and activation of T lymphocytes, including cytotoxic cells.[18] BCG has been used with success in the treatment of melanoma, hepatoma, and leukemia. Although most studies have involved cancer therapy, experimental results also indicate that BCG has potential in the treatment of other illnesses involving immunodeficiency states. Severe allergic reactions and shock have occurred infrequently during BCG treatments. Another bacterial species, *Corynebacterium parvum,* is also being studied as an immunostimulant.

Levamisole is an antihelminthic drug that possesses nonspecific immunostimulatory properties. In deficient animals and humans, it restores many different immunologic functions, suggesting that it acts on multiple populations of cells, including polymorphonuclear leukocytes, macrophages, and T lymphocytes (but not B lymphocytes). Pharmacologically, levamisole has been demonstrated to have a dual effect, inducing both cAMP- and cGMP-mediated processes.[21] Its effects on the immune response and its pharmacologic activity indicate that levamisole is a thymomimetic agent.

Levamisole has shown promise in the treatment of tumors and other diseases in which there are manifestations of immune dysfunction, including rheumatoid arthritis and Crohn's disease. Several investigators have used it successfully in the treatment of recurrent aphthous stomatitis and herpes labialis. In the former, in which autoimmunity may be involved, it has been suggested that the therapeutic effect results from enhancement of suppressor T lymphocytes, which normally prevent autoimmune responses.[17]

IMMUNOSUPPRESSIVE AGENTS

Despite its fundamentally protective nature, the immune response must sometimes be suppressed intentionally. Organ transplantation is the best example of an instance in which immunosuppression is needed. Graft rejection mechanisms are immunologic, and a successful operation requires that the immune response to transplanted tissue antigens be prevented. Other uses of immunosuppression are in the treatment of autoimmune diseases or allergies. Antilymphocytic sera (ALS), cytotoxic drugs, and irradiation are the most frequently used agents.[19]

ALS is produced in rabbits and horses by immunization with human thymocytes. Such sera lyse or agglutinate human lymphocytes in vitro and produce lymphocytopenia in vivo. They decrease CMI responses and prolong survival of allografts. Although the mechanism of action appears to be obvious, that is, death of lymphocytes, it is much more complex and not completely understood. For example, ALS does not affect B lymphocytes, and it shows selectivity in its action against T lymphocytes (some T cell subpopulations are quite resistant). Like most immunosuppressive agents, the effects of ALS are transient, and it must be given repeatedly. However, since ALS is in itself antigenic, these treatments can induce an immune response leading to serum sickness, a systemic immune complex hypersensitivity. This potential allergenicity has been reduced by using only the γ-globulin fraction of the sera.

Cytotoxic drugs are the most frequently used immunosuppressive agents. There are two classes of drugs: the first kills lymphocytes; the second interferes with the proliferative stage of the response. The lympholytic drugs are most effective if given before antigen administration. They include corticosteroids and alkylating agents, such as cyclophosphamide and phenylalanine mustard. Cyclophosphamide is active primarily against humoral immunity, whereas the steroids act on CMI. In addition to their lympholytic effects, steroids may interfere with macrophage processing by stabilization of macrophage cell membranes.

The second group of cytotoxic drugs, which are active against rapidly dividing or metabolizing cells, includes the purine antagonists mercapto-purine and azathioprine, the pyrimidine antagonist floxuridine, and methotrexate, a folic acid antagonist. These agents are given with, or within 48 hours of, antigen administration and inhibit cellular proliferation and initial differentiation, usually through inhibition of DNA and RNA synthesis. Originally developed for cancer therapy, these drugs can affect any group of rapidly proliferating cells and, because they are particularly toxic to hematopoietic tissues, may induce anemia or thrombocytopenia.

X-radiation is selective in its suppressive effects on the immune response. Sublethal doses (300 to 500 R), given before antigen administration, will suppress the primary immune response, especially humoral immunity. The secondary response is much more resistant to radiation than is the primary. This difference may simply be a matter of cell numbers rather than cell resistance, the nonprimed animal having many fewer reactive lymphocytes. The antilymphocytic effects result from unknown alterations of the lymphocytes' DNA, which, unlike that of most other mammalian cells, is sensitive to radiation during cell interphase. At higher doses, both primary and secondary responses are suppressed, and only memory cells survive. At supralethal doses (900 R), all immunologic cells are destroyed, and the immune system must be reconstituted using bone marrow transplants.

A new immunosuppressant, cyclosporine (cyclosporin A), is currently receiving much study.[5] A cyclic undecapeptide of fungal origin, the drug inhibits the generation of helper T lymphocytes without affecting the function of the suppressor T lymphocytes or the B cells and with minimum myelotoxicity. During the past few years, cyclosporine has been used successfully to prevent rejections of nonmatched cadaver kidney, liver, heart, heart-lung, bone marrow, and pancreas transplants. In fact, it can be said that this drug, which has increased the first-year survival of liver transplants from 35% to 65% or 70%, has revolutionized the field of transplantation. Some other uses for the drug currently under investigation are the autoimmune form of uveitis, juvenile diabetes, and parasitic diseases.

Cyclosporine has proved to be a highly selective immunosuppressant that is also relatively safe. The major adverse effect is a dose-related renal toxicity that occurs in 25% to 38% of patients. Other side effects include gingival hyperplasia, hirsutism, mild tremor, and hepatotoxicity.

The immunosuppressive agents described above (with the partial exception of cyclosporine) all pose the same problem—nonspecificity. They may suppress the response to all antigenic stimuli, and as a result the host cannot mount a response against the transplanted tissue, nor can it respond to the antigens of an infectious agent. Thus, the immunosuppressed patient is constantly in danger of developing life-threatening infectious diseases, in many cases caused by microorganisms that are harmless to normal individuals. Suppressed patients usually receive heavy antibiotic therapy, but even this may not be sufficient.

Much research has been carried out in the field of specific immunosuppression, but there is only one method, the prevention of Rh disease, that is of any significance clinically. A major cause of hemolytic disease of the newborn, or erythroblastosis fetalis, Rh disease occurs when an Rh-negative woman—one whose red blood cells (RBCs) do not contain the $Rh_O(D)$ antigen—becomes sensitized to the antigen by the exposure to the blood of her Rh-positive fetus. On subsequent pregnancies, the mother's anti-Rh antibody will pass through the placenta and cause massive destruction of the fetal erythrocytes.

Prevention of Rh disease involves injection of anti-Rh antibody into Rh-negative mothers who give birth to an Rh-positive child.[1] This treatment is based on the fact that high titers of specific antibody will inhibit the immune response to an antigen. Two possible mechanisms of action have been proposed for these immunosuppressive effects. The large quantities of specific antibody may act as a feedback mechanism that turns off the immune response before it is initiated. Such an inhibitory effect has been demonstrated in laboratory animals. A second mechanism may be that when the antibody reacts with the fetal RBCs in the mother, it coats the cells completely and hinders the antigen recognition process of the mother's immune system, or it induces immunologic clearance of the fetal cells, which may prevent normal macrophage processing. Antiserum to the Rh antigen is produced in Rh-negative male volunteers. The γ-globulin fraction containing anti-Rh antibody must be given within hours of parturition, because the fetal RBCs carrying the Rh antigen enter the mother's body at this time and induce the immune response that will cause problems in subsequent pregnancies. This specific immunosuppressive treatment has been very successful in preventing Rh disease, and it is now used routinely.

THERAPY FOR ALLERGIC REACTIONS

Allergic reactions are classified according to their immunologic mechanisms. Types I, II, and III are mediated by immunoglobulins, whereas type IV is mediated by CMI.

Type I reactions are the classic allergic reactions, anaphylaxis and atopy. Hay fever, asthma, and penicillin and food allergies are among the most common type I reactions. The reaction is initiated when an antigen combines with immunoglobulin E (IgE) on the membrane of a mast cell or basophil. Formation of this complex causes a decrease in intracellular cAMP, with subsequent degranulation and release of histamine and other pharmacologically active compounds. Treatment is primarily directed toward preventing release, neutralizing, or reversing the effects of histamine. Antihistaminic drugs that competitively block the actions of histamine are described in Chapter 23. Sympathomimetic amines, which act as physiologic antagonists to histamine and other mediators of allergy and which inhibit the release of these compounds from mast cells by stimulating formation of cAMP are discussed in Chapters 6 and 32. Another drug that prevents mast cell degranulation is cromolyn sodium. This drug stabilizes the adenylate cyclase–cAMP system, but it has no direct effect on the actions of histamine and related autacoids. Cromolyn sodium is useful only as a local agent; it is generally used as a powder that is insufflated as an aerosol or deposited directly in the nostrils. It has also been used in preliminary trials in patients with ulcerative colitis, a disease in which the immune process may be altered.

Type II allergies are called cytotoxic or antitissue reactions because they injure cells directly. Transfusion reactions, drug-induced hemolytic anemias, and certain autoimmune diseases are included here. The reaction occurs when antibodies (IgG or IgM) react with antigens in or adsorbed to cell membranes. Fixation of complement by bound antibodies can then lead to cytolysis, agglutination, or phagocytosis of the antigen-bearing cells, or all three. Immunosuppressive agents that inhibit autoantibody production and phagocytosis are used to treat severe type II autoimmune reactions. Corticosteroids and either azathioprine or methotrexate are often employed in combination.

Type III reactions, the immune complex allergies, are involved in acute poststreptococcal glomerulonephritis, chronic serum hepatitis, rheumatoid arthritis, and serum sickness. The complex formed when antigen reacts with antibody activates the inflammatory components of complement. Injury is caused by lysosomal enzymes released by polymorphonuclear leukocytes that infiltrate the area. Corticosteroids are useful in the treatment of immune complex allergies, primarily because of their antiinflammatory properties. In severe cases, azathioprine or cyclophosphamide may be administered to suppress the immune response and allow use of reduced quantities of steroids.

Type IV allergies, the CMI reactions, may involve cytotoxic cells or lymphokines, or both. Graft rejection is an example of the influence of cytotoxic lymphocytes. Patients receiving grafts are treated with combined immunosuppressive agents. For example, one regimen for treating heart transplant patients includes prednisone, azathioprine, and ALS.[13] In addition, radiation therapy may be used to suppress the activities of antigen-sensitive lymphocytes. Treatment of contact dermatitis, the dermal manifestation of CMI allergy, is symptomatic. Either local or, in severe cases, systemic corticosteroid treatments are used to control inflammation.

MONOCLONAL ANTIBODIES

Monoclonal antibodies, antibodies of a defined class, avidity, and specificity, were once associated only with myelomas. Better understanding of the cell membrane, especially intercellular membrane fusion, has led to the production of artificially induced monoclonal antibodies, molecules with much potential in research, diagnosis, and therapy.[11] Fusion of a normal plasma cell and myeloma cell results in the formation of a hybrid with the antibody-forming properties of the plasma cell and the proliferative properties of the myeloma cell.

Such hybrid cells are produced by mixing plasmacytes from an immunized animal and myeloma cells in the presence of a fusing agent (polyethylene glycol). The fused cells are then cultured under conditions that will allow survival of only those hybrid cells sharing the desired properties of both cell lines, that is, antibody formation and "immortality." When grown in tissue culture, the resultant hybridomas are capable of almost unlimited production of monoclonal antibodies. These compounds of exquisite immunologic specificity are being tailored for immunotherapy, the delivery of drugs to specific cells, serodiagnosis, immunohistology, affinity chromatography, and other uses.

Drugs used in immunotherapy

Nonproprietary name	Proprietary name
Agents for active immunization	
BCG vaccine	—
hepatitis B vaccine	Heptavax-B
tetanus toxoid	—
Agents for passive immunization	
immune globulin, (human)	Gammar
hepatitis B immune globulin (human)	H-BIG
Immunostimulants	
BCG vaccine	—
levamisole*	Ketarax
Immunosuppressants	
antilymphocytic sera (ALS)*	—
azathioprine	Imuran
cyclophosphamide	Cytoxan
cyclosporine	Sandimmune
floxuridine	FUDR
melphalan	Alkeran
mercaptopurine	Purinethol
methotrexate	Mexate
prednisone	Deltasone, Meticorten
Rho(D) immune globulin (human)	RhoGAM
Therapy for allergic reactions	
antihistamines (see Chapter 23)	
cromolyn sodium	Intal

*Not currently approved for use in the United States.

CITED REFERENCES

1. Ascari, W.Q. Prevention of erythroblastosis fetalis. In Queenan, J.T., ed. Modern Management of the Rh Problem, ed. 2. New York, Harper & Row, Publishers, Inc., 1977.
2. Ascher, M.S., Gottlieb, A.A., and Kirkpatrick, C.H., eds. Transfer Factor: Basic Properties and Clinical Applications. New York, Academic Press, Inc., 1976.
3. Bach, J., Bach, M., Charreire, J., Dardenne, M., and Pleau, J. The mode of action of thymic hormones. In Friedman, H., ed. Subcellular Factors in Immunity. New York Academy of Sciences, 1979.
4. Benenson, A.S., ed. Control of Communicable Diseases in Man, ed. 12. Washington, D.C., American Public Health Association, 1975.
5. Borel, J.F. Cyclosporin-A: Present experimental status. Transplantation Proceedings **13**:344-348, 1981.
6. Bowen, W.H., Genco, R.J., and O'Brien, T.C., eds. Immunologic Aspects of Dental Caries. Washington, D.C., Information Retrieval Inc., 1976.
7. Cohen, L., Holzman, R.S., Valentine, F.T., and Lawrence, H.S. Leucocyte dialysates require precommitted, antigen-reactive cells to augment lymphocyte proliferation. In Ascher, M.S., Gottlieb, A.A., and Kirkpatrick, C.H., eds. Transfer Factor: Basic Properties and Clinical Applications. New York, Academic Press, Inc., 1976.

8. Collected recommendations of the Public Health Service Advisory Committee on Immunization Practices. Morbidity and Mortality Weekly Report, **21** (suppl.), 1972.

9. Galant, S.P., Lundak, R.L., and Eaton, L. Enhancement of early human E-rosette formation by cholinergic stimuli. Journal of Immunology **117:**48-51, 1976.

10. Gershon, R.K. T-cell control of antibody production. Contemporary Topics in Immunology **3:**1-40, 1974.

11. Goding, J.W. Antibody production by hybridomas. Journal of Immunological Methods **39:**285-308, 1980.

12. Goldstein, A.L., Low, T.L.K., McAdoo, M., McClure, J., Thurman, G.B., Rossio, J., Lai, C.Y., Chang, D., Wang, S.S., Harvey, C., Ramel, A.H., and Meienhofer, J. Thymosin α_1: isolation and sequence analysis of an immunologically active thymic polypeptide. Proceedings of the National Academy of Sciences of the United States of America **74:**725-729, 1977.

13. Griepp, R.B., Stinson, E.B., and Shumway, N.E. Transplantation of the heart. Surgery Annual **8:**47-62, 1976.

14. Inactivated hepatitis B virus vaccine. Morbidity and Mortality Weekly Report **31:**317-328, 1982.

15. Landsteiner, K., and Chase, M.W. Studies on the sensitization of animals with simple chemical compounds. VII. Skin sensitization by intraperitoneal injections. Journal of Experimental Medicine **71:**237-245, 1940.

16. Lawrence, H.S. The transfer in humans of delayed skin sensitivity to streptococcal M substance and to tuberculin with disrupted leukocytes. Journal of Clinical Investigation **34:**219-230, 1955.

17. Lehner, T., Wilton, J.M.A., and Ivanyi, L. Double blind crossover trial of levamisole in recurrent aphthous ulceration. Lancet **2:**926-929, 1976.

18. Mitchell, M.S., Kirkpatrick D., Mokyr, M.B., and Gery, I. On the mode of action of BCG. Nature **243:**216-218, 1973.

19. Parker, C.W., and Vaura, J.D. Immunosuppression. Progress in Hematology **6:**1-81, 1974.

20. Russell, R.R.B., Beighton, D., and Cohen, B. Immunization of monkeys *(Macaca fascicularis)* with antigens purified from *Streptococcus mutans.* British Dental Journal **152:**81-84, 1982.

21. Symoens, J., and Rosenthal, M. Levamisole in the modulation of the immune response: the current experimental and clinical state. Journal of the Reticuloendothelial Society **21:**175-204, 1977.

40 Antineoplastic drugs

Samuel Dreizen

The antineoplastic drugs have added a new dimension to the ever broadening fight against cancer. They have become the treatment of choice for many widely disseminated malignancies that cannot be reached by surgery or are beyond the limits of safety of radiotherapy. They are also used as adjuncts to surgery and irradiation in the prevention of metastatic spread from locally treated primary tumors. In the past 30 years there has been a striking increase in the number of clinically active anticancer drugs and in the types of cancer that have proved to be drug sensitive. Pharmacologically, the antineoplastic drug spectrum currently includes alkylating agents, antimetabolites, antibiotics, plant alkaloids, steroids, and miscellaneous compounds (Table 40-1).

HISTORY OF CANCER CHEMOTHERAPY

The modern history of cancer chemotherapy began during World War II with the demonstration that several nitrogen mustard compounds acting as alkylating agents were effective in the treatment of Hodgkin's disease, malignant lymphomas, chronic leukemias, and allied disorders.[13] In 1944, the glucocorticoids were shown to have a profound effect on the volume, structure, and function of lymphoid tissue.[4] Subsequently this effect was utilized in the control of human leukemia.[9] In the intervening years, prednisone and prednisolone have replaced ACTH, cortisone, and hydrocortisone in drug protocols designed to ablate lymphoproliferative and myeloproliferative diseases.

In 1948, Farber and associates[8] obtained temporary remissions in children with acute leukemia who were given the folic acid antagonist 4-aminopteroylglutamic acid (aminopterin). This specially tailored molecule was the first antimetabolite to produce unequivocally beneficial results in a human neoplastic disease. The folate antagonist approach led to the development of competitive inhibitors of purines and pyrimidines that interfered with the synthesis of nucleic acids in rapidly multiplying neoplastic cells to a degree that was demonstrably tumor suppressive.[16,17]

The first antibiotic with activity against human tumors was actinomycin D. Introduced as an anticancer agent in 1952,[25] dactinomycin (actinomycin D) today is curative in many patients with Wilms' tumor and uterine choriocarcinoma. The anticancer effects of the vinca alkaloids, extracted from the periwinkle plant *(Vinca rosea),* were demonstrated initially in animals with experimental leukemia in 1960.[20] In the same year, vinblastine was found to be of value in the treatment of acute leukemias, Hodgkin's disease, and adenocarcinoma of the colon.[18] The earliest reports of the use of carmustine (BCNU), the prototype of the nitrosourea group of cytotoxic compounds, against human malignancies appeared in 1966.[19]

In 1967, the enzyme L-asparaginase was found to produce remissions in some patients with acute leukemia.[22] The first of the heavy metal complexes to have significant success in the treatment of human cancer was cisplatin, introduced in 1969.[24] For the most part, other miscellaneous anticancer drugs have a similarly short history of human application.

PRINCIPLES OF CANCER CHEMOTHERAPY

All antineoplastic drugs kill or impair susceptible tumor cells by blocking a drug-sensitive biochemical or metabolic pathway. Some, like the cell-cycle specific antimetabolites, act by inhibiting DNA synthesis and are most effective against rap-

Table 40-1. Classification of antineoplastic drugs

Class or type	Nonproprietary name	Proprietary name	Adverse effects*	Stomato-toxicity†	Used in treatment of
Alkylating agents					
Alkyl sulfonate	Busulfan	Myleran	*Myelosuppression*, pulmonary fibrosis, dermatotoxicity, hypotension, cataract formation, gynecomastia	0	Chronic myelocytic leukemia, polycythemia vera
Nitrogen mustards	Chlorambucil	Leukeran	*Gastroenterotoxicity, myelosuppression*, dermatotoxicity, hepatotoxicity	0	Chronic lymphocytic leukemia, lymphosarcoma, Hodgkin's disease, seminoma, ovarian carcinoma
	Cyclophosphamide	Cytoxan	*Immunosuppression, myelosuppression, gastroenterotoxicity, dermatotoxicity*, hemorrhagic cystitis, hepatotoxicity	+	Hodgkin's disease, lymphomas, lymphocytic leukemia, multiple myeloma, neuroblastoma, rhabdomyosarcoma, carcinoma of breast, ovary, lung, and bladder
	Estramustine	Emcyt	Gastroenterotoxicity, cardiovascular accidents, gynecomastia, dyspnea	0	Metastatic or progressive carcinoma of the prostate
	Mechlorethamine (nitrogen mustard)	Mustargen	*Myelosuppression, gastroenterotoxicity, tissue necrosis*, neurotoxicity, menstrual irregularities, teratogenicity	0	Hodgkin's disease, lymphomas, mycosis fungoides, pulmonary carcinoma
	Melphalan	Alkeran	*Myelosuppression*, gastroenterotoxicity, teratogenicity	0	Multiple myeloma, ovarian carcinoma
	Uracil mustard	—	*Myelosuppression*, gastroenterotoxicity, dermatotoxicity	0	Non-Hodgkin's lymphomas, chronic lymphocytic and myelocytic leukemias, polycythemia vera
Ethyleneimine derivative	Thiotepa	Thiotepa	*Myelosuppression, dermatotoxicity, gastroenterotoxicity*, infertility, teratogenicity, neurotoxicity	0	Carcinoma of breast, ovary, and bladder, Hodgkin's disease, lymphomas, sarcomas
Piperazine derivative	Pipobroman	Vercyte	*Myelosuppression*, gastroenterotoxicity, teratogenicity	0	Chronic myelocytic leukemia, polycythemia vera
Triazene derivative	Dacarbazine	DTIC-Dome	*Gastroenterotoxicity, myelosuppression*, fever, dermatotoxicity	0	Malignant melanoma, Hodgkin's disease, soft-tissue sarcoma
Nitrosoureas	Carmustine (BCNU)	BiCNU	*Myelosuppression*, gastroenterotoxicity, hepatotoxicity, nephrotoxicity	0	Hodgkin's disease and other lymphomas, brain tumors, melanoma, myeloma
	Lomustine (CCNU)	CeeNU	*Myelosuppression*, gastroenterotoxicity, hepatotoxicity, nephrotoxicity	0	Hodgkin's disease, brain tumors, multiple myelomas, melanoma
	Streptozocin	Zanosar	*Gastroenterotoxicity, nephrotoxicity, hepatotoxicity*, teratogenicity	0	Islet cell carcinoma of the pancreas

Antimetabolites

				Toxicity	
Folic acid analogue	Methotrexate	Mexate	++	*Myelosuppression, gastroenterotoxicity, pleuritic pain, hepatotoxicity, pulmonary fibrosis, dermatoxicity, photosensitivity, teratogenicity, nephrotoxicity, neurotoxicity*	Choriocarcinoma, trophoblastic tumors, testicular tumors, lymphocytic leukemia, lymphosarcoma, osteosarcoma, carcinoma of head, neck, breast, and lung, psoriasis
Purine analogues	Mercaptopurine	Purinethol	+	*Myelosuppression, hepatotoxicity, hyperuricemia, gastroenterotoxicity, immunosuppression*	Acute leukemias, chronic myelocytic leukemia
	Thioguanine	Tabloid Brand Thioguanine	++	*Myelosuppression, gastroenterotoxicity, hepatotoxicity, hyperuricemia*	Acute leukemias, chronic myelocytic leukemia
Pyrimidine analogues	Cytarabine	Cytosar-U	+	*Myelosuppression, hepatotoxicity, gastroenterotoxicity, dermatotoxicity, thrombophlebitis, teratogenicity*	Acute lymphocytic and myelocytic leukemias
	Fluorouracil	Adrucil	++	*Gastroenterotoxicity, myelosuppression, dermatotoxicity, neurotoxicity*	Gastrointestinal adenocarcinomas, carcinoma of breast, ovary, prostate, cervix, and bladder
	Floxuridine	FUDR	++	*Gastroenterotoxicity, myelosuppression, dermatotoxicity, neurotoxicity*	Hepatic metastases from gastrointestinal adenocarcinoma, carcinoma of head and neck

Antibiotics

	Bleomycin	Blenoxane	+	*Gastroenterotoxicity, pulmonary toxicity, dermatotoxicity, fever*	Squamous cell carcinoma of head, neck, esophagus, skin, and genitourinary tract, testicular carcinoma, lymphomas
	Dactinomycin (actinomycin D)	Cosmegen	++	*Gastroenterotoxicity, myelosuppression, tissue necrosis, dermatotoxicity*	Wilms' tumor, rhabdomyosarcoma, Ewing's sarcoma, neuroblastoma, testicular carcinoma, choriocarcinoma
	Daunorubicin	Cerubidine	++	*Myelosuppression, cardiotoxicity, gastroenterotoxicity, alopecia*	Acute nonlymphocytic leukemia
	Doxorubicin	Adriamycin	++	*Myelosuppression, gastroenterotoxicity, cardiotoxicity, dermatotoxicity, phlebitis, tissue necrosis*	Acute myelocytic and lymphocytic leukemias, sarcoma, lymphoma, neuroblastoma, transitional cell carcinoma of urinary tract, carcinoma of lung, ovary, thyroid, and breast
	Plicamycin (mithramycin)	Mithracin	++	*Hepatotoxicity, nephrotoxicity, myelosuppression, gastroenterotoxicity, hemorrhagic diathesis, dermatotoxic fever, neurotoxicity*	Embryonal testicular tumor, testicular choriocarcinoma, Wilms' tumor, tumor-associated hypercalcemia
	Mitomycin	Mutamycin	++	*Gastroenterotoxicity, myelosuppression, tissue necrosis, pulmonary toxicity, neurotoxicity, alopecia*	Carcinoma of head, neck, gastrointestinal tract, breast, and cervix, some lymphomas

For a full description of the toxicity and disease treated, refer to the text.

*MYELOSUPPRESSION—suppression of the blood cell–forming elements in the bone marrow resulting in leukopenia, anemia, and thrombocytopenia. GASTROENTEROTOXICITY—disturbances of the alimentary tract manifested as nausea, vomiting, diarrhea, mucosal inflammation, and mucosal ulceration. DERMATOTOXICITY—cutaneous disturbances manifested as alopecia, pigmentation, rashes, erythema, or exfoliation. NEUROTOXICITY—neurologic disturbances manifested as pain, paresthesias, paralysis, altered sensorium, diminished sensory acuity, or paralytic ileus. HEPATOTOXICITY—liver dysfunction caused by drug-induced hepatitis, parenchymal degeneration, cholangitis, or bile stasis. NEPHROTOXICITY—disturbances of kidney function caused by drug-induced renal tubular necrosis or renal insufficiency.

Italic type indicates frequently occurring toxicity. Roman type indicates moderate or occasional problems.

†0 = rare or not at all, + = occasional, ++ = frequent or common.

Continued.

Table 40-1. Classification of antineoplastic drugs—cont'd

Class or type	Nonproprietary name	Proprietary name	Adverse effects*	Stomatotoxicity†	Used in treatment of
Vinca alkaloids	Vinblastine	Velban	*Myelosuppression, gastroenterotoxicity,* dermatotoxicity, neurotoxicity	+	Hodgkin's disease, other lymphomas, choriocarcinoma, testicular tumors
	Vincristine	Oncovin	*Neurotoxicity,* dermatotoxicity	+	Hodgkin's disease, acute leukemia, Wilms' tumor, neuroblastoma, testicular tumors, palliation of carcinoma of breast, ovary, and lung
Hormone agonists and antagonists					
Adrenal corticosteroids	Prednisolone	Delta-Cortef	Peptic ulcer, hypokalemia, psychoses, osteoporosis, skin striae, susceptibility to infections	0	In combination with other antineoplastic drugs for Hodgkin's disease, acute leukemias, lymphomas, myeloma, breast carcinoma, bony metastases with hypercalcemia
	Prednisone	Deltasone			
Androgens	Dromostanolone	Drolban	Virlism, hirsutism, edema, alopecia, increased libido, acne, hypercalcemia, fluid retention	0	Disseminated carcinoma of breast, especially postmenopausal
	Fluoxymesterone	Halotestin			
	Testolactone	Teslac			
Estrogens	Clorotrianisene	TACE	Gynecomastia, breast tenderness, fluid retention, edema, nausea, anorexia, changes in libido, hypercalcemia	0	Postmenopausal carcinoma of breast, carcinoma of prostate
	Diethylstilbestrol	Stilphostrol			
	Ethinyl estradiol	Estinyl			
	Polyestradiol	Estradurin			
Progestins	Hydroxyprogesterone	Delalutin	Edema, local reactions, alopecia, hirsutism, genitourinary toxicity	0	Metastatic endometrial carcinoma, renal and breast carcinoma
	Medroxyprogesterone	Depo-Provera			
	Megestrol	Megace			
Adrenal suppressant	Aminoglutethimide	Cytadren	Myelosuppression, fever, dermatotoxicity, hypotension, masculinization	0	Carcinoma of the adrenal cortex, Cushing's syndrome
Antiestrogen	Tamoxifen	Nolvadex	Gastroenterotoxicity, hot flashes, vaginal discharge	0	Postmenopausal carcinoma of the breast
Miscellaneous	Asparaginase	Elspar	*Acute allergic reactions,* fever, gastroenterotoxicity, hepatotoxicity, coagulation defects	0	Acute lymphocytic leukemia
	Cisplatin	Platinol	*Nephrotoxicity, ototoxicity, gastroenterotoxicity,* myelosuppression, neurotoxicity, acute allergic reactions	0	Carcinoma of testis, ovary, bladder, and head and neck
	Etopside	VePesid	Myelosuppression, gastoenterotoxicity, dermatotoxicity, acute allergic reactions	+	Carcinoma of testis and lung
	Hydroxyurea	Hydrea	Myelosuppression, gastroenterotoxicity, dermatotoxicity	+	Myelocytic leukemia, melanoma
	Mitotane	Lysodren	*Gastroenterotoxicity, neurotoxicity,* dermatotoxicity, hematuria, cystitis	0	Carcinoma of the adrenal cortex
	Procarbazine	Matulane	*Gastroenterotoxicity,* myelosuppression, CNS depression, dermatotoxicity	+	Hodgkin's disease, multiple myeloma

idly dividing cells. Others, like the alkylating agents, act by interfering with nucleic acid function and protein production irrespective of the cell division cycle and are thus effective against both proliferating and resting cells. All are extremely potent and have only a slight margin of safety between tumoricidal and toxic doses.

Key considerations that together constitute the governing principles of cancer chemotherapy include the following.

1. The tumor must be susceptible to the drug selected for treatment. Not all tumors are responsive to the same agent.

2. The drug or method of administration must not have intolerable local or systemic toxicity that would prevent the completion of an adequate course of treatment.

3. The drug must come into contact with the tumor cells and be present in sufficient concentration during the critical periods of the cell metabolic cycle.

4. The therapeutic potential of the antineoplastic drugs may be enhanced by active antitumor defense mechanisms in the host. Immunotherapy given with chemotherapy, either concurrently or sequentially, may bolster the tumoricidal impact of the drugs.

5. The administration of combinations of antineoplastic drugs with different modes of action can increase the collective antitumor effect without a concomitant increase in undesirable side effects. Combined drug chemotherapy widens the range of antitumor activity and permits the use of lower doses, thereby diminishing the toxicity of each component. Only drugs that are partially effective when used alone should be combined.

6. Cancer chemotherapy is more effective when the tumor mass is small than when the tumor cell burden is high. Anticancer drugs kill cells according to first-order kinetics. Even a drug that destroys 99.99% of the tumor cells will leave a substantial number intact if the initial quantity was large. Because survival of few or perhaps even a single malignant cell may lead to tumor regrowth and eventually to death of the patient (host defenses often being ineffective against neoplastic cells), it becomes the goal of therapy to achieve total cancer cell destruction.[26]

7. Cancer cells may build up a resistance to a previously effective drug and become completely unresponsive. Such resistance has been ascribed to a variety of causes, including decreased drug penetration resulting from a reduction in tumor blood supply, drug-provoked mutations, enzyme alterations, and acquired resistance through natural selection of tumor cells insensitive to the drug.

8. The major tumor cell burden is often contained in the primary tumor mass. Removal of the primary tumor mass by surgery or destruction by irradiation gives chemotherapy a better chance of producing a cure because the micrometastases have a higher growth fraction and contain smaller numbers of drug-resistant cells than the primary tumor mass.

PHARMACOLOGIC EFFECTS
Antineoplastic alkylating agents

The alkylating agents, consisting of the nitrogen mustards (including chlorambucil, cyclophosphamide, mechlorethamine, and melphalan), busulfan, thiotepa, dacarbazine, pipobroman, and the nitrosoureas, have the common chemical characteristic of liberating alkyl radicals on degeneration. The alkyl radicals form covalent linkages with nucleophilic moieties such as phosphate, sulfhydryl, hydroxyl, carboxyl, amino, and imidazole groups.[12] They react with organic compounds essential for cell metabolism and prevent cell division by cross-linking strands of DNA. Except for cyclophosphamide, which also inhibits DNA synthesis, the alkylating agents are not cell-cycle specific. (See Figure 40-1 for a review of the cell division cycle.) Because they produce irreversible changes in the DNA molecule, the alkylating agents are mutagenic, teratogenic, and carcinogenic in addition to being oncolytic. The alkylating agents are also radiomimetic because they produce morphologic damage in cells that is similar to that caused by radiation injury. They vary greatly in lipid solubility, membrane transport, and pharmacokinetic properties, however, and therefore differ in clinical use. The molecular structures of representative alkylating agents are shown in Figure 40-2.

Busulfan. Busulfan, developed by Haddow and Timmis,[14] is used almost exclusively in the treatment of chronic myelocytic leukemia and polycythemia vera. A slow-acting sulfur mustard that is well absorbed after oral administration, busulfan is rapidly cleared from the blood and excreted in the urine as methane-sulfonic acid. Like other antineoplastic alkylating drugs, busulfan causes bone marrow depression manifested by leukopenia and thrombocytopenia. Additional busulfan-specific toxic manifestations include pulmonary fibrosis,

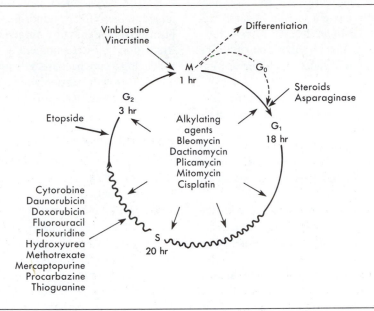

Figure 40-1. Cell cycle and probable point of action of antineoplastic drugs. G_1 = period before DNA synthesis, during which enzymes necessary for DNA synthesis are synthesized, S = period during which DNA is replicated for the various chromosomes, G_2 = period of specialized protein and RNA synthesis and manufacture of mitotic spindle apparatus, M = mitosis, G_0 = resting state when cells are not cycling and are not affected by many drugs.

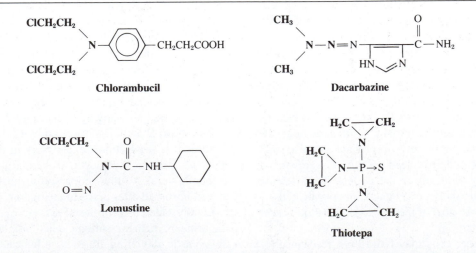

Figure 40-2. Structural formulas of representative alkylating agents. The portion of each molecule involved in alkylation reactions is shown in boldface type.

skin pigmentation, hypotension, gynecomastia, and cataract formation.

Chlorambucil. Chlorambucil is given orally for chronic lymphocytic leukemia, lymphosarcoma, Hodgkin's disease, seminoma, and carcinoma of the ovary. The drug is well absorbed and rapidly metabolized, but its route of excretion is uncertain. High doses cause nausea and vomiting. The major toxic manifestation is myelosuppression. Dermatitis and hepatotoxicity have been encountered in some patients.

Cyclophosphamide. Cyclophosphamide is a cyclic mustard that resulted from attempts to produce an alkylating agent with greater selectivity for neoplastic tissues than the original nitrogen mustard, mechlorethamine. Cyclophosphamide is of value in remission induction and maintenance therapy for Hodgkin's disease and other lymphomas, acute lymphocytic leukemia, multiple myeloma, neuroblastoma, rhabdomyosarcoma, and carcinoma of the breast, ovary, lung, and bladder. The drug is rapidly absorbed from the gastrointestinal tract after oral administration and is converted to active compounds by the liver. Intermediate metabolites have been identified in the urine; less than 15% of the drug is excreted unchanged by the kidneys. The catabolic products may produce a hemorrhagic cystitis and dysuria that are minimized by a high rate of fluid intake and urine flow. Cyclophosphamide is a powerful immunosuppressant and myelosuppressant. Nausea, vomiting, and alopecia are common side effects. Drug-associated stomatitis, hepatotoxicity, diarrhea, and skin pigmentation have been noted in occasional patients.

Estramustine. A recent addition to the alkylating antineoplastic drugs, estramustine is formed by combining nornitrogen mustard with estradiol. The estrogen moiety imparts some selectivity to the action of estramustine inasmuch as the drug is preferentially taken up by tissues with estrogen receptors. Currently, estramustine is approved for palliative treatment of prostate carcinoma. The selective distribution of estramustine may lower somewhat the severity of adverse reactions to alkylating agents; however, undesirable estrogenic side effects may also occur.

Mechlorethamine. Mechlorethamine was the first nitrogen mustard and the progenitor of the antineoplastic alkylating agents, and it is still used systemically in the treatment of Hodgkin's disease and other lymphomas. The drug is a vesicant that produces severe local tissue necrosis unless administered through a running intravenous infusion. This irritant effect is used to control intractable pleural effusions caused by intrapleural malignancies. In such instances, the drug is injected intracavitarily. The acute side effects of nitrogen mustard are nausea and vomiting, and these usually begin within 30 minutes after injection and persist for up to 8 hours. Mechlorethamine produces bone marrow suppression. Very high doses cause nerve deafness, brain damage, and convulsions.

Melphalan. Melphalan is a phenylalanine mustard that is administered orally or intravenously in the treatment of multiple myeloma and carcinoma of the ovary. Melphalan is readily absorbed from the gastrointestinal tract and remains in the blood for about 6 hours. The route and form of excretion are unknown. Drug metabolites are localized in the cytoplasm of liver, kidney, and spleen cells. Bone marrow depression, nausea, and vomiting are the principle toxic manifestations.

Thiotepa. This compound has definite value in controlling malignant pleural effusions and malignant ascites, since the drug does not cause the intense inflammatory reaction characteristic of nitrogen mustard. Thiotepa has produced favorable results in breast and ovarian carcinoma and in some lymphomas and sarcomas. It is used in the treatment of cancer of the bladder, where it is instilled directly into the lumen. Routes of administration for other malignancies are oral, intravenous, intraarterial, intramuscular, intratumor, and intracavitary. Absorption from the gastrointestinal tract is uncertain. After intravenous infusion, most of the drug is excreted unchanged in the urine. Toxicity is manifested by bone marrow depression, nausea and vomiting, fever, skin rashes, infertility, alopecia, and mental depression.

Dacarbazine. Dacarbazine is an artificially synthesized congener of the naturally occurring purine precursor 5-aminoimidazole-4-carboxamide. Two methyl groups are substituted in the triazeno chain. Originally developed as an antimetabolite, dacarbazine is N-demethylated in the liver to yield an effective alkylating derivative. Gastrointestinal absorption is incomplete and variable. After intravenous administration, the initial, distributive half-life is about 20 minutes. After 6 hours, 43% of the dose is excreted in the urine as the unchanged product or as 5-aminoimidazole-4-carboxamide.

The drug is most effective in malignant melanoma and is also active in Hodgkin's disease and in soft-tissue sarcomas. The predominant side effect is nausea and vomiting, and this is most prominent during the first day, diminishing thereafter. Myelosuppression in the form of thrombocytopenia and leukopenia may occur 20 to 40 days after therapy. Another toxic manifestation of dacarbazine is a flu-like syndrome characterized by fever, myalgia, and headache.

Nitrosoureas. The nitrosoureas carmustine (BCNU) and lomustine (CCNU) decompose in the body to yield reactive intermediates that act as classic alkylating agents in causing strand breaks and cross-links in DNA. They also produce isocyanates that inhibit DNA repair and alter the maturation of RNA. Carmustine must be administered intravenously, whereas lomustine is an oral preparation. Both are rapidly metabolized and slowly excreted in the urine. They are lipid soluble and able to cross the blood-brain barrier into the spinal fluid. Both are effective in advanced Hodgkin's disease,

brain tumors, myeloma, and melanoma. Each produces nausea and vomiting within 4 to 6 hours after administration and delayed bone marrow depression that becomes apparent in 3 to 6 weeks and lasts for 2 to 3 weeks. Renal and hepatic toxicity has occurred in occasional patients.

Streptozocin, a naturally occurring nitrosourea, has a similar mode of action to the synthetic drugs described above. Unlike carmustine and lomustine, however, streptozocin does not readily cross the blood-brain barrier nor is it strongly myelosuppressive. Streptozocin is unique in its special affinity for the islet cells of the pancreas. The drug is diabetogenic in animals and highly effective against metastatic insulinomas in humans. Intravascular routes are used for administering streptozocin; dosages are often limited by potentially fatal renal toxicity and severe nausea and vomiting.

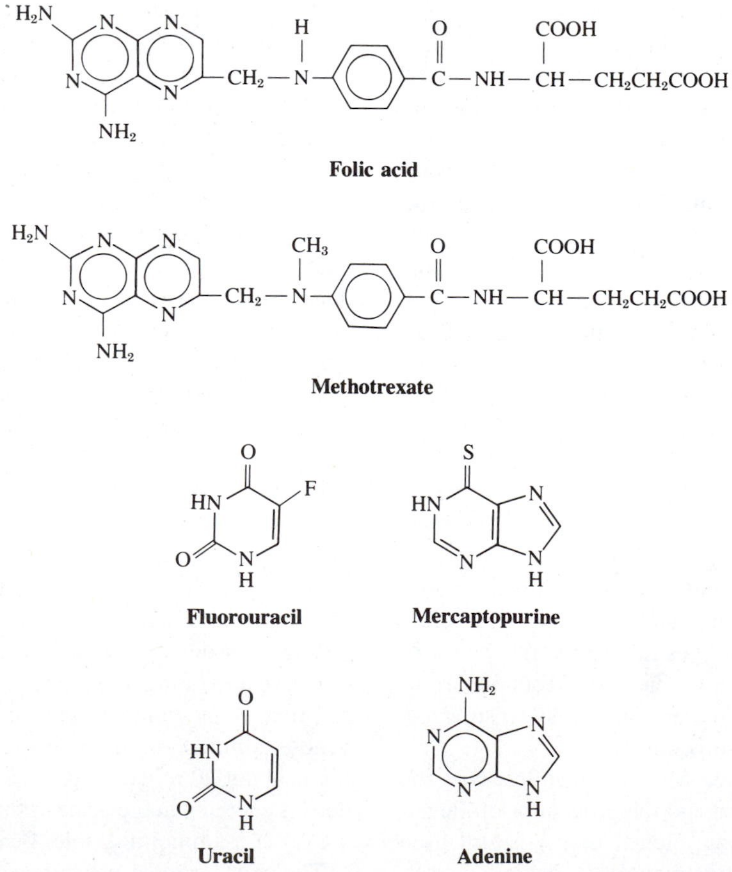

Figure 40-3. Structural relationships between several antimetabolites and their respective natural analogues.

Antimetabolites

The antimetabolites bear a marked structural resemblance to folic acid and to the purine and pyrimidine bases involved in the synthesis of DNA, RNA, and certain coenzymes (Figure 40-3). They differ in molecular arrangement from the corresponding metabolite to a degree sufficient to serve as competitive inhibitors. The inhibitory effect is reaction-specific and often may be reversed by providing an excess of the displaced metabolite or by supplying the product of the suppressed reaction. The antimetabolites characteristically interfere with growth of rapidly proliferating cells throughout the body. The bone marrow, lining of the alimentary tract, germinal cells, hair follicles, and developing fetus are most severely affected. Oral manifestations are an especially prominent feature of the toxicity of these agents.

Folic acid analogues. Folic acid is an essential vitamin that is converted into metabolically active tetrahydrofolic acid by the enzyme dihydrofolate reductase. Tetrahydrofolic acid participates in the synthesis of purines, pyrimidines, and ultimately nucleic acids by combining with a one-carbon unit and delivering the unit to metabolites requiring methylation.

The folate antagonist methotrexate and its 4-amino congeners bind tightly and almost irreversibly to dihydrofolate reductase, thereby inhibiting formation of the DNA precursor thymidylic acid.[23] Methotrexate inhibits cell division in the S phase of the cell cycle. The drug is readily absorbed from the gastrointestinal tract, more rapidly from an empty than from a full stomach. Delayed absorption increases the duration of action. The distributional plasma half-life of methotrexate is less than 1 hour, and 50% is bound to plasma proteins. More than 80% is excreted in the urine within 48 hours, and a small amount is excreted in the feces via the biliary tract.

Methotrexate is a valuable therapeutic agent in acute lymphocytic leukemia and choriocarcinoma. Intrathecal and intraarterial routes are used for meningeal leukemia and head and neck cancer, respectively. Methotrexate is sometimes effective in treating Hodgkin's disease, lymphosarcoma, acute myelocytic leukemia, chronic lymphocytic leukemia, testicular tumors, and carcinoma of the breast and lung. The drug is also included as postoperative adjuvant therapy in osteosarcoma, where it is given in very high doses followed by folinic acid "rescue."

The toxic reactions to tumoricidal doses of methotrexate are bone marrow depression manifested by leukopenia and thrombocytopenia that are conducive to secondary infections and hemorrhages, a very painful stomatitis with mucosal and epithelial ulceration, pharyngitis and dysphagia, esophagitis, gastroenterocolitis, and proctitis with an associated watery and bloody diarrhea. Pleuritic pain and pulmonary fibrosis, skin erythema and photosensitivity, and alopecia may also occur. Transient disturbances of liver function expressed by elevated transaminase activities are common. Large doses are nephrotoxic.

Purine analogues. The most commonly used purine analogues in cancer chemotherapy are mercaptopurine and thioguanine. The mechanisms of action of these thiopurines have not yet been fully established. Presumably these compounds affect the incorporation of purine derivatives into nucleic acids. The analogues are converted to the ribonucleotide form, which interferes with the conversion of inosinic acid (hypoxanthine ribonucleotide) to the ribotides of adenine and guanine.[7] They also inhibit *de novo* biosynthesis of purines from the small molecule precursors glycine, formate, and phosphate.

Orally administered mercaptopurine is rapidly absorbed. Half the dose is excreted in the urine in 24 hours. After intravenous injection, the half-life is about 90 minutes. There is a high level of cell uptake and rapid renal excretion of the drug and metabolic by-products. The drug is metabolized by methylation in the liver and by the hepatic enzyme xanthine oxidase. Currently, mercaptopurine is used mainly for remission maintenance in acute lymphocytic leukemia. The chief toxic effect is myelosuppression. Hepatotoxicity associated with bile stasis and rarely with hepatic necrosis has been reported. Hyperuricemia may follow rapid cell lysis in patients treated with this drug.

The purine analogue thioguanine has activity similar to that of mercaptopurine. Its major clinical use is in the treatment of acute myelocytic and acute lymphocytic leukemia in combination with other agents. The drug inhibits purine synthesis and is incorporated into fraudulent DNA. Toxicity is manifested by myelosuppression and occasionally by gastrointestinal intolerance.

Pyrimidine analogues. A number of pyrimidine congeners have been examined for antineoplastic activity. Of these fluorouracil, floxuridine, and cytarabine are currently marketed.

Fluorinated derivatives. The fluorinated pyrimidines, fluorouracil and floxuridine, are prepared by substituting a stable fluorine atom for hydrogen in position 5 of the uracil and deoxyuridine molecules, respectively.[15] These compounds are potent antimetabolites that link with thymidylate synthetase to block formation of thymidylic acid and impair DNA synthesis. Because of the unavailability of thymidine for cell replication and DNA production, the cells undergo a "thymineless death."

Fluorouracil is used most often in the treatment of gastrointestinal adenocarcinomas, breast cancer, and ovarian cancer. Activity has also been reported in bladder and prostate cancer. The drug is usually given intravenously, since oral absorption is unpredictable and incomplete. There is a rapid fall in blood concentration within 2 hours after administration, followed by a much slower decline. The drug is distributed throughout the body, with the greatest concentrations in liver and tumor tissue. It becomes active on enzymatic conversion to the nucleotide monophosphate. Metabolic degradation occurs in the liver, where fluorouracil is broken down stepwise into urea, carbon dioxide, and ammonia. These are excreted in the urine and expired air.

Floxuridine exerts a much more direct inhibition of thymidylate synthetase than does fluorouracil. The drug has to be given by continuous infusion because it is rapidly catabolized in vivo. Floxuridine administered intraarterially is indicated for gastrointestinal adenocarcinomas metastatic to the liver and has produced beneficial results in the treatment of head and neck carcinoma.

The adverse effects of the fluorinated pyrimidines may be quite severe. Stomatitis, pharyngitis, dysphagia, enteritis, diarrhea, anorexia, nausea, and vomiting frequently accompany the use of these drugs. The fluorinated pyrimidines suppress the bone marrow, leading to leukopenia and thrombocytopenia. Rarer side effects include erythematous and pigmented dermatitis, alopecia, and a reversible cerebellar ataxia.

Cytarabine. Cytarabine (cytosine arabinoside) is an analogue of 2-deoxycytidine that inhibits DNA synthesis by interfering with DNA polymerase.[3] It is also incorporated into fraudulent DNA and is primarily a cell-cycle S-phase specific agent. Cytarabine is not active when administered orally. When given intravenously, the drug is rapidly cleared from the blood and metabolized in the liver, where it is converted by cytidine deaminase to uracil arabinoside and excreted as such in the urine.

Cytarabine is used mainly in the treatment of acute myelocytic leukemia in combination with other agents. In fact, it is the most active single drug available for the treatment of this condition in adults, producing about a 25% incidence of complete remission. It has some modest activity against lymphomas. The major side effects are myelosuppression and megaloblastic anemia. High doses produce nausea and vomiting. Occasional patients may develop gastrointestinal disturbances, stomatitis, hepatic dysfunction, local thrombophlebitis, or dermatitis, or any combination of these symptoms.

Antibiotics

A number of substances originally isolated as antibiotics have been found to exert antineoplastic activity because of their cytotoxic properties. These substances, produced naturally by various *Streptomyces* species, operate by binding with DNA to produce irreversible complexes that inhibit cell division. Semisynthetic derivatives of some of the antibiotics are being prepared and tested clinically in an effort to reduce toxicity but retain the oncolytic potency of the parent compound.

Dactinomycin. Dactinomycin (actinomycin D) is a crystalline antibiotic composed of a phenoxazone chromophore and two cyclic peptide chains (Figure 40-4). The drug binds to DNA, forming a stable complex that prevents DNA-dependent RNA synthesis by impeding the progress of RNA polymerases along the DNA template.[10] Almost all of the drug is removed from the circulation within 2 minutes after intravenous injection. The highest concentrations are found in the submaxillary glands, liver, and kidneys. Approximately 50% is excreted unchanged in the bile and 10% in the urine within 24 hours.

Dactinomycin is the main agent for the treatment of Wilms' tumor and is of considerable value against choriocarcinoma and testicular tumors. It is also effective in embryonal rhabdomyosarcoma, neuroblastoma, and Ewing's sarcoma. Occasional responses are seen in melanoma, breast carcinoma, and gastrointestinal carcinoma. Nausea and vomiting occur within a few hours after administration. Extravasation from the vein causes severe tissue necrosis. Mucositis characterized by oral ulcerations and diarrhea often necessitates limiting the dose. Erythema, hyperpigmentation, and desquamation may develop in previously irradiated skin.

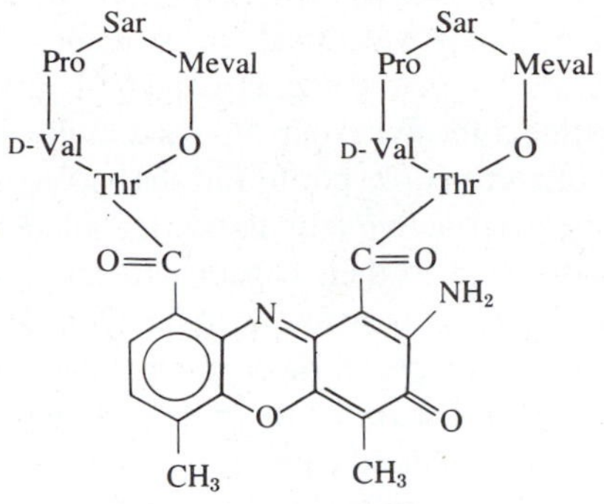

Figure 40-4. Structural formulas of dactinomycin and doxorubicin. Sar = sarcosine, Meval = N-methylvaline.

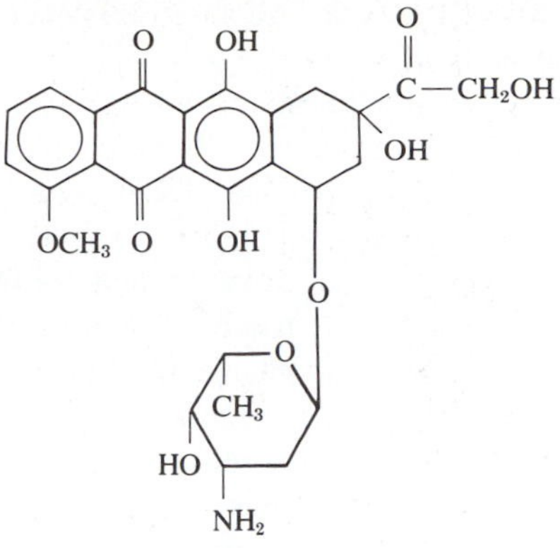

The drug suppresses all bone marrow elements.

Daunorubicin. Daunorubicin hydrochloride is the salt of a cytotoxic anthracycline antibiotic produced by *Streptomyces peucetius*. The drug combines with DNA in an intercalative mode by slipping into the helical structure between stacked bases. The killing effect of daunorubicin is at a maximum in the DNA-synthetic S phase of the cell cycle.

The drug is most useful in the treatment of acute myelocytic leukemia. Following intravenous injection, 25% of the dose is eliminated in an active form by urinary excretion, and 40% is lost through biliary excretion. The common toxic manifestations of daunorubicin are nausea, vomiting, alopecia, stomatitis, and extensive myelosuppression. Other toxic reactions are dose-dependent cardiomyopathy, manifested by acute congestive heart failure, and local necrosis from extravasation at the injection site. Minor effects include facial flush, fever, hyperpigmentation, skin rash, and drowsiness.

Doxorubicin. Doxorubicin is an anthracycline glycoside antibiotic formed by the *Streptomyces peucetius* var. *caesius*. Doxorubicin acts by intercalating into DNA and inhibiting both DNA and RNA synthesis.[1] The drug also damages preformed DNA and inhibits DNA repair. Although nearly identical to daunorubicin in structure, doxorubicin has a much broader spectrum of antineoplastic activity. The drug is extremely active against acute myelocytic and acute lymphocytic leukemia and many tumors that are resistant to most other che-motherapeutic agents, notably sarcomas, transitional cell carcinoma of the urinary tract, thyroid carcinoma, and some lung cancers. It has also proved effective in breast cancer, lymphomas, and neuroblastoma.

Doxorubicin is a vesicant that is always given intravenously. It is rapidly cleared from the plasma and concentrated in the tissues. Urinary excretion is low, rarely accounting for more than 10% of the administered dose. In contrast, biliary excretion is high. Plasma concentrations of doxorubicin and its metabolites are markedly elevated and the rate of elimination is greatly prolonged in the presence of severely impaired liver function.

The major toxic effects are alopecia that is often total but always reversible, nausea and vomiting that begin shortly after drug administration and last 2 to 3 days, fever on the day of administration, and phlebitis at the site of injection. Extravasation of the drug produces soft tissue necrosis. Myelosuppression, primarily granulocytopenia, is maximal 10 to 14 days after drug administration. Mucositis manifested mainly as soreness of the mouth with ulcerations occurs in almost all patients. Cardiomyopathy expressed as congestive heart failure becomes a serious risk in patients given a total dose exceeding 550 mg/m^2.

Bleomycin. Bleomycin is an antibiotic complex of several glycopeptides derived from *Streptomyces verticillus*. The cytotoxic action of bleomycin has been attributed to DNA scission and fragmentation with inhibition of the usual DNA repair mechanisms.[27] Bleomycin is rapidly cleared from the blood and concentrated in the liver, spleen, kidneys, and epithelial tissue. About 80% is excreted in the urine within 24 hours.

The main clinical applications of bleomycin are in the treatment of squamous cell carcinoma, testicular tumors, and lymphomas. Head and neck, esophageal, skin, vulvar, penile, anal, and cervical cancers may also respond. Toxicity includes fever with a flu-like syndrome, nausea, vomiting, alopecia, stomatitis, and skin changes manifested by hyperpigmentation, rash, ulceration, and exfoliation. An additional complication is interstitial pneumonitis that might progress to pulmonary fibrosis and fatal pulmonary insufficiency. Bleomycin does not cause any major myelosuppression.

Plicamycin. An antibiotic produced by *Streptomyces plicatus,* plicamycin (formerly mithramycin) binds with DNA to interfere with separation at the time of division and also impairs production of RNA by blocking formation of transfer RNA from DNA.[29] The drug is rapidly taken up from the blood, with maximal concentration in the kidneys and liver. Plicamycin is effective against embryonal carcinoma of the testis. Some beneficial results have been reported in testicular choriocarcinoma, Wilms' tumor, and carcinoma of the breast. Plicamycin is also used to treat tumor-associated hypercalcemia because of its action in suppressing the peripheral effect of parathyroid hormone.

This agent is toxic to the liver, kidneys, and bone marrow. Leukopenia and thrombocytopenia are common. The combination of thrombocytopenia and depressed hepatic synthesis of blood coagulation factors can produce severe gastrointestinal bleeding. Other common side effects are nausea, vomiting, fever, malaise, stomatitis, hypocalcemia, azotemia, and facial erythema.

Mitomycin. Mitomycin, derived from *Streptomyces caespitosus,* was found originally in soil near Tokyo, Japan, in 1955.[28] After intracellular activation, mitomycin inhibits DNA synthesis by reacting with DNA in the manner of the alkylating agents. The drug has a low order of antineoplastic activity when given alone. When combined with fluorouracil or the nitrosoureas, mitomycin has been effective against gastrointestinal, head and neck, breast, cervix, and lung carcinomas as well as some lymphomas. Severe toxicity to the bone marrow (neutropenia and thrombocytopenia) and to the alimentary tract (nausea, vomiting, oral ulceration, and diarrhea) are the limiting factors in the use of this drug.

Vinca alkaloids

Vinblastine and vincristine, the two alkaloids in clinical use, are asymmetrical dimeric compounds that are almost identical in structure (Figure 40-5). Vinblastine contains a methyl group and vincristine a formyl group attached to the nitrogen in the dihydroindole portion of the molecule. The antineoplastic activity of the vinca alkaloids has been attributed to their capacity to interfere with the synthesis of transfer RNA and to arrest cell division in metaphase by binding to the microtubular protein that forms the mitotic spindle.[11]

The vinca alkaloids are cleared from the blood within 30 minutes after intravenous administration. The drugs are excreted mainly via the biliary and intestinal tracts, with less than 5% appearing in the urine. Vinblastine is of major value in Hodgkin's disease, other lymphomas, choriocarcinoma, and testicular tumors. Vincristine is used in the treatment of acute leukemia, Hodgkin's disease, Wilms' tumor, neuroblastoma, and testicular tumors and in the palliation of ovarian, breast, and pulmonary carcinoma.

The most common toxic manifestation of vinblastine is leukopenia. High doses induce gastrointestinal disturbances denoted by nausea, vomiting, diarrhea, and anorexia. Partial alopecia, headache, paresthesias, mental depression, mild peripheral neuropathy, and phlebitis at the injection site are other side effects of this drug. Vincristine produces neurotoxicity that is dose related. Mild toxicity is manifested by vomiting, constipation, and abdominal cramps; moderate toxicity by alopecia and peripheral neuropathy; and severe toxicity by sensory loss, paresthesias, headache, slapping gait, loss of deep tendon reflexes, ataxia, and paralysis of cranial nerves II, III, VI, and VII. Marrow toxicity is generally mild, with anemia and reticulocytopenia the most prominent manifestations. Phlebitis may also occur.

Steroids

Adrenocorticosteroids, estrogens, antiestrogens, androgens, and progestational agents each have a role in cancer control. Prednisone is widely used in combination with other antineoplastic drugs in acute leukemia, Hodgkin's disease, lymphoma, and multiple myeloma and for reducing hypercalcemia associated wtih bony metastases. The estrogens are useful in the treatment of advanced prostatic carcinoma and postmenopausal carcinoma of the breast. Although the mode of action is unknown, the therapeutic response in breast cancer

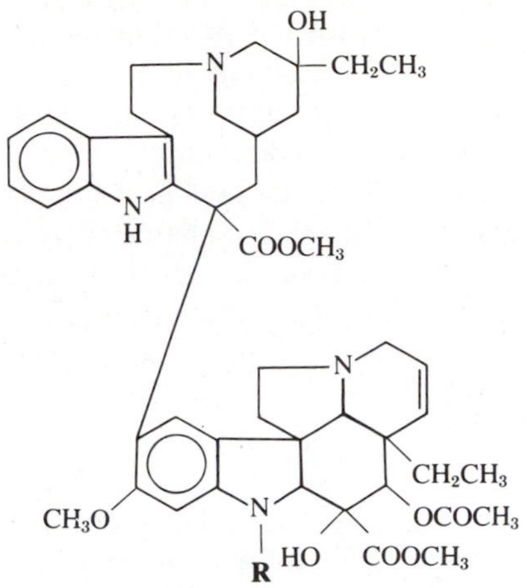

OH

N—CH₂CH₃

N
H

COOCH₃

R = CH₃ **Vinblastine**
R = CHO **Vincristine**

N

CH₂CH₃
CH₃O
OCOCH₃
N
R HO COOCH₃

Figure 40-5. Structural formulas of vinca alkaloids.

is correlated with the presence of estrogen-binding receptor sites in the tumor. The antiestrogen tamoxifen is beneficial in patients whose adenocarcinoma of the breast is dependent on estrogen for growth. Androgens are effective in some cases of metastatic breast cancer. The progestational agents are effective in metastatic endometrial, breast, and renal cell carcinoma. The pharmacology of this drug group is detailed in Chapters 22 and 35.

Three drugs have been found to suppress adrenocortical secretion—mitotane, metapyrone, and aminoglutethimide. Mitotane, as can be seen from Table 40-1, is classified with miscellaneous antineoplastic drugs. Aminoglutethimide inhibits the conversion of cholesterol to 2α-hydroxycholesterol, thereby reducing synthesis of corticosteroids. It has been used in patients with adrenal tumors, those with hypersecretion arising from ectopic production of ACTH, or, in combination with metapyrone, in patients with Cushing's disease.

Miscellaneous antineoplastic drugs

Asparaginase. Asparaginase catalyzes the hydrolysis of L-asparagine to L-aspartic acid and ammonia. It inhibits protein synthesis in tumor cells by depriving them of the amino acid asparagine. Clinical use is confined at present to acute lymphocytic leukemia. The drug has essentially no bone marrow toxicity but may produce acute anaphylaxis with hypotension, sweating, bronchospasm, and urticaria. Other side effects are chills, fever, nausea, vomiting, liver dysfunction, blood coagulation defects, pancreatitis, and immuno-

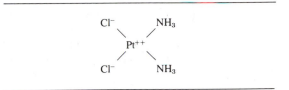

Figure 40-6. Structural formula of cisplatin.

suppression with depressed cell-mediated and humoral immunity.

Cisplatin. Cisplatin (cis-diamminedichloroplatinum or CDPP) is a heavy metal complex containing a central atom of platinum surrounded by two chloride ions and two amino groups in the cis position (Figure 40-6). The compound has biochemical properties similar to bifunctional alkylating agents in that it produces interstrand and intrastrand cross-links in DNA, thereby inhibiting its synthesis. Cisplatin is apparently not cell-cycle specific because it also interferes with RNA and protein synthesis. The drug has proved most effective in the treatment of carcinoma of the testis and ovary, transitional cell bladder neoplasia, and head and neck cancer. After intravenous injection cisplatin concentrates in the liver, kidneys, spleen, and intestinal wall. Up to 50% is excreted in the urine; the other excretory pathways are undetermined. Nephrotoxicity expressed as renal tubular necrosis is the major dose-limiting side effect. The agent is also ototoxic, causing initially high frequency and later complete hearing loss, and gastroenterotoxic, inducing nausea and vomiting. Long-term use produces peripheral neuropathy and high doses are severely leukopenic.

Etopside. Etopside is a new anticancer drug indicated for the treatment of advanced testicular cancer. It is also active against Kaposi's sarcoma and certain forms of lung cancer and lymphoma. A cell-cycle specific drug, etopside is unique in that it is most active in the G_2-phase of the cycle. The drug appears to prevent cell division by damaging DNA. Leukopenia and nausea and vomiting are the most common adverse effects; thrombocytopenia, other gastrointestinal disturbances, alopecia, stomatitis, and allergic reactions have also been reported.

Hydroxyurea. Hydroxyurea inhibits DNA synthesis by blocking the action of ribonucleoside reductase.[21] Hydroxyurea is readily absorbed from the alimentary tract. Plasma concentrations peak in 2 hours and fall to zero in 24 hours. Up to 80% of the drug is excreted in the urine within 12 hours.

Hydroxyurea is used to treat busulfan-resistant chronic myelocytic leukemia and to lower rapidly rising peripheral blast counts in acute leukemia. High doses most often produce myelosuppression and megaloblastic anemia and occasionally severe stomatitis, diarrhea, and alopecia.

Procarbazine. Procarbazine, a derivative of methylhydrazine, suppresses mitosis and produces chromosomal defects. It is an MAO inhibitor that possesses teratogenic and carcinogenic properties in addition to antineoplastic activity. Procarbazine is rapidly absorbed from the alimentary tract, quickly metabolized by the liver, and excreted in the urine mainly in the form of a metabolic breakdown product.

Procarbazine is most active against Hodgkin's disease and is modestly effective in the other lymphomas and multiple myeloma when given in combination with alkylating agents and vinca alkaloids. The toxic effects are nausea and vomiting with high doses, leukopenia and thrombocytopenia within 3 to 4 weeks, lethargy, drowsiness, fever, myalgia, and arthralgia.

COMBINATION CHEMOTHERAPY

Combination chemotherapy has a number of advantages over single drug therapy in the eradication of drug-responsive malignancies:

1. Most human neoplasms contain biologically and biochemically heterogeneous cell types that have different sensitivities to chemotherapeutic drugs. Consequently antitumor activity may be increased by use of mixtures of drugs with dissimilar mechanisms of cytotoxic action.

2. Repopulation of cell lines that have become insensitive to one drug may be prevented by the use of another drug.

3. Drugs used in cancer chemotherapy generally act at specific phases of the cell cycle. Combining an agent or agents effective against mitotically active cells with drugs effective against resting cells may result in an additive or synergistic antitumor effect.

4. One drug in a combination may interfere with the enzymatic destruction or delay the excretion of another drug, thus producing an additive effect.

5. Two or more drugs in a multidrug protocol may act on different receptor or enzyme sites in neoplastic cells, producing a more intense blockade of a metabolic process than would be attainable with a single agent.

6. Drugs used in cancer chemotherapy are characteristically quite toxic, and the doses used (and therefore the drugs' efficacy) are limited by that toxicity. Combining two toxic drugs (with different toxicities) provides an increase in the effectiveness of the combination without increasing damage to host tissues.

Combination chemotherapy has proved to be very effective in a number of cancers, including acute leukemia, Hodgkin's disease, non-Hodgkin's lymphomas, and osteogenic sarcoma. For example, in generalized Hodgkin's disease, the so-called MOPP regimen (mechlorethamine, vincristine [Oncovin], procarbazine, and prednisone) has become the treatment of choice and produces remissions in at least 80% of patients. A combination known as ABVD (doxorubicin [Adriamycin], bleomycin, vinblastine, and dacarbazine) has also been used successfully in Hodgkin's disease.

IMPLICATIONS FOR DENTISTRY

A rate of cell proliferation comparable to that of fast-growing tumors and a trauma-intense environment combine to make the mouth a frequent target for the toxic actions of the tumoricidal drugs. Some act directly by metabolic interference with the growth, maturation, and replication of the oral mucosal cells; others act indirectly by inducing myelosuppression, immunosuppression, or nerve damage. Direct effects in the mouth are expressed clinically by denudation and ulceration of the mucosa; indirect effects by bleeding, infections, pain, and paresthesias.[6]

Antitumor drugs cannot distinguish between malignant cells and normal cells and are thus potentially damaging to both. The prime purpose of cancer chemotherapy is to destroy the greatest number of cancer cells and the least number of normal cells. Although the oral reactions to the stomatotoxic antineoplastic drugs are, in general, dose related and duration related, cancer patients differ greatly in their capacity to tolerate a given amount of a particular drug or combination of drugs. There is considerably more interpatient than intrapatient variability in this regard. Those who develop oral toxicity during the first course of treatment will almost predictably demonstrate identical side effects during each subsequent course unless the drugs are changed or the doses are modified.

Drug-induced stomatitis

Stomatitis that is manifested chiefly as a mucositis of the lips, tongue, gingiva, buccal mucosa, palatal mucosa, or floor of the mouth is a common complication of therapy with many of the antineoplastic drugs. The folic acid, purine, and pyrimidine antimetabolites, the antibiotics, hydroxyurea, and procarbazine are the most culpable in this respect. Clinically, the stomatitis is characterized by reduced mucosal thickness and keratinization, superficial sloughing, intense reddening, and traumatic and atraumatic ulcerations. Pain is intense and unremitting. The manifestations begin shortly after treatment is instituted, peak within a week after course completion, and then slowly recede unless complicated by infection, hemorrhage, or repeated drug administration.

The oral mucosal reactions to the anticancer drugs may be local or general in distribution and acute to subacute in course. They are highly individualistic in pattern and are indistinguishable as to specific etiology. Their morphology is often altered by physical, chemical, and microbial trauma. The damage is reversible and usually totally reparable after drug withdrawal. Treatment is essentially palliative, involving topical anesthetics and analgesics, topical protectants, and cleansing mouthwashes (see Chapter 45). Prevention and control of nosocomial infections until tissue integrity is fully restored are of paramount importance in the management of these patients.

Drug-induced oral hemorrhages

The antineoplastic drugs so depress bone marrow activity that thrombocytopenia, leukopenia, and anemia are almost an inevitable part of treatment. The most prominent myelosuppressants are the alkylating agents, antimetabolites, antibiotics, vinca alkaloids, and several "miscellaneous" drugs: cisplatin, hydroxyurea, and procarbazine. Thrombocytopenia is the most frequent cause of mouth bleeding in patients receiving cancer chemotherapy. Although such episodes are rare at platelet counts above 50,000/mm^3, the incidence at counts below 20,000/mm^3 exceeds 50%.

Thrombocytopenic bleeding can originate in any part of the mouth exposed to trauma sufficient to injure the capillary beds. The bleeding is usually oozing and intermittent, as soft blood clots form, break away, and reform. Thrombocytopenic hemorrhages are best controlled by transfusions of fresh platelets until bone marrow recovery restores platelet production to effective levels.

Oral bleeding may also result from a reduction in blood clotting factors, because thromboplastic substances released during the rapid destruction of white blood cells by tumoricidal drugs use up other clotting factors. Bleeding problems may also arise from the inhibition of fibrinogen synthesis by asparaginase. Clinically, such bleeding mimics that of thrombocytopenia. Episodes of oral bleeding are differentiated on the basis of the blood fibrinogen, fibrin split product, and clotting factor titers.

Drug-induced oral infections

Because most of the antineoplastic drugs are both myelosuppressive and immunosuppressive, susceptibility to infection by the recipient is greatly increased. Profound and prolonged neutropenia and lymphocytopenia deprive the host of a substantial part of the protection afforded by the immune system. The neutropenia-related reduction in phagocytic activity is compounded by an abolition of antibody production, inhibition of delayed hypersensitivity, and blockade of the mononuclear cell phase of the inflammatory reaction by some of the drugs. Cyclophosphamide, methotrexate, mercaptopurine, fluorouracil, cytarabine, dactinomycin, the vinca alkaloids, asparaginase, the corticosteroids, and procarbazine each suppress one or more stages of the immune response.[2]

Drug-induced immunosuppression and oral mucosal changes that deplete the local tissue barriers to infection make the mouth a common site of microbial attack during cancer chemotherapy. The great preponderance of bacterial oral infections that develop during treatment with the antineoplastic drugs are caused by gram-negative bacilli, notably species of *Pseudomonas, Klebsiella, Serratia, Enterobacter, Proteus,* and *Escherichia.*[5] Oral staphylococcal and streptococcal infections are not nearly as numerous as before the advent of the semisynthetic penicillinase-resistant penicillins. The most frequent oral fungal infection in patients receiving cancer chemotherapy is candidiasis; the most frequent oral viral infection is herpes labialis. Candidiasis can blanket extensive areas of the oral mucosa; herpes can erode large portions of the lips and extend onto the circumoral skin. Every bacterial, fungal, and viral oral infection in these patients is potentially lethal, because the mouth may serve as a portal of entry for widespread dissemination. Each oral infectious agent must be rapidly identified and vigorously treated wth appropriate antibiotics to prevent fatal consequences.

Drug-induced oral nutritional deficiencies

Antineoplastic chemotherapeutic regimens that include folate antagonists often produce a folic acid–deficiency stomatitis. Interference with the production of metabolically active tetrahydrofolic acid impedes the production and maturation of the epithelial cells lining the oral mucosa, leading to atrophy and extinction of the lingual papillae and an extremely painful denudative and ulcerative mucositis. Similarly, regimens containing fluorouracil, a metabolic antagonist of uracil, prompt the development of a thymine-deficiency stomatitis manifested by unbalanced growth, cell death, sloughing, and ulceration of the mucosa.

In addition to the direct effect of the antimetabolites, the antineoplastic drugs compromise the nutritional status of the patient by (1) producing nausea and anorexia leading to a reduced food intake, (2) causing vomiting and diarrhea resulting in excessive nutrient losses, (3) inducing gastroenterocolitis and malabsorption, and (4) impairing liver function and thereby obstructing nutrient utilization. Such patients are particularly prone to develop deficiencies of protein and of the water-soluble vitamins that affect the oral structures. They require daily supplements of crystalline vitamins and, in some instances, intravenous hyperalimentation to prevent nutritional decompensation.

Drug-induced oral pain and paresthesias

The antineoplastic drug with a special propensity for neurotoxicity is vincristine. Toxicity is mani-

fested by mixed sensory and motor neuropathies involving the somatic and autonomic nerves. Vincristine-associated trigeminal and facial nerve aberrations, signaled by jaw pain mimicking a toothache, circumoral numbness, and tingling and weakness of the facial muscles, have been encountered in some patients. These symptoms start to subside when the drug is discontinued and disappear completely when the integrity of the drug-damaged nerve is fully restored.

Antineoplastic drugs

See Table 40-1.

CITED REFERENCES

1. Bachur, N.R. Adriamycin-daunorubicin cellular-pharmacodynamics. Biochemical Pharmacology **23**:207-216, 1974.
2. Bodey, G.P., Hersh, E.M., Valdivieso, M., Feld, R., and Rodriguez, V. Effects of cytotoxic and immunosuppressive agents on the immune response. Postgraduate Medicine **58**:67-74, 1975.
3. Chabner, B.A. Antimetabolites. In Pinedo, H.M., ed. Cancer Chemotherapy 1979. New York, Elsevier North Holland, Inc., 1979.
4. Dougherty, T.E., and White, A. Influence of hormones on lymphoid tissue structure and function: role of pituitary adrenotrophic hormone in regulation of lymphocytes and other cellular elements of the blood. Endocrinology **35**:1-14, 1944.
5. Dreizen, S., Bodey, G.P., and Brown, L.R. Opportunistic gram-negative bacillary infections in leukemia: oral manifestations during myelosuppression. Postgraduate Medicine **55**:133-139, 1974.
6. Dreizen, S., Bodey, G.P., and Rodriguez, V. Oral complications of cancer chemotherapy. Postgraduate Medicine **58**:75-82, 1975.
7. Elion, G.B., and Hitchings, G.H. Metabolic basis for the actions of analogs of purines and pyrimidines. Advances in Chemotherapy **2**:91-177, 1965.
8. Farber, S., Diamond, L.K., Mercer, R.D., Sylvester, R.F., and Wolff, J.A. Temporary remissions in acute leukemia in children produced by folic acid antagonist, 4-aminopteroylglutamic acid (aminopterin). New England Journal of Medicine **238**:787-793, 1948.
9. Fessas, P., Wintrobe, M.M., Thompson, R.B., and Cartwright, G.E. Treatment of acute leukemia with cortisone and corticotropin. Archives of Internal Medicine **94**:384-401, 1954.
10. Franklin, R.M. The inhibition of ribonucleic acid synthesis in mammalian cells by actinomycin D. Biochimica et Biophysica Acta **72**:555-565, 1963.
11. George, P., Journey, L.J., and Goldstein, M.N. Effect of vincristine on the fine structure of HeLa cells during mitosis. Journal of the National Cancer Institute **35**:355-375, 1965.
12. Golding, P.R. The clinical pharmacology of cytotoxic drugs. In Bagshawe, K.D., ed. Medical Oncology:Medical Aspects of Malignant Disease. Oxford, England, Blackwell Scientific Publications, 1975.

13. Goodman, L.S., Wintrobe, M.M., Dameshek, W., Goodman, M.J., Gilman, A., and McLennan, M.T. Nitrogen mustard therapy; use of methyl-bis (β-chloroethyl) amine hydrochloride and tris (β-chloroethyl) amine hydrochloride for Hodgkin's disease, lymphosarcoma, leukemia, and certain allied and miscellaneous disorders. Journal of the American Medical Association **132:**126-132, 1946.

14. Haddow, A., and Timmis, G.M. Myeleran in chronic myeloid leukaemia: chemical constitution and biologic action. Lancet **1:**207-208, 1953.

15. Heidelberger, C., and Ansfield, F.J. Experimental and clinical use of fluorinated pyrimidines in cancer chemotherapy. Cancer Research **23:**1226-1243, 1963.

16. Heidelberger, C., Chaudhuri, M.K., Danneberg, P., Mooren, D., Griesbach, L., Duschinsky, R., Schnitzer, R.J., Pleven, E., and Scheiner, J. Fluorinated pyrimidines, a new class of tumour inhibitory compounds. Nature **179:**663-666, 1957.

17. Hitchings, G.H., Elion, G.B., Falco, E.A., Russell, P.B., and VanderWerff, H. Studies on analogs of purines and pyrimidines. Annals of the New York Academy of Sciences **52:**1318-1335, 1950.

18. Hodes, M.E., Rohn, R.J., and Bond, W.H. Vincaleukoblastine. I. Preliminary clinical studies. Cancer Research **20:**1041-1049, 1960.

19. Iriarte, P.V., Hananian, J., and Cortner, J.A. Central nervous system leukemia and solid tumors of childhood: treatment with 1,3-bis (2-chloroethyl)-1-nitrosourea (BCNU). Cancer **19:**1187-1194, 1966.

20. Johnson, I.S., Wright, H.F., Svoboda, G.H., and Vlantis, J. Antitumor principles derived from Vinca rosea Linn. I. Vincaleukoblastine and leurosine. Cancer Research **20:**1016-1022, 1960.

21. Krakoff, I.H., Brown, N.C., and Reichard, P. Inhibition of ribonucleoside diphosphate reductase by hydroxyurea. Cancer Research **28:**1559-1565, 1968.

22. Oettgen, H.F., Old, L.J., Boyse, E.A., Campbell, H.A., Philips, F.S., Clarkson, B.D., Tallal, L., Leeper, R.D., Scwartz, M.K., and Jae, H.K. Inhibition of leukemias in man by L-asparaginase. Cancer Research **27:**2619-2631, 1967.

23. Osborn, M.J., Freeman, M., and Heunnekens, F.M. Inhibition of dihydrofolic reductase by aminopterin and amethopterin. Proceedings of the Society for Experimental Biology and Medicine **97:**429-431, 1958.

24. Rosenberg, B., Van Camp, L., Trosko, J.E., and Mansour, V.H. Platinum compounds: a new class of potent antitumour agents. Nature **222:**385-386, 1969.

25. Schulte, G. Erfahrungen mit neuen zytostatischen Mitteln bei Hämoblastosen und Karzinomen und die Abrenzung ihrer Wirkungen gegen Röntgentherapie. Zeitschrift für Krebsforschung und Klinische Onkologie **58:**500-503, 1952.

26. Skipper, H.T., and Schabel, F.M., Jr. Quantitative and cytokinetic studies in experimental tumor models. In Holland, J.F., and Frei, E., III, eds. Cancer Medicine. Philadelphia, Lea & Febiger, 1973.

27. Suzuki, H., Nagai, K., Yamaki, H., Tanaka, N., and Umezewa, H. On the mechanism of action of bleomycin: scission of DNA strands in vitro and in vivo. Journal of Antibiotics (Tokyo) **22:**446-448, 1969.

28. Wakaki, S. Recent advances in research on antitumor mitomycins. Cancer Chemotherapy Reports **13:**79-86, 1961.

29. Yarbro, J.W., Kennedy, B.J., and Barnum, C.P. Mithramycin inhibition of ribonucleic acid synthesis. Cancer Research **26:**36-39, 1966.

GENERAL REFERENCES

Bagshawe, K.D., ed. Medical Oncology: Medical Aspects of Malignant Disease. Oxford, England, Blackwell Scientific Publications, 1975.

Cancer chemotherapy. Medical Letter on Drugs and Therapeutics **25:**1-8, 1983.

Carter, S.K., Bakowski, M.T., and Hellman, K. Chemotherapy of Cancer, New York, John Wiley & Sons, Inc., 1977.

De Vita, V.T., Jr., Hellman, S., and Rosenberg, S.A., eds. Cancer. Principles and Practice of Oncology. Philadelphia, Lea & Febiger, 1982.

Holland, J.F., and Frei, E., III, eds. Cancer Medicine, ed. 2. Philadelphia, Lea & Febiger, 1982.

41 Aliphatic alcohols

Roy Aston

The aliphatic alcohols of clinical interest are methyl, ethyl, and isopropyl alcohol. The main use of ethyl and isopropyl alcohol, topical disinfection, is discussed in detail in Chapter 43. Methanol has no therapeutic indications and is of toxicologic interest only. Ethanol has limited clinical application, but as the most common intoxicant in Western civilization it is of immense importance because of its potential for abuse and dependence and because it is a major contributing factor to both individual and social ills in the United States and other nations.

CHEMISTRY, CLASSIFICATION, AND MECHANISM OF ACTION

Alcohols are hydroxyl derivatives of aliphatic hydrocarbons (Table 41-1). They are clear, colorless, flammable liquids that are completely miscible with water and most organic solvents. The aliphatic monohydroxy alcohols form a homologous series and, with increasing numbers of carbon atoms, display increasing potency as nonselective CNS depressants. Dihydroxy alcohols (glycols) have similar CNS properties, whereas trihydroxy derivatives lack depressant effects.[20]

Ethyl alcohol can be obtained as anhydrous alcohol (100% ethanol), as neutral spirits (95% ethanol), and as denatured alcohol. Denatured alcohol, intended primarily for industrial use, is ethanol with some substance added to render it unfit for consumption, such as methanol, benzene, diethyl ether, or kerosene.

ETHYL ALCOHOL

Over 700 million gallons of ethanol are produced annually in the United States, supplying over 95 million drinkers. The ethanol content of some common alcoholic beverages is given in Table 41-2. In this country, 18% of adults are classified as heavy drinkers, and about 10% are considered to be alcohol-dependent (chronic alcoholics). About 12% of male and 8% of female drinkers develop health problems related to alcohol.[4] Cirrhosis of the liver is the third major cause of death in urban areas in persons 25 to 65 years of age.[17]

The social costs of alcohol abuse are staggering. Alcohol-related industrial losses, caused by absenteeism and job inefficiency, welfare costs, and property damage related to alcohol exceed $40 billion annually. At least 800,000 automobile accidents with 28,000 traffic fatalities each year are alcohol related. Drinking aggravates criminal behavior.[4] Alcohol is found to be involved in one third of suicides and rapes, one half of assaults, and one half to two thirds of homicides.

Alcohol has inconsistent effects on the neurotransmitters in the brain.[3] Most actions of ethanol appear attributable to the drug itself, but in many instances alcohol's effects may be due to its primary oxidative metabolite, acetaldehyde, acting through two postulated mechanisms. First, acetaldehyde may enhance synaptosomal release of norepinephrine and inhibit its active neuronal reuptake.[4] Second, acetaldehyde forms condensation products with catecholamines to yield tetrahydroisoquinolines, and with indoleamines (e.g., serotonin) to yield tetrahydro-β-carbolines.[4,12,27] The former products increase alcohol consumption in rats,[28] whereas the latter bear a chemical resemblance to hallucinogens.

Nerve activity is enhanced by low concentrations of ethanol but inhibited by higher concentrations. The inhibition is attributed to an ethanol-induced fluidization of cell membrane phospholipids, similar to that produced by inhalation anesthetics.[10,32] Long-term ethanol ingestion, however, is accompanied by an adaptive alteration in phospholipid composition with an increased proportion of cho-

Table 41-1. Aliphatic alcohols

	Synonyms	Chemical formula
Methyl alcohol	Methanol, carbinol, wood alcohol, wood spirit	CH_3OH
Ethyl alcohol	Ethanol, grain alcohol	CH_3CH_2OH
Isopropyl alcohol	Isopropanol, 2-propanol, secondary propyl alcohol	H_3C $\diagdown$ $CHOH$ $\diagup$ H_3C

Table 41-2. Equivalents of alcoholic beverages

Form of alcohol	Classification of drinker — Sex	Classification of drinker — Age (years)	Potential resulting blood ethanol level (mg/dl)*
Beer (12 fl. oz., 4% ethanol†)	Male	17-34	33.0
		57-86	37.1
	Female	20-31	39.3
		60-82	43.6
Distilled spirits (1 fl. oz., 50% ethanol)	Male	17-34	30.5
		57-86	34.3
	Female	20-31	36.4
		60-82	40.3

*Calculated on the basis of lean body mass of 140 lb (63.5 kg).
†American proof number is twice the percentage of ethanol by volume.

lesterol. This causes greater lipid rigidity and therefore resistance to the disordering effects of ethanol and of halothane on membrane lipids; it may be the basis of ethanol tolerance and of cross-tolerance to anesthetic agents.

Pharmacologic effects

Central nervous system. In general, ethanol may be considered a typical nonselective, membrane-active CNS depressant, similar to the sedative-hypnotics and anesthetic agents, with a primary action on the reticular formation.[3] With low doses of alcohol, the EEG displays a reduced frequency and increased amplitude of alpha waves and, with high doses, an enhanced delta activity similar to a deep sleep pattern. Ethanol's effects are dose related and progress through the typical sequence of reduction in anxiety, sedation, hypnosis, anesthesia, and death. Because of the variability of absorption of different alcoholic beverages, the effects of ethanol are most commonly correlated with blood alcohol concentration (BAC) (Table 41-3).

At a BAC below 50 mg/dl, binocular fusion is impaired, and blurred vision occurs. Handwriting deteriorates, fine-motor coordination is reduced, and complex sensorimotor tasks begin to show impairment. The Romberg "standing steadiness" test reveals marked unsteadiness and increased body sway at a BAC of 30 mg/dl.[4]

At a BAC between 50 and 100 mg/dl, a drinker displays reductions in anxiety, critical judgment, and self-criticism, with enhanced sociability and self-esteem in group situations. Disinhibition, with talkativeness and a feeling of elation, occurs at the same time that mild sedation is produced, along with relaxation, drowsiness, and reduced alertness. Speech, movement, and simple reaction times are

Table 41-3. Correlates of blood alcohol concentration (BAC)

BAC (mg/dl)	Risk of multiple road accidents*	Percentage of persons "drunk"*†	Clinical state‡
50	2:1	15	Delightfully dizzy
100	6-7:1	45	
150	25:1	75	Drunk and disorderly
200	50:1	94	
300	Extremely high	98	Dazed and dejected
400		100	Dead drunk
500		100	Death's door

*Data from AMA Committee on Medicolegal Problems. Alcohol and the Impaired Driver. Chicago, American Medical Association, 1968.
†Percentage of persons exhibiting objective signs of intoxication, (e.g., ataxia, slurred speech, labile mood).
‡Classification modified from Gaddum, J.H. Pharmacology, ed. 5. New York, Oxford University Press, 1968.

slowed. Fear is reduced, and impulsive risk-taking behavior becomes evident. Most performance tasks are unaltered at a BAC of 50 mg/dl, but most are impaired at 100 mg/dl.[3] Sexual motivation may be enhanced at lower BACs through a reduction in anxiety and muscular tension,[4] and maximum penile diameter, in response to visual stimulation, is increased at a BAC of 25 mg/dl, though reduced at levels above 50 mg/dl.[3] In the male beagle, ejaculation is slowed, and ataxia makes intromission difficult at higher concentrations.[4]

At a BAC of 100 to 200 mg/dl, nausea, vomiting, and loss of self-control are common in an inexperienced drinker, whereas the experienced inebriate speaks and moves with exaggerated care.

Subjective time passes more slowly. Speech becomes slurred, and ataxia with staggering gait occurs. A unique positional alcohol nystagmus is produced in which, with the head tilted to the side, the eyes drift slowly upward and then jerk rapidly downward.[3] Alcohol produces deficits in both short- and long-term memory, and retrograde amnesia ("blackouts") may occur. At a BAC of about 150 mg/dl, there is a reduction in the length, though not in the number, of episodes of rapid eye movement (REM) sleep throughout the night, together with reduced movement during sleep.[4] Alcohol increases assertive or aggressive behavior and may precipitate a rage release reaction, especially if the initial mood of the drinker is unpleasant.[3] Significant analgesia is also produced.

In the range of 300 mg/dl ethanol, there may be mydriasis, sweating, hypotension, hypothermia, and loss of consciousness. At a BAC of 400 to 500 mg/dl medullary paralysis and death are likely to occur.

Autonomic nervous system. Acute alcohol administration results in an elevated catecholamine concentration in blood and urine, perhaps as a result of fluidization of membranes in noradrenergic nerve terminals and adrenal chromaffin cells. Adrenal monoamine release is accompanied by compensatory increases in the activity of medullary tyrosine hydroxylase, dopamine-β-hydroxylase (DBH), and phenylethanolamine-N-methyl transferase. Vascular smooth muscle exhibits hyperreactivity to norepinephrine at low ethanol concentrations and hyporeactivity at high concentrations. The latter effect may be caused by ethanol-induced facilitation of neuronal monoamine uptake,[1] because α-adrenergic receptor sensitivity is unaltered by ethanol. β_2-Adrenoceptor activity, however, is lessened by ethanol. Long-term ethanol administration causes an apparent reduction in the number of β_1-adrenoceptors on the heart. In addition, fluidization of cell membrane phospholipid results in blockade of calcium channels with a reduction in cellular calcium influx. This, in turn, reduces basal vascular tone and the contractile response of smooth muscle to endogenous catecholamines.

Cardiovascular system. The direct actions of ethanol on vasomotor tone, coupled with its complex adrenergic effects and centrally mediated influences, produce variable cardiovascular responses. In general, coronary blood flow is slightly enhanced, but there is no concomitant increase in myocardial oxygen uptake. Indeed, myocardial contractility is depressed by ethanol. Direct vasoconstriction has been observed in cerebral and renal vascular beds in vitro, but in vivo the effect of ethanol, occurring only at large doses, is an increase in blood flow to the brain and kidneys.[30] Mesenteric blood flow also appears to be increased.

One of the more consistent cardiovascular effects of alcohol ingestion is cutaneous vasodilation. The increased blood flow to the skin provides a feeling of warmth. In cold environments heat loss may be greatly accentuated, and alcohol is generally to be avoided in treating the hypothermic individual.

The ethanol metabolite acetaldehyde (which causes catecholamine release) produces tachycardia, increased cardiac output, and increased arterial blood pressure in man, all of which are abolished by adrenoceptor blockade. However, the amounts of acetaldehyde normally resulting from ingested ethanol have no cardiovascular effects.

Other effects. Small oral doses of ethanol temporarily enhance both salivary and gastric acid secretion, the increased salivation probably caused by a conditioned reflex. Large doses of alcohol reduce salivation.[3] Alcohol is a gastric irritant, producing inflammation of the stomach wall in concentrations greater than 15%. Ingestion of solutions of over 21% ethanol results in increased gastric mucus secretion and in petechial hemorrhage and ulceration.[38] Alcohol retards gastric emptying and inhibits absorption of glucose, amino acids, folic acid, thiamine, and vitamin B_{12} from the small intestine.[4]

Diuresis occurs as BAC rises, probably as a result of inhibition of the release of antidiuretic hormone from the posterior pituitary gland. Urinary sodium, potassium, and chloride are reduced, whereas magnesium and norepinephrine are increased.[4] Adrenal activation results in increased blood concentrations of corticosteroids, epinephrine, and glucose.

One of the potential salutary effects of ethanol is its influence on lipid metabolism. Intake on the order of one drink before dinner increases the ratio of high-density to low-density lipoproteins in the plasma, an effect inversely correlated with the incidence of coronary heart disease.[40]

Absorption, fate, and excretion

Ethanol is readily absorbed from the stomach and small intestine. The rate of gastric absorption is reduced by about half in the presence of food or fluid in the stomach, with a resultant lowering of peak BAC. Alcohol in the form of beer, which has a high food value, produces a BAC that is only half that produced by an equivalent amount of alcohol in the form of spirits.[11] Higher concentrations of alcohol inhibit absorption, however, and maximum blood concentrations are achieved by ingestion of 20% in water.

About 62% of inspired ethanol vapor is absorbed through the lungs, and intoxication can be achieved by this route. Percutaneous absorption can also occur and has led to death when infants were wrapped in ethanol-soaked cloth to treat hyperthermia.[3]

Ethanol is uniformly distributed throughout the total body water. Therefore, tissue alcohol concentration is proportional to both lean body weight and tissue water content. Considering the BAC as unity, the relative concentration of ethanol is 1.35 in urine, 1.17 in brain, 1.16 in blood plasma, 1.12 in saliva, 0.05 in alveolar air, and 0.02 in fat. The Widmark ratio, which expresses the concentration of ethanol in the whole body with respect to that in the blood, is 0.68 for men and 0.55 for women, a difference resulting from the higher adiposity of women. This ratio can be used to calculate the total body store of alcohol from a known BAC, and vice versa. Table 41-2 illustrates the influence of alcoholic beverage, age, and sex on BAC.

Over 90% of ingested ethanol is metabolized, mostly by a three-phase hepatic oxidation. Initially, ethanol is converted to acetaldehyde by alcohol dehydrogenase, which requires nicotinamide adenine dinucleotide (NAD) as a hydrogen acceptor:

$$CH_3CH_2OH + NAD^+ \rightleftharpoons NADH + H^+ + CH_3CHO$$

The binding of substrate and coenzyme to alcohol dehydrogenase involves sites on the enzyme containing zinc and sulfhydryl groups. Human alcohol dehydrogenase also oxidizes methanol, isopropyl alcohol, and ethylene glycol. This alcohol dehydrogenase reaction is the rate-limiting step in the metabolism of alcohol.

The second phase, conversion of acetaldehyde to acetate, occurs in liver and other tissues and is catalyzed by aldehyde dehydrogenase, which has a much greater affinity for acetaldehyde than does alcohol dehydrogenase:

$$CH_3CHO + NAD^+ + OH^- \rightleftharpoons CH_3CO_2^- + NADH + H^+$$

In the third step, acetate, as acetyl CoA, is further oxidized through the Krebs cycle to carbon dioxide and water.

The excess hydrogen from alcohol oxidation upsets hepatic chemistry and results in reduced gluconeogenesis and enhanced triglyceride and lactate formation.[17] Heavy bouts of drinking can therefore cause hypoglycemia; lactic acidosis; hyperuricemia (since lactate interferes with renal elimination of uric acid), which can precipitate gout; hyperlipemia; and fatty liver.

Two alternate pathways exist for alcohol oxidation. One utilizing catalase and a hydrogen peroxide–generating system, seems to be of little physiologic significance. The second, involving the microsomal enzyme–oxidation system (MEOS), becomes an important factor in alcohol elimination at high BACs,[17] in which it may account for 10% to 25% of ethanol metabolism.

Ethanol elimination follows zero-order kinetics (it is linear with respect to time) down to a BAC of 10 mg/dl, when it becomes first-order. The rate of decline of BAC, in the average human, is 16 mg/dl/hr, equivalent to about two thirds of a fluid ounce of 100 proof whiskey per hour.

About 2% to 8% of absorbed alcohol is excreted unchanged, largely through the lungs and kidneys. Minor amounts are detectable in saliva, tears, sweat, and feces.[3]

Drug interactions

Alcohol produces additive effects with all CNS depressants and potentiates the hypotensive effects of most vasodilators.[8,17] Long-acting drugs, such as diazepam, may cause additive depression with alcohol ingested as long as 24 hours after the drug was given.[19]

The use of alcohol influences the in vivo disposition of many drugs.[19] Short-term alcohol ingestion increases, although long-term alcoholism reduces, the oral absorption rate of diazepam. Alcohol inhibits the absorption and enhances the breakdown of penicillins in the stomach for up to 3 hours after alcohol intake.[16] Aspirin promotes gastric bleeding when combined with alcohol and can cause massive gastric hemorrhage in alcoholics who suffer from alcoholic gastritis.[9]

At high BACs, ethanol, by competing for the MEOS, inhibits the metabolism of, and exhibits supraadditive effects with, CNS depressants.[8,17] For the same reasons, short-term alcohol ingestion may result in exaggerated clinical responses to oral anticoagulants and hypoglycemic agents. Chloral hydrate, which is biotransformed by alcohol dehydrogenase, is markedly potentiated by alcohol.

In the chronic alcoholic without liver damage, continued alcohol intake results in induction of cytochrome P-450 and MEOS activity. Increased enzyme activity appears after about 3 weeks of heavy drinking and lasts 4 to 9 weeks after the cessation of drinking.[19] A significant reduction in plasma half-life of, and clinical response to, many drugs occurs (e.g., intravenous anesthetics, barbiturates, and antianxiety drugs). Enzyme induction may also enhance the toxicity arising from acetaminophen overdose. In long-term alcoholism, however, the development of hepatic damage offsets the effects of enzyme induction, and drug sensitivity may return to normal.[17,26]

General therapeutic uses

Ingestion of moderate amounts of alcohol is of value in improving the mood, appetite, and digestion of convalescent or geriatric patients. Recent studies suggest that it may also help prevent atherosclerosis by virtue of its previously discussed effects on plasma lipids. Alcohol may be used to treat syncope by raising the blood pressure reflexly through irritation of the mouth and throat. Topically applied 70% ethanol is employed as a rubefacient, anhidrotic, and antiseptic and as a means to cool the skin in cases of fever. Ethanol hardens the skin by protein precipitation and is used to prevent decubitus ulcers in bedridden patients. Ethyl alcohol is a solvent for the irritating principle of poison ivy, and its early use on affected skin can markedly reduce resulting dermatitis.

Absolute alcohol has been injected to destroy nerves or ganglia in treating intractable pain arising from conditions such as trigeminal neuralgia and inoperable cancer. Inhalation of ethanol vapor is of value in attacks of acute pulmonary edema, owing to its antifoaming action.

Therapeutic uses and implications for dentistry

The dental uses of ethanol as an antiseptic and disinfectant are discussed in Chapter 43. Alcohol has been employed as a desiccant and cleaning solution for cavity preparations; however, it does produce pain when applied to the unanesthetized pulp. Alcoholic beverages may be employed for sedation. In some patients, a glass of wine may be as effective as another CNS depressant in tablet form and be much more enjoyable. The dentist

administering this or any sedative must, of course, be mindful of drug interactions associated with alcohol.

The dentist can expect to encounter alcoholic patients in everyday practice. Alcoholics usually exhibit signs of deficient oral hygiene, such as coated tongue and heavy plaque and calculus deposits. They have twice the rate of tooth loss of the general population, commonly lack the mandibular and maxillary first molars, and frequently suffer from advanced chronic periodontitis.[34] Chronic asymptomatic enlargement of the parotid, and sometimes submandibular, glands may be observed. The dentist should be aware of the increased incidence of oral leukoplakia in alcoholics and be familiar with its appearance, particularly the erosive form, since 6% of such persons develop carcinoma, especially of the tongue, within 9 years of diagnosis of the lesion. Postoperative healing time is prolonged in alcoholics. This may be related to a marked increase in collagenase activity, which has been observed in the liver of alcoholics.[22]

Alcohol dependence

Abuse characteristics. Alcoholism is similar in all respects to dependence on CNS depressants, except that alcohol produces unique direct neurologic and muscular toxicity. Because alcohol can provide a major source of dietary calories, it also promotes malnutrition in the chronic drinker. Alcohol dependence is characterized by marked psychic and physical dependence, moderate tolerance, and a wide range of pathologic sequelae. Crosstolerance and cross-dependence with other general CNS depressants are observed.

Psychic dependence on alcohol is severe. The alcoholic develops a compulsion to obtain and use the drug to the extent that all other activities become secondary, and deterioration of personal and social concerns ensues. The typical alcoholic is indistinguishable from the average young drinker until his middle to late 20s, when the average drinker tends to decrease alcohol intake. The alcoholic continues to drink heavily, with periodic abstinence; the first major alcohol-related problem will occur at age 28 to 33. Personal, social, and medical problems increase through the 40s until death, usually in the middle 50s.[34] Alcoholism has a partial genetic basis, with a degree of heritability about equal to that of diabetes mellitus.

Tolerance to and physical dependence on ethanol probably depend on a common mechanism, inasmuch as they develop simultaneously and both reach a maximum that is not increased by additional alcohol intake.[5] Apart from the theories of cellular adaptation discussed in Chapter 46, tolerance and dependence may be caused by an adaptive increase in membrane phospholipid rigidity and a reversible resistance to ethanol-induced fluidization of the lipid bilayer.[10] The involvement of such a lipophilic site in the development of tolerance and dependence is corroborated by the observation that the relative severity of withdrawal symptoms from ethanol and tertiary butanol parallel their respective lipid solubilities.[24]

Alcohol abstinence syndrome. The severity of the acute alcohol abstinence syndrome correlates with the amount and duration of preabstinent alcohol intake. The mildest form is the tremulousness and nausea experienced "the morning after," which is readily reversed by "taking a hair of the dog" (i.e., a small amount of alcohol). The most severe abstinence syndrome, delirium tremens, is seen after 1 to 2 weeks of drinking at a level of about 15 quarts of beer, or 50 ounces of liquor, per day.[21] Severe withdrawal symptoms appear 6 to 8 hours after drinking ceases, peak at 48 to 96 hours, and generally resolve in about 2 weeks.[2]

Moderate abstinence results in anorexia, nausea, epigastric upset, tremulousness, sweating, apprehension, and insomnia. In more severe abstinence, additional symptoms of diarrhea, vomiting, nightmares, and agitation occur, together with autonomic signs of tachycardia, hyperpnea, and fever. Frank delirium tremens, if it occurs, is manifested by all the preceding symptoms together with possible psychosis, seizures, and hyperthermia.[2] Psychotic manifestations include muttering, delirium, paranoia, delusions, and auditory, visual, and tactile hallucinations of a threatening nature.[23] The individual usually displays agitation, confusion, disorientation, and panic. The hallucinatory symptoms appear to be a result of excessive rebound REM sleep that, suppressed during the drinking phase, spills over into the waking state during withdrawal.[14] Neuromuscular hyperexcitability is manifested by gross tremors and grand mal convulsions (with a marked sensitivity to stroboscopically induced seizures),[2] both of which correlate with a rapid urinary excretion of magnesium and a resultant hypomagnesemia during withdrawal.[25,39] Autonomic hyperactivity of abstinence leads to hyperthermia and circulatory collapse, the most dangerous aspects of withdrawal.[37]

Pathologic sequelae of alcoholism. Chronic alcoholism is associated with a number of severe physical complications, primarily of the nervous and gastrointestinal systems and of the skeletal and cardiac muscle.[2,9,27] These complications are summarized in Table 41-4.

Changes in the nervous system are related in part to malnutrition, and most respond to thiamine administration. Both central and peripheral nerve degeneration occur, resulting in a wide range of neurologic disorders involving psychologic and personality changes as well as peripheral neuritis, sensory loss, and muscle atrophy.

The inflammatory effects of alcohol on the gastrointestinal tract lead to esophagitis and chronic gastritis frequently associated with intense episodes of vomiting, which may lead to gastric laceration and hematemesis. There is a high correlation between heavy drinking and cancer of the mouth and throat. Peptic ulcers and pancreatitis are common among alcoholics.

Alcoholic liver damage is now regarded as a direct consequence of ethanol toxicity rather than of malnutrition.[18] It is heralded by the appearance of steatosis, or fatty liver, which is a benign and reversible syndrome seen almost universally among heavy drinkers. Hepatomegaly is associated with this early phase of liver disease. About half of the liver enlargement is probably caused by lipid accumulation, with the rest probably caused by intracellular protein that builds up in response to a disruption of the microtubular system. The accumulation of intracellular protein results in water retention and "ballooning" of hepatocytes. The fatty liver phase of liver damage can progress to generalized hepatic inflammation and "florid" alcoholic hepatitis, a condition that has a 10% to 30% mortality rate. In 10% to 15% of heavy drinkers, fatty liver progresses to Laennec's cirrhosis.

Direct toxic effects of alcohol on skeletal muscle may produce acute alcoholic myopathy characterized by muscular cramps, weakness, and swelling, which resolve after a few weeks of alcohol abstinence. In severe cases, extensive muscle degeneration results in myoglobinemia, hyperkalemia, and renal failure. A chronic form of alcoholic myopathy ultimately produces marked muscular atrophy, usually of the pelvic girdle and thighs.

Cardiomyopathy of alcoholism appears to result from the direct toxic effects of ethanol or acetaldehyde on the heart.[33] It is most common in men 25 to 50 years of age who have been long-term

Table 41-4. Pathologic sequelae of alcoholism

System or organ	Syndrome	Cause	Signs and symptoms
Nervous system	Wernicke's syndrome	Malnutrition	Confusion, amnesia, confabulation, peripheral neuropathy, diplopia, nystagmus, tremor, ataxia
	Korsakoff's psychosis	Malnutrition	Disorientation, amnesia, confabulation, peripheral neuritis
	Cerebral atrophy	Malnutrition	Irreversible degeneration of frontal lobe cortical cells with premature senility, dementia, personality disintegration
	Cerebellar atrophy	Malnutrition	Irreversible ataxia
	Peripheral neuropathy	Thiamine deficiency	Diminished tendon reflexes, sensory loss in feet or legs, muscle atrophy
Gastrointestinal tract	Esophagitis and gastritis	Inflammatory effects of alcohol	Heartburn, vomiting, gastric ulceration, hematemesis
	Peptic ulcers	Inflammatory effects of alcohol	Epigastric pain, anorexia, vomiting
	Pancreatitis	Inflammatory effects of alcohol	Weight loss, abdominal pain, blood loss, shock
Liver	Steatosis or fatty liver	Direct toxicity of ethanol	Enlarged liver
	Alcoholic hepatitis	Direct toxicity of ethanol	Anorexia, vomiting, weakness, jaundice, ascites, enlarged spleen and liver
	Laennec's cirrhosis	Direct toxicity of ethanol	Jaundice, portal hypertension, mental deterioration, renal failure, coma
Skeletal muscle	Alcoholic myopathy	Direct toxicity of ethanol	Cramping, weakness, edema, and atrophy of muscle
Cardiac muscle	Cardiomyopathy	Direct toxicity of ethanol or acetaldehyde	Weakness, shortness of breath, congestive heart failure, pulmonary congestion
Fetus	Fetal alcohol syndrome	Direct toxicity of ethanol	Microcephaly, reduced IQ, facial, cardiac, and genital defects

heavy users of alcohol. The myocardium reveals degenerative changes, and the early clinical signs include fatigue, weakness, dyspnea on exertion, sinus tachycardia, and palpitations. The disease progresses to cardiomegaly and frank congestive heart failure with ventricular arrhythmias and pulmonary congestion. The injury is irreversible in these later states. Treatment is the same as for other types of congestive heart failure, coupled with prolonged bed rest and permanent abstinence from alcohol.

The fetal alcohol syndrome (FAS) is a cluster of physical and mental defects occurring in children of women who consume alcohol during pregnancy. In over 90% of cases of FAS there is growth deficiency, microcephaly, and short palpebral fissures.[22] Fine motor dysfunction and midfacial hypoplasia are common, and about one half of cases exhibit epicanthic folds and cardiac defects. The degree of dysmorphogenesis correlates with mental deficiency, with mean IQs ranging from 82 down to 55.[9] Neither the dysmorphic nor intellectual aspects of the syndrome improve with age. The biochemical basis of FAS appears to result from the low fetal hepatic alcohol dehydrogenase activity, which in the 2-month fetus is only 3% to 4% of adult activity. Pregnant patients should be advised to avoid alcoholic beverages and to be aware of the alcoholic content of food and drugs.[36]

Treatment of alcoholism. The treatment of alcoholism involves the detoxification of the acutely intoxicated individual, medication to prevent severe symptoms of abstinence, and long-term rehabilitation.[27] To a large extent, the rate of detoxification will be determined by the rate at which the liver disposes of the alcohol, but the nature of the withdrawal period also depends on the environment, the nutritional status of the patient, and the medical personnel supervising the withdrawal. The symptoms associated with abstinence are usually treated with a long-acting benzodiazepine (e.g., chlordiazepoxide or diazepam), but phenobarbital, paraldehyde, and other drugs have been employed. Supplemental dietary thiamine, magnesium, and potassium are given.

Disulfiram (Antabuse) is employed in avoidance therapy for alcoholics.[35] The drug inhibits aldehyde dehydrogenase through the formation of a covalent disulfide bond between an enzymic thiol group and the drug. Disulfiram also inhibits other enzymes, notably DBH and oxidases of the microsomal enzyme system.

Oral doses of 250 mg per day have an onset of action of about 12 hours, and the effects are evident for up to a week after treatment is stopped. The protracted duration of action is based on the irreversible nature of disulfiram binding. Only with the synthesis of new enzyme does the metabolism of alcohol return to normal. Disulfiram itself commonly causes drowsiness and in daily doses in excess of 500 mg may cause paresthesias and muscle weakness. It may exaggerate schizophrenia or depression, possibly through alteration of central monoamine concentrations caused by the inhibition of DBH.

If alcohol is ingested during disulfiram treatment, the individual experiences symptoms of acetaldehyde poisoning.[35] Drinking 1.2 oz of 80 proof liquor causes flushing, tachycardia, palpitations, and tachypnea, all lasting about 30 minutes. Ingestion of more than 1.6 oz of 80 proof liquor produces intense palpitations and dyspnea, nausea, vomiting, and headache lasting up to 90 minutes. Unconsciousness, hypotensive shock, and sudden myocardial infarction may occur. For this reason, the drug must be employed only under strict medical supervision.

Disulfiram will inhibit oxidative biotransformation of diazepam, but not the conjugation of oxazepam or lorazepam.[35] Hypotensive episodes may occur during general anesthesia as a result of DBH inhibition and depletion of neuronal norepinephrine. However, even 500 mg per day of disulfiram fails to alter the cardiovascular response to pressor amines either of the direct- or indirect-acting variety.[31] Paraldehyde, because of its metabolic conversion to acetaldehyde, will produce toxic reactions in patients taking disulfiram.

METHYL ALCOHOL

Methyl alcohol is widely employed as an industrial solvent, as a denaturing agent for ethanol, and in "canned heat." Poisoning occurs when substances containing methanol are used as beverages in place of licit alcohol or when industrial workers are exposed to atmospheres containing methanol vapor.[7]

The metabolism of methanol involves the same enzyme systems as that of ethanol. Its elimination follows zero-order kinetics, but at a much slower rate than ethyl alcohol. This accounts for the delay in symptoms of methanol poisoning, which are caused by its oxidized metabolites, formaldehyde and formic acid.

Symptoms of methanol poisoning include early mild inebriation followed in 6 to 30 hours by dizziness, headache, vertigo, and occasional nausea and vomiting. As acidosis is produced by the accumulation of formic acid, extreme abdominal pain develops, respirations increase in depth and frequency, and the patient lapses into coma.[6] Visual symptoms are characteristic of methanol intoxication. Blurred vision, with spots or gray mist, photophobia, and eye tenderness commonly occur. The pupils are dilated, and the light reflex becomes sluggish. Permanent blindness is not uncommon even if the victim recovers completely otherwise. Visual damage develops because of the high rate of retinal oxidation of methanol, leading to formaldehyde accumulation with edema and permanent damage to ganglion cells.[7]

Death follows ingestion of 2 to 8 fluid ounces of methanol and is associated with blood concentrations of 74 to 110 mg/dl methanol and 9 to 68 mg/dl formic acid.[7] Urinary methanol concentration is about twice that in blood and is diagnostic of methyl alcohol poisoning.[6] The direct cause of death is cessation of respiration.[13] Breathing becomes shallow and slow, tonic seizures develop, and the victim dies with a marked terminal inspiratory gasp.

The treatment of choice is hemodialysis,[15] which provides rapid recovery without residual effects. Peritoneal dialysis, though also indicated, is less efficient. Acidosis is treated with intravenous infusions of sodium bicarbonate solution. Because ethanol is oxidized in vivo preferentially to methyl alcohol, the administration of ethyl alcohol inhibits the formation of toxic methanol metabolites. Therefore, ethyl alcohol should be administered intravenously or given orally to maintain a BAC of 100 mg/dl.

ISOPROPYL ALCOHOL

Isopropyl alcohol is employed as an antiseptic and disinfectant in dentistry. In a concentration of 70%, it is used as rubbing alcohol, and it is present in many hand lotions. Isopropyl alcohol is oxidized in vivo to acetone, which is largely excreted in expired air at about 10 times the rate of the alcohol itself.[7]

Toxicity arises from the use of isopropanol as a beverage. Symptoms are similar to those of ethanol intoxication but are marked by nausea, vomiting, abdominal pain, hematemesis, and melena. Severe renal dysfunction for 2 to 3 weeks is seen in survivors. Extensive hemorrhagic inflammation and edema of the bronchopulmonary tree are observed in fatal cases. Hemodialysis is the treatment of choice in isopropanol poisoning.[7] Ethanol appears to increase, rather than reduce, the toxic effects of isopropanol.[29]

CITED REFERENCES

1. Altura, B.M., Ogunkoya, A., Gebrewold, A., and Altura, B.T. Effects of ethanol on terminal arterioles and muscular venules: direct observations on the microcirculation. Journal of Cardiovascular Pharmacology **1**:97-113, 1979.
2. Aston, R. Characteristics of drug dependence to barbiturates, alcohol, and tranquilizers. In Mulé, S.J., and Brill, H., eds. Chemical and Biological Aspects of Drug Dependence. Cleveland, Chemical Rubber Company Press, 1972.
3. Barry, H. Alcohol. In Pradhan, S.N., and Dutta, S.N., eds. Drug Abuse: Clinical and Basic Aspects. St. Louis, The C.V. Mosby Co., 1977.
4. Brodie, H.K.H. The effects of ethyl alcohol in man. In National Commission on Marihuana and Drug Abuse, Second Report. Drug Use in America: Problems in Perspective, vol. 1. Washington, D.C., U.S. Government Printing Office, 1973.
5. Cicero, T.J. Tolerance to and physical dependence on alcohol: behavioral and neurobiological mechanisms. In Lipton, M.A., DiMascio, A., and Killam, K.F., eds. Psychopharmacology: A Generation of Progress. New York, Raven Press, 1978.
6. Closs, K., and Solberg, C.O. Methanol poisoning. Journal of the American Medical Association **211**:497-499, 1970.
7. Couri, D., and Nachtman, J.P. Toxicology of alcohols, ketones, and esters—inhalation. NIDA Research Monograph 15. Washington D.C., Department of Health, Education, and Welfare, 1977.
8. Dutta, S.N. Drug interactions in abusers. In Pradhan, S.N., and Dutta, S.N., eds. Drug Abuse: Clinical and Basic Aspects. St. Louis, The C.V. Mosby Co., 1977.
9. Eckardt, M.J., Harford, T.C., Kaebler, C.T., Parker, E.S., Rosenthal, L.S., Ryback, R.S., Salmoiraghi, G.C., Vanderveen, E., and Warren, K.R. Health hazards associated with alcohol consumption. Journal of the American Medical Association **246**:648-666, 1981.
10. Goldstein, D.B., and Chin, J.H. Interaction of ethanol with biological membranes. Federation Proceedings **40**:2073-2076, 1981.
11. Haggard, H.W., Greenberg, L.A., and Lolli, G. The absorption of alcohol with special reference to its influence on the concentration of alcohol appearing in the blood. Quarterly Journal of Studies on Alcohol **1**:684-726, 1941.
12. Hunt, W.A. Neurotransmitter function in the basal ganglia after acute and chronic ethanol treatment. Federation Proceedings **40**:2077-2081, 1981.
13. Hussey, H.H. Methanol poisoning. Journal of the American Medical Association **229**:1335-1336, 1974.
14. Johnson, L.C., Burdick, J.A., and Smith, J. Sleep during alcohol intake and withdrawal in the chronic alcoholic. Archives of General Psychiatry **22**:406-418, 1970.
15. Keyvan-Larijarni, H., and Tannenberg, A.M. Methanol intoxication: comparison of peritoneal dialysis and hemodialysis treatment. Archives of Internal Medicine **134**:293-296, 1974.
16. Kitto, W. Antibiotics and the ingestion of alcohol. Journal of the American Medical Association **193**:411, 1965.
17. Lieber, C.S. The metabolism of alcohol. Scientific American **234**:25-33, 1976.
18. Lieber, C.S. Pathogenesis and early diagnosis of alcoholic liver injury. New England Journal of Medicine **298**:888-893, 1978.
19. Linnoila, M., Mattila, M.J., and Kitchell, B.S. Drug interactions with alcohol. Drugs **18**:299-311, 1979.
20. Mardones, J. The alcohols. In Root, W.S., and Hofmann, F.G., eds. Physiological Pharmacology, vol. 1. New York, Academic Press, Inc., 1963.
21. Marjot, D.H. The length of the drinking bout preceding alcohol withdrawal states. British Journal of Addiction **64**:307-313, 1970.
22. Maruyama, K., Feinman, L., Fainsilber, Z., Nakano, M., Okazaki, I., and Leiber, C.S. Mammalian collagenase increases in early alcoholic liver disease and decreases with cirrhosis. Life Sciences **30**:1379-1384, 1982.
23. Marvin, T.R. Acute alcoholic withdrawal syndrome. Minnesota Medicine **53**:999-1003, 1970.
24. McComb, J.A., and Goldstein, D.B. Quantitative comparison of physical dependence on tertiary butanol and ethanol in mice: correlation with lipid solubility. Journal of Pharmacology and Experimental Therapeutics **208**:113-117, 1979.
25. Mendelson, J.H., Ogata, M., and Mello, N.K. Effects of alcohol ingestion and withdrawal on magnesium states of alcoholics: clinical experimental findings. Annals of the New York Academy of Sciences **162**:918-933, 1969.
26. Mezey, E. Ethanol metabolism and ethanol-drug interactions. Biochemical Pharmacology **25**:869-875, 1976.
27. Moore, R.A. Dependence on alcohol. In Pradhan, S.N., and Dutta, S.N., eds. Drug Abuse: Clinical and Basic Aspects, St. Louis, The C.V. Mosby Co., 1977.
28. Myers, R.D., and Melchior, C.L. Alcohol drinking: abnormal intake caused by tetrahydropapaveroline in brain. Science **196**:554-556, 1977.
29. Peterson, D.I., Peterson, J.E., and Hardinge, M.G. Protection by ethanol against the toxic effects of monofluoroethanol and monochloroethanol. Journal of Pharmacy and Pharmacology **20**:465-468, 1968.
30. Ritchie, J.M. The aliphatic alcohols. In Gilman, A.G., Goodman, L.S., and Gilman, A., eds. Goodman and Gilman's The Pharmacological Basis of Therapeutics, ed. 6. New York, Macmillan, Inc., 1980.
31. Rogers, W.K., Benowitz, N.L., Wilson, K.M., and Abbott, J.A. Effect of disulfiram on adrenergic function. Clinical Pharmacology and Therapeutics **25**:469-477, 1979.
32. Rubin, E., and Rottenberg, H. Ethanol-induced injury and

adaptation in biological membranes. Federation Proceedings **41:**2465-2471, 1982.

33. Sanders, M.G. Alcoholic cardiomyopathy: a critical review. Quarterly Journal of Studies on Alcohol **31:**324-368, 1970.
34. Schuckit, M.A. Overview of alcoholism. Journal of the American Dental Association **99:**489-493, 1979.
35. Sellers, E.M., Naranjo, C.A., and Peachey, J.E. Drug Therapy: Drugs to decrease alcohol ingestion. New England Journal of Medicine **305:**1255-1262, 1981.
36. Surgeon General's advisory on alcohol and pregnancy. F.D.A. Drug Bulletin **11:**9-10, 1981.
37. Victor, M. The alcohol withdrawal syndrome: theory and practice. Postgraduate Medicine **47:**68-72, 1970.
38. Williams, A.W. Effects of alcohol on gastric mucosa. British Medical Journal **1:**256-259, 1956.
39. Wolfe, S.M., and Victor, M. The relationship of hypomagnesemia and alkalosis to alcohol withdrawal symptoms. Annals of the New York Academy of Sciences **162:**973-984, 1969.
40. Yano, K., Rhoads, G.G., and Kagan, A. Coffee, alcohol and risk of coronary heart disease among Japanese men living in Hawaii. New England Journal of Medicine **297:**405-409, 1977.

GENERAL REFERENCES

Eneanya, D.I., Bianchine, J.R., Duran, D.O., and Andresen, B.D. The actions and metabolic fate of disulfiram. Annual Review of Pharmacology and Toxicology **21:**575-596, 1981.

Hawkins, R.D., and Kalant, H. The metabolism of ethanol and its metabolic effects. Pharmacology Reviews **24:**67-157, 1972.

Israelstam, S., and Lambert, F., eds. Alcohol, Drugs, and Traffic Safety. Toronto, Addiction Research Foundation of Ontario, 1975.

Kissin, B., and Begleiter, H., eds. The Biology of Alcoholism. Biochemistry, vol. 1. New York, Plenum Press, 1971.

Kissin, B., and Begleiter, H., eds. The Biology of Alcoholism. Clinical Pathology, vol. 3. New York, Plenum Press, 1974.

Kricka, L.J., and Clark, P.M. Biochemistry of Alcohol and Alcoholism. New York, Halsted Press, 1979.

Mello, N.K., and Mendelson, J.H. Alcohol and human behavior. In Iversen, L.L., Iversen, S.D., and Snyder, S.H., eds. Drugs of Abuse. Handbook of Psychopharmacology, vol. 12. New York, Plenum Press, 1978.

National Institute on Alcohol Abuse and Alcoholism. First Special Report to the United States Congress on Alcohol and Health. Washington, D.C., Department of Health, Education, and Welfare, 1971.

National Institute on Alcohol Abuse and Alcoholism. Second Special Report to the United States Congress on Alcohol and Health. Washington, D.C., Department of Health, Education, and Welfare, 1974.

Pirola, R.C. Drug Metabolism and Alcohol. Baltimore, University Park Press, 1978.

Symposium: Cardiovascular effects of alcohol and alcoholism. Federation Proceedings **41:**2437-2464, 1982.

42 Anticaries and antiplaque agents

Harold R. Englander

Odontolysis (dental caries, cavitation) results from an infection that attacks and destroys the crowns of teeth in persons of all ages and may even affect root surfaces in adults with gingival recession. During the last decade, there has been evidence of declining caries prevalence rates in the United States and Western Europe, but in areas without adequate fluoridation, fewer than five persons in 100 escape the disease. Statistics on the incidence of dental decay, extractions of carious teeth, and costs of restorations and prosthetic replacements are staggering. The total annual amount spent by Americans for dental care has surpassed $12 billion. Even so, Americans have accumulated at least a billion untreated cavities. Although dental restorations halt the progression of active carious lesions, they do little to prevent new ones. Within the next 20 years it is anticipated that an improper distribution of dentists throughout the century will make it impossible to manage the rapidly accumulating restorative needs of our population. Because of the ever-widening gap between the need and the provision of dental care, effective therapeutic approaches need to be developed to prevent dental caries infections. If, by such means, the number of new carious lesions could be reduced significantly and economically, the oral health needs of our nation could be met by only moderate shifts in dental manpower.

The scientific literature on dental caries is voluminous. There has been much controversy regarding its causes, partly because some researchers have not considered the many factors leading to odontolysis. Nonetheless, sufficient knowledge and insights do exist to provide a basis for practical and highly effective programs of prevention and control.

The principal purposes of this chapter are to (1) outline the salient etiologic features associated with odontolysis, (2) discuss the rationale for prophylactic and therapeutic measures, and (3) suggest or prescribe several promising anticaries agents and their regimens of application that can be used in the home and in schools and dental offices under the supervision of dentists and auxiliaries.

ETIOLOGY OF DENTAL CARIES

Odontolysis results from biologic interactions of microflora colonizing on the teeth (commonly called plaque), dietary carbohydrates, and anatomical characteristics and biochemical properties of the teeth. These factors may also be modified by a person's physiologic and behavioral characteristics, and such modification even occurs in experimental animals. Figure 42-1 depicts the interrelationship of these three factors. Activity of infection and severity of cavitation are affected by subfactors within each factor that can vary greatly. Scientists have found from numerous laboratory studies with experimental animals that certain conditions must exist before odontolysis will develop and progress. There is no reason to assume that human conditions are less complex.

Microbial pathogens

Carious lesions will not form unless bacteria contact tooth surfaces. Although it has been established that acidogenic bacteria are necessary for the formation of these lesions, experiments have shown that not all oral acidogenic bacteria are associated with caries, that not all carbohydrates are caries-conducive, and that proteolytic bacteria are not necessarily involved in the caries process.

Emphasis has been placed on the lactobacilli[37] as the primary causative agents of dental caries because they are both highly acidogenic and aciduric; that is, they produce acidic metabolites (e.g., lactic acid) and are able to tolerate an acid envi-

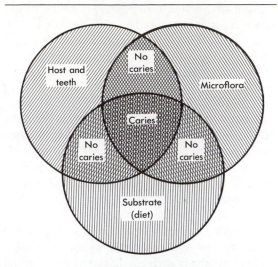

Figure 42-1. Etiology of dental caries. The overlapping circles depict the relationships among the three factors leading to dental caries. The many variables in each parameter make an assessment of its total contribution difficult. All three factors must be active to produce an infection; however, when there is no infection, it is often difficult to know whether one factor is solely responsible. (From Keyes, P.H. International Dental Journal **12**:443-464, 1962.)

ronment well. Lactobacilli tend to increase in dental plaques before the clinical appearance of caries, and they usually can be isolated from various depths of carious lesions. Indeed, so much importance has been attached to their role that tests of caries activity have been based on the lactobacillus count in spittle. Although their role is not fully understood, it seems likely that they are more than innocent bystanders in the caries process.

Seventy-five years ago it was thought that dental caries was a nonspecific disease caused by numerous species of acidogenic microorganisms.[32] However, evidence has increasingly shown that streptococci are a primary cause of odontolysis, particularly on smooth coronal surfaces of the teeth. Streptococci were initially connected with dental caries because (1) they were found in the vanguard of the advancing lesion and have been isolated from inflamed pulpal tissue beneath carious dentin, (2) they were shown to be the predominant forms of bacteria in plaque covering incipient carious lesions and in the early stages of dentinal invasion before gross cavitation of the enamel, (3) gram-positive cocci were observed invading carious enamel in histologic sections of human teeth, and (4) caries-like lesions were produced in extracted human teeth that had been incubated in liquid culture media containing carbohydrates and streptococci.

Ever since *Streptococcus mutans* was isolated from human carious lesions by Clarke[7] in 1924, accumulated evidence has incriminated it as a specific odontopathogen for caries of the enamel, particularly that occurring on smooth enamel surfaces of the teeth. Much of this information has been derived from experiments with rats, hamsters, and monkeys. For instance, Syrian hamsters that are infected with hamster or human strains of *S. mutans* and fed a diet high in sucrose accumulate dental plaque on their molar surfaces within 7 to 10 days, and within 30 to 50 days dental caries has destroyed the crowns.[16] Studies with monoinfected gnotobiotic rats have shown that dental caries follows inoculations with strains of *S. mutans* originally isolated from human carious lesions.[22] In summary, overwhelming evidence has accumulated implicating *S. mutans* as an important odontopathogen fulfilling Koch's postulates.

Within the past 20 years, work with hamsters and rats has linked the acidogenic filament-forming actinomyces with root surface lesions that are initiated in cementum after gingival recession has occurred. Human actinomycotic strains (e.g., *A. naeslundi* and *A. viscosus*) form dense, tenacious plaques at gingival margins and on root surfaces when animals consume fine-particle diets high in sucrose, glucose, or starch.[22,25] These gram-positive filaments have also been found invading the root surfaces of human teeth, and their prevalence in cervicoradicular plaques associated with destructive periodontitis and root surface cavitation is convincing circumstantial evidence of their importance in the etiology of root caries. The widespread occurrence and distribution of root lesions and periodontal disease throughout the world today[39,43] and in the teeth of ancient human skulls discovered in Great Britain indicate that actinomycotic infections have caused more dental disease than have streptococci.

Microbial products

The acidogenic properties of bacteria in dental caries have been emphasized, but acidogenesis is only part of the story. Laboratory studies have shown that dental caries does not always occur in experimental animals, even though they may harbor many types of acid-producing organisms. The acid by-products of microorganisms that do not colonize and form adhesive masses on the teeth are probably relatively harmless to enamel because the acids are dispersed and neutralized in the saliva.

Why then are strains of *S. mutans* cariogenic? The answer appears to lie in their ability to form adhesive extracellular gums in addition to acid after they are exposed to sucrose. These streptococci secrete an enzyme, dextransucrase (a glucosyl transferase), that is capable of promoting the polymerization of sucrose to yield high molecular weight, dextran-like, sticky polysaccharides called *polyglucans* or *mutans*. It is these extracellular polysaccharides that allow the cells of this streptococcal species to adhere to one another and to colonize and attach to the smooth surfaces of teeth.[23]

Plaque. Dental plaque generally consists of a variety of microbes in an intermicrobial dextranoid matrix that clings to tooth surfaces. Its color varies from white to yellowish gray. Plaque has been referred to by a variety of names, including bacterial plaque, gelatinous plaque, microcosm, oral debris, sordes, and zooglea (living glue). To a varying degree, plaque harbors a multitude of streptococci, including *S. mutans, S. sanguis,* and *S. salivarius,* a variety of lactobacilli, *Actinomyces* and related genera, spirochetes together with a constellation of other motile microbes, *Bacteroides melaninogenicus,* and a variety of additional gram-positive and gram-negative bacteria.[36] Many of these microorganisms are capable of producing acids. Plaque also contains salivary mucin, epithelial cells, biochemical constituents derived from saliva, and dissolved food residues. Greater quantities of plaque tend to accumulate on the sheltered, less accessible enamel surfaces, and rinsing with water alone usually will not dislodge it. It is particularly difficult to remove plaque from pits and fissures. As the microorganisms multiply and more polyglucan is produced, the mass of plaque quickly increases, and in a few days the mass becomes more noxious to the tooth and supporting structures.

Acids. The enzyme systems of acid-producing microorganisms in plaque are capable of producing large quantities of lactic and other organic acids by the fermentation of certain types of residual carbohydrates of dietary origin. Lactic acid, however, is the predominant acid produced by the anaerobic metabolic activity of cariogenic microorganisms, and repeated attacks of this acid on tooth substance lead to disintegration (demineralization) of the inorganic elements of the enamel surface and eventually to cavitation.

Normally, before eating, the pH of the plaque on tooth surfaces exposed to saliva is close to neutrality (pH 6.5 to 7.0). Acid is formed in plaque soon after foods containing high concentrations of glucose, sucrose, or other readily fermentable carbohydrates are eaten. The greatest concentration of acid (lowest pH) occurs in about 5 to 15 minutes. The rate of acid production depends on the characteristics and number of acidogenic microorganisms and on the concentration, chemical structure, and physical form of the carbohydrate ingested. A pH of 5.5 or below is considered harmful because the enamel and dentin begin to demineralize at this level of acidity.[42] The acid may be dissipated by the buffering and washing action of saliva, but too often this does not happen before irreversible etching of the tooth surfaces has occurred. Dental plaque tends to act as a diffusion barrier and to nullify the protective effect of saliva. When sufficient acids are produced in plaque, the tooth will be damaged because the hydrogen ion combines with the phosphate that has been incorporated in its crystalline hydroxyapatite mineral to form soluble phosphate salts.[11] Simultaneously, the lactate anion promotes demineralization by sequestering the calcium in hydroxyapatite.

Dietary substrates and nutrition

For decades there has been convincing evidence that dental caries cannot be initiated unless carbohydrate residues are available for metabolism by acidogenic microorganisms on the teeth. The relationship between consumption of refined carbohydrates and caries activity is no longer questioned.

Coronal caries that develops on the enamel surfaces of teeth is essentially a disease of modern origin; historically, its prevalence paralleled the introduction of sucrose into the Western world. Indeed, evidence of highly active lesions has seldom been found in ancient human remains, in persons living under primitive conditions, or in those who ingest natural, unrefined foodstuffs. Root surface caries, however, has been observed frequently in primitive people subsisting on diets high in certain types of starchy foods and may be the only kind of lesions seen. These lesions are associated with gingival recession and destructive periodontal disease. Increased coronal caries is observed frequently in persons who change from a diet of meat, fish, milk, fruits, and coarser cereals to one that includes substantial amounts of highly refined cereals, sugars, and other processed foods containing readily fermentable carbohydrates.

Often, individuals with inadequate or near starvation diets do not have dental caries because the caries-inducing microorganisms are deprived of sufficient caries-conducive substrates. This phenomenon has been seen in western Europe and in prisoners of war during World War II,[44] in children in war-torn or occupied countries, in famine areas of India, in protein-deficient natives of Nigeria, and in other underdeveloped countries where malnutrition is common. Little or no coronal caries occurs in Polynesians and New Guineans, but periodontal disease and root surface lesions (senile caries) are found in almost all older members of these populations. On the other hand, in some of the Scandinavian countries dental caries is not only highly prevalent but often severe. Reports have suggested that the high per capita ingestion of sugar is responsible for this elevated caries rate.

From a variety of experiments with animals, in vitro tests involving the growth of microbial plaque on nichrome wires, and studies in which plaque growth has been observed in humans, the following insights have emerged.

1. Animals can have diets containing adequate amounts of nutrients for normal growth, development, systemic health, and satisfactory reproduction and yet experience cavitation.

2. Diets differ widely in their cariogenic potential. Some favor lesions that are initiated in pits and fissures, others favor activity on smooth surfaces, and still others favor cemental changes. There can also be mixed activity with certain dietary and microbial combinations.

3. The quantity of food eaten, its texture and physical consistency, the concentration of carbohydrate in the diet, and the frequency of eating all affect the activity of odontolysis.

4. Negligible caries develops if watery diets are consumed or if they are intubated directly into the stomach.

5. The chemical structure of the carbohydrates consumed is also important. Caries is less active when substrates consisting of monosaccharides (glucose, fructose, and lactose) are substituted for sucrose.

6. In hamsters, plaque virtually disappears and existing carious lesions in enamel and dentin turn black and become arrested when sucrose in the diet is replaced by glucose, fructose, sorbitol, or starch.

7. Luxuriant, plaque-like growths quickly form on nichrome wires that are incubated in broth cultures of *S. mutans* containing sucrose, but they are not prone to form with monosaccharides or starch.

8. Frequent ingestion of sucrose promotes the rapid growth of plaque on the teeth of persons who abstain from toothbrushing. The plaque resembles the growth of microcolonies of *S. mutans* seen on agar culture. This phemonenon does not occur with the consumption of only glucose or starch.

9. Persons who are born with a condition known as hereditary fructose intolerance and must avoid foods containing sucrose are not prone to plaque formation and do not experience smooth surface caries.

Although acid production by strains of *S. mutans* may not be changed appreciably when sucrose is replaced as the carbohydrate substrate by monosaccharides and starches, there is less tendency toward plaque formation. As a result, the acid produced is not concentrated on tooth surfaces but is dispersed rapidly in the mouth and swallowed or neutralized. In addition, the number of *S. mutans* recovered from the teeth declines precipitously when sucrose is withdrawn from the diet.

In Sweden, Finland, and the United States, the sugar alcohols (xylitol, sorbitol, and mannitol) are being used to replace sucrose.[40] Animal studies have indicated that very little plaque and no caries develop as a result of diets containing these substances. Furthermore, the results of human studies have shown that bacterial fermentation of these substances occurs slowly and that the high terminal acidities in plaque associated with sucrose are prevented (Figure 42-2).

Frequent consumption of sugar, especially between meals, is associated with increased dental caries activity. Studies have shown that dental caries activity in the primary dentition is directly related to the frequency of between-meal eating of foods with high sugar content.[45] Caries activity has also been shown to increase when sugar is consumed in caramels, taffy, or other sticky forms, compared with ingestion of sugar solutions that are rapidly cleared from the teeth and mouth.[17] These findings are confirmed by results obtained with experimental animals.

Host factors

Few host factors have been identified that affect caries activity. It has never been shown, for example, that caries-free persons exhibit higher serum, saliva, and plaque antibodies against *S. mutans*, lactobacilli, or other acidogens than do persons who are caries prone. The possibility of developing and perfecting an effective and acceptable anticaries and antiplaque vaccine within the

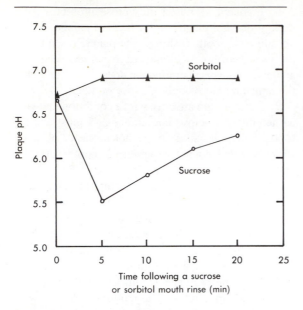

Figure 42-2. Plaque acidity (pH) in a typical caries-active person given a 1-minute sucrose and later a sorbitol mouth rinse. The pH values were measured before and at 5, 10, 15, and 20 minutes after the mouth had been rinsed for 1 minute. There was a precipitous drop in plaque pH after the sucrose rinse, whereas no acid was produced when the mouth had been rinsed with the nonfermentable sugar substitute sorbitol. If anything, the pH increased slightly after sorbitol because the sweet taste stimulated salivary flow and buffering action.

next 20 years is remote because such a polyvalent vaccine would have to be active against numerous strains of streptococci, actinomyces, and lactobacilli. Moreover, the antigenic properties of all microorganisms associated with dental caries have not been identified and characterized sufficiently as yet, and the practicability of producing secretory antibodies by injecting vaccines around or into human salivary glands can also be questioned.

Large differences in the rate of saliva flow have not been associated clearly with increased caries susceptibility in normal individuals because there is usually more than a sufficient amount of secretion to satisfy normal buffering and washing needs. In xerostomic persons suffering from Sjögren's syndrome and in those whose salivary glands have been destroyed by radiation therapy, however, there is little or no secretion from the salivary glands; therefore, only the tooth, and not the saliva, is able to neutralize the acids formed in plaque, and caries is prevalent. The shape or arrangement of the teeth may influence slightly the distribution of lesions in

infected persons, because crowded, malaligned teeth may favor microbial and food retention. It should be emphasized that calcium cannot be withdrawn from the enamel of fully formed teeth via the bloodstream. Endocrine disturbances, diseases affecting blood and bone metabolism, vitamin D deficiency, and pregnancy cannot directly mobilize mineral from erupted teeth to cause an increase in dental caries. Any increase in caries activity that may occur during pregnancy results from a change to undesirable eating patterns rather than from absorption of calcium from the teeth by dental pulp or saliva.

EFFECTS OF FLUORIDE

The anticaries effect of fluoride present in enamel is one host factor that is impressive and widely recognized. The discovery of the relationship between fluoride salts occurring naturally in drinking water and resistance to dental caries was an important advance in preventive dentistry. Persons who from birth regularly consume water containing approximately 1 part per million (ppm) or more of fluoride develop about 60% fewer cavities than those who do not. Studies that disclosed the benefits of fluoride began with surveys in communities where an enamel defect, enamel fluorosis (mottled enamel), was endemic. It was observed that although mottled teeth might be discolored and were sometimes structurally defective, they were far less susceptible to tooth decay. Mottling of the teeth such that appearance is impaired, however, was not prevalent unless the water contained more than 2 ppm fluoride and did not occur in persons who consumed high levels of waterborne fluoride after their teeth had been formed completely. Enamel fluorosis is not caused by the posteruptive topical effect of fluoride but by its effect on ameloblasts as they produce enamel.

Fluoridated water supplies

Numerous studies on child and adult populations consistently have shown the anticaries benefits and the safety of 0.7 to 1 ppm fluoride administered in communal water.[30] In warmer climates, slightly less than 1 ppm fluoride can provide the same amount of protection because more water is consumed. Important protection is conferred on the pits and fissures, but the smooth coronal surfaces of the teeth, especially in the anterior part of the mouth, receive even greater protection. Fluoride in low concentrations in drinking water exerts its

Table 42-1. Distribution of dental caries; experience of 1878 adolescents according to mean numbers of tooth surface sites

	Mean ± SE of total DMFS*	Proximal surfaces	Occlusal surfaces	Buccolingual surfaces	Anterior surfaces
Boston, Mass. (fluoride-deficient)	13.96 ± 0.59	3.52	6.92	3.52	1.12
Danvers, Mass. (fluoridated)†	8.60 ± 0.43	1.55	4.76	2.29	0.26
Mecklenburg County, N.C. (fluoride-deficient)	7.20 ± 0.54	1.28	4.08	1.84	0.31
Kalamazoo, Mich. (fluoridated)	5.12 ± 0.27	0.69	3.11	1.32	0.13
Stickney, Ill., (fluoridated)	4.51 ± 0.29	0.70	2.65	1.16	0.15
Charlotte, N.C. (fluoridated)	4.41 ± 0.32	0.42	2.74	1.25	0.08
Midland, Tex. (5 to 7 ppm fluoride)	2.40 ± 0.21	0.31	1.2	0.83	0.04

From Englander, H.R., and DePaola, P.F. Enhanced anticaries action from drinking water containing 5 ppm fluoride. Journal of the American Dental Association **98**:35-39, 1979.

*Proximal, occlusal, and buccolingual tooth surfaces; DMFS = decayed, missing, filled surfaces.

†Analysis of water showed 0.67 ppm fluoride.

NOTE; The mean difference between each fluoridated city versus Boston and between Midland versus every city is statistically significant (P < 0.01).

greatest anticaries effect when it can act both before and after eruption. When it acts after mineralization but before the eruption of the teeth, the pits and fissures are not protected, but the smooth surfaces become somewhat less vulnerable to cavitation. When the action is entirely posteruptive, the benefits are even less. Whereas the effect of fluoride in drinking water persists into adulthood, the effect is less for adults who consumed fluoridated water only during the first 8 years of life, that is, during tooth formation and mineralization.

The continuing beneficial effect of waterborne fluoride has been assessed from dental examinations conducted on almost 2000 adolescents, aged 12 to 15 years, living in seven cities in five states.[10] Important anticaries benefits were derived from water fluoridation at 1 ppm fluoride. Those exposed to water containing 5 to 7 ppm of naturally occurring fluoride experienced even more protection. A breakdown of the caries experienced by the kind of surface site attacked revealed an important and consistent anticaries effect of waterborne fluoride on all surfaces recorded (Table 42-1). Although the greatest anticaries effect was observed on proximal surfaces, a slightly smaller but still significant protective effect could be observed on occlusal and buccolingual surfaces. For example, when the mean DMFS (decayed, missing, filled surfaces) scores for children in Midland, Texas, with 5 to 7 ppm fluoride, were compared with those for children in fluoride-deficient Boston, there was a difference as high as 91% for proximal surfaces and 82% for occlusal surfaces. In Midland, virtually none of the smooth surfaces or lingual pits of the anterior teeth had been attacked by caries. Addi-

tional insight can be gained by distributing the children into groups according to individual dental caries experience ranging from 0 to 24 DMFT (decayed, missing, filled teeth; Table 42-2). Only 2% of the children in Boston had never experienced cavitation compared with a range of 9% to 27% for each of the four groups of children living in conventionally fluoridated communities. In contrast, approximately half the children who had consumed very high levels of natural fluoride in Midland were caries free. Fluoridating communal water to concentrations higher than 1 to 2 ppm fluoride, however, is not suggested because of the high risk of producing unaesthetic enamel fluorosis. But the very low dental caries activity found in Midland provokes speculation about the use of fluoride supplements in fluoridated areas and the development of imaginative preventive programs. Although the low caries record of nonfluoridated Mecklenburg County, North Carolina may be explained by the fact that beverages prepared with fluoridated water in nearby Charlotte were frequently ingested, it should also provoke speculation about additional anticaries substances besides fluoride that may be distributed on an uneven geographical basis.

Mechanisms of fluoride action

Although all details are not understood completely, the anticaries potential of fluoride stems from its ability to alter the physicochemical properties of the teeth and their environment and to affect adversely microorganisms in plaque.[4,26]

Effects on mineral structure. Numerous studies with powdered enamel and intact tooth surfaces have shown that exposure to fluorides renders the

Table 42-2. Distribution of 1878 adolescents according to dental caries experience in seven communities in five states

Number DMFT*	Boston, Mass.		Danvers, Mass.		Mecklenburg County, N.C.		Kalamazoo, Mich.		Stickney, Ill.		Charlotte, N.C.		Midland, Tex.	
	No.	%	No.	%	No.	%	No.	%	No.	%	No.	%	No.	%
0	6	1.9	28	9.1	13	10.8	62	19.7	83	26.6	54	25.4	153	49.2
1-5	99	32.8	163	53.4	73	60.8	189	60.0	183	58.7	124	58.2	140	45.0
6-10	120	39.7	103	33.8	29	24.2	60	19.0	38	12.2	31	14.6	18	5.8
11-24	77	25.5	11	3.6	5	4.2	4	1.3	8	2.6	4	1.9	0	0
TOTAL	302	100.0	305	100.0	120	100.0	315	100.0	312	100.0	213	100.0	311	100.0

From Englander, H.R., and DePaola, P.F. Enhanced anticaries action from drinking water containing 5 ppm fluoride. Journal of the American Dental Association **98**:35-39, 1979.
*Decayed, missing, filled teeth.

mineral components of the crown less soluble in acids. The reasons for this phenomenon are not entirely known. If the apatite crystals in enamel and bone contain fluoride, they appear to be larger and more perfectly formed, a property that is believed to reduce the solubility of crystalline materials. Enamel that contains optimum amounts of fluoride appears white and glassy, perhaps because its crystal structure is also better. Exposure of enamel to fluoride promotes formation of less soluble fluorapatite from the more soluble hydroxyapatite.

Insight into the protective action of fluoride may be gained by noting that saliva normally is supersaturated with respect to fluorapatite and hydroxyapatite. As the pH is lowered by acid, saliva becomes undersaturated to hydroxyapatite at about pH 5; however, it remains supersaturated to fluorapatite until the pH falls below about 4. Accordingly, enamel crystals that contain a relatively high concentration of fluorapatite are more resistant to etching and subsequent cavitation because they can withstand higher plaque acidities. More attention has been focused on the potential of fluoride to reduce the solubility of enamel than on its ability to protect cementum and dentin from the deleterious effects of acids. This could be a serious oversight, since many adults without coronal caries may experience root caries.

Inhibition of decalcification potential of plaque acids. It is generally not realized that fluoride can also completely inhibit the potential of acids to solubilize enamel. All the enamel on a tooth can be extensively decalcified within 24 hours by solutions of either organic or inorganic acids. This effect does not occur if the solutions contain adequate amounts of fluoride salts or hydrofluoric acid. The fluoride concentration of plaque can exceed 50 ppm by weight in persons who consume waterborne fluoride or rinse their mouths with fluoride solutions. Inasmuch as the distribution of fluoride varies between the organic and inorganic constituents of plaque, it is impossible to predict how much of it serves as a reservoir capable of inhibiting the decalcification potential of plaque acids. It is possible that frequently applied fluoride preparations could help maintain sufficient concentrations of fluoride in plaque to diminish the odontolytic potential of bacterial acids.

Enhancement of remineralization of enamel. An important action of fluoride is its ability to enhance the remineralization of enamel. The removal of acidogenic plaques, however, is probably essential before remineralization can occur.

Bactericidal and bacteriostatic effects. The following antibacterial effects may result from the presence of fluoride in plaque: (1) some of the bacteria may be killed, (2) normal bacterial growth and metabolic activity may be disturbed by disruption of enzyme systems, and (3) microorganisms at the interface of highly resistant enamel and cementum may be deprived of carbonate, phosphate, and other constituents of teeth essential for normal bacterial growth and well-being.

Substantial laboratory evidence from a variety of studies shows that fluoride can suppress *S. mutans* and other plaque microorganisms associated with coronal caries, periodontal lesions, and root caries. The amount of suppression depends on the type and concentration of the fluoride compound used, the pH of the solution, the duration of contact of the solution with bacteria, and the species of the exposed microorganisms. It has been reported that concentrations as low as 1 ppm fluoride can inhibit acid production, but concentrations in excess of 250 ppm fluoride are needed to affect the growth of streptococci and lactobacilli.

Numerous reports also have shown that acid production from microbial glycolysis can be inhibited by fluoride. Sufficient amounts of fluoride can be released from intact enamel surfaces in vitro to cause a marked inhibition of acidogenesis. The extent to which enzyme systems are affected will depend on the concentration of fluoride in solution, the pH, and other growth conditions of the experiments. It has been widely accepted that the enolase activity in glycolysis is especially sensitive to fluoride. Other researchers have postulated that fluoride may interfere with the transfer of metabolites (glucose) through cell walls or may even interfere with enzymes involved in the synthesis of polyglucan. High concentrations might interfere with phosphatases and possibly even some of the proteolytic enzymes.

Considerably less plaque forms on the teeth of experimental animals that have been treated with solutions containing sodium and stannous and amine fluorides. Under these conditions, cavitation has been very well controlled, often completely, and periodontal lesions have been less severe.

Depletion of crystalline material in teeth. Some of the anticaries effect of fluoride may be related to its unique ability to deplete the crystalline material in teeth essential to the vitality of invasive bacteria. The enamel surface containing fluoride may affect bacterial activity adversely because the noxious acids produced by sugar fermentation are not neutralized by the enamel surface. The survival, reproduction, and normal metabolic activity of acidogenic microbes also may be hindered because the necessary phosphate, carbonate, calcium, magnesium, and other substances are not released by the demineralization process.

Function and development of mammals. Data now available support the hypothesis that fluoride is a micronutrient essential for optimum development and function of mammals and perhaps all vertebrates. The possibility that it may help stabilize the mineral components of osseous tissues has led to its systemic administration to patients, especially postmenopausal women with osteoporosis. The reproductive capacity of animals is superior when the diet contains small amounts of fluoride, and recent studies have shown that fluoride favors the biologic processes conducive to growth, normal function, and improved pigmentation of incisor teeth.

CONTROL AND PREVENTION OF DENTAL CARIES AND PLAQUE

Highly effective control of odontolysis depends partly on measures that reduce or eliminate the responsible bacteria and plaque, protect against injurious acidic by-products, or prevent demineralization of the teeth. In laboratory animals, excellent control can be attained by producing changes in each of the factors illustrated in Figure 42-1. Beneficial results can be demonstrated by (1) reducing the frequency of eating and limiting the intake of readily fermentable carbohydrates, (2) enhancing the resistance of tooth surfaces with fluoride and possibly other agents, and (3) suppressing cariogenic bacteria and plaque with antibiotics and antibacterial agents or with mechanical measures. In humans, comparable results have been observed, although it is harder to regulate conditions for humans than for animals. In order to achieve highly effective control of human odontolysis, it probably will be necessary to employ several therapeutic measures that simultaneously influence diet, bacteria and plaque, and tooth resistance. Cases of rampant caries may require that all factors be controlled.

After a brief review of nonpharmacologic methods for preventing dental caries, the remainder of this chapter will be devoted to a discussion of fluoride and other agents that are currently used in the control of plaque formation and odontolysis.

Dietary recommendations

The rationale for dietary regulations has been discussed earlier. Coronal dental caries can be controlled by the virtual elimination of fermentable sugars, and the substitution of high protein diets has been recommended. Cases of rampant caries can be controlled for long periods by periodic restriction of carbohydrates. Jay and his associates[20] have devised a diet that many patients find more acceptable than one that requires continuous restriction of foods containing sucrose. It consists of three 2-week diet plans, each 2-week period having a different carbohydrate restriction. An alternative to a rigid diet is a sensible eating program that reduces the intake of food to three times a day, eliminates eating between meals, and limits intake of sugars to once daily, preferably with meals. In addition, it may be possible to substitute sugarless chewing gums and candies sweetened with sorbitol, mannitol, or xylitol. Other sugar substitutes are being sought and investigated.

Antiplaque measures and oral hygiene

In experimental animals, odontolysis will not occur if the teeth remain free from bacterial deposits, regardless of the diet consumed. Theoretically, if it were possible to keep human teeth free from plaque, odontolysis would not occur, and periodontal disease would be minimal. Accordingly, much can be achieved in plaque control by mechanical means with proper oral hygiene devices and techniques. These regimens involve recognition of plaque and its removal with brushes, effective dentifrices, dental floss, and rinsing. A disclosing solution may be a valuable aid in recognizing plaque.

For many years dentifrices were considered primarily as toiletries and cosmetic agents, but today many brands are recommended as therapeutic agents in anticaries programs. When plaque deposits are not adequately cleared from tooth surfaces by flosses, brushes, and other devices, some type of anticaries agent incorporated into a dentifrice could be valuable provided it diminishes plaque or delivers enough fluoride to tooth surfaces. Fluoride compounds may retard odontolysis even when applied in toothpastes that for the most part are used rather haphazardly.

Compounds other than those with fluoride have been incorporated into dentifrices to help eliminate plaque, render it harmless, increase tooth resistance, or to do all of these. The mode of action or rationale for the use of these substances varies: hexachlorophene, penicillin, tyrothricin, and other antibacterial agents reduce the number of acidogenic bacteria by antiseptic or germicidal action; urea, proteolytic enzymes, and oxidizing agents dissolve or denature plaque; various enzyme inhibitors, such as sodium-N-lauroyl sarcosinate, prevent or retard production of acid; and milk of magnesia and alkalinizing agents neutralize acids in plaque. For the most part these attempts have not proved fruitful.

Plastic pit and fissure sealants

Sealing caries-susceptible pits and fissures with self-curing or ultraviolet light–cured plastic sealants prevents bacterial colonization at these sites. It has been demonstrated that sealants can no longer be considered a temporary measure. They can be effective in prevention of caries for 6 years after a single application and are very effective in dental practices where reapplication of lost material can be done routinely. Sealant protection depends on sealant retention. When occlusal pits or fissures remain sealed they are protected against microbial invasion and odontolysis.[31]

Oral administration of fluorides

Fluoridation of community water. Fluoridation of community water supplies is an excellent public health measure, because it is safe, effective, economical, and requires no additional effort other than drinking the water. In a typical fluoridated city, one might expect to find several dental health benefits in individuals who from birth consume fluoridated water containing 1 ppm fluoride. The average person has about two-thirds fewer decayed, missing, or filled permanent teeth, and the protection provided the primary dentition of young children is similar. Protection of the permanent teeth persists throughout adulthood. There is a striking reduction in lesions affecting the proximal surfaces of posterior teeth; therefore, fewer complicated multisurface restorations are required. There is also important protection of the pits and fissures, and a very high percentage of the anterior teeth remain caries free. Finally, caries-free persons are commonly found, the teeth appear whiter and more perfectly formed (fewer enamel ''opacities'' and other defects are evident), and because there is lower tooth mortality, fewer adults are edentulous.

Fluoridation of school water. In some areas, children who do not have access to municipal waterborne fluoride have been provided with school water supplies that have been fortified with 2 to 7 ppm fluoride (3 to 7 times the concentrations found in municipal systems).[35] The higher concentrations in school water are supposed to compensate for the availability of fluoride only during school hours. Because these children generally do not drink the fluoridated water until the age of 6, at which time the crowns of almost all the permanent teeth have formed, fluorosis is not likely to be a problem. Studies have shown that the incidence of odontolysis is reduced in children treated wtih fluoridated school water, but not as much as in those with community fluoridation. Furthermore, the benefits of fluoridation do not persist after graduation from school.

Fluoride supplements. In recent years, fluoride has been dispensed in tablets, table salt, vitamin preparations, and other products to infants and children who do not have access to fluoridated water. These supplements are usually administered daily soon after birth and continued through the preeruptive maturation of the permanent teeth and thereafter. Clinical trials have not yet shown the benefits of such fluoride supplementation to be as great as from water fluoridation.

For those areas where the natural fluoride in drinking water is less than 0.2 ppm, the Council on Dental Therapeutics has recommended a schedule for fluoride supplementation in the diet as follows: for children less than 2 years of age, one tablet containing 1 mg fluoride should be added to each quart of water used for drinking and preparing food or formula, or alternatively, 0.25 mg fluoride should be administered daily; for children between 2 and 3 years of age, 0.5 mg fluoride should be administered daily; and for children 3 years of age and older, 1.0 mg fluoride should be given daily.

Topical application of fluorides

The value of topically applied fluorides has been supported by numerous studies of enamel from extracted human teeth and of experimental animals. There appears to be merit in almost all topical fluoride formulations and techniques of application. Benefits may be expected when the fluoride is used in mouthwashes, water-soluble gels, pastes, chewing gum, and table salt or when it is administered

by iontophoretic methods. It is thought that enhanced protection occurs if the teeth are exposed to fluoride shortly after eruption, because the enamel surface is very reactive at this time and absorbs additional fluoride rapidly.

A number of fluoride salts and formulations containing fluoride have been assessed, including fluorides of tin, lead, zirconium, ammonium, titanium, and vanadium, as well as monofluorophosphate and organic fluorides. Opinion is divided as to whether any of these compounds is superior to sodium fluoride in producing a more caries-resistant enamel. Sodium fluoride has the advantage of being inexpensive, readily available, stable, and not unpleasant tasting. Furthermore, it does not stain the teeth.

Topical applications with an aqueous solution acidified to approximately pH 3.2 and containing sodium fluoride and 0.1 M orthophosphoric acid are superior to treatments with plain sodium fluoride or stannous fluoride, because enamel surfaces treated with acidified fluoride phosphate solution acquire more fluoride. Apparently the formation of uncharged hydrofluoric acid at low pH favors the penetration of fluoride into enamel. The addition of orthophosphate promotes the formation of stable fluorapatite and tends to depress enamel dissolution and undesirable calcium fluoride formation. Enamel containing very high concentrations of permanently bound fluoride is very resistant to etching by acids. Recent studies have shown that mild etching of the enamel with 0.01 M phosphoric acid or pretreatment with 0.2 M aluminum nitrate before topical applications of sodium fluoride solutions appears to improve enamel fluoride uptake. Apparently aluminum is a strong complexing agent that can bind up to five ions of fluoride, and introduction of Al^{+++} followed by F^- into the enamel brings about a dual bonding of aluminum with apatite phosphate and the applied fluoride, thereby increasing the retention of fluoride.

Amine fluorides (e.g., oleylamine–hydrofluoric acid) have been used in an attempt to combine the protective effect of fluoride with the physicochemical protection afforded by long-chain aliphatic amines against enamel demineralization. Topical applications have been recommended with amine fluoride solutions containing approximately 1% fluoride. These compounds reduce enamel acid solubility more effectively than does stannous fluoride, and in vivo fluoride deposition and retention after topical treatments appear similar to that obtained from treatments with acidulated phosphate fluoride.

Frequency of application. Although the infrequent application of fluoride preparations may lead to a brief antibacterial effect, a slight reduction in the solubility of tooth surfaces, and the formation of surfaces that are slightly less susceptible to invasion by odontolytic microorganisms, there is no convincing evidence that any kind of infrequent fluoride treatment has a significant impact on the control of microbial plaque diseases. However, fluoride compounds can be applied frequently to teeth in toothpastes, in mouthwashes, in plastic trays coated with gels, in solutions with brushes, and by other devices. Such regular application of appropriate preparations should have an adverse effect on microorganisms in dental plaques. It should also make the mineral components of teeth highly resistant to demineralization, inhibit the decalcifying potential of plaque acids, and promote posteruptive maturation of enamel and remineralization. There is now a convincing body of evidence that the daily application of properly formulated fluoride preparations can arrest and prevent odontolysis, even in patients who have lost normal function of their salivary glands from radiation treatments and Sjögren's syndrome. Today, failure to control invasion and destruction of teeth can be attributed either to failure of clinicians to provide adequate intensive fluoride therapy or to patient indifference.

Fluoride in mouthwashes. The daily use of mouthwashes containing fluoride can be helpful in the control of odontolysis, but their use should be supervised carefully for three reasons: (1) the right amount must be used after the teeth have been cleared of food residues and plaque, (2) swallowing must not occur, and if it does the use of the mouthwash must be stopped, and (3) the mouth must be rinsed afterward. Addition of hydrogen peroxide (3%) will give a solution that has an acceptable taste and is difficult to swallow without gagging and will confer a foaming property on the mouthwash, thus making it possible to detect whether any residue remains in the mouth.

For more than 20 years Weisz[46] has supplemented his recommendations for the home care of children with a mouthwash containing 0.25% sodium fluoride. The ingredients used to prepare the mouthwash are dispensed in small packets. To prepare a concentrated stock solution, parents add water and flavoring agents according to the directions on the packets. The concentrate should be kept in a plastic bottle with a safety dispensing cap and stored out of the reach of young children. One tablespoon of the concentrate is added to half a glass of water. Patients are advised to rinse vigorously with it both morning and evening. The instructions on the packet clearly state "do not swallow." No adverse side effects have been observed in children so treated, and caries activity has been arrested in patients who follow this program.

There is evidence that stannous fluoride has a greater bactericidal effect than sodium fluoride, especially against microbial motility in plaque and gingival crevices. A mouthwash is now available that patients prepare by mixing equal parts of glycerine containing stannous fluoride and an acidulated aqueous solution of sodium fluoride. Teeth soaked in this preparation are not as well protected from the demineralizing effects of acids as are teeth that have been treated with a mixture of sodium fluoride and hydrogen peroxide.

Application of water-soluble gels. Experiments with both hamsters and school children have demonstrated great benefits from the daily application of sodium fluoride gels to the teeth.[12,13,15] It has also been found that application of fluoride gels may abate or arrest lesions in patients with highly odontolytic plaques associated with loss of salivary gland function as a consequence of irradiation for head and neck cancer[9] or other diseases. In fact, this arrest of cavitation occurs in spite of the fact that the irradiated patients continue to harbor large numbers of *S. mutans*.[3]

Fluoride gels are now available commercially for use by patients at home. They can be prepared easily, however, in the dental office by mixing a few ingredients and dissolving the mixture in distilled water. An inexpensive scale, food blender, and plastic bottles are the only equipment needed. A formula similar to that provided to Peace Corps volunteers calls for 10 gm sodium fluoride, 10 gm dibasic sodium phosphate, 1000 ml distilled water, and enough sodium carboxymethylcellulose to thicken the fluid mixture slightly (the exact amount will vary with the brand used). In mixing, the carboxymethylcellulose powder is added slowly to the vortex of the fluid until the desired consistency is obtained. Flavoring is optional, since the unflavored gel does not have an unpleasant taste. It can be flavored, however, with a few drops of lemon or orange extract together with saccharin (0.2 gm).[24]

The fluoride gel can be applied to custom-fitted maxillary and mandibular "toplicators" fashioned by vacuum-drawing heat-treated sheets of polyvinyl over plaster models of the jaws. There are several advantages of using toplicators for the administration of gels containing fluoride or other agents:

1. High concentrations of fluoride preparations can be held in intimate contact with the teeth and marginal gingiva for specific periods.

2. Saliva can be excluded from the field of application, thereby preventing dilution of an effective concentration of the active agent in the gel.

3. Intermittent biting pressure on the plastic toplicators tends to pump the medicine into pits, fissures, proximal surfaces, and other inaccessible regions of the dentition.

4. Since less than 0.5 ml of gel is usually applied in a thin layer to each toplicator, only a minimum amount of fluoride can be swallowed accidentally.

5. After the toplicators have been constructed, it is possible to simultaneously treat many children or other patients under supervision.

The gel-loaded toplicators should be worn for 5 to 10 minutes after as much plaque as possible has been cleared from all tooth surfaces. Any gel exuding from the tray should be expectorated, and

the mouth should be rinsed carefully after each treatment. This treatment has produced no reports of adverse reactions and should provide all of the attainable benefits of fluoride. Fluoride gels should be stored in plastic bottles sealed with safety caps out of the reach of children.

When additional carboxymethylcellulose is used to thicken the gel, it can be applied to the teeth with the fingers or with a toothbrush moistened with hydrogen peroxide, a pleasant mixture for toothbrushing. The effects of this procedure as an antiplaque and anticaries measure have not been described, but, in light of what is known, it would be more effective than many dentifrices that contain low concentrations of fluoride and other irritating flavoring agents. Not all persons need the intensive therapy described. The decision to use these methods will depend on the patient's concern for dental health and on the clinician's judgment.

The potential of the aforementioned fluoride treatment measures to control dentobacterial plaque and cavitation has been estimated in Table 42-3.

Toxicity of fluorides

More than 110 million people in the United States are currently drinking water that contains an

Table 42-3. Estimations of the potential of various fluoride treatment measures to control dentobacterial plaque and cavitation

Therapeutic goal	Communal water	School water	Table salt or drops	Slowly dissolved tablets	Occasional topicals*	Frequent or daily applications		
						Rinses	Gels†	Tooth-pastes‡
To prevent bacterial colonization	None	None	None	None	None	None	None	None
To disintegrate plaques rapidly	None	None	None	None	None	None	None	None
To kill bacteria in plaques	None	none	None	None	Moderate briefly	Moderate	Strong	Weak?
To inhibit bacterial metabolism	Slight	?	?	Weak	Moderate briefly	Strong	Strong	Weak?
To fortify enamel against lysis	Moderate	Weak	Weak	Weak	Weak	Strong	Strong	Weak
To fortify cementum against lysis	?	?	?	?	?	Moderate	Strong	Weak?
To prevent acids from decalcifying	Weak	?	?	Weak	None	Strong	Strong	?
To promote remineralization of lesions	Weak	?	?	Moderate	Moderate briefly	Strong	Strong	Weak

From Keyes, P.H., and Englander, H.R. Fluoride therapy in the treatment of dentomicrobial plaque disease. Journal of the American Society of Preventive Dentistry **5:**16-21, 36-38, 40, 1975.
*Solutions, prophylactic pastes, and gels.
†Gels in vinyl plastic trays, "toplicators."
‡Containing low concentrations of fluoride.

optimum concentration of controlled fluoride (0.7 to 1.2 ppm) for caries prevention or an equal or higher concentration of the naturally occurring trace element. Countless children are receiving fluoridated water at school, and various fluoride preparations are being topically applied in dental offices and homes. The extensive use of fluoride highlights its wide margin of safety. Long-term ingestion of water containing more than twice the optimum concentration of fluoride or long-term exposure to fluoride-containing materials can cause enamel fluorosis, if the exposure occurs during the period of tooth development. Osteosclerosis of the spine and pelvis can occur with the ingestion of drinking water containing 18 ppm fluoride or higher and is usually asymptomatic. Controlled water fluoridation rarely causes enamel fluorosis.

Acute toxicity from fluorides can result from the accidental ingestion of solutions that contain fluorides, such as insecticides, rodenticides, and preparations intended for topical application to teeth. The lethal dose for adults is said to be about 4 to 5 gm; for children, the lethal dose is much lower, about 0.3 to 0.5 gm. Signs of poisoning include symptoms resulting from the action of fluorides on the gastrointestinal tract (nausea, vomiting, increased salivation, diarrhea, abdominal pain), on the central nervous system (hyperreflexia, tonic and clonic convulsions, paresthesias), and on miscellaneous organs and systems (muscle pains, cardiovascular and respiratory depression). Many of these effects are indirect, resulting from a fluoride-induced decrease in the plasma concentration of free calcium ions; others are caused by inhibition of various enzyme systems. If these effects continue unchecked, death may result from cardiovascular or respiratory failure.

Treatment should be instituted immediately, starting with the administration of emetics to induce vomiting. Fluids containing calcium, for example, limewater (0.15% calcium hydroxide solution), should be introduced into the intubated stomach, or, if the patient is not vomiting, milk or limewater can be taken orally. Calcium gluconate (4 to 10 ml of a 10% solution) should be administered at the first sign of tetany and repeated if necessary. Simultaneously, appropriate measures should be taken to support respiration and circulation.

Although the normal procedures followed in the topical application of fluoride solutions does not normally pose a risk of acute toxicity, in order to minimize the possibility of accidental poisoning in young children no more than 80 mg of fluoride in liquid preparations or 100 mg in tablet form should be dispensed.

Antimicrobial agents

Methods for treating microbial plaques to control caries-conducive bacteria can be traced to Bunting and Palmerlee,[5] who applied methaphen and aniline dyes to tooth surfaces to check bacterial overgrowth. It is well recognized that the bacterial ecology of the mouth is difficult to change permanently, partly because it is highly dependent on eating habits. Although various components of the oral microflora can be reduced by adequate local contact with antibacterial drugs, these bacteria tend to reestablish themselves rapidly when the drug is discontinued.

Because an important infectious component is involved in the process of odontolysis, it might seem reasonable to employ chemotherapy in the control of microbial factors, as is customary in the treatment of other infections. There is particular concern for mentally and physically handicapped persons, many of whom are unable to use conventional oral hygiene measures. As mentioned earlier, persons who suffer from inadequate salivary gland function because of irradiation or surgery for facial tumors or because of degeneration of the glands have serious problems with plaque control and odontolysis. Persons incapacitated by heart disease and stroke also may have comparable oral hygiene problems. Although fluoride gels have helped immeasurably, the proper administration of antibiotics or other antibacterial agents to such patients could be beneficial in the control of odontopathic plaque and its sequelae. In cases of rampant caries, it would seem desirable to suppress the microbes colonizing on the teeth while other anticaries measures are carried out.

Antiplaque therapy and odontolysis control should not be based on haphazard, indiscriminate, or unsupervised use of powerful broad-spectrum antibacterial agents but on these chemotherapeutic guidelines: (1) selecting drugs that are nonallergenic, nonirritating, and nontoxic, (2) developing agents that are selective against the odontopathic gram-positive *S. mutans,* filaments, and other acidogens that thrive in plaque while having little effect on the normal oral flora, (3) using drugs that are inactive or not absorbed in the gastrointestinal tract, (4) prescribing drugs that do not produce imbalances in the normal oral ecology and overgrowth of other potential pathogens, such as *Candida albicans,* (5) applying antibiotics to ensure sufficient concentrations for an adequate time, (6) using synergistic or additive combinations of antibiotics to minimize the possibility of developing resistant strains of microorganisms, and (7) selecting the proper patients for whom other modes of therapy might not be adequate.

In 1940 it was reported that the use of daily mouth rinses containing organic mercurials would lead to the arrest and disappearance of plaques and dental caries.[18] The significance of this work was questioned, but in recent years there have been an increasing number of reports on the use of antimicrobial agents to control oral microorganisms and plaque. Penicillin was assessed in clinical trials but was soon discarded for this purpose when it was found that sensitivity could result. At the present time, a number of antimicrobial agents can be considered for topical use in the mouth.

Antibiotics. The antibiotics that show good potential for inhibiting plaque, dental caries, periodontal disease, or combinations thereof after topical or systemic administration include spiramycin, tetracycline, vancomycin, kanamycin, and actinobolin. Tyrothricin has also been studied as a plaque inhibitor, but its relatively low efficacy and high toxicity contraindicate its clinical use.

Spiramycin. Spiramycin, a macrolide antibiotic produced by *Streptomyces ambofaciens,* has the unusual property of being excreted in high salivary concentrations that equal or exceed those of the serum after oral administration. Its antibacterial spectrum is similar to erythromycin's, and it is bactericidal at about 4 times its bacteriostatic concentration. Spiramycin is especially effective against gram-positive streptococci and staphylococci and also against some gram-negative organisms and acts by inhibiting protein synthesis. It has been prescribed extensively for the treatment of human plaque and periodontal disease in Canada and Europe, but its use has not been approved in the United States. It shows good antiplaque and anticaries activity in experimental animals when applied topically or administered in the diet or drinking water. Harvey[19] has reported excellent results in the treatment of plaque diseases when 250 mg capsules of spiramycin were administered orally every 4 hours for 4 or 5 days together with subgingival scaling and curettage. Spiramycin is well tolerated, does not irritate the gastric mucosa, and has less effect on the intestinal microflora than many other commonly used antibiotics.

Tetracycline. The tetracyclines are a group of bacteriostatic antimicrobials that are derived from several varieties of *Streptomyces.* All have a common hydronaphthacene nucleus and are active against a wide variety of gram-positive and gram-negative bacteria, rickettsiae, and large viruses by inhibiting protein synthesis before peptide bond formation. Dampened tetracycline powder applied with a brush for several minutes daily to the teeth of experimental animals has been very effective in eliminating plaque, preventing dental caries, and arresting existing carious lesions. When administered in the animal's food or drinking water, it is effective in preventing plaque-related diseases. Long-term therapy with chlortetracycline has proved effective in the treatment of human periodontal diseases associated with severe plaque infections.[38] The usual dose prescribed has been one 250 mg capsule every 6 hours for 1 to 2 weeks. Recently, Keyes and his associates[27,28] have achieved excellent results with long-term tetracycline therapy in the treatment of dental plaque diseases. A 2-week course of tetracycline hydrochloride, 250 mg every 6 hours, is prescribed for patients with periodontal disease whose plaque samples show spirochetes and other motile microorganisms under phase-contrast microscopy. The antibiotic is either discontinued or reduced to two capsules per day for 10 weeks, depending on the disappearance of these motile forms. Such a yearly regimen of therapy together with local periodontal treatment and home care has resulted in effective control of destructive periodontal disease and dental caries over periods of several years.

When tetracyclines are prescribed, patients should be advised not to eat or drink for at least an hour before or after taking the antibiotic to prevent interference with absorption. Although the tetracyclines are relatively nontoxic antibiotics, they occasionally cause gastric disturbances and sequelae that result from suppression of the normal flora in the mouth and alimentary tract. Tetracycline therapy should be supervised carefully, and patients should be monitored for the development of oral superinfections with *C. albicans* and diarrhea and other changes in bowel habits.

Vancomycin. A rapidly bactericidal glycopeptide produced by *Streptomyces orientalis,* vancomycin has had considerable trial as a topical solution, ointment, or paste in animal and human studies of plaque inhibition. It blocks the cell wall mucopeptide synthesis of gram-positive bacteria and is especially effective against *S. mutans*. Infectious dental plaque, cavitation, and periodontal destruction can be inhibited completely in hamsters when a 10% to 15% aqueous solution of vancomycin is applied topically to the teeth for 2 minutes daily.[14] Human plaque and gingivitis can be controlled with the daily application of an ointment containing 1% vancomycin to the teeth and gingivae.[33,34] Furthermore, there is evidence that plaque, *S. mutans,* and dental caries can be reduced in children by daily 5-minute topical applications of a 3% vancomycin gel.[8,21] Vancomycin should not be given parenterally for plaque control because it is toxic. However, it is not absorbed from the gastrointestinal tract and is safe for topical use. An easily removable brown pellicle may develop on the teeth after repeated topical applications. The development of resistant strains of oral microorganisms has not been a problem in any clinical studies.

Kanamycin. Kanamycin is a bactericidal aminoglycoside antibiotic that was recovered from culture filtrates of *Streptomyces kanamyceticus*. It inhibits microbial protein synthesis and is a relatively weak inhibitor of streptococci in vitro. Kanamycin has been tested successfully as a human antiplaque agent at a 5% concentration in Orabase.[29] Inhibitory effects on plaque persist for several weeks after kanamycin is discontinued, and intermittent use results in good plaque control. Kanamycin can be applied topically in high concentrations with no toxic effects. It can be used as a 5% topical ointment apparently without danger of developing resistant organisms.

Actinobolin. Actinobolin is a lincomycin-related antibiotic that inhibits protein synthesis in susceptible gram-positive and gram-negative plaque bacteria. It possesses chelating properties enabling it to bind to enamel surfaces while retaining antibacterial activity. Animal assays indicate good anticaries activity at concentrations of 20 ppm. The potential of actinobolin as a caries inhibitor in humans is limited because it is bacteriostatic rather than bactericidal, and resistant microorganisms may emerge that are also resistant to lincomycin. It has a large margin of safety between toxic and therapeutic levels and is not absorbed after oral administration. This drug is not used for any other human infections.

Nonantibiotic agents. The most promising agents for the clinical control of plaque infections appear to be the bisbiguanides chlorhexidine and alexidine.

Chlorhexidine. Chlorhexidine has an established history of topical antimicrobial effectiveness for a variety of uses. It has been shown to be safe when applied to the skin, mucous membranes, and eye and has been used in throat lozenges in Europe. Chlorhexidine adheres strongly to teeth and dentobacterial plaque while retaining its antibacterial effects against a wide variety of gram-positive and gram-negative microorganisms. Chlorhexidine gluconate inhibits caries in rats, and mouthwashes containing 0.1 or 0.2% greatly inhibit the growth of human plaque.[41] Its powerful bactericidal effects after single daily topical applications delay the return of plaque for at least a week after topical applications have been discontinued. Two daily mouth rinses with 0.2% chlorhexidine gluconate or one daily topical application of a 2% solution completely inhibits the growth of human dental plaque. Topical chlorhexidine can prevent radiation caries in monkeys.[2] It has been shown that toothbrushing with 0.15%, 0.10%, and 0.05% chlorhexidine gluconate solutions prevents plaque and gingivitis.[1] The principal disadvantages of chlorhexidine are the formation of a readily removable stained pellicle on the teeth, tongue discoloration, an unpleasant taste at high concentrations, irritation of the oral mucosa, and taste disturbances. Intensity of tooth discoloration is directly related to chlorhexidine concentration. Toothbrushing with a 0.15% solution minimizes the oral mucous membrane reactions observed when mouth rinsing is used. Chlorhexidine has not been officially approved for this use in the United States.

Alexidine. Most of the remarks about chlorhexidine also apply to its diethyl analogue, alexidine. It can be used in lower concentrations than chlorhexidine because it has greater bactericidal activity.[6] The use of alexidine in the United States has not yet been approved.

SUMMARY

The knowledge available today makes it possible to develop a preventive program that will effectively control odontolysis, but some effort by the patient, dentist, dental hygienist, and auxiliary is required. It appears unlikely that there will be a simple agent to eradicate this infection. The best possible prophylactic and therapeutic results will follow the simultaneous application of the principles described in this chapter; no one factor should be employed to the exclusion of the others. Because it generally is difficult to attain the maximum benefit from a single therapeutic approach, clinicians should strive to achieve as much as they can from diet regulation, oral hygiene (deplaquing), fluoridation, topical fluorides, and, when indicated, antibacterial measures. In the management of rampant dental caries associated with plaques containing high populations of *S. mutans,* the dental therapist may have to proceed as follows: (1) advise reducing the frequency of eating all sugars to once a day, (2) instruct patients in how to disperse tenacious plaques with flosses, brushes, and other armamentaria, (3) prescribe frequent, even daily, intensive fluoride treatments, preferably with toplicators, (4) treat tooth surfaces frequently with appropriate antimicrobial agents (when they become available for such use), (5) prophylactically seal caries-free pits and fissures routinely in caries-susceptible persons, and (6) immediately excavate all carious lesions and seal dentin with temporary or permanent restorations.

CITED REFERENCES

1. Bay, L.M. Effect of toothbrushing with different concentrations of chlorhexidine on the development of dental plaque and gingivitis. Journal of Dental Research **57:**181-185, 1978.
2. Bowen, W.H., Thomson, L., Little, W., Cole, M., Swain, P., and Englander, H. The effects of irradiation on dental caries in primates *(M. mulatta).* 24th Orca Congress. Caries Research **12:**112, 1978.
3. Brown, L.R., Dreizen, S., Handler, S., and Johnston, D.A. Effect of radiation-induced xerostomia on human oral microflora. Journal of Dental Research **54:**740-750, 1975.
4. Brudevold, F. Fluoride therapy in improving dental practice through preventive measures. In Bernier, J.L., and Muhler, J.C., eds. Improving Dental Practice Through Preventive Measures, ed. 3. St. Louis, The C.V. Mosby Co., 1975.
5. Bunting, R.W., and Palmerlee, F. The role of *Bacillus acidophilus* in dental caries. Journal of the American Dental Association **12:**381-413, 1925.
6. Carlson, H.C., Porter, K., and Alms, T.H. The effect of an alexidine mouthwash on dental plaque and gingivitis. Journal of Periodontology **48:**216-218, 1977.
7. Clarke, J.K. On the bacterial factor in the aetiology of dental caries. British Journal of Experimental Pathology **5:**141-147, 1924.
8. DePaola, P.F., Jordan, H.V., and Soparkar, P.M. Inhibition of dental caries in school children by topically applied vancomycin. Archives of Oral Biology **22:**187-191, 1977.
9. Dreizen, S., Brown, L.R., Daly, T.E., and Drane, J.B. Prevention of xerostomia-related dental caries in irradiated cancer patients. Journal of Dental Research **56:**99-104, 1972.
10. Englander, H.R., and DePaola, P.F. Enhanced anticaries action from drinking water containing 5 ppm fluoride. Journal of the American Dental Association **98:**35-39, 1979.
11. Englander, H.R., and Keyes, P.H. Dental caries: etiological factors, pathological characteristics, therapeutic measures. In Steele, P.F., ed. Dimensions of Dental Hygiene. Philadelphia, Lea & Febiger, 1966.
12. Englander, H.R., and Keyes, P.H. The prevention of dental caries in the Syrian hamster after repeated topical application of sodium fluoride gels. Journal of the American Dental Association **73:**1342-1347, 1966.
13. Englander, H.R., and Keyes, P.H. Acid production in the dental plaque of hamsters protected from dental caries with sodium fluoride. Journal of Oral Therapeutics and Pharmacology **4:**382-387, 1968.
14. Englander, H.R., and Keyes, P.H. Control of *Streptococcus mutans,* plaque, and dental caries in hamsters with topically applied vancomycin. Archives of Oral Biology **16:**469-472, 1971.
15. Englander, H.R., Keyes, P.H., Gestwicki, M., and Sultz, H.A. Clinical anticaries effect of repeated topical sodium fluoride applications by mouthpieces. Journal of the American Dental Association **75:**638-644, 1967.
16. Fitzgerald, R.J., and Keyes, P.H. Demonstration of the etiologic role of streptococci in experimental caries in the hamster. Journal of the American Dental Association **61:**9-19, 1960.
17. Gustafsson, B.E., Quensel, C.E., Lanke, L.S., Lundquist, C., Grahńen, H., Bonow, B.E., and Krasse, B. The Vipeholm dental caries study. The effect of different levels of carbohydrate intake on caries activity in 436 individuals observed for five years. Acta Odontologica Scandinavica **11:**232-364, 1954.
18. Hanke, M.T. Studies on the local factors in dental caries. I. Destruction of plaques and retardation of bacterial growth in the oral cavity. Journal of the American Dental Association **27:**1379-1393, 1940.
19. Harvey, R.F. Clinical impressions of a new antibiotic in periodontics: spiramycine. Journal of the Canadian Dental Association **27:**576-585, 1961.
20. Jay, P., Beeuwkes, A.M., and Husbands, J. Dietary Program for the Control of Dental Caries. Ann Arbor, Mich., The Overbeck Co., 1964.
21. Jordan, H.V., and DePaola, P.F. Effect of prolonged topical application of vancomycin on human oral *Streptococcus mutans* populations. Archives of Oral Biology **22:**193-199, 1977.
22. Jordan, H.V., Keyes, P.H., and Bellack, S. Periodontal lesions in hamsters and gnotobiotic rats infected with actinomyces of human origin. Journal of Periodontal Research **7:**21-28, 1972.
23. Keyes, P.H. Research in dental caries. Journal of the American Dental Association **76:**1357-1373, 1968.
24. Keyes, P.H. Present and future measures for dental caries control. Journal of the American Dental Association **79:**1395-1404, 1969.
25. Keyes, P.H. Microbiology as a tool in preventive dentistry. In Bernier, J.L., and Muhler, J.C., eds. Improving Dental Practice Through Preventive Measures, ed. 3. St. Louis, The C.V. Mosby Co., 1975.

26. Keyes, P.H., and Englander, H.R. Fluoride therapy in the treatment of dentomicrobial plaque disease. Journal of the American Society of Preventive Dentistry **5**:16-21, 36-38, 40, 1975.

27. Keyes, P.H., Wright, W.E., and Howard, S.A. The use of phase-contrast microscopy and chemotherapy in the diagnosis and treatment of periodontal lesions—an initial report. Part I. Quintessence International **9**:51-56, 1978.

28. Keyes, P.H., Wright, W.E., and Howard, S.A. The use of phase-contrast microscopy and chemotherapy in the diagnosis and treatment of periodontal lesions—an initial report. Part II. Quintessence International **9**:69-76, 1978.

29. Loesche, W.J., Hockett, R.N., and Syed, S.A. Reduction in proportions of dental plaque streptococci following a 5-day topical kanamycin treatment. Journal of Periodontal Research **12**:1-10, 1977.

30. McClure, F.J. Water Fluoridation: The Search and the Victory. Bethesda, Md., U.S. Department of Health, Education, and Welfare, National Institutes of Health, National Institute of Dental Research, 1970.

31. Mertz-Fairhurst, E.J., Fairhurst, C.W., Williams, J.E., Della-Giustina, V.E., and Brooks, J.D. A comparative clinical study of two pit and fissure sealants: six-year results in Augusta, Ga. Journal of the American Dental Association **105**:237-239, 1982.

32. Miller, W.D. The Micro-organisms of the Human Mouth. Philadelphia, S. S. White Dental Manufacturing Co., 1890.

33. Mitchell, D.F., and Holmes, L.A. Topical antibiotic control of dentogingival plaque. Journal of Periodontology **36**:202-208, 1965.

34. Mitchell, D.F., Holmes, L.A., Martin, P.W., and Sakurai, E. Topical antibiotic maintenance of oral health. Journal of Oral Therapeutics and Pharmacology **4**:83-92, 1967.

35. Newbrun, E., ed. Fluorides and Dental Caries: Contemporary Concepts for Practitioners and Students. Springfield, Ill., Charles C Thomas, Publisher, 1975.

36. Nolte, W.A. The oral microflora. In Nolte, W.A., ed. Oral Microbiology, ed. 4. St. Louis, The C. V. Mosby Co., 1982.

37. Rosebury, T. The parasitic lactobacilli. Archives of Pathology **38**:413-437, 1944.

38. Roth, L.H. A report of long sustained therapy with chlortetracycline. Antibiotics and Medicine **1**:13-19, 1955.

39. Schamschula, R.G., Barmes, D.E., Keyes, P.H., and Gulbinat, W. Prevalence and interrelationships of root surface caries in Lufa, Papua New Guinea. Community Dentistry and Oral Epidemiology **2**:295-304, 1974.

40. Scheinin, A. Caries control through the use of sugar substitutes. International Dental Journal **26**:4-12, 1976.

41. Schiøtt, C.R., Löe, H., Jensen, S.B., Kilian, M., Davies, R.M., and Glavind, K. The effect of chlorhexidine mouthrinses on the human oral flora. Journal of Periodontal Research **5**:84-89, 1970.

42. Stephan, R.M. Intra-oral hydrogen ion concentrations associated with dental caries activity. Journal of Dental Research **23**:257-266, 1944.

43. Sumney, D.L., Jordan, H.V., and Englander, H.R. The prevalence of root surface caries in selected populations. Journal of Periodontology **44**:500-504, 1973.

44. Toverud, G., Rubal, L., and Wiehl, D.G. The influence of war and post-war conditions on the teeth of Norwegian school children. The Milbank Memorial Fund Quarterly **39**:489-539, 1961.

45. Weiss, R.L., and Trithart, A.H. Between-meal eating habits and dental caries experience of pre-school children. American Journal of Public Health **50**:1097-1104, 1960.

46. Weisz, W.S. Sodium fluoride mouthwash—can it help? Journal of Dentistry for Children **27**:267-272, 1960.

GENERAL REFERENCES

Cariostatic mechanisms of fluorides. Proceedings of a Workshop by the American Dental Association and the National Institute of Dental Research. In Caries Research, vol. 11, suppl. 1, 1977.

Driscoll, W.S., and Horowitz, H.S. A discussion of optimal dosage for dietary fluoride supplementation. Journal of the American Dental Association **96**:1050-1053, 1978.

Englander, H.R., Kesel, R.G., and Gupta, O.P. The Aurora-Rockford, Ill., study II. Effect of natural fluoride on the periodontal health of adults. American Journal of Public Health **53**:1233-1242, 1963.

Englander, H.R., Reuss, R.C., and Kesel, R.G. Roentgenographic and clinical evaluation of dental caries in adults who consume fluoridated versus fluoride-deficient water. Journal of the American Dental Association **68**:14-19, 1964.

Englander, H.R., Shklair, I.L., and Fosdick, L.S. The effects of saliva on the pH and lactate concentration in dental plaques. Journal of Dental Research **38**:848-853, 1959.

Flötra, L., Gjermo, P., Rölla, G., and Waerhaug, J. Side effects of chlorhexidine mouth washes. Scandinavian Journal of Dental Research **79**:119-125, 1971.

Fosdick, L.S., Englander, H.R., Hoerman, K.C., and Kesel, R.G. A comparison of pH values of in vivo dental plaque after sucrose and sorbitol mouth rinses. Journal of the American Dental Association **55**:191-195, 1957.

Gibbons, R.J., and Socransky, S.S. Intracellular polysaccharide storage by organisms in dental plaques: its relation to dental caries and microbial ecology of the oral cavity. Archives of Oral Biology **7**:73-79, 1962.

Glass, R.L., ed. The first international conference on the declining prevalence of dental caries: the evidence and the impact on dental education, dental research, and dental practice. Journal of Dental Research **61**:1304-1383, 1982.

Hardwick, J.L. The incidence and distribution of caries throughout the ages in relation to the Englishman's diet. British Dental Journal **108**:9-17, 1960.

Hartzell, T.B., Henrici, A.T., and Grey, W.A. Report of the Mouth-Infection Research Corps of the National Dental Association. Journal of the National Dental Association **3**:333-334, 1916.

Heifetz, S.B., Horowitz, H.S., and Driscoll, W.S. Effect of school water fluoridation on dental caries: results in Seagrove, N.C. after eight years. Journal of the American Dental Association **97**:193-196, 1978.

Hibitane (chlorhexidine). Alderley Park, Macclesfield, Cheshire, England, Pharmaceuticals Division, Imperial Chemical Industries Limited, 1973.

Löe, H., and Schiøtt, C.R. The effect of suppression of the oral microflora upon the development of dental plaque and gingivitis. In McHugh, W.D., ed. Dental Plaque. Edinburgh, E. & S. Livingstone, Inc., 1970.

Löe, H., Theilade, E., Jensen, S.B., and Schiøtt, C.R. Experimental gingivitis in man. III. The influence of antibiotics on gingival plaque development. Journal of Periodontal Research **2:**282-289, 1967.

Manly, R.S., and Harrington, D.P. Solution rate of tooth enamel in an acetate buffer. Journal of Dental Research **38:**910-919, 1959.

McClure, F.J. Fluoride drinking waters. Public Health Service publication no. 825. Washington, D.C., U.S. Government Printing Office, 1962.

Moulton, F.R., ed. Fluorine and Dental Health. Washington, D.C., American Association for the Advancement of Science, 1942.

Moulton, F.R., ed. Dental Caries and Fluorine, Washington, D.C., American Association for the Advancement of Science, 1946.

Orland, F.J., Blayney, J.R., Harrison, R.W., Reyneirs, J.A., Trexler, P.C., Ervin, R.F., Gordon, H.A., and Wagner, M. Experimental caries in germfree rats inoculated with enterococci. Journal of the American Dental Association **50:**259-272, 1955.

Preventive Dentistry Research Workshop Proceedings. Naval Medical Research and Development Command, Bethesda, Maryland, 1982.

43 Antiseptics and disinfectants

Roger R. Deuben

Antiseptics and disinfectants are used to reduce the number of microorganisms on epithelial tissues and inanimate objects, respectively. At present there is no substance commercially available that has all of the criteria necessary for ideal antisepsis or disinfection. Those available have an incomplete spectrum of microbicidal activity, or they are unacceptably toxic to the host, or their use is too time-consuming to be practical. A thorough understanding of the activities and limitations of currently available agents will help the clinician choose the regimen most appropriate for a particular use.

Before the clinician can make a rational selection, the properties of an ideal antiinfective must be considered. An ideal germicide would rapidly destroy all forms of infectious organisms without causing toxic or allergic reactions in the host. The agent must be active in the presence of such biologic substances as blood, saliva, and pus and be noncorrosive to such materials as plastic, chrome, stainless steel, and rubber. Finally, the compound should be inexpensive enough to allow its routine use in clinical practice.

A reduction in the number of pathogenic bacteria to which the patient is exposed is extremely critical in the practice of dentistry.[1,6,11] It must be emphasized that the chemicals discussed in this chapter are only adjuncts to the procedures necessary for the prevention of infection. They are not a substitute for classic sterilization techniques (such as autoclaving) but serve only to assist in the reduction of microorganisms on those objects to which it is impractical or impossible to apply steam, dry heat, or toxic gases. They are useful in the reduction of both resident and transient organisms on the practitioner's hands, the patient's skin, and objects used during routine operating procedures; however, they cannot substitute for accepted techniques of surgical asepsis.

The local antiinfectives have three basic mechanisms of action: denaturation of cellular protein, osmotic disruption of the cell by decreasing the surface tension of the surrounding media, and interference with metabolic processes. The first two modes of action are usually considered germicidal, because their effects are lethal to existing microbes. Germistatic substances, however, act by interfering with metabolic pathways, and although they may not kill organisms directly, they act effectively to reduce microbial survival by inhibiting their reproductive capacity.

When selecting an antiinfective, the clinician must take into account the class of organism that is to be eradicated. For example, a particular chemical may be bactericidal but have little or no effect on viruses or fungi. The spectrum of activity against a specific form of microorganism must also be considered. An agent such as benzalkonium chloride is lethal to many oral bacteria, but it does not significantly affect the survival of the tubercle bacillus. Even within the same species, different forms of the organism might be affected differently. Generally, the vegetative forms of bacteria are much more susceptible to chemical agents than are spores. For example, glutaraldehyde is extremely effective in rapidly killing vegetative forms but may require 10 hours or more to kill spores.

Two important contemporary concerns in the practice of dentistry are the transmission of tuberculosis and viral hepatitis. It has been estimated that in a large dental school clinic at least two active cases of tuberculosis appear each year.[1] When one considers that tuberculosis is a very serious illness, it is apparent that such a contact may have grave ramifications. The incidence of hepatitis B

Table 43-1. Spectrum of antimicrobial activity of different classes of antiseptics and disinfectants

Class of antiinfective	Gram-positive bacteria	Gram-negative bacteria	Bacterial spores*	Tubercle bacilli	Viruses	Fungi
Alcohols	+	+	−	+	±	±
Aldehydes	+	+	+	+	+	+
Phenols	+	+	±	+	−	+
Halogens	+	+	±	±	+	+
Biguanides	+	+	−	−	−	±
Surface-acting agents						
Anionic	+	−	−	−	−	−
Cationic	+	±	−	−	−	+
Heavy metals	+	±	−	−	±	+

Key: + = sensitive, ± = moderately sensitive, − = resistant.
*May require prolonged exposure, elevated temperature, or greater than normal antiinfective concentration.

is reported to be significantly higher in dental practitioners (14%) than in the general population (2.4%), and in those practitioners involved in soft-tissue surgery an even greater incidence (27%) is observed.[2] The organisms responsible for these two diseases are among the most resistant to the lethal effects of chemical disinfectants. However, it should be emphasized that significantly reducing the number of viable organisms a person is exposed to vastly improves the chances that the person's own defense mechanisms will eradicate the remainder.

Table 43-1 presents in summary form the antimicrobial activity of the classes of antiinfectives discussed below.

ALCOHOLS

The alcohols are probably still the most widely used local antiinfectives today. The two alcohols that are of primary practical importance are ethanol and isopropanol (isopropyl alcohol). Both agents are bactericidal, rapidly acting, and inexpensive. They are highly volatile and do not leave a residual film. These latter attributes result in an extremely short contact time after topical application, often too brief to afford more than partial antisepsis or disinfection. Their major uses are as skin antiseptics and as solvents for other antiseptic and disinfecting compounds. Because bacterial spores, viruses, and fungi are not significantly affected by these agents, alcohols cannot be solely relied on for the sterilization of surgical instruments.

These agents appear to exert their effects by denaturing proteins. Both are commonly used in solutions that are 70% alcohol by weight, but ethanol and isopropyl alcohol are sometimes more efficacious in lower and higher concentrations, respectively. Against some microbes, ethyl alcohol loses activity in concentrations greater than 70% because its protein denaturing and precipitating action requires water for optimal effect.

These drugs are somewhat caustic to human cells, and long-term use may result in excessive drying and irritation of tissues. Application to open wounds results in sensations of pain and coagulation of the tissue, under which bacterial proliferation can subsequently occur.

Isopropyl alcohol induces vasodilation when applied to the skin surface overlying blood vessels. This property can be advantageous when one is seeking to visualize a vessel for venipuncture, but it can also be disadvantageous in that the puncture may cause excessive bleeding.

ALDEHYDES

Formaldehyde is a strong germicide but is extremely toxic to tissues at effective concentrations (2% to 8%). Its value lies only in its disinfectant capabilities. Dilute solutions have been incorporated into some mouthwash preparations, but at the concentrations tolerated by the mucous membranes, formaldehyde exerts little or no effect on microbial viability. Repeated contact with this substance may cause sensitization, possibly resulting in severe eczematoid dermatitis. The use of formaldehyde is not recommended for surgical instruments because of its corrosive properties.

Glutaraldehyde is a superior disinfectant when compared with formaldehyde in that it is 2 to 8 times more effective against bacterial spores. Used in an alkalinized 2% aqueous solution, it retains activity against tubercle bacilli, spores, viruses, and fungi for up to 30 days. Glutaraldehyde is not greatly affected by the presence of organic material and is relatively nonirritating, nonallergenic, and noncorrosive. It has been advocated for cold sterilization of those instruments (rubber, plastic goods, etc.) that cannot tolerate the conventional methods. Although 10 minutes may be sufficient to kill most microorganisms, inactivation of certain highly resistant spores may require 10 or more hours of exposure. Acid-stabilized solutions of glutaraldehyde combine the advantages of the alkaline-buffered forms with a much longer active life and a more rapid (1 hour) sporicidal effect. However, these preparations must be heated to ensure the destruction of resistant spores.

PHENOLS AND RELATED COMPOUNDS

Phenol was one of the earliest agents used for surgical disinfection, having been introduced for this purpose by Sir Joseph Lister in 1867. Because of its extreme toxicity, its use as an antiinfective has been essentially replaced by more effective and less toxic substances. Alkyl substitutions on the phenol molecule greatly increase germicidal efficacy without appreciably affecting toxicity. Phenolic agents form weak complexes with tissue and microbial proteins, resulting in denaturation.

Many of these compounds are currently used in dentistry primarily for their destructive action rather than for their antimicrobial potential. If a phenol-treated area (such as a root canal) is covered, preventing the escape of the phenolic compound, the agent will be released from the denatured protein only to react with adjacent tissues. This progressive action can result in deep burns and extensive tissue damage. These compounds also possess local anesthetic activity, thus enhancing their appeal in the treatment of dental problems in which pain is a complicating factor.

Generally, the phenols have the advantage of retaining their antimicrobial effectiveness in the presence of organic material, which makes them useful when the removal of tissue and debris is impossible or impractical.

Cresol is the collective term for the orthomethylated, metamethylated, and paramethylated products of phenol. The active constituent of coal tar, cresol is 2 to 4 times as effective as phenol while retaining approximately the same toxicity. Various

cresol derivatives have been used in the treatment of pulpal and periapical infections, but because of their destructive nature, they have largely been replaced by safer agents. A 50% solution of cresol in saponified vgetable oil is marketed under the trade name of Lysol. This formulation is primarily reserved for the disinfection of large inanimate objects.

Guaiacol is the methyl ester of *o*-hydroxyphenol and is the predominant active constituent of beechwood creosote. It is used in the treatment of pulpal pain because of its rapid and direct analgesic properties. This agent is considerably less toxic than phenol, but it is also less effective as an antimicrobial.

Eugenol (2-methoxy-4-allylphenol) is a common ingredient in various dental pastes, where its antiseptic activity is quite low. Its most useful property, like that of guaiacol, is analgesia. If sealed into the pulpal cavity, as was once a common practice, it may produce severe tissue damage that may remain asymptomatic for a considerable period. Eugenol is the active phenolic constituent in oil of cloves.

HALOGENATED SUBSTITUTIONS OF PHENOLS

Parachlorophenol, as a 1% aqueous solution, is a very effective root canal antiseptic. Evidence has been presented to indicate that this concentration may be equal, in root canal therapy, to the much stronger and more toxic preparation of camphorated parachlorophenol.[4]

Hexachlorophene is probably the most important of the phenolic derivatives for skin antisepsis. It has been widely used as a surgical scrub primarily because of its long-lasting and cumulative antiseptic properties. Repeated washing results in maximum antimicrobial activity in approximately 3 days, at which time the resident bacterial concentration may be reduced by 95% to 99%.[5] A single scrub with a hexachlorophene soap immediately before surgery, however, is no more effective than soap alone. This agent is primarily effective against gram-positive bacteria, which constitute the majority of skin pathogens. It has little activity against the tubercle bacillus or hepatitis virus.

The incidence of adverse reactions from cutaneous absorption of this agent is very low. Proper repeated use in adults has not been reported to produce systemic or local toxicity. Animal studies have indicated that repeated whole-body washing

2 to 3 times daily with a 3% solution of hexachlorophene may result in neurotoxicity to newborn infants. This information coupled with reports of adverse reactions in neonates resulted in the removal by the FDA of products containing hexachlorophene from OTC sales. These items are still available, however, for presurgical use and remain very effective for this purpose.

HALOGENS AND HALOGEN-RELEASING COMPOUNDS

The halogens and halogen-releasing compounds include some of the most effective antiseptics available. The active principle appears to be the free halogen itself, with iodine and chlorine being the more effective and bromine and fluorine less active.

Sodium hypochlorite solution is one of a number of preparations (known as chlorophors) that release chlorine in the form of hypochlorous acid. These agents are potent germicides and bleaching agents, and they readily dissolve blood clots and necrotic debris. Several hypochlorite solutions have gained much popularity in dentistry, especially for the debridement of root canals. Chlorine compounds are corrosive to many metals and are quite irritating to tissues when used in high concentrations. Hypochlorous acid is moderately effective against hepatitis virus, but tubercle bacilli appear somewhat resistant.

Chloramine-T is a compound formed when an organic residue, sodium 4-toluenesulfonamide, is combined with hypochlorous acid. This agent is less corrosive and produces less tissue irritation than sodium hypochlorite solution; however, it does not have the ability to dissolve blood clots and necrotic debris. It is suggested that application of a 1% solution of chloramine-T to the surgical area before extraction of a tooth significantly reduces postsurgical bacteremia.[10]

Iodine compounds are probably still the most efficient antiseptics available to modern medicine. The germicidal spectrum includes all forms of vegetative pathogens: bacteria, viruses, protozoa, and fungi. Spores are somewhat resistant but are killed on extended exposure. For example, a 1:20,000 iodine solution is bactericidal within 1 minute and sporicidal against hydrated spores in approximately 15 minutes. (Dry spores may require higher concentrations and considerably longer exposure times to be destroyed.) Elemental iodine is available (with sodium or potassium salts added to increase solubility) in aqueous solutions or as a tincture (with 50% ethanol). Iodine compounds in general are not inhibited by the presence of organic material, are noncorrosive, and have a very low toxicity. Allergic reactions are rarely encountered. These agents will stain clothing and skin and, especially with the tincture, may cause skin irritation.

Iodophors are organic molecules complexed with iodine. They have the property of releasing iodine over a prolonged period. A common preparation, povidone-iodine, is claimed to have all the advantages of elemental iodine, including antitubercular activity. The added benefits of these substances are that they do not produce staining and are far less irritating than the elemental iodine preparations.

BIGUANIDES

Chlorhexidine, the first of the antibacterial biguanides to be employed clinically, was approved for use in the United States in 1976. As a 4% solution, chlorhexidine is an effective surgical scrub, combining the rapid action of povidone-iodine with the long-lasting effect of hexachlorophene.[7] The agent exerts several antimicrobial actions, but cell death is most probably the result of protein denaturation. Chlorhexidine is highly effective against gram-positive bacteria, less so against fungi and gram-negative bacteria, and ineffective against tubercle bacilli, spores, and hepatitis viruses.

The untoward effects of chlorhexidine are generally mild. Local tissue damage can occur if the drug is applied to abraded epithelium. On the other hand, chlorhexidine has a low allergenic potential, and the drug is poorly absorbed from the gastrointestinal tract, limiting systemic toxicity if ingested. Chlorhexidine applied intraorally, normally in concentrations of 0.2% to 1%, causes staining of the teeth, a bitter taste, and occasional swelling of the parotid glands. The use of chlorhexidine and another biguanide, alexidine, is discussed in Chapter 42.

SURFACE-ACTING AGENTS

Anionic agents are very weak antiseptics that are effective almost exclusively against gram-positive bacteria. The common soaps (e.g., green soap) are included in this group of antiseptics.

Cationic agents, the prototype for which is benzalkonium chloride, have traditionally been mislabeled as "cold sterilizing solutions." Although benzalkonium chloride is relatively effective against fungi and gram-positive and gram-negative bacilli, it is almost totally ineffective against spore-forming bacteria, tubercle bacilli, and viruses. In fact, benzalkonium chloride has been used experimentally to isolate tubercle bacilli from mixed cultures of bacteria. In general, the cationic agents are rapidly inactivated in the presence of soap, alcohol, and hard water, and their activity is virtually lost within weeks after their initial preparation. As a result, their routine use in modern dental practice should be discontinued.[3]

HEAVY METALS

Mercurials are bacteriostatic compounds that have been largely replaced by more effective agents. Their spectrum is limited to gram-positive bacteria and fungi; they show very limited activity against gram-negative organisms. Bacterial spores, tubercle bacilli, and viruses are insensitive.

Silver compounds have a relatively specialized use in the treatment of the particularly susceptible gonococcal organisms. The preparations are caustic and astringent. They must be prepared fresh and used with caution to prevent tissue damage and permanent skin discoloration (argyria). Tissue fluids and other organic materials impair the effectiveness of these compounds.

OXIDIZING AGENTS

A wide variety of oxidizing agents are available as antiseptics, varying from mild to quite strong. Among the substances that have been investigated for use in dentistry are molecular oxygen (including hyperbaric oxygen), 3% hydrogen peroxide, sodium perborate, zinc peroxide, calcium hypochlorate, sodium peroxide, and several extremely strong agents such as potassium permanganate and chromic trioxide.

With the recognition that anaerobic gram-negative rods may be implicated in periodontal disease,[9] much attention has been directed toward the possibility that the oxidizing agents might alter the subgingival environment sufficiently to make it aerobic. Although the oxidizing agents are effective against anaerobic microorganisms, they also produce undesired tissue changes, including edema, epithelial vacuolation, and sloughing.[8]

Hydrogen peroxide is a weak antiseptic when applied to tissues. The abundance of peroxidases associated with tissues rapidly inactivates the peroxide, concomitantly releasing gaseous oxygen. Probably the only value of hydrogen peroxide in wound antisepsis is from the effervescent oxygen loosening trapped debris and bacteria.

Table 43-2. Indications for use and effective concentrations of selected antiinfectives*

Agent	Indication	Concentration
Alcohol	Skin or mucosal antisepsis, solvent for other agents	70% wt/vol
Formaldehyde	Instrument disinfection	1%-2% aqueous solution, 3%-4% in 70% isopropyl alcohol
Glutaraldehyde	Instrument disinfection	Activated 2% solution
Parachlorophenol	Root canal, periapical infections	1%-98%
Cresol	Instrument disinfection	50%
Eugenol	Pulpal pain	Variable
Guaiacol	Pulpal pain	Variable
Hexachlorophene	Skin antisepsis and surgical scrub	0.75%-3% repeated application
Chlorhexidine	Skin antisepsis and surgical scrub	4%
Sodium hypochlorite	Root canal irrigation	5%
	Mucous membrane antisepsis	Neutral 0.5% solution
Chloramine-T	Topical skin antisepsis	0.1%-4%
	Mouthwash antisepsis	1%
Tincture of iodine	Skin, mucous membrane, tooth, and rubber dam disinfection	2% iodine and 2.4% sodium iodide in 50% aqueous alcohol
Iodine solution	Disclosing solutions	8%-9% iodine, other salts variable
Povidone-iodine	Skin and mucosal antisepsis	Solution containing 1% available iodine
Hydrogen peroxide	Tooth bleaching	30% solution
	Wound cleansing	3% solution

*This list includes only products listed by the Council on Dental Therapeutics of the American Dental Association.

USES IN DENTISTRY

Antiseptics and disinfectants play a major role in the practice of modern dentistry. The battle to abolish infection continues and must be pursued by all available means. The dentist can do much to reduce the presence of pathogenic organisms and thereby greatly enhance the potential for an uneventful recovery from dental procedures. Disinfectants should be part of an overall sanitation program that includes good housekeeping and routine disinfection of the operatory. In addition, all objects that come into contact with the patient and cannot be sterilized by conventional methods (e.g., the practitioner's hands, high-speed handpieces) should be adequately treated with chemical agents. Table 43-2 lists the indications for the use of specific antiseptics and the concentrations in which they are readily available.

Antiseptics and disinfectants

Nonproprietary name	Proprietary name
Alcohols	
alcohol (ethanol)	—
isopropyl alcohol	—
Aldehydes	
formaldehyde	Formalin, Formaldehyde Solution
glutaraldehyde, acidic	Wavicide-01
glutaraldehyde, alkaline	Cidex 7, Sporicidin
Phenols and related compounds	
chlorothymol	—
creosote	
cresol	Lysol
eugenol	Red Cross Tooth Ache Medication
guaiacol	—
hexachlorophene	Septisol, pHisoHex
hexylresorcinol	S.T.37
orthophenylphenol	—
parachlorometaxylenol	Metasep, nu-FLOW
parachlorophenol	—
phenol	—
resorcinol	—
thymol	—
triclosan	—
Halogens	
Chlorine	
chloramine-T	—
chloroazodin	—
diluted sodium hypochlorite solution	—
oxychlorosene	Clorpactin
sodium hypochlorite solution	—

Nonproprietary name	Proprietary name
Iodine	
iodine solution	—
iodoform	—
poloxamer-iodine	Prepodyne
povidone-iodine	Betadine
thymol iodide	—
tincture of iodine	—
Biguanides	
chlorhexidine gluconate	Hibiclens, Hibitane
Surface-acting agents	
benzalkonium chloride	Zephiran
benzethonium chloride	Phemerol
cetylpyridinium chloride	Ceepryn
green soap	—
methylbenzethonium chloride	Diaparene
Heavy metals	
Organic mercurials	
hydroxyphenyl mercuric chloride	—
merbromin	Mercurochrome
mercocresols	Mercresin
nitromersol	Metaphen
phenylmercuric nitrate	Phe-Mer-Nite
thimerosal	Merthiolate
Silver compunds	
silver nitrate	—
silver protein	Argyrol S.S. 10%
toughened silver nitrate	
Oxidizing agents	
benzoyl peroxide	—
hydrogen peroxide	—
potassium permanganate	—

CITED REFERENCES

1. Crawford, J.J., ed. Clinical Asepsis in Dentistry, Dallas, Tex., Baylor School of Dentistry, 1974.
2. Crawford, J.J. Office sterilization and asepsis procedures in endodontics. Dental Clinics of North America **23:**717-735, 1979.
3. Council on Dental Therapeutics. Quaternary ammonium compounds not acceptable for disinfection of instruments and environmental surfaces in dentistry. Journal of the American Dental Association **97:**855-856, 1978.
4. Harrison, J.W., and Madonia, J.V. Antimicrobial effectiveness of parachlorophenol. Oral Surgery, Oral Medicine, and Oral Pathology **30:**267-275, 1970.
5. Kundsin, R.B., and Walter, C.W. The surgical scrub—practical consideration. Archives of Surgery **107:**75-77, 1973.
6. Leinbach, R.C. Bacterial endocarditis prophylaxis: a comparison of current theory and practice. Journal of Dental Medicine **20:**66-71, 1965.
7. Lowbury, E.J.L., and Lilly, H.A. Use of 4% chlorhexidine detergent solution (Hibiscrub) and other methods of skin disinfection. British Medical Journal **1:**510-515, 1973.

8. Martin, J.H., Bishop, J.G., Guentherman, R.H., and Dorman, H.L. Cellular response to prolonged application of dilute hydrogen peroxide. Journal of Periodontology **39:**208-210, 1968.

9. Newman, M.G., Socransky, S.S., Savitt, E.D., Propas, D.A., and Crawford, A. Studies of the microbiology of periodontics. Journal of Periodontology **47:**373-379, 1976.

10. Sweet, J.B., Gill, V.J., Chusid, M.J., and Elin, R.J. Nitroblue tetrazolium and *Limulus* assays for bacteremia after dental extraction: effect of topical antiseptics. Journal of the American Dental Association **96:**276-281, 1978.

11. Winslow, M.B., and Millstone, S.H. Bacteremia after prophylaxis. Journal of Periodontology **36:**371-374, 1965.

GENERAL REFERENCES

Bain, M.J. Chlorhexidine in dentistry—review. New Zealand Dental Journal **76:**49-54, 1980.

Block, S.S. Disinfection, Sterilization, and Preservation, ed. 2. Philadelphia, Lea & Febiger, 1977.

Cooley, R.L., and Lubow, R.M. Hepatitis B—A review of the problem for the dentist. Clinical Preventive Dentistry **3:**16-18, 1981.

Council on Dental Therapeutics. Accepted Dental Therapeutics, ed. 39. Chicago, American Dental Association, 1982.

Davis, J.M., and Dineen, P. Local antiseptics. In Modell, W., ed. Drugs of Choice, St. Louis, The C. V. Mosby Co., 1984.

Gilmore, O.J.A. A reappraisal of the use of antiseptics in surgical practice. Annals of the Royal College of Surgeons **59:**73-103, 1977.

Gurney, B.F. Review of phenol. Dental Digest **78:**204-207, 1972.

Gurney, B.F. Substituted phenols 1. Hydroxy phenols, guaiacol, eugenol. Dental Digest **78:**260-262, 1972.

Gurney, B.F. Substituted phenols 2. Cresols, cresylacetate, formo-cresol. Dental Digest **78:**314-316, 1972.

Harvey, S.C. Antiseptics and disinfectants; fungicides; ectoparasiticides. In Gilman, A.G., Goodman, L.S., and Gilman, A., eds. Goodman and Gilman's The Pharmacological Basis of Therapeutics, ed. 6. New York, Macmillan, Inc., 1980.

Topical antiseptics and antibiotics. Medical Letter on Drugs and Therapeutics **19:**83-84, 1977.

SPECIAL SUBJECTS IN PHARMACOLOGY AND THERAPEUTICS

44 Management of pain and anxiety

John A. Yagiela
Stanley F. Malamed

"The threat and fear of pain constitutes one of the greatest obstacles to the acceptance of dental services in the United States."[18] This quote from the National Institute of Dental Research underscores an indisputable fact; dental treatment produces at least some degree of anxiety in the majority of the population. Apprehension is in all likelihood the leading contributor to untoward reactions in the dental chair; it is also the most common reason given for avoiding dental care by the 40% to 50% of the population who routinely do so.[5] Fear of the dentist may evolve from many sources, including past traumatic experiences, concerns about physical loss and disfigurement, observing anxiety in others (particularly one's mother), and exposure to "horror stories" by friends or the mass media.[31]

Studies on the palliation of nociceptive inputs within the central nervous system by nonnoxious stimuli,[20,25] inhibitory pathways and neurotransmitters,[36] and placebo responses[22] provide cogent examples of the mind's ability to modulate incoming signals and to interpret and respond to them in the context of the individual's environs, background, and emotional state. An important feature of anxiety is that it can markedly lower the pain tolerance.[31] Thus, stimuli that might otherwise be mildly discomforting cause suffering and overt reactions when experienced in a threatening environment by an anxious person. The increased pain that is felt in turn magnifies the level of anxiety, and a vicious cycle is born.

Local anesthetics, by providing a highly efficient means of blocking nociceptive transmissions from reaching the central nervous system, revolutionized the practice of dentistry in the twentieth century. Not even the most successful local anesthetic, however, can eliminate all painful stimuli from the dental experience. Indeed, the process of injecting the anesthetic solution is itself viewed by many patients as the most unpleasant aspect of restorative dentistry. Because local anesthetics do not relieve anxiety directly, they cannot ease the stress in a dental phobic nor calm the fears of an unruly child.

It is clear that to be maximally effective a comprehensive program for pain control must address all of the factors that influence the pain reaction. Local anesthetics and the analgesic drugs are used to block nociception specifically and are discussed, respectively, in Chapter 17 and in Chapters 20 and 21. Various techniques to provide a nonthreatening dental environment and to psychologically allay fear and apprehension are of unquestioned importance but lie beyond the scope of this textbook. In this chapter are described the pharmacologic approaches to the management of anxiety in the dental patient.

EVOLUTION OF PAIN AND ANXIETY CONTROL

As is recounted in Chapter 18, two dentists, Horace Wells and William Morton, were largely responsible for the introduction of general anesthesia into medical practice. That dentists should have played so prominent a role in the discovery of anesthesia is understandable in that more surgical procedures, however minor, were performed in the 1840s by dentists than by other health professionals. General anesthesia was thus the earliest method of pain control in dentistry, and it remained the most popular until the widespread adoption of local anesthesia in the late 1920s.

Although general anesthesia was employed successfully for many years, the dangers associated

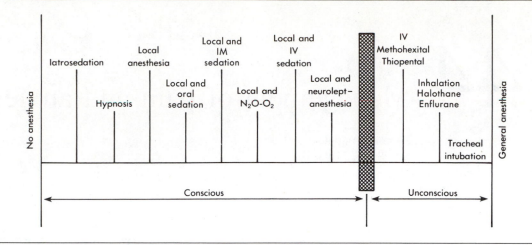

Figure 44-1. Total spectrum of pain and anxiety control in dentistry.

with its use were unacceptable to many dentists and to their patients. The American Society of Dental Surgeons went so far as to forbid anesthesia for minor operations, such as dental extractions.[18] Realizing that subhypnotic amounts of chloroform could provide analgesia and a calming effect in the conscious patient, Austin Hewitt became, in the late 1800s, one of the first clinicians to employ what would now be recognized as a form of conscious sedation. Another pioneer, W.H. DeFord, advocated, in an anesthesia textbook for dentistry published in 1908, the use of nitrous oxide as a sedative.[6] His recommendation had apparently little impact, however, for nitrous oxide continued to be used primarily as a general anesthetic for three more decades. The usual method consisted of administering 100% nitrous oxide until consciousness was lost, quickly performing the requisite dental procedure (''smash and grab''), and then giving 100% oxygen until the patient recovered. The loss of consciousness was induced not so much by the nitrous oxide as it was by the state of anoxia accompanying its use without oxygen.

The modern form of nitrous oxide and oxygen conscious sedation evolved in the 1940s and 1950s. After achieving widespread use in Denmark and other countries in the late 1950s, the technique was popularized in the United States by Harry Langa and other dentists who offered postgraduate courses on the subject. Eventually, nitrous oxide sedation became a standard component of the undergraduate dental curriculum.

The intravenous administration of drugs for pain and anxiety control began about 1932, with the use of hexobarbital for general anesthesia by the English dentist S.L. Drummond-Jackson. Through the pioneering work of John Lundy and others, thiopental was introduced for oral surgical procedures a few years later. The first refined method for intravenous conscious sedation is generally credited to Niels Jorgensen, who began using in 1945 what later became known as the Loma Linda (or Jorgensen) technique.[19]

SPECTRUM OF PAIN AND ANXIETY CONTROL

Currently, a large number of drugs and techniques are available to obtund the pain reaction. Taken together, these various approaches constitute the spectrum of pain and anxiety control in dentistry (Figure 44-1).

Conscious sedation versus general anesthesia

A vital distinction must be drawn between conscious sedation methods of pain control, which permit a patient to remain awake, and general anesthetic regimens, which render the individual comatose. Conscious sedation may be defined as ''a depressed level of consciousness that retains the patient's ability to independently and continuously maintain an airway and respond appropriately to physical stimulation or verbal command,'' whereas ''general anesthesia is a controlled state of unconsciousness, accompanied by partial or complete loss of protective reflexes, including inability to independently maintain an airway and respond pur-

Table 44-1. Comparison of conscious sedation versus general anesthesia for pain and anxiety control

Conscious sedation	General anesthesia
Patient conscious, cooperative	Patient unconscious
Protective reflexes intact	Protective reflexes absent
Vital signs stable	Vital signs labile
Risk very low	Risk relatively high
No special patient preparation necessary	Preoperative medication, fasting, laboratory testing required
Operator may perform sedation	Nonoperating anesthetist needed
Recuperation often rapid	Recuperation often prolonged, recovery area necessary
Suitable for the dental office	Best performed in the hospital
May be ineffective for some patients	Uniformly effective

posefully to physical stimulation or verbal command.''[29] By definition, general anesthesia represents a much greater intrusion on body functions; Table 44-1 lists the salient clinical differences that derive from this fact.

Conscious sedation coupled with local anesthesia is inherently quite safe and effective. Unfortunately, overzealous medication can convert a conscious sedation case into one of general anesthesia, with all of its attendant risks. A review of life-threatening reactions to ''sedation'' in dental patients[12] indicates that the following is a prescription for potential disaster: (1) administering greater than maximum recommended doses, multiple CNS depressants, or both in attempts to sedate the difficult patient; (2) failing to properly monitor the patient intraoperatively and postoperatively; and (3) lacking the training and resources to recognize and effectively treat adverse drug effects that may occur.

In oral and maxillofacial surgery, several forms of ''ultralight'' anesthesia are employed for short surgical procedures.[10,24] These intravenous (IV) techniques blur the distinctions between sedation and anesthesia as represented in Table 44-1. Although possessing an enviable record of safety,[1] ultralight anesthesia may cause respiratory depression[7] and lead to cardiac arrhythmias[32]; thus, practitioners who use it must be fully trained in outpatient general anesthesia for dentistry.[10]

Indications for use

The decision to use a pharmacologic method of pain and anxiety control in addition to, or in lieu of, local anesthesia should be based on careful consideration of the patient's medical history, his current psychologic and physical state, and the procedure that is planned. Obviously, a primary indication for use of conscious sedation or general anesthesia is the apprehensive patient. Such techniques are also invaluable for controlling motor disturbances, whether they be the uncoordinated writhing of a patient with cerebral palsy or the gagging of a susceptible person during the taking of an impression. Sedative and analgesic drugs may be particularly indicated to relieve the physical and emotional stress of treatment in an intolerant individual (e.g., a patient with cardiovascular disease, adrenal insufficiency, or asthma) or in a healthy person when the stress is likely to be great (e.g., extraction of bone-impacted third molars). Finally, these methods of pain control may be essential in cases of local anesthetic failure or with very small children or mentally retarded patients.

The remainder of this chapter is devoted to a discussion of the agents in current use, their routes of administration, and the advantages and disadvantages of each. Space limitations prohibit consideration of all individual drugs useful in comprehensive pain control, but sufficient examples of effective drug regimens are provided to cover virtually all situations amenable to conscious sedation and pain control. Several forms of ultralight anesthesia used for short surgical procedures in dentistry will also be mentioned.

ORAL SEDATION

The oral route is generally the safest and most frequently employed route of drug administration. It possesses advantages over parenteral routes that make it quite useful in selected situations calling for the management of pain and anxiety. There are also significant drawbacks that limit its routine use.

Advantages

The advantages of oral medication include almost universal acceptability, low cost, ease of administration, and relative safety. Patients are accustomed to taking drugs by mouth, so the dentist will rarely encounter an adult patient objecting to this method of sedation (or premedication as it is often referred to). However, the young child may be an unwilling recipient of orally administered drugs. Overdosage, idiosyncrasy, allergy, and other side effects may occur whenever drugs are administered, but such reactions are less likely to arise when drugs are given orally, and if they do develop they are normally less intense. Even so, a cavalier attitude toward oral sedation must be avoided, because potentially fatal reactions have occurred with even the safest of drugs.[2]

Disadvantages

The disadvantages of oral sedation include delayed onset, unreliable drug absorption, inability to easily regulate the intensity of drug effect, and often a prolonged duration of action.

Orally administered drugs must be absorbed from the stomach and small intestine in order to reach the systemic circulation. For most drugs used in conscious sedation, clinical effects are not evident for approximately 30 minutes, a delay known as the "latent period." As drug absorption continues, a peak blood concentration equivalent to the greatest degree of clinical effectiveness (most profound pain or anxiety relief) is reached. With most drugs, this maximal effect occurs about 60 minutes after ingestion.

The inability to titrate is another major disadvantage of the oral route. Titration is defined as the administration of small increments of a drug until a desired clinical effect is observed. The ability to titrate enhances the control that the person administering the drug has over its ultimate effect, there being no need to guess the correct dose for a particular patient. Figure 3-1 shows the frequency with which increasing doses of a drug elicit a stated response. A quantal dose-response curve such as this provides information on the minimum dose of a drug that will evoke the desired effect in a given proportion of the population. It should be noted that approximately 70% of subjects will show a response to a very narrow range of doses but that 15% of subjects will need a higher dose to experience the same effect and 15% would react at a lower dose. Titration permits the clinician to adjust for individual patient responsiveness.

Because of the prolonged latent period, titration is not feasible with oral administration. The practitioner must instead administer a predetermined dose, based on information obtained from the patient (medical history, previous drug reactions, age, weight) and from clinical experience (degree of anxiety or pain control required). Once a drug is taken orally, it is inconvenient to provide additional medication should the initial dose produce an inadequate response. A second dose may be given, but the 30-minute latent period makes this an unattractive option. Should the patient exhibit clinical signs of drug overdose after oral administration, there is usually no effective way of reversing the effect.

Another disadvantage of oral administration is the prolonged duration of action, which for many drugs is approximately 3 to 4 hours. This duration is often unacceptable for dental therapy because the patient will remain under the influence of the drug postoperatively and be unable to leave the dental office unescorted. Patients receiving oral medications for pain and anxiety control before or after surgery must be cautioned against ingesting alcohol or driving or operating potentially dangerous machinery for up to 24 hours.

Clinical applications

Oral drugs may be employed safely and effectively for the management of pain in the postoperative period and for the control of anxiety. Because of differences in patient responsiveness and the inability to titrate, the oral route is best reserved for the following applications:

1. Sedation the night before dental therapy to ensure restful sleep.

2. Preoperative anxiety reduction. If prescribed to be taken at home before the appointment, the dosage should be light enough to permit the patient to reach the dental office without difficulty, at which time more profound sedation may be achieved with more controllable techniques. If the medication is to be administered in the dental office, a light to moderate level of sedation may be sought.

3. Preoperative and postoperative pain relief. A large number of drugs are commonly administered via the oral route for the reduction of anxiety in dental practice. The majority of these are classified as either antianxiety drugs or sedative-hypnotics. Some of the most clinically useful of these agents are discussed below.

Antianxiety drugs. A number of benzodiazepine derivatives are currently available for use as antianxiety agents. There is very little difference in clinical effectiveness between these drugs, but important pharmacokinetic dissimilarities have caused several agents to be used more than others.

Diazepam is the most frequently employed benzodiazepine in dental practice. Available in 2, 5, and 10 mg tablets, it reaches maximal clinical effectiveness in approximately 1 hour. The average dose for a 70 kg patient is 5 to 10 mg. Elderly patients appear to be unusually sensitive to diazepam, and a halving of the dose is often indicated. Conversely, children appear to be resistant to the drug when the dose is calculated as a fraction of the adult dose on the basis of age, body weight, or surface area. A proper dose for young children is 0.2 to 0.5 mg/kg.[33]

Chlordiazepoxide is somewhat less rapidly absorbed than is diazepam, and it is not employed as frequently for preoperative anxiety reduction. Available in 5 mg tablets and in 5, 10, and 25 mg capsules, chlordiazepoxide is the only benzodiazepine currently sold under its nonproprietary name, making it the least expensive agent in this group. From 5 to 25 mg may be administered to the adult patient, depending on the degree of apprehension. Chlordiazepoxide has not been used much in young children, and it is not recommended for pediatric patients under the age of 6.

Flurazepam and temazepam are benzodiazepines classified as sedative-hypnotics. Both drugs are available in 15 and 30 mg capsules and are useful for treating insomnia the evening before dental therapy or as a means of achieving more intense (or perhaps more obvious) sedation before the scheduled appointment. A 30 mg capsule is usually administered 1 hour before bedtime; the 15 mg form is given to elderly or debilitated patients. Flurazepam has a faster onset of action and a longer history of clinical use; temazepam is not transformed to active metabolites and therefore may cause less drug hangover.

A number of other benzodiazepines are available for treatment of anxiety; of these, clorazepate and alprazolam compare favorably with diazepam and chlordiazepoxide in rate of onset and should be useful for conscious sedation in dentistry.

Sedative-hypnotics. Until the advent of the benzodiazepines, the barbiturates were the most commonly employed drugs for the management of anxiety. Although they are still employed in dentistry, their use has declined in recent years. The barbiturates are usually classified according to their duration of clinical activity after oral administration. Only the short-acting and ultra-short-acting barbiturates are of use in the management of preoperative anxiety. Short-acting drugs include pentobarbital and secobarbital. Although most of the ultra-short-acting barbiturates, such as thiopental and methohexital, are reserved for intravenous administration, hexobarbital is marketed in an oral dosage form. Pentobarbital and secobarbital are available in 50 and 100 mg capsules and are used for anxiety reduction the evening before the dental appointment and 1 hour before dental therapy if a more profound level of CNS depression than would be obtained with the benzodiazepines is desired. (Pentobarbital is also available in a 30 mg capsule and in an 18.2 mg/5 ml elixir, secobarbital in a 100 mg tablet and in a 22 mg/5 ml elixir.) The usual dosage for a 70 kg patient is 100 mg of either drug and 2 to 3 mg/kg for children. Hexobarbital is supplied in 260 mg tablets. Advantages to its use include a relatively rapid onset of action (15 minutes), a maximal effect achieved within 30 minutes, and a short duration of action (30 to 90 minutes). Hexobarbital is useful when rapid relief of anxiety is necessary for dental therapy and other more controllable techniques (inhalation, IV) are unavailable. The usual dose for an adult is one tablet 30 minutes before the appointment.

Chloral hydrate is a nonbarbiturate sedative-hypnotic most often used in pediatric dentistry. Although it may be effective in adults, chloral hydrate offers no significant advantage over other sedative-hypnotics, and it is rarely prescribed for adult dental patients. For use in children, the agent is available as a 500 mg/5 ml solution. The usual dose for a child is between 25 and 75 mg/kg up to a maximum of 1 gm. The agent has a margin of safety between therapeutic and lethal doses similar to that of the barbiturates.

For reasons largely other than pharmacologic, ethanol in the form of an alcoholic beverage can be of particular use in the apprehensive adult. Most adults are familiar with the soporific effect of ethanol and with their own required dose for sedation (normally the equivalent of 1 ox of pure, or 200 proof, ethanol). Perhaps as tranquilizing as the drug itself is the warm ambience that a glass or two of wine can lend to the dental waiting room.

Antihistamines. Hydroxyzine and promethazine are also commonly prescribed agents for the relief of anxiety in dental situations. Both drugs are classified as antihistamines and possess antiemetic and anxiolytic actions. Hydroxyzine is one of the most popular premedicants in pediatric dentistry. Rapidly absorbed from the gastrointestinal tract, hydroxyzine has an onset of action of 15 to 30 minutes, with a maximal effect occurring within 2 hours. Hydroxyzine hydrochloride is available in 10, 25, 50, and 100 mg tablets and as a syrup of 10 mg/5 ml, and the pamoate salt is available in 25, 50, and 100 mg capsules and as a 25 mg/5 ml suspension. Dosage will vary between 10 and 100 mg, depending on the size, emotional state, and activity of the patient. The incidence of adverse reactions with hydroxyzine is extremely low, and fatal overdosage has never been reported with its administration. Promethazine is a phenothiazine derivative. As with hydroxyzine, promethazine finds particular usefulness in pediatric dentistry, where it is employed as a single agent or in combination with an opioid analgesic. When used as the sole agent for sedation, promethazine is indicated for the management of mildly apprehensive patients. Given orally or parenterally in combination with meperidine or alphaprodine, this drug is employed for the management of disruptive children. The oral dosage range of promethazine is from 12.5 to 50 mg, based on the age or weight of the patient.

INTRAMUSCULAR ROUTE

Intramuscular (IM) administration is a parenteral technique possessing advantages over the oral route of administration, which makes it useful in certain circumstances for pain and anxiety control in dentistry. However, IM administration suffers in comparison with inhalation and IV techniques, and it is the least employed of the four routes discussed in this chapter.

Advantages

The advantages of IM administration over the oral route include its more rapid onset of action and the shorter time for maximal drug effect to develop. In addition, the absorption of drugs into the circulatory system will usually be more reliable than is the case with oral ingestion. Thus, a given dose of a drug will produce a more consistent clinical effect. Patient cooperation is not as essential as it is with other techniques described in this chapter. This advantage is important in management of the recalcitrant child or handicapped individual. The patient need only be restrained momentarily while the drug is administered.

Disadvantages

The disadvantages of the IM route include the latent period (10 minutes or more depending on the drugs used), which makes titration impossible, the inability to retrieve the drug should signs of toxicity develop, poor patient acceptance of injections, a prolonged duration of action, which requires that the patient be escorted from the dental office by a responsible adult, and the possibility of local tissue injury from either the drug or the injection. There are several anatomical locations available for IM injection: (1) the mid-deltoid region, the most commonly used site in adults, (2) the upper outer quadrant of the gluteal region, and (3) the anterolateral aspect of the thigh, the site of choice for children and an excellent spot for all IM injections. Before using any site, however, the administrator should become familiar with the anatomical structures in the region and be capable of avoiding them during injection.

Clinical applications

Because of the significant disadvantages of the IM route, it is not widely used in clinical dentistry. Although the route can be used to administer drugs for the control of pain and anxiety, the inability to titrate agents accurately makes it unwise to attempt to reach deep levels of sedation unless the administrator is trained in general anesthesia. In adult patients, there are few indications for giving drugs by the IM route. In the handicapped patient and in the recalcitrant child, however, techniques that require cooperation (inhalation, IV injection) may prove impossible, and the IM route may be the only effective means of conscious sedation available.[16] Thus, IM injection is best indicated for (1) light to moderate sedation in uncooperative patients, and (2) pain control only for patients in whom it is difficult to achieve adequate analgesia with local anesthetics.

Sedative and antianxiety drugs. The use of diazepam by the IM route is not generally recommended because tissue irritation may occur and because diazepam is one of the few drugs that is less effective and less reliable clinically after IM injection than after oral administration.[13,21]

The usual adult dose of pentobarbital is 100 to 200 mg IM. The dose for children (up to 25 kg) is 2 to 4 mg/kg. Barbiturates, particularly in low doses, may increase the responsiveness to painful stimuli. Adequate pain control is therefore essential for these patients. Overdosage produces respiratory depression.

Hydroxyzine and promethazine are each administered to children in a dose of 1 mg/kg. For adults, the dose of promethazine is 25 to 50 mg and that of hydroxyzine 50 to 100 mg.

Opioid analgesics Opioids are primarily used alone for the management of intense pain, because their effectiveness as sedatives is inconsistent and their side effects in large doses make them potentially hazardous. Nevertheless, they are often combined with one or more CNS depressants for sedation, especially in pediatric dentistry. Meperidine is frequently used in combination with the barbiturates to help overcome their tendency to produce hyperalgesia and with other drugs (e.g., promethazine) to produce a state resembling neuroleptanalgesia (see Chapter 19). The usual adult dose is between 50 and 100 mg, but the pediatric dose should vary with the weight of the patient (1 to 2 mg/kg).

Alphaprodine is a phenylpiperidine derivative related to meperidine in both molecular structure and pharmacologic profile. Alphaprodine has gained some popularity in dentistry, especially in pedodontics, because it is rapidly effective after parenteral administration and because it has a relatively short duration of action (1 to 2 hours). Commensurate with the drug's fast onset is the rate at which undesirable effects such as respiratory depression may develop.[27] The dentist must be aware of this problem and be prepared to respond quickly should an adverse reaction occur. (Opioid-induced respiratory depression may be readily reversed with 0.01 mg/kg naloxone preferably given intravenously.) The conventional adult dose is 40 to 60 mg; for children 0.3 to 0.6 mg/kg alphaprodine is commonly injected by pediatric dentists-submucosally in the mouth. This route avoids the unreliable intramuscular absorption of alphaprodine, promotes a rapid onset of effect, and may lead to more profound sedative and respiratory depressant effects. Promethazine or hydroxyzine is generally administered in the same syringe or as oral premedication.

Ketamine. First marketed in 1970, ketamine has not been extensively used in dentistry. Although a high incidence of delirium and other side effects are limiting insofar as the adult population is concerned, strong analgesia, minimal respiratory depression, and preservation of protective airway reflexes theoretically recommend it for use in pedodontics.[9,26] An IM injection of 3 to 4 mg/kg provides conscious dissociation for about 30 minutes (after a 5-minute latent period). Oral premedication with an antianxiety agent and inhalation of nitrous oxide and oxygen effectively double the working time. Atropine is generally administered with or before the ketamine to reduce salivary secretions.

INHALATION ROUTE

A variety of agents are administered via inhalation in order to produce general anesthesia. In dental practice, however, the inhalation route is synonymous with the use of nitrous oxide (N_2O) and oxygen (O_2). The first general anesthetic for conscious sedation, N_2O has been in use since 1844 in both medicine and dentistry. The advantages and disadvantages discussed below relate to the inhalation route in general and to the use of N_2O-O_2 in particular.

Advantages

The latent period for the inhalation route may be quite short. Drugs travel rapidly from the mouth or nose, through the lungs, and into the bloodstream. With some agents, like N_2O, clinical effects may become apparent as early as 15 to 30 seconds after inhalation. This short latent period can be used to advantage to permit titration of the drug. The administrator initially gives a small concentration of N_2O (10% to 15%) to the patient, waits 1 to 1½ minutes to judge clinical effectiveness, and then, if necessary, administers more N_2O in increments until the patient demonstrates the desired clinical signs and symptoms. The ease of titration is one reason inhalation sedation with N_2O-O_2 is considered by many to be the ideal sedative technique. Should a patient inadvertently receive too much or too little drug, the drug's effect can be rapidly (within 30 seconds) altered. The inhalation route is the only one in which the actions of a drug can be quickly adjusted in either direction. With IV administration, drug action can be enhanced very quickly, but it is not possible to lighten the degree of drug effect unless a specific pharmacologic antagonist is available.

When administration by inhalation ceases, recovery can be very rapid, which is a significant advantage in dentistry. Jastak and Orendurff[15] demonstrated that after the administration of 100% oxygen for a minimum of 3 to 5 minutes after N_2O-O_2 there is normally no residual effect on the patient's ability to operate a motor vehicle or other machinery. Patients need not be escorted home, and they may return to work or any other activity without restriction. It should be noted that there are stringent safety standards that must be met by the inhalation sedation units, including color coding of compressed gas cylinders, a pin index or other safety system to preclude the accidental switching of gases, minimum O_2 flow (e.g., 2 L), and an O_2 fail-safe valve to shut the machine off should O_2 delivery be interrupted. However, all mechanical devices can fail, and the administrator of N_2O is strongly urged not to rely solely on these fail-safe devices.[35] Careful technique and continuous observation of the patient will prove more effective in prevention of accidents than reliance on mechanical safe-guards. The reader is referred elsewhere for a more thorough discussion of safety features.[34]

Disadvantages

The disadvantages of inhalation sedation with N_2O-O_2 are few. Those that must be noted are the lack of potency of N_2O, the requirement for patient cooperation, the cost of and space needed for the equipment, the need for additional training of the dentist and staff, and occupational health hazards from trace anesthetic gases. When N_2O is used in conjunction with at least 30% oxygen, there will be a certain small proportion of patients in whom this technique will fail to produce its desired effect. However, to ensure against hypoxia, in no circumstances should this minimum concentration of oxygen be lessened. The vast majority of patients (75% to 80%) will experience the desired clinical effect between 30% and 40% N_2O, another 5% to 10% require between 40% and 50% N_2O, and the remaining 10% to 20% need either less than 30% or more than 50% N_2O.

A degree of patient cooperation is required for N_2O-O_2 to be effective. Success with this technique entails two factors: the ability of the patient to breathe through the nose and willingness to leave a nasal hood in place throughout the procedure. Difficulties arise in patients with chronic or acute sinus congestion, in mouth breathers, and in patients (e.g., claustrophobes and apprehensive children) who do not feel comfortable with the nasal hood in place.

Two minor disadvantages of the inhalation route are the size of the equipment and the additional training and expense required to safely administer N_2O-O_2. It is critically important that the dentist using this technique be well trained in all aspects of its clinical application. For this reason, it is strongly recommended that all dental staff using N_2O-O_2 sedation be properly trained according to the guidelines established by the American Association of Dental Schools.[4]

The possibility that chronic exposure to trace amounts of N_2O is deleterious to health has evoked considerable interest and concern on the part of the dental profession and has led to recommendations for minimizing the hazard.[17] Evidence concerning the toxic potential of N_2O in relation to long-term exposure is reviewed in Chapter 18.

Clinical applications

N_2O-O_2 by inhalation is the technique of choice for dental procedures of any length that require intraoperative anxiety control. Pain control, however, is not consistently obtained when N_2O-O_2 is employed as a single agent, and its use as an analgesic drug in lieu of local anesthesia is not recommended because of the high degree of effectiveness of local anesthetics and the increased incidence of unwanted side effects of N_2O that may accompany the increased concentration of N_2O required to produce profound analgesia. Inhalation sedation with N_2O-O_2 is highly effective in children and handicapped patients. It may also be useful as an adjunct to conscious sedation given by another means.

INTRAVENOUS ROUTE

The IV route represents the most effective method of ensuring predictable and adequate sedation in virtually all patients, for it makes possible the rapid attainment of blood concentrations at which drugs are clinically effective.

Advantages

The advantages of IV administration include a very short latent period, which ranges from approximately 10 to 30 seconds, the ability to titrate drugs, and the ability to enhance drug action rapidly. In clinical practice, the administrator will require 2 to 5 minutes to titrate a drug to a desired clinical level. An additional advantage of many intravenously administered drugs is that they produce variable periods of amnesia. Advantage may be taken of this amnesic period to carry out procedures that are feared by the patient, such as local anesthetic injection.

Disadvantages

The disadvantages of IV administration include the inability to reverse the actions of the drugs once they have been administered. Although it is possible to reverse the effects of some drugs (e.g., opioids and anticholinergics) through the use of specific antagonists, such is not the case with most agents. Another disadvantage of this route is that the rapid onset of action and the accentuated drug effects likely to be observed tend to magnify problems associated with drug overdosage or other side effects. Because of these factors, the dentist and dental staff must be well trained in the recognition and management of adverse reactions. Increasingly, states are requiring evidence of advanced training of one kind or another in anesthesiology before granting a permit to use IV sedation in clinical practice.

Patients must be cooperative if they are to receive drugs by the IV route; if they are not, venipuncture becomes very difficult. Many children will not permit venipuncture to be performed, and therefore IV sedation of children is often not desirable or even possible. A normal child who allows venipuncture probably does not require as profound a technique as IV sedation for dental treatment. Intraoral injection of local anesthetics may be administered with a little patience, and perhaps another technique of anxiety and fear reduction (for instance, inhalation) may be used in place of IV sedation. Handicapped (both physically and mentally) patients, on the other hand, are usually good candidates for IV drugs. These patients may prove to be unable to cooperate during dental therapy, but once they have received IV drugs they become readily manageable. Medical consultation before the contemplated procedure is usually recommended.

IV drug administration may not be suitable for all dentists. Although most dentists are uncomfortable during their early experiences with the technique, they gradually become more at ease as they gain clinical exposure and experience. However, a small percentage of practitioners will remain apprehensive about IV sedation and will be unable to provide dental care of normal quality. It is important to remember that regardless of the route of drug administration or the drug employed, the quality of dental care should never be compromised.

Indeed, it should be equal to or better than that expected without the use of drugs.

No technique of conscious sedation is a panacea, and IV administration is no exception. Although it is the most effective conscious sedation technique currently available, an occasional patient will be encountered in whom IV drugs will prove ineffective. Of course, agents can be administered intravenously until they do prove effective, but in many cases this course of action would constitute general anesthesia, and unless the dentist is well trained in the management of the unconscious patient, significant complications could develop.

Clinical applications

The IV route of administration is most frequently employed as a technique for management of the highly anxious dental patient. Drugs and techniques are available that permit effective anxiety control for varying lengths of time. In addition, with the increasing use of continuous IV infusion, it is easy to retitrate a drug should more time be needed to complete treatment.

IV drugs can sometimes be used for patients in whom it is difficult to achieve adequate pain control with local anesthesia alone. Although the use of IV opioid analgesics as the sole agent for pain control during dental therapy is usually unwarranted since high doses are required for this effect, smaller doses of opioids used in conjunction with local anesthesia will produce adequate pain control without significant increased risk to the patient.

Benzodiazepines. Diazepam administered via the IV route is a popular and effective technique for pharmacologic management of the anxious dental patient.[11] Available in a solution containing 5 mg/ml, it is administered *slowly* (5 mg/min) until the desired sedation level is attained. The dosage range is from 2 to 20 mg, with the average adult patient requiring approximately 15 mg. The duration of sedation is usually from 45 to 60 minutes. In more than 65% of all cases, an amnesic period, about 10 minutes in duration, is present at the onset of the procedure.[8,14] Diazepam is formulated in a viscous liquid and may irritate veins, leading to pain or thrombosis or both in up to 48% of patients receiving it.[28] Preparing the drug in an emulsified oil solvent appears to be an effective answer to this problem.[30]

Midazolam, a new water-soluble benzodiazepine, promises to supplement and possibly even replace diazepam for IV sedation when it becomes available for general use.[23] Midazolam combines all of the advantages of diazepam with three additional desirable attributes: little tendency to cause thrombophlebitis, a superior amnesic effect, and a very short elimination half-life (1.7 hours). The drug is about 50% more potent than diazepam and has a shorter duration of action.

Barbiturates. When administered intravenously, pentobarbital has a clinical action lasting from 2 to 3 hours. It is useful, therefore, for lengthy dental procedures. Barbiturates have the undesirable property of lowering a patient's pain reaction threshold, thereby making the patient overreact to pain. For this reason, pentobarbital is commonly employed with an opioid (e.g., meperidine) when used intravenously. Pentobarbital solution is available in a concentration of 50 mg/ml; when titrated (50 mg/min), 50 to 200 mg is usually required for adequate sedation.

Opioids. Meperidine is the most commonly used opioid analgesic in dentistry. Available in many dosage forms (e.g., 25, 50, and 100 mg/ml), it is often diluted with sterile saline to a 10 mg/ml solution before injection. It should be administered after the primary drug (diazepam or pentobarbital). When used in this way, only minimal doses of meperidine (25 to 50 mg) are necessary for increased analgesia and sedation. Adverse effects observed in ambulatory patients include nausea, vomiting, and orthostatic hypotension. They are dose related and are observed only infrequently when 50 mg of meperidine or less is employed.[3,18] Opioids used in addition to meperidine include alphaprodine, butorphanol, fentanyl, and pentazocine.

Anticholinergics. Scopolamine is sometimes used during IV sedation to inhibit salivary secretion, enhance the sedative action of other drugs, and produce amnesia. The dose is usually 0.3 to 0.6 mg. Scopolamine may produce disorientation and delirium in a small percentage of individuals, an effect that can be reversed by injection of physostigmine. Because of the increased likelihood of these unwanted effects in children and the elderly, scopolamine is infrequently employed in patients under age 6 or above age 65.

Multiple drug regimens. Several techniques of IV sedation involving two or more medications have been devised over the last 4 decades. Of these, the method popularized by Neils Jorgensen deserves special comment. The Jorgensen technique employs a combination of three drugs administered intravenously: pentobarbital, meperidine, and scopolamine. This technique has been employed by many dentists throughout the world, and it has proved to be a highly effective and safe procedure for management of the anxious dental patient requiring 2 to 4 hours of sedation.[18,19] Although indications for its clinical use today are decreasing, it still remains one of the more valuable techniques of IV sedation available.

The first drug, pentobarbital, is infused at a rate of 20 mg per minute until a basal level of sedation is attained. Then, an additional increment of 10% of the sedative dose is injected. Finally, a 5 ml solution of 25 mg meperidine and 0.32 mg scopolamine is administered at a ratio of 1 ml/20 mg pentobarbital (up to 5 ml).

GENERAL ANESTHESIA

General anesthesia was the first technique of pain and anxiety control introduced into dental and medical practice. Although still employed extensively in medicine, the use of general anesthesia in dentistry has been declining since the introduction of conscious sedation in the 1950s. There are several advantages to the use of general anesthesia—rapid onset of action, high efficiency, and reliability. Its disadvantages, however, greatly outweigh its advantages for the general practitioner. These include an increased risk to the patient and the requirement of an intensive training program in general anesthesia to prepare the dentist to safely manage the unconscious patient. Most general anesthetics employed today in dentistry are used for oral surgical procedures. Whenever general anesthesia is used, a team approach is necessary. In this approach, the dentist serves as the surgeon, performing the dental procedure, while a second person assumes the role of anesthesiologist, maintaining the patient's airway and monitoring vital signs throughout the procedure. On many occasions, a third person is engaged as the surgical assistant, responsible for suctioning and assisting whenever necessary.

Methohexital is an ultra-short-acting barbiturate that is frequently employed to induce general anesthesia or provide ultralight general anesthesia suitable for removal of impacted third molars. This agent has been included in several conscious sedation techniques, but its use for this purpose should be carefully scrutinized.[10] Because of the drug's potent CNS depressant actions, it is recommended that the use of methohexital be limited to those dentists who have completed at least 1 year of training in general anesthesia.

The most common method of using methohexital as a single agent is called the *minimal incremental technique*.[24] A dose of 1 mg/kg is given intravenously, which provides anesthesia of several minutes' duration. Afterward, small increments of drug (e.g., 20 mg) are injected to maintain deep sedation or ultralight general anesthesia. In order to avoid drug cumulation, this method is best limited to 200 mg drug and to 20 minutes of operating time.

A popular offshoot of the incremental technique is to employ drugs such as diazepam and meperidine (or fentanyl) for a base level of conscious sedation and then to inject small amounts of methohexital as needed for stressful manipulations in the course of a procedure. This approach provides a longer duration of sedation and less need for the ultra-short-acting barbiturate. It is advisable to administer local anesthetics for pain relief and oxygen to help prevent hypoxia with all such methods of deep sedation and general anesthesia.

SUMMARY

By means of one or more of the techniques described earlier for conscious sedation plus local anesthesia, it is possible for the dentist to manage 99% of all patients seeking treatment. These techniques will prove successful only if the patient suffers no adverse effects from them and if the quality of dental care provided during these procedures is not compromised. The ultimate goal in patient management should be to eliminate the need for the use of these techniques. To achieve this, the dentist and staff must make a conscious effort to make the patient comfortable through their actions and attitudes in the dental office. The drugs and techniques discussed in this chapter, when employed as described, can produce effective sedation or analgesia, or both, in most dental patients. All drugs, however, can cause undesirable reactions, most of which are unpleasant and some of which may be dangerous. In an effort to minimize these effects, the least profound route of administration that is effective for a given patient should be employed. Table 43-2 summarizes the recommended techniques of conscious sedation.

Table 44-2. Common routes of administering sedation in the dental office

Route	Control		Recommended safe sedation levels
	Titrate	*Rapid reverse*	
Oral	No	No	Light only
IM	No	No	Adults—light, moderate
			Children—light, moderate, profound
IV	Yes	No (most drugs)	Adults—light, moderate, profound
		Yes (opioids)	Children—light, moderate, profound*
Inhalation	Yes	Yes	Any level of sedation

From Malamed, S.F. Handbook of Medical Emergencies in the Dental Office, ed. 2. St. Louis, The C.V. Mosby Co., 1982.
*There is little need for intravenous sedation in normal, healthy children. Most children who accept a venipuncture will also permit a local anesthetic to be administered intraorally. Intravenous sedation is of great benefit, however, in the management of handicapped children.

CITED REFERENCES

1. ASOS anesthesia morbidity and mortality survey. Journal of Oral Surgery **32:**733-738, 1974.
2. Berger, R., Green, G., and Melnick, A. Cardiac arrest caused by oral diazepam intoxication. Clinical Pediatrics **14:**842-844, 1975.
3. Ceravolo, F.J., Meyers, H., Baraff, L.S., and Bennett, C.R. Full dentition periodontal surgery utilizing intravenous conscious-sedation. Journal of Periodontology **51:**462-464, 1980.
4. Curricular guidelines for comprehensive control of pain and anxiety in dentistry. Journal of Dental Education **44:**279-286, 1980.
5. Curson, I., and Coplans, M.P. The need for sedation in conservative dentistry: An investigation in the inner London area. British Dental Journal **128:**19-22, 1970.
6. DeFord, W.H. Lectures on General Anesthetics in Dentistry. Kansas City, Mo., John T. Nolde Mfg. Co., 1908.
7. Dionne, R.A., Driscoll, E.J., Gelfman, S.S., Sweet, J.B., Butler, D.P., and Wirdzek, P.R. Cardiovascular and respiratory response to intravenous diazepam, fentanyl, and methohexital in dental outpatients. Journal of Oral Surgery **39:**343-349, 1981.
8. Driscoll, E.J., Smilack, J.S., Lightbody, P.M., and Fiorucci, R.D. Sedation with intravenous diazepam. Journal of Oral Surgery **30:**332-343, 1972.
9. Duperon, D.F., and Jedrychowski, J.R. Preliminary report on the use of ketamine in pediatric dentistry. Pediatric Dentistry **5:**75-78, 1983.
10. Foreman, P.A. Control of the anxiety/pain complex in dentistry. Oral Surgery, Oral Medicine, and Oral Pathology **37:**337-349, 1974.
11. Foreman, P.A., Neels, R., and Willetts, P.W. Diazepam in dentistry. Anesthesia Progress **15:**253-259, 1968.
12. Goodson, J.M., and Moore, P.A. Life-threatening reactions after pedodontic sedation: an assessment of narcotic, local anesthetic, and antiemetic drug interaction. Journal of the American Dental Association **107:**239-245, 1983.
13. Greenblatt, D.J., and Shader, R.I. Benzodiazepines in Clinical Practice. New York, Raven Press, 1974.
14. Gregg, J.M., Ryan, D.E., and Levin, K.H. The amnesic actions of diazepam. Journal of Oral Surgery **32:**651-664, 1974.
15. Jastak, J.T., and Orendurff, D. Recovery from nitrous sedation. Anesthesia Progress **22:**113-116, 1975.
16. Jensen, S.T., Coke, J.M., and Cohen, L. Intramuscular sedation technique. Journal of the American Dental Association **100:**700-702, 1980.
17. Jones, T.W., and Greenfield, W. Position paper of the ADA ad hoc committee on trace anesthetics as a potential health hazard in dentistry. Journal of the American Dental Association **95:**751-756, 1977.
18. Jorgensen, N.B., and Hayden, J., Jr. Sedation, Local and General Anesthesia in Dentistry, ed. 3. Philadelphia, Lea & Febiger, 1980.
19. Jorgensen, N.B., and Leffingwell, F.E. Premedication in dentistry. Journal of the Southern California State Dental Association **21:**25-30, 1953.
20. Kerr, F.W.L. Pain: a central inhibitory balance theory. Mayo Clinic Proceedings **50:**685-690, 1975.
21. Kortilla, K., and Linnoila, M. Absorption and sedative effects of diazepam after oral administration and intramuscular administration into the vastus lateralis muscle and the deltoid muscle. British Journal of Anaesthesia **47:**857-862, 1975.
22. Levine, J.D., Gordon, N.C., and Fields, H.L. The mechanism of placebo analgesia. Lancet **2:**654-657, 1978.
23. Maisel, G.M. Midazolam: second generation benzodiazepine. Anesthesia Progress **27:**159-160, 1980.
24. McDonald, D. Methohexitone in dentistry. Australian Dental Journal **25:**335-342, 1980.
25. Melzack, R., and Wall, P.D. Pain mechanisms: a new theory. Science **150:**971-979, 1965.
26. O'Brien, D.N., and Kim, K.C. An evaluation of ketamine, droperidol, and nitrous oxide in pedodontic outpatients. Journal of Dentistry for Children **42:**31-36, 1975.
27. Okuji, D.M. Hypoxic encephalopathy after the administration of alphaprodine hydrochloride. Journal of the American Dental Association **103:**50-52, 1981.
28. Olesen, A.S., and Hüttel, M.S. Local reactions to I.V. diazepam in three different formulations. British Journal of Anaesthesia **52:**609-611, 1980.
29. Report—meeting of ADA Council on Dental Education Ad Hoc Committee on Anesthesiology. Anesthesia Progress **29:**24-25, 1982.
30. Rosenbaum, N.L. A new formulation of diazepam for intravenous sedation in dentistry: a clinical evaluation. British Dental Journal **153:**192-193, 1982.
31. Scott, D.S., and Hirschman, R. Psychological aspects of dental anxiety in adults. Journal of the American Dental Association **104:**27-31, 1982.
32. Tolas, A.G., Pflug, A.E., and Halter, J.B. Neurohumorally induced cardiac dysrhythmias during nitrous oxide-oxygen-thiopental anesthesia. Journal of Oral and Maxillofacial Surgery **41:**649-652, 1983.
33. Trapp, L.D. Pharmacologic management of pain and anxiety. In Stewart, R.E., Barber, T.K., Troutman, K.C., and Wei, S.H.Y., eds. Pediatric Dentistry, St. Louis, The C.V. Mosby Co., 1981.
34. Trieger, N. Pain Control. Berlin, Quintessence Books, 1974.
35. Upton, L.G., and Robert, R.C., Jr. Hazard in administering nitrous oxide analgesia: report of case. Journal of the American Dental Association **94:**696-697, 1977.
36. Wilson, P.R., and Yaksh, T.L. Pharmacology of pain and analgesia. Anaesthesia and Intensive Care **8:**248-256, 1980.

GENERAL REFERENCES

Allen, G.D. Dental Anesthesia and Analgesia (Local and General), ed. 3. Baltimore, Williams & Wilkins, 1984.

Bennett, C.R. Conscious-Sedation in Dental Practice, ed. 2. St. Louis, The C.V. Mosby Co., 1978.

Bennett, C.R. Monheim's General Anesthesia in Dental Practice, ed. 4. St. Louis, The C.V. Mosby Co., 1974.

Jorgensen, N.B., and Hayden, J., Jr. Sedation, Local and General Anesthesia in Dentistry, ed. 3. Philadelphia, Lea & Febiger, 1980.

Langa, H. Relative Analgesia in Dental Practice: Inhalation Analgesia and Sedation with Nitrous Oxide, ed. 2. Philadelphia, W.B. Saunders Co., 1976.

45 Treatment of oral complications of cancer radiotherapy

Samuel Dreizen

Because most primary oral malignancies are radiosensitive squamous cell carcinomas, irradiation is the treatment of choice when the neoplasm cannot be readily or fully resected. The aim of radiotherapy is to eradicate the tumor by doses of ionizing radiation that, ideally, will be well tolerated by the surrounding structures. In practice, some degree of transient or permanent tissue damage invariably accompanies the use of tumoricidal radiation, and the oral complications of such treatment can be physically and psychologically devastating unless the patient is properly forewarned and the side effects are efficiently and effectively managed.

The oral complications of cancer radiotherapy stem from radiation injury to the salivary glands, oral mucosa, oral musculature, and alveolar bone. These injuries directly or indirectly create a cluster of clinical consequences, including xerostomia, rampant dental decay, mucositis, taste loss, osteoradionecrosis, infection, trismus, and nutritional stomatitis. The manifestations vary in pattern, duration, and intensity, and all do not affect every patient. The purpose of this chapter is to describe the way in which these manifestations may be handled therapeutically.

PHARMACOLOGIC THERAPIES
Xerostomia

The secretion of saliva declines drastically when the major salivary glands are included in the radiation fields. The reduction is related to the dose and the duration of therapy and reflects the progression of radiation-induced inflammatory and degenerative changes in the acinar and ductal cells.

The normal cellular arrangement is replaced in the irradiated gland by ductal remnants and loose fibrous connective tissue moderately infiltrated with lymphocytes and plasma cells.

Radiation-induced xerostomia is rapid in onset, pronounced, persistent, and irreversible. In 42 patients with oral cancer who were given a tumor dose of 200 rads per day 5 days per week through parallel opposed fields, the average salivary flow rate in response to masticatory stimulation dropped 57% after the first week of therapy, 76% after 6 weeks of treatment, and 95% 3 years after irradiation. Some of these patients reported subjective improvement in mouth dryness in the months following radiotherapy, but measurement of flow rates showed no increase in saliva production.[4]

The treatment of radiation-induced xerostomia is essentially palliative and accommodative. Glycerin-containing mouth rinses[9] and troches[5] and saliva substitutes made of carboxymethylcellulose, sorbitol, and salts[8] provide relief by coating and lubricating the mucosa (Table 45-1). Most patients with xerostomia accommodate to the shortage of saliva by moistening and thinning foods with sauces, gravies, milk, and other fluids to facilitate chewing and swallowing.

Xerostomia also deprives the teeth of an important natural defense against dental decay. The decrease in saliva production is accompanied by (1) the emergence of a highly cariogenic microflora that replaces noncariogenic microorganisms, (2) a sharp decrease in the total daily output of caries-protective salivary electrolytes and immunoproteins, and (3) a change in food consumption patterns to frequent, nondetergent, high carbohydrate meals. These microbial, chemical, immunologic, and dietary changes add up to an enormous increase in the caries challenge.

Adapted from Dreizen, S., Daly, T.E., Drane, J.B., and Brown, L.R. Oral complications of cancer radiotherapy. Postgraduate Medicine **61**(2):45-92, 1977.

Table 45-1. Commercial saliva substitutes for relief of xerostomia

Proprietary name	Ingredients
Saliva Substitute (solution)	Sorbitol, sodium carboxymethylcellulose, methyl paraben
Orex, Xero-Lube (solution or pump spray)	Calcium, magnesium, potassium, and sodium chlorides, potassium phosphate (monobasic and dibasic), sodium fluoride, sorbitol, sodium carboxymethylcellulose, methylparaben
Moi-Stir (pump spray)	Calcium, magnesium, potassium, and sodium chlorides, potassium phosphate (dibasic), sorbitol, sodium carboxymethylcellulose, methylparaben and propylparaben
Salivart (spray)	Calcium, magnesium, potassium, and sodium chlorides, potassium phosphate (dibasic), sorbitol, carboxymethylcellulose, nitrogen (as propellant)

Regardless of the patient's caries history, the development of xerostomia is inevitably followed by rampant dental decay unless stringent protective steps are taken. Caries can start on any surface of the tooth and progress rapidly to total destruction of the crown. Cariogenesis is so greatly accelerated that frank lesions may appear within 3 months after radiotherapy.

The ravages of dental decay in the irradiated patient can be almost completely prevented with daily application of a 1% sodium fluoride gel containing a red, plaque-disclosing dye. The gel is applied by means of flexible plastic carriers that are custom fabricated on stone casts prepared from alginate impressions of the dental arches. Clenching the carriers pumps the gel onto and between the teeth. The gel must remain in contact with the teeth for at least 5 minutes. When the carriers are removed and the gel is rinsed off, the plaques are stained red and they can be removed by brushing and flossing.[3]

To be maximally effective, this preventive program must be instituted at the beginning of radiotherapy and continued every day. This regimen not only keeps decay from starting but also arrests caries caused by xerostomia in previously unprotected patients. Because of the tremendous and ever present risk of caries, only diligent, lifelong cooperation by the patient will ensure prevention.

Oral mucositis

The oral mucosa responds to irradiation by a series of changes that are related to the dose and the duration of therapy. Initially, the mucosa in the path of radiation appears reddened and swollen as a result of irritative hyperemia and edema. As treatment continues, the mucosa becomes denuded, ulcerated, and covered with a fibrinous exudate. Pain, burning, and discomfort are commonly present at rest and are greatly intensified by contact with coarse or highly seasoned foods. Involvement of the pharyngeal mucosa produces difficulties in swallowing and speaking.

Oral mucositis persists throughout radiotherapy and for several weeks thereafter, and then spontaneous remission begins unless secondary infection has occurred. In many patients, lidocaine viscous, swished in the mouth 30 minutes before mealtimes to produce topical anesthesia, makes eating without discomfort possible.

Taste loss

Patients undergoing radiotherapy for oral cancer quickly lose their sense of taste. Conger[2] found that the rate of loss is exponential up to an accumulated dose of about 3,000 rads and then slows as acuity approaches zero. Damage to the microvilli and outer surface of the taste cells has been proposed as the principal mechanism for loss of the sense of taste.

In most instances, taste acuity is partially restored within 20 to 60 days after completion of radiotherapy and is fully restored within 60 to 120 days. Some patients, however, are left with residual hypogeusia. In such patients, partial to complete return to taste acuity has been obtained by treatment with zinc ion (25 mg of elemental zinc given orally as 110 mg of zinc sulfate heptahydrate 4 times a day).[6] Because zinc ion may produce some gastrointestinal toxicity, the zinc sulfate must be administered with each meal and with a snack at bedtime. Patients who were given zinc ion before radiotherapy have experienced fewer gustatory complaints and have not had as severe hypogeusia as nontreated patients.

Radiation necrosis

Radiotherapy impairs the viability of the oral mucosa at the primary site of irradiation by inducing fibrosis and a decrease in blood supply. Necrotic ulcers may develop in these areas 2 to 3 months after completion of radiotherapy and any time thereafter. The ulcers are usually precipitated by trauma, are extremely painful, heal slowly, and enlarge rapidly unless treated quickly and energetically. Early, superficial necrotic ulcers are best managed with sprays or irrigations of warm, mild solutions of salt or soda. The spread of necrosis can be controlled and healing can be promoted by application of a paste containing zinc peroxide, carboxymethylcellulose, and hydrogen peroxide or a spray of 0.5% prednisolone sodium phosphate with neomycin sulfate.[7]

Trauma before or after heavy irradiation to tooth-bearing bone produces conditions that predispose the tissue to bone exposure, infection, and necrosis. Conservative treatment with zinc peroxide packs or applications of 1% neomycin solution should be tried first in every patient with osteoradionecrosis. Adjunctive measures include gentle removal of loose bone spicules; flushing with mild, warm solutions of hydrogen peroxide, salt, or soda; strict oral hygiene; and appropriate systemically administered antibiotics when needed for gross infection. Surgical intervention should not be attempted unless a proper, persistent trial of the conservative measures has proved ineffectual.

Oral infections

The most common oral infection in patients who have had radiotherapy for cancer of the mouth is candidiasis. It has been suggested that irradiation exerts a detrimental effect on the oral tissues, creating a more favorable environment for the growth of the fungus.[1] Candidal infection of the oral mucosa produces symptoms of burning, tenderness, and dryness and is characterized by soft, white, creamy patches or streaks that often enlarge and coalesce. Removal of the growth exposes a superficially ulcerated mucosal surface.

All patients with oral candidiasis should be treated promptly to prevent hematogenous spread and seeding of the esophagus with swallowed organisms. Most mild cases of oral candidiasis respond to nystatin suspension used as a mouth rinse 3 to 4 times a day. Extensive and nystatin-resistant infections are best treated with intravenously administered amphotericin B.

The factors most likely to lead to bacterial infection of the oral cavity are radiation caries, radiation mucositis, radiation necrosis of the soft and hard tissues, debilitation, and malnutrition. All acute and subacute bacterial infections should be treated with organism-specific antibiotics as soon as culture and sensitivity studies have been completed, regardless of the stage of cancer care.

Carious teeth should not be extracted after radiotherapy because of the extremely high risk of osteoradionecrosis developing in the extraction sites; instead, they should be treated endodontically or allowed to exfoliate. If extraction is unavoidable, the amount of trauma should be kept to a minimum, and large doses of antibiotics should be given prophylactically. Extractions should be limited to no more than two or three teeth at a time and must be performed with utmost care and removal of all sharp bony edges, necrotic bone, and debris. The extraction sites must be sutured to promote primary wound healing.

NONPHARMACOLOGIC THERAPIES

The treatment of two other complications of radiotherapy is nonpharmacologic, and only a few words will be said about these.

Trismus

Trismus, a condition in which tonic spasms of the masticatory muscles limit opening of the mouth, may develop during or after radiotherapy if these muscles are included in the treatment fields. Patients whose masticatory muscles are to be heavily irradiated should be instructed to exercise them by opening the mouth as wide as possible 20 times at least 3 times daily. If trismus has already developed, exercises and various prosthetic appliances may prove helpful.

Nutritional stomatitis

Many patients who undergo radiotherapy for oral cancer become nutritional casualties. Profound loss of appetite is an early and sustained reaction to radiation-provoked soreness, xerostomia, taste loss, dysphagia, nausea, and vomiting. Eating becomes a pleasureless and painful chore, and food selection is restricted to items that do not aggravate the oral discomfort, often at the expense of adequate nutrition. When prolonged and severe enough, lack of nutrients can precipitate a nutritional-deficiency stomatitis.

Nutritional complications can be avoided by modifying the texture and consistency of the diet, by adding between-meal snacks to increase protein and caloric intake, and by administering vitamin and mineral supplements.

SUMMARY

The stomatologic complications of radiotherapy for oral cancer are physical and physiologic in nature, transient or lasting in duration, and reversible or irreversible in type. It is noteworthy that some of these complications can be treated pharmacologically, although some respond, at least limitedly, to physical and nutritional measures.

CITED REFERENCES

1. Chen, T.Y., and Webster, J.H. Oral monilia study on patients with head and neck cancer during radiotherapy. Cancer **34**:246-249, 1974.
2. Conger, A.D. Loss and recovery of taste acuity in patients irradiated to the oral cavity. Radiation Research **53**:338-347, 1973.
3. Daly, T.E., and Drane, J.B. Management of Dental Problems in Irradiated Patients. Refresher course. Chicago, Radiological Society of North America, 1972.
4. Dreizen, S., Brown, L.R., Daly, T.E., and Drane, J.B. Prevention of xerostomia-related dental caries in irradiated cancer patients. Journal of Dental Research **56**:99-104, 1977.
5. Dykes, P., Harris, P., and Marston, A. Treatment of dry mouth. Lancet **2**:1353, 1960.
6. Henkin, R.I. Prevention and treatment of hypogeusia due to head and neck irradiation. Journal of the American Medical Association **220**:870-871, 1972.
7. MacComb, W.S. Necrosis in treatment of intraoral cancer by radiation therapy. American Journal of Roentgenology, Radium Therapy, and Nuclear Medicine **87**:431-440, 1962.
8. Matzker, J., and Schreiber, J. Synthetischer Speichel für Therapie der Hyposialien, inbesondere bei der radiogenen Sialadenitis. Zeitschrift für Laryngologie, Rhinologie, Otologie und Ihre Grenzgebiete **51**:422-428, 1972.
9. Robinson, J.E. Dental management of the oral effects of radiotherapy. Journal of Prosthetic Dentistry **14**:582-587, 1964.

46 Drug abuse

Roy Aston

A comprehensive history of drug abuse is not within the scope of this chapter, but a review of trends in drug abuse within the United States since 1850 will provide a perspective from which to evaluate the current drug abuse scene.

Other than alcohol (which is considered separately in Chapter 41), the first major drugs of abuse in the United States were cocaine and the opioids. Throughout the nineteenth century, unregulated opium production led to a plethora of patent medicines containing opium derivatives. As a result, many middle-class Americans became dependent on opium because of promiscuous use of such preparations. Social attitudes toward drug abuse, nevertheless, remained relaxed until the Civil War, when widespread use of morphine for dysentery, malaria, and pain resulted in such large numbers of morphine-addicted veterans that morphine dependence became known as the "soldier's disease."[6] In 1884, Sigmund Freud suggested that the recently isolated alkaloid cocaine would be useful in treating opium dependence, as well as depression, asthma, and loss of libido. In the same year, William Halsted, known as the father of modern surgery, introduced the use of cocaine for nerve block. By 1890, evidence of toxicity had dampened European enthusiasm for the use of cocaine as a general nostrum, but in the United States, unrestricted application of cocaine products for the treatment of a variety of disorders, from corns to venereal disease, continued until 1902, when the manufacturers of Coca-Cola ceased to employ cocaine-containing syrup in their soft drink.[30]

Between 1900 and 1920, the mass media developed the myth of cocaine-crazed black renegades committing heinous crimes against an innocent white community.[30] Opioid dependence was still prevalent, and morphine was the major opioid of abuse. In 1914, a federal law, the Harrison Narcotic Act, placed domestic regulation of cocaine and opioids under the jurisdiction of the U.S. Internal Revenue Service and provided penalties of up to $2000 or 5 years in prison for violation of its statutes. Later amendments to this act in 1922, 1951, and 1956 further increased these penalties. By the 1930s, the increased cost and reduced availability of street cocaine led to the rise of amphetamine as a stimulant drug of abuse. During this period, intravenous heroin use was becoming popular, and by 1935 it was as widely abused as morphine. Although the number of opioid addicts did not increase significantly in the United States between World Wars I and II, addiction began to be equated with criminality.[6] Nowhere was this association more evident than with the use of marijuana. Sensationalized accounts of murders perpetrated by ethnic minorities under the influence of the "killer weed" led to the passage of the Marihuana Tax Act of 1937, which banned its production, distribution, and sale.

After World War II, opioid addiction reached major proportions, especially among ghetto dwellers who had come from rural areas of the South and Puerto Rico.[6] The wave of drug abuse reached its peak in the 1960s with a marked rise in illegal drug use in the white, middle-class community, involving marijuana, LSD, amphetamine, barbiturates, and heroin. In 1970, the Comprehensive Drug Abuse and Control Act, administered by the Department of Justice, replaced previous federal laws and amendments in this area. This act classifies drugs into five schedules according to their abuse liability and provides a graded set of penalties for violation of regulations relating to manufacture, sale, prescription, and record-keeping of drugs of abuse. All states have passed legislation, similar to the federal law, regulating intrastate drug traffic.

The 1970s and 80s have witnessed the emergence of an increasingly drug-oriented society; in addition to the socioeconomically deprived ''hard'' drug users, successful people from the middle and upper classes have been experimenting with and becoming dependent on a variety of what are sometimes referred to as recreational drugs. The popularity and prominence of these drugs varies from moment to moment and may be influenced by such factors as the availability of heroin,[15] the emergence of new drugs (e.g., methaqualone), style or chic (e.g., cocaine), and easy illegal synthesis (e.g., phencyclidine). There has developed also a pattern of polydrug use in which opposite effects of different classes of drugs are successively sought. The responsible lay press has been calling attention to the pervasiveness of the drug problem and its possible adverse effects on industrial productivity, the judgment of middle-management workers, and the functioning of high-level professionals. Although heroin continues to be widely abused, other drugs that have become prominent, chiefly for their recreational use, are cocaine, phencyclidine, amyl nitrite and related vasodilators, various volatile solvents, and methaqualone. It would probably be fair to say that use of marijuana is ubiquitous.

TERMINOLOGY OF DRUG ABUSE

Drug abuse is defined by the World Health Organization Expert Committee on Drug Dependence as ''persistent or sporadic excessive drug use inconsistent with or unrelated to accepted medical practice.''[41] Certain terms are used in connection with drug abuse, and these too must be defined. The term *drug dependence* was introduced to replace such terms as addiction and habituation, which were difficult to define and carried many nonscientific connotations. This term refers to a ''state, psychic and sometimes physical, resulting from the interaction between a living organism and a drug, characterized by behavioral and other responses that always include a compulsion to take the drug on a continuous or periodic basis in order to experience its psychic effects and sometimes to avoid the discomfort of its absence.''[41] In order for drug dependence to exist, there must be a psychologic compulsion to continue drug administration either to produce pleasure or to avoid discomfort. Additional characteristics of drug dependence, which may or may not be present, are physical dependence and tolerance. Physical dependence is

Table 46-1. Abuse characteristics of drug groups

	Psychic dependence	Physical dependence	Tolerance
Opioid analgesics	+ + +	+ + +	+ + +
CNS depressants	+ +	+ + +	+ +
Amphetamines	+ + +	+	+ + +
Cocaine	+ +	0	+
Hallucinogens			
LSD	0	0	+ +
Phencyclidine	+ +	0	+ + +
Marijuana	0	+	+

Key: + + + = marked, + + = moderate, + = slight, 0 = absent.

a state that ''leads to the appearance of a characteristic and specific group of symptoms, termed an abstinence syndrome, when the administration of the drug is discontinued or—in the case of certain drugs—significantly reduced.''[20] Tolerance exists when ''repetition of the same dose of a drug has progressively less effect,'' or when ''the dose needs to be increased to obtain the same degree of pharmacological effect as was caused by the original dose.''[20] Cross-tolerance may be observed among drugs of similar or different chemical types.

On the basis of a commonality of characteristics and the phenomena of cross-tolerance and cross-dependence, the major drugs of abuse can be placed into relatively distinct categories: (1) narcotic analgesics, or opioids, (2) general depressants of the central nervous system, including sedative-hypnotics, antianxiety drugs, and alcohol, (3) amphetamines and related psychomotor stimulants, (4) cocaine, (5) hallucinogens, and (6) marijuana.

Table 46-1 lists the major abuse characteristics of these six drug groups; that is, the degree of psychic and physical dependence and tolerance development commonly associated with the abuse of each drug group. Table 46-2 lists some of the common slang or ''street'' names used for these drugs.

In the following discussion, each group will be described in terms of four factors: the symptoms produced by a prototype substance, the abuse characteristics of the drug, the abstinence syndrome, and the symptoms and treatment of acute overdosage with the drug or others from that group. At the end of the chapter, the implications of drug abuse for the dentist will be considered.

OPIOID ANALGESICS

The group of opioid analgesics includes heroin, morphine, and the various synthetic and semisyn-

Table 46-2. Slang terms for some drugs of abuse

Drug	Slang equivalent
Heroin	Blanco, chip, dope, H, horse
Morphine	Gunk, hocus, monkey, pink
Barbiturates	Barbs, candy, Christmas trees, downers, goofballs
Secobarbital	Lilly, M and M's, red devils
Amobarbital	Blue angel, blue devils, blue heavens, jack up
Pentobarbital	Nebbies, yellow jackets
Methaqualone	Ludes, paris, quads, soapers
Racemic amphetamine	Beans, bennies, peaches
Methamphetamine	Crystal, doe, love drug, meth, speed
Cocaine	C, coke, Charlies, Cadillac, girl, gold dust, her, junk, snow
LSD	Acid, cubes, dot, purple haze, white lightning
Mescaline	Mesc
Psilocybin	Mushrooms, silly putty
Phencyclidine	Angel dust, animal tranquilizer, elephant, mist, peace, PCP
Marijuana	Acapulco gold, bhang, grass, Panama gold, pot, weed

thetic derivatives, all of which have similar abuse characteristics but differ from each other in the duration of their actions, in the intensity of their effects, and to some extent in the pattern of their use. In the discussion that follows, morphine will be considered the prototype for this group, unless another drug is specifically mentioned.

Pharmacologic effects

A mixture of excitatory and sedative effects results from acute morphine administration in the dependent individual.[27] Stimulant effects include a feeling of increased energy with talkativeness ("soap boxing"). This alternates with periods of relaxation or tranquility ("coasting") and mental clouding. The addict appears to be asleep, but only the head and facial muscles are relaxed ("nodding"). When sleep occurs there is depression of rapid eye movement (REM) and stage 4 sleep, with an increase in the duration of lighter states of sleep. Although the stimulant effects are prominent initially, they are eventually replaced by reduced anxiety and social interaction, overt drowsiness, hypochondria, and irritability. The addict experiences itchy skin, miosis, constipation, sweating, xerostomia, and urinary retention. There is a slight increase in blood pressure, pulse rate, body temperature, and urinary catecholamine excretion; in contrast, respiratory rate is reduced. Meperidine

produces a unique picture of arousal with agitation, tremor, and possible acute delirium.

Abuse characteristics

Psychic dependence on opioids is marked, as exemplified by the high relapse rate among addicts after withdrawal. Drug-seeking behavior (purposive symptoms of abstinence) is manifested by pleas, complaints, demands, and other activities directed toward obtaining the drug. Such behavior becomes prominent shortly after the next expected dose; it increases for 36 to 72 hours, until physical abstinence symptoms are maximal, and subsides thereafter. For a period of about 6 months after acute withdrawal, the addict displays a secondary abstinence syndrome, the behavioral components of which include hyperresponsiveness to stress, overconcern about discomfort, and a poor self-image, all of which tend to promote the taking of drugs. An additional factor in opioid relapse is "conditioned abstinence," in which a former addict, after a long drug-free period, may experience symptoms of acute abstinence if exposed to an environment or stimulus associated wtih previous withdrawal symptoms.[27] The relapse rate is lowest in patients who have been drug-free for over 6 months.

Physical dependence on opioids is manifested on abrupt drug withdrawal as an acute, or primary, abstinence syndrome lasting 1 or more weeks, followed by a chronic, or secondary, syndrome lasting about 6 months. Acute abstinence may be precipitated by the administration of opioid antagonists, such as naloxone, or agonist-antagonists, such as pentazocine, after only 2 days of opioid administration. The severity of withdrawal is proportional to the daily dose of drug, with minimal abstinence signs occurring after 30 to 40 mg per day of morphine sulfate and near maximal signs associated with a daily dose of 240 mg. In general, short-acting narcotic analgesics produce the most severe abstinence signs on withdrawal of the drug. The onset of morphine withdrawal symptoms occurs after 8 to 12 hours of abstinence; the acute symptoms peak at 48 to 72 hours and end in 7 to 10 days. With meperidine these times are approximately halved, whereas with methadone they are about 7 times longer.[27]

Symptoms of acute morphine abstinence are similar to a bad case of influenza and reflect hyperactivity of both the central and autonomic nervous systems.[27,32] Within the first 12 hours of abstinence, the addict exhibits yawning, lacrimation, rhinor-rhea, and a restless sleep ("yen"). After the first day there is increasing anxiety, insomnia, and violent yawning. Abdominal cramps occur with nausea, vomiting, and diarrhea, which together with anorexia and sweating may lead to weight loss, dehydration, ketosis, and acid-base imbalance. In spite of hyperglycemia, there is a craving for sweets, but there is an aversion to tobacco. Muscles, bones, and joints ache; muscle spasms cause involuntary kicking movements ("kicking the habit"). The addict displays periodic piloerection ("cold turkey") and experiences hot and cold flashes. Blood pressure, pulse and respiratory rate, body temperature, and pupillary diameter all increase. Occasionally, cardiovascular collapse may occur, but withdrawal is rarely fatal in healthy individuals. During the succeeding 6 months, residual symptoms of secondary abstinence are seen. These are similar to those observed during chronic morphine dependence.

Tolerance to opioids is a cellular rather than a drug disposition tolerance and develops to different drug effects at different rates.[27,32] Pronounced tolerance to analgesia, euphoria, respiratory depression, hypotension, and lethality is observed in humans. Tolerance is less marked to the sedative and miotic effects, and no tolerance appears to develop to the constipating and convulsive actions of opioids. Cross-tolerance occurs among all opioids. Tolerance to all opioid effects, except those of emesis and hypothermia, is rapidly lost during abstinence, and death may result if an addict returns to the previously maintained dosage after withdrawal has been completed.

The development of opioid tolerance appears to be inseparable from that of physical dependence, and it is probable that there is a common mechanism involved. Most theories of tolerance and dependence invoke the development, during chronic opioid use, of compensatory alterations in central neurotransmission that, when uncovered by withdrawal of the drug, lead to central hyperactivity and enhanced autonomic tone.[40] Postulated changes include reduced dopamine turnover (resulting in diminished central inhibition), increased synaptic vesicular Mg^{++}-dependent ATPase and Ca^{++} (resulting in enhanced neurotransmitter release), and enhanced serotonergic or reduced cholinergic activity. Tolerance and dependence have also been ascribed to a reduction in the release of endogenous peptide opioids[36] and to increases in

central adenylate cyclase activity. The latter may relate to the observed amelioration or suppression of the narcotic withdrawal syndrome by the central α_2-receptor agonist, clonidine.[10]

Acute toxicity

In acute opioid overdose, the classic triad of coma, respiratory depression, and pinpoint pupils is common to all opioid agonists (except meperidine, in which case the pupils may be dilated in tolerant individuals). Hypoventilation leads to marked hypoxemia and cyanosis, and acute pulmonary edema with pink, frothy sputum may be seen, especially with heroin. Nausea and vomiting may be prominent. Hypotension, as a result of cerebral ischemia, develops gradually but may eventually lead to irreversible shock. Convulsions do not occur with most opioids, although they have been reported in children suffering from codeine overdose, in addicts in response to meperidine, and in cases of propoxyphene poisoning.

The treatment of choice is rapid intravenous administration of 0.4 mg naloxone, repeated if necessary at 2- to 3-minute intervals. Dramatic improvement occurs within minutes, with enhanced ventilation and dilation of the pinpoint pupils. The patient must be closely monitored, since the antagonist's effect lasts only 1 to 4 hours. This is especially important with methadone overdose because respiratory depression may last up to 48 hours. If vital signs return to normal, no attempt should be made to arouse the patient with additional naloxone because, if the patient is an opioid addict, large doses of the antagonist may precipitate an acute abstinence syndrome.

GENERAL CNS DEPRESSANTS

Barbiturates, nonbarbiturate sedatives, and antianxiety agents can be grouped into a single pharmacologic category because they share the same abuse characteristics. In the discussion that follows, the characteristics of barbiturate abuse will be covered separately from those of the nonbarbiturate and antianxiety drugs.

Barbiturates

Pharmacologic effects. The signs of barbiturate intoxication are similar to those produced by alcohol. Single doses of 150 mg secobarbital produce disinhibition and lightheadedness. There is prolongation of simple and complex reaction times, ataxia, and impairment of mental processes. Drowsiness, slurred speech, and lack of emotional control occur. These symptoms last for about 2 hours. Single doses of short-acting barbiturates, in the range of 400 to 700 mg, produce signs of severe intoxication or even light coma within 30 to 45 minutes, which terminate in 4 to 5 hours.[3] The next day the individual suffers from nervousness, tremor, anorexia, and headache, a picture similar to that of an alcohol hangover.

Abuse characteristics. Psychic dependence is most commonly associated with abuse of the short- or intermediate-acting barbiturates, such as secobarbital, butabarbital, and pentobarbital. Dependence on long-acting agents is less common, and dependence occurs only rarely with the intravenously administered ultra-short-acting members of the class. Primary barbiturism usually arises when the drugs are prescribed for long-term sedation or when alcoholics discover that these drugs provide a state of intoxication similar to that of alcohol but easier to conceal and less irritating to the gastrointestinal tract.

Unlike opioids, barbiturates do not induce physical dependence unless increasing doses are taken over a period of a month or longer. Minimum abstinence symptoms are elicited by abrupt withdrawal from long-term use of daily doses of 400 to 500 mg pentobarbital or secobarbital, 800 mg amobarbital, or 1200 mg barbital.[16] With long-term use of increasing doses, progressively more severe symptoms of abstinence can be precipitated, even by abruptly reducing the accustomed dose by half. Although withdrawal from daily doses of 600 to 800 mg secobarbital after 1 or 2 months produces a relatively minor abstinence syndrome, withdrawal from 800 to 900 mg per day after 60 days or more will produce major abstinence symptoms.

The barbiturate abstinence syndrome has some resemblance to that seen after alcohol withdrawal.[3,22] After a usually symptomless period (8 to 18 hours), the individual exhibits increasing symptoms of anxiety, insomnia, agitation, and confusion. Anorexia, nausea and vomiting, sweating, weakness, and significant weight loss are common. Coarse tremors in the face and hands, as well as dilation of the pupils and increases in respiratory rate, heart rate, and blood pressure, may arise. Orthostatic hypotension and syncope may also be elicited. These symptoms become more severe during the first 24 to 30 hours of abstinence, at which time the major manifestations of abstinence may

develop (i.e., convulsions, delirium, and hyperthermia).

Muscle fasciculations and enhanced deep reflexes may progress to frank seizures on the second to eighth day after withdrawal. One or more grand mal convulsions of less than 3 minutes' duration may occur, with consciousness being regained within 5 minutes. In some cases, however, status epilepticus may ensue. The prolonged postictal stupor, typical of epileptic seizures, is not seen, but there may be confusion for 1 or 2 hours.

Delirium develops gradually over 2 to 4 days and is heralded by a period of insomnia. Delirium is characterized by confusion, disorientation of time and place, nightmares, and vivid auditory and visual hallucinations. Paranoid delusions with extreme fear and agitation may develop, especially at night ("night terrors"). The symptoms terminate spontaneously after a prolonged period of sleep. It has been suggested that this withdrawal psychosis may be caused by rebound REM sleep which, having been suppressed during the period of intoxication, intrudes into the waking state.[3] During the phase of delirium, body temperature is elevated. A continuous marked hyperthermia is a life-threatening problem that, if not immediately and vigorously treated, may (along with agitation) lead to fatal exhaustion and cardiovascular collapse.[3] After the acute abstinence syndrome, recovery is gradual but complete after about 8 days, although residual weakness may be noted for 6 to 12 weeks. It should be emphasized that abrupt withdrawal from large doses of barbiturates or related depressants (e.g., antianxiety drugs) can precipitate a severe and life-threatening withdrawal syndrome that carries a significant mortality rate.

Tolerance to barbiturates is low-grade; there is only a 25% to 60% increase in anesthetic dose requirement.[3] Tolerance is usually complete to doses of short-acting barbiturates of up to 500 mg per day, but doses of greater than 800 mg per day are always associated with signs of intoxication. The onset of tolerance occurs in humans in about 3 days and is maximal in about 1 week.[22] Duration of tolerance, however, has not been accurately determined; it appears to be about 1 to 2 weeks. Unlike the opioids, barbiturate tolerance is demonstrable in individuals who have developed no signs of physical dependence,[16] indicating separate mechanisms for these two phenomena. Although cellular tolerance can be demonstrated, it appears that most of the tolerance to large doses of short-acting barbiturates is associated with hepatic enzyme induction,[22] which results in enhanced barbiturate elimination. Thus, there should be an increased barbiturate ED50 (from decreased drug accumulation during repeated administrations) but no concomitant change in acute LD50 (little or no alteration in the peak concentration obtained with a single dose). Indeed, there is evidence from animal studies that hepatic tolerance may coexist with central barbiturate intolerance, which could actually enhance the acute lethality of these drugs during a period of apparent tolerance.[4]

Acute toxicity. Ingestion of 15 or more hypnotic doses of a barbiturate is life-threatening. Coma is preeminent, with progressive deterioration of respiration and blood pressure. The victim exhibits hypoxia and cyanosis, cardiovascular shock, hypothermia, and anuria. Death is normally caused by cerebral anoxia; if respiratory death is avoided by artificial ventilation, the patient may succumb to complications such as cardiovascular shock, renal failure, or pulmonary or cerebral edema. Treatment of acute barbiturate poisoning is discussed in Chapter 14. It is sufficient to say here that therapy is mainly supportive, consisting of oxygen administered by artificial respiration, fluids or pressor agents or both to maintain circulation, and osmotic diuretics with sodium bicarbonate to alkalinize the urine and hasten elimination of the drug.

Nonbarbiturate sedative-hypnotics

Various depressants may be classified according to chemical structure into aldehyde derivatives (chloral hydrate, paraldehyde), propanediol carbamates (meprobamate, tybamate), and heterocyclics (glutethimide, methyprylon, methaqualone). All drugs in this group produce patterns of intoxication, tolerance, and psychic and physical dependence that are, with few exceptions, similar to those produced by barbiturates and ethanol. All exhibit some degree of cross-tolerance and can suppress the abstinence symptoms of other depressants of the central nervous system. Several authors have reviewed the abuse characteristics of these agents.[3,22]

The abstinence syndrome consists of restlessness, insomnia, and anxiety that progress to confusion and disorientation and may develop into delirium with paranoid delusions, hallucinations, and thought disorders. As with the barbiturates, grand mal seizures and hyperthermia may occur.

Symptoms of intoxication with nonbarbiturate drugs are similar to those seen with barbiturates and ethanol. Extreme overdose leads to coma and death from respiratory failure. Overdose of methaqualone, a much abused drug, is characterized by convulsions, impairment of blood coagulation, and gastric hemorrhage, in addition to coma.[3]

Benzodiazepine antianxiety drugs

Benzodiazepines elicit a pattern of dependence that is similar to that associated with hypnotics; both exhibit cross-tolerance and can suppress abstinence symptoms brought on by withdrawal of one or the other class of drug.[3] This commonality of dependence characteristics may be related to barbiturate receptors that have been reported to form a functional macromolecular complex with benzodiazepine receptors, GABA receptors, and the chloride ionophore.[38]

Psychic dependence on diazepam frequently occurs with abuse, though it is usually less severe than that seen with barbiturates. Physical dependence develops with daily doses as low as 15 to 30 mg diazepam taken for several weeks.[9] Barbiturate-like withdrawal signs, including insomnia, depression, hallucinations, psychosis, and convulsions have all been reported. Withdrawal agitation and insomnia may occur following prolonged therapeutic use of as little as 3 mg per day of diazepam. Onset of the abstinence syndrome, however, is delayed for 1 to 2 weeks because the long elimination half-lives of diazepam (54 hr) and its active metabolite desmethyldiazepam (92 hr) lead to slow loss of the drug from the body.[19] The delay of withdrawal signs is also true of other benzodiazepines that are biotransformed to long-acting metabolites, such as flurazepam, clorazepate, and halazepam. The short-acting 3-hydroxybenzodiazepines, such as oxazepam, lorazepam, and temazepam, which are directly conjugated and excreted, are associated with earlier and more severe abstinence symptoms.[9]

Acute benzodiazepine toxicity is characterized by coma, cardiovascular depression, and, ultimately, apnea. However, individuals taking up to 300 mg of diazepam orally recover uneventfully without the need for assisted respiration.[17] Disorientation, profound depression, and hypoventilation from benzodiazepine overdose may be treated by intravenous administration of physostigmine (2

mg), together with the anticholinergic drug gly-
copyrrolate (0.2 mg) to prevent the peripheral side
effects of the physostigmine.[7]

AMPHETAMINE AND RELATED PSYCHOMOTOR STIMULANTS

Psychomotor stimulants include analogues of
phenylethylamine (*d*-amphetamine and methamphetamine) and a group of amphetamine derivatives in which the terminal amine nitrogen is part
of a heterocyclic group (methylphenidate, phenmetrazine) or a diethylated group (diethylpropion).
Several of these drugs are shown in Figure 46-1.
Amphetamines and methylphenidate are generally
reserved for treatment of narcolepsy and childhood
hyperkinesis; phenmetrazine and diethylpropion
are anorectics with high and low levels of abuse
liability, respectively. Amphetamine is the most
widely abused member of this class, and its abuse
characteristics will be emphasized as a prototype.
The other central stimulants have similar actions
and abuse syndromes.

It is difficult to distinguish the general effects of
these drugs from those of cocaine, except that cocaine induces no remarkable tolerance. Although
tolerance to amphetamine is extreme, cross-tolerance to the effects of cocaine does not occur.

Pharmacologic effects

Single oral doses of 5 to 20 mg amphetamine
produce wakefulness, reduced fatigue and reaction
times, and improved performance of psychomotor
tasks, especially in sleep-deprived individuals.
There are feelings of enhanced well-being, moderate exhiliration, euphoria, and gregariousness.
Judgment is impaired, and irrational behavior may
occur. Peripherally, amphetamine causes a rise in
blood pressure, tachycardia, mydriasis, sweating,
and constipation. These effects probably result
from the release of norepinephrine from central and
peripheral neurons.

High oral doses of amphetamine induce feelings
of cleverness, enhanced abilities, aggressiveness,
and fearlessness. Single doses of 50 to 200 mg
cause a manic ''high,'' paranoid rage, and violent
diarrhea and vomiting. These reactions constitute
the ''Sunday syndrome'' observed among certain
professional football players who employ amphetamine to enhance their game performance.[26] Intravenous use results in a markedly pleasurable
''flash'' described as an ''expanding, flashing, vi-
brating feeling,'' or a ''total body orgasm,'' fol-

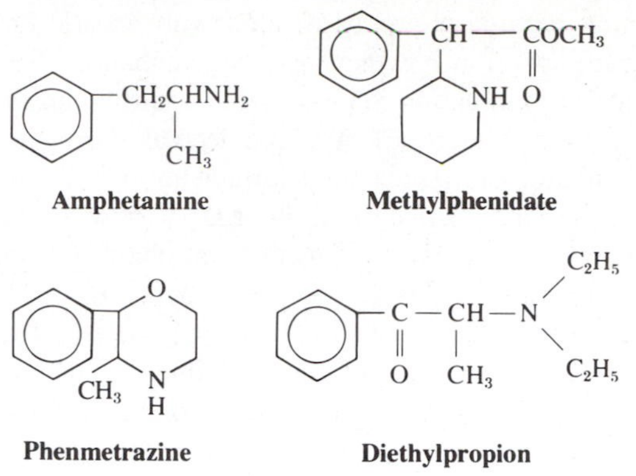

Figure 46-1. Structural formulas of amphetamine and some related stimulant drugs.

lowed by rebound depression, dysphoria, and restlessness.

Long-term amphetamine abuse leads to stereotypy, psychosis, and overt violence. Stereotypy is
characterized by pleasurable curiosity and fasci-
nation with detail. Compulsive, repetitive activity
develops, such as cleaning an immaculate home or
disassembling and reconstructing mechanical objects. Amphetamine psychosis develops within 1 to
5 days of drug use, and usually lasts 6 to 7 days;
the psychotogenic dose varies from 30 mg in non-
tolerant to 1500 mg in tolerant individuals. The
reaction is one of paranoid schizophrenia but without the thought disorder seen in the endogenous
form of the disease. The most common symptoms
are delusions of persecution, auditory, tactile, and
especially visual hallucinations, and hyperactivity.
Anxiety, agitation, aggressiveness, and depression
are often observed. Paranoia, hallucinations, and
terror reactions lead to hostility and difficulty in
controlling rage. Amphetamine abusers display a
high incidence of unpremeditated, unprovoked,
and bizarre acts of violence, assaultive behavior,
and even homicidal behavior. After amphetamine
is discontinued, confusion, delusions, and loss
of memory may persist for several weeks or
months.

Although possibly difficult to identify, the long-
term amphetamine abuser typically shows a picture
of anxiety, akathisia, volatile mood, headaches,
and cramps. In addition, the abuser frequently displays signs of mental and physical fatigue, poor

personal hygiene, facial twitching, skin excoriations, and worn teeth and a chewed tongue as a result of continuous oral movements.[15] Signs of increased peripheral adrenergic activity, such as mydriasis, sweating, xerostomia, hyperreflexia, and paroxysmal atrial tachycardia, may also be exhibited.

Abuse characteristics

The degree of psychic dependence and abuse potential is very high for all the drugs in this group, except diethylpropion. Many habitual users begin as occasional users: students wanting to study through the night, truck drivers needing to stay awake for long hauls, housewives suffering from depression. Marked tolerance to the stimulant effects of amphetamine develops. Whereas the therapeutic dose of amphetamine is 10 to 15 mg, abusers may inject intravenously up to 2 gm per day. Such self-administration may occur in "runs" of 3 to 6 days without any sleep. The mechanism of tolerance is unknown but has been attributed to an enhanced excretion of amphetamine in urine made acidic by anorexia and ketosis and to the depletion of central catecholamine stores with replacement by *p*-hydroxynorephedrine, a metabolite of amphetamine that may function as a false transmitter.

Physical dependence on amphetamine is not readily demonstrable. However, withdrawal from the drug after a full "run" is followed by a prolonged sleep of up to 3 days' duration (with increased REM activity during sleep lasting for 2 weeks), succeeded by a ravenous appetite, apathy, and depression.[15] This complex of symptoms is interpreted as evidence of true physical dependence by some authors. Human abstinence depression is correlated with a central reduction in 3-methoxy-4-hydroxyphenylglycol, a norepinephrine metabolite, which provides support for the hypothesis that amphetamine withdrawal symptoms are the result of central catecholamine depletion.[15]

Acute toxicity

Acute severe overdose, although uncommon, is characterized, especially in children, by central and cardiovascular stimulation. Coma and convulsions occur, which may develop into status epilepticus. Cardiac arrhythmias and hypertension, occasionally precipitating subarachnoid hemorrhage or intracerebral hematomas, may lead to cardiovascular collapse. Typically, hyperpyrexia is induced and, if pronounced, must be treated vigorously with chlorpromazine and whole-body cooling. Seizures may be controlled with intravenous diazepam. It has been shown that acidification of the urine with ammonium chloride increases the rate of urinary excretion of unchanged amphetamine and causes rapid clearing of psychotic symptoms.[2]

COCAINE

Cocaine is a local anesthetic that produces adrenergic effects by blocking neuronal reuptake of norepinephrine.[39] The leaves of the Bolivian and Peruvian coca plant, which contain up to 1.8% of the pure alkaloid, are the source of cocaine paste (30% to 90% cocaine). The paste is converted to pure cocaine hydrochloride, primarily in Colombia, from whence it is shipped to illicit markets. In 1980, this illicit traffic involved 45 metric tons of cocaine worth about $30 billion. Most "street" cocaine appears to be the pure drug, but up to 30% of samples contain adulterants such as amphetamine, mannitol, or lidocaine. Procaine shares some "desirable" characteristics with cocaine and can produce a high. It is not surprising, therefore, that procaine powder is frequently used to cut cocaine and, mixed with mannitol or lactose, is sold as cocaine. The drug, as the hydrochloride salt, is used orally, intravenously, and most frequently intranasally ("snorting"). When the hydrochloride is converted to a more combustible form, known as the free base, the drug can be smoked. In this form, there is a rapid onset and a more intense high. Cocaine paste is also smoked, particularly by abusers in South America. Regular users of cocaine take 1 gm or more per month, whereas heavy abusers may inject as much as 2 gm every day.

Pharmacologic effects

As a recreational drug, cocaine uniformly causes euphoria and signs of CNS stimulation, as for example, garrulousness and alertness. Thus, the drug facilitates social interaction in group settings. There is a subjective feeling of greater mental agility and immunity to fatigue and hunger. This essentially pleasant "high" is produced by doses of about 100, 25, and 10 mg of cocaine by the oral, intranasal, and IV routes, respectively,[34] and it lasts from 1 to 5 hours depending on the route. In these doses, cocaine causes a moderate mydriasis and an increase in systolic blood pressure with tachycardia, but no effects on respiration or body temperature are elicited.[34] Often, hypersexuality occurs, especially in women, though larger doses tend to reduce libido, and the orgasmic "rush" produced by intravenous cocaine may become a substitute for coitus.

With intensified use, the euphoric effects of the drug are replaced by restlessness, anxiety, and irritability. Anxiety becomes intense, the abuser loses the ability to concentrate, stereotyped compulsive behavior and paranoid delusions supervene, and hallucinations develop that are typically tactile, with sensations of insects burrowing under the skin or snakes crawling over the body. Frequent intranasal use of cocaine leads to chronic rhinitis and rhinorrhea, and perforation of the nasal septum may occur secondarily to chronic ischemia.

Abuse characteristics

Employed intranasally as a low-dose recreational drug, cocaine exhibits moderate or no psychic dependence liability, whereas intravenous use of higher doses over prolonged periods produces marked compulsive dependence. Physical dependence does not occur, but prolonged dose-related reactive depression, fatigue, anxiety, and a desire for more cocaine follow withdrawal from large doses of the drug. Oral diazepam has been useful in treating anxiety; psychotherapy or cautious use of tricyclic antidepressants is recommended for prolonged depression. Tolerance does not develop during low-dose use, but with long-term heavy use there is rapid and marked tolerance to the stimulant effects of cocaine.

Acute toxicity

Severe overdose may occur even after "snorting" the drug. Initially, there is excitement and apprehension, nausea, vomiting, and abdominal pain. Muscle twitching is observed, together with tachycardia, elevated blood pressure, and skin pallor. Tonicoclonic seizures, ventricular arrhythmias, and hyperpnea progressing to dyspnea and cyanosis develop. Death, if it occurs, is rapid, usually within 5 hours. The patient loses consciousness, becomes areflexic, and suffers terminal convulsions with respiratory and cardiovascular failure.

Treatment of cocaine overdose is symptomatic. Central stimulation can be treated with IV diazepam, ventricular arrhythmias with IV lidocaine, and respiratory depression with oxygen and positive pressure ventilation.

HALLUCINOGENS

Hallucinogens are defined as drugs that alter perception, mood, and thought without changes in consciousness or orientation.[31] These drugs are also referred to as *psychotomimetics,* because their effects mimic naturally occurring psychoses, or as *psychedelics* because of their use by people to induce mystical experiences. Many other names have been applied to this drug class, none of which is totally suitable; the plethora of nomenclature reflects the wide range of effects experienced by individuals using these compounds and the fact that these drug-induced experiences cannot readily be described. Here, these drugs will be categorized as psychedelic and deliriant hallucinogens.

Psychedelic hallucinogens

The psychedelic hallucinogens may be divided into three chemical classes (Table 46-3), all of which bear some structural similarity to the indole nucleus characteristic of 5-hydroxytryptamine and the rauwolfia alkaloids.[31] The first class is derived from lysergic acid and includes the potent hallucinogen *d*-lysergic acid diethylamide (LSD) and acetyl-LSD. The effective hallucinogenic oral dose of these drugs is 1 to 2 μg/kg. The second chemical group is derived from tryptamine; it includes dimethyltryptamine, diethyltryptamine, and dipropyltryptamine (DMT, DET, DPT) and their hydroxylated derivates bufotenine and psilocin, as well as the phosphorylated analogue of the latter, psilocybin. The effective human dose of psilocybin is 100 to 200 μg/kg orally. The third class of psychedelics is derived from amphetamine and includes mescaline (TMA), dimethoxyamphetamine (DMA), and dimethoxymethylamphetamine (DOM). The amphetamine derivatives are the least potent group of hallucinogens, the effective oral dose for humans being 5000 to 10,000 μg/kg. The exception is DOM, the potency of which approaches that of LSD. In the discussion of abuse of these drugs, LSD is considered the prototype.

Pharmacologic effects. The subjective effects of LSD are enormously dependent on the set (psychologic makeup of the subject) and the setting (environmental influences at the time of the drug experience), the expectations of the subject and the observer, and the size of the dose. Symptoms of the LSD syndrome occur sequentially, with somatic symptoms developing first, followed by perceptual

Table 46-3. Chemical classification and structures of some hallucinogenic drugs

Drugs	Derived from	Structural formula
Lysergic acid diethylamide (LSD) Acetyl-LSD	 **Lysergic acid**	 **Lysergic acid diethylamide**
Dimethyltryptamine (DMT) Diethyltryptamine (DET) Dipropyltryptamine (DPT) Bufotenine Psilocin Psilocybin	 **Tryptamine**	 **Dimethyltryptamine** **Psilocin**
Dimethoxyamphetamine (DMA) Trimethoxyamphetamine (TMA, mescaline) Dimethoxymethylamphetamine (DOM)	 **Amphetamine**	 **Mescaline**

and mood changes and then by psychic or psychedelic phemonena.[33,35]

Within a half hour of ingestion of 0.1 mg LSD, a feeling of inner tension develops, often relieved by laughing or crying. This release is accompanied by somatic symptoms of mild sympathetic stimulation and motor alterations. The individual feels dizzy, weak, vaguely numb, and nauseated. Marked mydriasis is accompanied by a rise in blood pressure and pulse rate, tremor, hyperreflexia, and, at high doses, ataxia. These somatic effects are soon submerged by perceptual and psychic effects, which begin about 45 minutes after the drug is taken. Emotional changes vary markedly. Some individuals experience euphoria, elation, serenity, or ecstasy, whereas in others the initial tension may progress to anxiety and depression, evoking a panic reaction. Still others may shift from a feeling of high spirits to one of deep depression. Occasionally, a paranoid rage reaction occurs, though most subjects tend to be passive, quiet, and withdrawn.

Distortion of sense perception is the most specific symptom of the LSD syndrome, affecting all modalities, but especially vision. Colors seem unusually bright and vivid, and objects appear distorted and seem to undulate and flow. Fixed objects appear to shift from near to far, fine surface details appear in deep relief, and colorful, dreamlike images occur as vivid streaming filmstrips even with the eyes closed. Frank visual hallucinations are rare, but visual illusions are not uncommon, as when a spot on the wall is mistaken for a face. There are distortions of body image, enhanced auditory perception, and, more rarely, alteration of other sensory modalities. Time sense is distorted; it is often described as stopping or going backward. Synesthesias are common, so that music may be experienced visually, or colors may be "heard."

Changes in sensory perception are soon followed by psychic changes in ego function. This phase constitutes the psychedelic "trip." Subjects may experience depersonalization, ego boundaries dissolve, and the separation between self and environment melts away. There is a sense of union with the infinite universe, accompanied by feelings of profound insight, revelation, and expanded consciousness. This loss of self is interpreted as a "good trip" by psychedelic drug users, but, on occasion, loss of control and fear of self-disintegration foster panic and even attempts at self-destruction. The individual remains oriented and alert throughout the experience and often remembers all events during the "trip" even months later.

Although all psychedelics mimic the effects of LSD, certain differences are observed.[31] Mescaline produces more perceptual effects and less euphoria than LSD. It also has a slower onset and a longer duration of action. Psilocybin produces more euphoria than LSD and is of shorter duration. One of the shortest-acting hallucinogens is DMT, which must be inhaled or injected. Its effects last only 45 to 60 minutes and have been described as the "businessman's trip."

Adverse reactions to LSD are primarily psychic. Panic reactions can be treated with calm reassurance or oral diazepam in doses of 15 to 30 mg. For severe reactions, oral or intramuscular chlorpromazine may be required. It has been estimated that 1 in 20 LSD users experience "flashbacks," in which spontaneous recurrences of the LSD experience take place during abstinence from the drug. They may occur months after the previous "trip" and last from a few minutes to a few hours. The recurrences may take perceptual, somatic, or emotional forms and are treated in the same way as panic reactions. In addition, prolonged psychotic states may be precipitated by LSD use, requiring in some instances long-term hospitalization. It has been suggested that LSD causes chromosomal damage in users and may be teratogenic. However,

most investigations of this possible effect do not support the claim.[31]

Abuse characteristics. In general, use of these drugs is not associated with physical or compulsive psychic dependence, although tolerance evidently develops, and cross-tolerance is seen among members of this class (but not to amphetamine itself). With repeated use, tolerance to LSD develops within 1 week but lasts only a few days after discontinuance of the drug.

Acute toxicity. The adult human lethal dose of LSD has been estimated to be 2 mg/kg. However, to date no deaths caused directly by LSD overdosage have been reported.[33] Ingestion of up to 50 mg results in hyperactivity, psychosis, amnesia, upper gastrointestinal tract bleeding, and coma.

Deliriant hallucinogens

The deliriant hallucinogens include anticholinergic drugs, such as the belladonna alkaloids, and phencyclidine (PCP). Administration of these drugs produces a state characterized by confusion, delirium, drowsiness, dysphoria, unpleasant hallucinations, loss of memory, and agitation. In the following discussion, PCP will be considered the prototype of the deliriant hallucinogens.

PCP, originally investigated as an anesthetic agent in humans but subsequently abandoned because of severe dysphoric and psychotomimetic side effects, is currently marketed only for anesthetic use in nonhuman primates. A related drug, ketamine, is used in humans as a "dissociative anesthetic." PCP was introduced into the illicit street trade about 1967. More recently, primary abuse of PCP has become widespread, with the drug being smoked (in treated tobacco, parsley, or marijuana), swallowed, sniffed, and occasionally injected. The relative ease of synthesizing PCP has led to a rash of illicit but profitable manufacturing operations.

Pharmacologic effects. In low doses, PCP produces a state similar to alcohol intoxication, characterized by drowsiness, extreme agitation, incoordination, and ataxia. In addition, distortions of body image occur together with disordered thought processes, feelings of estrangement, and hostility. The subject exhibits a blank stare and is often unable to speak. Catatonic muscle rigidity occurs, with blurred vision, nystagmus, sweating, and generalized numbness. No genuine hallucinations are seen at lower doses. Amnesia of the episode may occur.

Psychotomimetic sequelae are seen during recovery from acute overdose and may develop as a delayed reaction some days or weeks later. These alarming symptoms may even follow a small, otherwise asymptomatic dose of PCP. The episode mimics schizophrenia and, because of drug-induced paranoia and superhuman feelings, may cause violent antisocial acts if the subject is confronted with any perceived threat.

Abuse characteristics. Psychic dependence, not observed with other hallucinogens, reportedly may become appreciable in long-term users of PCP, but signs of physical dependence are consistently absent. Marked tolerance, however, does occur, with the dose requirement for intoxication increasing from 5 to 10 mg in naive users to as high as 200 to 500 mg in long-term abusers.

Acute toxicity. Symptoms of acute intoxication occur at oral doses greater than 20 mg, appearing 15 to 30 minutes after ingestion. At these doses, marked analgesia with shivering, hypersalivation, vomiting, hyperpnea, and hyperpyrexia result. Focal seizures may occur, developing into convulsions at doses greater than 70 mg, which also produce deep and prolonged coma with loss of protective reflexes. Death has been attributed to intracranial hemorrhage, status epilepticus, and respiratory failure.

Treatment of acute intoxication centers on acidification of the blood and urine to reduce the entry of PCP into the brain and hasten its renal excretion. Additional measures include gastric suction, sensory deprivation, IV diazoxide for hypertensive crisis, and IV diazepam to control seizures. Other central depressants must be avoided during the acute phase of toxicity.

MARIJUANA

Marijuana, or cannabis, refers to the material obtained from the hemp plant, *Cannabis sativa,* which is usually smoked in the form of cigarettes. Delta-9-tetrahydrocannabinol (Δ^9-THC), one of many constituent cannabinoids of hemp, appears to be the main psychoactive ingredient, with an effective dose of 50 to 200 µg/kg by oral ingestion or 25 to 50 µg/kg when smoked.[28] When smoked, the onset of action is rapid, with a peak effect occurring in 15 to 30 minutes. Blood concentration kinetics show a biphasic decline, reflecting an initial half-life of 30 minutes and a secondary half-life of several days because of enterohepatic recycling and sequestration in fat.[29] Liver, brain, and other organs hydroxylate the drug to 11-hydroxy-Δ^9-THC, a highly psychoactive metabolite that may play a major role in the effects of marijuana.[28] Δ^9-THC and its metabolites are excreted largely in the feces but also in urine, a process that takes more than a week after a single administration.

Pharmacologic effects

The mechanism of action of Δ^9-THC is unknown. Moderate doses of marijuana produce autonomic responses consisting of xerostomia, conjunctival injection, tachycardia with reduced peripheral resistance, and, in large doses, orthostatic hypotension. No changes are seen in pupillary diameter, respiratory rate, blood glucose concentrations, or deep tendon reflexes.[28] The drug produces subjective relaxation, euphoria and disinhibition, improved sense perception, stronger imagery, and impaired short-term memory. The most consistent behavioral effect is a feeling that time is passing slowly, associated wtih a greater concentration on the concrete present. Hostility and aggressiveness are reduced. The drug stimulates appetite and may cause a signficant weight gain in casual, as well as heavy, users. Impaired driving ability occurs with low doses of the drug and is related to its effects on reaction time and distance and time estimation, as well as to increased steering errors and reduced attentiveness to peripheral stimuli (e.g., another car emerging from a side street).

Larger doses of marijuana (i.e., four or more cigarettes) induce psychotomimetic effects similar to those of LSD.[28] Acute anxiety and panic may occur, most commonly in inexperienced users or those under stress. These feelings may last for several hours and be manifested by the subject assuming a prostrate form and showing obvious agitation or depression. Even severe panic states, however, appear to be treatable with authoritative reassurance. IV doses of Δ^9-THC frequently result in dysphoria, panic, and paranoia. Prolonged reactions to marijuana have been reported but are not well documented. They include flashbacks, psychotic reactions, and a long-term amotivational syndrome with apathy and reduced work output.[28]

There is no evidence of any irreversible brain damage occurring in heavy long-term marijuana use. Marijuana leaf, however, has a greater carcinogenic hydrocarbon content than does tobacco. *Aspergillus* contamination of marijuana cigarettes may be a significant source of infection in smokers developing pulmonary aspergillosis.[21]

Studies of the potential clinical utility of marijuana show it to be effective in the treatment of glaucoma and of some value in the relief of nausea and vomiting resulting from cancer chemotherapy. It is of questionable value as a bronchodilator, anticonvulsant, or analgesic.[25] Some derivatives of Δ^9-THC may prove to be more useful clinically than the parent drug, which, particularly in the older patient, is limited by the occurrence of drowsiness, the marijuana high, and occasional psychotomimetic effects.

Abuse characteristics

There is no evidence that long-term marijuana use produces psychic dependence to any degree. The occurrence of physical dependence is also questionable, though abrupt withdrawal following long-term heavy use (up to 210 mg/day) has been reported to lead to insomnia, rebound REM sleep, tremor, irritability, anorexia, diarrhea, and weight loss, which peak at 25 to 36 hours and last 3 to 4 days.[28] This abstinence syndrome is similar to that seen with most general CNS depressants. Dose-related tolerance develops to both the behavioral and physiologic effects of the drug, with no cross-tolerance to opioid analgesics or to LSD.

Acute toxicity

Acute marijuana toxicity has been reported occasionally after IV use of impure extracts.[23] The symptoms include extreme thirst, shaking chills, fever, tachycardia, and generalized aching pains. Prolonged hypotension and a reversible renal insufficiency may also develop. However, even massive doses of Δ^9-THC fail to produce anesthesia in humans.[29]

POLYDRUG ABUSE

Drug abuse problems are often compounded by the practice of taking two or more drugs in combination or in sequence.[14] The polydrug abuser may seek additive or potentiated effects (e.g., with the simultaneous use of alcohol and sedatives) or the modulation or termination of effects (e.g., with the sequential use of amphetamines and barbiturates). About 20% of chronic alcoholics abuse other drugs, especially barbiturates, antianxiety drugs, and marijuana. Primary heavy users of marijuana frequently employ amphetamines or psychedelic agents, whereas heroin addicts are particularly apt to abuse amphetamine, cocaine, hallucinogens, and barbiturates. The majority of patients in methadone

maintenance programs appear to be polydrug abusers.

Complications of polydrug abuse include an increased incidence of medical problems, such as hepatitis, bacterial endocarditis, and cardiac conduction defects.[14] When multiple physical dependence develops, the withdrawal syndrome becomes difficult to treat and is associated with significantly enhanced mortality.

DENTAL IMPLICATIONS OF DRUG ABUSE

It is often claimed that drug abusers, in particular opioid addicts, have a history of poor employment and academic adjustment and have difficulty with interpersonal relationships. They are characterized as egocentric, immature, impulsive, and self-deprecating and are said to suffer from psychologic needs for approval, respect, and appreciation. Drugs of abuse are employed to reverse this state by producing euphoria or to submerge it by eliminating unwanted thoughts.

Certain signs may alert the clinician to the possible parenteral abuse of drugs. Telltale cutaneous lesions may result from the chronic hypodermic administration of drugs of abuse.[42] These lesions include acute septic complications, such as subcutaneous abscesses, cellulitis, and thrombophlebitis, as well as chronic cutaneous complications, including skin "tracks," "pop" scars, and infected lesions, which occur most commonly in the thigh or antecubital or deltoid regions. Skin "tracks" result from frequent, multiple injections that produce chronic tissue inflammation. These are typically erythematous linear or bifurcated lesions, which become indurated and hyperpigmented. "Pop" scars, resulting from intradermal (subcutaneous) injections in inexperienced users, are irreversible, circular, depressed, atrophic, and hyperpigmented lesions, usually about 1 to 3 cm in diameter. Another sign that may alert the clinician to the problem of drug abuse is the presence of an ill-defined febrile illness. This often reflects a low-grade bacteremia resulting from the injection of drugs.[37]

In ascertaining whether a patient is abusing drugs, the dentist cannot depend on being able to identify a particular personality type, to recognize cutaneous lesions (which may be concealed under clothing), or to diagnose a mild febrile illness. Rather, the dentist must rely on careful and thorough questioning of the patient and on the skillful use of a well-designed medical history questionnaire.

Drug abuse is a subject of considerable importance to dentists because of their occasionally being the unwitting target or victim of the drug abuser's need to secure drugs, the long history of drug abuse among health professionals, the number of medical and dental abnormalities associated with drug abuse, and the interactions between drugs dentists customarily prescribe and those the patient is abusing.

Dentist as target of drug abusers

It is inevitable that drug abusers will, through pretense and subterfuge, attempt to obtain drugs from dentists. Therefore, the dentist should be aware of any patient who complains of pain from pulpitis or an abscess and who refuses immediate endodontic or surgical intervention, particularly if the patient exhibits yawning, sneezing, miosis, and an unusual thirst. The opioid abuser will frequently claim to be allergic to codeine or pentazocine in an effort to obtain stronger drugs such as meperidine, morphine, or hydrocodone.[1] As a general defense against drug abusers, the dentist should never let patients know where such drugs are kept, never leave prescription pads out where they may be taken, and avoid the use of prewritten prescription forms.

Drug use among dentists

Dentists are not immune to the hazards of drug abuse; in fact, like physicians, they may be in greater danger of developing drug dependencies than the general population because of the ready accessibility of narcotic analgesics and general CNS depressant drugs. Indeed, it is commonly agreed that narcotic addiction among medical personnel is 10 times that of the general population.

One form of abuse common among dentists and other health professionals is the "sniffing" of nitrous oxide (Chapter 19). Such "recreational" inhalation over periods of several months has been associated with peripheral neuropathy characterized by a distal loss of sensation and vibratory sense, hypoactive tendon reflexes, electric shock sensations traveling upward from the feet on flexion of the neck, and a sensation of a tight abdominal band.[24] Partial improvement of symptoms occurs on abstinence from nitrous oxide for 4 to 6 months. Although no abstinence symptoms have been reported in individuals withdrawn from nitrous oxide

abuse, the possibility of a true opioid-like psychic dependence on the drug is enhanced by reports that nitrous oxide analgesia in rats is antagonized by naloxone and by chronic morphinization.[5]

Medical and dental complications of drug abuse

The most common and serious medical complications in the drug-abusing patient are endocarditis and hepatitis. Bacterial endocarditis in the drug abuser is most commonly caused by *Staphylococcus aureus,* which appears to derive from an increase in endogenous pathogens in the addict rather than from contaminated drugs or drug paraphernalia.[37] In drug-abusing patients the disease often affects the tricuspid valve, which is unusual in nonabusers. Murmurs are frequently absent, and the patient's initial symptoms usually appear to be simply a case of staphylococcal bacteremia. A predominance of respiratory symptoms is indicative of tricuspid valve involvement. The disease is usually acute, with rapid destruction of valves and progression to heart failure. *Pseudomonas* endocarditis, though less common, involves primarily the tricuspid valve and has an overall mortality of 50%. *Candida albicans* infects the left-sided valves and is almost invariably fatal. Secondary staphylococcal infections include an exfoliative (scalded skin) syndrome, septic arthritis and vertebral osteomyelitis, meningitis or metastatic brain abscesses (associated with facial paresis, hemiplegia, delirium, or coma), renal cortical abscesses, glomerulonephritis, nephrosis, and lung abscesses.

Viral hepatitis is frequently seen among drug abusers and is probably transmitted via contaminated needles.[8] Hepatitis B antigen is, however, often absent in the one third of drug abusers who experience recurring episodes of infection. The disease is usually mild, but individuals displaying early signs of elevated prothrombin time, fever, elevated leukocyte count, or encephalopathy have a poor prognosis. In 50% to 80% of cases, the acute infection results in a chronic inflammatory hepatic disease.

Intravenous drug abusers are a population at risk of acquired immune deficiency syndrome (AIDS); other groups at risk are homosexual males, Haitian immigrants, and hemophiliacs. Prodromal symptoms include unexplained prolonged fever, fatigue, weight loss, and generalized lymphadenopathy. Lymphopenia and skin test anergy are common. Opportunistic infections later develop, including

Kaposi's sarcoma, *Pneumocystis carinii* pneumonia, and oral candidiasis or herpes zoster. The disease may prove to be fatal to many who acquire it. It is believed to be caused by a subgroup of the human T-cell leukemia virus family, designated HTLV-III. The U.S. Centers for Disease Control have recommended that clinicians avoid direct contact with blood, excretions, secretions, or tissues of patients exhibiting any of the above symptoms who are from any of the known groups at risk of AIDS.

Specific dental complications of drug use include rampant caries and rapidly progressing periodontal disorders resulting from nutritional deficiencies and neglect of personal hygiene.[42] Self-mutilation has occurred among drug abusers; teeth may be deliberately damaged in an effort to obtain drugs. As mentioned earlier, chronic amphetamine abusers typically develop facial tics and bruxism, which result in a traumatized tongue and worn teeth.[15] These subjects may also chronically rub the tongue along the inside of the lower lip, producing ulcers on the abraded tissues.[11] Xerostomia is a common finding in those who chronically abuse opioids, amphetamines, and marijuana. Chronic amphetamine users are also prone to cardiac arrhythmias,[11] particularly paroxysmal atrial tachycardia.

Drug interactions in drug abuse

Drug interactions exhibited by abusers are not unique but depend on the drug of abuse.[12,13] Because sedative-hypnotic agents (barbiturates and glutethimide in particular) induce hepatic microsomal activity, abusers of such substances may be resistant to the therapeutic effects of corticosteroids, digitoxin, oral anticoagulants, and other CNS depressants. Chloral hydrate may exacerbate the effects of oral anticoagulants, such as warfarin, by being metabolized to trichloroacetic acid, which competes with warfarin for plasma protein binding sites. Paraldehyde may increase the risk of sulfonamide crystalluria by acidifying the urine.

Opioid abusers will generally show tolerance to other opioid analgesics. The dentist should beware of giving pentazocine to such patients, since this agonist-antagonist may precipitate an acute abstinence syndrome in opioid-dependent patients.

Methylphenidate reportedly inhibits drug biotransformation and may potentiate the effects of other agents, such as barbiturates and phenytoin.[12]

Marijuana, though considered a minor drug of abuse in terms of social acceptance, intensifies the CNS depression produced by barbiturates and general anesthetics.[29] Atropine administered to marijuana smokers may precipitate prolonged periods of tachycardia.[18] It has also been reported that physostigmine given to marijuana-intoxicated subjects can produce profound depression with suicidal feelings.[13]

CITED REFERENCES

1. Abbott, L. Don't be deceived by a drug addict. American Medical Association News **19:**1-4, 1976.
2. Änggård, E., Jönsson, L.E., Hogmark, A.L., and Gunne, L.M. Amphetamine metabolism in amphetamine psychosis. Clinical Pharmacology and Therapeutics **14:**870-880, 1973.
3. Aston, R. Chemical, pharmacological, and dependence characteristics of hypnosedatives and minor tranquilizers. In National Commission on Marihuana and Drug Abuse, Second Report. Drug Use in America: Problem in Perspective, vol. 1, Washington, D.C., U.S. Government Printing Office, 1973.
4. Aston, R. Mechanisms contributing to barbiturate intolerance in the rat. British Journal of Pharmacology **49:**527-533, 1973.
5. Berkowitz, B.A., Ngai, S.H., and Fink, A.D. Nitrous oxide "analgesia": resemblance to opiate action. Science **194:**967-968, 1976.
6. Brill, H. The treatment of drug dependence: a brief history. In National Commission on Marihuana and Drug Abuse, Second Report. Drug Use in America: Problem in Perspective, vol. 4. Washington, D.C., U.S. Government Printing Office, 1973.
7. Caldwell, C.B., and Gross, J.B. Physostigmine reversal of midazolam-induced sedation. Anesthesiology **57:**125-127, 1982.
8. Cherubin, C.E. Hepatic complications. In Pradhan, S.N., and Dutta, S.N., eds. Drug Abuse: Clinical and Basic Aspects, St. Louis, The C.V. Mosby Co., 1977.
9. Choice of benzodiazepines. Medical Letter on Drugs and Therapeutics **23:**41-43, 1981.
10. Clonidine for opiate withdrawal. Medical Letter on Drugs and Therapeutics **21:**100, 1979.
11. Connell, P.H. Clinical manifestations and treatment of amphetamine type of dependence. Journal of the American Medical Association **196:**718-723, 1966.
12. Davis, J.M., Sekerke, H.J., and Janowsky, D.S. Drug interactions involving the drugs of abuse. In National Commission on Marihuana and Drug Abuse, Second Report. Drug Use in America: Problem in Perspective, vol. 1. Washington, D.C., U.S. Government Printing Office, 1973.
13. Dutta, S.N. Drug interactions in abusers. In Pradhan, S.N., and Dutta, S.N., eds. Drug Abuse: Clinical and Basic Aspects. St. Louis, The C.V. Mosby Co., 1977.
14. Dutta, S.N., and Kaufman, E. Multiple drug abuse. In Pradhan, S.N., and Dutta, S.N., eds. Drug Abuse: Clinical and Basic Aspects. St. Louis, The C.V. Mosby Co., 1977.
15. Ellinwood, E.H., and Petrie, W.M. Dependence on amphetamine, cocaine, and other stimulants. In Pradhan, S.N., and Dutta, S.N., eds. Drug Abuse: Clinical and Basic Aspects. St. Louis, The C.V. Mosby Co., 1977.

16. Fraser, H.F., Wikler, A., Essig, C.F., and Isbell, H. Degree of physical dependence induced by secobarbital or pentobarbital. Journal of the American Medical Association **166**:126-129, 1958.

17. Greenblatt, D.J., Allen, M.D., Noel, B.J., and Shader, R.I. Acute overdosage with benzodiazepine derivatives. Clinical Pharmacology and Therapeutics **21**:497-514, 1977.

18. Gregg, J.M., Campbell, R.L., Levin, K.J., Ghia, J., and Elliott, R.A. Cardiovascular effects of cannabinol during oral surgery. Anesthesia and Analgesia; Current Researches **55**:203-213, 1976.

19. Hillestad, L., Hansen, T., and Melsom, H. Diazepam metabolism in normal man. II. Serum concentration and clinical effect after oral administration and cumulation. Clinical Pharmacology and Therapeutics **16**:485-489, 1974.

20. Isbell, H., and Chrusciel, T.L. Dependence liability of ''non-narcotic'' drugs. Bulletin of the World Health Organization **43**(suppl):1-111, 1970.

21. Kagen, S.L. *Aspergillus:* an inhalable contaminant of marihuana. New England Journal of Medicine **304**:483-484, 1981.

22. Kalant, H., LeBlanc, A.E., and Gibbins, R.J. Tolerance to, and dependence on, some non-opiate psychotropic drugs. Pharmacological Reviews **23**:135-191, 1971.

23. King, A.B., and Cowen, D.L. Effect of intravenous injection of marihuana. Journal of the American Medical Association **210**:724-725, 1969.

24. Layzer, R.B., Fishman, R.A., and Schafer, J.A. Neuropathy following abuse of nitrous oxide. Neurology **28**:504-506, 1978.

25. Lemberger, L. Potential therapeutic usefulness of marijuana. Annual Review of Pharmacology and Toxicology **20**:151-172, 1980.

26. Mandell, A.J., Stewart, K.D., and Russo, P.V. The Sunday syndrome: from kinetics to altered consciousness. Federation Proceedings **40**:2693-2698, 1981.

27. Mansky, P.A. Opiates: human psychopharmacology. In Iversen, L.L., Iversen, S.D., and Snyder, S.H., eds. Drugs of Abuse. Handbook of Psychopharmacology, vol. 12. New York, Plenum Press, 1978.

28. Meyer, R.E. Behavioral pharmacology of marihuana. In Lipton, M.A., DiMascio, A., and Killam, K.F., eds. Psychopharmacology: A Generation of Progress. New York, Raven Press, 1978.

29. Paton, W.D.M. Pharmacology of marijuana. Annual Review of Pharmacology **15**:191-220, 1975.

30. Petersen, R.C. History of cocaine. In Petersen, R.C., and Stillman, R.C., eds. Cocaine: 1977. N.I.D.A. Research Monograph No. 13. Rockville, Md., U.S. Department of Health, Education, and Welfare, 1977.

31. Pradhan, S.N. LSD and other hallucinogens. In Pradhan, S.N., and Dutta, S.N., eds. Drug Abuse; Clinical and Basic Aspects, St. Louis, The C.V. Mosby Co., 1977.

32. Pradhan, S.N., and Dutta, S.N. Narcotic analgesics. In Pradhan, S.N., and Dutta, S.N., eds. Drug Abuse: Clinical and Basic Aspects. St. Louis, The C.V. Mosby Co., 1977.

33. Pradhan, S.N., and Hollister, L.E. Abuse of LSD and other hallucinogenic drugs. In Pradhan, S.N., and Dutta, S.N., eds. Drug Abuse: Clinical and Basic Aspects. St. Louis, The C.V. Mosby Co., 1977.

34. Resnick, R.B., Kestenbaum, R.S., and Schwartz, L.K. Acute systemic effects of cocaine in man: a controlled study by intranasal and intravenous routes. Science **195**:696-698, 1977.

35. Snyder, S.H. Hallucinogens. In National Commission on Marihuana and Drug Abuse, Second Report. Drug Use in America: Problem in Perspective, vol. 1. Washington, D.C., U.S. Government Printing Office, 1973.

36. Terenius, L. Endogenous peptides and analgesia. Annual Review of Pharmacology and Toxicology **18**:189-204, 1978.

37. Tuazon, C.U., and Sheagren, J.M. Septic complications. In Pradhan, S.N., and Dutta, S.N., eds. Drug Abuse: Clinical and Basic Aspects. St. Louis, The C.V. Mosby Co., 1977.

38. Valdes, F., Fanelli, R.J., and McNamara, J.O. Barbiturate and GABA receptors coupled to benzodiazepine receptors in rat hippocampal formation: a radiohistochemical study. Life Sciences **29**:1895-1900, 1981.

39. Van Dyke, C., and Byck, R. Cocaine. Scientific American **246**:128-141, 1982.

40. Way, E.L., and Glasgow, C. Recent developments in morphine analgesia: tolerance and dependence. In Lipton, M.A., DiMascio, A., and Killam, K.F., eds. Psychopharmacology: A Generation of Progress. New York, Raven Press, 1978.

41. World Health Organization Expert Committee on Drug Dependence, Sixteenth report. World Health Organization Technical Report Series, no. 407, Geneva, 1969.

42. Young, A.W. Cutaneous manifestations. In Pradhan, S.N., and Dutta, S.N., eds. Drug Abuse: Clinical and Basic Aspects. St. Louis, The C.V. Mosby Co., 1977.

GENERAL REFERENCES

Braude, M.C., and Szara, S., eds. The Pharmacology of Marihuana. New York, Raven Press, 1976.

Domino, E.F., ed. PCP (Phencyclidine): Historical and Current Perspectives. Ann Arbor, Mich., NPP Books, 1981.

Martin, W.R., ed. Amphetamine, psychotogen, and marihuana dependence. In Drug Addiction. Handbook of Experimental Pharmacology, vol. 45. New York, Springer-Verlag, 1977.

Martin, W.R., ed. Morphine, sedative-hypnotic, and alcohol dependence. In Drug Addiction. Handbook of Experimental Pharmacology, vol. 45. New York, Springer-Verlag, 1977.

Nahas, G.G., and Paton, W.D.M., eds. Marijuana; Biological Effects. New York, Pergamon Press, 1980.

Petersen, R.C., ed. Marihuana Research Findings: 1976. N.I.D.A. Research Monograph No. 14, Rockville, Md., U.S. Department of Health, Education, and Welfare, 1977.

Smith, E.E., Wesson, D.R., Buxron, M.E., Seymour, R.B., Ungerleider, J.T., Morgan, J.P., Mandell, A.J., and Jara, G., eds. Amphetamine Use, Misuse and Abuse: Proceedings of the National Amphetamine Conference, 1978. Boston, G.K. Hall & Co., 1979.

Spotts, J.V., and Spotts, C.A., eds. Use and Abuse of Amphetamine and Its Substitutes. NIDR Research Issues 25. Rockville, Md., U.S. Department of Health, Education, and Welfare, 1980.

47 Toxicology

Wyatt R. Hume
William Warner
John A. Yagiela

Toxicology is the science of poisons, including their detection, nature, and effects on biologic systems, humans in particular. Toxic effects may result from exposure to chemicals in the environment, substances used or produced in industry, household products, foodstuffs, and drugs. Obviously, toxicology is a broad discipline, one encompassing a number of subspecialties. Among the concerns of toxicologists are the identification of adverse effects and the elucidation of their mechanisms, the proper management of untoward reactions, the analysis of toxic agents in the environment and in various body compartments and fluids, the environmental influences of industrial chemicals and pollutants, forensic investigations and other medicolegal problems, and government regulations. Much of these areas lies beyond the scope of a survey of pharmacology.

The toxicology of individual drugs or groups of drugs is an integral part of their pharmacology and is therefore described in the appropriate chapters of this book. Here, the general principles of toxicology will be reviewed, along with the toxicology of some common substances that are not described elsewhere in the text. The prevention and management of acute poisoning will also be outlined.

GENERAL PRINCIPLES

All chemicals can kill cells, organs, or individuals if they reach high enough concentrations in a given part of the body and remain there for an appropriate time. However, only those chemicals that can reasonably do so are considered toxic; thus, water, nitrogen, and oxygen are not listed as toxins even though each can be lethal in special circumstances. Despite such limitation, the number of potential toxins is vast.

One primary concern of toxicology is the evaluation of risk. With every chemical, be it a drug, food additive, or industrial solvent, a balance must be struck between the benefits of using that agent and its attendant risk. This task can be accomplished in part by determining the answers to several questions. First, what adverse effects are associated with exposure to the agent, and what is the expected incidence of these effects? The answers to these queries are scientific in nature and can usually be gleaned from toxicologic studies. The next question that must be answered is whether or not the risk is acceptable. Unlike the previous questions, this one addresses social, economic, and ethical values not amenable to easy analysis.

In a clinical setting, the benefits of all possible regimens must be compared to the risks involved. Likewise in the area of environmental toxicology, the economic benefits that are realized by permitting the release of a pollutant must be compared to the biologic risks that are thus assumed. It should be noted that the term *safety* was not used in the above discussion. Safety suggests to some individuals that a course of action is free of hazard. Certainly, exposure to any substance must be considered to be associated with some risk.

Dose-response relationships

Most toxic chemicals display some degree of organ specificity, usually affecting a limited number of target organs. In general, toxicologic studies are designed to demonstrate the dose-response relationship that is associated with each of those actions. Aside from providing information concerning the amount of a chemical that is required to produce a specific effect, dose-response curves also provide evidence that a causal relationship exists between the observed effect and the chemical being investigated.

Toxicity is readily quantified when simple criteria of response, such as death, are used. If the percentage of a test population killed is plotted against the dose for a given route of administration, then the median lethal dose, LD50, may be calculated; this and other indices of lethality are useful for comparisons between chemicals (see Chapter 3). The death of individual cells is also relatively easy to measure, using such indicators as the loss of ability to exclude dye or the release of labeled cell contents, or by measuring cessation of metabolic function. It is often useful, however, to know more than the acute lethal dose. Various measurements of enzyme function, histochemical staining, and electron microscopic examination of subcellular structure may all give information useful in the prediction of later and more dramatic pathologic changes.

The doses that are used in toxicologic studies are often well above those that can be practically administered to humans. The reason for such high doses becomes evident when considering the statistical problems associated with the use of a small number of animals to predict what will happen during large scale human exposure. As already mentioned in Chapter 3, any large population contains individuals with markedly differing sensitivities to the effects of biologically active agents. When designing a toxicologic study, the use of high doses provides an assurance of obtaining a measurable response even if the experimental group is composed entirely of relatively insensitive individuals. Although this procedure will overestimate the incidence of some toxicities, it is considered to be an acceptable compromise.

Factors that alter dose-response relationships

As with all pharmacologic effects, dose-response relationships of toxic substances can be altered by a variety of factors. For instance, different species may react differently to the same compound. Even within a species, each strain may react differently. An analogous situation occurs with human populations. For example, members of some ethnic groups produce erythrocytes that are deficient in the enzyme glucose-6-phosphate dehydrogenase. This enzyme is an integral part of a system that provides reducing equivalents for the protection of cellular enzymes and membranes. When individuals with a deficiency of this enzyme are exposed to oxidants, metabolic functions may be impaired, and methemoglobinemia and hemolysis may occur.[10]

Because many compounds are converted into metabolites with either enhanced or diminished biologic activity, factors that alter the metabolic rate may affect the toxicity of some substances. Studies have demonstrated that males frequently have higher metabolic rates than females. Consequently, the actions of some drugs, such as the barbiturates, may be diminished in males. This effect can be reversed by pretreating males with estrogen.[15]

Toxicities may be altered by disease states, dietary status, age, and weight. Gastrointestinal contents at the time of administration can also have a significant effect on toxicity. Many substances appear to be less toxic when they are administered after a meal (usually as a result of diminished absorption), whereas other compounds are more toxic or, in the case of some phenothiazine derivatives, may interact with dietary constituents to produce substances of greater toxicity than the parent compound. The ability of a chemical to produce toxic effects may also vary with such factors as the time and frequency of administration, the physical form of the chemical, and even the season of the year during which the study is being conducted. Even this partial list provides some insight into the numerous variables that must be considered when evaluating toxicologic data.

Acute and chronic toxicities

Toxicities are often classified according to the amount of time that must pass before they become evident. Acute toxicities develop shortly after a single or small number of exposures, whereas chronic toxicities may take multiple exposures or even years to develop. Acute intoxication with ethanol is an example of the former reaction, and cirrhosis of the liver is representative of the latter. In the case of a carcinogen, decades may pass before a tumor is produced. Other toxicities, for example those of the reproductive system, might occur early in childhood but remain undetected for years, until sexual maturation is attained. Even then, the complex feedback mechanisms that control the function of all endocrine systems make abnormalities in many of these organs difficult to detect.

Cells may survive brief contact with a given concentration of a toxic chemical but die with prolonged exposure, if the mechanism of action is reversible inhibition of an essential metabolic pathway. For example, the cyanide–cytochrome oxidase complex is dissociable, and cyanide poisoning may therefore be overcome with no harm to the individual (if treatment is rapid) by administration of drugs that promote its removal from vital enzymes and eventual elimination from the body. On the other hand very brief initial contact will cause prolonged tissue presence and major effects if binding is less reversible, as occurs with mercury and sulfhydryl enzymes or with the organophosphate insecticides and cholinesterase enzymes.

Exposure to subtoxic concentrations of chemicals that accumulate in the tissues, if repeated at intervals less than the clearance time, will lead to the eventual development of toxic concentrations. Repeated exposures to sublethal concentrations of toxins may also cause cumulative damage to tissues. Of clinical relevance to dentists is the response of the pulp to repeated episodes of chemical trauma, as occurs in frequent replacement of restorations. The pulp survives a given degree of insult initially, with the death of some cells and some loss of vascularity; it is then less well equipped to deal with a subsequent insult.

When chronic toxicities develop, they often have no relationship to the acute effects of the same substances. For example, organophosphate pesticides produce an immediate cholinomimetic effect, but repeated exposure to low concentrations of the same compounds may result in a slowly developing neuronal degeneration.[1] Another example of differences between acute and chronic toxicity is provided by the organochlorine pesticides, for example DDT. The immediate toxicities of these compounds reflect their actions on the central and peripheral nervous systems,[6] whereas reproductive toxicities have become apparent in a number of species that concentrate the compounds over a long period of time.[11]

Chemical by-products as toxicants

When a dose-dependent effect is demonstrated, further studies are often conducted to investigate the possibility that the biologically active agent might be a contaminant or metabolite of the substance that was under study. Many toxicities are known to be caused by metabolites, frequently of only minor quantitative importance, of the chemicals that were originally suspected as being harmful. For example, most of the environmental pollutants that are suspected of exhibiting carcinogenic activity are actually procarcinogens. Conversion of these substances in the body to highly reactive electrophiles must proceed before cellular damage can occur. These active metabolites are often so unstable that if they were injected directly into a test animal they would be inactivated before producing their biologic effect.

If the substance under investigation is not pure, as is usually the case with commercial products, each individual component or contaminant may have its own biologic activity. An illustration of the importance of this principle is provided by the chemical that is commonly called dioxin. This compound is formed during the manufacture of a number of herbicides and is consequently a contaminant of the commercial products. Only as a result of studies on purified dioxin was it realized that the teratogenic effect that had previously been associated with the herbicides was actually caused by this contaminant.[4] This information led to a reduction in the maximum allowable content of dioxin in commercial products.

When a substance undergoes chemical transformation during use, the parent compound and its reaction products may have different biologic effects. This factor has greatly impeded investigation of the toxic effects of cigarette smoke, a mixture of up to 5000 compounds. The chemical composition of cigarette smoke has been found to vary according to such factors as the source of the tobacco, the temperature of combustion, the type of paper used in the cigarette, and the density of tobacco packing. Failure to consider such seemingly minor details can complicate the interpretation of toxicologic data.

A related problem has been encountered when studies are performed on chemicals that may burn under extraordinary conditions. For example, plastics used to construct electrical conduits, or as components of the interiors of automobiles and airplanes, may release a variety of combustion products when they are exposed to high temperatures. Obviously, if a substance may undergo chemical transformation during use, failure to assess the hazard posed by products of pyrolysis may result in a serious underestimation of risk.

Local versus systemic toxicity

Toxic effects may be local (at or near the applied site) or remote. With local effects, the toxic agent reaches a concentration dependent on that applied minus diffusion away from the site, clearance into the blood, dilution by local secretions such as saliva, gastric fluid, or tears, and local metabolism of the toxin. If the site of application is a short distance from the target tissue, as in the case of a chemical diffusing through epidermis to dermis, or through dentin to pulp, then a concentration gradient will also be established across the intervening tissue, according to the nature of the medium, molecular size of the toxin, and binding affinities to tissue constituents.

Remote toxic effects usually depend on blood absorption and transport. The concentration developed in a tissue at a particular time will vary with the rate of absorption into blood, the distribution to other tissues and fluids, the rate of metabolism and excretion (all of which influence the blood concentration) and the affinity between the target tissue and the toxin. Portals of entry into the body are the lungs, the skin, the gastrointestinal tract, and other mucous membranes; chemicals may also reach internal tissues and blood directly by trauma or intentional injection. As is discussed in Chapter 2, substances with high lipid solubility move readily across membranes, and their uptake is generally more rapid than that of water-soluble chemicals. Metabolic breakdown of toxins occurs primarily in the liver, and excretion in the urine or bile. Of note is the possibility of toxic effects in the liver or kidney during these processes, caused either by concentration of the toxin or by the formation of toxic metabolites. Toxic substances may reach any tissue, with transfer to the cerebrospinal fluid, to the fetus, and even to the nursing infant via milk being possible.

Principal target organs

Central nervous system. The tissues that are most often affected by toxicants are those of the central nervous system. The high metabolic rates of individual neurons, and their inability to rely on anaerobic glycolysis, make these cells very susceptible to the actions of a large number of chemicals. Any substance that interferes with cellular respiration, or that can compromise pulmonary ventilation or cerebral circulation, can produce irreversible damage to central neurons.

Among the most sensitive cells in the central nervous system are small sensory fibers. Sensory neuropathies, such as paresthesias and altered perceptions of sound and light, can result from exposure to a large variety of chemicals. Alternatively, ataxia, tremor, and diplopia usually indicate a damaged motor pathway.

Such undesirable effects can develop despite the presence of the blood-brain barrier. Although this complex barrier excludes many substances from the brain (see Chapter 2), it can be disrupted by trauma or by exposure to some chemicals, for example, mercury. Even when intact, the blood-brain barrier does not effectively restrict entry of compounds of great lipid solubility, a group that includes many drugs, pesticides, and industrial chemicals. Furthermore, the "barrier" offers no protection from the hypoxia and hypercapnia that can result from effects on tissues outside of the central nervous system.

Cardiovascular system. The cardiovascular and hematopoietic systems are also frequent targets of toxic substances. For example, a variety of chemicals (including drugs, industrial solvents, and venoms) can produce hemolytic anemia. This effect provides an excellent illustration of how an action on one cell type can be reflected in a number of different ways. Aside from the obvious loss of oxygen-carrying capacity, a cluster of signs and symptoms may appear that relate back to the primary event. Hemolysis is associated wtih fever and pain in the extremities. As the number of intact erythrocytes diminishes, immature blood cells are released into the circulation. The liver and spleen, organs that normally destroy damaged red blood cells, become enlarged. The catabolic conversion of large quantities of hemoglobin into bile pigments results in jaundice, and, in severe cases, hemoglobin may appear in the urine.

Another toxicity affecting erythrocytes is the development of methemoglobinemia. This condition arises when oxidizing substances enter erythrocytes and convert the iron within the hemoglobin molecule into the ferric form. The result is easy fatigability, sensory disturbances, and cyanosis.

Exposure to certain substances may diminish the ability of bone marrow to produce adequate numbers of blood cells. The result can be inadequate oxygenation, bleeding abnormalities, or compromised immune function. For example, a reduction in the number of circulating granulocytes is associated with an abnormally great susceptibility to infection. A much more serious blood dyscrasia, agranulocytosis is characterized by the absence of neutrophils from bone marrow and peripheral tissues. The most serious toxic reaction of the hematopoietic system is aplastic anemia. In this condition the bone marrow loses its ability to produce any cellular elements.

Visceral organs. The liver and kidney are often the targets of toxic substances. Hepatotoxicity is frequently manifested as necrosis with either highly localized or widespread cellular destruction. With the loss of liver cells the body may become more susceptible to the biologic actions of other compounds. A reduction in the activity of hepatic microsomal enzyme systems may prolong the half-life of many drugs, and the reduced concentration of blood proteins may exaggerate the toxicity of substances that normally demonstrate a high degree of protein binding. Another form of hepatotoxicity that is occasionally observed is cholestatic hepatitis. In this condition, which is known to be caused by a variety of drugs, bile flow is disrupted and jaundice develops.

The great blood supply that is received by the kidney and its ability to concentrate solutes, in both the urine and the tubule cells, make this organ particularly prone to the actions of poisons. Adverse changes in renal function may be manifested as alterations in the chemical composition of urine or its rate of formation. However, such indices of renal injury are sometimes difficult to detect. The kidney has a remarkable ability to compensate for malfunctions. Consequently, if renal function is not continuously monitored the signs of toxicity may be missed.

Even though a substance might have a direct effect on a visceral organ, the toxicity may be indirectly manifested at other sites. For example, if liver function is compromised, the resultant increase in the blood concentration of ammonia will cause confusion and facial grimacing. Likewise, the uremia that results from renal insufficiency will also produce CNS, cardiovascular, and endocrine abnormalities.

PREVENTION AND MANAGEMENT OF ACUTE POISONING

The prevention of chemical toxicity is a responsibility of the entire community. Governmental agencies and private corporations must act in concert to minimize toxic hazards in the workplace and the environment. In the home, it is the responsibility of parents and older siblings to protect young children from harm as they actively explore their surroundings. Numerous good sources of information are available to aid families in protecting themselves against accidental poisoning. Several steps can also be taken by practitioners to limit the possibility of accidental poisoning. Patients should be encouraged to keep all medications out of the reach of children. Drugs should always be kept in child-resistant containers. Transferring medications to more convenient receptacles is to be condemned; not only does this practice increase the accessibility of drugs to inquisitive youngsters, it also promotes accidental ingestion by adults. Information reproduced on the label of a prescribed drug should be understandable and include the name of the agent and the purpose of medication. This procedure will help reduce confusion between drugs in the medicine cabinet and permit, in the case of accidental ingestion, the rapid identification of the compound involved. Patients should be warned not to attempt self-medication with drugs left over from previous courses of therapy but to discard any unused medication.

Although the diagnosis and treatment of poisoning is rightfully the purview of the physician, the principles of therapy will be summarized here, since they apply to the management of any drug overdose. Moreover, a dentist may well be called on to provide emergency treatment of acute poisoning within the practice environment or because of his or her background as a health professional.

1. *Summon help*. In the event of acute poisoning, whether from a drug or other chemical, the community poison control center can be of invaluable service. These centers are equipped with extensive files describing the signs and symptoms of poisoning and the recommended method of treatment for most toxic substances distributed within the United States. Such centers can be reached by telephone on a 24-hour basis. Obviously, if the toxic reaction is serious, expert medical assistance should be sought immediately.

2. *Supportive therapy*. Because hypoxia and shock are two common manifestations of serious toxicity, it is imperative that respiration and circulation be monitored and assisted if required. For convulsions, physical protective measures may suffice, along with the administration of oxygen to help avoid hypoxia. IV diazepam is the drug of choice for pharmacologic control of continuing seizures. Aspirin and some other agents may produce life-threatening disturbances in body temperature

or in water and electrolyte balance that require symptomatic treatment as well.

3. *Identify cause.* Proper therapy aimed at eliminating exposure to the toxin or reversing its effects depends on identifying the poison. Questioning the victim or the victim's associates, searching for empty containers, or looking for telltale physical signs on the patient (miosis or needle tracks for opioid overdose; burn marks in the mouth for ingestion of caustic chemicals) all may be important in establishing the cause of the poisoning.

4. *Terminate absorption.* For a chemical in contact with the skin, repeated washing with soap and water is indicated. With ingested compounds other than petroleum products and corrosive substances, vomiting should be induced in the conscious patient. Syrup of ipecac is normally the agent of choice because, although it requires about 20 minutes to act, its effect is self-limiting, the drug being regurgitated with the poison. For home use, a small volume of ipecac can be purchased without a prescription. Depending on body weight, 15 to 30 ml followed closely by a glass of warm water will be sufficient. In the unresponsive patient, the induction of vomiting is proscribed, but gastric lavage can be employed by qualified personnel if care is taken to avoid aspiration of stomach contents by the victim. The binding of many drugs within the gastrointestinal tract can be achieved by activated charcoal (10 to 50 gm in water); cathartics may be employed to hasten the exit of drugs from the intestine.

5. *Specific therapy.* Specific antidotes are available to treat poisoning by certain classes of compounds. Antidotes may be useful in preventing the absorption of ingested agents (e.g., calcium salts for fluoride ion), increasing their rate of elimination (e.g., dimercaprol for inorganic mercury), or blocking their toxic activity (e.g., naloxone for morphine). One specific antidote should be remembered by dentists. For ingestion of toxic amounts of fluoride, as may occur in the home with prescribed tablets or in the dental operatory with topical liquids or gels, the local antidote to prevent absorption is calcium (in milk, calcium lactate, calcium gluconate, or lime water). If necessary, 2 to 10 ml of 10% calcium gluconate may be injected intravenously to bind fluoride and overcome hypocalcemia. Of course, dentists who employ opioid analgesics for conscious sedation must be familiar with the use of naloxone to reverse opioid-induced respiratory depression (see Chapter 20).

6. *Enhance elimination.* Measures to hasten elimination of toxicants are in the realm of poison centers and emergency-care physicians; they are mentioned here for the sake of completeness. The renal excretion of weak electrolytes can often be accelerated by appropriate modification of urinary pH. Administration of large volumes of water in conjunction with an osmotic diuretic is helpful in promoting urinary excretion and in reducing the renal concentration of nephrotoxic poisons. In some instances, peritoneal dialysis or hemodialysis with an artificial kidney may be necessary.

SPECIFIC POISONS

In addition to prescribed or OTC drugs, there are a number of household products and environmental toxicants that are commonly implicated in poisoning. The major compounds of interest include the heavy metals, carbon monoxide and other air pollutants, organic solvents, and pesticides.

Mercury and other heavy metals

Heavy metal poisoning has been recognized since antiquity. Arsenic has been used with both therapeutic and lethal intent for many millenia, and it is considered possible that the fall of the Roman empire was hastened by the pervasive contamination of the water supply by lead. Today, arsenic, chromium, lead, mercury, and other metals are being released into the environment as a consequence of burning fossil fuels, mining operations, metal processing, and other industrial activities. Occasional catastrophies, such as the death of 46 people in Minamata, Japan (from consuming fish contaminated with methylmercury by the effluent of a local chemical plant), are stark reminders of the potential toxicity of these substances and of the need for vigilance with regard to their use.[13]

As a class, heavy metals have an affinity for functional groups, particularly sulfhydryl moieties, that are essential for the physiologic function of various enzymes and other proteins. Although toxic responses vary, because of differences in the distribution and binding affinities of the different metals, gastrointestinal disturbances, blood dyscrasias, neurologic disorders, and dermatologic changes are common manifestations of heavy metal poisoning. Because of its importance to dentistry, only mercury poisoning will be discussed in detail; information concerning the other metals may be found elsewhere.[9]

Chemical forms of mercury. Three general forms of mercury exist that have the potential for toxicity: elemental (metallic) mercury, as a liquid or vapor, which is present in the dental environment as an essential component of dental amalgam; inorganic mercury compounds including the metal-mercury complexes of amalgam; and organic compounds of mercury, which are found in nature in low concentrations and are produced industrially. Some mercury compounds have been used in medicine as diuretics and as antiseptics, but their use is now rare. The body is affected differently by each of these groups; in dentistry it is the first two that are of primary concern.

Absorption, fate, and excretion. Elemental mercury is a liquid that vaporizes readily at room temperature. Vaporization is facilitated by agitation, which produces fine droplets and therefore increases surface area, and by heat. Mercury vapor is readily absorbed via the lungs, as it consists of individual molecules that are relatively lipid soluble. Approximately 80% of inhaled mercury vapor reaches the blood. Elemental mercury may also be absorbed when it is rubbed on the skin, again a consequence of its lipid solubility. In the gastrointestinal tract, because of elemental mercury's very low solubility in water and its tendency to remain in large droplets (with a resultant small surface area), little of the metal is absorbed. Oxidation in the stomach causes some surface dissolution, but the resultant mercurous and mercuric ions are mostly fixed in the chyme and mucosa. The bulk of ingested metallic mercury is excreted unchanged in the feces.

Compounds of mercury are variably absorbed. Some organic mercurials, such as the notable environmental toxin methylmercury and the mercurial antiseptics thimerosol and mercurochrome, are highly lipid soluble and are almost totally absorbed from the gastrointestinal tract. As evidenced by instances of systemic toxicity, when these antiseptics were applied to large abraded areas of skin, transcutaneous uptake can also occur. A small percentage of mercuric chloride but almost no mercurous chloride gains access to the systemic circulation. Fine particles of inorganic mercury compounds, as are produced in cutting and grinding dental amalgam, lodge in the alveoli and are slowly dissolved and absorbed. Ingested amalgam particles, however, are essentially inert relative to their rate of passage through the gastrointestinal tract and pose little or no threat to the patient.

The oxidation of elemental mercury from vapor to the mercurous and mercuric ions in the blood and tissues takes several minutes.[7] During this time nonionized mercury may cross the blood-brain barrier, high lipid solubility being required for such passage. Subsequent oxidation produces mercuric ions, which then tend to be retained in the central nervous system. Fast movement into and slow clearance from the brain and spinal cord (and presumably the fetus as well) therefore occur with exposure to mercury vapor. Ionized mercury from whatever source binds to proteins in blood and to the cell membranes and hemoglobin of red cells. It slowly reaches equilibrium with similar binding sites in various tissues; those tissues in which secretion occurs tend to have the highest mercury concentrations. In general descending order, inorganic mercury accumulates in the pancreas, kidney, liver, and spleen at concentrations greater than blood and then in the brain and other tissues. Organic mercury compounds differ in the pattern of distribution according to their chemical structure and lipid solubility. Methylmercury readily penetrates capillary walls, including those of the brain, and reaches similar concentrations in all tissues.

Inorganic mercury is excreted via the kidneys and the gastrointestinal tract. The half-time for clearance from most tissues is about 60 days, with the central nervous system and kidneys having longer retention times. Repeated exposure at intervals of less than a month leads to accumulation; thus, hazardous concentrations may be reached following multiple low-level exposures. Methylmercury is poorly excreted by the kidneys; its biologic half-life is 2 to 3 months, and the potential for accumulation is even greater than with exposure to inorganic or elemental mercury.

Mercury toxicity. Mercury forms covalent bonds with sulfur and therefore inactivates sulfhydryl-containing enzymes and precipitates proteins. At low mercury concentrations cellular metabolism is depressed, and at higher concentrations the cells die. Acute exposure of epithelial surfaces to high mercury titers causes local necrosis by protein coagulation.

Inhalation of mercury vapor may directly damage the lungs, with initial symptoms resembling an acute onset of influenza and, in the worst scenario, death from pulmonary edema within a few days. Chronic exposure to lower amounts of vapor leads primarily to CNS toxicity. Motor disturbances include "intention" tremors during fine motor tasks, then more generalized muscle spasms and loss of major motor control, such as the ability to walk, as a result of cerebellar ataxia. Insomnia, loss of appetite, diarrhea, depression, fatigue, and a decline in mental activity and memory are all considered to be part of the syndrome of chronic mercury poisoning. Stomatitis, a metallic taste and foul breath, blue pigmentation of the gingival margin, and necrosis of the alveolar process suggest that mercury is excreted in the saliva and crevicular fluid. Renal tubular lesions may lead initially to a toxic diuresis, followed later by a progressive fall in urine output. Brown or yellow discoloration of the anterior capsule of the lens may also occur.

Both acute and chronic poisoning can occur with organic and highly dissociated inorganic mercury compounds. Symptoms of acute poisoning include damage to the alimentary tract and kidney; chronic effects are similar to those described above.

Mercury hygiene in dentistry. There is considerable evidence that mercury poisoning is a potential hazard in dentistry. An extreme example of this danger is provided by a case report of a 42-year-old dental assistant who died of acute renal failure associated with high concentrations of mercury in the kidneys (measured at autopsy).[2] The report stated that she had "handled mercury in compounding dental amalgam" for at least 20 years. The onset of nephrotoxicity without concomitant CNS symptoms as occurred in her case would be consistent with the uptake of mercury through the skin (and hence conversion to the ionic form before it could reach the brain) rather than via the lungs. It is possible that the victim's handling of amalgam may have included hand-mulling. Although the details of this report were not sufficient to rule out contact with mercury other than in the dental office, it is obvious that exposure of dentists, their staffs, and their patients to hazardous forms of mercury should be minimized. The following are recommendations published by the Council on Dental Materials and Devices of the American Dental Association, with a few amendments added to reflect more recent information on mercury hygiene.[3,7,12]

1. Store mercury in unbreakable, tightly sealed containers.
2. Perform all operations involving mercury over areas that have impervious and suitably lipped surfaces so as to confine and facilitate recovery of spilled mercury or amalgam.
3. Clean up any spilled mercury immediately.

Before doing so, however, sprinkle powdered sulfur on the mercury to reduce its ability to vaporize. Droplets may be picked up with narrow bore tubing connected (via a wash-bottle trap) to the low-volume aspirator of the dental unit.

4. Use tightly closed capsules during amalgamation.
5. Use a no-touch technique for handling the amalgam.
6. Salvage all amalgam scrap and store it in a tightly sealed, dry pot with powdered sulfur. Although storage under water has been recommended, it has also been argued that the water soon becomes saturated with mercury, which then may escape into the environment by vaporization.[12]
7. Work in well-ventilated spaces.
8. Avoid carpeting dental operatories as decontamination is not possible.
9. Eliminate the use of solutions containing mercury.
10. Avoid heating mercury or amalgam.
11. Use water spray and suction when grinding dental amalgam. Also use facemasks to reduce the chance of inhaling amalgam particles.
12. Use conventional dental amalgam compacting procedures, manual and mechanical, but do not use ultrasonic amalgam condensors.
13. Perform yearly mercury determinations on all personnel regularly employed in dental offices, remembering that blood mercury titers are a reasonable index of recent exposure but that they do not give information on the amount of mercury accumulated in the brain or kidney.
14. Have periodic mercury vapor determinations made of the air in operatories. Local health authorities should be able to perform such tests. The clinical threshold for safety is uncertain, but concentrations below 1 ng/m^3 probably pose no risk. A significant increase in psychosomatic disturbances may occur after long-term exposure to concentrations in excess of 10 ng/m^3.[7] It should be noted that instruments available for measuring mercury vapor are not highly accurate.[12]
15. Alert all personnel involved in handling of mercury, especially during training or in-

doctrination periods, of the potential hazard of mercury vapor and the necessity for observing good mercury hygiene practices.

Treatment of poisoning—heavy metal chelators. Acute poisoning by oral ingestion is treated by prompt removal of the ingested compounds. Sulfhydryl-rich protein, as contained in milk or eggs, is administered in combination with gastric lavage. For inorganic mercury that gains access to the bloodstream, chelating agents are the mainstays of therapy. Dimercaprol and penicillamine are the two drugs currently marketed for promoting the excretion of mercury (Figure 47-1); a few other agents are available for the treatment of poisoning by other heavy metals (e.g., edetate calcium disodium for lead, deferoxamine for iron).

Dimercaprol, formerly known as British antilewisite or BAL, was developed during World War II as an antidote for the arsenical gas lewisite. As such, it represents one of the few drugs tailor-made for a specific purpose. Subsequently, dimercaprol was found to be an active chelator of a variety of heavy metals.

Dimercaprol is prepared in an oily vehicle and must be injected intramuscularly. It is maximally effective when given shortly after an acute exposure to mercury; however, it is of some value even in chronic mercurialism. The drug is usually injected 2 to 3 times a day initially, with doses tapering off to once or twice a day over a course of therapy that lasts about 10 days. The dimercaprol-mercury complex (actually two dimercaprol molecules to a single mercury atom) is excreted in the urine, which must be kept alkaline to avoid dissociation of the conjugate.

Penicillamine is a highly effective chelator of copper and is of primary importance in the management of Wilson's disease (hepatolenticular degeneration). Although less effective against other metals, penicillamine is often the agent of choice for asymptomatic patients with a moderate body burden of metal because it is orally effective. Generally, 1 to 2 gm per day is administered as needed for therapy of mercury poisoning. The penicillamine-mercury complex (also involving two drug molecules for each mercury atom) is excreted in the urine.

Neither dimercaprol nor penicillamine is very effective in the treatment of chronic poisoning by methylmercury, and other strategies (involving hemodialysis, L-cysteine infusion, and polythiol resin administration) must be employed.

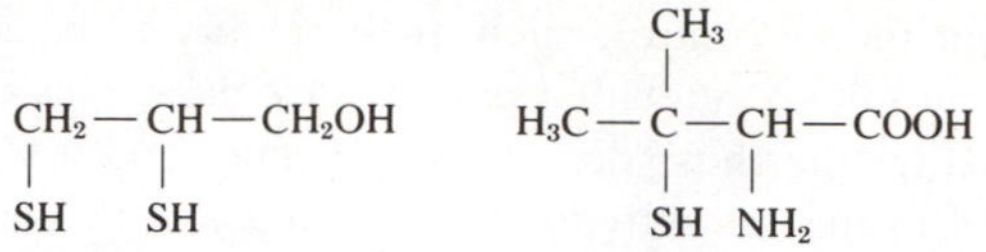

Figure 47-1. Structural formulas of dimercaprol and penicillamine.

Carbon monoxide and other air pollutants

Three "progressive" trends of human civilization—urbanization, industrialization, and mechanical transportation (primarily the automobile)—have combined to foul the air we breathe. In descending order of importance, the major air pollutants are carbon monoxide, sulfur oxides, hydrocarbons, particulate matter, and nitrogen oxides. Although all of these substances are potentially toxic, consideration here will be limited to carbon monoxide, because it accounts for one half of the air pollution in the United States and because it is the leading cause of death in fires, a common instrument for suicide, and a causative factor of heart disease in cigarette smokers.

Carbon monoxide is produced during the incomplete combustion of organic fuels (wood, gasoline, etc.). Inadequate ventilation permits carbon monoxide to accumulate, an event that is not easily detected because the gas is odorless, tasteless, colorless, and nonirritating. Moreover, even if an individual notices signs and symptoms of carbon monoxide poisoning, confusion often precludes an effective response, such as seeking fresh air.

The acute toxicity of carbon monoxide is a result of its ability to compete with oxygen for binding to hemoglobin. The affinity of hemoglobin for carbon monoxide is over 200 times that for oxygen. Not only does carbon monoxide reduce the oxygen-carrying capacity of the blood directly, it compounds the deficit by distorting the dissociation curve for the remaining oxygen binding sites (Figure 47-2).

The signs and symptoms of the functional anemia imposed by carbon monoxide are dose dependent. Beginning with a 10% concentration of carboxyhemoglobin and continuing until about 50%, at which point consciousness is lost, there is progressively severe headache and development of weakness, nausea and vomiting, and cardiovas-

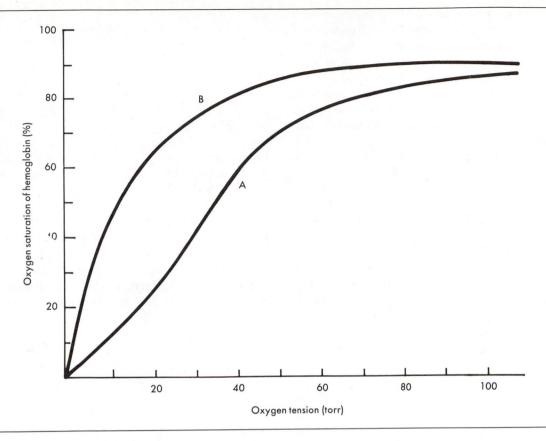

Figure 47-2. Effect of carbon monoxide on oxygen dissociation. Curve A represents the normal desaturation curve for oxyhemoglobin and shows that half of the bound oxygen is made available to tissues as the oxygen tension (P_{O_2}) falls to a little over 30 torr. In the presence of 50% carboxyhemoglobin, the P_{O_2} must drop to a hypoxic value of 10 torr before a similar percentage of oxygen is released from its hemoglobin binding sites.

cular instability. Respiration is increased but less than one might expect, because the arterial P_{O_2} is unaffected by carbon monoxide. As the percentage of carboxyhemoglobin advances beyond 50%, coma, convulsions, and finally cardiopulmonary collapse ensue.

Treatment of carbon monoxide poisoning is aimed at eliminating the gas from the body. The victim must be moved into fresh air. Respiration should be closely monitored and artificial ventilation provided if necessary. Because the antagonism between oxygen and carbon monoxide is competitive, 100% oxygen is essential in combating hypoxia and hastening elimination of the poison. Hyperbaric chambers with oxygen at 2 to 3 atmospheres pressure is indicated for the unconscious patient.

Long-term exposure to low concentrations of carbon monoxide, as experienced by cigarette smokers, has several effects on the cardiovascular system. A reactive polycythemia may occur, there may be accelerated development of atherosclerosis, and blood flow to the major organs is increased. The fetus is particularly sensitive to the hypoxic effects of carbon monoxide; infants born to women smokers are more likely to suffer from subtle neurologic deficits. Obviously, abstinence from cigarettes is necessary to avoid this form of air pollution.

Organic solvents and vapors

Volatile organic compounds are widely used in industry as solvents, fuels and lubricants, and chemical reactants. Concerns about occupational hazards have led to adoption by regulatory agencies of maximum allowable standards (or threshold limit values) for exposure to many of these airborne poisons. In the home, occasional inhalation of low concentrations of gasoline, nail polish, and other vapors is normally innocuous; of much greater concern is accidental ingestion of toxic liquids, especially by young children. Many of these compounds are sold commercially in child-resistant containers. Transfer of these liquids to unlabeled and easily opened vessels (sometimes even milk or soft drink bottles) is a dangerous but all too common practice.

There are several different categories of organic liquids in widespread use: aliphatic and aromatic hydrocarbons (in gasoline, paint thinner, and glues), halogenated hydrocarbons (chloroform, dichloromethane, and formerly carbon tetrachloride), and alcohols and glycols (isopropyl alcohol and ethylene glycol). Although these agents make up a diverse array of chemicals with many different properties, important generalizations can be drawn regarding their toxicology. All of these compounds are CNS depressants and can be thought of as toxic general anesthetics. Thus, sedation, confusion, excitement, delirium, unconsciousness, and finally respiratory arrest are caused by increasing degrees of poisoning. As with some of the volatile anesthetics, sensitization of the heart to catecholamines is a prominent feature of exposure. Hepatotoxicity and nephrotoxicity are likely to be caused by the halogenated hydrocarbons, and these dangers are the reason chloroform was abandoned as a general anesthetic and carbon tetrachloride is no longer found in household products.

Treatment of poisoning is generally supportive. Because of their low surface tensions, organic solvents as a group are more likely to be aspirated after ingestion than are other poisons. Also, aspiration is more dangerous than normal because these substances can cause a chemical pneumonitis leading to hemorrhagic pulmonary edema and death. For these reasons, emesis is not induced, and gastric lavage (with endotracheal intubation to protect the airway) is performed only when a potentially lethal quantity of organic liquid may have been swallowed. Sympathomimetic amines with β-adrenergic activity should not be used to support the circulation because ventricular fibrillation may ensue.

In dentistry, the only organic solvent of concern is methyl methacrylate monomer. Fortunately, this common pollutant of dental laboratories and offices is of relatively low toxicity. Prolonged inhalation of the vapor causes both lung and liver damage in various experimental animals. Methyl methacry-

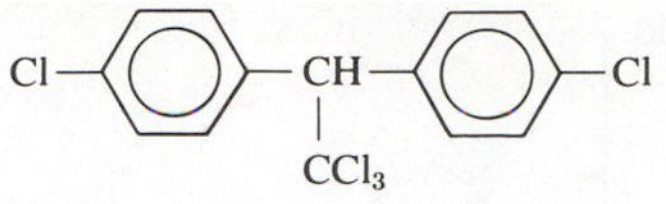

Figure 47-3. Structural formula of DDT.

late causes respiratory arrest when inhaled or ingested in sufficient doses (10 ml/kg is the oral LD50 in rats).[14] There does not appear to be recorded evidence of toxicity in humans; however, a variety of vague complaints (nausea, fatigue, irritability) have been ascribed to inhalation of vapor in concentrations from 0.5 to 150 ppm.[8] It should also be noted that local toxic responses can arise from methyl methacrylate leaching out of newly polymerized plastic and that the risk of contact sensitivity to the monomer is high.[5]

Pesticides

An impressive arsenal of poisons is used to protect humans and domestic livestock from animal-borne diseases, buildings and parkways from infestations, and agricultural products from blights and pests. By the nature of their use, these substances are dispersed throughout the environment. They are variably toxic; the safest agents capitalize on differences between humans and target organisms for selective toxicity; other compounds are nonselective but enjoy widespread use anyway because of desirable physical properties or because suitable alternatives are not available. Two agents, DDT and cyanide, will be discussed because of their historical significance and because they illustrate different aspects of the toxicology of pesticides.

DDT. DDT, otherwise known as chlorophenothane, is an organochlorine insecticide (Figure 47-3). Soon after its introduction in the 1940s, DDT was being used throughout the world for the suppression of malaria (mosquito vector) and to increase agricultural yield. DDT has numerous advantages: it is inexpensive, highly effective, and safe. To date there has not been a single fatality proved to be caused by DDT alone. When toxic manifestations do occur, they are primarily of a central excitatory nature: hyperreactivity to stimuli, irritability, tremors, and convulsions.

In 1972, however, DDT was largely banned from use in the United States, and many other countries

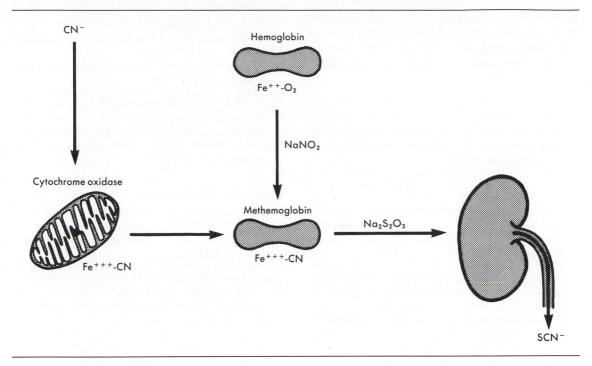

Figure 47-4. Treatment of cyanide poisoning. Cyanide, whether inhaled or ingested, combines with ferric ions (Fe^{+++}) in cytochrome oxidase to inhibit cellular respiration. Therapy is aimed at eliminating cyanide from the cells by a two-step process: (1) Sodium nitrite ($NaNO_2$) is administered intravenously to oxidize the iron in hemoglobin from the ferrous (Fe^{++}) to the ferric state; the methemoglobin then competes for the bound cyanide, freeing cytochrome c oxidase. (2) Cyanide is inactivated by the administration of sodium thiosulfate to yield thiocyanate, which is readily excreted in the urine. Experimentally, these steps reduce the lethal potency of cyanide by 80%.

subsequently imposed similar limitations. These actions were taken because of concern about the possible carcinogenic potential of DDT and because of its effects on beneficial wildlife. DDT has an extremely high lipid/water partition coefficient and is resistant to metabolic degradation. These attributes allow DDT to accumulate, particularly in body fat. DDT is also concentrated as it moves up the food chain, an effect dependent on its retention and stability in animal tissues. Although studies have not found increased cancer rates in humans based on long-term exposure, hepatic tumors have been shown to occur in rats. Of greater importance is the effect of DDT on birds, especially the large predatory varieties.[11] Although not lethal per se, DDT causes a thinning of the eggshell and increased breakage of eggs. To a large extent, DDT and related organochlorine insecticides have now been replaced by the organophosphates (Chapter 8), which are more toxic to humans but less per-

sistent in the environment and therefore less likely to be carcinogenic and detrimental to wildlife.

Cyanide. No discussion of toxicology would be complete without at least a brief mention of cyanide poisoning. Hydrogen cyanide gas is one of the most rapidly acting poisons, which is why it is used as a fumigant and for executions. Cyanide is also a natural component of fruit seeds and nuts and is widely used in metal finishing. The toxic potential of ingested cyanide was underscored in 1978 by the murder-suicide of more than 900 religious cultists in Guyana.

The cyanide ion has a high affinity for iron in the ferric state. Mitochrondrial cytochrome c oxidase, which is the terminal cytochrome in the respiratory chain, is inactivated by the binding of cyanide to the ferric ion in the heme portion of the molecular complex. The signs and symptoms of cyanide poisoning are like those of acute hypoxia. Hyperpnea, headache, and hypertension are early signs of poisoning; hypoxic convulsions presage death by respiratory arrest. The treatment of cyanide poisoning is directed at removing cyanide from cytochrome c oxidase and is reviewed in Figure 47-4.

CITED REFERENCES

1. Abou-Donia, M.B. Organophosphorus ester-induced delayed neurotoxicity. Annual Review of Pharmacology and Toxicology **21:**511-548, 1981.
2. Cook, T.A., and Yates, P.O. Fatal mercury intoxication in a dental surgery assistant. British Dental Journal **127:**553-555, 1969.
3. Council on Dental Materials and Devices, American Dental Association. Recommendations in mercury hygiene, February 1974. Journal of the American Dental Association **88:**391-392, 1974.
4. Courtney, K.D., and Moore, J.A. Teratology studies with 2,4,5-trichlorophenoxyacetic acid and 2,3,7,8-tetrachlorodibenzo-*p*-dioxin. Toxicology and Applied Pharmacology **20:**396-403, 1971.
5. Danilewicz-Stysiak, Z. Experimental investigation on the cytotoxic nature of methyl methacrylate. Journal of Prosthetic Dentistry **44:**13-16, 1980.
6. Doherty, J.D. Insecticides affecting ion transport. Pharmacology and Therapeutics **7:**123-151, 1979.
7. Gerstner, H.B., and Huff, J.E. Clinical toxicology of mercury. Journal of Toxicology and Environmental Health **2:**491-526, 1977.
8. Innes, D.L., and Tansy, M.F. Central nervous system effects of methyl methacrylate vapor. Neurotoxicology **2:**515-522, 1981.
9. Klaassen, C.D. Heavy metals and heavy-metal antagonists. In Gilman, A.G., Goodman, L.S., and Gilman, A., eds. Goodman and Gilman's The Pharmacological Basis of Therapeutics, ed. 6. New York, Macmillan, Inc., 1980.
10. Marks, P.A., and Banks, J. Drug-induced hemolytic anemias associated with glucose-6-phosphate dehydrogenase deficiency: a genetically heterogeneous trait. Annals of the New York Academy of Sciences **123:**198-206, 1965.
11. Peakall, D.B. Pesticides and the reproduction of birds. Scientific American **222:**72-78, 1970.
12. Roydhouse, R.H. Mercury hazard. Australian Dental Journal **24:**273-274, 1979.
13. Smith, W.E., and Smith, A.M. Minimata. New York, Holt, Reinhart & Winston, 1975.
14. Spealman, C.R., Main, R.J., Haag, H.B., and Larson, P.S. Monomeric methyl methacrylate: studies on toxicity. Industrial Medicine **14:**292-298, 1945.
15. Streicher, E., and Garbus, J. The effect of age and sex on duration of hexobarbital anesthesia in rats. Journal of Gerontology **10:**441-444, 1955.

GENERAL REFERENCES

Albert, A. Selective Toxicity: The Physicochemical Basis of Therapy, ed. 6. London, Chapman and Hall, 1979.

AMA Drug Evaluations, ed. 5. Chicago, American Medical Association, 1983.

Clarkson, T.W. The pharmacology of mercury compounds. Annual Review of Pharmacology **12:**375-406, 1972.

Doull, J., Klaassen, C.D., and Amdur, M.O., eds. Casarett and Doull's Toxicology: The Basic Science of Poisons, ed. 2. New York, Macmillan, Inc., 1980.

Jensen, L.B. Poisoning Misadventures: Narrative Excerpts on Food-Borne Diseases and Poisoning for the Physician, Microbiologist, Attorney, and Nutritionist. Springfield, Illinois, Charles C Thomas, Publisher, 1970.

Kaye, S. Handbook of Emergency Toxicology: A Guide for the Identification, Diagnosis, and Treatment of Poisoning, ed. 3. Springfield, Illinois, Charles C Thomas, Publisher, 1970.

Klaassen, C.D. Toxicology. In Gilman, A.G., Goodman, L.S., and Gilman, A., eds. Goodman and Gilman's The Pharmacological Basis of Therapeutics, ed. 6. New York, Macmillan, Inc., 1980.

Smyth, R.D., and Hottendorf, G.H. Application of pharmacokinetics and biopharmaceutics in the design of toxicological studies. Toxicology and Applied Pharmacology **53:**179-195, 1980.

48 Geriatric pharmacology

Enid A. Neidle
Anthony Picozzi

Geriatric pharmacology is perhaps the youngest subspecialty of pharmacology. Although it has long been obvious that because children are smaller than adults some reduction of drug dosage is appropriate, it was not understood until recently how the elderly patient differed from younger adults. (In fact, there were some widely held misconceptions about aging, for instance, that senility or a steady and significant rise in blood pressure is a normal concomitant of aging.) Nor did the field of geriatric pharmacology emerge out of a specific incident, as occurred with thalidomide, which made it clear that the fetus represents an area of special concern for the pharmacologist. Rather, the field of geriatric pharmacology has developed out of changes in demography that have been accompanied by an increasing knowledge of and sensitivity to the special physiologic, pharmacologic, pathologic, psychologic, economic, and emotional problems of the elderly.

In 1950, the elderly, usually defined as 65 years of age or older, represented 8% of the population; by 1980, they represented 11%, and it is predicted that by 2030 this percentage will have grown to 18%.[29] In absolute numbers, the over-65 population is expected to expand from 25 million in 1980 to 30 million in 1990, an increase of 20%. Of special interest to the dentist is the fact that because of advances in preventive dentistry the incidence of dental caries has declined and will continue to do so, more people will retain their teeth into old age, and the mix of dental services required by the elderly will change. Even in recent years, the rate of edentulousness in those aged 65 has declined 3% to 4% (to a figure of 46%), while the incidence of periodontal disease and the need for restorative dentistry has likewise grown.[9] This trend means that an increasing number of elderly will be needing the kind of dental treatment that was formerly rare in the elderly patient, treatment that will require among other things antianxiety drugs, analgesics, anesthesia, and antiinflammatory drugs. It also means that the dentist will be confronted by an increasing number of so-called medically compromised patients.

The growing field of geriatric physiology has documented that the healthy elderly individual is substantially and measurably different from his younger counterpart. And more recently, pharmacologists have begun to appreciate how these changes affect the pharmacokinetics and pharmacodynamics of drugs.

As people age, of course, they fall prey to a variety of diseases for which they take a multiplicity of often highly "important" drugs, that is, drugs that are strong in effect and potentially quite toxic. The elderly also take a considerable number of self-administered OTC drugs. The number of drugs taken by older people has been variably estimated in a great number of studies to be anywhere from four in the healthy 65-year old[23] to as many as 11 in the same-aged person just prior to hospitalization.[27] As is shown in Chapter 4, the potential for adverse drug interactions increases exponentially with the number of drugs taken (see Figure 4-1), so it is obvious that the elderly patient who is taking multiple medications may present a pharmacologic problem. It is also increasingly evident that the pathologic status of the patient may affect responses to drugs, irrespective of the number of drugs being taken. Large multicenter drug surveillance studies, which have proved so valuable in tracking the epidemiology of adverse drug reactions, have been able to document the special drug problems that are likely to be encountered among the aging. Finally, many segments of our society, not the least important of which is the health care provider, have become sensitized to the nonmedical problems common among the elderly (loneliness, depression, poverty, poor nutritional status) and have come to understand how these can complicate the therapeutic management of the elderly.

This chapter presents a contemporary view of geriatric pharmacology; it deals mainly with alterations in drug responsiveness that can be attributed directly to aging and only in passing with those sociopsychologic problems that indirectly have an impact on how the elderly use and react to drugs.

PHYSIOLOGIC CHANGES ASSOCIATED WITH AGING

Although some of the changes associated with aging (gray hair, changes in posture, wrinkled skin) have very little impact on pharmacology, many do have the potential for influencing all aspects of the body's response to drugs. The differences in residual physiologic functions between an average 30-year old man and an average 70-year old man are shown in Table 48-1. It can be seen that the changes, involving virtually all physiologic parameters, range from relatively small (a 10% decline in nerve conduction velocity) to relatively large (a reduction of 50% in renal plasma flow). Table 48-1 also shows the alterations that occur in body weight, plasma volume, total body water, and the proportion of body fat to body weight. Inevitably, these alterations affect the distribution, biotransformation, excretion, and sequestration of drugs; the specific features of these changes will be considered shortly.

There is a well-documented decline in homeostatic competence in the elderly that accounts for the increased incidence of postural hypotension with age,[3] the increasing sluggishness of thermoregulation, and the fact that the elderly are less able to compensate rapidly for the hypotensive effects, for instance, of an antihypertensive drug.[18] It should be noted that the elderly undergo physiologic changes that could be characterized as normal accompaniments of the aging process, but that they also, to a greater or lesser extent, suffer changes that are pathologic or related to disease states, as well as those that are economic, psychologic, and sociologic. Physiologic and chronologic aging often proceed at different rates, and this makes the elderly population more heterogeneous than, for instance, a population of children between birth and puberty.[41]

Table 48-1. Physiologic functions and tissue distributions in the healthy elderly adult (aged 70s) compared with those of a healthy young adult (aged 30s)*

Lean body weight	↓
Body fat/body weight	↑ ↑
Brain weight	↓ ↓
Brain blood flow	↓
Nerve conduction velocity	↓
Cardiac output	↓ ↓
Diastolic blood pressure	↑
Peripheral resistance	↑ ↑
Total kidney glomeruli	↓ ↓
Glomerular filtration rate	↓ ↓
Renal plasma flow	↓ ↓ ↓
Hepatic blood flow	↓ ↓
Hepatic weight	↓
Hepatic weight/body weight	↓
Pulmonary vital capacity	↓ ↓
Oxygen uptake during exercise	↓ ↓ ↓
Basal metabolic rate	↓
Plasma volume	↓
Total body water	↓
Plasma albumin concentration	↓

*↓ = decrease of 15 to 24%; ↓ ↓ = decrease of 25 to 49%; ↓ ↓ ↓ = decrease of 50% or more; ↑ = increase of up to 25%; ↑ ↑ = increase greater than 25%.

NONPHYSIOLOGIC ASPECTS OF AGING
Multiple disease states

The elderly suffer from more diseases then the young. Some of these are degenerative (e.g., cataracts, detached retina), others are caused by cumulative exposure to environmental contaminants (e.g., cancer, in all likelihood), and still others are the consequences of essentially normal processes of aging (e.g., the postmenopausal osteoporosis that is related to decrease in estrogen secretion). Among the elderly there is increased incidence of all varieties of heart disease (arrhythmias, myocardial infarction, valvular disease), atherosclerosis, the arthritides, diabetes, osteoporosis, a variety of gastrointestinal problems, declines in both humoral- and cell-mediated immune responses (that lead to an increased sensitivity to infectious diseases), and various sensory and musculoskeletal impairments. It has been estimated that 80% of the elderly have at least one chronic illness and usually more; the Federal Council on Aging put the figure as high as 86%. It is not unexpected, then, that although the elderly represent only 11% of the population, they account for 30% of the adult patient population in hospitals and for 25% of the total expenditure on drugs.[16] A study of 200 geriatric hospital admissions showed that 78% suffered from at least four major diseases.[45] It is also noteworthy that the symptoms of disease in the elderly may often be misleading. Infections are sometimes manifested not by fever but by tachycardia; the elderly patient is often less sensitive to (or more stoic about) pain; symptoms may be forgotten, misreported, or misinterpreted.

Multiple medications

It follows logically that if the elderly suffer more diseases than do the young, so also do they take more medications. Many studies have been done in this area, and collectively they show that (1) 25% of patients over 65 discharged from the hospital receive six or more drugs daily[37]; (2) the elderly average 13 prescriptions a year[22]; (3) in 1971 Medicare patients received an average of 10 drugs each day[27]; (4) in a group of 151 patients 75 years or older, almost 90% took drugs regularly, and 37% took three to four each day[23]; and (5) a very high percentage of psychotropic medications are prescribed for the elderly.[40] This high level of drug use among the elderly is compounded by the fact that 70% of older people regularly used OTC medications, in contrast to only 20% of the adult population.[20] Actually, 40% of all the drugs used by the elderly are OTC, and more than 55% of these are analgesics.[6]

The use of multiple medications in the elderly brings with it problems, many of them wholly predictable. There has been extensive documentation of the fact that adverse drug reactions (ADRs) are more common both among the elderly per se and among those who take many medications at the same time. For instance, in a study of 700 hospitalized patients, drug-induced illness was found in 25% of those over 70 years and in only 12% of those aged 41 to 50.[34] In an extended study of over 6000 hospital admissions, 58% of illnesses that were clearly drug-induced occurred in patients aged 50 to 80. One third of these drug-induced illnesses were traceable to eight drugs; aspirin, digoxin, warfarin, hydrochlorothiazide, prednisone, vincristine, norethindrone, and furosemide. This study also showed that many patients could not correctly identify their medications, that nearly half received prescriptions from two or more physicians or dentists (who presumably did not know what the other was prescribing), and that over 10% took medications that had been prescribed for someone else.[4] The loss of homeostatic competence in the elderly has been alluded to already. In a group of 266

patients hospitalized for ADRs to propranolol, one third of which were life-threatening, the majority were over 60 years of age but there was no evidence of a dose-response relationship for toxicity.[18] Adverse drug effects to flurazepam are 4 times more common in people over 60 and 20 times more common in those over 70 than they are in the general adult population.[35] This finding no doubt reflects the increased sensitivity of the aging patient to central nervous depressants.

Adverse drug reactions are most commonly encountered in the treatment of arthritis, congestive heart failure, diabetes, hypertension, prostatic hypertrophy, urinary tract infections, and respiratory tract infections. The most commonly prescribed drugs for the elderly are cardiovascular agents (digitalis, diuretics, and antihypertensives), psychotropic drugs, and analgesics. Among the OTC products, the most popular are analgesics, laxatives, antacids, and vitamins. A large study in an ambulatory elderly population showed that the top five nonprescription drugs were aspirin, multiple vitamins, vitamin E, multiple vitamins with minerals, and vitamin C.[24] There is no evidence that specific disease states predispose to ADRs, but the nature of the medications taken for these diseases and the prevalence of polypharmacy among the old provides an acceptable explanation for their high incidence. Common ADRs include cardiotoxicity from digitalis brought about by the simultaneous use of potassium-depleting diuretics; peptic ulcers from adrenal cortical steroids and nonsteroidal antiinflammatory drugs; respiratory depression from opioid analgesics; and stupor, confusion, and even excitement from sedatives and antianxiety drugs. It has already been noted that the incidence of adverse reactions increases exponentially with the number of drugs taken; it is also true that the average hospital stay and the mortality rate increase in the same fashion.[38]

One manifestation of polypharmacy that may confront the dentist is xerostomia. Antimuscarinic side effects are common to a diverse array of drugs used to treat afflictions more prevalent in the elderly than in other age groups. Centrally mediated influences and changes in extracellular fluid and electrolytes may also contribute to the drug-induced xerostomia. Table 48-2 lists those drugs that may adversely affect the production of saliva and the indications for their use. Although the antisialic effect of any single agent might be tolerable, or even negligible, combinations of drugs can cause a variety of problems. In the geriatric patient with

Table 48-2. Some drugs that cause xerostomia and the indications for their use

Drug group	Examples	Indications for use
Anticholinergics	Trihexphenidyl	Parkinson's disease
	Isopropamide	Peptic ulcer (adjunctive therapy)
	Thiphenamil	Spastic conditions of the gastrointestinal and genitourinary tracts
Antidepressants	Amitriptyline	Mood disorders
Antihistamines	Orphenadrine	Parkinson's disease
	Promethazine	Sedation
	Chlorpheniramine	Relief of cold symptoms, hay fever
Antipsychotics	Chlorpromazine	Psychiatric disorders
Benzodiazepines	Diazepam	Anxiety relief
	Flurazepam	Sedation and hypnosis
Centrally acting adrenergic drugs	Methyldopa	Hypertension
Diuretics	Chlorothiazide	Hypertension and congestive heart failure

a removable prosthesis, dry mouth can impair denture retention, make speech difficult, and reduce patient acceptance of the appliance. Frictional trauma and a fall in intraoral pH (from the relative lack of salivary lubrication and buffering) predispose the patient to candidal infection. In its most extreme, xerostomia can lead to rampant dental caries and periodontal disease.

Patient compliance

Patient compliance is assumed to be a major source of medication errors and therefore adverse drug reactions. Ample evidence exists that a substantial percentage of the elderly make serious or potentially serious medication errors.[17,28,33] Dose errors consist of omitting medications, use of medications not prescribed by the physician or dentist, and errors of dosage, sequence, and timing. A study in which the digoxin serum concentration was used as a measure of compliance demonstrated that age is less of a deterrent to compliance than are regimens involving the use of several drugs.[44] Noncompliance can arise for a variety of reasons, many of which are described in Chapter 3. Problems especially identified with the elderly that contribute to noncompliance include poor comprehension and memory, deficits in vision and hearing, financial strictures, inability to cope with the environment, self-neglect, cultural attitudes, and physical obstacles to getting medications out of the bottle (particularly the child-resistant kind) and self-administering them.

Psychosocioeconomic factors

Any discussion of geriatric pharmacology would be incomplete without mention of the various psychologic, sociologic, and economic problems that frequently confront the elderly. Although it is no longer true that the elderly inevitably suffer a serious reduction in income, 14% are in poverty, and elderly single women are worse off than men or couples (21% are below the poverty line). The elderly also live in increasing isolation, away from families, children, and spouses, and suffer from depression, loneliness, and sometimes senility. And, they receive 3 times as many prescriptions for psychotropic drugs as do younger people even though they are more vulnerable to the adverse effects of these drugs and take twice as long to recover from them as do young patients.[21] This constellation of factors in the elderly can bring with them a host of sequelae—inadequate diet, poor nutrition, loss in weight, forgetfulness and inattention to medical and pharmacologic needs, and an inability or lack of desire to fill prescriptions and to take them as directed. One widely held belief about the elderly is that their nutritional status is compounded by losses in salivary secretory ability and taste acuity that are presumed to occur with aging and would naturally interfere with the enjoyment of food. Although there have been some studies that showed a diminution in the parotid gland flow rate and a decreased concentration of salivary amylases,[25] recent studies have shown that there is no diminution in stimulated parotid saliva flow in older individuals and that the decline in gustatory function is at most modest among the elderly, principally related to a small decrease in the number of taste buds.[1] On the other hand, it cannot be denied that pathologic aging may have an adverse effect on salivary function and that many of the drugs and treatments to which the older person is subject will cause xerostomia of varying degrees of severity.

PHARMACOLOGIC CHANGES ASSOCIATED WITH AGING

The response to a drug is ultimately determined by the amount that reaches the receptors, the speed with which it reaches them, the sensitivity and/or number of receptors, and the duration of the drug's sojourn in the body. These factors are in turn affected by pharmacokinetic processes—the absorption, distribution, biotransformation, and excretion of drugs—and pharmacodynamic factors, principally the number of available receptors and their receptivity to particular drugs. Changes occurring during the aging process can affect any of the sites shown in Figure 2-1 and are likely to have an impact on the body's response to drugs. It is probably fair to say that the principal concerns of geriatric pharmacology are in the fields of pharmacokinetics and pharmacodynamics. The changes that have been discovered in these areas will be discussed in the following two sections of the chapter.

Pharmacokinetic changes

The evidence that there are alterations in pharmacokinetics during aging is relatively substantial. Most of these changes translate into increased drug susceptibility; a few confer decreased responsiveness.

Absorption of drugs. A number of well-documented changes in the gastrointestinal tract could have an impact on the absorption of drugs taken by the oral route. These changes include an increase in gastric pH,[2] a reduced rate of gastric emptying,[14] a decrease in gastrointestinal motility and surface area, a decline in the number of absorptive cells, decreased effectiveness of active transport processes, decreased splanchnic blood flow, or some combination of all of these.[26] Probably, the most important of these factors is gastric pH, because most drugs are absorbed by passive diffusion, and even if reduced the surface available for absorption remains relatively vast. Although experiments point to a slower rate of absorption in the elderly, the net amount absorbed tends to remain the same.[8,36] And for some drugs, as for instance oxazepam and diazepam, age appears to have no effect on either the rate or completeness of absorption. It is currently believed that age alone does not bring about clinically important changes in absorption.

Distribution. There are four well-documented alterations during aging that can affect the distribution of drugs. First, there is a decrease in total body water and weight. Second, there is an increased ratio of fat/lean body mass. Third, there is a fall in cardiac output but an increase in the fraction of that output going to the brain and heart. Fourth, there is, as shown in Table 48-1, a decrease in plasma albumin available for the binding of drugs.

These age-related changes have the potential for bringing about the following effects in drug distribution: a greater sequestration in the body fat of lipid-soluble drugs and a lower plasma concentration of these drugs; a smaller volume of distribution of water-soluble drugs (as has been demonstrated for acetaminophen),[11] which is magnified in elderly women because of their higher fat/lean body ratio; a higher proportion of lipophilic drugs given intravenously (thiopental by design, local anesthetics by accident) presented to the brain; a higher concentration of free drug in the plasma (with drugs that are normally significantly protein bound). Theoretically, at least, therapeutic and toxic effects should be achieved at lower plasma concentrations for drugs that are extensively protein bound, and the elderly are more susceptible to drug interactions and ADRs when several protein-bound drugs are administered simultaneously.[43] This should merit consideration of modified dosage schedules for the elderly patient. It is worthwhile to note that for some drugs there has been no documented age-related difference in protein binding; three of these are diazepam, salicylate, and penicillin G.[7]

Metabolism. The biotransformation of drugs may be affected by changes in hepatic blood flow, the functional liver mass, and the efficiency of the hepatic enzymes responsible for phase I and phase II reactions. The latter could result from decreases in the number of enzyme molecules, their activity, or both.

As indicated in Table 48-1, hepatic blood flow decreases steadily with age. It has been estimated that this decline occurs at the rate of 0.3% to 1.5% a year.[15] Between ages 25 and 65 this would amount to a 40% to 45% reduction in liver blood flow. Part of this drop is a reflection of the documented decrease in cardiac output, which amounts to about 30%. Liver weight is clearly related to body weight, and both begin to decline at about age 50.[30] There is, however, a significant reserve capacity of the liver, and it is not clear whether these changes in total weight or hepatic blood flow or even the declines in enzyme systems as estimated by animal studies significantly affect the capacity of the aging but otherwise healthy liver to handle normal drug intake.

A number of studies have shown that the rate of clearance of some drugs that undergo phase I biotransformation is reduced with age. Such drugs are diazepam, chlordiazepoxide, alprazolam, quinidine, propranolol, and nortriptyline.[19] On the other hand, the oxidation of agents like lidocaine, warfarin, ethanol, and prazosin are not affected. Drugs that are transformed by phase II conjugation, such as lorazepam, oxazepam, and isoniazid, also show negligible age-related changes in half-life or clearance rates.

At this time it is felt that the most significant factor influencing drug metabolism in the elderly is the decline in hepatic blood flow.

Excretion. Table 48-1 makes it clear that virtually all components of the renal excretory system are affected by age. The decline in kidney function, which begins around age 40, is manifested by a steady rise in blood urea nitrogen, which goes from 12.9 mg/dl at maturity to 21.2 mg/dl at age 70. Drugs such as penicillin, digoxin, cimetidine, and lithium that are excreted unchanged by the kidney show a decreased renal clearance with age.[8,12] The kidney is a site not only of physiologic age-related changes but also a focus of many disease processes and, significantly, a primary route of excretion for many cytotoxic drugs and drug metabolites. It follows that serious consideration must be given to renal excretory capacity in prescribing drugs for the elderly. As is pointed out in Chapter 3, measurement of creatinine clearance is a good way of assessing the status of kidney function. In the event that there is a significant drop in creatinine clearance, it is customary either to increase the interval between doses of the drug or to reduce the dosage. Although there is certainly a diminution in renal function that is related to age, kidney disease is, of course, not restricted to the elderly.

A good example of the role played by the renal excretory mechanism is provided by a recent study of two groups of patients, one older than 75 years and the other aged 25 to 60, whose recovery from a single bolus injection of pancuronium was studied. Although the dose-response curve for both groups was essentially the same, the recovery time for the older group was significantly prolonged, and this was attributed to delayed renal excretion

of the drug, not to changes in sensitivity to pancuronium. The elimination half-life for the younger patients was 107 minutes, as compared wtih 201 minutes for the elderly patients.[13]

Pharmacodynamic changes

There are three possibilities for pharmacodynamic alterations in drug reactivity with aging—a change in the number of receptors, a change in their affinity for the drug, or a change in tissue responsiveness to drug-receptor binding. Discovering which of these possibilities accounts for a particular reaction is difficult because it requires a knowledge of receptor number, binding affinity, and quantitation of the sequential steps following the drug-receptor interaction to the final observed response. Nevertheless, experimental evidence exists that one or more of these changes do occur with several groups of drugs.

Decreases in sensitivity to β-adrenergic agonists and antagonists have been reported in a number of studies. Using the production of cAMP by lymphocytes as an indicator of responsiveness to isoproterenol in the young and old, it was found that there is a decrease in adenylate cyclase in normal subjects aged 67 to 90 as compared with those of 18 to 27 years.[10] An age-related decline in β-adrenergic receptors and in alprenolol binding has also been demonstrated.[32]

Increased sensitivity to CNS depressants is a recognized fact. In tests involving nitrazepam, age-related decrements in psychomotor performance were described and linked to pharmacodynamic, not pharmacokinetic, changes.[5] Elderly patients who were given diazepam for a surgical procedure required lower doses than younger patients to reach the same level of sedation.[31] This observation has been confirmed in other studies for both diazepam and temazepam.[39] Determination of the minimum alveolar concentration for isoflurane showed an 18% drop in anesthetic requirement between young adults (19 to 30 years) and 55-year olds; similar results have been obtained with other anesthetics.[42]

IMPLICATIONS FOR DENTISTRY

It should be clear that the elderly patient differs from the younger adult in ways that have the potential for affecting responses to drugs. Changes potentially affecting pharmacokinetics and pharmacodynamics occur during aging, and these would tend to prolong the half-lives of some drugs, decrease the rate of biotransformation and renal excretion of others, alter the pattern and volume of distribution and the sequestration of drugs in body fats, and interfere with the normal binding of drugs by plasma proteins. It is possible, too, to hypothesize a decreased receptor sensitivity to some drugs and to others an increased sensitivity, perhaps related in some instances to decreased homeostatic competence. At this stage in the development of the science of geriatric pharmacology, there are remarkably few documented instances of problems with drugs that arise directly out of pharmacokinetic and pharmacodynamic changes. On the other hand, it is well known that responses to drugs in the elderly are confounded by multiple medications, by pathologic states, by compliance errors, and by a variety of psychosocioeconomic factors that beset older people. Some precautions appropriate to dentistry are listed below:

1. The elderly usually take more drugs, both prescription and nonprescription, than the general adult population, and drug interactions as well as adverse drug reactions are likely to occur in this polypharmaceutical setting. This makes it important that the dentist take careful histories of the patient's medical and pharmacologic status at regular intervals during treatment.

2. The elderly are more sensitive than are young adults to the CNS-depressant effects of drugs. It may be necessary to reduce the dosages of analgesics, antianxiety drugs, sedative-hypnotics, and general anesthetics.

3. The elderly appear to be less sensitive to pain, and, in view of this and the documented sensitivity to the depressant effects of the opioid analgesics, it may be wise to consider limiting the use of such drugs.

4. Because of the known loss in homeostatic competence, drugs that alter blood pressure, heart rate, and smooth muscle tone should be used with caution in the elderly. Conversely, immunosenescence may dictate a more aggressive antibiotic therapy than normal for the prevention and treatment of infections.

5. The elderly are more susceptible to orthostatic hypotension than younger adults. Special attention is called for when they go from a reclining posture in the dental chair to a standing position.

6. There is a well-known decline in renal function in the healthy elderly patient and an even greater decrease in patients with kidney disease. This fact should be taken into consideration when prescribing drugs whose principal route of excretion is the kidney. Conventionally, dosage intervals are increased in such circumstances, but the dose of the drug or drugs may have to be reduced.

7. The dentist should be aware of the psychosocioeconomic status of the patient and sensitive to such problems as the expense of the medications and the possibility of forgetfulness and poor compliance. Special packaging, clear labeling, and simplified dose regimens may improve compliance, as may having a responsible relative or friend monitor drug therapy.

CITED REFERENCES

1. Baum, B.J. Current research on aging and oral health. Geriatric Dentistry **1**:105-109, 1981.
2. Bender, A.D. Effect of age on intestinal absorption: implications for drug absorption in the elderly. Journal of the American Geriatrics Society **16**:1331-1339, 1968.
3. Caird, F.I., Andrews, G.R., and Kennedy, R.D. Effect of posture on blood pressure in the elderly. British Heart Journal **35**:527-530, 1973.
4. Caranasos, G.J., Stewart, R.B., and Cluff, L.E. Drug-induced illness leading to hospitalization. Journal of the American Medical Association **228**:713-717, 1974.
5. Castleden, C.M., George, C.F., Marcer, D., and Hallett, C. Increased sensitivity to nitrazepam in old age. British Medical Journal **1**:10-12, 1977.
6. Chien, C.P., Townsend, E.J., and Ross-Townsend, A. Substance use and abuse among the community elderly: the medical aspect. Addictive Diseases **3**:357-372, 1978.
7. Crooks, J., O'Malley, K., and Stevenson, I.H. Pharmacokinetics in the elderly. Clinical Pharmacokinetics **1**:280-296, 1976.
8. Cusack, B., Kelly, J., O'Malley, K., Noel, J., Lavan, J., and Horgan, J. Digoxin in the elderly: pharmacokinetic consequences of old age. Clinical Pharmacology and Therapeutics **25**:772, 1979.
9. Dental manpower. Interim Report of the American Dental Association's Special Committee on the Future of Dentistry. Chicago, American Dental Association, 1982.
10. Dillon, N., Chung, S., Kelly, J., and O'Malley, K. Age and beta adrenoceptor-mediated function. Clinical Pharmacology and Therapeutics **27**:769-772, 1980.
11. Divoll, M., Abernethy, A.B., and Greenblatt, D.J. Acetaminophen kinetics in the elderly. Clinical Pharmacology and Therapeutics **31**:151-156, 1982.
12. Drayer, D.E., Romankiewicz, J., Lorenzo, B., and Reidenberg, M.M. Age and renal clearance of cimetidine. Clinical Pharmacology and Therapeutics **31**:45-50, 1982.
13. Duvaldestin, P., Saada, J., Berger, J.L., D'Hollander, A., and Desmonts, J.M. Pharmacokinetics, pharmacodynamics, and dose-response relationships of pancuronium in control and elderly subjects. Anesthesiology **56**:36-40, 1982.
14. Evans, M.A., Triggs, E.J., Cheung, M., Broe, G.A., and Creasey, H. Gastric emptying rate in the elderly: implications for drug therapy. Journal of the American Geriatrics Society **29**:201-205, 1981.
15. Geokas, M.C., and Haverback, B.J. The aging gastrointestinal tract. American Journal of Surgery **117**:881-892, 1969.

16. Gibson, R.M., Mueller, M.S., and Fisher, C.R. Age differences in health care spending, fiscal year 1976. Social Security Bulletin **40:**3, 1977.

17. Gillum, R.F., and Barsky, A.J. Diagnosis and management of patient noncompliance. Journal of the American Medical Association **228:**1563-1567, 1974.

18. Greenblatt, D.J., and Koch-Weser, J. Adverse reactions to propranolol in hospitalized medical patients: a report from the Boston Collaborative Drug Surveillance Program. American Heart Journal **86:**478-484, 1973.

19. Greenblatt, D.J., Sellers, E.M., and Shader, R.I. Drug disposition in old age. New England Journal of Medicine **306:**1081-1088, 1982.

20. Guttmann, D. Patterns of legal drug use by older Americans. Addictive Diseases **3:**337-356, 1977.

21. Lamy, P.P. Prescribing for the Elderly. Littleton, Mass., John Wright PSG, Inc., 1981.

22. Lamy, P.P., and Vestal, R.E. Drug prescribing for the elderly. Hospital Practice **11:**111-118, 1976.

23. Law, R., and Chalmers, C. Medicines and elderly people: a general practice survey. British Medical Journal **1:**565-568, 1976.

24. May, F.E., Stewart, R.B., Hale, W.E., and Marks, R.G. Prescribed and nonprescribed drug use in an ambulatory elderly population. Southern Medical Journal **75:**522-528, 1982.

25. Meyer, J., Spier, E., and Neuwelt, F. Basal secretion of digestive enzymes in old age. Archives of Internal Medicine **65:**171-184, 1940.

26. Montgomery, R., Haeney, M.R., and Ross, I.N. The ageing gut: a study of intestinal absorption in relation to the elderly. Quarterly Journal of Medicine **47:**197-211, 1978.

27. Nitham, C.J., Parkhurst, Y.E., and Sommers, E.B. Physicians' prescribing habits: effects of Medicare. Journal of the American Medical Association **217:**585-587, 1971.

28. Parkin, D.M., Henney, C.R., Quirk, J., and Crooks, J. Deviation from prescribed drug treatment after discharge from hospital. British Medical Journal **2:**686-688, 1976.

29. Projections of the Population of the United States 1977 to 2050. Washington, D.C., U.S. Bureau of the Census, No. 704, July 1977.

30. Rasmussen, S.N., Hansen, J.M., Kapmann, J.B., Sköbstad, L., and Bach, B. Drug metabolism in relation to liver volume and age. Scandinavian Journal of Gastroenterology **11:**86, 1976.

31. Reidenberg, M.M., Levy, M., Warner, H., Coutinho, C.B., Schwartz, M.S., Yu, G., and Cheripko, J. Relationship between diazepam dose, plasma level, age, and central nervous system depression. Clinical Pharmacology and Therapeutics **23:**371-374, 1978.

32. Schocken, D.D., and Roth, G.S. Reduced β-adrenergic receptor concentrations in ageing man. Nature **267:**856-858, 1977.

33. Schwartz, D., Wang, M., Feitz, L., and Goss, M.E.W. Medication errors made by elderly, chronically ill patients. American Journal of Public Health **52:**2018-2029, 1962.

34. Seidl, L.G., Thornton, G.F., Smith, J.W., and Cluff, L.E. Studies on the epidemiology of adverse drug reactions. III. Reactions in patients on a general medical service. Bulletin of the Johns Hopkins Hospital **119:**299-315, 1966.

35. Sellers, E.M. Clinical pharmacology and therapeutics of benzodiazepines. Canadian Medical Association Journal **118:**1533-1538, 1978.

36. Shader, R.I., Greenblatt, D.J., Harmatz, J.S., Frankie, R.I., and Koch-Weser, J. Absorption and disposition of chlordiazepoxide in young and elderly male volunteers. Journal of Clinical Pharmacology **17:**709-718, 1977.

37. Smith, C.R. Use of drugs in the aged. Johns Hopkins Medical Journal **145:**61-64, 1979.

38. Smith, J.W., Seidl, L.G., and Cluff, L.E. Studies on the epidemiology of adverse drug reactions. V. Clinical factors influencing susceptibility. Annals of Internal Medicine **65:**629-640, 1966.

39. Swift, C.G., Haythorn, J.M., Clarke, P., and Stevenson, I.H. The effect of ageing on measured responses to single doses of oral temazepam. British Journal of Clinical Pharmacology (suppl. 1):413-414, 1981.

40. Thompson, T.L., II, Moran, M.G., and Nies, A.S. Psychotropic drug use in the elderly. New England Journal of Medicine **308:**134-138, 1983.

41. Vestal, R.E. Drug use in the elderly: a review of problems and special consideration. Drugs **16:**358-382, 1978.

42. Wade, J.G., and Stevens, W.C. Isoflurane: an anesthetic for the eighties. Anesthesia and Analgesia **60:**666-682, 1981.

43. Wallace, S., Whiting, B., and Runcie, J. Factors affecting drug binding in plasma of elderly patients. British Journal of Clinical Pharmacology **3:**312-330, 1976.

44. Weintraub, M., Au, W.Y.W., and Lasagna, L. Compliance as a determinant of serum digoxin concentration. Journal of the American Medical Association **224:**481-485, 1973.

45. Wilson, L.A., Lawson, I.R., and Braws, W. Multiple disorders in the elderly. A clinical and statistical study. Lancet **2:**841-843, 1962.

GENERAL REFERENCES

Finch, C.E., and Hayflick, L., eds. Handbook of The Biology of Aging. New York, Van Nostrand Reinhold Co., 1977.

Lamy, P.P. Prescribing for the Elderly. Littleton, Mass., John Wright PSG, Inc., 1981.

Masoro, E.J., Adelman, R.C., and Roth, G.S., eds. CRC Handbook of Physiology in Aging. Boca Raton, Fla., CRC Press, Inc., 1981.

Roberts, J., Adelman, R.C., and Cristofalo, V.J., eds. Pharmacological Interventions in the Aging Process. Advances in Experimental Medicine and Biology, vol. 79. New York, Plenum Press, 1978.

49 Prescription writing and drug regulations

Anthony Picozzi
Norton M. Ross

THE PRESCRIPTION

A prescription is a written or verbal order for medication to be used for the diagnosis, prevention, or treatment of a specific patient's disease by a licensed physician, dentist, podiatrist, or veterinarian. It is a legal document for which the prescriber and pharmacist are both responsible; if it is given verbally, therefore, the pharmacist should immediately reduce it to writing. A prescription may also be written for a drug to be used in a clinician's practice by designating it "for office use." Prescriptions are subject to state, federal, and local regulations.

As determined by the FDA, a legend drug is one that requires a prescription in order to be dispensed by a pharmacist, in contrast to an OTC drug, which can be purchased without a prescription. Legend drugs include agents with abuse liability that are under the control of the Drug Enforcement Administration (DEA) of the Department of Justice, as well as drugs that are not specifically controlled, such as antibiotics, local anesthetics, some antihistamines, and systemic corticosteroids. Agents permitted to be sold over the counter are deemed to be safe and effective when used without professional guidance and include such preparations as nonnarcotic analgesics, antacids, cold remedies, vitamins, topical antibiotics, topical corticosteroids, and others. Many OTC cough preparations, as Schedule V drugs, are controlled by the DEA but do not require a prescription. OTC or nonprescription medications are manufactured under the same quality control standards that apply to prescription drugs; their safety and effectiveness are also monitored by the FDA.

A simple prescription is one written for a preparation with only one active ingredient, the agent that produces the desired effect (e.g., codeine phosphate, 30 mg tablets), as compared with a compound prescription, which calls for a preparation with more than one active ingredient (e.g., aspirin, 227 mg; caffeine, 32 mg; phenacetin, 162 mg; and codeine phosphate 30 mg). Most such formulations are available precompounded in a single dosage form and may be prescribed as a single drug (e.g., Tabloid APC with codeine tablets). When the combination is a rational one (as is the compounding of aspirin with codeine for enhanced pain relief), the ease of prescribing and using the preparation may justify its selection. All too frequently, however, unnecessary drugs (e.g., caffeine) or inappropriate combinations (such as the mixing of two nonnarcotic analgesics) are employed. Because such formulations are prepared in fixed proportions by the manufacturer and thus are not subject to adjustment to suit the needs of the individual patient, their utility is further restricted. Therefore, fixed combinations, with few exceptions, should not be employed; when more than one drug is required, each should be individually prescribed in accordance with the therapeutic requirements of the patient.

Drug names

As discussed in Chapter 3, any drug may be identified by more than one designation in various references, texts, and package inserts. Of special interest here are the nonproprietary and proprietary names. The nonproprietary name, sometimes referred to as the common, usual, or generic name, is selected by the United States Adopted Names Council. Since, with few exceptions, any given drug will have only one nonproprietary name in the United States (the designation may differ in other countries), it is this name by which the drug is primarily identified. The same agent, however, may have many proprietary or trade names, which are given to it by the various manufacturers or marketers of the drug and used for promotional purposes. In all advertisements and labeling using the trade name, the nonproprietary name of the drug must also be prominently identified. In recent years, there has been a strong tendency on the part of governmental regulatory agencies to encourage or even mandate the prescribing and dispensing of drugs by their nonproprietary names. At this writing, 49 states and the District of Columbia have repealed their existing antisubstitution laws and replaced them with drug substitution laws permitting or, in some states, requiring the pharmacist to dispense ''generic'' drugs (preparations containing the same active chemicals in identical amounts but sold by different companies) unless specifically prohibited by the prescriber. Also, the Federal Government has instituted maximum allowable cost programs in an effort to contain the cost of prescription drugs to the consumer by limiting the prescription use of proprietary names. These programs require the prescriber to certify the necessity of prescribing a specific brand of drug rather than its nonproprietary counterpart. Questions of whether the consumer ultimately realizes a saving and whether there is therapeutic equivalence among generically equivalent drugs are controversial issues still under debate. Also being debated are the effects, if any, these programs have on the pharmaceutical industry, particularly in regard to investment in the development of new drugs.

Equivalence: chemical, pharmaceutical, biologic, and therapeutic

Drug products that contain the same amounts of the same active ingredients in the same dosage forms and that meet present official compendium standards are considered chemical equivalents. Pharmaceutical equivalents are drug products that contain the same amounts of the same therapeutic or active ingredients in the same dosage form and that meet standards based on the best currently available technology. This means that pharmaceutical equivalents will be formulated identically and will have to pass certain laboratory tests for equivalent activity, including dissolution tests where appropriate, by standards that have not as yet been established for all classes of drugs. Bioequivalent drugs are those that, when administered to the same

individual in the same dosage regimen, will result in comparable bioavailability. (Bioavailability refers to the extent and rate of absorption of a dosage form as reflected by the time-concentration curve of the administered drug in the systemic circulation.) With proper testing methods, it is hoped that pharmaceutical equivalence will ensure biologic equivalence, at least insofar as the extent of absorption is concerned.

Therapeutic equivalents are chemical or pharmaceutical equivalents that, when administered to the same or comparable individuals in the same dosage regimen, provide essentially the same efficacy (and toxicity). Achieving therapeutic equivalence among various brands of the same drug is the goal of pharmaceutical testing. The only way that therapeutic equivalency can be satisfactorily demonstrated is by properly controlled human clinical trials, which are expensive and time-consuming. At the present time, scientists assume that those drugs that, in the absence of contradictory clinical evidence, are bioequivalent will also be therapeutically equivalent. It was also once widely assumed that chemically equivalent drugs would have comparable bioavailability. That this latter assumption is not necessarily true, however, has been demonstrated for many categories of drugs that have identical formulations but apparently have different bioavailabilities or do not demonstrate therapeutic equivalence.

Problems of bioequivalence can arise from many areas. First, although the amounts of the therapeutic ingredients may be the same in identical dosage form, the preparations may contain different binders, excipients, diluents, stabilizers, preservatives, or a variety of other inactive ingredients in order to give them their physical form. Second, the force by which the preparation mixture is compressed into the tablet or capsule dosage form, or the manner in which the granules or aggregates are dissolved, dispersed, or suspended in a liquid formulation, may also differ. Third, the quality control or the age, purity, and physical consistency of any of the chemical constituents contained in different formulations of chemically equivalent products can differ. All of these various and sometimes poorly controlled factors can influence the rate at which the product disintegrates, deaggregates, or dissolves in the gastrointestinal tract, thereby affecting absorption of the active ingredients. The rate at which or the degree to which breakdown products of the active ingredients are formed may also differ, affecting either the stability (shelf life) or possibly the potential toxicity of the product. Unfortunately, current standards to not ensure the bioequivalence or therapeutic equivalence of all drugs, and variations in bioavailability have been shown to be responsible for some treatment failures with certain drug categories. Nevertheless, requirements by the FDA for bioavailability testing of new drugs and disintegration and dissolution measurements for existing agents (e.g., tetracyclines) have made and will continue to make significant inroads into the problem of therapeutic inequivalence of chemically identical drug products.

As a major step toward facilitating the wider use of generic drugs to slow the rising cost of health care, the FDA has formulated a list of all FDA-approved drugs that it regards as therapeutically equivalent in order to guide states in identifying less expensive generic alternatives that pharmacists can substitute for more expensive brand name products. This list indicates which drugs are considered therapeutically equivalent (''positive formulary''), which drugs may not be therapeutically equivalent (''negative formulary''), and those about which the agency has not yet made a determination. It is the policy of the FDA to consider pharmaceutically equivalent drugs as therapeutically equivalent unless there is scientific evidence to the contrary.

Although it is true that FDA ''recalls'' of generic drugs greatly outnumber those of brand name drugs, the vast majority of American pharmaceutical firms follow Good Manufacturing Practice regulations and are inspected periodically by the FDA for compliance with quality control standards. Additionally, many generic name products are manufactured and distributed by the same company that markets the brand name drug. For these reasons it should not be assumed that a generic name product is necessarily inferior to its brand name counterpart. In fact, it has been shown that in most cases generic brands are bioequivalent and that occasionally they may even be superior. It is therefore left to the practitioner to know the properties of the drugs employed and to decide whether to prescribe by trade or nonproprietary name. As a guide in making this decision, however, it should be recognized that differences in bioequivalence between brand and generic drugs may exist but that they are probably minor. When the condition being treated is not serious or life-threatening, when the therapeutic index of the drug category being prescribed is not critical, when there is some assurance that the savings realized by prescribing according to nonproprietary name is actually being passed on to the patient (which cannot always be assumed), and unless there is evidence that the generic preparations are biologically inequivalent, a drug should be prescribed by its nonproprietary name.

Components of the prescription

A complete, ideal prescription is made up of several parts, each of which provides specific information about the prescriber, the patient, and the drug.

The name and full address of the prescriber are necessary. The telephone number is not required but is usually included as a convenience to the pharmacist.

The patient's full name and address are required on prescriptions for DEA-controlled substances; the patient's age is optional but is desirable on prescriptions for children under 12, permitting the pharmacist to confirm the dosage.

The date that the prescription is written and signed is always desirable and is required on prescriptions for DEA-controlled substances.

The symbol ℞, known as the superscription, is generally understood to be an abbreviation of the Latin *recipe,* meaning ''take thou,'' but was probably derived from the ancient Roman symbol for Jupiter and used in the physician's prayer for the survival of the patient.

The inscription provides specific information about the drug preparation: (1) the name of the drug, which can be either the nonproprietary or the proprietary name, or both, with the proprietary name following the nonproprietary in parentheses, for example, pentazocine (Talwin), and (2) the unit dosage or amount of the drug in milligrams (as with penicillin V) or in units (as with penicillin G). If the prescription is for a liquid preparation, the individual unit of dosage is usually contained in each teaspoonful or 5 ml. The pharmacist's responsibility to both the patient and the practitioner dictates that the prescription be checked for possible errors in dosage.

The subscription is the prescriber's directions to the pharmacist with regard to fulfilling the inscription. Because almost all drugs used by dentists are available in precompounded form, the subscription is usually brief, including only:

1. The quantity and dosage form of the drug to be dispensed; that is, the number of tablets or capsules or the volume of a liquid preparation. This

direction is written, preferably in arabic numerals, for an appropriate amount of the drug as determined by the manner in which it will be used by the patient, the amount the patient will need, the toxicity and abuse potential of the drug, and the cost to the patient. Especially with drugs subject to abuse, the quantity should be both placed in parentheses and written out (in English, not Latin) to avoid alteration. (Without this precaution, for example, 15 is easily changed to 45, 75, or 150). In any prescription, no greater quantity of drug than is needed should be ordered.

2. The number of authorized refills of the prescription. The number and its time limitations are specified for DEA-controlled drugs but are otherwise left to the discretion of the practitioner. If refill directions are not specified by the prescriber, no prescription may be refilled. With controlled substances, care should be taken to devise a refill authorization system that is not easily altered, such as crossing out all except the desired number in a series (e.g., Ø, 1, 2̶, 3̶).

3. Directions to the pharmacist to list the medication on the container label. The current trend in most states is to require the pharmacist to identify medications on the label unless such identification is not considered to be in the patient's best interest and specifically prohibited by the prescriber. Identifying the drug could prevent allergic reactions or adverse interactions with other medications and-misuse of the unused portion of the prescription. It may be especially helpful in directing the management of victims of drug poisoning.

The transcription or signature (from the Latin *signa*, meaning "label" or "let it be labeled"), indicated on the prescription by "Label:" or "Sig:", is the prescriber's directions to the patient that will appear on the medicine container. At one time, such directions were uniformly written in Latin, but modern practice is to use English. Latin abbreviations are still employed by many clinicians in order to save time; however, such gains are undoubtedly trivial in most dental practices and may be accompanied by some loss of accuracy (e.g., q. 4.h. instead of q.i.d. represents a 50% dosage error) and compromised patient compliance. Figure 49-1 depicts the same prescription for an analgesic medication, one written entirely in English and the other in Latin abbreviations with their Latin equivalents and English translations.

Since relatively few patients will be able to recall oral instructions accurately, the labeled directions

Label: Take two tablets immediately. Take one or
two tablets every 4 hours as needed for
relief of pain.

Sig: Tab 2 stat. Tab 1 or 2 q. 4 h., p.r.n. for
relief of pain.

Figure 49-1. Sample of the same prescription written in English and in Latin.

should be specific, not merely "use as directed." Indeed, failure to be specific can, in some states, provide the basis for malpractice suits.

A subject of current interest with regard to directions on prescriptions is patient compliance or, more accurately, noncompliance. As discussed in Chapter 3, 25% to 60% of all patients fail to take medications as intended by their doctors. Noncompliance includes such practices as improper or inappropriate timing of doses or premature discontinuation of the medication. The many possible reasons for patient noncompliance may involve a lack of knowledge or understanding of the drug or the purpose for which it was prescribed, misinformation from nonmedical sources, negative patient attitudes toward illness or "taking drugs," development of an adverse effect, economic factors, or inadequate communication (instruction and emphasis) by the practitioner.

Patient compliance is probably improved when the prescriber explains the condition for which the patient is being treated, what the alternative treatment regimens are, the probable or anticipated benefits, adverse reactions, and side effects, and the importance of following the medication instructions accurately. This should then be reinforced by complete, detailed instructions on the prescription. Perhaps the most important aspect of a prescription is that it is a means of communication which is likely to be ignored if written perfunctorily but can enhance the doctor-patient relationship and contribute to patient compliance if care is used in presenting it. Writing a prescription in English and in the patient's presence and then explaining it may, in addition to improving compliance, equip the patient to detect any errors that may occur in filling the prescription.

Patient compliance may also be improved by selecting drugs that need to be taken only once or twice daily over agents that have to be administered more frequently. When multiple drug therapy is necessary, combination products, when appropriate, are helpful in reducing the "confusion over pill profusion," as is prescribing drugs with distinctive physical characteristics (e.g., a red tablet, a white tablet, and a capsule instead of three white tablets).

The signature and degree of the prescriber convey the authority of the prescriber to order the medication and of the pharmacist to fill the prescription. Although all prescriptions should be signed, a signature is actually required by law only for certain controlled substances (Schedule II drugs), since other prescriptions can be phoned in without a signature and be put into writing by the pharmacist. When it appears, the signature is followed by the prescriber's professional degree rather than preceded by "Dr.," as the abbreviation for "Doctor." Most state dental practice acts specify that prescriptions may be written only for patients under active care. Many state laws stipulate that only those classes of drugs directly involved with dental treatment may be prescribed.

Finally, the prescriber's DEA registration number must appear on any prescription for a controlled or scheduled drug, in compliance with the Controlled Substances Act of 1970. This number, however, should not routinely be entered on prescriptions that do not require it, in order to prevent its use by potential abusers who may have access to blank prescription pads.

Many states additionally have their own controlled dangerous substances (or similar) act. Should state, federal, or local regulations governing any drug or procedure differ, the most stringent of the regulations applies. Both the state and federal certificates of registration must be renewed annually. DEA registration is not required of practitioners in the military or the Public Health Service nor of recent graduates in internship or residency programs, in which case the institutional DEA registration number may be used.

Prescription writing and format

Prescriptions should be written concisely, accurately, and legibly. Ink, indelible pencil, or typing is required for prescriptions for Schedule II drugs and is preferable for all prescriptions. With the advent of safe and effective drugs, consumer education, and the concept of informed consent, the need for therapeutic mysticism of an illegible prescription written in a foreign language no longer

Table 49-1. Latin abbreviations frequently used in prescription writing

Abbreviation	Latin	English
ad lib.	ad libitum	at pleasure
a.c.	ante cibum	before meals
aq.	aqua	water
b.i.d.	bis in die	twice a day
caps.	capsula	capsule
c̄	cum	with
d.	dies	a day, daily
disp.	dispensa	dispense
gtt.	guttae	drops
h.	hora	hour
h.s.	hora somni	at bedtime
non rep.	non repetatur	do not repeat
no.	numerus	number, amount
p.c.	post cibum	after meals
p.r.n.	pro re nata	as needed
q.h.	quaque hora	every hour
q. 4 h.	quaque quarta hora	every 4 hours
q.i.d.	quater in die	4 times a day
Sig.	signa	let it be labeled, label
stat.	statim	immediately
tab.	tabella	tablet
t.i.d.	ter in die	three times a day

exists. Furthermore, similarity between the names of some highly active and potentially toxic drugs makes illegibility all the more indefensible.

Blank printed prescription pads should not have the name of a pharmacy or pharmaceutical company imprinted anywhere on the form, because such an implicit endorsement may direct the patient to a particular pharmacy or manufacturer's product. Pads should also be kept in a drawer or under similar cover when not in use to avoid loss or theft of prescription blanks by a potential drug abuser. Should theft of a prescription pad be suspected, such loss should be reported to the state drug control agency. Additionally, for good dental practice as well as for medicolegal reasons, a duplicate of each prescription or a record thereof should be kept in the patient's file.

Figure 49-2 presents a typical preprinted prescription form used, with minor variations, by most practitioners. In those states with laws permitting or, as in some instances, mandating the substitution of a generic preparation for a proprietary drug, the prescription form may have a space to allow the clinician to indicate when a substitution is or is not permitted. Figure 49-3 presents two sample prescriptions. The first, for antibiotic prophylaxis be-

John R. Brown, D.M.D.
123 Main St.
Metropolis, N.J.
Phone: 625-7846

For_____   Age_____

_____   Date_____

R̸

Substitution
  ☐ permitted
  ☐ not permitted
_____

Signature

Label ☐   Refill 0 1 2 3

DEA #_____

Figure 49-2. Typical prescription form.

fore dental therapy, is written by nonproprietary name; the second, for postoperative pain relief, is written by trade name. In the latter case, the dosage is implicit in the particular formulation selected (i.e., acetaminophen 325 mg; codeine 30 mg).

Posology

The dosage of a prescribed drug may vary according to several factors: the degree or severity of the condition for which it is being prescribed; the age, weight, or temperament of the patient; the route, frequency, or timing of administration; concurrent medication; patient suggestibility (placebo effect), habits, sensitivities, or previous medication history (hyperreaction or hyporeaction); and the systemic health of the patient.

The manufacturer's package insert, pharmacology texts, and various compendia list the "official," "average," or "usual" adult dose for a drug. A listed dose or dosage range is a guide for prescription purposes, and although it does not carry the weight of a regulation, it does have medicolegal implications should there be an adverse effect. Practitioners are well advised to stay within the recommended dosage range unless they have a sound reason to go beyond it. Sources especially useful in providing dosages include the *Physicians' Desk Reference, Facts and Comparisons, Accepted*

Dental Therapeutics, and *AMA Drug Evaluations.* Brief resumés of these sources of drug information are provided in Chapter 3.

For dosage determination, "an adult" is usually interpreted to mean an individual 18 years or older and weighing approximately 70 kg (150 pounds). Children and many underweight, diseased, or aged patients require a dosage of pharmacologically active agents that is lower than normal. Very large or obese patients frequently require a higher dose.

Several rules have been proposed for computing the dosage of a drug for children:

1. Clark's rule,

$$\frac{\text{Weight in lbs}}{150}, \text{ or } \frac{\text{Weight in kg}}{70}$$

equals the fraction of the adult dose for the child. This fraction, multiplied by the adult dose, equals the child's dose.

2. Young's rule,

$$\frac{\text{Age of patient}}{\text{Age} + 12}$$

equals the fraction of the adult dose for the child. Again, this fraction multiplied by the adult dose yields the child's dose.

3. Surface area (in meters^2) extrapolated from the patient's height and weight, is divided by 1.73

℞

Penicillin V potassium 500 mg
Dispense 12 tablets

Sig: Take 4 tablets with water 1 hour before dental appointment. Take 1 tablet every 6 hours thereafter for 8 doses.

Substitution
☒ permitted
☐ not permitted

Label ☒   Refill ☒☒ 2 ☒

_____
Signature

DEA #_____

℞

Tylenol with Codeine #3
Dispense sixteen (16) tablets

Sig: Take 1 or 2 tablets every 4 hours as needed for relief of pain.

Substitution
☒ permitted
☐ not permitted

Label ☒   Refill 0 ☒☒☒

_____
Signature

DEA #__AB1234567_____

Figure 49-3. Sample prescriptions. The one at the bottom indicates that the substitution of a generic drug is permitted.

(the average adult surface area) to determine the fraction of the adult dose. This method is seldom, if ever, used in dentistry. However, simple dosage tables or graphs, such as Table 49-2, are available that obviate time-consuming calculations.

Of these methods, Clark's rule is the most widely used. Young's rule is perhaps the most subject to error. However, because physiologic functions dealing with drug disposition are generally proportional to body surface area, the last method is probably the most accurate of the three. This distinction is rather dubious, though, because drug responses in children, especially the very young, are modified by factors other than body size (see Chapter 3). When dosage information is unavailable and one of these methods has to be employed to estimate the child dose, it is important to monitor the patient carefully to ensure that therapeutic effects are obtained and that toxic reactions are held to a minimum.

Weights and measures

Two systems of designating weights and measures of drugs and preparations are the apothecaries' and the metric systems. Although many attempts have been made to promote the use of the much preferred metric system, the older apothecaries' measures are still employed by some clinicians. Roman numerals are generally used with the apothecaries' system and arabic numbers with the metric.

The grain is the unit of weight and the minim is the unit of liquid measure (volume) in the apothecaries' system. There are 480 grains in 1 ounce

Table 49-2. Determination of child dose by surface area

Weight (lb)	Fraction of adult dose	Weight (kg)

The fraction of the adult dose (center scale) is determined by reading across from the weight in pounds (left scale) or kilograms (right scale). For this scale, surface area was estimated as the 0.7 power of the weight (in pounds) times 0.055. The fraction of the adult dose was determined by dividing the surface area by 1.73 (the average adult value).

and 480 minims in a fluid ounce. The gram is the unit of weight and the milliliter is the unit of volume in the metric system. One gram equals 1000 milligrams, and 1000 milliliters constitutes 1 liter. Some approximate equivalents between the two systems are given in Table 49-3.

Household measures are commonly encountered when liquid preparations are prescribed. If the directions call for the patient to take a certain volume of drug solution, the pharmacist converts the metric value given into its household equivalent, as indicated in Table 49-4. Unfortunately, utensils likely to be employed by patients may yield different volumes of medicine than were initially intended. To circumvent this problem, many commercial products are provided with calibrated measuring devices; patients should be encouraged to use these when taking their medications.

DRUG LAWS

Various federal, state, and local laws have been enacted to control the manufacture, sale, and dispensing of drugs. In order to comply with these regulations, the clinician should be aware that the most stringent of these laws takes precedence, whether it be federal, state, or local.

Table 49-3. Approximate apothecaries' and metric equivalents

Apothecaries'	Metric
Weight	
1/65 grain	1 mg
1 grain	65 mg
15 grains	1 gm
1 dram	4 gm
1 ounce	30 gm
Volume	
1 minim	0.06 ml
16 minims	1 ml
1 fluid dram	4 ml
1 fluid ounce	30 ml
1 pint	480 ml

Table 49-4. Metric equivalents of some common household measures

Household measure	Metric volume
1 drop	0.05 ml
1 teaspoon	5 ml
1 tablespoon	15 ml
1 teacup	120 ml
1 glass	240 ml
1 pint	480 ml

Historical development of drug legislation

Throughout history, nations have attempted to regulate the commerce and usage of drugs. One of the major concerns has always been the establishment of criteria for drug identity and purity, and to this end, the development of pharmacopeias has proved invaluable. A pharmacopeia is a written description of the source, identification, and preparation of medicinal agents. The first pharmacopeia to gain legal status was one adopted by the city-state of Nürnberg in the early sixteenth century.

After the American Revolution, the only pharmacopeias available in the United States were of European authorship. To remedy this, in 1820 a group of physicians, pharmacists, and chemists met in Philadelphia to prepare a new pharmacopeia for the country. This first U.S. Pharmacopeial Convention established certain policies, notably that only drugs of proven merit would be included in *The United States Pharmacopeia* (USP) and that regular revisions of the document would be issued.

The USP published in 1980 is the twentieth edition.

Because most multiple drug entities and various commonly prescribed nostrums and remedies were excluded from the USP, the need remained for a compendium to promote the standardization of these medicinals. Thus, in 1888, the American Pharmaceutical Association began to publish *The National Formulary of Unofficial Preparations,* later to be abbreviated to *The National Formulary* (NF). Like the USP, the NF was periodically revised, until 1975, after which it was merged with the USP.

Around the turn of the twentieth century, a growing public clamor and indignation over the quality, purity, and safety of food and drug products led to the passage of the Food and Drug Act of 1906. In this legislation, the USP and NF were given legal status with respect to defining the purity and quality of drugs. Standards were also established for the labeling of medicinal products. In the years that followed, these standards were extended by court decisions and congressional actions to cover promotional materials in addition to the products themselves.

Before 1937, the testing of drugs and ingredients used in the preparation of medications was not necessary before marketing. In that year a relatively new solvent, diethylene glycol, was employed to prepare an "Elixir of Sulfonamides." This agent caused the death of over 100 people, mostly children, and was responsible for the swift passage of the Federal Food, Drug, and Cosmetic Act of 1938. This act required manufacturers to provide the FDA with evidence of drug safety in the form of a New Drug Application before distributing the agent. Unless the application was disapproved within 60 days, the pharmaceutical company was then free to market the compound. The act of 1938 also introduced the principle of separating drugs into prescription and nonprescription categories by requiring companies selling OTC drugs to furnish purchasers with the information necessary for their safe and effective use. Questions concerning which drugs could be sold over the counter and which had to be reserved for prescription use were not resolved, however, until passage of the Durham-Humphrey Amendment in 1951 (see below).

In response to the thalidomide tragedy in Europe, Congress passed the Kefauver-Harris Amendment of 1962. This amendment to the 1938 act required manufacturers of new drugs to proceed along set standards of animal and human pharmacologic and toxicologic testing, the data from each step to be reviewed by the FDA. Requirements for evaluating efficacy and studying chronic and fetal toxicity were specific omissions of the 1938 act that were corrected by this legislation. (The various stages of testing of drugs are reviewed in Chapter 3.) Also included in the Kefauver-Harris Amendment was a requirement that all prescription and OTC medications approved since 1938 be reviewed for their safety and efficacy.

In addition to laws regulating drugs in general, special legislation has been enacted pertaining to drugs of abuse. The historical development of these laws is presented in Chapter 46.

Rules and regulations governing prescription drugs

The two federal laws controlling prescription drugs are the Durham-Humphrey Amendment (Section 503B) of 1951 to the Food, Drug, and Cosmetic Act of 1938 and the Comprehensive Drug Abuse Prevention and Control Act (Controlled Substances Act) of 1970. The Durham-Humphrey law restricted the dispensing of certain types of drugs (antibiotics, corticosteroids, and other agents whose unsupervised use may not be safe) to the prescription order of a licensed practitioner. These drugs are known as legend drugs since they are required to bear the label "Caution: Federal law prohibits dispensing without prescription." Under this law, a prescription for these drugs may not be refilled unless authorized by the prescriber. Many prescription drugs are currently being reviewed by the FDA to determine if they would be safe for OTC use. The FDA has the responsibility for reviewing the labeling and advertising of the use of drugs, both legend and OTC. This review, based on documented clinical studies, limits the labeled indications and uses of the product, but does not necessarily limit the practitioner to use the drug only in these situations. The FDA recognizes the need to explore new uses for approved drugs. The practitioner, however, can be liable under civil law for mishaps that occur with unlabeled uses of a drug. Although the federal government has set no standards concerning which legend drugs a dentist may employ clinically, many state laws regulating the practice of dentistry restrict drugs used to those associated with dental treatment. A typical law of this kind states that dentists can "diagnose, treat, operate, or prescribe for any disease, pain, injury, deficiency, deformity, or physical condition of the

Table 49-5. Classification of controlled substances

Schedule	Criteria for inclusion	Examples of drugs
I	High abuse potential, no currently accepted medical use, may lead to severe dependence	LSD, marijuana, tetrahydrocannabinols, mescaline, peyote, heroin
II	High abuse potential, accepted medical use, may lead to severe dependence	Amphetamines, methadone, meperidine, methaqualone, methylphenidate, morphine, codeine, oxycodone, cocaine, pentobarbital, secobarbital
III	Abuse potential less than drugs in Schedules I or II, accepted medical use, moderate to low dependence liability relative to drugs of Schedule II	Benzphetamine, glutethimide, methyprylon, mixtures of codeine with aspirin or acetaminophen, paregoric
IV	Low abuse potential compared with drugs in Schedule III, accepted medical use, limited dependence liability relative to drugs in Schedule III	Phenobarbital, meprobamate, chlordiazepoxide, ethchlorvynol, diazepam, propoxyphene, chloral hydrate
V	Abuse potential less than drugs in Schedule IV, accepted medical use, limited dependence liability relative to drugs in Schedule IV	Cough preparations containing codeine or similar opioid derivatives

human teeth, alveolar process, gums, or jaws.''

Control of the distribution of depressant and stimulant drugs (e.g., opioids, barbiturates, and amphetamines) and other classes of drugs designated as possessing abuse potential by the DEA is regulated by the Controlled Substances Act. The act divided opioid and other drugs into five schedules based on the drugs' potential for abuse, their medical usefulness, and the degree to which they may lead to physical or psychologic dependence. The criteria for inclusion within the five schedules are presented in Table 49-5.

In order to prescribe controlled substances, the licensed practitioner must register with the DEA. The registration must be renewed annually, and the certificate of registration must be retained and displayed by the practitioner. If controlled drugs are to be administered to patients in the practitioner's office, they can be obtained only on special order forms that are available from the DEA. A record of the dates of acquisition and dispensing of such drugs must be kept, and a biennial inventory of controlled substances on hand must be filed with the DEA.

Schedule I drugs may not be prescribed and are made available only for specific, approved research projects. With the exception of prescriptions for Schedule II products, which may not be refilled, controlled drug prescriptions can be refilled up to 5 times within 6 months, assuming that the prescriber authorizes these refills. After the final permitted refill, a new prescription for the product must be obtained.

Drugs in Schedule V, which consist of preparations containing limited quantities of certain opioids agents, may be sold without a prescription, assuming that the drug is dispensed by a pharmacist to a purchaser who is at least 18 years of age and that a record of the transaction be kept by the pharmacist.

A pharmacist is permitted to fill oral prescriptions for any drug except Schedule II products, provided they are subsequently committed to writing and filed by the pharmacist. The law does allow for the dispensing of verbal prescriptions for opioid and other Schedule II drugs in emergency situations, but the quantity must be limited to the amount needed for the emergency, the prescription must be put in writing by the pharmacist, and the prescriber must furnish the pharmacist with a signed written prescription within 72 hours. The labeling of prescriptions for all controlled substances must contain the warning ''Caution: Federal law prohibits the transfer of this drug to any person other than the patient for whom it was prescribed.''

Information and applications for registration may be obtained from the Drug Enforcement Administration, P.O. Box 28083 Central Station, Washington, D.C. 20005, or from the DEA Regional Office in the area in which the applicant practices.

The DEA offers the following suggestions for writing prescriptions for controlled substances:

1. Keep prescription blanks in a safe place where they cannot be stolen easily. Minimize the number of prescription pads in use.

2. Write prescription orders for Schedule II

drugs in ink or indelible pencil, or use a typewriter. They must be signed by the clinician. Prescribing controlled substances by telephone is discouraged unless the patient is familiar or the validity of the request can be substantiated.

3. Write out the actual amount prescribed, in addition to giving an arabic number or roman numeral, in order to discourage the alteration of prescription orders.

4. Avoid writing prescription orders for large quantities of medications, especially controlled drugs, unless it is determined that such quantities are necessary.

5. Maintain only a minimum stock of controlled drugs in the office.

6. Keep all controlled drugs under lock.

7. Be cautious when a patient says that another clinician has been prescribing a specific controlled drug product or claims that only one product "works" for him or her. Consult the clinician or the hospital records, or else examine the patient thoroughly and decide independently if the drug product should be prescribed.

8. Prescription blanks should be used only for writing prescription orders, not for notes or memos. A drug abuser could easily erase the message and use the blank to forge a prescription order.

9. Never sign prescription blanks in advance.

10. Maintain an accurate record of controlled drug products that have been dispensed or administered, as required by the Controlled Substances Act of 1970 and its regulations.

11. Assist the pharmacist who telephones in verifying information about a prescription order. A corresponding responsibility rests with the pharmacist who dispenses the prescribed medication.

12. Telephone the nearest office of the DEA to obtain or to furnish information. Calls will be held in the strictest confidence.

Glossary of abbreviations

All elements that commonly exist in ionic form will be referred to as Na^+, Ca^{++}, H^+, K^+, Cl^-, etc.

Å	Ångstrom units
Ab	antibody
ABVD	doxorubicin, bleomycin, vinblastine, dacarbazine
ACh	acetylcholine
ACH	adrenal cortical hormone
AChE	acetylcholinesterase
AChR	acetylcholine receptor
ACTH	adrenocorticotropic hormone
ADA	American Dental Association
ADH	antidiuretic hormone
ADR	adverse drug reaction
ADT	*Accepted Dental Therapeutics*
Ag	antigen
AHG	antihemophilic globulin
AIDS	acquired immune deficiency syndrome
ALS	antilymphocytic sera
AMA	American Medical Association
ANUG	acute necrotizing ulcerative gingivitis
6-APA	6-aminopenicillanic acid
APAP	acetaminophen
APC	aspirin-phenacetin-caffeine
APD	action potential duration
ARAS	ascending reticular activating system
ASA	aspirin
ATP	adenosine triphosphate
ATPase	adenosine triphosphatase
A-V	atrioventricular (node)
BAC	blood alcohol concentration
BAL	dimercaprol (British antilewisite)
BCG	bacillus Calmette-Guérin
BCNU	carmustine
BuChE	butyrocholinesterase
C_6	hexamethonium
C_{10}	decamethonium
cAMP	cyclic adenosine 3'-5'-monophosphate
CCNU	lomustine
CEB	calcium entry blocker
ChAc	choline acetylase
ChE	cholinesterase
CGH	chorionic gonadotropin
cGMP	cyclic guanosine 3″-5″-monophosphate
CHL	cholesterol
CMI	cell-mediated immunity
CNS	central nervous system
CoA	coenzyme A
COMT	catechol-O-methyltransferase
CTZ	chemoreceptor trigger zone
DBH	dopamine-β-hydroxylase
DCI	dichloroisoproterenol
DDT	chlorophenothane
DEA	Drug Enforcement Administration
DES	diethylstilbestrol
DET	diethyltryptamine
DFP	isoflurophate (formerly diisopropylfluorophosphate)
dl	deciliter
DMA	dimethoxyamphetamine
DMFS	decayed, missing, filled surfaces
DMFT	decayed, missing, filled teeth
DMPP	dimethylphenylpiperazinium
DMSO	dimethyl sulfoxide
DMT	dimethyltryptamine
DNA	deoxyribonucleic acid
DOM	dimethoxymethylamphetamine
Dopa	dihydroxyphenylalanine
DPT	dipropyltryptamine or Demerol, Phenergan, Thorazine
E	Epinephrine
EAMG	experimental autoimmune myasthenia gravis
ECG	electrocardiogram
ED	effective dose
ED_{50}	dose that produces half-maximal response
ED50	median effective dose
EDTA	ethylenediaminetetraacetic acid
EEG	electroencephalograph
EPP	endplate potential
EPSP	excitatory postsynaptic potential
ERP	effective refractory period

ETEC	enterotoxigenic *Escherichia coli*	**NDA**	New Drug Application
FAS	fetal alcohol syndrome	**NE**	norepinephrine
FDA	Food and Drug Administration	**NF**	National Formulary
FSH	follicle-stimulating hormone	**N₂O**	nitrous oxide
GABA	γ-aminobutyric acid	**NSAID**	nonsteroidal antiinflammatory drug
GDP	guanosine diphosphate	**NTS**	nucleus tractus solatarius
GI	gastrointestinal	**OSHA**	Occupational Safety and Health Administration
GMP	guanosine monophosphate		
GTH	growth hormone	**OTC**	over the counter
GTP	guanosine triphosphate	**PABA**	*p*-aminobenzoic acid
GU	genitourinary	**PAG**	periaqueductal gray
H	histamine (receptor)	**PAM**	pralidoxime
HBsAg	hepatitis B surface antigen	**Pa$_{O_2}$**	arterial blood oxygen tension
HDL	high density lipoproteins	**PAS**	*p*-aminosalicylic acid
HDN	hemolytic disease of the newborn	**P$_{CO_2}$**	partial pressure of carbon dioxide
HSV	herpes simplex virus	**P$_{O_2}$**	partial pressure of oxygen
5-HT	5-hydroxytryptamine	**PCP**	phencyclidine
Hz	Herz	**PDR**	Physicians' Desk Reference
IgA	immunoglobulin A	**P-F**	phosphofluoride (linkage)
IgE	immunoglobulin E	**PG**	prostaglandin
IgG	immunoglobulin G	**PGI₂**	prostacyclin
IgM	immunoglobulin M	**pH**	$-\log H^+$ concentration
ILDL	intermediate low density lipoproteins	**PI**	Pharmacopeia Internationalis
IM	intramuscular	**PMN**	polymorphonuclear (leukocyte)
IND	Notice of Claimed Investigational Exemption for a New Drug	**PNMT**	phenylethanolamine-N-methyltransferase
INH	isoniazid (isonicotinic acid hydrazide)	**PO**	per os (by mouth)
IPSP	inhibitory postsynaptic potential	**PO/IM**	oral/intramuscular potency ratio
ISA	intrinsic sympathomimetic activity	**PPM**	parts per million
IV	intravenous	**PRA**	plasma renin activity
LD	lethal dose	**PSI**	pounds per square inch
LDL	low density lipoproteins	**PTH**	parathyroid hormone
LH	luteinizing hormone	**PTT**	partial thromboplastin time
LPH	lipotropin	**R**	resistance factor
LSD	lysergic acid diethylamide	**RBC**	red blood cell
LT	leukotrienes	**REM**	rapid eye movement (sleep)
MAC	minimum alveolar concentration	**RH**	releasing hormone
MAO	monoamine oxidase	**RIA**	radioimmunoassay
MAOI	monoamine oxidase inhibitor	**RNA**	ribonucleic acid
MBD	minimal brain dysfunction (syndrome)	**RT**	resistance transfer factor
mChR	muscarinic receptor	**S**	Svedberg units
MDP	maximum diastolic potential	**S-A**	sinoatrial (node)
MEOS	microsomal enzyme–oxidation system	**SAR**	structure-activity relationship
MEPP	miniature endplate potential	**SBE**	subacute bacterial endocarditis
MG	myasthenia gravis	**SC**	subcutaneous
MH	malignant hyperthermia	**SIF**	small intensely fluorescent (cells)
MIC	minimum inhibitory concentration	**SRS**	slow-reacting substance
MLC	minimum lethal concentration	**SRS-A**	slow-reacting substance of anaphylaxis
mV	millivolt	**T₃**	triiodothyronine
NAD(H)	nicotinamide adenine dinucleotide (reduced)	**T₄**	thyroxine (tetraiodothyronine)
		TBC	tetrahydro-β-carboline
NADP(H)	nicotinamide adenine dinucleotide phosphate (reduced)	**TBG**	thyroxine-binding globulin
		TEA	tetraethylammonium
Na,K-ATPase	sodium, potassium adenosine triphosphate	**TF**	transfer factor
		Δ^9-THC	delta-9-tetrahydrocannabinol
NAPA	N-acetylprocainamide	**TI**	therapeutic index
nChR	nicotinic receptor	**TIQ**	tetrahydroisoquinolines

TMA	mescaline	**USAN**	United Stated Adopted Name (Council)
TMJ	temporomandibular joint	**USP**	United States Pharmacopeia
TMP-SMZ	trimethoprim-sulfamethoxazole	**USPDI**	United States Pharmacopeia Dispensing Information
TRH	thyrotropin-releasing hormone		
TSH	thyroid-stimulating hormone	V_d	volume of distribution
TX	thromboxane	**VLDL**	very low density lipoproteins
TXA$_2$	thromboxane A$_2$	**VMA**	vanillylmandelic acid
		VRG	vessel rich group

Index

A

Abbokinase; *see* Urokinase
Abdominal distention, gastrointestinal stimulants for, 492
Abel, John, 2
Abscesses
  central nervous system, 571
  surgical intervention and antibiotics for, 528
Absence seizures, 225
Absolute alcohol, 624
Absorbable gelatin film, 462, 471
Absorbable gelatin sponge, 462, 471
Absorption, 24-31
  in drug interactions, 81, 82
  in elderly, 707
  and elimination, kinetics of, 49-51
Abstinence syndrome
  alcohol, 625
  barbiturate, 678
  marijuana, 686
  opioid, 676-677
  sedative-hypnotic, 679
ABVD regimen for Hodgkin's disease, 616
Abuse, drug: *see* Drug abuse
Abuse potential of benzodiazepines, 198
Accelerated allergic reactions, 550
Accelerated angina, 409
Accepted Dental Remedies, 2
Accepted Dental Therapeutics (ADT), 76-77, 716
Accumulation, drug, time course of, 52
Acebutolol, 433, 439
Acecainide, 391
Acenocoumarol, 471
Acetaldehyde, 620, 622, 627
Acetaminophen
  absorption, fate, and excretion of, 321
  and alcohol, interaction of, 624
  and aspirin, differences between, 314
  chemistry and classification of, 320
  half-life of, 50
  mechanism of action of, 320
  pharmacologic effects of, 320-321
  and related aniline derivatives, 320-323
  in renal failure, 58
  in saliva, 34
  structure of, 321

Acetaminophen—cont'd
  therapeutic uses of
    in dentistry, 322
    general, 321-322
  toxic reactions and side effects of, 322-323
Acetanilid, structure of, 321
Acetazolamide
  as anticonvulsant, 233, 235
  as diuretic, 416, 417, 418-419, 423, 424
Acetohexamide, 501, 508
Acetophenazine, 190
Acetyl coenzyme A, 101
Acetylcarbromol, 223
Acetylcholine (Ach), 137, 138, 143, 147
  absorption, fate, and excretion of, 142
  and acetylcholinesterase, interaction of, 139
  antagonists of, mechanism of action of, 150-151
  in cholinergic transmission, 101
  in ganglionic transmission, 159
  identification of, 93-94
  inhibition of, by atropine, 16
  in myasthenia gravis, 144
  and neuromuscular blocking agents, 165, 166
  receptors for, 7-8
    interaction of, 10-11
  structure of, 138
Acetylcholine receptor in myasthenia gravis, 144-145
Acetylcholinesterase, 139
Acetylcysteine
  for acetaminophen overdose, 323
  as mucolytic, 482
N-Acetylprocainamide, 387, 391
Acetylsalicylic acid; *see* Aspirin
Achromycin; *see* Tetracycline(s)
Acid-base equilibrium, aspirin effects on, 316
Acidic glutaraldehyde, 650, 653
Acidity, plaque, 632, 633, 634
Acidogenic bacteria in dental caries, 630-631
Acidosis, lactic, 501
Acids in dental plaque, 632
  decalcification potential of, 636
Acne, 565
Acquired immune deficiency syndrome, (AIDS), 687-688
Acrisorcin, 592
Actidil; *see* Triprolidine

Interactions—cont'd
  of antipsychotics, 182
  of aspirin, 319, 320
  of cardiac glycosides, 405, 406
  of centrally acting muscle relaxants, 206
  classification of, 80
  in drug abuse, 688
  enzyme induction in, 46
  factors influencing, 85
  of ganglionic blocking agents, 163
  mechanisms of, 80-85
  of monoamine oxidase inhibitors, 132
  of neuromuscular blocking agents, 171-172
  of opioids, 311
  with receptor, 7-12
  of sedative-hypnotics, 215-216, 217
  of tetracyclines, 567
  useful in pharmacotherapeutics, 85
Intermediate coronary syndrome, 409
Intermediate low density lipoproteins, 442, 443
Interstitial cystitis, 31
Intestinal candidiasis, 587
Intestine; *see also* Gastrointestinal tract
  absorption in, 24-25
    iron, 452
  pH of, 25
Intraarterial injections, 30
Intramuscular injection, 29
Intramuscular sedation in dentistry, 662-663
Intraocular pressure, reduction of, 114, 126, 127, 423
Intraperitoneal infusion of fluids, 30
Intravascular injection of local anesthetics, 261
Intravenous drug administration, 28-29
Intravenous sedation in dentistry, 664-666
Intrinsic activity, 14
Intrinsic factor, 451
Intrinsic pathway of blood coagulation, 460, 461
Intrinsic sympathomimetic activity, 125
Intropin; *see* Dopamine
Inulin, 32
  volume of distribution of, 35
Inversine; *see* Mecamylamine
Investigational Exemption for New Drug, Claimed, Notice of, 72
Iodine, 651, 652, 653
  for hyperthyroidism, 503
Iodine solution, 652, 653
Iodinated glycerol, 482
Iodoform, 653
Iodophors, 651
Iodotope; *see* Sodium iodide I-131
Ionic bonds, 9
Ionic permeability and local anesthetics, 251
Iontophoresis, 31
Ipecac, syrup of, 482, 487, 493, 695
Iprindole, 183, 187
Iproniazid, 176
Iris and lens, adhesions between, 154
Iron, 451-453
Iron deficiency anemia, 450, 451-453
Iron dextran, 453, 458
Iron poisoning, 453

Iron polysaccharide, 458
Irreversible α-adrenoceptor blockers, 123-124
Ischemia, cardiac
  adrenergic drugs and, 115
  lipid-lowering drugs and, 448
  streptokinase and, 466
Ischemic necrosis, norepinephrine and, 258
Islet cells, streptozocin effect on, 610
Islets of Langerhans, 498
Ismelin; *see* Guanethidine
Ismotic; *see* Isosorbide
Isobucaine, 265
Isocaine; *see* Mepivacaine
Isocarboxazid, 190
Isoetharine, 119, 477, 482
  structure of, 108
Isoflurane, 279, 283, 293
  and aging, 708
  partition coefficients of, 276
  structure of, 286
Isoflurophate, 138, 143
  structure of, 141
Isomers, optical, differences in, 11
Isoniazid, 49, 176, 529, 580-581, 582
  and aging, 708
  interaction of, with antimuscarinic drugs, 156
  side effects of, 63
  toxicity of, 532
Isopropamide, 157
Isopropyl alcohol, 627-628, 649, 653
  toxicity of, 700
Isoproterenol, 57, 111, 119, 121
  aerosol administration of, 28
  and aging, 708
  for asthma, 370, 477, 482
  inactivation of, 27
  pharmacologic effects of, 112
  and phenylephrine, 119
  structure of, 108
Isoptin; *see* Verapamil
Isopto; *see* Carbachol
Isopto Carpine; *see* Pilocarpine
Isopto Eserine; *see* Physostigmine
Isopto P-Es; *see* Pilocarpine and physostigmine
Isordil; *see* Isosorbide dinitrate
Isosorbide, 416, 424
Isosorbide dinitrate, 410, 411, 414
  structure of, 411
Isoxazolyl derivatives, 552, 554-555
Isoxicam, 346, 359
Isoxsuprine, 109, 119
  structure of, 108
Isuprel; *see* Isoproterenol

J

Jackson, Charles T., 269
Jacksonian motor epilepsy, 226
Janimine; *see* Imipramine
Joint disease, degenerative, 342
Joint prosthesis, bacterial endocarditis prophylaxis for patients with, 535, 536
Jorgensen technique, 658, 666
Journal of the American Dental Association (JADA), 77